Renal Tubular Disorders

KIDNEY DISEASE

Editors

Volume 1 Proteinuria: An Integrated Review, *Amadeo J. Pesce and Martin Roy First*

Volume 2 The Aminoglycosides: Microbiology, Clinical Use, and Toxicology, *edited by Andrew Whelton and Harold C. Neu*

Volume 3 Hepatorenal Disorders, *S. P. Wilkinson*

Volume 4 Acute Renal Failure: Correlations Between Morphology and Function, *edited by Kim Solez and Andrew Whelton*

Volume 5 Renal Tubular Disorders: Pathophysiology, Diagnosis, and Management, *edited by Harvey C. Gonick and Vardaman M. Buckalew, Jr.*

Volume 6 Potassium in Cardiovascular and Renal Medicine: Arrhythmias, Myocardial Infarction, and Hypertension, *edited by Paul K. Whelton, Andrew Whelton, and W. Gordon Walker*

Other Volumes in Preparation

Renal Tubular Disorders

Pathophysiology, Diagnosis, and Management

Edited by

HARVEY C. GONICK

Cedars-Sinai Medical Center
and University of California at Los Angeles
School of Medicine
Los Angeles, California

VARDAMAN M. BUCKALEW, JR.

Bowman Gray School of Medicine
of Wake Forest University
Winston-Salem, North Carolina

Marcel Dekker, Inc. **New York and Basel**

Library of Congress Cataloging in Publication Data

Main entry under title:

Renal tubular disorders.

(Kidney disease ; v. 5)
Includes index.
1. Renal tubular transport, Disorders of.
I. Gonick, Harvey C. II. Buckalew, Vardaman M., Jr.
III. Series. [DNLM: 1. Kidney Diseases. 2. Kidney Tubules--physiopathology. W1 KI586R v.5 / WJ 301 R39353]
RC918.T73R46 1985 616.6'1 85-16084
ISBN 0-8247-7371-3

MARCEL DEKKER, INC.
270 Madison Avenue, New York, New York 10016

Current printing (last digit):
10 9 8 7 6 5 4 3 2 1

PRINTED IN THE UNITED STATES OF AMERICA

To Gloria and Sherry,
without whose support
this volume would not have been possible

About the Series

This book is the fifth in a series of texts on nephrology intended to cover all aspects of that discipline. Nephrology has grown at a great rate over the past decade, and the available knowledge has outstripped the texts available. The discipline has, however, attained such maturity that a description of any one of its parts becomes more than ephemeral—or worse, outdated before it even appears. We aim to fill some of the many gaps that exist, not only for the specialist in nephrology, but also for the general physician interested in nephrology. In this description, we include the study and management of hypertension, since these two are interwoven at so many points. We welcome comments on the series as it evolves, or suggestions for topics that might be considered for future volumes.

J. Stewart Cameron
London, England

Andrew Whelton
Baltimore, Maryland

Richard J. Glassock
Torrance, California

Charles van Ypersele de Strihou
Brussels, Belgium

Preface

Renal tubular disorders have captured the imagination of the nephrologist and renal physiologist to a degree far disproportionate to the incidence of these disorders in clinical medicine. This may be due to the fact that it is possible to relate clinical manifestations of some of these conditions to pathophysiology and, ultimately, to defects at the molecular biology level.

The concept of renal tubular disorders developed following the demonstration in 1921 by A. N. Richards that urine formation resulted from glomerular filtration, tubular reabsorption, and secretion, followed by the development of methods for measuring glomerular filtration rate in man by Homer Smith and Donald Van Slyke. The recognition that an abnormality in tubular function alone could lead to a complex clinical syndrome resulted from the work of Fanconi and de Toni in the early 1930s. These investigators demonstrated that a renal loss of phosphate could lead to metabolic bone disease, which they called "renal rickets." Using the newly developed concepts of Richards, Smith, and Van Slyke, they showed that these patients had normal glomerular filtration rates. This demonstration implied that renal phosphate wasting was due to some abnormality in renal tubular function, although this concept was not clearly stated in the original articles.

Over the intervening years, a number of clinical syndromes have been recognized as being due to hereditary abnormalities in renal tubular function. Although the classic hereditary disorders of renal tubular function are rare, the insights achieved by detailed study of isolated tubular abnormalities have contributed substantially to the understanding of major clinical disorders such as renal calculi, metabolic acidosis, metabolic bone disease, and failure to thrive in infants, most of which may be frequently seen by practitioners of general medicine. Moreover, acquired renal tubular disorders are being recognized with increasing frequency, usually as a result of nephrotoxic drugs.

Developments in renal physiology over the past few decades have made it possible to pinpoint the specific tubular segment responsible for a given isolated defect in tubular transport. For example, glucose and amino acids are known to be reabsorbed predominantly in the first (S_1) segment of the proximal tubule. Thus, one might anticipate that abnormal function of that segment would be required to explain renal glycosuria or aminoaciduria.

At the same time, increased understanding of membrane transport has made possible the development of molecular theories of how a hereditary process could affect function of a specific segment of the nephron. Thus, transport abnormalities could develop in a number of ways, including: (1) an abnormality in a specific carrier protein at either the luminal or contraluminal membrane; (2) diminished activity of one or more enzymes involved in cellular energy production; (3) accumulation of inhibitors of enzymes involved in transport or in energy production, secondary to another defect in intermediary metabolism; (4) abnormalities in synthesis of hormones critical to normal tubular function; and finally, (5) abnormalities in receptors for these hormones or in the "second message" system. Acquired diseases could affect transport function in isolated nephron segments in much the same way.

While it is possible to theorize about molecular mechanisms, our knowledge of certain aspects of the transport process, such as specific carrier proteins and hormone receptors, is still fragmentary. Thus, delineation of "*the* molecular defect" of any tubular disorder is, at best, incomplete. For example, it is generally considered that different carriers exist for different classes of amino acids, and the kinetic aspects of these presumed carriers are fairly well established. However, identification of the normal carrier proteins and the abnormal structure that may cause disease has not yet been accomplished. Within the various hereditary phosphaturias, at least one is probably due to defective synthesis of the active metabolite of vitamin D_3, with production of secondary hyperparathyroidism. Another may be due to defective synthesis of the receptor for this vitamin D metabolite. Again, our knowledge of the structure and function of the receptor is so preliminary that no molecular theory is yet possible to explain the lack of response to vitamin D.

With regard to Fanconi syndrome, both human and animal studies have emphasized the generalized nature of the proximal tubular transport defect. Accordingly, theories have been developed that attempt to explain these observations on the basis of a defect in a common transport mechanism. Biochemical studies of animal models have suggested that this abnormality might reside in either a defective membrane permeability or impairment of the ability of the Na-K-ATPase enzyme transport system to maintain the normal sodium gradient across the cell. Although such studies have not yet been possible in the human disease, Fanconi syndrome in animals is the only tubular disorder that can likely be attributed to a specific enzymatic defect.

It is our expectation that, as techniques improve and new concepts develop, eventually the specific genetic defects of most renal tubular disorders will be characterized. For the present, we have developed a comprehensive survey of the classic renal tubular disorders, including experimental background and pathophysiology, genetic characterization, clinical features, and treatment. We believe this is the first time such a comprehensive collection of information on this topic has been attempted. To the extent we have been successful, our thanks are due in large part to our colleagues who prepared the individual papers.

Harvey C. Gonick
Vardaman M. Buckalew, Jr.

Contributors

Daniel C. Batlle, M.D. Associate Professor, Department of Medicine, University of Illinois College of Medicine, and Chief, Nephrology Section, West Side Veterans Administration Hospital, Chicago, Illinois

Edward G. Biglieri, M.D. Professor, Department of Medicine, Clinical Study Center, University of California at San Francisco, San Francisco, California

Gregory L. Braden, M.D.* Research Fellow, Renal-Electrolyte Section, Department of Medicine, University of Pennsylvania School of Medicine, Philadelphia Veterans Administration Medical Center, and Hospital of the University of Pennsylvania, Philadelphia, Pennsylvania

Eileen D. Brewer, M.D. Assistant Professor, Department of Pediatrics, University of Utah School of Medicine, Salt Lake City, Utah

Vardaman M. Buckalew, Jr., M.D. Professor, Section on Nephrology, Department of Medicine, and Department of Physiology and Pharmacology, Bowman Gray School of Medicine of Wake Forest University, Winston-Salem, North Carolina

Ruth Ellen Bulger, Ph.D.† Professor, Department of Pathology and Laboratory Medicine, University of Texas Health Science Center, Houston, Texas

Ralph J. Caruana, M.D. Associate Professor, Section on Nephrology, Department of Medicine, Bowman Gray School of Medicine of Wake Forest University, Winston-Salem, North Carolina

---

Current affiliation
*Assistant Professor, Department of Medicine, Tufts University School of Medicine, Boston, and Director, Renal Laboratory, Baystate Medical Center, Springfield, Massachusetts
†Professor, Graduate School of Biomedical Sciences, University of Texas Health Science Center, Houston, Texas

Russell W. Chesney, M.D. Professor, Department of Pediatrics, University of Wisconsin Center for Health Sciences, Madison, Wisconsin

Malcolm Cox, M.D. Associate Professor, Department of Medicine, University of Pennsylvania School of Medicine, Chief, Renal-Electrolyte Section, Medical Service, Philadelphia Veterans Administration Medical Center, and Hospital of the University of Pennsylvania, Philadelphia, Pennsylvania

Dennis C. Dobyan, Ph.D. Assistant Professor, Department of Pathology and Laboratory Medicine, University of Texas Health Science Center, Houston, Texas

Chester M. Edelmann, Jr., M.D. Associate Dean for Clinical Affairs and Professor, Department of Pediatrics, Albert Einstein College of Medicine of Yeshiva University, New York, New York

Leon G. Fine, M.D. Professor of Medicine and Chief, Division of Nephrology, Department of Medicine, Center for the Health Sciences, University of California at Los Angeles School of Medicine, Los Angeles, California

John W. Foreman, M.D. Assistant Professor, Department of Pediatrics, University of Pennsylvania School of Medicine, Philadelphia, Pennsylvania

John R. Gill, Jr., M.D. Chief of Service, Hypertension-Endocrine Branch, National Heart, Lung and Blood Institute, National Institutes of Health, Bethesda, Maryland

Harvey C. Gonick, M.D. Clinical Chief, Division of Nephrology, Department of Medicine, Cedars-Sinai Medical Center, and Adjunct Professor, Department of Medicine, University of California at Los Angeles School of Medicine, Los Angeles, California

Henry N. Hulter, M.D. Division of Nephrology, Department of Medicine, University of California at San Francisco, San Francisco, California

Rolf Kinne, M.D.* Chairman, Department of Physiology and Biophysics, Albert Einstein College of Medicine of Yeshiva University, New York, New York

Thomas F. Knight, M.D.† Assistant Professor, Department of Internal Medicine, Veterans Administration Medical Center and Baylor College of Medicine, Houston, Texas

Herbert J. Kramer, M.D. Professor of Medicine, Medizinische Poliklinik, University of Bonn, Bonn, Federal Republic of Germany

---

Current affiliation

*Director, Department of Physiology II, Max-Planck-Institut für Systemphysiologie, Dortmund, Federal Republic of Germany

†Associate Professor, Department of Internal Medicine, University of Nebraska College of Medicine, Omaha, Nebraska

Ira Kurtz, M.D., F.R.C.P.(C)* Research Fellow, Renal Division, Department of Medicine, University of California at San Francisco, San Francisco, California

Neil A. Kurtzman, M.D.† Professor of Medicine and Physiology and Chief, Section of Nephrology, Department of Medicine, University of Illinois College of Medicine, Chicago, Illinois

Terry Maher, M.D.†† General Clinical Research Center and Renal Division, Department of Medicine, University of California at San Francisco, San Francisco, California

R. Curtis Morris, Jr., M.D. Professor of Medicine and Pediatrics and Director, General Clinical Research Center, University of California at San Francisco, San Francisco, California

Floyd C. Rector, Jr., M.D. Professor, Departments of Medicine and Physiology, Cardiovascular Research Institute, University of California at San Francisco, San Francisco, California

Morris Schambelan, M.D. Professor, Department of Medicine, Chief, Division of Endocrinology, and Associate Director, General Clinical Research Center, University of California at San Francisco, San Francisco, California

Anthony Sebastian, M.D. Professor, Department of Medicine, and Co-Director, General Clinical Research Center, University of California at San Francisco, San Francisco, California

Stanton Segal, M.D. Professor, Departments of Pediatrics and Medicine, University of Pennsylvania School of Medicine, Philadelphia, Pennsylvania

Harry O. Senekjian, M.D.** Assistant Professor, Renal Section, Department of Internal Medicine, Veterans Administration Medical Center, and Baylor College of Medicine, Houston, Texas

Irwin Singer, M.D. Professor, Department of Medicine, University of Pennsylvania School of Medicine, Philadelphia Veterans Administration Medical Center, and Hospital of the University of Pennsylvania, Philadelphia, Pennsylvania

---

Current affiliation

*Assistant Professor, Division of Nephrology, Department of Medicine, University of California at Los Angeles, Los Angeles, California

†Professor of Medicine and Physiology and Chairman, Department of Internal Medicine, Texas Tech University Health Sciences Center, Lubbock, Texas

††Nephrology Medical Group, Inc., San Pablo, California

**Clinical Associate Professor, Department of Internal Medicine, University of Utah, Salt Lake City, Utah

Edward J. Weinman, M.D.* Professor, Division of Nephrology, Department of Internal Medicine, Veterans Administration Medical Center and Baylor College of Medicine, Houston, Texas

Sung-Feng Wen, M.D. Professor, Nephrology Section, Department of Medicine, University of Wisconsin Center for Health Sciences, Madison, Wisconsin

Norimoto Yanagawa, M.D.† Assistant Professor, Department of Medicine, University of California at Los Angeles School of Medicine, Los Angeles, and Sepulveda Veterans Administration Medical Center, Sepulveda, California

---

Current affiliation
*Professor of Internal Medicine and Director, Division of Nephrology, Department of Internal Medicine, University of Texas School of Medicine at Houston, Houston, Texas
†Assistant Professor, Department of Medicine, Sepulveda Veterans Administration Medical Center/University of California at Los Angeles School of Medicine/San Fernando Valley Program, Sepulveda, California

Contents

Renal Tubular Disorders

1

Biochemical Aspects of Tubular Transport

ROLF KINNE*
Albert Einstein College of Medicine of Yeshiva University, New York, New York

I. THE MEMBRANE MOLECULAR APPROACH TO STUDY EPITHELIAL TRANSPORT PROCESSES

The membrane molecular approach can be considered as a method to study epithelial transport by investigating transport-related properties of isolated plasma membranes. Thus, there are two steps to this method, first the isolation of membranes, and second the investigation of transport-related properties.

A. Isolation of Plasma Membranes from the Kidney

To study membrane transport processes under well-defined biochemical and biophysical conditions it is of advantage to separate the membranes from their natural intracellular and extracellular environment. After isolation both the former extracellular and the former intracellular (cytoplasmic face) of the membrane are accessible for experimental modification and can be exposed to solutions of known and constant composition. In isolating plasma membranes from the kidney—or from epithelia in general—the following aspects are important: The plasma membranes should be derived from defined tubular segments or defined tubular cells and defined areas of the cell surface. Only when these criteria are fulfilled can reliable correlations between the results obtained with isolated membranes in vitro and the function of a tubular segment in vivo be established.

Luminal Membrane of the Proximal Tubule

Cortical nephrons

The apical membranes of cortical proximal tubules were the first to be isolated in reasonable purity. Using thin slices of rat kidney cortex brush-border membranes can be isolated by differential centrifugation, free-flow electrophoresis, differential precipitation, or density centrifugation (see Ref. 1 for references). These methods are used separately or in combi-

Current affiliation: Max-Planck-Institut für Systemphysiologie, Dortmund, Federal Republic of Germany

nation and take advantage of the different size, different density, or different surface charge of the apical membrane compared to basal-lateral membranes and intracellular membranes. The brush-border membrane fractions have in common that the membranes show a high degree of vesiculation, the orientation of the membrane in the vesicles is almost exclusively right side out (2), i.e., the orientation of the membrane in the vesicle is identical to the orientation of the membrane in the intact cell. Depending on the homogenization and isolation procedure three different kinds of membrane fragments can be derived from the luminal surface of the proximal tubular cells, namely, brush-border fragments (3), microvilli (4), and pinocytic vesicles. Brush-border fragments are composed of several rodlike microvilli and the intermicrovillar crypts, and contain occasionally lateral plasma membranes, including the junctional complexes. In addition, the brush-border membrane fragments have trapped small vesicles–probably pinocytic vesicles (see Fig. 1). The "microvilli" represent short resealed fragments of the long microvilli. Part of the microvillus or the entire fragment has attained a spherelike appearance (see Fig. 2). These microvilli vesicles are the membrane fragments used currently most frequently for transport studies and biochemical investigations. The third fraction possible to obtain contains intervillous crypts and pinocytic vesicles. This fraction has been used for investigations of the transport of macromolecules across the tubular cell (5).

Deep nephrons and pars recta

By using the red outer medulla of rabbit kidney as starting material Turner and Dousa (6) isolated brush-border microvilli that are predominantly derived from pars recta and some early segments of the proximal tubules of juxtamedullary nephrons. Such fractions are a first useful step in dealing with tubular heterogeneity. Indeed, interesting differences in D-glucose transport and phosphate transport have been found between microvilli vesicles isolated from the cortical tubules and the pars recta.

Basal-Lateral Plasma Membranes of the Proximal Tubule

The contraluminal surface of the proximal tubule cells appears morphologically as a labyrinth structure with numerous infoldings of the plama membranes. For this membrane the term basal-lateral, antiluminal, or contraluminal membrane is used. The basal-lateral membrane fractions isolated so far by free-flow electrophoresis, differential precipitation, or density gradient centrifugation (see Ref. 1 and Fig. 3) thus contain the membrane areas of cell attachment to the basement membrane, the areas of infoldings, and the lateral membranes extending into the junctional regions. The membrane fractions are usually obtained from kidney cortex slices; they represent a mixture of plasma membranes derived from proximal tubular cells, distal cells, and others. According to studies about transport properties and marker enzymes, the membranes from proximal tubules seem to dominate (7). Further refinements of separation techniques such as electrophoretic cell separation (8) are necessary before basal-lateral plasma membranes derived exclusively from proximal tubule cells are available. The plasma membrane fractions contain membrane sheets as well as membrane vesicles. The membranes of the vesicles are usually randomly oriented; about an equal percentage is oriented right side out or inside out (9). In the latter orientation, the former cytoplasmic surface of the membrane is exposed to the incubation medium. Such vesicles have been a valuable tool for the studies of ATP-dependent transport processes in the basal-lateral membrane such as the ATP-dependent calcium transport (10) (see below).

Plasma Membranes from the Thick Ascending Limb of Henle's Loop

Isolation of plasma membranes from the thick ascending limb of Henle's loop has been achieved recently by first isolating a cell population from rabbit outer medulla (11) that

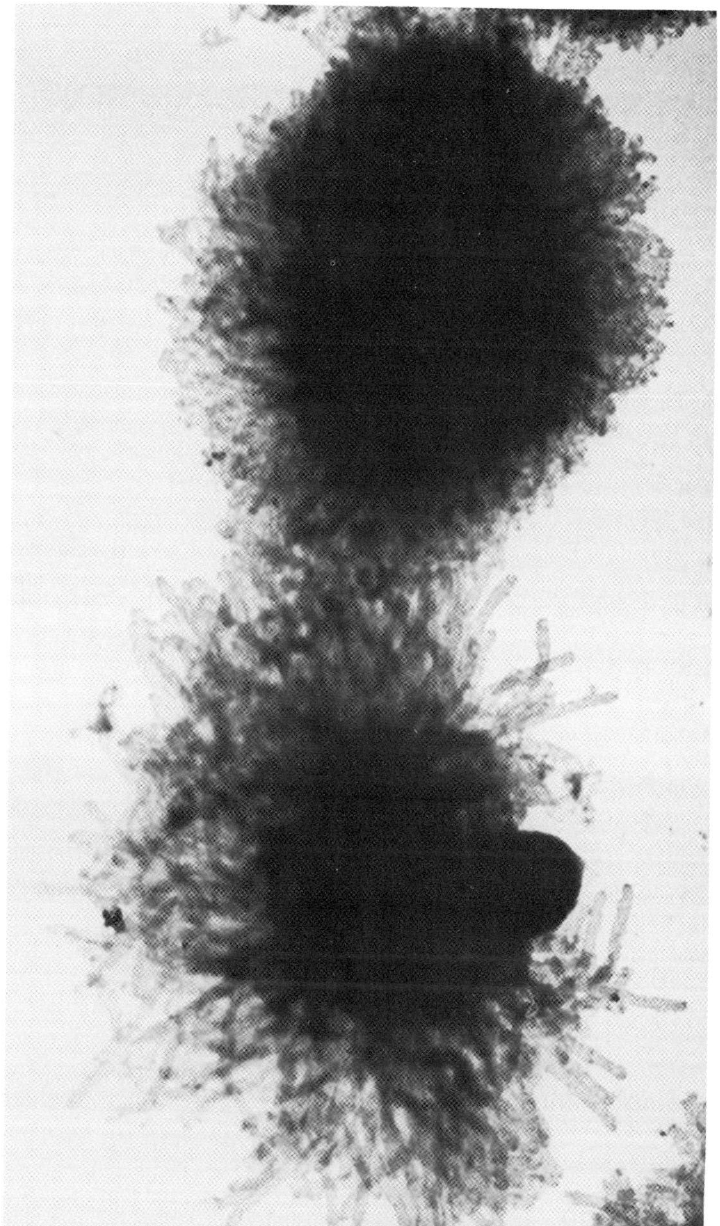

Fig. 1 Brush-border fragment isolated by differential centrifugation from rat kidney cortex. The brush-border fragment is composed of numerous fingerlike microvilli. Magnification ×23000. (From Ref. 3.)

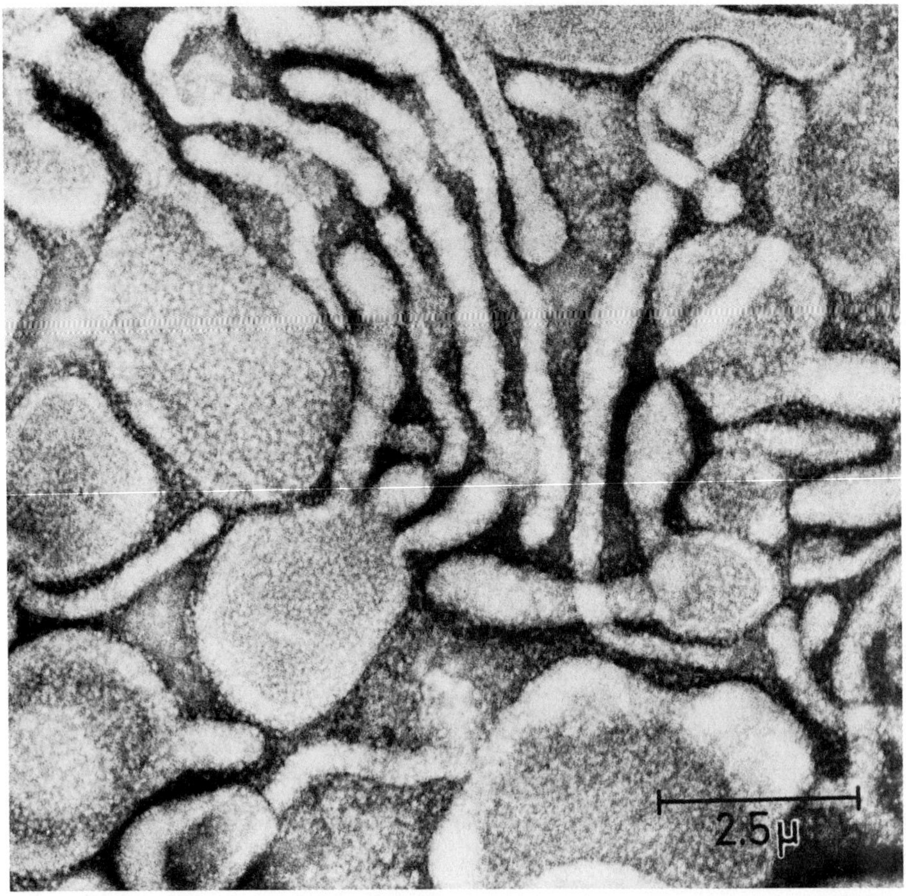

Fig. 2 Microvilli vesicles isolated from rat kidney by differential precipitation with calcium. The microvilli fragments are partially vesiculated. (From Ref. 4.)

according to morphological functional and enzymatic criteria contains 90-95% cells of thick ascending limb of Henle's loop. After isolation of the cells, a plasma membrane fraction is prepared by differential centrifugation. This fraction can in turn be subdivided into luminal and contraluminal membrane fragments by free-flow electrophoresis. The membrane fractions contain membrane sheets as well as vesicles; therefore enzymatic characterization and analysis of transport properties have been possible. It can be expected that these membranes will contribute markedly to our understanding of transport processes in this tubular segment. Although the method is currently limited by the low yield of membrane protein, cell culture techniques might overcome this problem not only for the thick ascending limb of Henle's loop but also for other tubule segments.

Plasma Membranes from the Papillary Collecting Duct

Taking advantage of the enrichment of a certain tubular segment in a particular anatomically defined area of the kidney, plasma membranes from the papillary collecting duct could be isolated (12). Using bovine white papilla as starting material luminal and contraluminal membranes could be separated by free-flow electrophoresis and their enzymatic composition could be determined. Transport studies with these fractions have been initiated but not

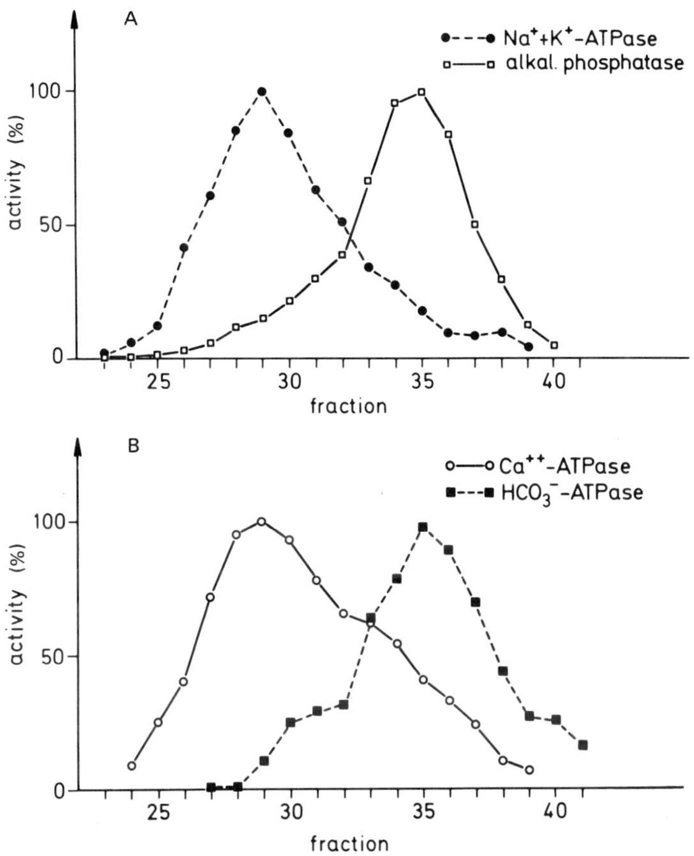

Fig. 3 Separation of luminal and contraluminal membranes from rat kidney cortex by free-flow electrophoresis. (A) The alkaline phosphatase indicates the distribution of microvilli, the ($Na^+ + K^+$)-ATPase indicates the distribution of the basal-lateral plasma membranes. (B) The distribution of the luminal bicarbonate stimulated ATPase and of the contraluminal Ca^{2+}-ATPase is shown. (From Ref. 198.)

pursued, hitherto. Plasma membrane fractions less well defined with respect to the cellular origin have also been isolated from renal medulla (13).

It is evident from the above discussion that currently only a few segments of the renal tubule are accessible for the membrane-molecular approach to investigate epithelial transport. Even the membranes prepared so far have to be considered as imperfect in one aspect or the other. In addition to problems of heterogeneity with respect to cellular and subcellular origin of the membranes—the variations of vesicle size, of vesicle permeability, and of membrane orientation still impose severe limitations on the experimental possibilities.

B. Transport-Related Parameters of Isolated Membranes

In essence four different transport-related properties can be investigated in isolated membranes: (1) Transport systems that are coupled to an enzymatic reaction, (2) permeability by simple diffusion, (3) carrier-mediated diffusion systems, (4) and membrane systems related in a broad sense to regulation of transport processes. A typical example of a transport system coupled to an enzymatic reaction is the Na-K-ATPase (14) enzyme, which can be studied by following the hydrolysis of ATP. Such studies have revealed remarkable details about the interaction of sodium, potassium, magnesium, and adenosine triphosphate (ATP) with the enzyme and about their role in various partial reactions; they have, however, provided only limited information about the ion translocation process per se. This is due to the fact that most of the studies were performed with membrane fragments where the asymmetrical ion distribution encountered in the living cell is no longer present and where it is not possible to measure ion fluxes simultaneously with the enzymatic reaction. This disadvantage does not apply to the red blood cell or red cell ghosts that can be preloaded with a defined solution and where ion translocation and ATP-hydrolysis can be determined simultaneously. The red cell ghosts are also an excellent model for the study of carrier-mediated diffusion processes by measuring ion fluxes across the membranes. Such measurements are also possible now with renal plasma membranes because almost all plasma membrane fractions isolated from renal cells vesiculate spontaneously. When a vesicle is formed the plasma membranes again separate two compartments, namely the artificially composed intravesicular and extravesicular compartment, and an analysis of diffusional and carrier-mediated solute transfer is possible. The first transport studies with epithelial plasma membrane vesicles were performed by Hopfer et al. (15); essentially the same techniques are used today in most of the experiments with renal plasma membrane vesicles. Additional techniques have been adopted from studies with bacterial membrane vesicles (16).

Plasma membrane properties related to transport regulation comprise hormone receptors —that alter transport properties directly or by activating a multiplier system such as the adenylate cyclase—mediator systems such as protein kinases, or enzymes that catalyze membrane lipid methylation or protein adenosylribosylation. The distribution of hormone-sensitive adenylate cyclases in the tubule has been defined in the laboratory of Morel et al. (17). As an example the distribution of the calcitonin-sensitive adenylate cyclase in the rabbit tubule is given in Fig. 2 of Chap. 2. The cyclase was stimulated significantly by calcitonin in the medullary ascending limb, cortical ascending limb, and distal cortical tubule. The degree of stimulation and the response differs from species to species. The interested reader should consult the particular literature (19-20). The studies have revealed again how heterogeneous the renal tubule is, an aspect that although evident from morphological studies was not perceived in its functional importance. Studies with isolated membranes have demonstrated that the adenylate cyclase of proximal tubule and collecting duct cells is exclusively localized in the contraluminal membranes of the cells (6,12). This localization holds probably for all segments, since peptide hormones elicit this action in low concentrations only from the peritubular site. The luminal membranes contain putative mediator systems such as protein kinases (12,20). In addition, membrane components are substrates for phosphorylation, methylation, and adenosylribosylation (21).

In general, the membrane molecular approach has yielded results that are compatible with the transport properties observed in the intact epithelium (22). The results are quantitatively in good agreement with the in vivo transport data. There are, however, also discrepancies. One is, for example, that chloride-hydroxyl ion exchange has been demonstrated in isolated rabbit kidney brush-border membranes (23), whereas in in vitro perfusion studies of proximal tubules no evidence for the operation of this system could be obtained (24). This discrepancy might be related to an activation of a transport system during isolation of the cell membrane. It is also possible that the brush-border membrane fraction contains membranes both from early and late proximal tubules, whereas the perfusion study was performed only in early proximal tubules. Late proximal tubules might possess the chloride-hydroxyl exchange system. The inhomogeneity of some of the membrane preparations lead also to the hypothesis that more than one D-glucose transport system is present in the brush-border membrane. This multiplicity has now been shown to be caused by the presence of membranes from the early and late parts of the proximal tubule (R. J. Turner).

The membrane molecular approach has further methodological limitations. Firstly, only the sequence of events comprising the transcellular movement of solutes can be investigated, the paracellular route is excluded, and any interaction between the two pathways is destroyed. In addition, intracellular factors such as the composition of the cytoplasm, the membrane potential, and cytoskeletal elements are lacking in the vesicles after the isolation. Most transport studies are performed for the sake of simplicity in unphysiological solutions. Only recently have attempts been made to mimic the composition of the intracellular fluid in brush-border membrane vesicles, and a strong effect of potassium, for example, on the transport of glutamic acid has been observed (25,26). In the future, such reconstitution experiments will bridge at least partially the gap between the transport studies with vesicles and the studies in intact tissue.

In the following, a summary of transport systems found in isolated plasma membrane vesicles will be provided. Since the field is developing rapidly, any omissions are unintentional. The section is arranged by tubular segments and where applicable the entry step, the exit step, and the rate-limiting step for a certain solute are considered.

II. ENERGETICS OF TUBULAR TRANSPORT

Transport of a solute across an epithelium can be described thermodynamically as the sum of active and passive transport processes. The active transport processes can be further subdivided into primary and secondary active processes. Passive transport processes are solute movements that occur due to physical driving forces such as concentration differences, electrical potential differences and by solvent drag. The relation between the various physical driving forces and the passive transport system is described in the following formula:

$$J_i = (1 - \sigma_i)\,\bar{c}_i\,J_v - P_i\,(\Delta c_i + \frac{ZF}{RT}\Delta\Psi \circ \bar{c}_i)$$

where P represents the permeability coefficient, σ the reflection coefficient, c the concentration difference, $\Delta\Psi$ the electrical potential difference, $\bar{c}_i$ the mean concentration, J_v the volume flow, and Z the valency, and R, T, and F have the usual meaning.

Primary active transport across a membrane has been defined as a transport process that is directly coupled to a chemical reaction providing the energy for transport of a solute against its electrochemical potential difference (37). One example of primary active transport is the sodium and potassium transport mediated by the Na-K-ATPase. If this definition is extended to an epithelium, the entry of a solute can be passive and the cellular exit be mediated by a primary active transport. The transcellular transport of the solute is then termed primary active (see Fig. 4).

Secondary active transport across an epithelium involves at least three components, transportate 1, transportate 2, and a cotransport system that translocates the two transportates simultaneously. During the translocation step transportate 1 (for example, sodium across the luminal membrane of the proximal tubule) moves down its electrochemical potential difference, whereas transportate 2 (e.g., D-glucose across the luminal membrane of the proximal tubule) is transported against its electrochemical potential difference. Transportate 1 is then removed actively from the cell by a primary active transport system (such as the Na-K-ATPase for sodium); the action of the primary active transport system main-

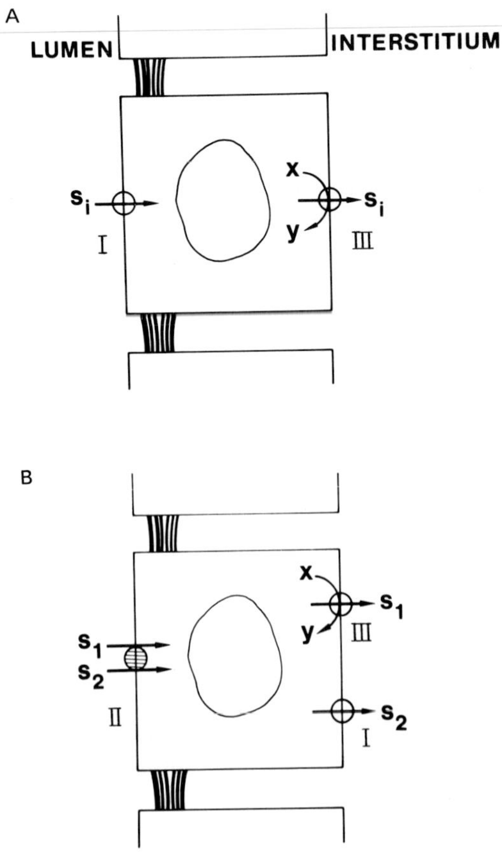

Fig. 4 Schematic representation of (A) primary active and (B) secondary active transport of solutes across an epithelium. For further explanation see text. I represents facilitated diffusion systems, II cotransport systems, and III primary active transport systems.

tains the electrochemical potential difference for transportate 1 (see Fig. 4). The coupling of the two transportates is governed by the following relation:

$$J_1 - L_{11} \Delta\mu_1 + L_{12} \Delta\mu_2$$

where L_{11} is the straight coefficient, L_{12} is the cross coefficient, and $\Delta\mu_1$ and $\Delta\mu_2$ are the electrochemical potential differences of transportate 1 and 2, respectively.

Important points of the coupled transport are electrogenicity and stoichiometry. The coupling of D-glucose and sodium flux, for example, makes the movement of D-glucose sensitive to the electrical potential difference across the luminal membrane of the proximal tubule (28). An anion such as lactate is transported across the brush-border membrane via a sodium cotransport system with a stoichiometry of two cations per anion; this stoichiometry leads to a net movement of a positive charge during sodium-lactate cotransport. Thereby, the intracellular negativity that opposes lactate entry into the cell is overcome and the chemical concentration difference for sodium becomes the main determinant for lactate uptake (27).

III. ENERGY SOURCES FOR TUBULAR TRANSPORT

A. Biochemical Driving Forces

Studying the biochemical reactions that provide the energy for tubular transport has two important aspects. On the one hand, it is of genuine interest to define the major metabolic pathways in the various segments of the tubule. The activity of these pathways determines the substrates that are used by the tubule and the metabolic end products. On the other hand, the elucidation of the energy metabolism was expected to yield information on the nature of the high-energy intermediates used for the transport processes. For example, for a long time it was not clear whether ATP is used as high-energy intermediate for transport in the proximal tubule; as a consequence, it was difficult to accept a major role for Na-K-ATPase in tubular transport.

The use of micromethods to determine enzyme activities, substrate levels, cofactors, and metabolic activity in microdissected tubular segments has recently provided important information on the biochemical pathways present in the tubular cells and about the concentration of high-energy intermediates. From these data and from data obtained on substrate oxidation by tubular segments one can delineate the following scheme for metabolic reactions in the various tubular segments (see Refs. 29 and 30 for references). The proximal tubule is high in oxidative metabolism via the citric acid cycle; it has a high gluconeogenetic capacity and a low glycolytic capacity. Transport in the proximal tubule can be supported by free fatty acids, acetate, lactate, pyruvate, and tricarboxylic acids. The relative rate of substrate uptake is determined, however, not only by the intracellular capacity of the metabolic pathways but also by the affinity and capacity of transport systems in the plasma membranes (31). The brush-border membrane has been demonstrated to contain highly active sodium cotransport systems for a variety of substrates such as lactate (32), citrate, succinate, and α-ketoglutarate (33). The exact interplay between the intracellular systems and the membrane transport systems remains to be determined; its understanding could shed light on the interesting question whether the energy metabolism of the cell—and in turn the transport properties—can be changed by regulation of the substrate uptake into the cell.

Another segment with a high oxidative metabolism is the thick ascending limb of Henle's loop. The concentration of tricarboxylic acid cycle enzymes is as high as in the proximal tubule; free fatty acids and acetate support the transport. In addition, however, this segment —especially the medullary portions—contains glycolytic enzymes and is capable of maintaining a high ATP level and transport activity in the presence of D-glucose and cyanide (34). The glycolytic capacity increases and the oxidative energy metabolism decreases when the tubular segments are located in the papilla. The collecting duct derives its energy almost exclusively from glycolysis. The ATP levels in this tubular segment are very similar to the ATP levels in other segments, indicating that the storage form of metabolic energy is always ATP independent from the metabolic reactions by which it is generated. One additional reaction system that has been postulated to energize amino acid transport system in Ehrlich's ascites tumor cells is the membrane-bound redox reaction. Similar systems have been observed in brush-border membranes; their role in transport has yet to be determined (35).

B. Physical Driving Forces

In addition to energy-rich intermediates that are driving forces for transport, physical driving forces also have to be considered. This was first realized in the field of mitochondrial transport and oxidative phosphorylation, where after a futile search for high-energy intermediates of oxidative phosphorylation, the electrochemical potential difference for protons was postulated to be the driving force established by the flow of electrons through the respiratory chain and used consecutively for the generation of ATP through the ATPase complex. This "chemiosmotic" theory by Mitchell had its congeners in the sodium gradient hypothesis established by Crane (36). The latter theory can be called the osmo-osmotic theory, since osmotic energy is used to perform osmotic work. The sodium gradient hypothesis postulated that transport systems exist that couple the movement of one transportate down its electrochemical potential difference to the uphill movement of another transportate, i.e., against its electrochemical potential difference. The basic principle of the sodium gradient hypothesis has been expanded since to include the membrane potential across plasma membranes and it is now well established that a large number of solutes are transported via such cotransport systems. It is therefore essential to include in the consideration of driving forces electrical potential differences and ion gradients across the membranes (27).

IV. TRANSPORT SYSTEMS IN THE PROXIMAL TUBULE

In the proximal tubule bulk reabsorption of inorganic and organic solutes takes place; in addition, some weak organic anions and cations are secreted. The transport mechanisms for a wide variety of solutes have been identified recently at the membrane level and will be discussed below. The majority of transport processes involves sodium cotransport systems and, thus, can be classified as secondary active.

A. Sodium Transport

The rat proximal tubule reabsorbs about 70% of the filtered load of sodium; about one-third of the transport is active and proceeds through the cell, and two-thirds of the transport is passive, driven by solvent drag and diffusion via the paracellular pathway (37). In the cellular passage of sodium mainly two systems are involved: Sodium cotransport systems at the luminal membrane mediate entry into the cell and Na-K-ATPase at the contraluminal membrane mediates sodium exit (see Fig. 5).

The Entry Step

Sodium enters the cell of the proximal tubule following a steep electrochemical potential difference. Sodium entry occurs via sodium cotransport systems such as the sodium-proton exchange systems and various other sodium-solute symport systems.

The sodium-proton exchange system has been studied extensively in rat kidney and rabbit kidney brush border (38-40). In both preparations it could be demonstrated that in the presence of a sodium gradient across the brush-border membrane ($Na_o > Na_i$) protons are extruded from the vesicles, as demonstrated either by recording the extravesicular pH with a pH-sensitive electrode or by following the alkalinization of the intravesicular compartment by means of the distribution of a weak acid. The Na-H exchanger is most probably electroneutral, facilitating a 1:1 exchange between sodium and protons, sodium and sodium, or sodium and ammonium. The affinity of the cation-binding site for sodium is about 6 mmol, for lithium 1.9 mmol, and for NH_4 4.3 mmol (39-41). Compounds with a high density of positive charges such as harmaline and amiloride (41,42) have been found to inhibit the Na-H exchange by competing with sodium for its binding site. The affinity of the Na-H exchanger for amiloride is 3×10^{-5} mol/liter; its action is relatively specific. Harmaline is rather unspecific; it affects not only the Na-H exchange but also the sodium glucose cotransport ($K_i \sim 0.2$ mmol), sodium-alanine cotransport, and renal ATPases (42,43).

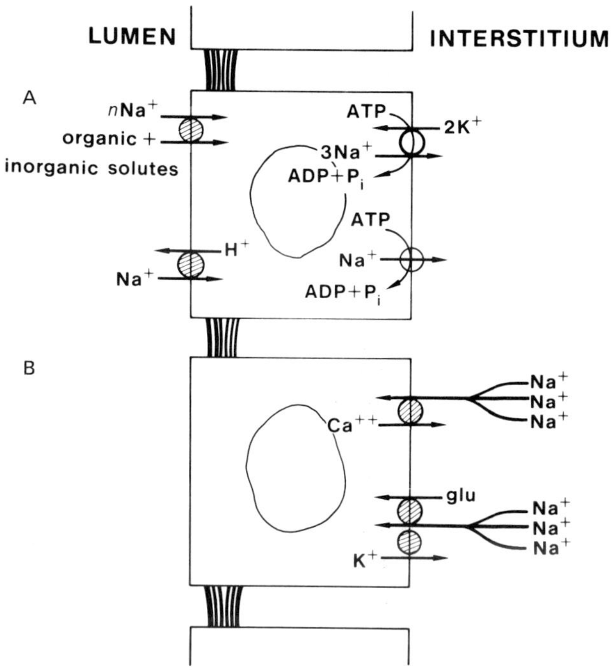

Fig. 5 Sodium transport systems in the proximal tubule. (A) The main pathways in transcellular absorption are indicated. (B) Leak pathways across the contraluminal membrane are shown.

With respect to the molecular nature of the Na-H exchange system, it has been demonstrated recently that carboxyl groups but not tyrosine groups are essential for the function of the transport system (44,45).

The second major pathway for sodium entry into the cell is the sodium symport systems, which will be discussed in detail below. The relative contribution of Na-H exchange and other sodium cotransport systems to the overall sodium entry across the luminal membrane varies from species to species. In the rabbit proximal tubule, as judged from microperfusion experiments (46), both pathways seem to contribute significantly to the sodium entry.

The Exit Step

The exit of sodium at the basal-lateral cell pole occurs against an electrochemical potential difference and thus requires energy. More and more evidence has accumulated that the predominant (if not only) system involved in active sodium transport across this membrane is the Na-K-ATPase (see Fig. 5). The first piece of evidence is that the enzyme is localized exclusively in the basal-lateral plasma membranes (47). It has been shown recently that if measured under optimum conditions, the specific activity of the enzyme found in the rabbit proximal tubule per millimeter of transporting epithelium is more than enough to explain the reabsorption of sodium. A ratio of 1.8 sodium ions transported per ATP hydrolyzed can be calculated from the overall sodium reabsorption observed in perfused tubules and the enzyme activity found in vitro (48).

A third point of concern with respect to the involvement of Na-K-ATPase in active sodium transport was an apparently very high Na/O_2 ratio in the kidney. As pointed out recently (29), if the appropriate corrections for passive ion movements are employed, the highly unlikely Na/O_2 ratio of 27 or Na/ATP ratio of 4.7 drops to 2.7 which is below the upper limit of the sodium/ATP ratio observed for the isolated, reconstituted Na-K-ATPase (14).

As a final point, another pathway for sodium exit should be discussed. Proverbio et al. (49) have described an ATPase in renal cortex plasma membranes that is stimulated by sodium (but not by potassium) and inhibited by ethacrynic acid (but not by ouabain). The authors (49) postulate a role of this enzyme in ethacrynic acid and furosemide inhibitable NaCl extrusion from the proximal tubular cell (50). In vitro, the specific activity of the Na-ATPase is about one-tenth of the Na-K-ATPase activity, suggesting that the pathway if operating in the intact cell contributes only to a small extent to the sodium transport across the basal-lateral membrane.

The basal-lateral plasma membrane of the proximal tubule contains in addition several sodium cotransport systems such as the sodium-calcium exchange system (10) and the sodium-glutamate symport system (51,52). These systems represent pathways through which sodium cycles that has been extruded from the cell (see Fig. 5).

The Rate-Limiting Step and Regulation of Sodium Transport

From the data presented above it is interesting to ask the question whether the entry or the exit step is rate limiting in the transcellular sodium transport in the proximal tubule. Two lines of evidence indicate that under normal conditions the rate of transcellular transport might be limited by the luminal entry step. When rabbit kidney proximal tubules are perfused with a solution containing no organic solutes, the rate of transepithelial sodium reabsorption is very low, whereas addition of organic solutes increases the reabsorption dramatically because sodium enters the cell via the sodium-solute cotransport systems (46). Another way to increase the sodium entry into the cell was used by Aronson et al. (53). The application of amphotericin B to the luminal membrane of rabbit proximal tubule increased transepithelial sodium transport by a factor of two (53). In addition, if the activity of the Na-K-ATPase found in isolated proximal tubules is considered, only about half of the enzyme activity seems to be operating under normal transport conditions. This figure can be derived from comparing the ratio of three sodium ions transported per one ATP hydrolyzed in the optimally coupled Na-K-ATPase reaction to the amount of sodium transported in the tubule per unit of enzyme (1.7 sodium ions per ATP hydrolyzed) activity. The latter ratio assumes that all sodium ions are transported actively. If one takes into account, however, that less than 50% of the transepithelial sodium transport in the proximal tubule is active, the ratio drops to 0.8. Assuming that the ratio of three sodium per ATP hydrolyzed holds in the intact tubule, the Na-K-ATPase is only used to about 27% of its capacity. Although comparing enzyme activities in vitro with the actual rate of enzymatic reactions in vivo is always problematic because effective ion concentrations, substrate concentration, and the concentrations of inhibitors are not known, the considerations presented above tend to indicate that the luminal entry step can be the rate-limiting step for sodium transport under conditions of normal ATPase and metabolic activities.

With respect to the hormonal regulation, only the exit step represented by the Na-K-ATPase has been investigated. The results obtained so far are equivocal. One study reported that adrenalectomy decreases sodium reabsorption and Na-K-ATPase in microdissected tubules (54). Treatment of rabbits with desoxycorticosterone (Doca), low salt diet, or short-term application of aldosterone, which increased transport activity, failed to increase enzyme activity (48). Similar results concerning the regulation of sodium transport and the Na-K-ATPase by thyroid hormones have been obtained. Thyroidectomy decreases isotonic volume reabsorption and reduced the Na-K-ATPase activity (55,56). Short-term treatment of the animals with low doses of triiodothyronine (T_3) increases isotonic volume reabsorption, but the ATPase activity in kidney cortex homegenates is initially not changed. The increase of ATPase occurs with a time lag and does not show a time course that is identical to the increase of transport. These observations also point to a possible regulation of transport both at the entry step and the exit step; short-term regulation might involve mainly the former, long-term regulation mainly the latter.

B. Proton Transport

Two transport systems have been found in the brush-border membrane that contribute to the acidification of the primary filtrate (see Fig. 6). One is the sodium-proton exchange system that plays an important role in sodium reabsorption as well as in proton secretion (38-41). The properties of this system have been described above. The other system is an ATP-driven proton pump that has been demonstrated recently in brush-border membrane vesicles. Vesicles loaded with ATP and an ATP-regenerating system show intravesicular ATP hydrolysis that is inhibited by a pH gradient ($pH_i > pH_o$) and stimulated by protonophors (57). The vesicles show also CFCCP-sensitive proton secretion. Both ATP-dependent proton secretion and intravesicular ATP hydrolysis are inhibited by dicyclocarbodiamide, Dio 9, and the cholesterol complexing agent filipin, but not by oligomycin (58). The latter findings indicate that the ATP-dependent proton transport in the brush-border membrane differs from the mitochondrial ATPase reaction. Further experiments are required to study how the ATP-driven proton pump is related to a Mg-ATPase activity in brush border membranes that is stimulated by oxyanions and that has been hypothesized to be involved in renal proton transport (51). Other unsolved questions concern the electrogenicity, stoichiometry, and capacity of the ATP-dependent proton transport system.

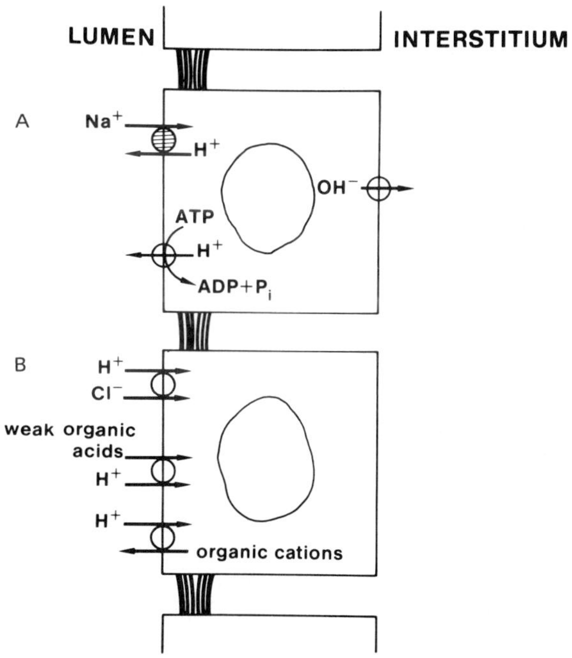

Fig. 6 Proton transport systems in the proximal tubule. (A) The main transcellular pathways for proton secretion (or bicarbonate reabsorption) are shown. (B) Proton entry mechanisms in the luminal membrane.

As indicated in Fig. 6, the luminal membrane contains additional transport systems by which protons recycle or are exchanged. According to some authors, *p*-aminohippurate uptake by brush-border membrane vesicles is stimulated by a pH gradient across the membrane (60), as is the efflux of organic cations (61). With respect to the exit step, no studies with plasma membrane vesicles are available. Electrophysiological studies point to the presence of a high conductivity pathway for OH ions in the basal-lateral membranes (62).

It should be mentioned in this context that both the brush-border membranes and the basal-lateral plasma membranes contain carbonic anhydrase activity, which appears to be closely associated with the membranes (63). The luminal carbonic anhydrase might be involved in the buffering of protons in the tubular fluid, but the role of the contraluminal enzyme is unclear. It is difficult at the present state of knowledge to define how much the Na-H exchanger and the proton ATPase contribute to the overall proton secretion of the tubule. According to micropuncture studies in the rat, about 80% of the proton secretion in the proximal tubule is sodium dependent (64,65). If one were to equate sodium dependence with the operation of the Na-H exchanger—recent studies indicate that the proton ATPase is sodium independent—in the rat about 80% of proton secretion would occur via the sodium-proton exchanger.

In view of the high intracellular buffer capacity the rate-limiting step for proton secretion is probably located in the luminal membrane. There is one report that in acidosis the brush-border membrane-bound anion-sensitive Mg-ATPase is increased in rat kidney brush borders (66). If this result can be confirmed, the ATPase—and thus probably the ATP-dependent proton pump—might be regulated by the acid-base status of the animal.

C. Calcium Transport

Calcium transport in the proximal tubule also involves a sodium-dependent exchange system and a sodium-independent ATP-driven transport system (see Fig. 7). Since the intracellular calcium activity is very low, calcium transport across the luminal membranes follows its electrochemical potential difference and the transfer across the contraluminal membrane requires energy. In rat brush-border vesicles calcium entry is saturable ($K_m \sim 5 \times 10^{-3}$ mol/liter) and strongly temperature dependent (10). The luminal membrane possesses also binding sites for calcium located probably both at the membrane surface and the cyto-

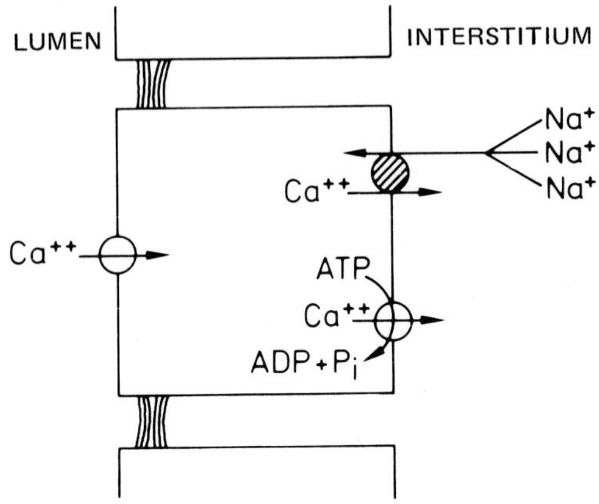

Fig. 7 Calcium transport systems in the proximal tubule. Only the transcellular pathways are indicated in the figure.

plasmic face of the membrane. The physiological role of these binding sites is not clear; they might be involved in membrane stabilization and regulation of membrane permeability. Experimental evidence for such a role has been obtained in studies where the sodium permeability of brush-border membrane vesicles isolated in the presence or absence of calcium has been compared. Rat kidney brush-border vesicles prepared in high calcium show a lower sodium permeability and appear to be more stable than membranes prepared without calcium (4).

At the contraluminal cell side a sodium-calcium exchange system and an ATP-driven calcium transport system exist. The sodium-calcium exchange system has been demonstrated in rat kidney basal-lateral plasma membranes (10). Calcium efflux from these vesicles was markedly stimulated by the presence of sodium in the incubation medium. The stimulatory effect of sodium was even more pronounced when the membrane was short circuited electrically by valinomycin and potassium. These results suggest that the system is electrogenic and more than two sodium ions are exchanged per one calcium ion. An even higher stoichiometry has to be assumed in order to explain the very steep calcium gradient of three orders of magnitude or more that can be maintained across the contraluminal membranes.

The apparent affinity of the exchange system for calcium has not yet been defined; with sodium a half maximal stimulation of calcium exchange (at 100 μmol Ca^{2+}) is achieved at about 30 mmol (10). Sodium-calcium exchange seems to be the main system involved in calcium reabsorption in the proximal tubule. This can be concluded from the finding that in the absence of sodium calcium transport in the proximal tubule is very low (67).

With respect to ATP-dependent calcium transport, basal-lateral plasma membranes were found to possess a Ca^{2+}-ATPase activity (68,69) and to accumulate calcium in the presence of Mg and ATP (10). The ATP-dependent calcium transport system has an apparent affinity for free calcium of about 1 μmol; it is inhibited by lanthanum, ruthenium red, and verapamil. The ATP-dependent transport system is most probably sodium independent. The relationship between the Ca^{2+}-ATPase activity and the ATP-dependent Ca^{2+} transport as well as the stoichiometry of the transport system remain to be determined. It is also not clear whether and how the two calcium transport systems in the basal-lateral membrane cooperate and how changes in the ATP-dependent transport system affect calcium transport in the proximal tubule.

D. Chloride Transport

The mechanism of chloride transport across the proximal tubule is far from being understood. In a phenomenological study in the rat Froemter et al. (37) concluded that transport of chloride in the proximal tubule is passive and probably proceeds via the paracellular route. In *Necturus* proximal tubule on the contrary, evidence was provided from measurements of intracellular ion activities that a NaCl cotransport system operates in the luminal membrane (70). In a study using rabbit kidney brush-border vesicles, chloride uptake was stimulated by intravesicular alkalinization and by an inside positive membrane diffusion potential (23). From these results it was concluded that the membranes contain a Cl-OH exchange system and a conductive pathway for chloride. The concerted action of the Cl-OH exchanger and Na-H exchanger could lead to a coupled transfer of NaCl, in agreement with the observations in the *Necturus* proximal tubule. On the other hand, Schwartz could not find evidence for the operation of a Cl-OH transport system in the early proximal tubule of rabbit kidney (24). As discussed above, there are several explanations for the discrepancies between the findings in vivo and the results of the vesicle studies—heterogeneity of the vesicles is the most probable one. Transport of chloride across the basal-lateral membrane has been studied in *Necturus* kidney. According to Shindo and Spring, chloride exit is accompanied by potassium movements (71).

E. Phosphate Transport

For a long time phosphate transport in the proximal tubule was poorly understood and transport models were highly speculative. This situation changed when the first studies with isolated plasma membrane vesicles were performed in which the transport across the membranes could be distinguished from metabolic reactions and mitochondrial transport events (72,73).

The Entry Step

Phosphate transport across the brush-border membrane is now generally assumed to involve a sodium-phosphate cotransport system (see Fig. 8). This is evident from studies with rat, rabbit, mice, and dog renal brush-border membranes in which phosphate uptake is stimulated

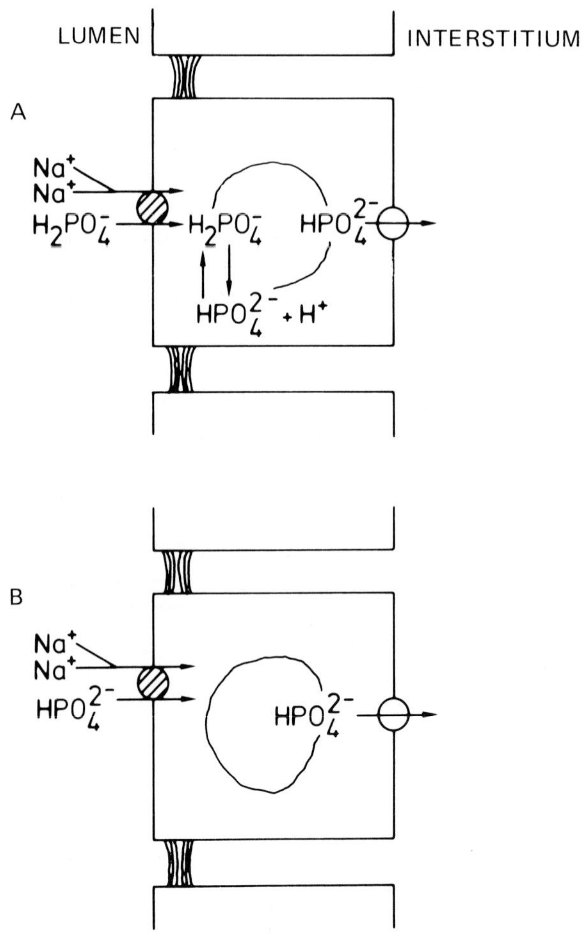

Fig. 8 Phosphate transport systems in the proximal tubule. (A) the absorption of primary phosphate, (B) the absorption of secondary phosphate is shown.

by the presence of sodium, and sodium uptake into the vesicles is enhanced by the presence of phosphate (74-77). Studies on the electrogenicity and the pH dependence of the transport revealed that the transport system accepts both primary and secondary phosphate with quite similar affinities and that always two sodium ions are cotransported with one phosphate ion (74,78). This stoichiometry leads to electroneutral sodium cotransport of secondary phosphate and an electrogenic (positive charge) sodium cotransport of primary phosphate.

Along the proximal tubule acidification takes place and the ratio of secondary to primary phosphate decreases. At a given sodium gradient and membrane potential across the luminal membrane the driving force for the cellular uptake of secondary phosphate consists of the concentration difference for sodium across the membrane, whereas the driving force for the uptake of primary phosphate includes both the concentration difference for sodium and the electrical potential difference. In the latter part of the proximal tubule, therefore, the reabsorption of primary phosphate can proceed against a steep concentration difference. In this part the pH difference between the tubular lumen and the cytosol may act as additional driving force for phosphate uptake (see Fig. 8). Primary phosphate translocated by the sodium-phosphate cotransport system across the luminal membrane dissociates into secondary phosphate and proton inside the cell, thus the intracellular concentration of primary phosphate is lowered, and consequently the concentration difference for primary phosphate increases, favoring cellular uptake. Such a mechanism has been demonstrated experimentally in rabbit brush-border vesicles (78).

With respect to the biochemical nature of the transport system, it has been hypothesized that alkaline phosphatase is involved in phosphate transport across the brush-border membrane (78). Studies with proteases and inhibitors of alkaline phosphatase revealed, however, that in the isolated membrane vesicles alkaline phosphatase and phosphate transport behave differently and that their activities can be dissociated (80,81). Alkaline phosphatase is, for example, much less sensitive to proteolytic digestion than the sodium-phosphate cotransport system, whereas ethylenediaminotetraacetic acid (EDTA) and phenylalanine inhibit alkaline phosphatase activity but not phosphate transport in rat brush-border membrane vesicles. Thus, it seems unlikely that alkaline phosphatase and the sodium-phosphate cotransport system are identical molecules.

The Exit Step

The molecular mechanisms involved in phosphate transport across the basal-lateral membrane of the proximal tubule are still poorly understood. The transfer is definitely different from the transport across the luminal membrane (74). As demonstrated in isolated rat basal-lateral plasma membranes, the sodium sensitivity is much lower (or even absent) and the transfer may be electrogenic—i.e., phosphate may be transported as an anion across the membrane (see Fig. 8).

The Rate-Limiting Step and Regulation of Phosphate Transport

The sodium-phosphate cotransport system is the main regulatory site for phosphate reabsorption in the proximal tubule. A parallel behavior of sodium-dependent phosphate uptake by isolated brush-border membranes and phosphate reabsorption in the proximal tubule has been observed in X-linked hypophosphatemia in mice, and after parathyroidectomy, parathyroid hormone (PTH) substitution, high phosphate diet, low phosphate diet, and 1, 25-dihydroxyvitamin D application in rats, dogs, and pigs (82-90). In all instances, V_{max} of the transport system is altered; the affinities of the transport system for phosphate and

–if tested–for sodium do not change. The latter finding is important because sodium increased the maximum velocity of phosphate uptake–thus an alteration of the affinity of the transport system for sodium could alter the maximal velocity of the sodium-phosphate cotransport. The molecular basis for the change in transport capacity remains to be elucidated. Phosphorylation of regulatory sites or regulatory proteins, ADP-ribosylation (21,91), alterations in the lipid surrounding, activation of latent sites, or insertion of transport sites into the membrane are feasible possibilities.

F. Sulfate-Thiosulfate Transport

Studies with rat kidney brush-border vesicles have shown that the uptake of sulfate into the vesicles is markedly stimulated by the presence of sodium (92). This effect of sodium is not due to the generation of a vesicle inside positive membrane potential because stimulation is also observed when the membrane has been short-circuited by the use of valinomycin and potassium. The sodium-dependent uptake is inhibited by thiosulfate and wolframate but not by phosphate (92).

When a membrane diffusion potential is generated across the brush-border membrane by means of salt gradients the sodium-dependent sulfate uptake is not affected, indicating that the transfer of sodium with sulfate is electroneutral. This result suggests that two cations (probably sodium) are translocated together with the divalent anion sulfate. All the results taken together lead to the conclusion that the brush-border membrane contains a sodium-sulfate cotransport system which is shared by thiosulfate and wolframate. In in vivo studies indeed a sodium-dependent reabsorption of sulfate has been found in rat proximal tubule (93). Interestingly enough, there is also a secretory pathway for thiosulfate. After removal of sodium from the tubular lumen the tubule secretes thiosulfate because the absorptive pathway is not operating.

The transport processes at the contraluminal membrane have not been investigated in vesicles. Microperfusion studies indicate that the secretory system for thiosulfate is inhibited by probenecid (93). This result is compatible with the assumption that the thiosulfate is transported by the weak organic acid transport system. Studies with isolated perfused rabbit tubules imply also the role of anion exchange systems in sulfate transport (94).

G. Sugar Transport

The membrane-molecular approach was first applied to the D-glucose transport in the proximal tubule. Phlorizin binding studies with isolated brush-border fragments provided the first information on the properties of the sodium-D-glucose cotransport system in this membrane (95). Transport studies with brush-border membranes as well as basal-lateral plasma membranes (96-114) confirmed this assumption and extended our knowledge markedly. Thus, today the sodium-D-glucose cotransport system can be considered as a model system for the investigation of biophysical and biochemical events in sodium cotransport systems in general (97).

The Entry Step

In brush-border membrane vesicles the uptake of D-glucose is stereospecific and markedly stimulated in the presence of sodium. In the presence of a sodium gradient across the membrane, D-glucose is accumulated inside the vesicles ("overshoot") (see Fig. 9). The time course of D-glucose uptake and the occurrence of the overshoot can be described in thermodynamic terms by the following equation:

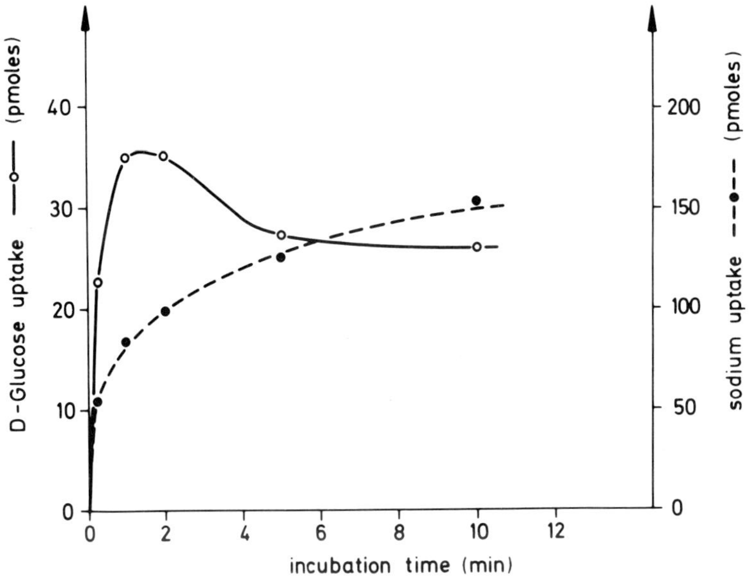

Fig. 9 Time course of D-glucose and sodium uptake into rat kidney microvilli vesicles. D-glucose uptake was investigated in the presence of a sodium chloride gradient across the membrane. (From Ref. 96.)

$$J_{glu} = L_{glu\,glu} \Delta c_{glu} + L_{glu\,Na} \Delta \mu_{Na}$$

where:

$$\Delta \mu_{Na} = \Delta \psi - 2.3 \frac{RT}{F} \log \frac{[Na]_o}{[Na]_i}$$

and the abbreviations have the following meaning:

J_{glu}	= glucose net flux
$L_{glu\,glu}$	= straight coefficient
$L_{glu\,Na}$	= cross coefficient
$\Delta \mu_{Na}$	= electrochemical potential difference for sodium across the membrane
Δc_{glu}	= concentration difference for glucose across the membrane
$\Delta \psi$	= electrical potential difference
$[Na]_o$	= sodium concentration in the incubation medium
$[Na]_i$	= sodium concentration inside the vesicles

The uptake of glucose into the vesicles (see Fig. 9) can be divided into four phases. In the initial uptake phase both Δc_{glu} and $\Delta \mu_{Na}$ are positive, since at the beginning of the experiment the inside of the vesicle contains essentially no sodium and no D-glucose. When the intravesicular D-glucose concentration becomes larger than the extravesicular D-glucose concentration and Δc_{glu} becomes negative, the only remaining driving force for D-glucose uptake is $\Delta \mu_{Na}$. Since at the same time sodium enters the vesicle via a D-glucose independent pathway–i.e., via Na^+-H^+ exchange–$\Delta \mu_{Na}$ is slowly dissipated (see Fig. 9). At the peak of the overshoot, the driving force residing in the residual sodium gradient and the opposing driving force exerted by Δc_{glu} cancel. Subsequently $\Delta \mu_{Na}$ becomes smaller than Δc_{glu} and efflux occurs. After 60 min of incubation all solutes are in equilibrium. When tested experimentally (110,111) the accumulation of D-glucose in the presence of defined sodium gradients was about 80% of the theoretical value indicating a close coupling between sodium gradient and glucose uptake (27).

In addition to a chemical gradient of sodium, the membrane potential is also capable of driving D-glucose accumulation in brush-border membrane vesicles. This has been demonstrated by imposing a diffusion potential across the membrane in the absence of a chemical sodium gradient (110,111).

Furthermore, the transfer of sodium across the brush-border membrane is stimulated by the presence of D-glucose (51,113). Sodium uptake into brush-border membranes is increased in the presence of D-glucose gradient. When vesicles preloaded with sodium are exposed to a sugar gradient the intravesicular sodium increases and a transient accumulation of sodium inside the vesicles is observed (see Fig. 10). Since the latter experiments are performed under conditions where electrical driving forces for sodium movement can be excluded, they indicate that the driving force related to the glucose gradient can be utilized by the cotransport system to accumulate sodium. This reciprocal behavior—a sodium gradient drives D-glucose accumulation and a D-glucose gradient drives sodium accumulation—is a very strong piece of evidence for a sodium solute cotransport system. If the two fluxes are compared quantitatively a stoichiometry of close to one is obtained (112).

The contribution of the chemical gradient of sodium and the electrical potential difference are additive although not equivalent (111,115). The membrane potential in addition affects the transport system itself, changing its kinetic parameters and affecting the binding of phlorhizin to the transport system (115,116). An inside negative membrane potential—that simulates the situation in vivo—stimulates D-glucose uptake and increases phlorhizin binding. The mechanism of the action of the membrane potential is not clear and still under investigation.

With regard to the biochemical characteristics of the transport system, the active site of the sodium-D-glucose cotransport system can be considered as being composed of a cation binding site, a sugar binding site, and a phlorhizin binding site. In sugar uptake studies an apparent K_m value for sodium of about 25 mmol was found (96) and the specificity for sodium is very high, while lithium—in contrast to some amino acid cotransport systems—

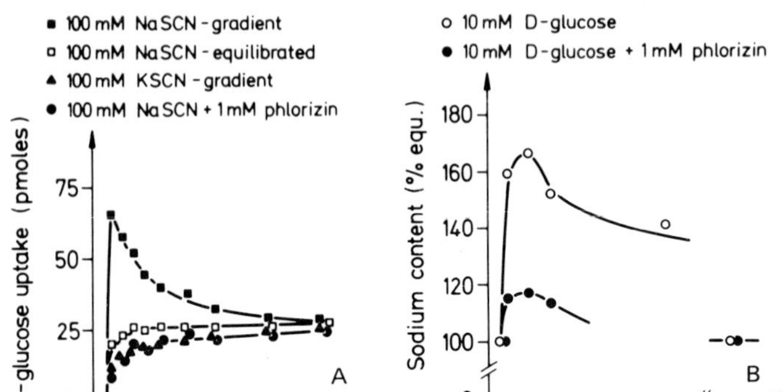

Fig. 10 Coupling between sodium and D-glucose flux in microvilli vesicles isolated from rat kidney cortex. (A) The effect of a sodium gradient on D-glucose uptake. (B) The effect of a D-glucose gradient on the sodium content. (From Ref. 51.)

cannot replace sodium. The interaction of sodium with the binding site is inhibited by harmaline (42). This hallucinogenic drug carries a strong positive charge and competes with sodium; its apparent affinity for the sodium site is about 2 mmol. If sodium binds to the transport system the affinity for D-glucose increases (95). In binding studies, similarly, the affinity for phlorhizin has been found to increase, whereas the maximum number of phlorizin binding sites remains constant (95).

The sugar binding site of the renal hexose transport system is, similar to the intestinal transport system (117,118), characterized by a high stereospecificity. As shown by Kleinzeller et al. (119), glucose interacts with the transport system via hydroxyl groups at C_1, C_2, C_3, probably C_4, and the ring oxygen. The D-glucoconfiguration is the preferred structure. At C_6 an interaction between a hydroxyl group and the binding site facilitates transport, but its presence seems not to be essential. The chemical nature of the interaction between the transportate and the transport system is not defined as yet, but studies with fluorinated glucose analogues suggest that hydrogen bonding is involved.

The above described structural requirements hold both for the transport of D-glucose across the brush-border membrane and for the interaction of sugars with the surface of the transport molecule exposed to the tubular lumen. This can be concluded from the similarity of the results obtained in D-glucose transport studies (with intact tissue or right side out oriented brush-border vesicles) and in phlorizin binding studies on isolated membranes (97,120).

In isolated vesicles the apparent affinity of the sugar binding site is 12 mmol under conditions where sodium is equilibrated across the membrane. Under conditions of a sodium gradient the affinity is about 1 mmol (97). The difference in affinity is probably due to the effect of the membrane potential on the glucose-sodium cotransport system.

The binding of phlorizin to the sodium-glucose cotransport systems involves an interaction with the sugar binding site via the glucose moiety of phlorizin and with an aglucone binding site via the phloretin moiety. Free hydroxyl groups and free rotation between ring A and ring B as well as proper spacing between the aglucone and the sugar residue (distance about 14 Å) are essential for an optimum binding of phlorizin to the transport system (97).

With respect to the molecular structure of the sodium-glucose cotransport system, we still have to rely mainly on hypothetical schemes, since no studies on the isolated transport system have been possible so far. The transport system is envisaged as a protein unit (monomer or dimer) spanning the membrane (121) and possessing two distinct, nonidentical surfaces, the outer surface facing the tubular lumen and an inner surface facing the cytoplasm. The two surfaces probably differ in their substrate specificity and in the number of SH groups that can be modified by *N*-ethylmaleimide (NEM) (97).

Several attempts have been made to purify the sodium-D-glucose transport system (122-131). These attempts have been only partially successful because the transport protein constitutes a minute portion of the total membrane protein. Recently, affinity chromatography has been used to enrich the transport activity (127). In reconstituted proteoliposomes the transport activity of the fraction that is retained by a phlorhizin column and can be eluted by a high concentration of glucose is enriched about 40-fold above the membrane fraction (127). Further purification with increased yield is necessary to make studies on the composition and the conformation of protein possible. With respect to amino acid side chains that are essential for the function of the transport system, SH groups seem to play an essential role. *N*-ethylmaleimide blocks glucose transport and phlorhizin binding in isolated vesicles; approximately three SH groups are protected by phlorhizin from the reaction with the transport protein (87), indicating a very close association of these groups to the active site. A similar substrate protection effect has been observed for sodium and tyrosine reactive reagents (135). This could indicate that a tyrosine group is located close to the sodium binding site.

The Exit Step

Transport studies with basal-lateral plasma membranes indicate that the sugar transport system in the contraluminal cellface is sodium independent, more sensitive to phloretin than to phlorhizin, inhibited by cytochalasin B, and shows a stereospecificity different from that of the sodium-glucose cotransport system in the brush-border membrane (51,96,106) (Fig. 11). A free OH group at C_1 is required, and sugars modified at the C_2-OH group such as 2-deoxy-D-glucose and mannose are transported (132). The translocation of the sugars across the basal lateral membrane is not associated with a phosphorylation step (133), although there is immediate intracellular phosphorylation of sugars that are taken up at the basal pole of the cell (134). This phosphorylation effectively reduces the efflux of these sugars out of the cell.

Another carbohydrate transport system present in the brush-border membrane is a transport system for myoinositol. In isolated brush-border membranes the transport of myoinositol is sodium dependent, electrogenic, and inhibited by phlorizin and D-glucose (136,137). D-Glucose is, however, not transported by the myoinositol system because D-glucose does not exchange with myoinositol in heterocounterexchange experiments (136).

H. Transport of Small Peptides

Physiologically important peptides such as angiotensin II and bradykinin are filtered and subsequently hydrolyzed at the brush-border surface to yield tripeptides, dipeptides, and

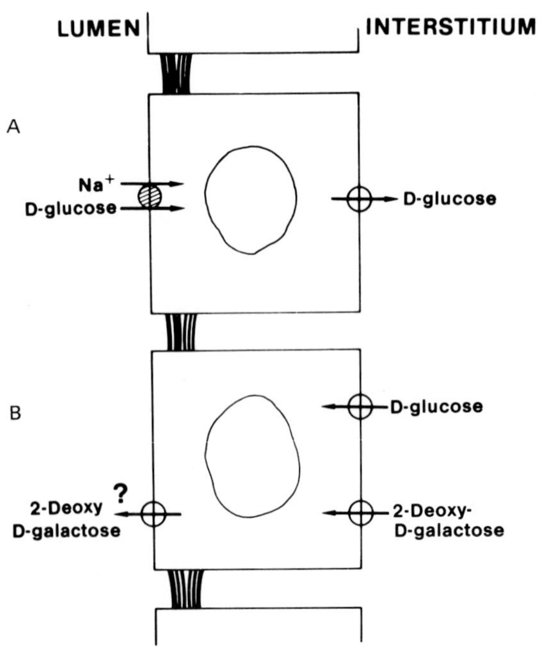

Fig. 11 Sugar transport systems in the proximal tubule. (A) relates to sugar absorption, (B) to sugar uptake at the contraluminal cell side.

free amino acids (138-144). The free amino acids are transported by the sodium cotransport systems discussed below. Some dipeptides, however, can be taken up in intact form into the cell by specific transport systems located in the brush-border membrane (145-147). For example, rabbit kidney brush border contains a transport system for glycyl-L-proline that is sodium independent, has a K_m of 1.1 mmol, and a V_{max} of 0.81 nmol/min per mg protein (145-147). L-Histidyl-L-proline, carnosine (β-alanyl-histidine), and L-leucyl-glycine compete with glycyl-L-proline for the transport system, while the corresponding free amino acids at the same concentration are ineffective. This indicates that the peptide bond and both amino acid residues are essential for the recognition of the substrate by the transport system. The proline residue is probably more essential than the glycyl-residue, since L-histidyl-proline is a very strong inhibitor of glycyl-L-proline transport. After transport into the cell the dipeptide is broken down by a cytoplasmic or membrane associated glycyl-L-proline hydrolase. The hydrolysis of the dipeptide reduces the intracellular concentration of the dipeptide and, thus, a favorable gradient for cellular uptake is maintained. Nothing is known about the transport of peptides across the basal-lateral plasma membranes.

The majority of the di- and tripeptides that are filtered, especially those without proline or hydroxyproline residue, are hydrolyzed completely and the amino acids are consequently taken up by the amino acid transport systems in the brush-border membrane. This has been demonstrated by microperfusion techniques in the intact tubule (140) and by in vitro studies with isolated membrane vesicles (145-147). The importance of these processes for the plasma clearance of peptides, whether physiologically active peptides or peptides taken up by the small intestine is evident.

I. Amino Acid Transport

The Entry Step

Studies with isolated brush-border membranes have essentially confirmed the presence of six different classes of transport systems (148,149) based on a different stereospecificity. The six systems are: a transport system for neutral amino acids, glycine, imino acids, basic amino acids, acidic amino acids, and β-amino acids (150-167). The results obtained so far with the isolated membranes are compiled in Table 1. In analyzing the data two areas of discrepancy can be noted. One concerns the presence of more than one transport system in the membrane fractions. It has to be determined in the future whether there indeed exist two transport systems in the same membrane or whether the high-affinity systems are related to binding reactions of the membrane. Since a strong axial heterogeneity of the tubule with respect to amino acid transport has been observed (22), it is also possible that the various transport systems are present in different parts of the proximal tubule (168-170). Another discrepancy concerns the sodium dependency of some of the transport systems, for example, for arginine. Technical problems such as binding of the amino acid to the membranes and pH changes inside the vesicle can make a clear-cut demonstration of sodium dependence difficult in isolated vesicles. Such difficulties can account for some of the discrepancies.

Despite the technical difficulties, sodium dependence has been observed for at least one transport system in each of the six classes, suggesting that at least six sodium-amino acid cotransport systems exist in the brush-border membrane. Sodium in most instances increases the apparent affinity of the transport system for the amino acid, whereas the apparant V_{max} remains constant. The affinity for sodium at low amino acid concentrations varies between 4.5 and 60 mmol. In comparison to the sodium-D-glucose cotransport system,

Table 1 Amino Acid Transport Systems in Isolated Brush-Border Membranes

Amino acid	Sodium dependence	Stereospecificity	K_m	V_{max}	Species	Reference
L-Phenylalanine	Yes	D-Phenylalanine shows countertransport	4 mmol (100 mmol NaCl gradient)	36 nmol/min per mg protein (100 mmol NaCl gradient)	Rat	(166)
L-Alanine	Yes	Alanine, glycine, imino acids	0.4 mmol (100 mmol NaCl	0.42 nmol/min per mg protein	Rabbit	(156)
Glycine 1	Yes	Shared with proline	4.0 mmol (200 mmol NaCl gradient)	26.4 nmol/min per mg protein (100 mmol NaCl gradient)	Rat	(150,151)
Glycine 2	Yes	Noncompetitively inhibited by proline	0.22 mmol (200 mmol NaCl gradient)	0.72 nmol/min per mg protein (100 mmol NaCl gradient)	Rat Rat	(150,151) (150,151)
Proline 1	Yes	Shared with glycine	0.067 mmol (100 mmol NaCl gradient)	7.04 nmol/min per mg protein (100 mmol NaCl gradient)	Rat	(150,151)
Proline 2	No	Only proline accepted	5.62 mmol	18.68 nmol/min per mg protein	Rat	(150,151,157)
Proline 3	?	?	?	?	Rabbit	(159)
β-Alanine	Yes	Shared with taurine	30 μmol (100 mmol NaCl gradient)	0.04 nmol/min per mg protein (100 mmol NaCl gradient)	Rabbit	(158)
Taurine	Yes	Shared with β-alanine, hypotaurine	17 μmol (100 mmol NaCl gradient)	0.456 nmol/min per mg protein (100 mmol NaCl gradient)	Rat	(163)
L-Arginine 1	Not clear	Accepts also ornithine, cystine, and lysine	70 μmol	6 nmol/min per mg protein	Rabbit	(152)
L-Arginine 2	Yes	Accepts also ornithine, cystine, lysine, and D-arginine	3.5 mmol (70 mmol NaCl gradient)	32 nmol/min per mg protein (70mmol NaCl gradient)	Rabbit	(153)
L-Cystine	?	Shared by basic amino acids	0.033 mmol	0.4 nmol/min per mg protein	Rat	(161)
L-Cystine	Yes	?	0.93 mmol (100 mmol NaCl gradient)	3.96 nmol/min per mg protein (100 mmol NaCl gradient)	Rat	(161)
Glutamic acid 1	Yes	Shared with phenylalanine and glutamine	0.016 mmol (100 mmol NaCl gradient)	0.8 nmol/min per mg protein (100 mmol NaCl gradient)	Rabbit	(164,165)
Glutamic acid 2	Yes	?	3.6 mmol	16 nmol/min per mg protein	Rabbit	(164,165)
Glutamic acid 3	Yes	?	?	?	Rat	(25,154,162)
Glutamine 1	Yes	Some overlap with neutral and basic amino acids	0.14 mmol (100 mmol NaCl gradient)	2.4 nmol/min per mg protein (100 mmol NaCl gradient)	Rat	(154)
Glutamine 2	Yes	?	8.5 mmol	68 nmol/min per mg protein	Rat	(154)
Glutamine 3	Yes	?	0.76 mmol (150 mmol NaCl gradient)	9.6 nmol/min per mg protein (150 mmol NaCl gradient)	Rat	(160,155)

amino acid cotransport systems show a lower specificity of the cation binding site. Lithium can effectively replace sodium in stimulating amino acid uptake into the brush-border vesicles.

There is another important difference between the sodium-D-glucose transport system and sodium-amino acid cotransport systems. Sodium-dependent L-glutamate uptake, for example, is stimulated by the presence of potassium at the inside of the brush border and L-glutamate efflux by the presence of potassium at the outside of the vesicle (162,164,165). It could be demonstrated that a potassium gradient directed from the inside to the outside of the vesicle can support an intravesicular accumulation of the amino acid. The results suggest that in the presence of sodium an exchange between L-glutamate and potassium occurs (Fig. 12). In rat kidney brush borders L-glutamate transport in the presence of potassium and sodium is electrogenic, i.e., involves the transfer of a positive charge (25,162). In order to explain the electrogenicity one has to assume that four cations move together with one divalent glutamate in exchange against one potassium. In rabbit kidney the transport seems to be electroneutral (165).

The Exit Step

In studies with basal-lateral plasma membranes from rat and rabbit kidney cortex the transport of neutral amino acids such as phenylalanine (166), histidine (51), and proline (106) was found to be sodium independent and to proceed via facilitated diffusion systems. The

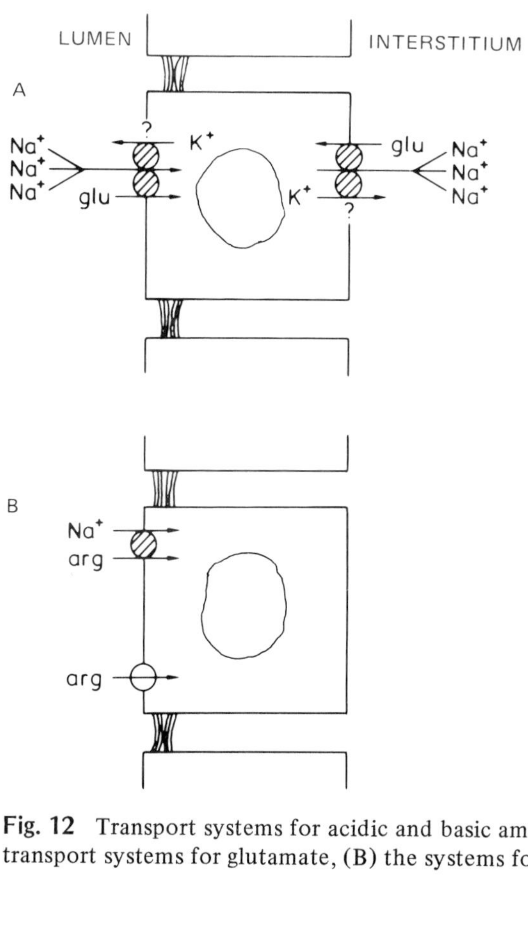

Fig. 12 Transport systems for acidic and basic amino acids in the proximal tubule. (A) the transport systems for glutamate, (B) the systems for arginine.

transport of glutamate, on the contrary, shows sodium dependence and is—similar to the brush-border membrane system—stimulated by a potassium gradient across the membrane (51,52). No studies concerning basic amino acid transport across the basal-lateral membranes have been performed hitherto. Thus, at least for the cortical parts of the proximal tubule, there seems to be an asymmetry of the cell with respect to sodium cotransport systems for neutral amino acids (see Fig. 13). Such an asymmetry has also been observed in electrophysiological studies and perfusion studies (148).

In the pars recta of the proximal tubule the basal-lateral plasma membrane probably contains sodium-dependent neutral amino acid transport systems. This can be concluded from the observations of Barfuss, Schafer, and Mays (168-170) that peritubular perfusion of pars recta segments from rabbit kidney with radioactively labeled amino acids leads to an intracellular accumulation of the amino acids. The accumulation is not observed if sodium is removed from the perfusion medium. Thus, it can be speculated that there is segmental inhomogeneity within the proximal tubule, not only with respect to brush-border transport functions but also with respect to basal-lateral membrane transport function. Further investigations of this important aspect of transport at the membrane level has not yet been possible because of the lack of suitable cell and membrane preparations. The physiological role of the sodium cotransport systems in the basal-lateral plasma membrane could be to provide the cells with the amino acids needed for the protein turnover in the cell. Since the luminal concentration of amino acids at the end of the proximal tubule is very low, the supply across the apical membrane is probably not sufficient.

J. Transport of Organic Anions

The proximal tubule handles organic anions in essentially two ways. A number of carboxylic acids that act as fuels for cellular energy production are reabsorbed by the tubular cell and

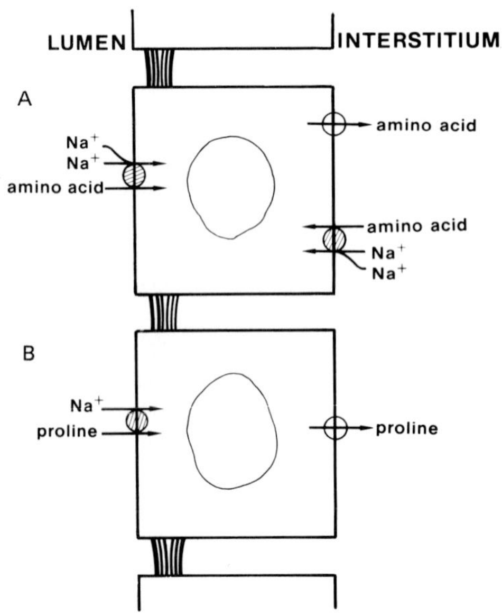

Fig. 13 Transport systems for neutral amino acids in proximal tubule. A stoichiometry of two sodium/one neutral amino acid is assumed for the cotransport system. This ratio may vary for the different sodium cotransport systems. The presence of the contraluminal sodium-dependent uptake system depends on the tubular segment investigated. For explanation of the symbols, see legend to Fig. 4.

subsequently metabolized; these include lactate, pyruvate, citric acid, α-ketoglutarate, and succinate. Other weak organic acids are secreted by the proximal tubule; these include p-aminohippuric acid, gluconic acid conjugates, glutathione conjugates of xenobiotics (171), and breakdown products of neurotransmitters such as vanillic acid. The analysis of the molecular mechanism and of the driving forces of tubular transport of the organic acids in the intact cell is complicated by intracellular metabolism and intracellular binding. Therefore, studies with vesicles were especially useful in defining and characterizing transport processes occurring at the plasma membrane level.

K. Transport of L-Lactate

Lactic acid will be discussed as a prototype for substrates taken up by the renal cell across the luminal brush-border membrane (33,172,173). In isolated brush-border membrane vesicles two pathways exist for lactate transport, a diffusional pathway and a sodium-lactate cotransport system (Fig. 14). At 1 mmol lactate the former contributes only about 10% to the total lactate uptake. The sodium-lactate cotransport system transports L-lactate and D-lactate with an apparent affinity of about 4 mmol and 5 mmol, respectively. The similar affinity of the transport system for D-lactate and for L-lactate is an interesting feature. Its molecular basis remains to be elucidated.

The uptake of the anion lactate is, in the presence of sodium, accompanied by a transfer of a positive charge, as evidenced by the stimulation of lactate uptake by an inside negative membrane potential. Such electrogenicity can be explained by the assumption that two cations (probably sodium) are cotransported with one lactate anion. As a consequence, in vivo, the electrical potential difference across the brush-border membrane (cell inside negative) favors the uptake of lactate via the sodium-lactate cotransport system, whereas it inhibits the uptake of the lactate anion. Nonionic diffusion does not seem to play a major

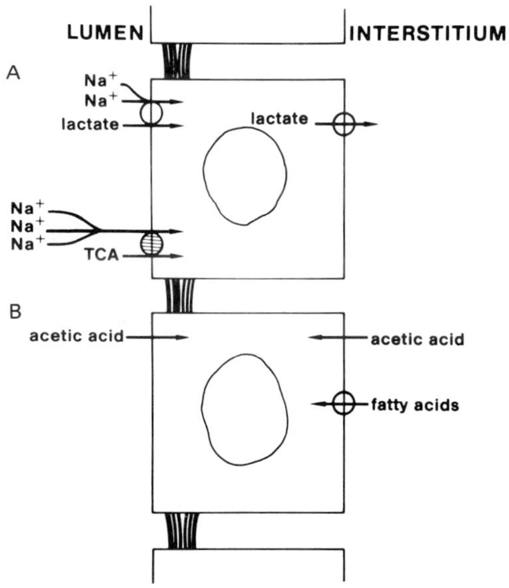

Fig. 14 Transport systems for metabolites in proximal tubule. (A) the transport system studied so far for lactate and tricarboxylic acids, (B) cellular tentative entry mechanisms for acetic acid and long chain fatty acids.

role in L-lactate uptake, and pH gradients established over the brush-border membrane do not affect L-lactate uptake significantly. This is also evident from micropuncture experiments (173).

L-lactate transfer in basal-lateral membrane vesicles is sodium independent and inhibited by SITS and probenecid (172). Lactate is probably transported as an anion across the membrane, since an inside positive membrane potential stimulates uptake into the vesicles. In vivo, exit from the cell is therefore favored by the electrical potential difference across the membrane. If the cellular lactate concentration is very low or if the membrane potential decreases, however, a situation can be imagined which favors the uptake of L-lactate across the basal-lateral membrane.

L. Transport of Tricarboxylic Acid Cycle Intermediates

In the brush-border vesicles the uptake of citrate, succinate, and α-ketoglutarate is stimulated by the presence of a sodium gradient (33,174). Similar to the L-lactate-sodium cotransport, sodium-dependent succinate cotransport is electrogenic and positive charges are transferred during the translocation. The stoichiometry of the transport system is probably three sodium per one succinate anion, although the question whether protons are also cotransported has not yet been clarified.

In an extensive study on the stereospecificity of this transport system it was found that the transport system interacts with citrate (but not *cis*-aconitate or isocitrate), α-ketoglutarate, succinate, fumarate, malate, and oxalacetate (174).

The only major metabolite whose transport in the kidney is poorly understood is pyruvate. Data in micropuncture experiments and in studies with isolated vesicles are conflicting. In micropuncture studies pyruvate inhibits D-lactate transport, but in brush-border vesicles pyruvate does not inhibit L-lactate uptake (32,172). Since it has been demonstrated that D- and L-lactate are transported by the same transport system, further experiments are required to resolve the discrepancies. One possibility would be that pyruvate, perhaps as enolate ($CH_2 = C(OH) - COOH$), can displace D-lactate from the carrier, but not L-lactate.

M. Glutamine Transport

In rat kidney brush-border membrane two transport systems for glutamine have been found (see Table 1) (154,155). Both are sodium dependent with a similar apparent K_m for sodium of 12 mmol. The high-affinity system (K_m 0.1 mmol, V_{max} = 0.62 nmol/15 sec per mg) also accepts L-phenylalanine, L-valine, L-ornithine, L-arginine, and L-lysine. In acidosis glutamine uptake across the brush-border membrane of rat kidney appears to be increased (155).

N. Transport of Fatty Acids

Small fatty acids such as acetate are transported across the brush-border membrane via the monocarboxylic acid-sodium cotransport system that also transports lactate (Ullrich et al., Pflügers Arch. 395:220-226, 1982). Long chain fatty acids, due to their binding to albumin, are not filtered and therefore do not appear in the primary urine. They are taken up at the contraluminal membrane probably via the transport system for weak organic acids. Evidence for such a mechanism was provided by Barac-Nieto and Cohen (175) in studies on the uptake of free fatty acids by the kidney. The uptake was inhibited by probenecid, the classic inhibitor of the weak organic acid transport system (175).

O. Transport of Nicotinic Acid

Nicotinic acid, an important vitamin, is also transported in a sodium dependent manner across the brush-border membrane ($K_m \sim 0.3$ mmol). The system requires one carboxyl group attached to a pyridine, pyrazine, or benzene ring (176). If an additional charged group is introduced into the ring, the ability of the compound to inhibit nicotinic acid uptake is markedly reduced. The sodium-nicotinic acid cotransport is apparently electroneutral, suggesting a stoichiometry of one sodium per one molecule of nicotinic acid.

P. Transport of Weak Organic Acids Such as *p*-Aminohippuric Acid

Although the transepithelial secretion of *p*-aminohippuric acid (PAH) has been studied extensively by a variety of techniques including plasma membrane vesicles, its biochemical and biophysical nature has remained obscure hitherto (177). There is general agreement that PAH is secreted by the renal proximal tubule and that the secretion can occur against steep electrochemical potential differences across the epithelium. It is also evident that PAH is accumulated inside the cell; it is, however, not clear how much PAH is bound to cellular constituents and how much is present in the free form. Despite this uncertainty the uptake of PAH across the basal-lateral membrane is considered to be active, while the exit step is assumed to be passive. With respect to the transport systems involved, the picture is only relatively clear for the transport across the basal-lateral membranes. Two studies performed with membranes from rat and dog kidney cortex agree that the basal-lateral membranes contain a transport system for PAH with an apparent affinity of 0.56 mmol and a V_{max} of 0.87 nmol/min per mg protein in dog kidney membranes (178) and of 0.54 mmol and of ~ 1.0 nmol/mg protein per 15 sec in rat kidney membranes (179). The transport system accepts probenecid with a fourfold to 10-fold higher affinity. None of the studies could detect a sodium-dependency of the transport. Ion gradient experiments indicated, however, that PAH crosses the membrane as an anion (179) (see Fig. 15).

With respect to the luminal exit step in flounder kidney brush-border membranes a stereospecific transport system for PAH has been demonstrated (180). The apparent affinity of the luminal transport system for PAH and probenecid is much lower than the affinity of the contraluminal transport system. Similar to the experiments with basal lateral membranes, transfer of PAH across the luminal transport system seems to occur in the form of an anion (180).

In rabbit kidney cortex and rat kidney brush-border membranes, PAH transport occurs primarily via nonionic diffusion (102,181). Additionally, a stimulation of probenecid-sensitive and probenecid-insensitive PAH uptake by a pH gradient ($pH_o < pH_i$) was observed (181). Thus, probably three pathways for PAH exist in the brush-border membrane: carrier-mediated transport as an anion, carrier-mediated transport together with a proton, and nonionic diffusion. In vivo, transfer of PAH as an anion across the luminal membrane (see Fig. 15) driven by the electrical potential difference would favor secretion. Nonionic diffusion on the other hand would at the given pH difference across the brush border (intracellular pH 7.4, intratubular pH 6.5) increase backleak of PAH into the cell. Thus, further studies are required to find the driving force for the contraluminal uptake and to define better the luminal exit step.

Q. Transport of Bile Acids

In micropuncture studies it was found that the absorption of taurocholate by the proximal tubule is active and depends on the presence of sodium (182). This suggested that a sodium-

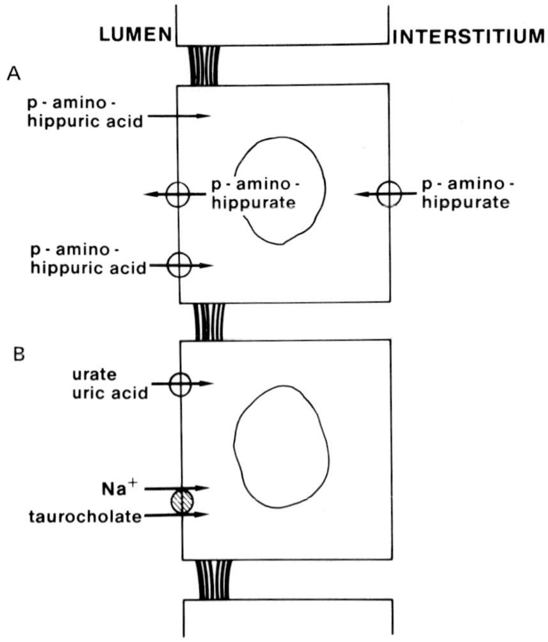

Fig. 15 Transport systems for organic anions in proximal tubule. (A) the various ways for the nondissociated *p*-aminohippuric acid and the anion *p*-aminohippurate are indicated, (B) the transport systems for urate and taurocholate are shown.

taurocholate cotransport system is involved in the absorptive process. Studies with isolated brush-border membrane vesicles showed that taurocholate uptake is sodium dependent and specific, i.e., glycocholate and cholate inhibit taurocholate uptake (182). The apparent K_m of the system (in the presence of 100 mmol NaCl gradient) is 0.33 mmol and the V_{max} 7.8 nmol/mg protein per min. The transport of taurocholate by the sodium cotransport system is electroneutral. The simplest explanation for the electroneutrality would be a 1:1 stoichiometry for sodium and the taurocholate anion. pH gradients are without effect on taurocholate uptake, indicating that nonionic diffusion plays no role in the transport across the brush-border membrane.

R. Transport of Uric Acid

The transport system for uric acid assumed to be present in the brush-border membrane (183) has not been well characterized hitherto. Studies with brush-border membranes from rabbit kidney indicate that a pH gradient ($pH_o > pH_i$) stimulates the uptake and that the transport is inhibited by pyranoic acid (181,184). The studies are in general complicated by the presence of enzyme activities in the membrane which lead to rapid formation of allantoin during or after the translocation of uric acid across the membrane. It seems premature to make any definite statements about the nature of the transport; nonionic diffusion as well as H^+ cotransport are possible, but their role in uric acid secretion or reabsorption has yet to be defined (181,184).

S. Transport of Organic Cations

Endogenous organic cations such as acetylcholine, creatinine, epinephrine, histamine, and thiamine (185-187) are secreted in the proximal tubule. The same transport system is involved in the renal elimination of amiloride, atropine, and morphine and its derivatives. Choline is at low plasma concentrations avidly reabsorbed and at high plasma concentrations secreted by the tubule. Studies on plasma membrane vesicles isolated from dog kidney indicate that both the luminal and the contraluminal membranes contain a transport system for organic cations. The systems have different K_m and V_{max} for *N*'-methylnicotinamide, the luminal system has a higher affinity (K_m = 1.6 mmol), and a higher maximal transport rate (V_{max} = 19.9 nmol/min per mg protein) than the contraluminal membrane (188).

On the basis of countertransport experiments it was proposed that the transport system in the brush-border membrane behaves like a symmetrical carrier, whereas the transport system at the contraluminal membrane has properties similar to a gated channel (188). Whether these assumptions are correct remains to be established. A protein fraction has been purified from renal membranes that after incorporation into the phospholipid vesicles facilitates the uptake of *N*'-methylnicotinamide (189). As judged by this assay the organic cation transport system is approximately 45-fold enriched in the protein fraction.

In order to elucidate the driving forces for the energy-requiring luminal secretion process, the effect of various cation gradients on the transport of *N*'-methylnicotinamide was investigated. It was found that a pH gradient (vesicle outside more acid than the vesicle inside) stimulated the efflux of *N*'-methylnicotinamide markedly, suggesting that a proton-*N*'-methylnicotinamide exchange system is present in the brush-border membrane (61). Such a system could operate well in vivo, where the intratubular pH is about 1 pH unit below the intracellular pH. The degree to which the pH gradient is indeed capable to maintain the steep apparent concentration difference for *N*'-methylnicotinamide across the brush-border membrane remains to be elucidated; a stoichiometry greater than 1 might provide the energetic coupling for a maximum 100-fold concentration difference.

V. TRANSPORT SYSTEMS IN THE THICK ASCENDING LIMB OF HENLE'S LOOP

A method has been developed to isolate a cell fraction from rabbit kidney outer medulla that is highly enriched in cells of the thick ascending limb of Henle's loop (11). The cells exhibit the highest rate of respiration in the presence of sodium chloride compared to sodium nitrate or lithium chloride. The sodium and chloride dependent respiration is inhibited by ouabain and by low concentrations of diuretics such as bumetanide and furosemide (34). Since active chloride transport in the isolated perfused thick ascending limb is also sodium dependent and inhibited by ouabain as well as by furosemide (190-192), the isolated cells seem to have retained the typical features of the active ion transport that is exhibited in the intact epithelium. Starting from these cells a plasma membrane fraction can be prepared by differential centrifugation that contains predominantly luminal plasma membranes. Identification of the luminal plasma membranes was achieved by iodinization of the cell surface of the isolated cells. The absence of contraluminal plasma membranes is indicated by a decreased activity of the Na-K-ATPase in the membrane fraction. This membrane fraction shows sodium uptake that is stimulated by chloride and potassium and inhibited by low concentrations of furosemide. The stimulatory effect of chloride is also observed in the absence of any ion gradient in vesicles preequilibrated with chloride. Since electrical driving forces can be excluded, the presence of a sodium-chloride cotransport system in these membranes can be postulated. In chloride flux measurements with this membrane fraction a stimulation of chloride uptake by sodium and potassium could be demonstrated, thus establishing the existence of a sodium-potassium chloride cotransport system. The affinity of the chloride-dependent sodium transport system for sodium is about 1 mmol in the presence of 100 mmol chloride and the affinity for chloride is about 30 mmol in the presence of 0.5 mmol sodium (193; F. Hannafin et al., unpublished data). In the presence of potassium the transfer of sodium together with chloride is not affected by diffusion potentials established across the membranes. The affinity of the transport system for bumetanide is in the same range as the sensitivity of the active chloride transport in the intact tubule (191,193). Since bumetanide in the perfused tubule acts only from the lumen (190-193), it can be assumed that the sodium-potassium chloride cotransport system is present in the luminal membranes. In support of this assumption, sodium uptake into basal-lateral membrane vesicles isolated from the thick ascending limb of Henle's loop cells shows a much lower stimulation by chloride than the uptake by the luminal membrane fraction (B. Koenig, unpublished observations).

These data provide evidence that the entry of chloride into the cells of the rabbit thick ascending limb is mediated by a sodium-potassium chloride cotransport system (see Fig. 16). This transport system is the target for the loop diuretics. Due to the presence of this cotransport system chloride would be accumulated inside the cell above the electrochemical

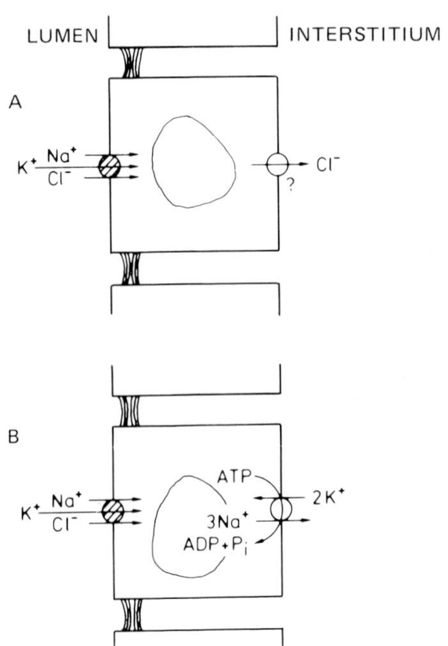

Fig. 16 Transport systems for chloride and sodium in the thick ascending limb of Henle's loop. (A) The transport systems involved in chloride transport, (B) the systems involved in sodium transport. The stoichiometry of the Na-K-Cl cotransport system is 1/1/2 and its presence has been firmly established in microperfusion studies (194).

equilibrium. At the contraluminal membrane, therefore, chloride could leave the cell following its electrochemical potential difference.

It also has been found that the luminal membrane of the cortical rabbit thick ascending limb contains a barium-sensitive potassium channel, that the contraluminal membrane possesses a high chloride conductivity, and that the lumen inside positive potential is mainly a result of the different permeabilities of the luminal and contraluminal membrane (194). Inhibition of chloride transport by barium indicates rapid cycling of potassium across the luminal membrane through the NaCl-KCl cotransporter and via the barium-sensitive potassium channel.

With respect to other transport related membrane functions, it should be mentioned that membranes of the thick ascending limb of Henle's loop cells contain a filipin-sensitive Mg-ATPase that in analogy with the proximal tubule (59) might be involved in luminal proton secretion, and an adenylate cyclase stimulated strongly by calcitonin and to a lesser extent by antidiuretic hormone (11).

The transport of sodium by the thick ascending limb of Henle's loop involves for the luminal entry step mainly the NaCl-KCl cotransport system. This is evident from the low effect of ouabain on cell respiration in the absence of chloride (34). Cell respiration doubles, however, when low concentrations of amphotericin are added to the incubation medium (P. Silva et al., unpublished observations). Amphotericin makes the membranes more permeable for sodium and thus bypasses the rate-limiting uptake via the sodium-chloride cotransport system. Exit of sodium from the cell is mediated by the Na-K-ATPase localized in the basal-lateral plasma membranes (see Fig. 16).

VI. TRANSPORT SYSTEMS IN THE DISTAL TUBULE

For the membrane molecular approach the distal tubule is terra incognita. This is due to the fact that no membrane fractions are available that can be classified as being derived from the distal tubule or parts of it. In addition, studies on the distribution of adenylate cyclase have indicated that there is a tremendous axial heterogeneity in this segment with respect to cell type and, thus, probably also cell function (19-21).

Two points of interest should be mentioned that deal with the transport of sodium by the distal tubule. Histochemical and immunochemical studies at the ultrastructural level revealed that the Na-K-ATPase in the distal tubule is localized in the basal-lateral plasma membrane. The amount of basal-lateral infoldings—and the total Na-K-ATPase associated with the cells increases when animals are treated with mineralocorticoids (195). The enzyme, therefore, undoubtedly plays a major role in transepithelial sodium transport and its regulation. The luminal sodium entry step is known to be inhibited by low concentrations of amiloride. Based on this observation, Cuthbert and Edwardton performed binding studies with radioactively labeled amiloride in rat kidney, and rabbit kidney cortex homogenates (196). Binding sites for amiloride with an apparent dissociation constant of 2.8 to 10 μmol were detected; this value is about 40 times higher than the K_i value observed for the inhibition of sodium transport in the distal tubule and 15 times smaller than the affinity of the sodium-proton exchanger for amiloride. The reason for this discrepancy lies in the inhomogeneity of the material used for the binding studies. Proximal tubules as well as distal tubules are present in the homogenate and the membranes from the distal tubule containing the high-affinity binding site probably constitute only a minor fraction of the total material.

VII. THE COLLECTING DUCT

Studies on properties of luminal and contraluminal membranes isolated from collecting duct cells have concentrated mainly on two transport-related parameters, the presence and distribution of ATPases tentatively identified as involved in sodium or proton transport, and the presence and distribution of membrane systems related to the action of antidiuretic hormone. Fractionation studies on the papillary collecting duct (12) indicated that the luminal membrane contains an anion-stimulated ATPase that, similar to the proximal tubule, might be involved in proton secretion of the collecting duct. The apical membrane contains also a cyclic AMP-dependent protein kinase. This enzyme, due to its predominant localization in the luminal membrane, has been postulated to be involved in the cAMP-mediated increase in luminal water permeability. The contraluminal membrane contains a calcium-activated ATPase and the Na-K-ATPase (13), which indicates a similar distribution of enzymes and pumps as in the proximal tubule (Fig. 17). The basal-lateral membrane is also the sole localization of the adenylate cyclase stimulated by antidiuretic hormone (12). Transport studies performed with luminal plasma membrane vesicles revealed that the glucose uptake into the vesicles is sodium independent—in contrast to the findings in the proximal tubule.

A new aspect of membrane-molecular analysis has been introduced recently in conjunction with experiments on the action of ADH on the tubule. Freeze fracture images of the luminal membrane revealed that after stimulation of the collecting duct with ADH particle aggregates appear in the membrane that are probably related to the increased water permeability of the membrane (197). Although the nature of the particles in biochemical terms is far from being understood, this approach is a fascinating tool for the identification of events occurring during regulation of transport processes.

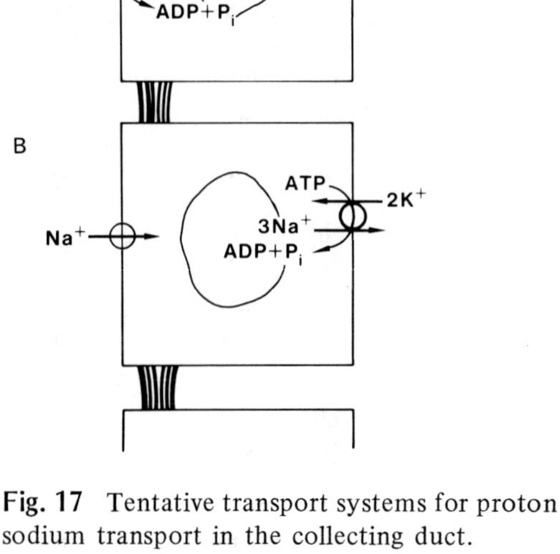

Fig. 17 Tentative transport systems for proton secretion (bicarbonate reabsorption) and sodium transport in the collecting duct.

ACKNOWLEDGMENT

I gratefully acknowledge the skillful and patient editorial work of Diane McDonnell and Alice Terner.

Part of the author's experimental work mentioned in the article has been supported by NIH grants AM 27441 and GM 27859.

REFERENCES

1. Murer, H.; and Kinne, R. The use of isolated vesicles to study epithelial transport processes. J. Membr. Biol. 55:81-95, 1980.
2. Haase, W.; Schaefer, A.; Murer, H.; and Kinne, R. Studies on the orientation of brush-border membrane vesicles. Biochem. J. 172:57-62, 1978.
3. Kinne, R.; and Kinne-Saffran, E. Isolierung und enzymatische Charakterisierung einer Buerstensaumfraktion der Rattenniere. Pflügers Arch. 308:1-15, 1969.
4. Evers, C.; Haase, W.; Murer, H.; and Kinne, R. Properties of brush border vesicles isolated from rat kidney cortex by calcium precipitation. Membr. Biochem. 1:203-219, 1978.
5. Bode, F.; Pockrandt-Hemstedt, H.; Baumann, K.; and Kinne, R. Analysis of the pinocytic process in rat kidney. I. Isolation of pinocytic vesicles from rat kidney cortex. J. Cell Biol. 63:998-1008, 1974.
6. Turner, S. I.; and Dousa, T. P. Differences in transport capacity for phosphate (P_i) of luminal brush border membrane (BBM) prepared from subcapsular (SC) and juxtamedullary (JM) cortex. 14th Ann. Meet. Am. Soc. Nephrol. Abstr.:14A, 1981.
7. Shlatz, L. J.; Schwartz, I. L.; Kinne-Saffran, E.; and Kinne, R. Distribution of parathyroid hormone-stimulated adenylate cyclase in plasma membranes of cells of the kidney cortex. J. Membr. Biol. 24:131-144, 1975.
8. Heidrich, H. G.; and Dew, M. E. Homogeneous cell populations from rabbit kidney cortex. Proximal, distal tubule, and renin-active cells isolated by free flow electrophoresis. J. Cell Biol. 74:780-788, 1977.
9. Kinne, R.; Keljo, D.; Gmaj, P.; and Murer, H. The energy source of glucose and calcium transport in the renal proximal tubule. In: New Aspects of Renal Function, vol. 6: Excerpta Medica Congress Series #422, Proc. 6th Workshop Conf. Hoechst, 1977, edited by Vogel, H. G., and Ullrich, K. J., Amsterdam, Oxford Press, 1978, pp. 41-47.
10. Gmaj, P.; Murer, H.; and Kinne, R. Calcium ion transport across plasma membranes isolated from rat kidney cortex. Biochem. J. 178(3):549-557, 1979.
11. Eveloff, J.; Haase, W.; and Kinne, R. Separation of renal medullary cells: Isolation of cells from the thick ascending limb of Henle's loop. J. Cell Biol. 87:672-681, 1980.
12. Schwartz, I. L.; Shlatz, L. J.; Kinne-Saffran, E.; and Kinne, R. Target cell polarity and membrane phosphorylation in relation to the mechanism of action of antidiuretic hormone. Proc. Natl. Acad. Sci. USA 71:2595-2599, 1974.
13. Iyengar, R.; Mailman, D. S.; and Sachs, G. Purification of distinct plasma membranes from canine renal medulla. Am. J. Physiol. 234(3):F247-F254, 1978.
14. Jørgensen, P. L. Sodium and potassium ion pump in kidney tubules. Physiol. Revs. 60: 864-917, 1980.
15. Hopfer, U.; Nelson, K.; Perrotto, J.; and Isselbacher, K. J. Glucose transport in isolated brush border membrane from rat small intestine. J. Biol. Chem. 248(1):25-32, 1973.
16. Kaback, H. R. Transport in isolated bacterial membrane vesicles. Methods Enzymol. 31:696-709, 1974.
17. Chabardes, D.; Imbert-Teboul, M.; Montegut, M.; Clique, A.; and Morel, F. Distribution of calcitonin-sensitive adenylate cyclase along the rabbit kidney tubule. Proc. Natl. Acad. Sci. USA 73:3608-3612, 1976.

18. Imbert, M. D.; Chabardes, D.; Montegut, M.; Clique, A.; and Morel, F. Adenylate cyclase activity along the rabbit nephron as measured in single isolated segments. Pflügers Arch. 354:213-228, 1975.
19. Morel, F.; Chabardes, D.; and Imbert, M. Functional segmentation of the rabbit distal tubule by microdetermination of hormone-dependent adenylate cyclase activity. Kidney Int. 9:264-277, 1976.
20. Kinne, R.; Shlatz, L. J.; Kinne-Saffran, E.; and Schwartz, I. L. Distribution of membrane-bound cyclic AMP dependent protein kinase in plasma membranes of cells of the kidney cortex. J. Membr. Biol. 24:145-159, 1975.
21. Yanagawa, N.; and Lang, D. ADP-Ribosylation of the luminal membrane inhibits phosphate transport across intact renal proximal tubule. 14th Ann. Meet. Am. Soc. Nephrol. Abstr.:15A, 1981.
22. Ullrich, K. J. Transport of organic solutes. In: Membrane Transport in Biology, vol. IV, edited by Giebisch, G., Tosteson, D. C., and Ussing, H. H. New York, Springer-Verlag, 1978, pp. 413-448.
23. Warnock, D. G.; and Yee, V. J. Chloride uptake by brush border membrane vesicles isolated from rabbit renal cortex. Coupling to proton gradients and K^+ diffusion potentials. J. Clin. Invest. 67(1):102-115, 1981.
24. Schwartz, G. Absence of Cl^--OH^- exchange in the rabbit proximal convoluted tubule. Clin. Res. 30:462a, 1982.
25. Burckhardt, G.; Kinne, R.; Stange, G.; and Murer, H. The effects of potassium and membrane potential on sodium-dependent glutamic acid uptake. Biochim. Biophys. Acta 599:191-201, 1980.
26. Sacktor, B.; and Schneider, E. G. The singular effect of an internal K^+ gradient ($K_1^+ > K^+$) on the Na^+ gradient ($Na^+ > Na^+$)-dependent transport of L-glutamate in renal brush border membrane vesicles. Int. J. Biochem. 12:229-234, 1980.
27. Heinz, E. Electrical Potentials in Biological Membrane Transport. New York, Springer-Verlag, 1981.
28. Aronson, P. S. Identifying secondary active solute transport in epithelia. Am. J. Physiol. 240(9):F1-F11, 1981.
29. Kinne, R. Metabolic correlates of tubular transport. In: Membrane Transport in Biology vol. IVA and B, Transport Organs, edited by Giebisch, G., Tosteson, D. C., and Ussing, H. H., New York, Springer-Verlag, 1978, pp. 529-562.
30. Guder, W. G.; and Wirthensohn, G. Renal turnover of substrates. In: Renal Transport of Organic Substances, edited by Greger, R., Lang, F., and Silbernagl, S., New York, Springer-Verlag, 1981, pp. 66-77.
31. Kippen, I.; Klinenberg, J. R.; and Wright, E. M. Effects of metabolic intermediates on sugar and amino acid uptake in rabbit renal tubules and brush border membrane. J. Physiol. (Lond.). 304:373-387, 1980.
32. Barac-Nieto, M.; Murer, H.; and Kinne, R. Lactate-sodium cotransport in rat renal brush border membranes. Am. J. Physiol. 239(5):F496-F506, 1980.
33. Kippen, I.; Hirayama, B.; Klinenberg, J. R.; and Wright, E. M. Transport of tricarboxylic acid cycle intermediates by membrane vesicles from renal brush border. Proc. Natl. Acad. Sci. USA 76(7):3397-3400, 1979.
34. Eveloff, J.; Bayerdoerffer, E.; Silva, P.; and Kinne, R. Sodium-chloride transport in the thick ascending limb of Henle's loop: Oxygen consumption studies in isolated cells. Pflügers Arch. 389:263-270, 1981.
35. Benavides, J.; Garcia, M. L.; Valdivieso, F.; and Giminez-Gallego, G. Ubiquinone, nonheme iron, and flavins in the renal brush border plasma membranes. Arch. Biochem. Biophys. 206(2):451-453, 1981.
36. Crane, R. K. The gradient hypothesis and other models of carrier mediated active transport. Rev. Physiol. Biochem. Pharmacol. 78:99-159, 1977.

37. Froemter, E.; Rumrich, G.; and Ullrich, K. J. Phenomenologic description of Na^+, Cl^-, and HCO_3^- absorption from proximal tubules of the rat kidney. Pflügers Arch. 343: 189-220, 1973.
38. Murer, H.; Hopfer, U.; and Kinne, R. Sodium/proton antiport in brush border membrane vesicles isolated from rat small intestine and kidney. Biochem. J. 154:597-604, 1976.
39. Kinsella, J. L.; and Aronson, P. S. Interaction of NH_4^+ and Li^+ with the renal microvillus membrane Na^+-H^+ exchanger. Am. J. Physiol. 241(10):C220-C226, 1981.
40. Kinsella, J. L.; and Aronson, P. S. Properties of the Na^+-H^+ exchanger in renal microvillus membrane vesicles. Am. J. Physiol. 238(6):F461-F469, 1980.
41. Kinsella, J. L.; and Aronson, P. S. Amiloride inhibition of the Na^+-H^+ exchanger in renal microvillus membrane vesicles. Am. J. Physiol. 241(10):F374-379, 1981.
42. Aronson, P. S.; and Bounds, S. E. Harmaline inhibition of Na-dependent transport in renal microvillus membrane vesicles. Am. J. Physiol. 238(3):F210-F217, 1980.
43. Samarazija, I.; Kinne-Saffran, E.; Baumann, K.; and Froemter, E. The mechanisms of action of harmaline on renal solute transport. Pflügers Arch. 368:83-88, 1977.
44. Burnham, C.; Muenzesheimer, T.; Rabon, E.; and Sachs, G. The Na^+/H^+ antiport in renal brush border vesicles. Fed. Proc. 40(3):462 (Abstract 1318), 1981.
45. Lin, J. T.; Stroh, A.; and Kinne, R. Involvement of tyrosine residues in sodium-transporter interaction. Biochim. Biophys. Acta 692:210-217, 1982.
46. Burg, M.; Patlak, C.; Green, N.; and Villey, D. Organic solutes in fluid absorption by renal proximal convoluted tubules. Am. J. Physiol. 231:627-637, 1976.
47. Heidrich, H.-G.; Kinne, R.; Kinne-Saffran, E.; and Hannig, K. The polarity of the proximal tubule cell in rat kidney: Different surface charges for the brush-border microvilli and plasma membranes from the basal infoldings. J. Cell Biol. 54:232-245, 1972.
48. Garg, L. C.; Knepper, M. A.; and Burg, M. B. Mineralocorticoid effects on Na-K-ATPase in individual nephron segments. Am. J. Physiol. 240:F536-F544, 1981.
49. Proverbio, F.; Condrescu-Guidi, M.; and Whittembury, G. Oubain-insensitive Na^+ stimulation of an Mg^{2+}-dependent ATPase in kidney tissue. Biochim. Biophys. Acta 394: 281-292, 1975.
50. Proverbio, F.; Robinson, J. W. L.; and Wittembury, G. Sensitivities of (Na^+-l)-ATPase and Na^+ extrusion mechanisms of oubain and ethacrynic acid in the cortex of the guinea-pig kidney. Biochim. Biophys. Acta 211:327-336, 1970.
51. Kinne, R.; and Murer, H. Recent advances in the understanding of renal amino acid and sugar transport. In: Proc. of the VIIth Intl. Cong. Nephrol., Montreal, 1978, pp. 601-608.
52. Sacktor, B.; Rosenbloom, I. L.; Liang, C.; and Cheng, L. Sodium gradient and sodium plus potassium gradient-dependent L-glutamate uptake in renal basolateral membrane vesicles. J. Membr. Biol. 60:63-71, 1981.
53. Aronson, P. S.; Haslett, J. P.; and Kashgarion, M. Dissociation of proximal tubular glucose and Na^+ reabsorption by amphotericin B. Am. J. Physiol. 236(5):F392-F397, 1979.
54. Doucet, A.; and Katz, A. I. Short-term effect of aldosterone on Na-K-ATPase in single nephron segments. Am. J. Physiol. 242(10):F273-F278, 1981.
55. DeSanto, N. G.; Capasso, G.; Paduano, C.; Carella, C.; and Giordano, C. Tubular transport processes in proximal tubules of hypothyroid rats. Micropuncture studies on isotonic fluid, amino acid and buffer reabsorption. Pflügers Arch. 384:117-122, 1980.
56. DeSanto, N. G.; Capasso, G.; Kinne, R.; Moewes, B.; Carella, C.; Anastasio, P.; and Giordano, C. Tubular transport processes in proximal tubules of hypothyroid rats. Lack of relationship between thyroidal dependent rise of isotonic fluid reabsorption and Na^+-K^+-ATPase activity. Pflügers Archiv. 394:294-301, 1982.
57. Kinne-Saffran, E.; Beauwens, R.; Kinne, R.; and Murer, H. Proton translocation systems in rat renal brush border membranes. In: Advances in Physiological Science, vol.

11, Kidney and Body Fluids. Edited by Takacs, L., Elmsford, N.Y., Pergamon Press, 1981, pp. 481-488.
58. Kinne-Saffran, E.; Beauwens, R.; and Kinne, R. An ATP driven proton pump in brush border membranes from rat renal cortex. J. Membr. Biol. 64:67-76, 1981.
59. Kinne-Saffran, E.; and Kinne, R. Further evidence for the existence of an intrinsic bicarbonate-stimulated Mg^{2+}-ATPase in brush border membranes isolated from rat kidney cortex. J. Membr. Biol. 49(3):235-251, 1979.
60. Kippen, I.; Hirayama, B.; Klinenberg, J. R.; and Wright, E. M. Effects of dibutyryl cyclic AMP on the transport of alpha-methyl-D-glucoside and alpha-amino isobutyric acid in separated tubules and brush border membranes from rabbit kidney. Biochim. Biophys. Acta 558(1):126-135, 1979.
61. Holohan, P. D.; and Ross, C. R. Mechanisms of organic cation transport in kidney plasma membrane vesicles. 2. WpH studies. J. Pharmacol. Exp. Ther. 216:294-298, 1981.
62. Froemter, E.; and Ullrich, K. J. Effect of inhibitors and the mechanisms of anion transport in the proximal renal tubule of rats. In: Anion and Proton Transport, edited by Brodsky, W. A., Ann. N.Y. Acad. Sci. 341:97-110, 1980.
63. Wistrand, J.; and Kinne, R. Carbonic anydrase activity of isolated brush border and basal-lateral membranes of renal tubular cells. Pflügers Arch. 370:121-126, 1977.
64. Chan, Y. L.; and Giebisch, G. Relationship between sodium and bicarbonate transport in the rat proximal tubule. Am. J. Physiol. 240:F222-F230, 1981.
65. Ullrich, K. J.; Rumrich, G.; and Baumann, K. Renal proximal tubular buffer (glycodiazine) transport: Inhomogeneity of local transport rate, dependence on sodium, effect of inhibitors and chronic adaptation. Pflügers Arch. 357:149-163, 1975.
66. Misanko, B. S.; and Solomon, S. Activity of HCO_3^--stimulated ATPase in the acidotic rat kidney. Miner. Electrolyte Metab. 6:217-236, 1981.
67. Ullrich, K. J.; Rumrich, G.; and Kloess, S. Active Ca^{++} reabsorption in the proximal tubule of the rat kidney. Dependence on sodium and buffer transport. Pflügers Arch. 364:223-228, 1976.
68. Kinne-Saffran, E.; and Kinne, R. Localization of a calcium-stimulated ATPase in the basal-lateral plasma membranes of the proximal tubule of rat kidney cortex. J. Membr. Biol. 17:263-274, 1974.
69. Katz, A. I.; and Doucet, A. Calcium-activated adenosine triphosphatase along the rabbit nephron. Int. J. Biochem. 12:125-129, 1980.
70. Spring, K. R.; and Kimura, G. Chloride reabsorption by renal proximal tubules of Necturus. J. Membr. Biol. 38(3):233-254, 1978.
71. Shindo, T.; and Spring, K. R. Chloride movement across the basolateral membrane of proximal tubule cells. J. Membr. Biol. 58(1):35-42, 1981.
72. Lang, F.; Greger, R.; Knox, F. G.; and Oberleithner, H. Factors modulating the renal handling of phosphate. Renal Physiol. 4(1):1-16, 1981.
73. Kleerekoper, M.; Bernstein, R. S.; Rao, D. S.; Frame, B.; Levin, N. W.; and Parfitt, A. M. Parathyroid hormone, phosphate and the kidney. Prog. Biochem. Pharmacol. 17: 190-198, 1980.
74. Hoffmann, N.; Thees, M.; and Kinne, R. Phosphate transport by isolated renal brush border vesicles. Pflügers Arch. 362(2):147-156, 1976.
75. Kinne, R.; Berner, W.; Hoffman, N.; and Murer, H. Phosphate transport by isolated renal and intestinal plasma membranes. Adv. Exp. Med. Biol. 81:265-277, 1977.
76. Cheng, L.; and Sacktor, B. Sodium gradient-dependent phosphate transport in renal brush border membrane vesicles. J. Biol. Chem. 256(4):1556-1564, 1981.
77. Kinne, R.; and Faust, R. G. Incorporation of D-glucose, L-alanine- and phosphate-transport systems from rat renal brush-border membranes into liposomes. Biochem. J. 168(2):311-314, 1977.

78. Sacktor, B.; and Cheng, L. Sodium gradient-dependent phosphate transport in renal brush border membrane vesicles. Effect of an intravesicular > extravesicular proton gradient. J. Biol. Chem. 256:8080-8084, 1981.
79. Kempson, S. A.; Kim, J. K.; Northrup, T. E.; Knox, F. G.; and Dousa, T. P. Alkaline phosphatase in adaptation to low dietary phosphate intake. Am. J. Physiol. 237(5): E465-E473, 1979.
80. Storelli, C.; and Murer, H. On the correlation between alkaline phosphatase and phosphate transport in rat renal brush border membrane vesicles. Pflügers Arch. 384(2): 149-153, 1980.
81. Tenenhouse, H. S.; Scriver, C. R.; and Vizel, E. J. Alkaline phosphatase activity does not mediate phosphate transport in the renal-cortical brush-border membrane. Biochem. J. 190(2):473-476, 1980.
82. Evers, C.; Murer, H.; and Kinne, R. Effect of parathyrin on the transport properties of isolated renal brush-border vesicles. Biochem. J. 172(1):49-56, 1978.
83. Stoll, R.; Kinne, R.; Murer, H.; Fleisch, H.; and Bonjour, J. P. Phosphate transport by rat renal brush border membrane vesicles: Influence of dietary phosphate, thyroparathyroidectomy, and a 1,25-dihydroxyvitamin D3. Pflügers Arch. 380(1):47-52, 1979.
84. Hruska, K. A.; and Hammerman, M. R. Parathyroid hormone inhibition of phosphate transport in renal brush border vesicles from phosphate-depleted dogs. Biochim. Biophys. Acta 645:351-356, 1981.
85. Kempson, S. A.; and Dousa, T. P. Phosphate transport across renal cortical brush border membrane vesicles from rats stabilized on a normal, high or low phosphate diet. Life Sci. 24(10):881-887, 1979.
86. Barrett, P. Q.; Gartner, J. M.; and Rasmussen, H. Effect of dietary phosphate on transport properties of pig renal microvillus vesicles. Am. J. Physiol. 239(4):F352-F359, 1980.
87. Tenenhouse, H. S.; and Scriver, C. R. Renal adaptation to phosphate deprivation in the Hyp mouse with X-linked hypophosphatemia. Can. J. Biochem. 57(6):938-944, 1979.
88. Tenenhouse, H. S.; and Scriver, C. R. Renal brush border membrane adaptation to phosphorus deprivation in the Hyp/Y mouse. Nature 281(5728):225-227, 1979.
89. Tenenhouse, H. S.; and Scriver, C. R. The defect in transcellular transport of phosphate in the nephron is located in brush-border membranes in X-linked hypophosphatemia (Hyp mouse model). Can. J. Biochem. 56(6):640-646, 1978.
90. Tenenhouse, H. S.; Scriver, C. R.; McInnes, R. R.; and Glorieux, F. H. Renal handling of phosphate in vivo and in vitro by the X-linked hypophosphatemic male mouse: Evidence for a defect in the brush border membrane. Kidney Int. 14(3):236-244, 1978.
91. Kempson, S. A.; Colon-Otero, G.; Ou, S. Y.; Turner, S. T.; and Dousa, T. P. Possible role of nicotinamide adenine dinucleotide as an intracellular regulator of renal transport of phosphate in the rat. J. Clin. Invest. 67(5):1347-1360, 1981.
92. Luecke, H.; Stange, G.; and Murer, H. Sulphate ion/sodium ion cotransport by brush border membrane vesicles isolated from rat kidney cortex. Biochem. J. 182:223-229, 1979.
93. Ullrich, K. J.; Rumrich, G.; and Kloess, S. Bidirectional active transport of thiosulfate in the proximal convolution of the rat kidney. Pflügers Arch. 387:127-132, 1980.
94. Brazy, P. C., and Dennis, V. W. Sulfate transport in rabbit proximal convoluted tubules: Presence of anion exchange. Am. J. Physiol. 241:(10):F300-F307, 1981.
95. Frasch, W.; Frohnert, P. P.; Bode, F.; Baumann, K.; and Kinne, R. Competitive inhibition of phlorizin binding by D-glucose and the influence of sodium: A study on isolated brush border membrane of rat kidney. Pflügers Arch. 320:265-284, 1970.
96. Kinne, R.; Murer, H.; Kinne-Saffran, E.; Thees, M.; and Sachs, G. Sugar transport by renal plasma membrane vesicles. Characterization of the systems in the brush border microvilli and basal-lateral plasma membranes. J. Membr. Biol. 21(3-4):375-395, 1975.

97. Kinne, R. 1976. Properties of the glucose transport system in the renal brush border membrane. In: Current Topics in Membrane and Transport, vol. 8, edited by Bronner, F., and Kleinzeller, A., New York, Academic Press, pp. 209-267.
98. Aronson, P. S.; and Sacktor, B. The Na^+ gradient-dependent transport of D-glucose in renal brush border membranes. J. Biol. Chem. 250(15):6032-6039, 1975.
99. Busse, D.; John, A.; and Steinmaier, G. Carrier-mediated transfer of D-glucose in brush border vesicles derived from rabbit renal tubules. Na^+-Dependent versus Na^+-independent transfer. Biochim. Biophys. Acta 401(2):231-243, 1975.
100. Crane, R. K.; and Dorando, F. C. On the mechanism of Na^+-dependent glucose transport. In: Function and Molecular Aspects of Biomembrane Transport, edited by Quagliariello, E., Amsterdam, Elsevier/North Holland, 1979, pp. 271-278.
101. DeSmedt, H.; and Kinne, R. Temperature dependence of solute transport and enzyme activities in hog renal brush border membrane vesicles. Biochim. Biophys. Acta 648: 247-253, 1981.
102. Kippen, I.; Hirayama, B.; Klinenberg, J. R.; and Wright, E. M. Transport of p-aminohippuric acid, uric acid and glucose in highly purified rabbit renal brush border membranes. Biochim. Biophys. Acta 556:161-174, 1979.
103. Mamelok, R. D.; Macrae, D. R.; Hittelman, K.; Hoefer, J. P.; and Prusiner, S. D. Kinetics of D-glucose transport into renal membrane vesicles: Measurements using a vacuum manifold apparatus. J. Biochem. Biophys. Methods 4:147-153, 1981.
104. Misfeldt, D. S.; and Sanders, M. J. Transepithelial transport in cell culture: D-Glucose transport by a pig kidney cell line ($LLC\text{-}PK_1$). J. Membr. Biol. 59:13-18, 1981.
105. Poiree, J. C.; Vannier, C.; Sudaka, P.; and Fehlmann, M. Glucose transport by horse kidney brush borders. I. Transport properties of brush border membrane closed vesicles. Biochimie 60(6-7):645-651, 1978.
106. Slack, E. N., Liang, C.-C. T., and Sacktor, B. Transport of L-proline and D-glucose in luminal (brush border) and contraluminal (basal-lateral) membrane vesicles from the renal cortex. Biochem. Biophys. Res. Comm. 77(3):891-897, 1977.
107. Turner, R. J.; and Silverman, M. Sugar uptake into brush border vesicles from dog kidney. I. Specificity. Biochim. Biophys. Acta 507(2):305-321, 1978.
108. Turner, R. J.; and Silverman, M. Sugar uptake into brush border vesicles from normal human kidney. Proc. Natl. Acad. Sci. USA 74(7):2825-2829, 1977.
109. Turner, R. J.; and Silverman, M. Sugar uptake into brush border vesicles from dog kidney. II. Kinetics. Biochim. Biophys. Acta 511(3):470-486, 1978.
110. Beck, J. C.; and Sacktor, B. Energetics of the Na^+-dependent transport of D-glucose in renal brush border membrane vesicles. J. Biol. Chem. 250(22):8674-8680, 1975.
111. Beck, J. C.; and Sacktor, B. The sodium-electrochemical potential-mediated uphill transport of D-glucose in renal brush border membrane vesicles. J. Biol. Chem. 253(15):5531-5535, 1978.
112. Kinne, R.; Barac, M.; and Murer, H. Sodium cotransport systems in the proximal tubule: current developments. In: Current Topics in Membrane and Transport, vol. 13, edited by Boulpaep, E.; Bronner, F.; and Kleinzeller, A., New York, Academic Press, 1980, pp. 303-313.
113. Hilden, S. A.; and Sacktor, B. D-Glucose-dependent sodium transport in renal brush border membrane vesicles. J. Biol. Chem. 254(15):7090-7096, 1979.
114. Sacktor, B. Electrogenic and electroneutral Na^+ gradient-dependent transport systems in the renal brush border membrane vesicle. In: Current Topics in Membrane and Transport, vol. 13, edited by Boulpaep, E.; Bronner, F.; and Kleinzeller, A., New York, Academic Press, 1980, pp. 291-300.
115. Toggenburger, G.; Kessler, M.; Rothstein, A.; Semenza, G.; and Tannenbaum, C. Similarity in effects of Na^+ gradients and membrane potentials on D-glucose transport by, and phlorizin binding to, vesicles derived from brush borders of rabbit intestinal mucosal cells. J. Membr. Biol. 40:269-290, 1978.

116. Aronson, P. S. Energy-dependence of phlorizin binding to isolated renal microvillus membranes. Evidence concerning the mechanism of coupling between the electrochemical Na^+ gradient and sugar transport. J. Membr. Biol. 42:81-89, 1978.
117. Barnett, J. E. G.; Jarvis, W. T. S.; and Munday, K. A. Structural requirements for active intestinal sugar transport. The involvement of hydrogen bonds at C-1 and C-6 of the sugar. Biochem. J. 109:61-67, 1968.
118. Barnett, J. E. G.; Jarvis, W. T. S.; and Munday, K. A. Structural requirements for active intestinal sugar transport. Spatial and bonding requirements at C-3 of the sugar. Biochem. J. 114:469-473, 1969.
119. Kleinzeller, A.; McAvoy, E. M.; and McKibbin, R. D. Active renal hexose transport: structural requirements. Biochim. Biophys. Acta 600:512-529, 1980.
120. Vick, H.; Diedrich, D. F.; and Baumann, K. Reevaluation of renal tubular glucose transport inhibition by phlorizin analogs. Am. J. Physiol. 224(3):552-557, 1973.
121. Hopfer, U.; and Groseclose, R. The mechanism of Na^+-dependent D-glucose transport. J. Biol. Chem. 255(10):4453-4462, 1980.
122. Crane, R. K.; Malathi, P.; and Preiser, H. Reconstitution of specific Na^+-dependent D-glucose transport in liposomes by Triton X-100-extracted proteins from purified brush border membranes of rabbit kidney cortex. FEBS Lett. 67(2):214-216, 1976.
123. Crane, R. K.; Malathi, P.; Preiser, H.; and Fairclough, P. Some characteristics of kidney Na^+-dependent glucose carrier reconstituted into sonicated liposomes. Am. J. Physiol. 234(1):E1-E5, 1978.
124. Fairclough, P.; Malathi, P.; Preiser, H.; and Crane, R. K. Reconstitution into liposomes of glucose active transport from the rabbit renal proximal tubule. Characteristics of the system. Biochim. Biophys. Acta 553(2):295-306, 1979.
125. DaCruz, M. Untersuchungen des Natrium D-Glucosekotransportsystems nach Rekonstitution in Liposomen. Thesis, Johann Wolfgang Goethe University, Frankfurt, 1984.
126. Koepsell, H.; Menuhr, H.; Wissmueller, T. F.; Ducis, I.; and Haase, W. Reconstitution of D-glucose transport and high-affinity phlorizin binding after solubilization of kidney brush border proteins. Anns. N.Y. Acad. Sci. 358:267-281, 1980.
127. Lin, J. T.; DaCruz, M. E.; Riedel, S.; and Kinne, R. Partial purification of hog kidney sodium-D-glucose cotransport system by affinity chromatography on a phlorizin polymer. Biochim. Biophys. Acta 640(1):43-54, 1981.
128. Malathi, P.; Preiser, H.; and Crane, R. K. Protease-resistant integral brush border membrane proteins and their relationship to sodium-dependent transport of D-glucose and L-alanine. Anns. N.Y. Acad. Sci. 358:253-266, 1980.
129. Poiree, J. C.; Mangual, R.; and Sudaka, P. Identification of a protein component of horse kidney brush border D-glucose transport system. Biochem. Biophys. Res. Commun. 90(4):1387-1392, 1979.
130. Tannenbaum, C.; Toggenburger, G.; Kessler, M.; Rothstein, A.; and Semenza, G. High-affinity phlorizin binding to brush border membranes from small intestine: Identity with (a part of) the glucose transport system, dependence on the Na^+-gradient, partial purification. J. Supramolec. Struct. 6:519-533, 1977.
131. Thomas, L. Isolation of N-ethylmaleimide-labelled phlorizin-sensitive D-glucose binding protein of brush border membrane from rat kidney cortex. Biochim. Biophys. Acta 291:454-464, 1973.
132. Kleinzeller, A.; Tam, I.; Kanter, R. K.; and McAvoy, E. M. The structural requirement for C_1-OH for the active transport of D-mannose and 2-deoxy-D-hexoses by renal tubular cells. Biochim. Biophys. Acta 373:397-403, 1974.
133. Keljo, D. J.; Kleinzeller, A.; Murer, H.; and Kinne, R. Is hexokinase present in the basal lateral membranes of rat kidney proximal tubular epithelial cells? Biochim. Biophys. Acta 508:500-512, 1978.
134. Kleinzeller, A.; and McAvoy, E. M. Transport and phosphorylation of 2-deoxy-D-galactose in renal cortical cells. Biochim. Biophys. Acta 455:126-143, 1976.

135. Lin, J. T.; Stroh, A.; and Kinne, R. Renal sodium-D-glucose cotransport system: Involvement of tyrosyl-residues in sodium-transporter interaction. Biochim. Biophys. Acta 692:210-217, 1982.
136. Hammerman, M. R.; Sacktor, B.; and Daughaday, W. H. myo-Inositol transport in renal brush border vesicles and its inhibition by D-glucose. Am. J. Physiol. 239(8): F113-F120, 1980.
137. Takenawa, T.; Wada, E.; and Tsumita, T. myo-Inositol binding and transport in brush border membranes of rat kidney. Biochim. Biophys. Acta 464:108-117, 1977.
138. Pullman, T. N.; Oparil, S.; and Carone, F. A. Fate of labeled angiotensin II microinfused into individual nephrons in the rat. Am. J. Physiol. 228(3):747-751, 1975.
139. Carone, F. A.; Pullman, T. N.; Oparil, S.; and Nakamura, S. Micropuncture evidence of rapid hydrolysis of bradykinin by rat proximal tubule. Am. J. Physiol. 230(5): 1410-1424, 1976.
140. Silbernagl, S. Intratubular splitting of peptides and their reabsorption as single amino acids from the proximal convolution of rat kidney: A microperfusion study. Kidney Int. 11:219, 1977.
141. Peterson, D. R.; Chrabasczcz, G.; Peterson, W. R.; and Oparil, S. Mechanism for renal tubular handling of angiotensin. Am. J. Physiol. 236(4):F364-F372, 1979.
142. Carone, F. A.; and Peterson, D. R. Hydrolysis and transport of small peptides by the proximal tubule. Am. J. Physiol. 238(3):F151-F158, 1980.
143. Stetler-Stevenson, M. A.; Flouret, G.; and Peterson, D. R. Handling of luteinizing hormone-releasing hormone by renal proximal tubular segments in vitro. Am. J. Physiol. 241(10):F117-122, 1981.
144. Benoit, F. L.; and Watten, R. H. Renal tubular transport of hydroxyproline peptides: Evidence for reabsorption and secretion. Metabolism 17(1):20-33, 1968.
145. Ganapathy, V.; Mendicino, J. F.; and Leibach, F. H. Transport of glycl-L-proline into intestinal and renal brush border vesicles from rabbit. J. Biol. Chem. 256(1):118-124, 1981.
146. Ganapathy, V.; Mendicino, J.; Pashley, D. H.; and Leibach, F. H. Carrier-mediated transport of glycyl-L-proline in renal brush border vesicles. Biochem. Biophys. Research Comm. 97(3):1133-1139, 1980.
147. Ganapathy, V.; Mendicino, J.; and Leibach, F. H. Evidence for a depeptide transport system in renal brush border membranes from rabbit. Biochim. Biophys. Acta 642: 381-391, 1981.
148. Froemter, E. Electrical aspects of tubular transport of organic substances. In: Renal Transport of Organic Substances, edited by Greger, R., Lang, F., and Silbernagl, S., New York, Springer-Verlag, 1981, pp. 30-44.
149. Silbernagl, S. Renal transport of amino acids and oligopeptides. In: Renal Transport of Organic Substances, edited by Greger, R., Lang, F., and Silbernagl, S., New York, Springer-Verlag, 1981, pp. 93-117.
150. McNamara, P. D.; Ozegovic, B.; Pepe, L. M.; and Segal, S. Proline and glycine uptake by renal brushborder membrane vesicles. Proc. Natl. Acad. Sci. USA 73(12):4521-4525, 1976.
151. McNamara, P. D.; Pepe, L. M.; and Segal, S. Sodium gradient dependence of proline and glycine uptake in rat renal brush-border membrane vesicles. Biochim. Biophys. Acta 556:151-160, 1979.
152. Busse, D. Transport of L-arginine in brush border vesicles derived from rabbit kidney cortex. Arch. Biochem. Biophys. 191(2):551-560, 1978.
153. Hilden, S. A.; and Sacktor, B. L-Arginine uptake into renal brush border membrane vesicles. Arch. Biochem. Biophys. 21:(1):289-297, 1981.
154. Weiss, S. D.; McNamara, P. D.; Pepe, L. M.; and Segal, S. Glutamine and glutamic acid uptake by rat renal brushborder membrane vesicles. J. Membr. Biol. 43:91-105, 1978.

155. Alleyne, G. A. O.; McFarlane, N.; Scott, A.; and Scott, B. Glutamine uptake by cortical slices and luminal brush border vesicles of rat kidney. Int. J. Biochem. 12:99-102, 1980.
156. Fass, S. J.; Hammerman, M. R.; and Sacktor, B. Transport of amino acids in renal brush border membrane vesicles. J. Biol. Chem. 252(2):583-590, 1977.
157. Goldmann, D. R.; Roth, K. S.; Langfitt, T. W., Jr.; and Segal, S. L-Proline transport by newborn rat kidney brush-border membrane vesicles. Biochem. J. 178(1):253-256, 1979.
158. Hammerman, M.; and Sacktor, B. Transport of β-alanine in renal brush border membrane vesicles. Biochim. Biophys. Acta 509:338-347, 1978.
159. Hammerman, M. R.; and Sacktor, B. Transport of amino acids in renal brush border membrane vesicles. Uptake of L-proline. J. Biol. Chem. 252(2):591-595, 1977.
160. McFarlane-Anderson, N.; and Alleyne, G. A. O. Transport of glutamine by rat kidney brush-border membrane vesicles. Biochem. J. 182:295-300, 1979.
161. McNamara, P. D. Transport interaction of cystine and dibasic amino acids in renal brush border vesicles. Science 197:169-171, 1977.
162. Murer, H.; Leopolder, A.; Kinne, R.; and Burckhardt, G. Recent observations on the proximal tubular transport of acidic and basic amino acids by rat renal proximal tubular brush border vesicles. Int. J. Biochem. 12:223-228, 1980.
163. Rozen, R.; Tenenhouse, H. S.; and Scriver, C. R. Taurine transport in renal brush-border membrane vesicles. Biochem. J. 180:245-248, 1979.
164. Schneider, E. G.; and Sacktor, B. Sodium gradient-dependent L-glutamate transport in renal brush border membrane vesicles. Effect of an intravesicular-extravesicular potassium gradient. J. Biol. Chem. 255(16):7645-7649, 1980.
165. Schneider, E. G.; Hammerman, M. R.; and Sacktor, B. Sodium gradient-dependent L-glutamate transport in renal brush border membrane vesicles. Evidence for an electroneutral mechanism. J. Biol. Chem. 255(16):7650-7656, 1980.
166. Evers, J.; Murer, H.; and Kinne, R. Phenylalanine uptake in isolated renal brush border vesicles. Biochim. Biophys. Acta 426:598-615, 1976.
167. Sacktor, B. Mechanisms and specifications of amino acid transport in proximal tubule luminal membrane vesicles. In: Renal Function, edited by Giebisch, G. H., and Purcell, E. F., New York, Josiah Macy, Jr. Foundation, 1978, pp. 221-229.
168. Barfuss, D. W.; and Schafer, F. A. Active amino acid absorption by proximal convoluted and proximal straight tubules. Am. J. Physiol. 236(5):F149-F162, 1979.
169. Barfuss, D. W.; Mays, J. M.; and Schafer, J. A. Peritubular uptake and transepithelial transport of glycine in isolated proximal tubules. Am. J. Physiol. 238(4):F324-F333, 1980.
170. Schafer, J. A.; and Barfuss, D. W. Membrane mechanisms for transepithelial amino acid absorption and secretion. Am. J. Physiol. 238(5):F335-F346, 1980.
171. Inoue, M.; Okajima, K.; and Morino, Y. Renal transtubular transport of mercapturic acid in vivo. Biochim. Biophys. Acta 641:122-128, 1981.
172. Murer, H.; Barac-Nieto, B.; Ullrich, K. J.; and Kinne, R. Renal transport of lactate. In: Renal Transport of Organic Substances, edited by Greger, R., Lang, F., and Silbernagl, S., New York, Springer-Verlag, 1981, pp. 210-223.
173. Hoehmann, P. P.; Frohnert, P. P.; Kinne, R.; and Baumann, K. Proximal tubular lactate transport in rat kidney: A micropuncture study. Kidney Int. 5:261-270, 1974.
174. Wright, S. H.; Kippen, I.; Klinenberg, J. R.; and Wright, E. M. Specificity of the transport system for tricarboxylic acid cycle intermediates in renal brush borders. J. Membr. Biol. 57:73-82, 1980.
175. Barac-Nieto, M.; and Cohen, J. J. Non-esterified fatty acid uptake by dog kidney: Effect of probenecid and chlorothiazide. Am. J. Physiol. 215:98-107, 1968.
176. Boumendil-Podevin, E. F.; and Podevin, R. A. Nicotinic acid transport by brush border membrane vesicles from rabbit kidney. Am. J. Physiol. 240(9):F185-F191, 1981.

177. Haeberle, D. A. 1981. Characteristics of p-aminohippurate transport in the mammalian kidney. In: Renal Transport of Organic Substances, edited by Greger, R., Lang, F., and Silbernagl, S., New York, Springer-Verlag, 1981, pp. 189-209.
178. Kinsella, J. L.; Holohan, P. D.; Pessah, N. I.; and Ross, C. R. Transport of organic ions in renal cortical luminal and antiluminal membrane vesicles. J. Pharmacol. Exp. Ther. 209:443-450, 1979.
179. Berner, W.; and Kinne, R. Transport of p-aminohippuric acid by plasma membrane vesicles isolated from rat kidney cortex. Pflügers Arch. 361(3):269-277, 1976.
180. Eveloff, J.; Kinne, R.; and Kinter, W. B. p-Aminohippuric acid transport into brush border vesicles isolated from flounder kidney. Am. J. Physiol. 237(4):F291-F298, 1979.
181. Blomstedt, J. W.; and Aronson, P. S. pH Gradient-stimulated transport of urate and p-aminohippurate in dog renal microvillus membrane vesicles. J. Clin. Invest. 65:931-934, 1980.
182. Wilson, F. A.; Burckhardt, G.; Murer, H.; and Rumrich, G. Sodium-coupled taurocholate transport in the proximal convolution of the rat kidney in vivo and in vitro. J. Clin. Inves. 67:1141-1150, 1981.
183. Lang, F. Renal handling of urate. In: Renal Transport of Organic Substances, edited by Greger, R., Lang, F., and Silbernagl, F., New York, Springer-Verlag, 1981, pp. 234-261.
184. Boumendil-Podevin, E. F.; Podevin, R. A.; and Priol, C. Uric acid transport in brush border membrane vesicles isolated from rabbit kidney. Am. J. Physiol. 236(6):F519-F525, 1979.
185. Rennick, B. R. Renal tubular transport of organic cations. In: Renal Transport of Organic Substances, edited by Greger, R., Lang, F., and Silbernagl, S., New York, Springer-Verlag, 1981, pp. 178-188.
186. Besseghir, K.; Pearce, L. B.; and Rennick, B. Renal tubular transport and metabolism of organic cations by the rabbit. Am. J. Physiol. 242(10):F308-F314, 1981.
187. Rennick, B. R. Renal tubule transport of organic cations. Am. J. Physiol. 240(9): F83-F89, 1981.
188. Holohan, P. D.; and Ross, C. R. Mechanisms of organic cation transport in kidney plasma membrane vesicles. I. Countertransport studies. J. Pharmacol. Exp. Ther. 215:191-197, 1980.
189. Holohan, P. D.; Pessah, N. I.; and Ross, C. R. Reconstitution of N'-methyl-nicotinamide and p-aminohippuric acid transport in phospholipid vesicles with a protein fraction isolated from dog kidney membranes. Pharmacol. 16:343-356, 1979.
190. Burg, M.; and Green, N. Function of the thick ascending limb of Henle's loop. Am. J. Physiol. 224:659-668, 1973.
191. Imai, M. Effect of bumetanide and furosemide on the thick ascending limb of Henle's loop of rabbits and rats perfused in vitro. Eur. J. Pharmacol. 41:409-416, 1977.
192. Rocha, A. S.; and Kokko, J. P. Sodium chloride and water transport in the medullary thick ascending limb of Henle. Evidence for active chloride transport. J. Clin. Invest. 52:612-623, 1973.
193. Koenig, B.; Ricapito, S.; and Kinne, R. Chloride transport in the thick ascending limb of Henle's loop: Potassium dependence and stoichiometry of the NaCl cotransport system in plasma membrane vesicles. Pflügers Arch. 399:173-179, 1983.
194. Greger, R.; and Schlatter, E. Properties of the basolateral membrane of the cortical thick ascending limb of Henle's loop of rabbit kidney. A model for secondary active chloride transport. Pflügers Arch. 396:325-334, 1983.
195. Wade, J. B.; O'Neil, R. G.; Pryor, J. L.; and Boulpaep, E. L. Modulation of cell membrane area in renal collecting tubules by corticosteroid hormones. J. Cell Biol. 81(2): 439-445, 1979.

196. Cuthbert, A. W.; and Edwardson, J. M. Attempts to define the amiloride receptor in kidney tissue. In: Epithelial Ion and Water Transport, edited by Macknight, A. D. C., and Leader, J. P., New York, Raven Press, 1981, pp. 35-42.
197. Harmanci, M. C.; Sterm, P.; Kachadorian, W. A.; Valtin, H.; and DiScala, V. A. Vasopressin and collecting duct intramembranous particle clusters: A dose-response relationship. Am. J. Physiol. 239(6):F560-F564, 1980.
198. Kinne, R. 1976. Renal HCO_3^--ATPase and Ca^{++}-ATPase. Are they involved in renal proton and calcium transport? In: Proceedings of the Sixth International Congress on Nephrology, Florence, 1975, edited by Giovannetti, S., Bonomini, V., and D'Amico, A. Basel, Karger, pp. 139-145.

(Note added in proof:) The references were compiled in 1981 and have only been updated where essential changes in our knowledge have occurred.

2

Transport in Individual Nephron Segments

LEON G. FINE
Center for the Health Sciences, University of California at Los Angeles School of Medicine, Los Angeles, California

NORIMOTO YANAGAWA
University of California at Los Angeles School of Medicine, Los Angeles, and Sepulveda Veterans Administration Medical Center, Sepulveda, California

I. METHODS OF STUDYING RENAL TUBULAR FUNCTION

A. Clearance Methods

A variety of clearance procedures have been used to study renal tubular function in intact animals and in man. The noninvasive nature of these methods makes them ideal for the investigation of tubular function in patients; however, the method has a number of inherent pitfalls. In order to determine the contributions of tubular reabsorption to overall kidney function a number of parameters have been studied, including fractional excretion of sodium and water, the excretion of substances reabsorbed principally in the proximal tubule (i.e., glucose, bicarbonate, phosphate, calcium, magnesium, urate, and lithium), free water clearance or free water reabsorption at a given rate of delivery of sodium chloride, and potassium and hydrogen ion excretion at a given rate of sodium delivery. These techniques have also been used to evaluate the site of action of a variety of pharmacological agents which act upon the renal tubule.

In treating the kidney as a "black box," evidence of tubular reabsorption or secretion is obtained by estimating fractional excretion rates. Fractional excretion rates of less than 100% indicate that substances are absorbed from the renal tubule, whereas a fractional excretion rate in excess of 100% is the only unequivocal evidence of tubular secretion. However, when substances are both reabsorbed and secreted, e.g., urate, a simple estimation of fractional excretion can obviously provide little information about the relative contributions of each process, unless highly specific inhibitors are employed to block one or other process.

The influence of a variety of physiological and pharmacological maneuvers on proximal tubular reabsorption in vivo has been based upon the measurement of changes in fractional water excretion during maximal water diuresis, i.e., V/GFR (1). The assumption is that the entire nephron from the beginning of the thick ascending limb to the end of the collecting tubule is essentially water impermeable during maximal water diuresis. An increase or decrease in flow, therefore, would indicate changes in fractional delivery out of the proximal tubule. A number of pitfalls are inherent in this approach. Firstly, the assumption that the collecting tubule is totally impermeable to water under these conditions is not necessarily correct. This may be due either to incomplete suppression of antidiuretic hormone (ADH) release or to the inherent properties of the collecting tubule. In fact, it has been estimated that fractional reabsorption of water by the collecting tubule under conditions of maximal diuresis is actually greater than that which obtains during hydropenic conditions (2). Ideal markers of proximal tubular reabsorption have been sought, but no such marker has yet been identified. Amongst the substances studied have been glucose, phosphate, urate, bicarbonate, calcium, and magnesium, but for all of these substances there is evidence of some tubular handling beyond the proximal tubule. It is possible that lithium could provide a useful marker of tubular sodium reabsorption by the proximal tubule, but until direct studies are performed on distal nephron segments, it remains unclear whether lithium, too, is handled by the distal nephron.

To evaluate the function of the ascending limb of Henle's loop, the assumption has been made that free water clearance is an approximate index of sodium chloride reabsorption in this segment. The generation of free water is due to the reabsorption of sodium chloride from the medullary and cortical portions of the ascending limb of Henle's loop. This approach does not take into account the fact that additional free water may be generated by solute reabsorption more distallly, i.e., in the distal convoluted tubule and in the collecting tubule. The contribution of these latter nephron segments is significantly less than that of the ascending limb. Free water clearance is influenced by the delivery of sodium chloride out of the proximal tubule and this may be increased or decreased depending on the rate of delivery of sodium chloride to the diluting segment. A variety of formulas have been proposed, including:

$$\frac{C_{H_2O}/GFR}{(C_{Na} + C_{H_2O})/GFR} \tag{1}$$

$$\frac{C_{H_2O}/GFR}{(C_{Cl} + C_{H_2O})/GFR} \tag{2}$$

$$\frac{C_{H_2O}/GFR}{V/GFR} \tag{3}$$

It is not the purpose of this chapter to examine the specific advantage of using one or other formula, other than to point out that the fact that a variety of approaches have been proposed is indicative of the complexity of the clearance approach in determining tubular reabsorption in a specific nephron segment.

Distal tubular reabsorption or secretion (i.e., the distal convoluted tubule and the collecting tubule) have been examined by expressing potassium excretion as a function of the rate of sodium excretion when the latter is augmented by hypertonic saline infusion. The assumption is made that potassium secretion is dependent upon sodium delivery to the distal nephron. Once again, these assumptions are not necessarily correct, since potassium reabsorption and secretion may also occur in the proximal tubule and in the ascending limb and the potassium secretory system, under normal circumstances, may be operating well below capacity.

B. Stop-Flow Methods

The stop-flow technique is a modification of the clearance technique which provides information about the functions of different segments of the nephron without complicated procedured other than ureteral catheterization.

After intravenous infusion of various markers (e.g., inulin, *p*-aminohippurate, or other solutes under study) urinary flow is stopped by clamping the ureteral catheter for short period of time. During this period of time, the urine will be exposed to the action of different nephron segments, and the concentrations of various solutes change in accordance with the direction of transport. The occlusion is then released and serial samples are collected from ureteral catheter. The first samples will represent the urine trapped in the most distal degments of the nephron, while the later samples are made up of the urine trapped in more proximal parts of the nephron.

The advantage of the technique is the ease with which the locus and the direction of the transport of various solutes can be determined. However, the disadvantage of this technique is apparent (3). First, during the stop-flow, there is probably sufficient time to allow the solutes to diffuse longitudinally. Second, samples from the proximal tubule probably are the result of the action of the proximal tubule during the period of stop-flow and the action of the distal tubule during the period of new outflow. Third, a more precise distinction than "proximal" or "distal" is impossible.

C. In Vivo Micropuncture

Although the clearance method allows the study of renal function without surgical intervention, it does not permit insight into the function of different nephron segments. In order to overcome the limitation of the clearance method, the micropuncture technique was first introduced by Richards and Wearn in 1923. Since then, micropuncture has been widely employed, and several modifications of the original method have been introduced.

1. Free flow micropuncture technique: Superficial proximal convoluted tubules and distal convoluted tubules are punctured with a micropipette under the microscope; the tubular fluid is collected at a constant rate so as to perturb flow as mininally as possible. Tubular fluid is then analyzed for various solutes. If an impermeable solute, such as inulin, is present in the plasma (P) and is completely filtered, absorption of water will concentrate the inulin within the tubular fluid (TF) and the concentration ratio, TF/P inulin, indicates the fraction of filtrate reabsorbed up to the site of puncture.
2. Split oil droplet method: A double-barreled micropipette is inserted into a superficial tubule and a drop of oil is injected through one barrel into the lumen of the tubule. Through the second barrel, a small amount of solution is injected so as to split the oil drop into two portions. The rate of tubular absorption of the solution can be determined by measuring the rate of the change in the length of the column of fluid separating the two oil droplets.
3. Continuous microperfusion method: A small drop of the oil is first introduced into the lumen of the tubule; a second pipette is then inserted distal to the oil drop, and the test solution is infused at a fixed rate through this pipette using an infusion pump. Contamination by newly formed filtrate is prevented by the proximal oil drop. With a third pipette inserted at a more distal site, the perfused fluid is collected and analyzed.

Using the micropuncture technique, the accessible parts of the nephron include the superficial proximal convoluted tubule and the distal convoluted tubules. In certain species the loops of Henle and the collecting ducts may also be accessible for micropuncture if the renal papilla extends into the renal pelvis and can be exposed. In the Wistar-Munich strain of rat the glomeruli can be studied directly because in these animals some glomeruli are located in the most superficial cortex.

Many segments of the nephron, including the late proximal convoluted tubule, the proximal straight tubule, the thick ascending limbs of the loop of Henle, the cortical and medullary collecting tubule, and most of the juxtamedullary nephrons, are inaccessible to micropuncture and, therefore, the function of these parts of the nephron can only be inferred indirectly. Microcatheterization techniques have been employed to sample fluid from the inner medullary collecting tubule.

Among the disadvantages of the micropuncture technique are the ease with which contamination of the collected sample by fluid from outside of the tubule and/or from a different part of the tubule can occur and the complications associated with surgical preparation, e.g., dehydration and anesthesia.

D. In Vitro Perfusion of Isolated Segments of the Rabbit Nephron

A significant advance in the understanding of renal tubular function was made by Burg and associates at the National Institutes of Health when they developed a method of studying isolated segments of the renal tubule by in vitro perfusion (4). The rabbit and mouse are the only experimental animals from which nephron segments can be conveniently dissected without the use of collagenase and they have been the most extensively studied species using this technique. The significant advantage of the technique lies in the ability to study nephron segments which were previously inaccessible to in vivo micropuncture study. In addition, both the lumen and the peritubular environment can be precisely manipulated so that specific transport processes can be studied with facility. The ease with which specific isotopes can be added either to the luminal or the peritubular environment allows measurements of unidirectional fluxes to be made.

The method consists of rapidly removing the kidney and transferring a slice of either cortex or medulla into a chilled medium and microdissecting a well-identified nephron segment under a dissecting microscope without the use of collagenase. The tubule is transferred to a temperature- and pH-controlled bath and one end is sucked into a holding pipette. The lumen is cannulated with a perfusing pipet. The perfusing pipet can also act as a reference electrode so that with an electrode in the peritubular bath fluid completing the circuit the transtubular potential difference (PD) can be measured throughout the course of an experiment. The other end of the tubule segment is sucked into a collecting pipet and samples of fluid emerging from the tubule are collected under mineral oil. More sophisticated methods have been used to measure transtubular electrical resistance (5) and, more recently, intracellular potentials (6). Not only have normal nephron segments been studied using the technique of in vitro perfusion, but, more recently, segments obtained from various models of disease have also been examined.

II. ANATOMICAL AND FUNCTIONAL SUBDIVISIONS OF THE MAMMALIAN NEPHRON

A. Structure of the Rabbit Nephron

The rabbit nephron has been more extensively studied in vitro than the nephrons of other species and may thus be used as a prototype of the mammalian nephron. A schematic representation of the subdivisions of the rabbit nephron is shown in Fig. 1. In almost all cases the segment is characterized not only by a distinctive cell type (or types) but also a pattern of function which distinguishes it from adjacent segments. The cell types are individually discussed below.

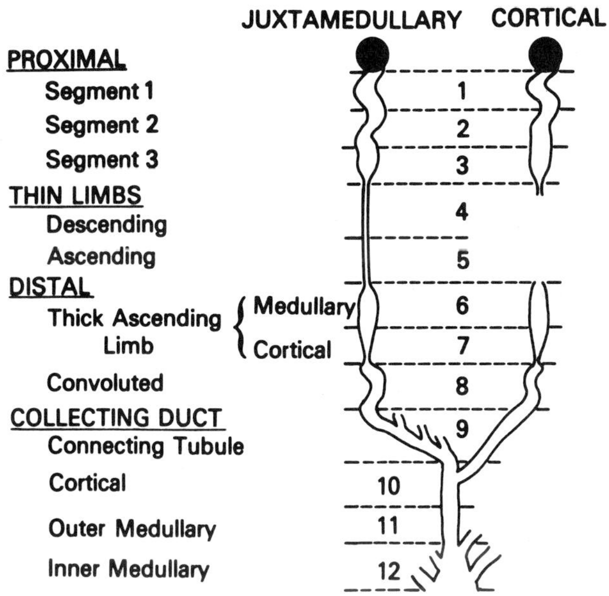

Fig. 1 Subdivisions of the rabbit nephron. (From Ref. 10.)

B. Distribution of Hormone-Sensitive Adenylate Cyclase

Morel and coworkers have successfully applied an additional method of characterizing the different segments of the nephron in the rabbit, rat, mouse, and human by examining hormone-dependent adenylate cyclase in collagenase-dispersed segments of the renal tubule (7). Fig. 2 shows that the subdivisions used by these workers are essentially similar to those shown in Fig. 1. However, both on the basis of the adenylate cyclase response and the appearance under the dissecting microscope the distal nephron has been further subdivided. The distal convoluted tubule is shown to have three sections, i.e., "bright, "granular and "light portions. The distal convoluted tubule includes segments between the macula densa and the first branching with another tubule. The cortical collecting tubule is also divided into granular and light portions, the former corresponding to collecting tubules which form arcades in the cortex, whereas the latter represents those which traverse the medullary rays.

As may be seen, each hormone studied has receptors in more than one segment of the nephron. That this pattern is not uniform among all species is typified by the distribution of vasopressin-sensitive adenylate cyclase in various species (Table 1). In all mammalian species studied, AVP acts predominantly on the cortical and medullary collecting tubule. In the rabbit it has a minimal effect on the medullary thick ascending limb. In the mouse and the rat a significant vasopressin response is elicited in the medullary thick ascending limb, whereas in man it is totally absent in this segment. Adenylate cyclase responsive to parathyroid hormone, calcitonin, isoproterenol, and arginine vasopressin have been described.

III. PROXIMAL TUBULE

The division of the proximal tubule into S_1, S_2, and S_3 segments (Fig. 3) appears to be a more physiologically significant subdivision than the conventional subdivision into convoluted and straight portions (8). The morphology of the proximal tubule throughout its

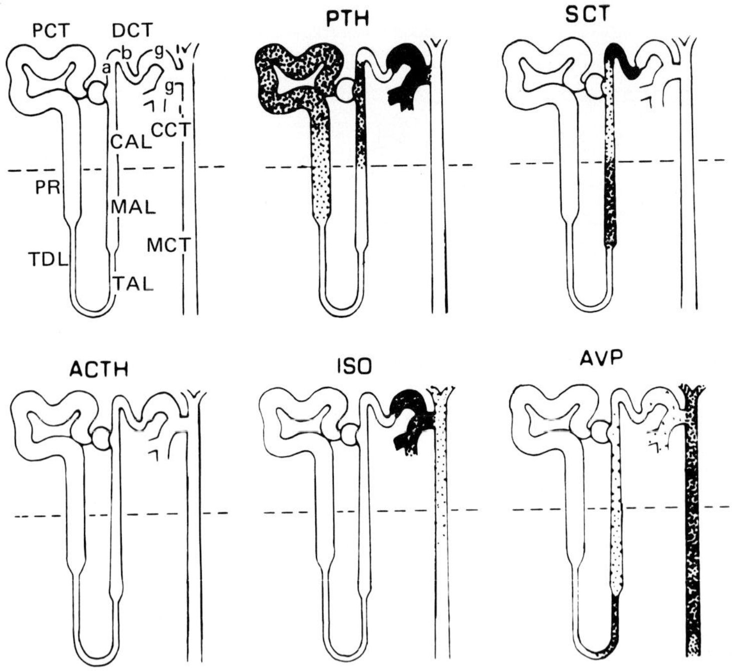

Fig. 2 Hormone-sensitive adenylate cyclase activity in the rabbit nephron. PCT and PR, proximal convoluted tubule and pars recta; TDL and TAL thin descending and ascending limbs of the loop of Henle; MAL and CAL, medullary and cortical thick ascending limbs; DCT, distal convoluted tubule, including a bright (b), granular (g), and light (l) portion; CCT, cortical collecting tubule, including a light (l) and granular (g) portion. MCT, medullary collecting tubule. Dot density is proportional to the increase in adenylate cyclase activity induced by the hormones. PTH, parathyroid hormone; SCT, calcitonin; ACTH, adenocorticotropin; ISO, isoproterenol; AVP, arginine vasopressin. (From Ref. 7.)

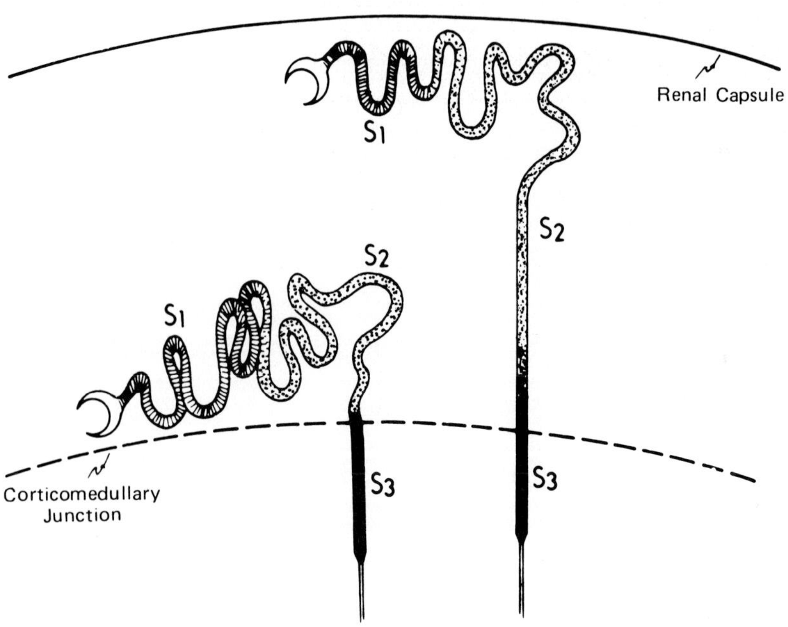

Fig. 3 Subdivisions of the rabbit superficial and juxtamedullary proximal tubules. (From Ref. 8.)

Table 1 Hormone-Sensitive Adenylate Cyclase in Mammalian Nephrons

Nephron segment	Parathyroid hormone			Vasopressin			Calcitonin			Isoproterenol	
	Rabbit	Rat	Man	Rabbit	Rat	Man	Rabbit	Rat	Man	Rabbit	Rat
Proximal convoluted	++	++	++	0	0	0	0	0	0	0	0
Proximal straight	+	+	+	0	0	0	0	0	0	0	0
Medullary thick Ascending limb	0	0	+	+	++	0	++	+	+	0	0
Cortical thick Ascending limb	+	++	+	+	+	0	+	++	+	0	+
Distal convoluted	0	++	++	0	0	0	++	++	++	0	+
Connecting tubule	++	++	++	0	0	0	0		++	++	+
Cortical collecting	0	0	0	++	++	++	0	+	++	+	+
Medullary collecting	0	0		++	++	++	0	0	0	+	0

Adenylate cyclase activity: 0, no stimulation; +, significant stimulation; ++, stimulation greater than 300 fmol/mm per hr.
Source: Compiled from Ref. 7.

length is relatively homogeneous, but the height of the brush border and the extent of the basal interdigitations decrease from S_1 through S_3. These segments reabsorb a large fraction of the glomerular filtrate, utilizing active sodium transport as the fundamental transport process.

A. Sodium Chloride, Water, Glucose, Amino Acid, and Organic Anion Transport

S_1 Proximal Tubule (Fig. 4)

The fluid entering the S_1 segment, which is the earliest portion of the proximal tubule (the first millimeter), is an ultrafiltrate of plasma formed by the glomerulus. The function of this segment has been studied both in vitro microperfusion and by in vivo micropuncture techniques. In this segment of the nephron, sodium, potassium, bicarbonate, glucose, amino acids, lactate, phosphate, and other metabolic intermediates are reabsorbed. As the glomerular filtrate courses through the segment, the chloride concentration increases. This increase is virtually complete within 1-2 mm of the glomerulus. Concomitantly, the concentrations of other solutes including bicarbonate, glucose, amino acids, and lactate decrease. Tubular reabsorption of water occurs isosmotically.

Sodium reabsorption in this nephron segment has been attributed predominantly to active processes, whereas, as will be shown later, sodium reabsorption in more distal segments of the proximal tubule appears to have both active and passive components (9). The isosmotic reabsorption of fluid appears to be coupled exclusively to the reabsorption of sodium, since when sodium is replaced by other cations such as lithium tetramethylammonium, or choline, fluid reabsorption ceases. On the other hand, replacement of chloride by nitrate or perchlorate does not appear to have a significant effect on fluid reabsorption (10).

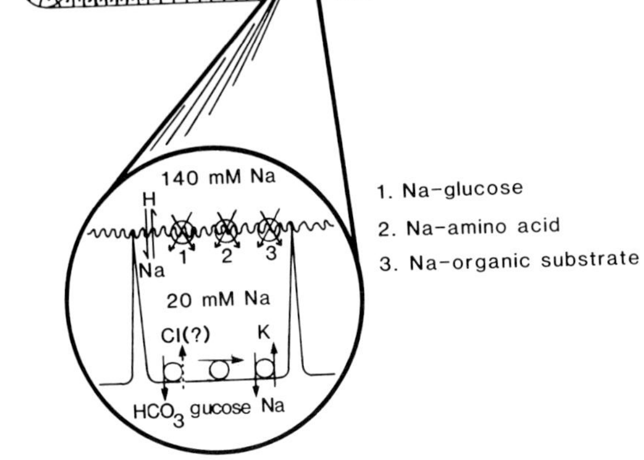

Fig. 4 Transport processes across the S_1 proximal tubule. (active transport; ---> diffusion down an electrochemical gradient; cotransport; ⇌ antiport.)

Evidence for active transport of sodium in this segment is based upon the fact that the movement of sodium occurs against an electrochemical gradient. Transepithelial voltage is negative in the lumen of the early proximal convoluted tubule perfused with an ultrafiltrate of serum (~ -4 mV) (11). Thus, sodium moves against an electrical gradient. When nonabsorbable substances such as mannitol or raffinose are present in the tubular fluid sodium chloride reabsorption proceeds without the concomitant reabsorption of water, thus lowering its luminal concentration to 30 meq/liter below the concentration in the peritubular capillary blood. The ability of this segment of the proximal tubule to establish such a concentration gradient is further evidence for active transport (10). Fluid reabsorption is inhibited by ouabain and by removal of potassium from the peritubular fluid (11). Both these maneuvers serve to inhibit the activity of sodium-potassium-activated ATPase (Na-K-ATPase) which is the sodium pump located in the basolateral cell membrane.

In the first 1-2 mm of the proximal tubule, sodium is preferentially reabsorbed with neutral organic solutes and with bicarbonate, acetate, phosphate, citrate, and lactate (9). These solutes are transported from the lumen into the cell across the brush border by specific carrier complexes which require the presence of sodium ions. The energy which drives the movement of the sodium-carrier complex across the brush border is derived from the electrochemical gradient for sodium ions which in turn is maintained by the Na-K-ATPase located in the basolateral cell membrane. The principal coupled-transport processes can be divided into: (1) cotransport of sodium with neutral organic solutes, (2) cotransport of sodium with anions such as phosphate, acetate, citrate, and lactate, and (3) countertransport of sodium and hydrogen ions.

Neutral Organic Solute-Sodium Cotransport

The dependence of sodium transport on the presence of organic solutes within the tubular lumen has been demonstrated by the removal of these substances during perfusion of isolated rabbit proximal tubules. A significant decrease in fluid (sodium chloride) reabsorption was demonstrated, whereas removal of the same solutes from the peritubular fluid had no effect (12). The reabsorption of sugars and amino acids by the proximal tubule likewise requires the presence of sodium in the tubular fluid and can be inhibited by ouabain (12). Studies on isolated brush-border membrane vesicles indicate that the organic solute-sodium-carrier complexes carry a net positive charge across the luminal membrane and in turn are influenced by the transmembrane potential difference. It has been concluded that the carrier combines with one sodium ion and one neutral organic solute molecule to effect this coupled transport (13). The depolarization of the luminal membrane which occurs contributes to the generation of a lumen negative potential.

Once the sodium ion has gained access to the peritubular surface it can either diffuse back into the lumen or it can lead to the passive movement of chloride ions out of the lumen through a paracellular pathway. It appears that the relative ionic conductances of the proximal tubular epithelium, i.e., the permselectivity to sodium and chloride, are the determinants of which process will predominate (9). Thus, if permeability to chloride is twice as great as that to sodium, two-thirds of the paracellular current flow will be in the form of chloride ions moving from lumen to peritubular surfaces and one-third in the form of sodium moving in the opposite direction. In contrast, if the permselectivity ratio is reversed, two-thirds of the current flow will be in the form of sodium ions moving from blood to lumen and one-third in the form of chloride moving in the opposite direction. In this regard, the fact that both the superficial and juxtamedullary early proximal convoluted tubule is sodium selective (14) means that there is probably significant recycling of sodium ions back into the lumen. In later segments of the superficial proximal tubule which are chloride selective (14) neutral organic solute reabsorption could lead to significant additional chloride reabsorption.

It appears that the interaction of glucose and amino acids with sodium is linked to transport rather than to the metabolism of these organic substances. It has been shown, for instance, that when glucose or alanine is added to a perfusate which is free of organic solutes the rate of fluid reabsorption increases significantly. Nonmetabolizable analogs such as α-methyl-D-glucoside have a similar effect, suggesting that these substances are cotransported rather than metabolized (12). The interaction of sodium with glucose and amino acids in the brush-border membrane is discussed more fully in Ch. 1.

Cotransport of Sodium with Organic Anions

Direct evidence for the existence of sodium lactate and sodium phosphate transport has been demonstrated in brush-border membrane vesicles (see Ch. 1 for details). Furthermore, the addition of citrate and lactate to the proximal tubular perfusate has been shown to result in an increase in the rate of fluid reabsorption. No change in transtubular PD was observed. These studies indicate that reabsorption of these salts is an electroneutral process. There is a possibility, however, that some sodium phosphate cotransport is electrogenic (15). This would occur if the sodium-phosphate carrier is associated with two sodium ions for each phosphate ion. At neutral pH, the bulk of phosphate reabsorption would be electroneutral, since HPO_4^{2-} is the predominant species, whereas the small amount of $H_2PO_4^-$, coupled in a 1:2 ratio with Na, would effect net transfer of positive charge.

Sodium-Hydrogen Countertransport

The principal ion reabsorbed with sodium in the early proximal tubule is bicarbonate. The reabsorption of sodium and bicarbonate are interdependent. If bicarbonate is removed from the perfusate and the peritubular fluid, fluid reabsorption is inhibited. Likewise, when sodium is removed from the bath or sodium transport is inhibited by ouabain, bicarbonate reabsorption is inhibited. This interdependence of sodium and bicarbonate transport also appears to reside in an interaction at the level of the brush border membrane, which involves a carrier that exchanges cellular hydrogen ions for luminal sodium ions (17). The hydrogen ions entering the lumen titrate the bicarbonate leading to net reabsorption of bicarbonate. The existence of these specific counter-transport processes has been definitively demonstrated in brush-border membrane vesicles (Ch. 1).

The transport of sodium from cell interior to peritubular surface across the basolateral membrane, which is mediated by Na-K-ATPase, is referred to as primary active transport. The generation of a low intracellular sodium concentration and a cell interior which is electrically negative create an electrochemical gradient for sodium entry across the luminal membrane. Once the organic solutes and anions have entered the cells, the permeability of the peritubular membrane and the presence of specific carriers in this membrane will regulate the efflux of these substances from the cell. The existence of a glucose carrier (18,19) and a specific bicarbonate transport mechanism, which is inhibited by acetazolamide and disulfonic stilbenes, has been demonstrated in the peritubular membrane (20,21).

The proximal tubule is regarded as a "leaky" epithelium comparable to the gallbladder and jejunum. This means that permeability to water, sodium, and chloride is high and that the reflection coefficient for sodium chloride is low. It is believed that permeation of sodium, chloride, and water occur through the lateral intercellular space. The presence of such an intercellular pathway was established by experiments in which a current was passed across the epithelium and the resistance of the epithelium was found to be significantly lower than the resistance calculated for the individual luminal and peritubular plasma cell membranes (22). This suggests that the high conductance pathway is between cells. Solutes which are generally regarded as impermeant, e.g., sucrose and raffinose, have been found to pass through the epithelium under certain circumstances.

If water reabsorption across the proximal tubule is isosmotic and is passive in nature, the question arises as to what the driving force for such passive movement could be. (The existence of lateral intercellular spaces provides the pathway for the movement of water.) One explanation has been that sodium enters the lateral intercellular spaces across the basolateral cell membrane and, since the concentration of sodium chloride is higher in these spaces than in the lumen or the general extracellular fluid space, this concentration difference causes the osmotic movement of water into the lateral spaces across cell membranes or through the tight junctions (23). Alternately, transport of solute out of the lumen may reduce the osmolality of luminal fluid very slightly. Since the water permeability of the proximal tubule is high, small osmotic presure differences would be sufficient to drive a significantly large amount of fluid. Finally, the driving force may relate to the differences in the reflection coefficients of glucose, bicarbonate, and non-chloride sodium salts across the epithelium. If the reflection coefficient of sodium chloride is lower than that of the other solutes, the removal of these solutes from the lumen and their transfer into the lateral intercellular space would create an *effective* osmotic pressure which is higher in the lateral intercellular space than in the lumen, despite the fact that the concentration of sodium in the lumen and peritubular space is the same.

S_2 Proximal Tubule (Late Proximal Convoluted Tubule and Early Proximal Straight Tubule (Fig. 5)

In superficial nephrons, the S_2 segment includes the later portion of the convoluted tubule and the early portion of the pars recta (proximal straight tubule). In juxtamedullary nephrons, it includes only the late proximal convoluted tubule, since the pars recta is much shorter in this nephron population (8). A number of differences between the S_1 and S_2 segments have been delineated. The function of the S_2 segment, in vivo, is dependent not only on its intrinsic properties, but on the composition of the tubular fluid which is delivered

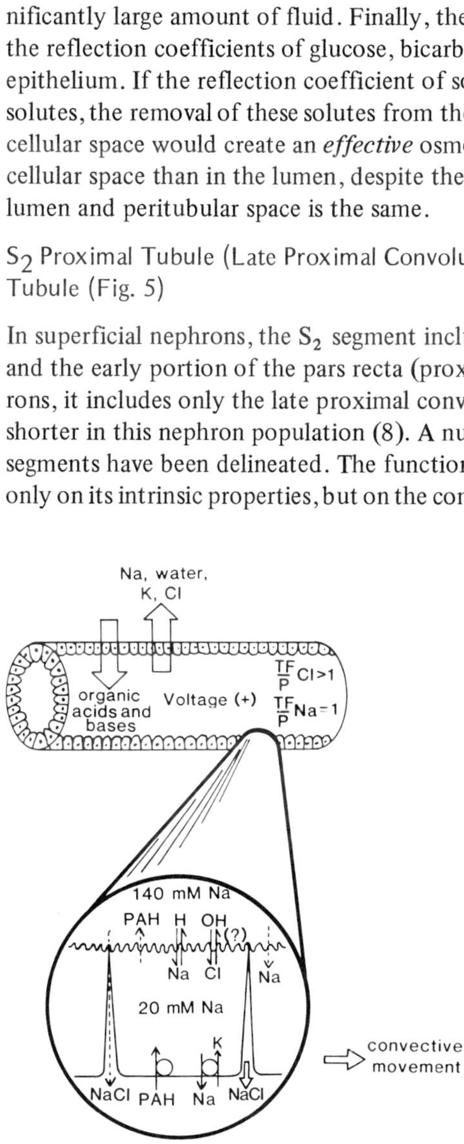

Fig. 5 Transport processes across the S_2 proximal tubule (symbols as for Fig. 4).

to it out of the S_1 segment. In the S_2 segment, the fluid reabsorptive rate is approximately 50% (24,25) and glucose reabsorption 10% (26) of that observed in the S_1 segment (8,27). In contrast, the secretion of organic anions, such as *p*-aminohippurate (PAH) by the S_2 segment is at least five times higher than in the S_1 segment. Bicarbonate reabsorption proceeds at about 25% the rate of that observed in the S_1 segment. The overall pattern therefore reflects a lower intrinsic rate of reabsorption, but a high intrinsic rate of tubular secretion (Table 2).

By the end of the S_1 proximal convoluted tubule the concentration of bicarbonate, glucose, amino acids, lactate, and other solutes has been significantly decreased. The concentration of chloride, on the other hand, is elevated above that of the peritubular fluid (30) and the pH of the tubular fluid has been lowered by hydrogen ion secretion. In vivo, the transepithelial voltage is lumen positive. This positive voltage predominantly reflects a chloride diffusion potential, since the tubule is permeable to chloride (14, 31-33) and the gradient for diffusion is from the lumen to the peritubular surface. If the bicarbonate permeability of the tubule were the same as the chloride permeability, this potential would be offset by a tendency for reabsorbed bicarbonate to diffuse from peritubular to luminal surfaces. However, since bicarbonate permeability is lower than chloride permeability, the net result is a lumen positive potential. By making the chloride concentrations and bicarbonate concentrations inside and outside the tubule equal the positive luminal potential is abolished. The existence of a luminal fluid containing a high concentration of chloride allows for a second mechanism of sodium chloride and volume reabsorption to occur, namely, passive paracellular sodium transport. Chloride moves down its concentration gradient and sodium moves passively together with chloride. Since the reflection coefficient for sodium chloride is less than that for sodium bicarbonate or glucose or amino acids (which are now present only on the peritubular surface), an effective osmotic pressure difference exists across the tubular epithelium. This osmotic pressure difference, which is capable of driving the osmotic flow of water, would result in additional convective sodium chloride reabsorption, i.e., transfer of sodium chloride by solvent drag. Thus, the passive transport process includes both convective and diffusive flows of sodium chloride. This mode of transport is confined to segments beyond the early proximal tubule (9).

It appears that passive transport mechanisms may not be the same in superficial and juxtamedullary proximal convoluted tubules (14,31,33). It has recently been demonstrated that passive forces play an important role in volume reabsorption in superficial nephrons, whereas this mode of transport is absent in the juxtamedullary segments. This may be related to the fact that in the juxtamedullary proximal tubule, the permeability to sodium greatly exceeds that to chloride, thus minimizing the tendency of chloride to move out of the lumen.

Table 2 Differences Between S_1 and S_2 Proximal Tubule Segments

Transport rate (mol/cm per sec $\times 10^{-12}$)	S_1	S_2
Fluid (nl/mm per min)	1.18 and 1.38	0.42 and 0.62
Glucose	13	1
p-Aminohippurate	-0.05	-0.25
Bicarbonate	13	3
Glycine	4.75	0.42

Source: Ref. 10.

In addition to passive paracellular sodium transport, active transport is also found in the S_2 segment. It should be pointed out that many of the studies initially performed on isolated perfused proximal tubules did not carefully draw the distinction between early and late proximal tubules, and it is assumed that the sampling included mainly, but not exclusively, S_2 segments.

In the presence of anion concentration gradient (increased chloride and decreased bicarbonate in the lumen), these tubules generate a small lumen-positive PD and reabsorb sodium chloride. Ouabain increases the lumen-positive potential of this segment in the rabbit superficial proximal convoluted tubule (35). If the transtubular PD is the sum of a positive chloride diffusion potential (lumen positive) and an electrogenic active sodium transport potential (lumen negative), obliteration of the latter by ouabain could explain the increase in luminal positivity. In contrast, it has been shown that in juxtamedullary proximal convoluted tubules perfused with high chloride solutions, the PD is lumen negative rather than positive and volume reabsorption is entirely abolished by ouabain in this segment (36).

Sodium chloride transport across this segment of the nephron could be the result of direct coupling of sodium and chloride transport or it could be effected by two ion exchangers, i.e., a sodium-hydrogen antiport system and a chloride-hydroxyl antiport system. These are discussed more fully in Ch. 1. It has recently been estimated that approximately 50% of the sodium delivered into the proximal tubule is reabsorbed by active mechanisms, 12% by passive mechanisms, and the remainder escapes reabsorption to be delivered downstream (9).

The cellular events in transepithelial sodium transport have been carefully studied in *Necturus* proximal tubule (37-40). In this species, salt and water are reabsorbed isosmotically. Reabsorption is not dependent on bicarbonate concentration in this species. By means of intracellular ion-specific electrodes and radioisotope tracers it has been possible to show that sodium is actively transported out of the proximal tubule across the peritubular border. This process serves to reduce intracellular sodium activity to approximately 30 mmol/liter. The voltage across the peritubular cell border is approximately 60 mV. The low intracellular sodium activity provides the driving force for entry of sodium across the luminal brush-border membrane and chloride entry into the cells occurs in an electroneutral fashion, i.e., chloride transport is a secondary active transport process, since it is driven by sodium transport. By this mechanism, chloride activity within the cells is higher than the expected value predicted by passive distribution according to the voltage. It is this high intracellular chloride activity which provides the driving force for its exit across the peritubular membrane. As noted above, it is uncertain whether secondary active chloride transport exists in the mammalian proximal tubule.

More recent studies in isolated perfused rabbit proximal tubules have shown the potential difference across the basolateral membrane to be approximately 50 mV (6). Ouabain and low bath potassium depolarizes the membrane, whereas removal of luminal glucose and alanine hyperpolarize it. These results are consistent with a potassium-selective basolateral membrane, since inhibition of the sodium-potassium pump should result in depolarization as cell potassium is lost. The hyperpolarization following glucose or alanine removal is due to decreased sodium transport into the cell via the sodium-glucose or sodium-amino acid cotransport system.

In summary, there are two principal mechanisms of sodium transport in the S_2 proximal tubule (Fig. 5). Two-thirds is transcellular, with sodium entering the cell by diffusion and sodium-hydrogen countertransport. This sodium leaves the cell by active transport. One third of sodium transport is paracellular driven either by the chloride diffusion gradient (secondary to the positive lumen potential) or by solvent drag (convective movement).

S_3 Proximal Tubule

The S_3 proximal tubule is located in the outer medulla and probably does not exceed 1 mm in length (8). It is the terminal part of the pars recta of the superficial proximal tubule and it is the only straight part of the juxtamedullary proximal tubule. The S_3 segment secretes PAH and other organic anions but at a slower rate than the S_2 segments. Other functional parameters have not been studied.

Regulation of Proximal Tubular Sodium Chloride Transport by Extrinsic Factors

Peritubular Physical Factors

The rate of net sodium and fluid reabsorption by the proximal tubule is affected by a number of physical factors which include peritubular hydrostatic pressure, peritubular oncotic pressure, and hematocrit. The glomerular ultrafiltrate is protein-free. The removal of this protein-free component from the plasma entering the glomerulus results in a plasma protein concentration in the efferent arteriole and peritubular capillaries which is higher than that in the systemic blood. The high colloid osmotic pressure generated by this concentration of the plasma proteins could promote the reabsorption of fluid into the peritubular capillaries by retarding backflux of fluid into the leaky proximal tubule. The hydrostatic pressure within the proximal tubule is higher than that in the interstitium and peritubular capillaries, and this too could serve as a driving force for fluid reabsorption from the tubule lumen. However, in order for these physical forces to be primary determinants of fluid reabsorption, the tubule would be required to have a water permeability which is significantly higher than that which has been measured. If either of these factors were directly responsible for fluid reabsorption, elevation of intratubular pressure should also increase net fluid reabsorption, whereas elevation of colloid osmotic pressure within the tubular fluid should retard fluid reabsorption. Neither of these experimental maneuvers has a direct effect on the rate of fluid reabsorption (41-43). It appears, therefore, that the physical factors act across the peritubular capillaries rather than across the tubular epithelium.

The forces favoring or retarding reabsorption (Fig. 6) are those which are distributed between the lumen of the peritubular capillary and the interstitial space surrounding the renal tubule. Net fluid reabsorption across the proximal tubule is the difference between the reabsorptive flux and the leak into the tubule. When peritubular capillary hydraulic pressure is increased or colloid is absent from the medium surrounding the tubule, the backflux component is presumably increased. Evidence in favor of this proposal is provided by the fact that large molecular-weight substances such as sucrose can penetrate the tubular epithelium under these conditions (44,45). Similarly, the electrical conductance of the epithelium also increases (22). It is believed that the pathway for this fluid movement is between cells rather than through cells. Until a direct method of measuring hydrostatic and colloid osmotic pressure in the interstitial and intercellular spaces is possible, it will be difficult to evaluate the mechanisms whereby these physical factors alter net fluid reabsorption.

Tubule Fluid Flow Rate

The method of *in vitro* perfusion has allowed this parameter to be evaluated with facility. By varying the perfusion rate in vitro, the direct effects of flow on net sodium chloride transport can be evaluated. In the proximal tubule perfused in vitro at flow rates comparable to those which obtain in vivo there is no relationship between perfusion rate, i.e., tubular fluid flow rate, and net fluid reabsorption. In contrast, in vivo experiments reveal that there is a direct relationship between flow into the proximal tubule (i.e., glomerular filtration rate) and sodium reabsorption (46). This relationship has been called glomerulotubular balance. The term refers to the fact that when single nephron filtration rate is varied a constant

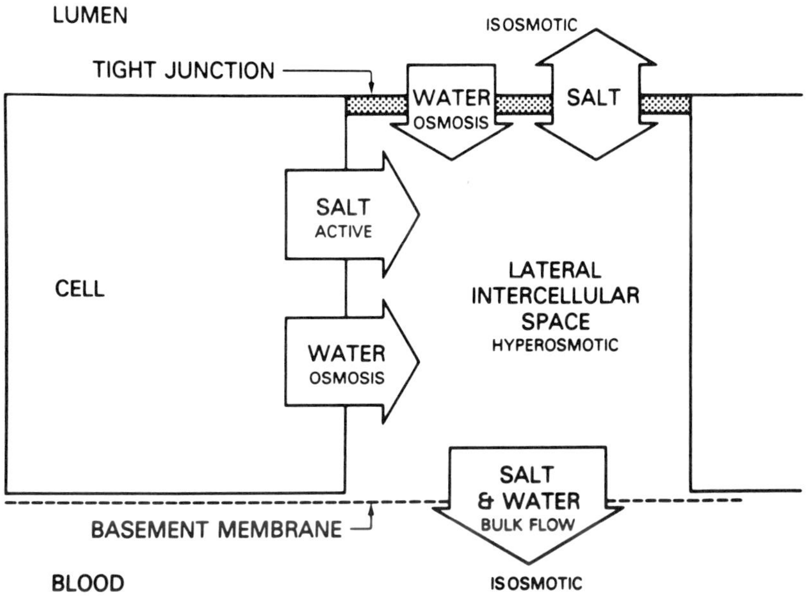

Fig. 6 Physical forces determining salt and water reabsorption across the proximal tubule. (From Ref. 10.)

fraction of the filtrate is reabsorbed up to a given point in the proximal tubule. Absence of an in vitro effect and the presence of an effect in vivo suggests that peritubular factors play an important role in glomerulotubular balance. If at a fixed single nephron plasma flow rate the rate of glomerular filtration increases (filtration fraction increases), the protein concentration in the peritubular capillaries will be raised. This increase in peritubular oncotic pressure would enhance net sodium and fluid reabsorption, so that the increase in glomerular filtration rate would be paralleled by an increased reabsorptive rate in the proximal tubule.

An additional mechanism which may be important in determining the rate of fluid reabsorption is the composition of the tubular fluid. When the tubular fluid contains organic solutes such as glucose and amino acids, the reabsorption of which is coupled to sodium, the rate of delivery of these solutes into the tubular lumen would become a determinant of the reabsorption rate of sodium. This would apply mainly to the earliest portion of the proximal tubule (S_1), since these substances are absent from the tubule lumen further downstream. An increased filtration rate would deliver organic solutes and sodium at an increased rate to the early proximal tubule. At any given reabsorption rate there would be less reduction in the concentration of these organic solutes in the luminal fluid, so that coupled organic solute-sodium transport would proceed over a greater length of the proximal tubule (10).

B. Potassium Transport

Sixty to seventy percent of the filtered potassium is reabsorbed along the length of the proximal tubule. Tubular fluid to plasma (TF/P) potassium ratios are close to unity, suggesting that potassium may be reabsorbed passively together with sodium chloride and water (49). However, in some experiments TF/P potassium ratios have been shown to fall below unity, suggesting that active potassium transport does occur (50,51). This can also be shown by inhibiting sodium, water, and hydrogen transport with azetazolamide, thus preventing the increase in chloride concentration along the proximal tubule and the development of a lumen-positive potential. Under these circumstances, potassium reabsorption is not inhibited. Thus, it appears as if a separate transport mechanism for potassium does exist in the proximal tubule. Additional evidence supporting an active transport mechanism across the luminal membrane is the finding of a potassium activity ratio (intracellular/intraluminal) which exceeds the measured electrical potential difference and which is reduced during perfusion of the tubule lumen with ouabain (52). In addition to the movement of potassium through the proximal tubular cells, it is reasonable to suppose that potassium reabsorption also proceeds through the paracellular pathway. This component of sodium chloride transport would be driven by solvent drag induced by the sodium-dependent fluid reabsorption.

C. Bicarbonate Transport

Bicarbonate reabsorption by the proximal tubule has been studied by in vitro perfusion of rabbit proximal tubules (28,29). The acid-base status of the animals does not influence the rate of reabsorption which is approximately 5 peq/cm per sec. Parathyroid hormone (PTH) decreases bicarbonate reabsorption by approximately 50% in the proximal straight tubule (16). PTH also decreases fluid reabsorption in the proximal convoluted tubule, a process that is bicarbonate-dependent (54).

D. Phosphate Transport

Both in vivo micropuncture (53) and in vitro perfusion studies (54) have shown that the early part of the proximal convoluted tubule, i.e., the S_1 segment, has a much greater capacity to reabsorb phosphate than the later part of the proximal tubule. Approximately 40% of the filtered phosphate is reabsorbed in the first few convolutions, whereas about 75% of the filtered phosphate will be reabsorbed by the end of the proximal convoluted tubule. (Fig. 7).

The rate of phosphate reabsorption by the S_2 segment has been shown to be approximately one-fourth of that by S_1 segment, i.e., 3.0 vs. 11.4 pmol/mm per min. Phosphate is reabsorbed by proximal straight tubule (S_3 segment) at an even slower rate (54). There is no difference in phosphate absorption rates between the superficial proximal convoluted tubule and the juxtamedullary proximal convoluted tubule (55). Internephron heterogeneity may exist because of the different ratio of S_1 to S_3 segment lengths in different subpopulations of nephrons and because of the differences in the filtered load of phosphate between the superficial and juxtamedullary nephrons.

Several pieces of evidence have appeared to suggest that most of the phosphate reabsorption in the proximal tubule is Na dependent. In isolated perfused rabbit proximal tubules, both phosphate and fluid reabsorption can be inhibited by adding ouabain to the bath, while phosphate absorption is not affected when fluid absorption is inhibited by adding raffinose to the perfusate (54). In brush-border membrane vesicles (56), phosphate uptake can be inhibited by removing Na from the medium and is a saturable process, i.e., phosphate uptake by the brush border of the proximal tubule is due to secondary active transport linked to primary active Na transport. It has been suggested that the coupling between Na and phosphate is in 2:1 ratio and can either proceed as an electroneutral process when phosphate is in the divalent form, or an electrogenic process carrying a positive charge when phosphate is in the monovalent form. The fact that glucose and alanine absorption competes with phosphate absorption suggests that the transport of these substances may occur through the same pathway.

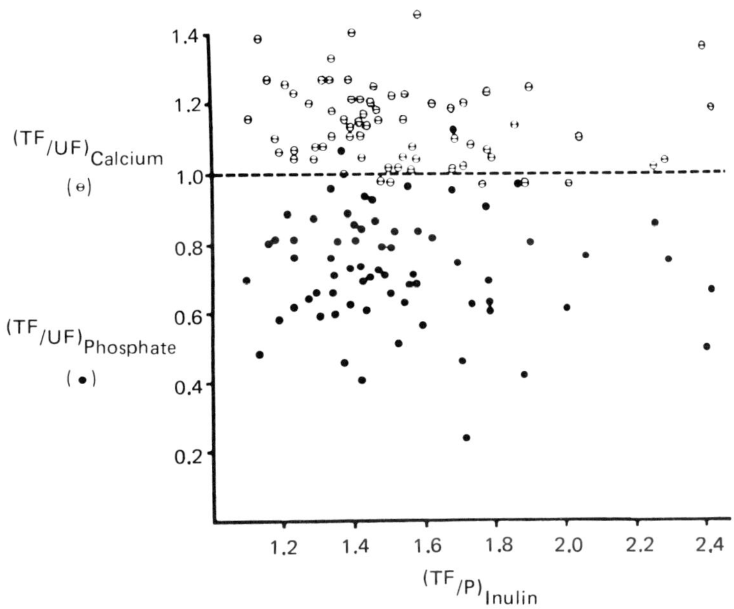

Fig. 7 Tubular fluid: Ultrafiltrate (TF/UF) ratios for calcium and phosphate along the proximal tubule of the hydropenic dog. (From Ref. 53.)

Phosphate transport across the basolateral membrane appears to be a Na-independent, passive process (157), being favored by the high intracellular phosphate concentration and the inside-negative membrane potential.

Factors Regulating Phosphate Transport in the Proximal Tubule

Proximal phosphate reabsorption can be inhibited by extracellular volume expansion (58), parathyroid hormone (59), high dietary phosphate intake (60), and a carbonic anhydrase inhibitory diuretic, e.g., acetazolamide (61). Alkalinization of the tubular fluid and/or increasing bicarbonate concentration of the tubular fluid have been shown to inhibit proximal phosphate reabsorption in micropuncture studies (62). Because the pK_a of phosphate is 6.9 at alkaline pH most of the phosphate will be in the divalent form, which is suggested to be less permeable than the monovalent form. However, this contention has not been supported by observations in isolated perfused tubules in which both alkalinization and acidification of the bath decreased proximal phosphate absorption (54). In brush-border membrane vesicles alkalinization of the medium actually increased phosphate uptake into the vesicles (56). In this regard, it has been hypothesized that the inhibitory effect of parathyroid hormone on phosphate reabsorption could be mediated through its inhibitory effect on bicarbonate reabsorption with consequent alkalinization of the tubule fluid (62), but there are data which do not support this hypothesis. In the isolated rabbit proximal tubule, it has been shown that parathyroid hormone acts only on late proximal convoluted and proximal straight tubules (59), segments which receive tubular fluid containing significantly reduced bicarbonate concentration.

Inhibition of phosphate reabsorption by extracellular volume expansion has been shown to be independent of filtered load, serum Ca concentration, and parathyroid hormone (63-65). The mechanism of this inhibition is most likely secondary to the decreased proximal Na reabsorption which accompanies volume expansion.

The mechanisms by which dietary phosphate intake affects proximal phosphate reabsorption are still obscure. It has been shown that this adaptation to phosphate intake occurs independently of parathyroid hormone, serum Ca, filtered load of phosphorus (60), and vitamin D (66). A correlation between tubular alkaline phosphatase activity and the tubular response to dietary phosphate alteration has been shown (67), although a temporal dissociation between these two events has recently been demonstrated (68).

E. Calcium Transport

Calcium reabsorption by proximal convoluted tubule seems to parallel fluid and Na reabsorption (69). Proximal tubule fluid/ultrafiltrate (TF/UF) Ca concentration usually is close to unity (Fig. 7). From microperfusion studies, it has been suggested that most of the Ca reabsorption occurring in the proximal convoluted tubule is due to a Na-dependent, passive mechanism. Only about 20% of the Ca reabsorbed is thought to be due to an active transport mechanism, which is also Na dependent (70).

With a low intracellular Ca concentration (71) and an inside-negative potential (72) Ca entry through the brush border membrane may occur passively. However, the exit of the Ca through the basolateral membrane has to be an active process for the same reason. This active extrusion of Ca may be mediated either by a Na-Ca countertransport mechanism (which would explain the Na dependence of active Ca transport) (73) or by a Ca-activated ATPase localized on the basolateral membrane of the proximal tubules (74) (see Ch. 1). Proximal convoluted tubules appear to be highly permeable to Ca, backflux of Ca being estimated to be approximately three times the net flux (75).

Since (TF/UF) Ca at the tip of the loop of Henle was found to be significantly lower than (TF/UF) Na (76), and because the descending limb of loop of Henle has been shown to be relatively impermeable to Ca (77), it has been postulated that Ca reabsorption either occurs along the proximal straight tubule, or that heterogeneity between superficial and juxtamedullary nephrons exists. The former possibility is supported by the finding that the proximal straight tubule is capable of actively reabsorbing substantial amounts of Ca against a transepithelial electrochemical gradient (78).

Extracellular volume expansion (79), hypercalcemia (80), hypermagnesemia (81), and increased concentration of anions (82) have been shown to inhibit proximal calcium reabsorption. The inhibitory effect of anions on calcium reabsorption is probably due to complex formation with calcium ions.

F. Magnesium Transport

In contrast to other cations, the ratio (TF/UF) Mg in the proximal convoluted tubules rises to as high as 1.5-2.2, indicating that only 15-30% of the filtered Mg is being reabsorbed (83). In vivo microperfusion studies have revealed a very low backleak of the Mg, suggesting that the proximal convoluted tubule is relatively impermeable to Mg, and that Mg reabsorption occurs via a transcellular rather than a paracellular route (84). The cellular mechanism of Mg transport is unknown. There is no information available on Mg transport in the proximal straight tubule.

Proximal Mg reabsorption can be inhibited by extracellular volume expansion (85). Hypermagnesemia reduces fractional reabsorption of Mg in the proximal tubules (84), whereas parathyroid hormone enhances Mg reabsorption (86)

G. Urate Transport

Urate handling by the proximal tubule varies considerably from species to species. In the rat there is both reabsorption and secretion of urate, the latter process occurring in the last portion of the superficial proximal tubule accessible to micropuncture (87-89). In the rabbit net reabsorption has been demonstrated by micropuncture and uphill secretion has been demonstrated in vitro (91). The secretory process is temperature-dependent and is inhibited by ouabain. Although it has not been studied rigorously, it is likely that the main site of urate secretion is the S_2 segment.

IV. THIN DESCENDING AND ASCENDING LIMBS OF HENLE'S LOOP

A. Sodium Chloride, Water, and Urea Transport

The thin descending and ascending limbs of Henle's loop play an important role in the urinary concentrating process. Most of the information about the function of the thin limbs is derived from micropuncture studies, conclusions being drawn from comparisons of fluid sampled from the end of the accessible proximal convoluted tubule and from the tip of the loop of Henle, both of which nephrons can be exposed during the puncture procedure. Inherent in this approach is the pitfall that different nephron populations are being sampled, i.e., the proximal tubules of superficial nephrons and the loops of Henle of the juxtamedullary nephrons. Thus, a comparison between the composition of tubular fluid at the two points does not necessarily reflect the function of any particular nephron population. A further problem with this approach lies in the fact that a significant segment of the proximal tubule, i.e., part of the S_2 and the entire S_3 segment, is interposed between the two micropuncture sites, so that the contribution of this segment to transport processes can confuse interpretation of the data.

In vitro studies have revealed no evidence for active sodium chloride transport in either the thin descending or thin ascending limb of Henle's loop (92-95). It was thus proposed that if sodium chloride or water are removed from the lumen, this must occur as a passive process. Water permeability in the thin descending limb is very high, whereas it is very low in the thin ascending limb. Permeabilities to sodium and urea are also different in the two segments (Table 3). In the descending limb both sodium and urea permeabilities are low, whereas in the ascending limb sodium permeability is considerably greater and exceeds the permeability to urea. Chloride permeability is also high in this segment. These differential permeability properties are adequate to explain the mechanism of water and sodium chloride removal by the loop of Henle according to passive processes (96).

Fluid is abstracted from the thin descending limb which courses through a hyperosmotic medulla and papilla so that sodium chloride concentration is elevated toward the tip of the loop. This has been demonstrated in descending limbs perfused in vitro. The concentration of sodium chloride is elevated primarily by water abstraction rather than by solute addition. Micropuncture studies in rats have shown that removal of water alone does not account for the concentrations of sodium chloride and urea at the bend of the loop of Henle, and it has therefore been proposed that, in this species at least, addition of sodium chloride and urea to the descending limb contributes to the high papillary-tip concentrations. Whether the entry of urea is due to passive diffusion into the tubular lumen or whether there is active secretion of urea by the pars recta has not been established with certainty.

Tubular fluid at the tip of the loop of Henle contains a high sodium chloride concentration and a lower urea concentration. In contrast, the interstitial fluid at the tip of the papilla

Table 3 Hydraulic Conductivity, Permeability to Water, Urea, and Sodium, and Reflection Coefficients for NaC1 and Urea in Mammalian Species

Segment	Hydraulic conductivity (L_p) (X 10^{-5} cm^3 cm^{-2} sec^{-1} atm^{-1})	Permeability (P) (X 10^{-5} cm sec^{-1})			Reflection coefficient σ		Animal	Method of perfusion
		Water	Urea	Na	NaCl	Urea		
Proximal tubule	18		11.1		0.68	0.79	Rat	In vivo
	15.5	560					Rat	In vivo
	2.9-6.3			9.3	0.68		Rabbit	In vitro P.T.
			5.3			0.91	Rabbit	In vitro P.T.
Descending limb	3.9	119	13		<0.50	<0.50	Rat	In vitro papilla
				47			Rat	In vitro papilla
	17		1.5			0.96	Rabbit	In vitro D.L.
				1.6	0.95		Rabbit	In vitro D.L.
Thin ascending limb	0.3	50	14		1.0	<0.50	Rat	In vitro papilla
				11			Rat	In vitro papilla
Thick ascending limb	0.1			6.3			Rabbit	In vitro T.A.L.
	0						Rabbit	In vitro T.A.L.
Distal tubule, no ADH	2.7						Rat	In vivo
			1				Rat	In vivo
	1.6	157					Rat	In vivo

Distal tubule, ADH	7.9						Rat	In vivo
present			1		0.52	0.67	Rat	In vivo
	6.3	327					Rat	In vivo
Cortical collecting	0.4	38	0.1				Rabbit	In vitro C.D.
tubule, no ADH	0.1	47	0		1.0	1.0	Rabbit	In vitro C.D.
	0.2						Rabbit	In vitro C.D.
Cortical collecting	1.6	97	0.1				Rabbit	In vitro C.D.
tubule, ADH present	1.4	142	0		1.0	1.0	Rabbit	In vitro C.D.
	1.3						Rabbit	In vitro C.D.
Papillary collecting	0.3	45	20				Rat	In vitro papilla
tubule, no ADH				5.4			Rat	In vitro papilla
Papillary collecting	2.0	87	30		0.9	0.4	Rat	In vitro papilla
tubule. ADH present				5.9			Rat	In vitro papilla
			4.7				Rat	In vivo
Vasa recta		>192	47				Rat	in vitro papilla
				39-82			Rat	In vitro papilla
				28-51			Hamster	In vivo

P.T., proximal tubule; D.L., descending limb; C.D., collecting duct, T.A.L., thick ascending limb.
Source: Jamison, R. L. Countercurrent systems. In: MTP International Review of Science, vol. 6, Kidney and Urinary Tract Physiology, edited by Thurau, K., 1979. (Reproduced with permission of Butterworth and Co., London.)

has a higher urea concentration than sodium chloride concentration due to reabsorption of urea from the medullary collecting ducts. Because the permeability of the thin ascending limb to sodium chloride is greater than to urea (Table 3) sodium chloride will diffuse out of the tubule at a rate which is greater than the entry of urea into the tubule. The net result will be transport of solute out of the tubular fluid and, since the segment is essentially impermeable to water, the osmolality of the tubular fluid will fall. This process can occur, therefore, without invoking an active transport mechanism. In addition to this passive mechanism, there are in vivo data in rats to suggest that active transport of sodium chloride may also occur in the thin ascending limb (100-102).

B. Potassium Transport

Recent evidence suggests that there is recycling of potassium from the medullary collecting tubule into the thin ascending limb (102). This can be inhibited by amiloride, which blocks potassium secretion in the collecting tubule. A high K diet enhances the recycling process, while a low K diet diminishes it.

C. Divalent Ion Transport

In isolated tubule perfusion studies (77) both thin limbs of the loop of Henle have been shown to be relatively impermeable to phosphate and calcium. There is no significant transport of these ions occurring in these segments of the nephron. Although there is no direct study of Mg transport in the thin limbs, the observed increase in (TF/UF) Mg at the tip of the loop of Henle (103) is thought to be due to water abstraction.

V. THICK ASCENDING LIMB OF HENLE'S LOOP

A. Sodium, Chloride, and Water Transport

The thick ascending limb is divided into a medullary and a cortical portion. The cells of the medullary portion are thicker than those of the cortical segment. Micropuncture studies in which tubular fluid was sampled from the early distal convoluted tubule revealed low sodium chloride concentrations, i.e., 30-60 meq/liter. From these observations it was deduced that sodium chloride was reabsorbed by the ascending limb and, since this process of tubular fluid dilution was independent of whether the final urine was concentrated or diluted, it suggested that the final process of urine concentration occurred in a more distal nephron segment.

Microperfusion studies of the thick ascending limb in vitro revealed that it is also virtually impermeable to water (104-105). Sodium chloride reabsorption in the medullary thick ascending limb (105) was significantly greater than in the cortical segments (104). The cortical segment, perfused at very slow perfusion rates, was able to maintain a steady-state luminal sodium concentration of 65 meq/liter, so that under conditions of slow tubular fluid transit this would be the concentration of sodium chloride entering the distal convoluted tubule. There is a direct correlation between the rate of sodium chloride reabsorption and tubule fluid flow rate in the thick ascending limb.

The transepithelial PD across both segments of the thick ascending limb was found to be lumen positive when the concentrations of sodium and chloride in bath and perfusate were equal (104,105). Chloride reabsorption, which occurs against an electrochemical gradient, was considered to be active. If chloride is removed from the perfusate, the positive voltage is inhibited. This does not occur when sodium is removed. When chloride is replaced by another anion such as nitrate net sodium chloride transport is inhibited. It was thus assumed that active chloride transport is the primary reabsorptive process and that sodium reabsorption occurs down its electrochemical gradient.

This interpretation has recently been called into question by studies which showed that under conditions of Na removal in vitro there is sufficient Na contamination of the tubular fluid to confuse the interpretation of the transport events. If sodium is rigorously removed, it can be shown that all active chloride reabsorption is Na dependent, suggesting that sodium and chloride are cotransported across the luminal membrane (106). The driving force for this process is provided by the downhill electrochemical gradient for Na across the luminal membrane which is generated by the basolateral Na pump. Chloride movement across the luminal membrane proceeds by secondary active transport; the consequent elevation of the intracellular chloride potential allows it to leave the cell across the basolateral membrane down its electrochemical gradient. Of interest is the fact that sodium chloride transport in the thick ascending limb can be inhibited by ouabain, which acts on the Na-K-ATPase associated with the basolateral membrane (Fig. 8). In this segment of the nephron, the specific activity of this enzyme is very high.

It has been demonstrated that luminal potassium is required for the transfer of Na and Cl across the luminal membrane (107). In addition, barium, which blocks the luminal K conductance, also decreases net NaCl transport. Based on these findings, the most current model of the thick ascending limb cell incorporates a 1 Na-1 K-2 Cl cotransport process in the luminal membrane as well as a high K conductance in this membrane, which recycles the K back into the lumen. The lumen-positive voltage which results drives Na through the paracellular pathway and, since basolateral chloride conductance is high, the net transfer of NaCl is effectively driven entirely by the basolateral Na-K pump.

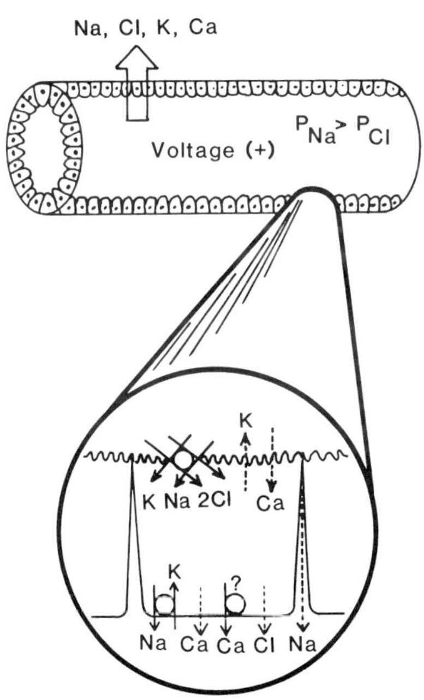

Fig. 8 Transport across the cortical and medullary thick ascending limbs of the loop of Henle (symbols as for Fig. 4).

The thick ascending limb is a relatively leaky epithelium and the relatively high electrical conductance is accounted for mainly by the high sodium permeability (108). The high permeability to sodium facilitates reabsorption of sodium down its electrochemical gradient. On the other hand, the lower permeability to chloride minimizes the backflux of chloride which has been transported out of the tubular lumen. The lumen-positive voltage, therefore, can be accounted for both on the basis of secondary active chloride transport and on the basis of a dilution potential. (Since the segment is more permeable to sodium than to chloride, passive movement of NaCl from the peritubular surface into the lumen down a concentration gradient will generate a lumen-positive potential.) As sodium chloride concentration in the lumen is lowered, the voltage increases. This high positive voltage is thought to be an important factor in driving the passive reabsorption of other cationic species such as potassium and calcium. At very slow perfusion rates the positive voltage is also significantly increased (104). This is due to the fact that continued sodium chloride reabsorption lowers the concentration of sodium chloride in the lumen to a minimal value and the dilution potential generated by a concentration difference between bath and lumen adds to the existing lumen-positive potential.

At slow perfusion rates, when close to steady-state conditions obtain, the measured sodium concentration difference between lumen and bath and the measured potential can be compared with the theoretical voltage which would be required for sodium distribution to be passive according to the Nernst equation. Comparisons such as these have shown that the measured and the theoretical voltages are in agreement, consistent with passive transport of sodium (104). However, the measured sodium flux ratio compared with the flux ratio which should obtain if the distribution of sodium were according to passive processes indicates that sodium transport may not occur exclusively by simple passive diffusion and that some active transport may be present (10).

NaCl transport in the thick ascending limb is altered by vasopressin and possibly by prostaglandins (see Sect. IX, below).

B. Potassium Transport

The potassium concentration at the tip of the loop of Henle in the exposed renal papilla is markedly increased above that of plasma (97,111-118). The fact that potassium concentration is higher than the inulin concentration indicates that there has been net entry of potassium into the descending limb. Whether this entry occurs in the descending limb per se or in the more proximal pars recta is uncertain. These observations have led to the proposal that there is recycling of potassium from the medullary collecting duct, into the interstitium, and thence into the descending limb (111,112). Potassium loading enhances this process and amiloride, which inhibits potassium secretion in the collecting tubule, decreases it.

Micropuncture studies have shown that approximately 10% of the filtered potassium enters the early distal tubule. Thus, in the superficial nephrons, at least, a significant amount of potassium must be reabsorbed somewhere in the loop of Henle. Potassium reabsorption by the thick ascending limb appears to be largely a passive process which is dependent upon the transepithelial voltage. When the positive voltage is increased net potassium efflux from the tubule is increased, whereas when voltage is decreased or is lumen negative, there is net potassium entry into the tubule (108).

C. Bicarbonate Transport

Bicarbonate reabsorption has been shown to be negligible in the cortical thick ascending limb of the rabbit, regardless of the acid-base status of the animals (16).

D. Phosphate Transport

Micropuncture studies in the desert rat have shown that the fractional delivery of phosphate to the superficial early distal tubule is higher than that to the tip of the loop of Henle, suggesting either that there is phosphate addition to the ascending limb or that there is internephron heterogeneity (119). Since the thick ascending limb has been shown to be impermeable to phosphate in vitro (77), it is likely that the increase in fractional delivery is due to the internephron heterogeneity (Fig. 9).

E. Calcium Transport

Since a large amount of Na is reabsorbed by the thick ascending limb coupled to active chloride transport, the close correlation between (TF/UF) Ca and (TF/UF) Na observed at the distal tubule from micropuncture studies (120) suggests similar transport mechanisms for Na and Ca in the ascending limb (120). Hence, a parallel increase in Na and Ca delivery to the distal tubule is observed when furosemide is given to inhibit chloride transport along the thick ascending limb. If, however, Ca is passively extruded by the positive luminal potential, it can be expected that the reabsorption of Ca, a divalent cation, should be greater than Na, a monovalent cation. The fact that this is not observed in micropuncture studies, has led to the suggestion that Ca is transported as a monovalent species such as $CaCl^+$. In the isolated thick ascending limb calcium transport is passive and Ca permeability is lower than Na permeability (121). It has been suggested that the close correlation between Ca and Na reabsorption by thick ascending limb can be explained by the low Ca permeability. On the other hand, other in vitro microperfusion studies have suggested that Ca reabsorption in the thick ascending limb is, at least partially, due to an active transport process (77, 122). Heterogeneity has been shown to exist along the thick ascending limb, since Ca reabsorption by the cortical segment is due to an active transport mechanism, whereas in the

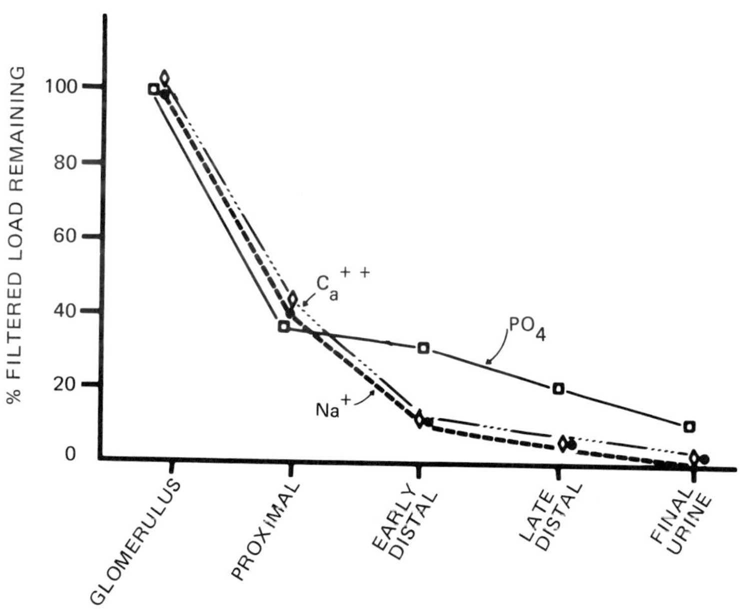

Fig. 9 Percent of the filtered load of calcium, phosphate, and sodium remaining at different nephron sites and in the final urine in the intact animal. (From Ref. 53.)

medullary segment Ca is reabsorbed passively (123). Discrepancies between results obtained by different investigators emphasize the need for additional studies in this area.

Parathyroid hormone has been shown to inhibit Ca reabsorption in the thick ascending limb in both micropuncture (124) and in vitro perfusion studies (125). The inhibitory effect of hypermagnesemia on Ca reabsorption in thick ascending limb may be partially PTH mediated (126).

F. Magnesium Transport

Micropuncture studies indicate that Mg is reabsorbed by the ascending limb (85). It has been estimated that about 50-60% of the filtered Mg is reabsorbed by this segment. The observation that hypermagnesemia retards Ca reabsorption, while hypercalcemia retards Mg reabsorption suggests a Ca-Mg interaction in the thick ascending limb. The rabbit thick ascending limb has a large reabsorptive capacity for Mg, and this Mg reabsorption is voltage dependent, consistent with the contention that Ca and Mg interact with each other (127).

Hypermagnesemia, hypercalcemia, calcitonin, and furosemide (128) have all been shown to inhibit Mg reabsorption. Parathyroid hormone may enhance Mg reabsorption in the thick ascending limb (86) as well as in the proximal tubule. This may be masked by the inhibitory effect of hypercalcemia associated with increased PTH secretion.

VI. DISTAL TUBULE

A. Sodium Chloride Transport

The distal tubule, as it is defined by the micropuncturist, is that segment of the nephron which lies between the macula densa and the first junction with another distal tubule to form a collecting duct. Ultrastructural studies and the different responses of the adenylate cyclase system of different parts of the distal nephron to hormone stimuli (see above) have led to a redefinition of the distal tubule. However, in order to correlate structure with function, it would be necessary to study specific segments by in vitro perfusion. This has been a difficult task, both because the definition of the origin of the segments under the dissecting microscope is imprecise and because the length of the segment (often less that 1 mm) is too short to provide meaningful information using these techniques.

From micropuncture studies, it is evident that continued sodium chloride reabsorption occurs along the distal convoluted tubule. This process continues to lower the osmolality of the tubular fluid in which sodium concentrations of 35 meq/liter are achieved by the end of the accessible distal convoluted tubule (129). The rate of sodium reabsorption in this segment is approximately 30% of that in the proximal tubule. The transepithelial voltage is not uniform in this segment and is shown to be dependent upon the precise site at which it is measured (130). In the earliest portion, i.e., closest to the macula densa, the voltage is close to zero, and this increases to approximately 50 mV toward the latter portion of the tubule.

Active sodium transport across the basolateral membrane is driven by Na-K-ATPase, with transport across the epithelium being against an electrochemical gradient, i.e., active transport. Chloride reabsorption is mostly passive, but there may be some active transport of chloride in addition. The fact that the distal tubule is able to establish steep concentration gradients for sodium chloride is related to its low permeability to sodium chloride. This is also reflected by a high transepithelial electrical resistance of about 180 ohm cm^2 (131). In the proximal tubule, the resistance is between 5 and 7 ohm cm^2.

It has always been difficult to understand why vasopressin has an unpredictable effect on water permeability in this segment of the nephron. Recently it has been shown that in different species of animals the micropuncturist's definition of the distal tubule actually includes segments which have a cellular morphology typical of the collecting tubule (132). The percent of nephrons with collecting tubule morphology varies from species to species, and since the collecting tubule epithelium is the site of action of vasopressin, it is only in those segments which include part of the collecting tubule that a vasopressin effect is seen. The increase in water permeability induced by vasopressin results in the osmotic reabsorption of water. The distal convoluted tubule is impermeable to urea. Thus, urea, which is delivered from the ascending limb and which originates either by recycling from the collecting tubule or by delivery out of the proximal tubule, remains within the tubular lumen and contributes to the osmolality of the tubular fluid. By acting as an effective osmotic agent urea retards the movement of water out of the lumen of the tubule and allows steep concentration gradients of sodium chloride to be generated.

In the distal convoluted tubule there is a direct correlation between the rate of sodium chloride reabsorption and the tubular fluid flow rate. The effect of the flow rate in this segment is mediated by the concentration of sodium within the tubular lumen. Increases in sodium concentration from 45 to 90 meq/liter causes sodium reabsorption to increase independently of the flow rate. Thus, the effect of flow on NaCl reabsorption seems to be as follows: At higher flow rates, the rate of sodium reabsorption does not lower tubular fluid sodium concentration as much as it does at lower flow rates and, thus, the *concentration* of sodium in the fluid delivered to subsequent segments will be higher over the remaining length of the tubule. Under these circumstances net sodium reabsorption increases (133).

B. Potassium Transport

Cellular Mechanisms of Potassium Transport

The high intracellular potassium concentration in the distal tubular cell is maintained by an energy-dependent active sodium-potassium exchange mechanism. Both the luminal and the basolateral cell membranes have finite permeabilities to potassium. Since it has been possible to measure the electrical potential difference across the peritubular membrane and the potassium activity within the cell using ion-selective electrodes, one can demonstrate that the measured potential cannot account for the distribution of potassium inside and outside the cell on a passive basis. Active transport across the peritubular membrane must occur (134). This is related to the extrusion of sodium from the cell, which is either a one-to-one neutral exchange pump or a rheogenic pump in which the number of sodium ions extruded exceeds the number of potassium ions entering the cell.

The sodium-potassium pump is now known to be the ouabain-sensitive Na-K-ATPase. Inhibition of the pump increases the concentration of sodium within the cell and lowers the potassium concentration. The coupling between sodium and potassium, however, appears to be quite variable (134). By providing more sodium to the pump, on the cellular side, the activity of the pump would increase and potassium entry to the cell would increase. It is this relationship which determines the fundamental link between increases in net sodium reabsorption in the distal nephron and increased potassium secretion. Since the net rate of transport of sodium chloride greatly exceeds that of potassium, only a small fraction of sodium reabsorption can be directly linked to potassium secretion.

The actual concentration of potassium within the cell has been difficult to determine. The potassium activity, which is the more relevant measurement in terms of establishing electrochemical gradients, can be determined by potassium-selective microelectrodes which can be inserted into single cells. Potassium activity in the distal tubules of amphibia and mammals reveals cellular potassium activities which are considerably lower than measured potassium concentrations (135). It is not clear why this difference exists, but it suggests that finite pools of potassium exist within the cell and that this compartmentalization may provide only a portion of the total potassium ions for transport across the epithelium.

Potassium secretion along the distal tubule is related to the transtubular potential difference along this nephron segment. In the earliest post-macula densa segment, the transtubular potential is low or lumen positive and potassium secretory rate is low. The luminal negativity increases toward the end of the distal convoluted tubule which has the greatest capacity for potassium secretion (133). The origin of the transtubular potential has not been fully established, but is increased by stimulating sodium transport and by the presence of poorly reabsorbable anions within the tubular lumen. The potential difference across the luminal membrane is lower than that across the peritubular membrane. Passive movement of potassium thus proceeds preferentially across the luminal membrane (49). On a low potassium diet, it is possible to demonstrate a reabsorptive pump for potassium in the luminal membrane. Under these conditions, net potassium secretion is converted to net reabsorption. Although the lumen negativity which persists under these conditions would favor entry of potassium into the lumen, the fact that net transport proceeds in the opposite direction suggests that there must be an active transport mechanism located in the luminal membrane.

Factors Modulating Potassium Transport

The distal nephron segments are the major sites of potassium secretion into the tubular fluid. Potassium secretion into the distal tubule of the rat is markedly influenced by the dietary intake of potassium (136). (Fig. 10). Thus, on a low potassium diet there is little entry of potassium along the distal tubule. If anything, potassium is reabsorbed with evidence of further reabsorption along the collecting tubule. Under conditions of potassium loading there is significant potassium secretion into the distal tubule and beyond this segment. Differences between the fractional excretion of potassium to the end of the distal convoluted tubule and the final urine can be attributed either to potassium secretion by the collecting tubule or to a different contribution of superficial and juxtamedullary nephrons to overall potassium excretion. On the basis of micropuncture studies the former explanation is considered the most likely (137,138). Apart from diet, a number of factors influence the rate of potassium secretion in the distal tubule. These include changes in acid base balance (Fig. 11), diuretics, adrenal steroids, and increased fluid and sodium delivery to the distal nephron.

Cellular Potassium Concentration

Since the total body potassium stores are confined primarily to the intracellular compartment, changes in dietary intake with excess or depletion of total body potassium reflect the intracellular content of potassium. Potassium deprivation is associated with a decrease in the potassium concentration in the renal tubular cells (135,139). As has been pointed out above, dietary intake determines whether net secretion or reabsorption of potassium occurs along the distal tubule. During potassium deprivation, the activity of potassium within the distal tubular cells is reduced as is the electrical potential difference across the tubule. Decreased uptake across the peritubular membrane has also been proposed, although in the net reabsorptive states, there may be stimulation of luminal potassium uptake by an active mechanism.

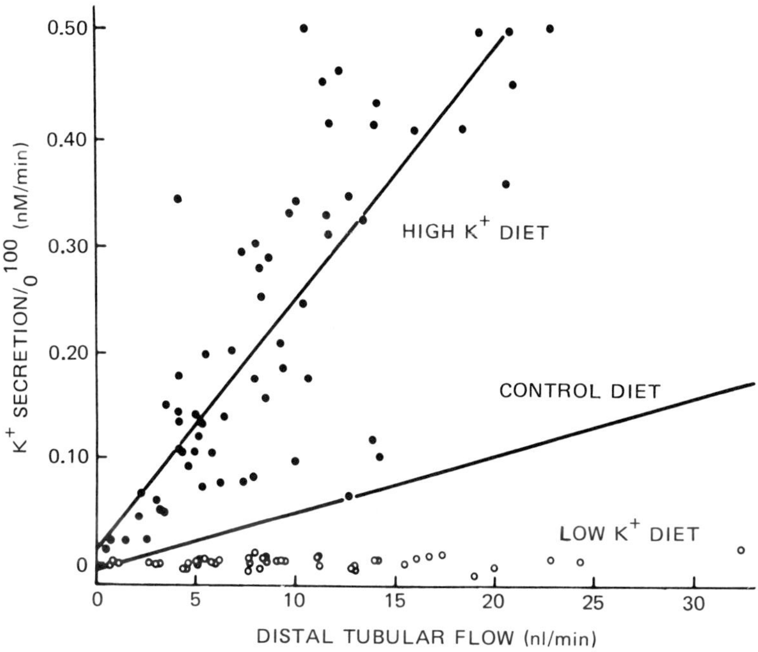

Fig. 10 Effect of control, low, and high potassium diets on potassium secretion in the distal tubule. Absolute rates of normalized (0-100%) distal tubular potassion secretion are expressed as a function of distal volume flow rate. (From Ref. 148.)

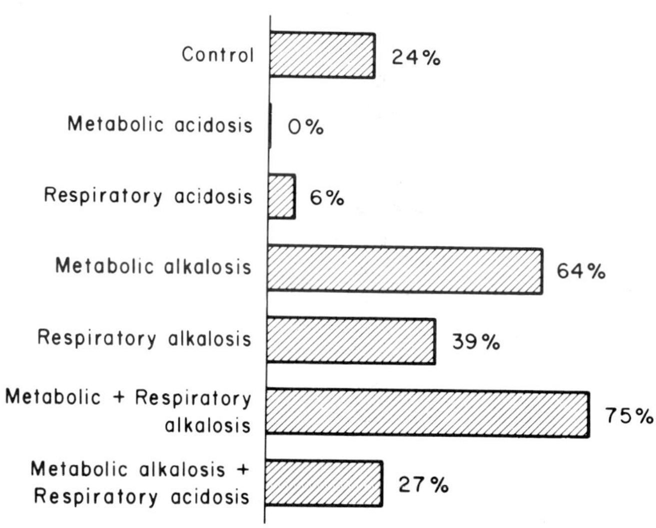

Fig. 11 Effects of alterations in acid-base balance on distal tubular potassium transport. (Modified from Ref. 49.)

In contrast to potassium deprivation, potassium loading leads to an augmentation of renal potassium excretion (140-142), a condition which has been called potassium adaptation. Under these circumstances, net potassium excretion increases dramatically due to enhanced secretion by the distal convoluted tubule and the cortical collecting tubule. Potassium uptake into the cells across the peritubular membrane is increased and potassium activity in the cells also increases. An increase in renal Na-K-ATPase has been demonstrated and this has been attributed to an increase in the number of pump sites in the peritubular membrane. It is possible that significant potassium loading is required to induce this change, since moderate increases in intake can result in increased secretion of potassium in the collecting tubule without a change in the specific activity of Na-K-ATPase in the cortical collecting tubule (143). Under conditions of significant potassium loading, the increase in the activity of this enzyme may be related to higher plasma aldosterone levels.

Tubule Fluid Flow Rate and Sodium Delivery

A critical determinant of the rate of potassium secretion appears to be the rate of delivery of sodium to the distal nephron (Fig. 10). Acute reduction of GFR decreases potassium excretion (144). Reduction of sodium intake also reduces potassium excretion (145,146). Under conditions of mineralocorticoid excess the kaliuresis can be attenuated by sodium deprivation. On the other hand, maneuvers which increase the delivery of sodium to the distal nephron increase the rate of potassium excretion. These include extracellular volume expansion, administration of diuretics acting on the proximal tubule and the loop of Henle, unilateral or subtotal nephrectomy, and administration of sodium salts with poorly reabsorbable anions. The influence of sodium on potassium secretion appears to occur beyond the end of the distal convoluted tubule (137). Micropuncture studies in hydropenic rats have shown that the fractional excretion of sodium into the urine is lower than that in the late distal tubule. When, however, saline is administered, this reduction in fractional excretion is reversed, suggesting that the influence of saline expansion is exerted somewhere beyond the end of the distal tubule, i.e., in the collecting tubule. No evidence of an altered contribution of juxtamedullary nephrons has been provided which could account for this phenomenon (138).

Additional evidence for the influence of sodium delivery on potassium secretion is provided by studies on isolated perfused cortical collecting tubules, in which it has been shown that reduction of luminal sodium concentration below 50 meq/liter will attenuate the rate of potassium secretion (147). The mechanism whereby luminal sodium exerts its effect on potassium secretion may be by increasing luminal negativity, hence favoring passive potassium movement from the cell into the lumen, or via carrier-mediated sodium-potassium exchange in the luminal membrane. Reduction in the lumen negativity or decreased activity of a carrier-mediated exchange would decrease the secretory flux and allow a reabsorptive flux to proceed unopposed. Thus, net secretion could be converted into net reabsorption. Under all conditions in which sodium delivery to the distal nephron is increased, flow rate is also increased. The rate of sodium reabsorption in the distal nephron is at least 10 times greater than the rate of potassium secretion, so that sodium reabsorption would have to be decreased to extremely low levels in order to impair potassium secretion. It thus appears likely that flow rate and the delivery of sodium to the distal nephron in some way interact to stimulate potassium secretion (133).

A number of elegant studies have been performed in which the influence of flow rate per se has been evaluated (148). These studies have demonstrated that the concentration of potassium within the distal tubular fluid is relatively constant regardless of the flow rate. This implies that there is extremely rapid equilibration between the potassium in the cell and in the lumen. This being the case, an increase in flow rate with a constant tubule fluid potassium concentration would result in an increase in the net delivery of potassium out of the tubule. This influence of flow on potassium secretion is modified according to the basal potassium secretion rate. Thus, the effect of the flow is greater in animals maintained on a high potassium diet than it is in animals maintained on a low potassium diet in which increasing tubular flow has only a minimal effect on net potassium delivery out of the tubule.

Because of the difficulty of separating flow from sodium delivery under standard free-flow conditions experiments have been performed in which distal tubules have been perfused in vivo in such a way as to vary flow and sodium concentration independently. Under these circumstances, it has been clearly shown that even when the rate of net sodium reabsorption is not changed, flow rate per se can alter the rate of potassium secretion (133).

Diuretics, which act upstream to the distal nephron (in the proximal convoluted tubule, azetazolamide; in the thick ascending limb, mercurials, ethacrynic acid, furosemide), exert their kaliuretic action by increasing the flow rate and the delivery of sodium to the distal nephron. Certain diuretics, such as spironolactone, triamterene, and amiloride, have a specific inhibitory effect on potassium secretion in the distal convoluted tubule and the cortical collecting tubule. The effects of amiloride are particularly interesting (149), since this diuretic blocks the entry of sodium ions through the apical membrane of anuran membranes and is thought to interfere with the entry of sodium across the luminal membrane of the distal nephron. This effect would reduce the luminal negativity and thus impair passive potassium entry into the lumen. The fact that it does not have a direct inhibitory effect on potassium secretion is demonstrated by the fact that amiloride does not change the permeability of the cortical collecting tubule to potassium and restoration of the lumen negativity by means of an external current can restore potassium secretion even in the presence of amiloride (150).

Mineralocorticoids

It has been pointed out above that endogenous mineralocorticoid excess stimulates sodium transport in the distal convoluted tubule and the cortical collecting tubule. The effects of mineralocorticoids in enhancing potassium secretion are dependent on the delivery of sodium to the distal nephron. There is, however, no direct coupling between sodium reabsorption and potassium secretion exerted by mineralocorticoids. In fact, during the "escape" phenomenon, when the sodium retaining effect of mineralocorticoid is overridden, significant kaliuresis persists. Mineralocorticoids appear to exert their effect on potassium secretion by increasing the permeability of the luminal membrane to potassium and by elevating intracellular potassium concentration (151-154). These inferences are drawn from observations on adrenalectomized animals in which both parameters were decreased and could be reversed by administering mineralocorticoids. Potassium secretion is stimulated in the cortical collecting tubule perfused in vitro by deoxycorticosterone acetate (Doca) pretreatment of the animals for approximately 2 weeks (155,156). These is no evidence of a direct in vitro effect of a mineralocorticoid on potassium secretion by the collecting tubule. The enhanced potassium secretory rate, stimulated by in vivo administration of Doca, is paralleled by an increase in the surface area of the basolateral membranes of the collecting tubule (157).

Acid-Base Balance

Acute metabolic alkalosis stimulates potassium excretion and acute metabolic acidosis depresses it. The effect of metabolic alkalosis is to increase bicarbonate delivery to the distal nephron. Since bicarbonate is essentially an unreabsorbable anion in the distal nephron, luminal negativity would increase and enhance potassium secretion. On the other hand, acute metabolic acidosis by lowering the luminal pH decreases potassium secretion (49). The relationship between cellular potassium and acid-base status is such that potassium ions are shifted into cells during alkalosis and exit from cells during acidosis. Since the renal tubular cells are no exception to this rule, the potassium content of the distal tubular cells would be an important determinant of the potassium secretory rate under these conditions. The influx of ^{42}K across the peritubular cell membrane has been measured directly and found to be enhanced in metabolic acidosis (658). Potassium activity measured with an ion-selective electrode is increased in the renal tubular cells during alkalosis and decreased in acidosis (13).

Chronic metabolic acidosis is different from acute acidosis in that it causes an increase in potassium excretion (159). The mechanism for this is not clear, but may be related to sodium and fluid delivery to the distal nephron. Reduction in filtered load of bicarbonate reduces the reabsorption of sodium and water in the proximal tubule and thus promotes increased distal delivery the same way as is observed in alkalosis. This effect is, of course, dependent upon whether the acidosis per se has reduced the intracellular potassium content of the distal tubular epithelial cells to a level which limits the rate of potassium secretion. The interplay between these two factors is what determines the final rate of potassium excretion.

C. Phosphate Transport

Micropuncture studies in thyroparathyroidectomized rats indicate that there is phosphate reabsorption in the distal tubule (160). This appears to be inhibited by PTH. It was suggested from these studies that the distal tubule may be critical in the final regulation of phosphate excretion. However, other stationary microperfusion and tracer-microinjection studies provided no evidence of distal phosphate reabsorption (161), indicating that internephron heterogeneity may be responsible for the observations made in free-flow micropuncture studies.

D. Calcium Transport

Approximately 9% of the filtered calcium is actively reabsorbed by the distal tubule (162). This have been confirmed in isolated distal convoluted and granular collecting tubules of the rabbit (163).

Uptake of Ca across the luminal membrane is likely to be a passive process which occurs down an electrochemical gradient. On the other hand, the extrusion of Ca through the basolateral membrane is probably an active process which occurs against an electrochemical gradient. Whether the energy required for this active transport is supplied from Ca-activated ATPase or from Ca-Na countertransport is not known.

VII. CORTICAL COLLECTING TUBULE

The cortical collecting tubule originates from the connecting tubule from which it is distinguished by a difference in cell type. The rabbit cortical collecting tubule has two cell types, i.e., the principal cell, which has extensive basolateral infoldings, and the intercalated cell. Most of the available information on the function of this segment is derived from in vitro studies of isolated collecting tubule segments.

A. Sodium Chloride Transport (Fig. 12)

Sodium reabsorption occurs by an active transport mechanism, whereas chloride is reabsorbed passively, driven by the negative luminal voltage. Considerable variation in the transtubular potential difference has been reported. Initially, this was thought to be due to random variation; however, it was subsequently observed that the voltage is linked to the endogenous mineralocorticoid status of the animal (155,156). In animals that have been maintained on a high potassium diet or been given Doca, the transepithelial potential in the collecting tubule is significantly greater than in control animals. This increase in voltage is paralleled by an increase in net sodium transport. The voltage is the sum of the negative potential generated by the absorption of sodium and the positive potential that results from potassium and hydrogen ion secretion. Potassium secretion is also increased under conditions of mineralocorticoid excess (151).

If both sodium and potassium transport are inhibited by removal of sodium from the perfusate and the bath, and by removal of potassium from the bath, or by addition of amiloride to the luminal surface or ouabain to the peritubular surface, the voltage becomes lumen-positive (149). This lumen-positive voltage has been presumed to be due to hydrogen ion secretion, since it is decreased by the administration of acetazolamide, which under conditions of normal sodium and potassium transport increases lumen negativity by reducing the contribution of hydrogen ion secretion to the potential. Net potassium secretion by the collecting tubule can be reduced by lowering the pH of the perfusate from 7.4 to 6.8. Under these conditions, transepithelial voltage becomes more negative.

The rate of sodium chloride reabsorption in the cortical collecting tubule is approximately 25% of that observed in the proximal convoluted tubule. Perfusion of the collecting tubule

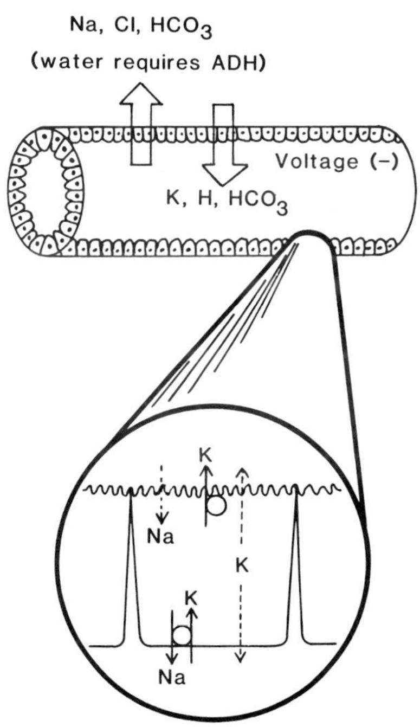

Fig. 12 Transport processes across the cortical collecting tubule (symbols as for Fig. 4).

at slow perfusion rates leads to a significant reduction in the concentration of sodium in the lumen and a significant elevation of luminal potassium concentration (147). The ability to generate these steep gradients is due to a low permeability to sodium and potassium. The flux ratio for sodium (lumen to bath/bath to lumen) is 6.7, so that the backflux component for sodium is low (149). As would be expected, the transepithelial electrical resistance is high, approximately 250 ohm cm^2.

B. Potassium Transport

The same factors which affect the transtubular potential difference in the distal convoluted tubule affect it in the cortical collecting tubule. In contrast to the distal convoluted tubule, however, the luminal potassium concentration in the collecting tubule can be raised to exceed the concentration predicted by the electrochemical potential difference across the luminal membrane (147). Thus, an active secretory pump for potassium must be present in the luminal membrane in the cortical collecting tubule. Potassium transfer across the luminal membrane appears to be electrogenic and reduces the lumen negativity associated with sodium transport.

In contrast to the medullary and papillary collecting tubules, the cortical collecting tubule has not been shown to reabsorb potassium even in animals on a low potassium diet.

C. Bicarbonate Transport

The cortical collecting tubule may reabsorb or secret bicarbonate depending on the acid-base status of the animal (16). Net secretion was observed in rabbits treated with sodium bicarbonate. With no pretreatment there was either a small amount of net reabsorption or net secretion, whereas ammonium chloride loading uniformly resulted in net reabsorption of bicarbonate.

D. Phosphate Transport

In isolated perfused rabbit collecting tubules absence of net phosphate transport has been shown in one study (59), whereas net phosphate absorption equivalent to 13% of the perfusion load was observed in another study confined to the light segment of cortical collecting tubule (165). Addition of PTH in the bath did not have effect on phosphate transport (59).

E. Calcium Transport

It was estimated that from 3 to 10% of the filtered calcium is reabsorbed beyond the end of the distal convoluted tubule. Whether this is due to further reabsorption by the collecting tubules or due to internephron heterogeneity is not clear. Net Ca reabsorption has been observed only in the granular segment of the collecting tubule (166). This Ca transport is enhanced when PTH is added to the bath, and it appears to be Na independent.

F. Magnesium Transport

There is no difference between the fractional delivery of Mg to the superficial distal tubule and fractional urinary Mg excretion (167), suggesting that there is no Mg reabsorption or secretion in the terminal nephron segments. When the light segment of the cortical collecting tubule was perfused in vitro no significant Mg transport was found (165), an observation consistent with micropuncture results.

G. Urate Transport

No evidence for urate secretion was found in the rabbit cortical collecting tubule (91). There also appears to be little or no urate reabsorption in the distal nephron where urate permeability is very low.

VIII. MEDULLARY COLLECTING TUBULE

A. Sodium Chloride Transport

Sodium chloride reabsorption proceeds at approximately the same rate in outer medullary collecting tubules as in the cortical collecting tubule (168). The transepithelial voltage is either lumen negative or lumen positive. As inner medullary collecting ducts course through the medulla they join to form the branched papillary collecting duct. This segment has been studied by retrograde microcatheterization and by direct micropuncture of the exposed papilla. The voltage has been observed to vary from −4 to −37 mV (10). The techniques used to study the voltage in vivo are not sufficiently accurate to allow conclusions to be drawn as to the relative active and passive components of sodium chloride transport in this segment. Continued reabsorption of sodium chloride can reduce the concentration in the tubular fluid to less than 10 meq/liter.

The transepithelial electrical resistance in this segment is high and this presumably corresponds to a low sodium chloride permeability. In the absence of vasopressin, water permeability is low. Vasopressin causes an increase in water permeability. Urea permeability, both in the presence and absence of vasopressin, is relatively high and exceeds that of the outer medullary collecting tubule and the medullary thick ascending limb.

B. Potassium Transport

There appears to be no active transport of either sodium or potassium across the inner stripe of the medullary collecting tubule, i.e., in the portion which lies nearest the inner medulla or papilla (169,170). In this segment, Na and K diffuse across the wall of the tubule down their respective concentration gradients. In vivo, these gradients probably effect some K absorption and Na secretion.

Data on potassium transport in the inner medullary and papillary collecting ducts has been derived exclusively from microcatheterization and micropuncture studies (171), which have been performed on the exposed rodent papilla. Although potassium secretion does occur along this segment, it is not of great magnitude under normal circumstances, but it can be stimulated under conditions of marked potassium loading. Delivery of potassium to the papillary base has been found to exceed that which is delivered to the end of the superficial distal tubule. Along the papillary collecting tubule, potassium content decreases. Thus, it appears as if there is secretion of potassium into the cortical collecting tubule and reabsorption in the medullary collecting tubule (138).

Mineralocorticoids appear to have their effect on Na, K, and Cl localized specifically to the cortical portion of the collecting tubule, there being no effect of the administration of Doca on the reabsorption or secretion of these ions in either the inner or outer medullary collecting tubule (172). It is thus of considerable interest that recent studies have demonstrated that mineralocorticoids stimulate H^+ secretion and HCO_3 reabsorption in the rabbit inner medullary collecting tubule and that this effect occurs in the complete absence of Na and is not inhibited by amiloride (173).

C. Divalent Ion Transport

Microcatheterization study in intact rats revealed no net phosphate transport in medullary collecting duct (174). There is no information available on Ca transport in medullary collecting tubule. Magnesium is not reabsorbed in the medullary collecting tubule of rats (175).

IX. HUMORAL AND NEUROGENIC CONTROL OF SODIUM CHLORIDE REABSORPTION

A. Parathyroid Hormone

Although parathyroid hormone appears to have receptors on a number of different sites on the nephron (see above), its action has best been studied in the proximal tubule. Apart from its more important effects on phosphate and calcium reabsorption, PTH inhibits salt and water reabsorption in the proximal tubule, as demonstrated by in vitro perfusion (176,177) and by micropuncture. This action is mimicked by exogenous cyclic-AMP analogs. Parathyroid hormone also appears to have an inhibitory effect on bicarbonate reabsorption by the proximal tubule (178). Since the net reabsorptive rates of a number of disparate solutes appear to be affected in an uniform manner, it is likely that parathyroid hormone and cyclic-AMP exert their effect not only on active transport mechanisms, but by increasing the backflux of a number of solutes into the tubules through the intercellular pathway. This has been confirmed by demonstrating that the flux of large molecules, which do not enter cells, is increased (179).

B. Prostaglandins

There is controversy as to whether prostaglandins exert a direct effect on tubular reabsorption of sodium chloride. There are data suggestive of the fact that active sodium transport is inhibited in the cortical collecting tubule (180,181) and that chloride transport is inhibited in the thick ascending limb. Additional other studies have failed to show a direct effect on these segments (168). It appears as if the presence or absence of serum in the bath is a determining factor in the response of the tubule to exogenous prostaglandins (182). Inhibition of endogenous prostaglandin synthesis in perfused tubules in vitro does not alter sodium chloride transport.

Recent studies suggest that the inhibitory action of vasopressin on net reabsorption of Na and Cl in the cortical collecting tubule may be exerted through stimulation of prostaglandin biosynthesis (183).

C. Antidiuretic Hormone

The primary action of antidiuretic hormone is to increase the permeability of the collecting tubules to water. In addition, antidiuretic hormone leads to a transient increase in transepithelial potential and sodium reabsorption in the isolated perfused cortical collecting tubule, similar to its effect on anuran membranes. This effect, however, is transient and is followed by a decrease in potential and net sodium chloride reabsorption (184). More recently it has been demonstrated that vasopressin stimulates chloride transport in the mouse thick ascending limb (182,183,185,186).

D. Aldosterone

The primary action of aldosterone is to enhance sodium reabsorption and potassium secretion in the distal nephron. It appears to act on the distal convoluted and the cortical (151,

155) and inner medullary collecting tubules. There is some evidence that it may have an effect on the proximal segments. A number of mechanisms have been proposed for the effect of aldosterone on sodium reabsorption (187,188). These include: (1) an increase in the permeability of the luminal membrane which enhances entry of sodium ions into the cells and increases their availability to the sodium pump on the basolateral membrane; (2) an increase in the activity of the sodium pump, i.e., Na-K-ATPase; and (3) an effect on oxidative metabolism in mitochondria to provide a greater amount of energy for active sodium transport.

In the cortical collecting tubule, the rate of sodium chloride reabsorption is greatly increased in animals pretreated with mineralocorticoids or in animals in which potassium intake has been increased (151,155). The latter would also increase endogenous mineralocorticoid secretion. No effect of glucocorticoids has been demonstrated. There also appears to be a direct relationship between the plasma aldosterone level and the rate of sodium reabsorption by this segment. In addition to its effect on the cortical collecting tubule, an effect on the distal convoluted tubule has also been shown in micropuncture experiments. Whether this effect is related to that portion of the distal convoluted tubule which is morphologically identical with the collecting tubule or whether the effect extends along the true distal tubule is controversial, but the bulk of evidence suggests a diffuse effect along the entire distal nephron. An increase in the area of the basolateral membrane has been observed in the principal cells of the cortical collecting tubule of rabbits treated with Doca (157).

E. Natriuretic Factor

The natriuretic substance derived from the serum and urine of uremic patients has been shown to inhibit the transtubular potential difference and active sodium transport in the cortical collecting tubule (189). This effect is observed only when this factor is applied to the peritubular surface. There is no effect on the passive permeability to sodium. The exact chemical nature of this natriuretic factor has not yet been determined.

F. Other Hormones

Other hormones including angiotensin, progesterone, estrogen, prolactin, glucagon, thyroid hormone, and calcitonin appear to have effects on tubular sodium reabsorption, but these have not been fully investigated.

G. Renal Nerves

Apart from the role of the renal nerves in mediating changes in vascular tone, adrenergic nerve endings directly impinge upon the proximal and distal tubules. It is obvious that in vitro these neurogenic connections are severed and thus the bulk of evidence relating sodium chloride reabsorption to the innervation of the kidney is derived from in vivo experiments. Stimulation of the renal nerves enhances sodium chloride reabsorption (190,192). Denervation leads to a natriuresis (192). These effects are blocked by α-adrenergic blockers such as phenoxybenzamine. Although the acute effects of denervation or stimulation of the adrenergic nerves on sodium chloride reabsorption can be demonstrated, these effects are absent in chronic experiments in conscious animals (193) and in denervated transplanted kidneys. In all these circumstances, sodium handling appears to be normal. In rabbit proximal convoluted tubules, both L-norepinephrine and isoproterenol stimulate fluid reabsorption (194). This appears to be a direct β-adrenergic effect, since it is blocked by propranolol, not by phenoxybenzamine. These results are surprising, since catecholamines are thought to work via the adenylate cyclase system and a catecholamine-sensitive adenylate cyclase has not been identified in the rabbit proximal tubule. Isoproterenal has recently been shown to stimulate chloride transport directly in the cortical collecting tubule (195).

X. IN VITRO PERFUSION OF ISOLATED NEPHRON SEGMENTS IN EXPERIMENTAL MODELS OF RENAL DISEASE

Tubular function in experimental models of renal disease has been studied by perfusion of isolated nephron segments in vitro. The advantage of using this approach is that the intrinsic alterations in tubular function imposed by the disease state can readily be distinguished from those which are dependent upon extratubular factors in the uremic milieu. Using this technique normal nephron segments may be compared with uremic nephron segments in either a normal or uremic milieu.

Using the remnant kidney model in the rabbit, volume reabsorption in superficial proximal straight tubule has been studied (196). Significant compensatory hypertrophy was found to occur after a period of approximately 3 weeks and this was associated with an increase in net volume reabsorption of about 60%. Superficial proximal straight tubules obtained from remnant kidneys in which the contralateral kidney was left in situ (i.e., animals that were not uremic) did not show the increase in volume reabsorption nor the compensatory hypertrophy. Subsequent studies on the late superficial proximal convoluted tubule (33), i.e., the S_2 segment, in both a remnant kidney model (which has an increase in single nephron glomerular filtration rate [SNGFR]) and kidneys embolized with microspheres (which have a decreased SNGFR), also revealed intrinsic alterations in proximal tubular function (Fig. 13). Net volume reabsorption and transtubular potential difference were significantly increased in the uremic-remnant kidney model, whereas these were decreased significantly in the embolized kidney model. Although an increase in tubular size and reabsorptive surface area could account for the increased reabsorptive rate observed in the remnant kidney model, no change in tubule size was observed in the segments obtained from the embolized kidney, suggesting that the "memory" of the in vivo reabsorptive pattern which was observed in vitro was not simply a function of tubule size. Associated with these

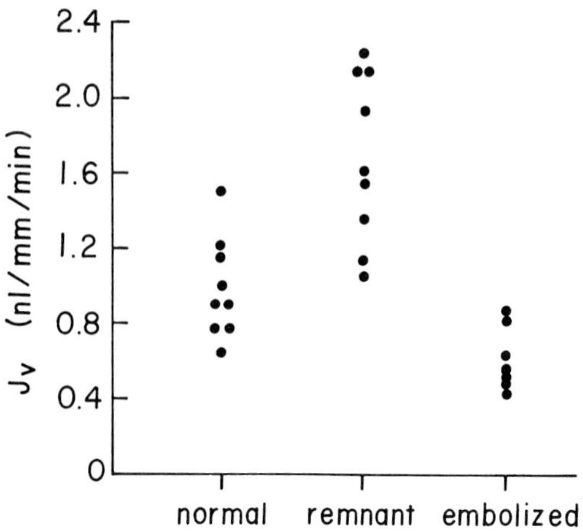

Fig. 13 Net volume reabsorption (J_V) by S_2 proximal convoluted tubules obtained from normal rabbits and rabbits with remnant kidneys and embolized kidneys. (From Ref. 33.)

changes was a reversal of the normal permselectivity of this nephron segment. The late superficial proximal convoluted tubule of the normal rabbit is more permeable to chloride than to sodium. In both the remnant and the embolized kidney model this permselectivity was found to be reversed.

Examination of collecting tubule function in the remnant kidney model also showed important intrinsic alterations in tubular function. The vasopressin response of the cortical collecting tubule is significantly blunted and this has been shown to be due to a decreased responsiveness of adenylate cyclase to vasopressin (197). However, since the effects could not be reversed with an exogenous cAMP analog, it must be presumed that the alteration in vasopressin responsiveness and/or sensitivity is due both to an alteration of the receptor-adenylate cyclase activation and a post-cAMP defect. Of interest is the fact that the uremic animals had endogenous vasopressin levels which were significantly elevated and the possibility of down-regulation of the vasopressin receptor must be considered as a partial explanation for this phenomenon.

Potassium adaptation in the cortical collecting tubule has likewise been shown to be significantly altered in the uremic remnant kidney (143). Net potassium secretion by isolated perfused cortical collecting tubules of normal rabbits was increased significantly when the animals were maintained on a high potassium diet (Fig. 14). This was associated with an increase in transtubular potential difference. In cortical collecting tubules from remnant kidneys of rabbits maintained on a normal potassium intake, the basal potassium secretory rate was twice as high as that of the normal collecting tubule. When these uremic rabbits were maintained on a high K diet, net potassium secretion was six times as great as the rate observed in the normal animals on a normal diet. Thus, significant intrinsic alterations in

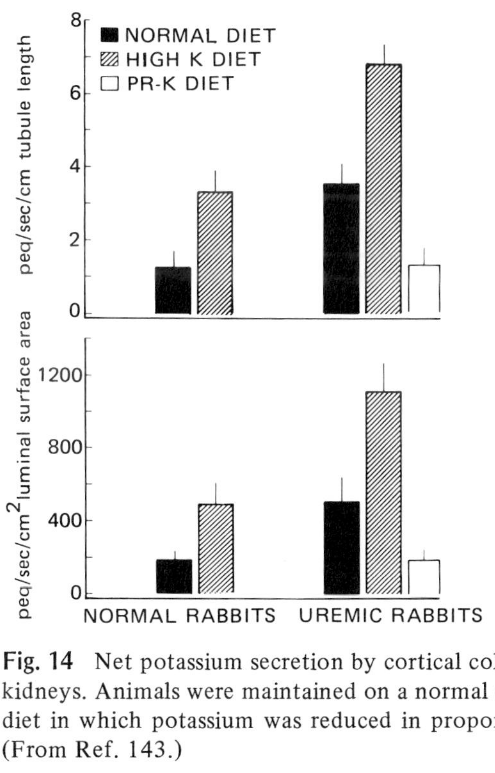

Fig. 14 Net potassium secretion by cortical collecting tubules from normal and remnant kidneys. Animals were maintained on a normal diet, a high potassium diet (high K), or a diet in which potassium was reduced in proportion to the reduction in nephron mass. (From Ref. 143.)

potassium secretion may be observed in the collecting tubule. In these animals, aldosterone levels were found to be significantly elevated only in the uremic rabbits on a high potassium diet. No increase in the specific activity of Na-K-ATPase was observed in the collecting tubules of normal or uremic animals maintained on the high potassium diet. The fact that increased Na-K-ATPase has been observed in other remnant kidney models may be related to the fact that significant potassium loading has been used to demonstrate this change, whereas in the collecting tubule studies described above, potassium intake was increased only twofold. Thus a dissociation between an increase in net potassium secretion and Na-K-ATPase can be shown.

Studies have been performed to elucidate the nature of the adaptation in phosphate transport in the proximal straight tubule of uremic rabbits with remnant kidneys (198,199). In these experiments, a dissociation between net volume reabsorption and net phosphate reabsorption could be demonstrated by altering dietary phosphorus. In addition, in uremic animals on a normal diet in which there was no evidence of secondary hyperparathyroidism, in vitro sensitivity of the proximal tubule PTH was increased, whereas in uremic animals with hyperparathyroidism, PTH sensitivity was decreased below normal. All of these changes indicate that intrinsic alterations in both reabsorptive rates and the sensitivity to hormones occur in experimental models of chronic renal failure.

Studies have also been performed on nephron segments obtained from rabbits with experimental acute renal failure induced by renal artery clamping for 60 min (200). In these studies, net volume reabsorption by the superficial proximal convoluted and the proximal straight tubule was decreased as was the ability of the cortical thick ascending limb of Henle's loop to reduce luminal chloride concentration. The hydro-osmotic response of the collecting tubule to a maximum vasopressin stimulus was similarly blunted. Prior treatment of the animals with either mannitol or furosemide obviated the decrease in volume reabsorption by the proximal tubule, but did not affect the function of the cortical thick ascending limb. Mannitol pretreatment did not prevent the blunting of the vasopressin responsiveness of the collecting tubule (201).

Nephron segments have also been studied in a rabbit model of bilateral and unilateral obstructive nephropathy (202). In unilateral obstruction, volume reabsorption by the superficial proximal convoluted tubule was not different from control. However, in juxtamedullary proximal convoluted tubules, it was reduced by approximately 30%. A similar reduction was observed in the pars recta. In the proximal straight tubule, the thick ascending limb and the cortical collecting tubule of bilaterally obstructed kidneys, the pattern of fluid reabsorption was virtually identical to that observed in unilateral obstruction, i.e., NaCl transport was uniformly decreased in these segments. The foregoing studies indicate that the use of isolated perfused nephron segments will continue to provide important insights into intrinsic defects or adaptations in tubular function in experimental models of disease.

ACKNOWLEDGMENTS

Part of the work cited in this chapter was supported by grant RO1 AM 25301 from the National Institutes of Health and a grant from the Philip Martin Renner Fund for Kidney Research. We acknowledge the assistance of Dr. M. A. Kirschenbaum, who provided the illustrations on tubule cell function.

REFERENCES

1. Seldin, D. W.; and F. C. Rector, Jr. Evaluation of clearance methods for localization of site and action of diuretics. In: Modern Diuretic Therapy in the Treatment of Cardiovascular Disease, edited by Lant, A. F., and Wilson, G. M., Amsterdam, Exerpta Medica, 1973, p. 97.

2. Jamison, R. L.; Buerkert, J.; and Lacy, F. B. A micropuncture study of collecting tubule function in rats with hereditary diabetes insipidus. J. Clin. Invest. 50:2444, 1971.
3. Orloff, J.; Pitfalls in the use of stop-flow for the localization of diuretic action with special reference to Na reabsorption. In: The Physiology of Diuretic Agents. Ann. N.Y. Acad. Sci. 132:344, 1966.
4. Burg, M. B.; Grantham, J. J.; Abranow, M.; and Orloff, J. Preparation and study of fragments of single rabbit nephrons. Am. J. Physiol. 210:1293, 1966.
5. Helman, S. I.; Grantham, J. J.; and Burg, M. B. Effect of vasopressin on electrical of renal cortical collecting tubules. Am. J. Physiol. 220:1825, 1971.
6. Biagi, B.; Kubota, T.; Sohtell, M.; and Giebisch, G. Intracellular potentials in rabbit proximal tubules perfused in vitro. Am. J. Physiol. 240:F200, 1981.
7. Morel, F. Sites of hormone action in the mammalian nephron. Am. J. Physiol. 240: F159, 1981.
8. Woodhall, P. B.; Tisher, C. C.; Simonton, C. A.; and Robinson, R. R. Relationship between para-aminohippurate secretion and cellular morphology in rabbit proximal tubules. J. Clin. Invest. 61:1320, 1978.
9. Berry, C. A.; and Rector, F. C., Jr. Active and passive sodium transport in the proximal tubule. Miner, Electrolyte Metab. 4:149, 1980.
10. Burg, M. B. Renal handling of sodium, chloride water, amino acids and glucose. In: The Kidney, edited by Brenner, B. M., and Rector, F. C., Jr. Philadelphia, Saunders, 1981, p. 328.
11. Burg, M. B.; and Orloff, J. Electrical potential differences across proximal convoluted tubules. Am. J. Physiol. 219:1714, 1970.
12. Burg, M. B.; Patlak, C.; Green, N.; and Villey, D. Organic solutes in fluid absorption by renal proximal convoluted tubules. Am. J. Physiol. 231:627, 1976.
13. Aronson, P. S.; and Sacktor, B. The Na^+ gradient dependent transport of D-glucose in renal brush border membranes. J. Biol. Chem. 250:6032, 1975.
14. Jacobson, J. R.; and Kokko, J. P. Intrinsic differences in various segments of the proximal convoluted tubule. J. Clin. Invest. 57:818, 1976.
15. Hoffman, N.; Thees, M.; and Kinne, R. Phosphate transport by isolated renal brush border vesicles. Pfluegers Arch. 362:147, 1976.
16. Burg, M. B.; and Iino, Y. Control of renal bicarbonate transport. In: Membrane Biochemistry, vol. 2, New York, Crane, Russak and Co., 1979, p. 405.
17. Kinsella, J. L.; and Aronson, P. S. Properties of the Na^+-H^+ exchanger in renal microvillus membrane vesicles. Am. J. Physiol. 238:F461, 1980.
18. Kinne, R. Properties of the glucose transport system in the renal brush border membrane. In: Current Topics in Membranes and Transport, edited by Bronner, F., and Kleinzeller, A., vol. 8, New York, Academic Press, 1976, p. 209.
19. Silverman, M. Glucose transport in the kidney. Biochim. Biophys. Acta 457:303, 1976.
20. Fromter, E.; and Sato, K. Electrical events in active H^+/HCO_3-transport across rat kidney proximal tubular epithelium. In: Gastric Hydrogen Ion Secretion, edited by Kasbekar, D., Sachs, G., and Rehm, W., New York, Marcel Dekker, 1974, p. 382.
21. Ullrich, K. J.; Capasso, G.; Rumrich, R.; Papavissiliou, F.; and Koss, S. Coupling between proximal tubular transport processes. Studies with ouabain, SITS, and HCO_3-free solutions. Pfluegers Arch. 368:245, 1977.
22. Boulpaep, E. Permeability changes of the proximal tubule of Necturus during saline loading. Am. J. Physiol. 222:517, 1972.
23. Diamond, J.; and Bossert, W. Standing-gradient osmotic flow. A mechanism for coupling of water and solute transport in epithelia. J. Gen. Physiol. 50:2061, 1967.
24. Kokko, J. P.; Burg, M. B.; and Orloff, J. Characteristics of NaCl and water transport in the renal proximal tubule. J. Clin. Invest. 50:69, 1971.
25. Hamburger, R.; Lawson, N.; and Dennis, V. Effects of cyclic adenosine nucleotides on fluid absorption by different segments of proximal tubule. Am. J. Physiol. 227:396, 1974.
26. Tune, B.; and Burg, M. Glucose transport by proximal tubules. Am. J. Physiol. 221: 580, 1971.

27. Tune, B. M.; Burg, M. B.; and Patlak, C. S. Characteristics of p-amminohippurate transport in proximal renal tubules. Am. J. Physiol. 217:1057, 1969.
28. Burg, M. B.; and Green, N. Bicarbonate transport by isolated perfused rabbit proximal convoluted tubules. Am. J. Physiol. 217:1057, 1969.
30. McKinney, T. D.; and Burg, M. B. Sodium, bicarbonate, and fluid absorption by renal proximal straight tubules, Kidney Int. 12:1, 1977.
30. Neumann, K. H.; and Rector, F. C., Jr. Mechanism of NaCl and water reabsorption in the proximal convoluted tubule of rat kidney. Role of chloride concentration gradients. J. Clin. Invest. 58:1110, 1976.
31. Kawamura, S.; Imai, M.; Seldin, D.; and Koko, J. Characteristics of salt and water transport in superficial and juxtamedullary straight segments of proximal tubules. J. Clin. Invest. 55:1269, 1975.
32. Berry, C. A.; Warnock, D. G.; and Rector, F. C., Jr. Ion selectivity and proximal salt reabsorption. Am. J. Physiol. 235:F2134, 1978.
33. Trizna, W.; Yanagawa, N.; Bar-Khayim, Y.; Houston, B.; and Fine, L. G. Functional profile of the isolated uremic nephron. Evidence of proximal tubular "memory" in experimental renal disease. J. Clin. Invest. 68:760, 1981.
34. Holmberg, C.; Kokko, J. P.; and Jacobson, H. R. Determination of chloride and bicarbonate permeabilities in proximal convoluted tubules. Am. J. Physiol. 241:F386, 1981.
35. Schafer, J.; Patlak, C.; and Andreoli, T. A component of fluid absorption linked to passive ion flows in the superficial pars recta. J. Gen. Physiol. 66:445, 1975.
36. Jacobson, H. R. Characteristics of volume reabsorption in rabbit superficial and juxtamedullary convoluted tubules. J. Clin. Invest. 63:410, 1979.
37. Spring, K. R.; and Giebisch, G. Kinetics of Na^+ transport in necturus proximal tubule. J. Gen. Physiol. 70:307, 1977.
38. Kimura, G.; and Spring, K. R. Luminal Na^+ entry into Necturus proximal tubule cells. Am. J. Physiol. 236:F295, 1979.
39. Spring, K. R.; and Kimura, G. Chloride reabsorption by renal proximal tubules of Necturus. J. Memb. Biol. 38:233, 1978.
40. Kimura, G.; and Spring, K. R. Transcellular and paracellular tracer chloride fluxes in Necturus proximal tubule. Am. J. Physiol. 235:F617, 1978.
41. Earley, L.; and Schrier, R. Intrarenal control of sodium excretion by hemodynamic and physical factors. In: Handbook of Physiology, section 8, Renal Physiology, edited by Orloff, J., and Berliner, R. W. American Physiological Society, Washington, D.C. 1973, p. 677.
42. Imai, M.; and Kokko, J. Transtubular oncotic pressure gradients and net fluid transport in isolated proximal tubules. Kidney Int. 6:138, 1974.
43. Green, R.; Windhager, E. E.; and Giebisch, G. Protein oncotic pressure effects on proximal tubular fluid movement in the rat. Am. J. Physiol. 226:265, 1974.
44. Bank, N.; Yarger, W.; and Aynedjian, H. A microperfusion study of sucrose movement across the rat proximal tubule during renal vein construction. J. Clin. Invest. 50:294, 1971.
45. Imai, M.; and Kokko, J. Effect of peritubular protein concentration on reabsorption of sodium and water in isolated perfused proximal tubules. J. Clin. Invest. 51:314, 1972.
46. Gertz, K. H.; and Boylan, J. Glomerulotubular balance. In: Handbook of Physiology, section 8, Renal Physiology, edited by Orloff, J., and Berliner, R. W., American Physiological Society, Washington, D.C., 1973, p. 763.
47. Brenner, B. M.; and Troy, J. L. Postglomerular vascular protein concentration–Evidence for a causal role in governing fluid reabsorption and glomerulotubular balance by the renal tubule. J. Clin. Invest. 50:336, 1971.
48. Brenner, B. M.; Troy, J. L.; Daugharty, T. M.; and MacInnes, R. M. Quantitative importance of changes in postglomerular colloid osmotic pressure in mediating glomerulotubular balance in the rat. J. Clin. Invest. 52:190, 1973.

49. Giebisch, G.; Malnic, G.; and Berliner, R. W. Renal transport and control of potassium excretion. In: The Kidney, edited by Brenner, B. M., and Rector, F. C., Jr., Philadelphia, Saunders, 1981, p. 408.
50. Diezi, J.; Michoud, P.; and Giebisch, G. Effects of nephrectomy on renal salt and water transport in the remaining kidney. Kidney Int. 10:450, 1976.
51. Beck, L. H.; Senesky, D.; and Goldberg, M. Sodium-independent active potassium reabsorption in proximal tubule of the dog. J. Clin. Invest. 52:2641, 1973.
52. Fujimoto, M.; Kubota, T.; and Kotera, K. Electrochemical profile of K and Cl ions across the proximal tubule of bullfrog kidneys. Contrib. Nephrol. 6:114, 1977.
53. Goldberg, M.; Agus, Z. S.; and Goldfarb, S. Renal handling of calcium and phosphorus. In: International Review of Physiology. Kidney and urinary tract physiology II, vol. II, edited by Thurnau, K. Baltimore, Maryland, University Park Press, 1976, p. 211.
54. Dennis, V. W.; Woodhall, P. B.; and Robinson, R. R. Characteristics of phosphate transport in isolated proximal tubule. Am. J. Physiol. 231:979, 1976.
55. Dennis, V. W. Studies in isolated perfused tubules. In: Symposium on the Regulation of P_i Transport. Abstracts of the American Society of Nephrology, 11th Annual Meeting, New Orleans, 1978, p. 15.
56. Hoffmann, N.; Thees, M.; and Kinne, R. Phosphate transport by isolated renal brush border vesicles. Pfluegers Arch. 362:147, 1976.
57. Kinne, R.; Berner, W.; Hoffman, N.; and Murer, H. Phosphate transport by isolated renal and intestinal plasma membranes. Adv Exp. Med. Biol. 81:265, 1977.
58. Frick, A. Proximal tubular reabsorption of inorganic phosphate during saline infusion in the rat. Am. J. Physiol. 223:1034, 1972.
59. Dennis, V. W.; Bello-Reuss, E.; and Robinson, R. R. Response of phosphate transport to parathyroid hormone in segments of rabbit nephron. Am. J. Physiol. 233:F29, 1977.
60. Steele, T. H.; and DeLuca, H. F. Influence of dietary phosphorus on renal phosphate reabsorption in the parathyroidectomized rat. J. Clin. Invest. 57:867, 1976.
61. Ullrich, K. J.; Rumrich, G.; and Kloss, S. Phosphate transport in the proximal convolution of the rat kidney. III. Effect of extracellular and intracellular pH. Pfluegers Arch. 377:33, 1978.
62. Bank, N.; Aynedjian, H. S.; and Weinstein, S. W. A microperfusion study of phosphate reabsorption by the rat proximal renal tubule. J. Clin. Invest. 54:1048, 1974.
63. Massry, S. G.; Coburn, J. W.; and Kleeman, C. R. The influence of extracellular volume expansion on renal phosphate reabsorption in the dog. J. Clin. Invest. 36:1236, 1957.
64. Hebert, C. S.; Rouse, D.; Eknoyan, G.; Martinez-Maldonado, M.; and Suki, W. N. Decreased phosphate reabsorption by volume expansion in the dog. Kidney Int. 2:247, 1972.
65. Cuche, J. L.; Ott, C. E.; Marchand, G. R.; and Knox, F. G. Lack of effect of hypocalcemia on renal phosphate handling. J. Lab. Clin. Med. 88:271, 1976.
66. Steel, T. H.; Engle, J. E.; Tanaka, Y.; Lorenc, R. S.; Dudgeon, K. L.; and Deluca, H. F. Phosphatemic action of 1,25-dihydroxyvitamin D_3. Am. J. Physiol. 229:489, 1975.
67. Kempson, S. A.; Donsa, T. P. Phosphate transport across renal cortical brush border membrane vesicles from rats stabilized on a normal high or low phosphate diet. Life Sci. 24:888, 1979.
68. Levine, B. S.; Hodsman, A.; Ho, K.; Shaw, H. F.; Hirayama, B.; Kippen, I.; Lee, D. B. N.; and Coburn, J. R. Early renal brush border adaptation to dietary phosphorus restriction. Kidney Int. 19:113, 1981.
69. Sutton, R. A. L.; and Dirks, J. H. The renal excretion of calcium: A review of micropuncture data. Can. J. Physiol. Pharmacol. 53:979, 1975.
70. Ullrich, K. J.; Rumrich, G.; and Kloss, S. Active Ca^{2+} absorption in the proximal tubule of the rat kidney. Dependence on sodium and buffer transport. Pfluegers Arch. 364:223, 1976.

71. Baker, P. F. Regulation of intracellular Ca and Mg in squid axons. Fed. Proc. 35:2589, 1976.
72. Khuri, R. N.; Agulian, S. K.; Bogharian, K.; Nassar, R.; and Wise, W. Intracellular bicarbonate in single cells of necturus kidney proximal tubule. Pfluegers Arch. 322:39, 1971.
73. Taylor, A.; and Windhager, E. E. Possible role of cytosolic calcium and Na-Ca exchange in regulation of transepithelial sodium transport. Am. J. Physiol. 236:F505, 1979.
74. Kinne-Saffran, E.; and Kinne, R. Localization of a calcium-stimulated ATPase in the basal-lateral plasma membranes of the proximal tubule of rat kidney cortex. J. Membr. Biol. 17:263, 1974.
75. Murayama, Y.; Morel, F.; and Le Grimellec, C. Phosphate, calcium and magnesium transfers proximal tubules and loops of Henle, as measured by single nephron microperfusion experiments in the rat. Pfluegers Arch. 333:1, 1972.
76. Jamison, R. L.; Frey, N. R.; and Lacy, F. B. Calcium reabsorption in the thin loop of Henle. Am. J. Physiol. 227:745, 1974.
77. Rocha, A. S.; Magaldi, J. B.; and Kokko, J. P. Calcium and phosphate transport in isolated segments of rabbit Henle's loop. J. Clin. Invest. 59:975, 1977.
78. Rouse, D.; and Suki, W. N. Active calcium absorption in the superficial pars recta (SPR). Abstracts of the 7th International Congress of Nephrology, 1978, p. E17.
79. Duarte, C. G.; and Watson, J. F. Calcium reabsorption in proximal tubule of the dog. Am. J. Physiol. 212:1355, 1967.
80. Le Grimellec, C.; Roinel, N.; and Morel, F. Simultaneous Mg, Ca, P, K, Na and Cl analysis in rat tubular fluid. III. During acute Ca plasma loading. Pfluegers Arch. 346:171, 1974.
81. Quamme, G. A.; and Dirks, J. H. Effects of magnesium (Mg) on calcium (Ca) and Mg transport in the rat: A microperfusion study. Abstracts of 7th Annual Meeting of the International Society of Nephrology, 1978, p. E12.
82. Le Grimellec, G.; Roinel, N.; and Morel, F. Simultaneous Mg, Ca, P, K, Na and Cl analysis in rat tubular fluid. I. During perfusion of either inulin or ferrocyanide. Pfluegers Arch. 340:181, 1973.
83. Quamme, G. A.; Wong, N. L. M.; Dirks, J. H.; Roinel, N.; de Rouffignac, C.; and Morel, F. Magnesium handling in the dog kidney: A micropuncture study. Pfluegers Arch. 377:95, 1978.
84. Quamme, G. A.; and Dirks, J. H. Intraluminal and contraluminal magnesium on magnesium and calcium transfer in the rat nephron. Am. J. Physiol. 238:F187, 1980.
85. Wen, S. F.; Evanson, R. L.; and Dirks, J. H. Micropuncture study of magnesium transport in proximal and distal tubule of the dog. Am. J. Physiol. 219:570, 1970.
86. Harris, C. A.; Burnatowska, M. A.; Seely, J. F.; Sutton, R. A. L.; Quamme, G. A.; and Dirks, J. H. Effects of parathyroid hormone on electrolyte transport in the hamster nephron. Am. J. Physiol. 236:F342, 1979.
87. Steele, T. H. Control of uric acid excretion. New Eng. J. Med. 287:1193, 1971.
88. Fanelli, G. M., Jr.; and Weiner, I. M. Pyrazinoate excretion in the chimpanzee. Relation to urate disposition and the actions of uricosuric drugs. J. Clin. Invest. 52:1946, 1973.
89. Abrahamson, R. G.; and Levitt, M. F. Micropuncture study of uric acid transport in rat kidney. Am. J. Physiol. 228:1597, 1975.
90. Roche-Ramel, F.; and Peters, S. Urinary excretion of uric acid in non-human mammalian species. In: Handbook of Experimental Pharmacology. Uric Acid, vol. 51, edited by Kelley, W. N., and Weiner, I. M. Berlin, Springer, 1978, p. 211.
91. Chonko, A. M. Water secretion in isolated rabbit renal tubules. Am. J. Physiol. 239: F545, 1980.
92. Imai, M.; and Kokko, J. Sodium, urea and water transport in the thin ascending limb of Henle. Generation of osmotic gradients by passive diffusion of solutes. J. Clin. Invest. 53:393, 1974.

93. Kokko, J. Sodium, chloride and water transport in the descending limb of Henle. J. Clin. Invest. 49:1838, 1970.
94. Imai, M. Function of the thin ascending limb of Henle of rats and hamsters perfused in vitro. Am. J. Physiol. 232:F201, 1977.
95. Imai, M.; and Kokko, J. P. Mechanism of sodium and chloride transport in the thin ascending limb of Henle. J. Clin. Invest. 58:1054, 1976.
96. Kokko, J. P.; and Rector, F. C., Jr. Contercurrent multiplication system without active transport in inner medulla. Kidney Int. 2:214, 1972.
97. De Rouffignac, C.; and Morel, F. Micropuncture study of water, electrolytes, and urea movements along the loops of Henle in Psammonys. J. Clin. Invest. 48:474, 1969.
98. Jamison, R.; Buerkert, J.; and Lacy, F. A micropuncture study of Henle's thin loop in Brattleboro rats. Am. J. Physiol. 224:180, 1973.
99. Pennell, J.; Lacy, F.; and Jamison, R. An in vivo study of the concentrating process in the descending limb of Henle's loop. Kidney Int. 5:337, 1974.
100. Marsh, D.; and Azen, S. Mechanism of NaCl reabsorption by hamster thin ascending limbs of Henle's loop. Am. J. Physiol. 228:71, 1975.
101. Johnson, P. A.; Battilana, C. A.; Lacy, F. B.; and Jamison, R. L. Evidence for a concentration gradient favoring outward movement of sodium from the thin limb of Henle. J. Clin. Invest. 59:234, 1977.
102. Arrascue, J. F.; Dobyan, D. C.; and Jamison, R. L. Potassium recycling in the renal medulla: Effects of acute potassium chloride administration to rats fed a potassium-free diet. Kidney Int. 20:348, 1981.
103. Brunette, M. G.; Vigneault, N.; and Carriere, S. Micropuncture study of magnesium transport along the nephron in the young rat. Am. J. Physiol. 227:891, 1974.
104. Burg, M.; and Green, N. Function of the thick ascending limb of Henle's loop. Am. J. Physiol. 224:659, 1973.
105. Rocha, A. S.; and Kokko, J. P. Sodium chloride and water transport in the medullary thick ascending limb of Henle. Evidence for active chloride transport. J. Clin. Invest. 52:612, 1973.
106. Greger, R. Chloride reabsorption in the rabbit cortical thick ascending limb of the loop of Henle. A sodium dependent process. Pfluegers Arch. 30:38, 1981.
107. Greger, R.; and Schlatter, E. Presence of luminal K^+, a prerequisite for active NaCl transport in cortical thick ascending limb of Henle's loop of rabbit kidney. Pflügers Arch. 392:92, 1981.
108. Burg, M. B.; and Bourdeau, J. E. Function of the thick ascending limb of Henle's loop. In: New Aspects of Renal Function, edited by Vogel, H. G., and Ullrich, K. G. Amsterdam, Excerpta Medica, 1978, p. 91.
109. Schmidt, U.; and Dubach, U. C. Activity of (Na^+, K^+) stimulated adenosine triphosphatase in the rat nephron. Pflügers Arch. 306:219, 1969.
110. Doucet, A.; and Katz, A. I. Renal potassium adaptation: Na-K ATPase activity along the nephron after chronic potassium loading. Am. J. Physiol. 238:F380, 1980.
111. Battilana, C. A.; Dobyan, D. C.; Lacy, F. B.; Bhattacharya, J.; Johnston, P. A.; and Jamison, R. L. Effect of chronic potassium loading on potassium secretion by the pars recta or descending limb of the juxtamedullary nephron in the rat. J. Clin. Invest. 62:1093, 1978.
112. Dobyan, D. C.; Lacy, F. B.; and Jamison, R. L. Suppression of potassium recycling in the renal medulla by short term potassium deprivation. Kidney Int. 16:704, 1979.
113. De Rouffignac, C.; and Morel, F. Micropuncture study of water, electrolytes, and urea movements along the loops of Henle in Psammomys. J. Clin. Invest. 48:474, 1969.
114. Jamison, R. L. Micropuncture study of segments of thin loop of Henle in the rat. Am. J. Physiol. 215:326, 1968.

115. Jamison, R. L. Micropuncture study of superficial and juxtamedullary nephrons in the rat. Am. J. Physiol. 218:46, 1970.
116. Jamison, R. L.; and Lacy, F. B. Effect of saline infusion on superficial and juxtamedullary nephrons in rat. Am. J. Physiol. 221:690, 1971.
117. Jamison, R. L.; Lacy, F. B.; Pennell, J. P.; and Sanjana, V. M. Potassium secretion by the descending limb of pars recta of the juxtamedullary nephron in vivo. Kidney Int. 9:323, 1976.
118. Marsh, D. J.; Solute and water flows in thin limbs of Henle's loop in the hamster kidney. Am. J. Physiol. 218:824, 1970.
119. De Rouffignac, C.; Morel, F.; Moss, N.; and Roinel, N. Micropuncture study of water and electrolyte movements along the loop of Henle in Psammomys, with special reference to magnesium, calcium and phosphorus, Pflugers Arch. 344:309, 1973.
120. Edwards, B. R.; Baer, P. G.; Sutton, R. A. L.; and Dirks, J. H. Micropuncture study of diuretic effects on sodium and calcium reabsorption in the dog nephron. J. Clin. Invest. 52:2418, 1973.
121. Bourdeau, J. E.; and Burg, M. B. Voltage dependence of calcium transport in the thick ascending limb of Henle's loop. Am. J. Physiol. 236:F357, 1979.
122. Imai, M. Calcium transport across the rabbit thick ascending limb of Henle's loop perfused in vitro. Pflugers Arch. 374:255, 1978.
123. Suki, W. N.; Rouse, D.; Ng, R. C. K.; and Kokko, J. P. Calcium transport in the thick ascending limb of Henle. Heterogeneity of function in the medullary and cortical segments. J. Clin. Invest. 66:1004, 1980.
124. Sutton, R. A. L.; Wong, N. L. M.; and Dirks, J. H. Effects of parathyroid hormone on sodium and calcium transport in the dog nephron. Clin. Sci. Molec. Med. 51:345, 1976.
125. Bourdeau, J. E.; and Burg, M. B. Effect of parathyroid hormone on calcium transport in the cortical thick ascending limb of Henle's loop. Clin. Res. 27:410A, 1979.
126. Buckle, R. M.; Care, A. D.; Cooper, C. W.; and Gitelman, H. J. The influence of plasma magnesium concentration on parathyroid hormone secretion. J. Endocrinol. 42:529, 1968.
127. Shareghi, G. R.; and Agus, Z. S. Magnesium transport in the rabbit cortical thick ascending limb (CTAL). Clin. Res. 27:430A, 1979.
128. Quamme, G. A. Effect of intraluminal furosemide on calcium and magnesium transport in the loop of Henle and the role of PTH. Kidney Int. 14:642, 1978.
129. Khuri, R. N.; Wiederholt, M.; Streider, N.; and Giebisch, G. Effects of graded solute diuresis on renal tubular sodium transport in the rat. Am. J. Physiol. 228:1262, 1975.
130. Wright, F. Increasing magnitude of electrical potential along the renal distal tubule. Am. J. Physiol. 220:624, 1971.
131. Bermudez, L.; and Windhager, E. E. Osmotically induced changes in electrical resistance of distal tubules of rat kidneys. Am. J. Physiol. 229:1536, 1975.
132. Woodhall, P.; and Tisher, C. Response of the distal tubule and cortical collecting duct to vasopressin in the rat. J. Clin. Invest. 53:3095, 1973.
133. Wright, F. S.; and Giebisch, G. Renal potassium transport: Contributions of individual nephron segments and populations. Am. J. Physiol. 235:F515, 1978.
134. Kubota, T.; Biagi, B.; and Giebisch, G. Intracellular potassium activity measurements in single proximal tubules of Necturus. In: Cellular Mechanisms of Renal Tubular Ion Transport. Current Topics in Membranes and Transport, vol. 13, edited by Boulpaep, E. New York, Academic Press, 1980, p. 63.
135. Khuri, R. N. Electrochemistry of the nephron. In: Membrane Transport in Biology, vol. IV, edited by Giebisch, G., Tosteson, D. C., and Ussing, H. H. New York, Springer-Verlag, 1979, p. 47.
136. Malnic, G.; Klose, R. M.; and Giebisch, G. Micropuncture study of renal potassium excretion in the rat. Am. J. Physiol. 206:647, 1964.

137. Reineck, H. J.; Osgood, R. W.; Ferris, T. F.; and Stein, J. H. Potassium transport in the distal tubule and collecting duct of the rat. Am. J. Physiol. 229:1403, 1975.
138. Reineck, H. J.; Osgood, R. W.; and Stein, J. H. Net potassium addition beyond the superficial distal tubule of the rat. Am. J. Physiol. 235:F104, 1979.
139. Khuri, R. N.; Agulian, S. K.; and Kalloghlian, A. Intracellular potassium in cells of the distal tubule. Pflugers Arch. 335:297, 1972.
140. Adam, W. R.; and Dawaborn, J. K. Potassium tolerance in rats. Aust. J. Exp. Biol. Med. Sci. 50:757, 1972.
141. Silva, P.; Ross, B. D.; Charney, A. N.; Besarab, A.; and Epstein, F. H. Potassium transport by the isolated perfused kidney. J. Clin. Invest. 56:862, 1975.
142. Thatcher, J. S.; and Radike, A. W. Tolerance to potassium intoxication in the albino rat. Am. J. Physiol. 151:138, 1947.
143. Fine, L. G.; Yanagawa, N.; Schultze, R. G.; Tuck, M.; and Trizna, W. Functional profile of the isolated uremic nephron. Potassium adaptation in the rabbit cortical collecting tubule. J. Clin. Invest. 64:1033, 1979.
144. Davidson, D. G.; Levinsky, N. G.; and Berliner, R. W. Maintenance of potassium excretion despite reduction of glomerular filtration during sodium diuresis. J. Clin. Invest. 37:548, 1958.
145. Malnic, G.; Klose, R. M.; and Giebisch, G. Micropuncture study of distal tubular potassium and sodium transport in rat nephron. Am. J. Physiol. 211:529, 1966.
146. Peterson, L.; and Wright, F. S. Effect of sodium intake on renal potassium excretion. Am. J. Physiol. 233:F225, 1977.
147. Grantham, J. J.; Burg, M. B.; and Orloff, J. The nature of transtubular Na and K transport in isolated rabbit collecting tubules. J. Clin. Invest. 49:1815, 1970.
148. Khuri, R. N.; Wiederholt, M.; Strieder, N.; and Giebisch, G. Effects of flow rate and potassium intake on distal tubular potassium transfer. Am. J. Physiol. 228:1249, 1975.
149. Stoner, L. C.; Burg, M. B.; and Orloff, J. Ion transport in cortical collecting tubule: Effect of amiloride. Am. J. Physiol. 227:453, 1974.
150. Garcia, E.; Malnic, G.; and Giebisch, G. Effects of changes in electrical potential difference upon tubular potassium transport. Am. J. Physiol. 238:F235, 1980.
151. Schwartz, G.; and Burg, M. Mineralocorticoid effects on cation transport by cortical collecting tubules in vitro. Am. J. Physiol. 235:F576, 1978.
152. Wiederhol, M.; Agulian, S.; and Khuri, R. N. Intracellular potassium in the distal tubule of the adrenalectomized and aldosterone-treated rat. Pflugers Arch. 347:117, 1974.
153. Wiederholt, M.; Schoormans, W.; Fischer, F.; and Behn, C. Mechanism of action of aldosterone on potassium transfer in the rat kidney. Pflugers Arch. 345:157, 1972.
154. Wiederholt, M.; Behn, C.; Schoormans, W.; and Hansen, L. Effect of aldosterone on sodium and potassium transport in the kidney. J. Steroid Biochem. 3:151, 1972.
155. O'Neil, R. G.; and Helman, S. I. Transport characteristics of renal collecting tubules: Influences of Doca and diet. Am. J. Physiol. 233:F544, 1977.
156. Helman, S. I.; and O'Neil, R. G. Model of active transepithelial Na and K transport of renal collecting tubules. Am. J. Physiol. 233:F559, 1977.
157. Kashgarian, M. Changes in cell membrane surface associated with alteration of transepithelial ion movement. In: Cellular Mechanisms of Renal Tubular Ion Transport. Current Topics in Membranes and Transport, vol. 13, edited by Boulpaep, E. New York, Academic Press, 1980, p. 149.
158. Clapp, J. R.; Rector, F. C.; and Seldin, D. W. Effect of unreabsorbed anions on proximal and distal transtubular potentials in the rat. Am. J. Physiol. 202:781, 1962.
159. Gennari, F. J.; and Cohen, J. J. The role of the kidney in potassium homeostasis. Lessons from acid-base disturbances. Kidney Int. 8:1, 1975.

160. Pastoriza-Munoz, E.; Colindres, R. E.; Lassiter, W. E.; and Lechene, C. Effect of parathyroid hormone on phosphate reabsorption in rat distal convolution. Am. J. Physiol. 235:F321, 1978.
161. Lang, F.; Greger, R.; Marchand, G. R.; and Knox, F. G. Stationary microperfusion study of phosphate reabsorption in proximal and distal nephron segments. Pflugers Arch. 368:45, 1977.
162. Lassiter, W. E.; Gottschalk, C. W.; and Mylle, M. Micropuncture study of renal tubular reabsorption of calcium in normal rodents. Am. J. Physiol. 204:771, 1963.
163. Shareghi, G. R.; and Stoner, L. C. Calcium transport across segments of the rabbit distal nephron in vitro. Am. J. Physiol. 235:F367, 1978.
164. Boudry, J.; Stoner, L.; and Burg, M. The effect of lumen pH on potassium transport in renal cortical collecting tubules. Am. J. Physiol. 230:239, 1976.
165. Shareghi, G. R.; and Agus, Z. S. Phosphate transport in the light segment of the rabbit cortical collecting tubule (CCT). Miner. Electrolyte Metab. 2:268, 1979.
166. Shareghi, G. R.; and Stoner, L. C. Calcium transport across segments of the rabbit distal nephron in vitro. Am. J. Physiol. 235:F367, 1978.
167. Le Grimellec, C.; Roinel, N.; and Morel, F. Simultaneous Mg, Ca, P, K, Na and Cl analysis in rat tubular fluid. II. During acute Mg plasma loading. Pflugers Arch. 340: 197, 1973.
168. Fine, L. G.; and Trizna, W. Influence of prostaglandins on sodium transport of isolated medullary nephron segments. Am. J. Physiol. 232:F383, 1977.
169. Stokes, J. B. Na and K transport across the cortical and outer medullary collecting tubule of the rabbit: Evidence for diffusion across the outer medullary portion. Am. J. Physiol. 242:F514, 1982.
170. Morgan, T.; Sakai, F.; and Berliner, R. In vitro permeability of medullary collecting ducts to water and urea. Am. J. Physiol. 214:574, 1968.
171. Hierholzer, K. Secretion of potassium and acidification in collecting ducts of mammalian kidney. Am. J. Physiol. 201:318, 1961.
172. Stokes, J. B.; Ingram, M. J.; Williams, A. D.; and Ingram, D. Heterogeneity of the rabbit collecting tubule: Localization of mineralocorticoid hormone action to the cortical portion. Kidney Int. 20:340, 1981.
173. Stone, D. K.; Seldin, D. W.; Kokko, J. P.; and Jacobson, H. R. Mineralocorticoid modulation of rabbit medullary collecting duct acidification. A sodium-independent effect. J. Clin. Invest. 72:77, 1983.
174. de Rouffignac, C.; Imbert, M.; and Roinel, N. Movements of Na, K, Cl, Mg, Ca, P, and urea along the papillary collecting ducts (CD) of Psammomys obesus (Abstract 78). Proceedings of the 6th International Congress of Nephrology, 1975.
175. Brunette, M. G.; Vigneault, N.; and Carriere, S. Micropuncture study of renal magnesium transport in magnesium-loaded rats. Am. J. Physiol. 229:1695, 1975.
176. Hamburger, R. J.; Lawson, N. L.; and Schwartz, J. H. Response to parathyroid hormone in defined segments of proximal tubule. Am. J. Physiol. 230:286, 1976.
177. Dennis, V. W. Influence of bicarbonate on parathyroid hormone-induced changes in fluid absorption by the proximal tubule. Kidney Int. 10:373, 1976.
178. Iino, Y.; and Burg, M. B. Effect of parathyroid hormone on bicarbonate absorption by proximal tubules in vitro. Am. J. Physiol. 236:F387, 1979.
179. Jacobson, H. R. Altered permeability in the proximal tubule response to cyclic AMP. Am. J. Physiol. 236:F71, 1979.
180. Stokes, J. B.; and Kokko, J. P. Inhibition of sodium transport by prostaglandin E_2 across the isolated, perfused rabbit collecting tubule. J. Clin. Invest. 59:1099, 1977.
181. Iino, Y.; and Imai, M. Effects of prostaglandins on Na transport in isolated collecting tubules. Pflugers Arch. 373:125, 1978.
182. Fine, L. G.; Kirschenbaum, M. Absence of direct effects of prostaglandins on sodium chloride transport in the mammalian nephron. Kidney Int. 19:797, 1981.

183. Holt, W. F.; and Lechene, C. ADH-PGE_2 interactions in cortical collecting tubule. I. Depression of sodium transport. Am. J. Physiol. 241:F452, 1981.
184. Frindt, G.; and Burg, M. B. Effect of vasopressin on sodium transport in renal cortical collecting tubules. Kidney Int. 1:224, 1972.
185. Hall, D. A.; and Varney, D. M. Effect of vasopressin on electrical potential difference and chloride transport in mouse medullary thick ascending limbs of Henle's loop. J. Clin. Invest. 66:792, 1980.
186. Hebert, S. C.; Culpepper, R. M.; and Andreoli, T. E. NaCl transport in mouse medullary thick ascending limbs. II. ADH enhancement of transcellular NaCl cotransport; origin of transepithelial voltage. Am. J. Physiol. 241:F432, 1981.
187. Ullrich, K. J.; and Papavassiliou, F. Sodium reabsorption in the papillary collecting duct of rats. Effect of adrenalectomy, low Na^+ diet, acetazolamide, HCO_3-free solutions, and amiloride. Pflugers Arch. 379:49, 1979.
188. Edelman, I. S. Candidate mediators in the action of aldosterone on Na^+ transport. In: Membrane Transport Processes, vol. 1, edited by Hoffman, J. F., New York, Raven Press, 1978, p. 125.
189. Fine, L. G.; Bourgoignie, J. J.; Hwang, K. H.; and Bricker, N. S. On the influence of the natriuetic factor from patients with chronic uremia on the bioelectric properties and sodium transport of the isolated mammalian collecting tubule. J. Clin. Invest. 58:590, 1976.
190. DiBona, G. F. Neurogenic regulation of renal tubule sodium reabsorption. Am. J. Physiol. 233:F73, 1977.
191. DiBona, G. F. Neural control of renal tubular sodium reabsorption in the dog. Fed. Proc. 37:1214, 1978.
192. Colindres, R. E.; and Gottschalk, C. W. Neural control of renal tubular sodium reabsorption in the rat: Single nephron analysis. Fed. Proc. 37:1218, 1978.
193. Lifshitz, M. D. Lack of a role for the renal nerves in renal sodium reabsorption in conscious dogs. Clin. Sci. Molec. Med. 54:567, 1978.
194. Bello-Reuss, E. Effect of catecholamines on fluid reabsorption by the isolated proximal convoluted tubule. Am. J. Physiol. 238:F347, 1980.
195. Iino, Y.; Troy, J. L.; and Brenner, B. M. Effects of catecholamines on electrolyte transport in cortical collecting tubule. J. Membr. Biol. 61:67, 1981.
196. Fine, L. G.; Trizna, W.; Bourgoignie, J. J.; and Bricker, N. S. Functional profile of the isolated uremic nephron. Role of compensatory hypertrophy in the control of fluid reabsorption by the proximal straight tubule. J. Clin. Invest. 61:1508, 1978.
197. Fine, L. G.; Schlondorff, D.; Trizna, W.; Gilbert, R. M.; and Bricker, N. S. Functional profile of the isolated uremic nephron. Impaired water permeability and adenylate cyclase responsiveness of the cortical collecting tubule to vasopressin. J. Clin. Invest. 61:1519, 1978.
198. Yanagawa, N.; and Fine, L. G. Intrinsic, PTH-independent phosphate (P) transport in the isolated uremic proximal tubule. Abstr. Am. Soc. Nephrol. 13:111A, 1980.
199. Yanagawa, N.; Houston, B.; and Fine, L. G. Altered parathyroid hormone (PTH) sensitivity of the uremic proximal tubule: Evidence for regulation of hormone-receptor interaction. Abstr. Am. Soc. Nephrol. 13:11A, 1980.
200. Hanley, M. J. Isolated nephron segments in a rabbit model of ischemic acute renal failure. Am. J. Physiol. 239:F17, 1980.
201. Hanley, M.; and Davidson, K. Prior mannitol and furosemide infusion in a model of ischemic acute renal failure. Am. J. Physiol. 10:F556, 1981.
202. Hanley, M. J.; and Davidson, K. Isolated nephron segments from rabbit models of obstructive nephropathy. J. Clin. Invest. 69:165, 1982.

3

Structure of the Kidney

DENNIS C. DOBYAN and RUTH ELLEN BULGER
University of Texas Health Science Center, Houston, Texas

Several new techniques such as scanning electron microscopy and transmission electron microscopy have extended our powers of observation so that morphological parameters of tissues and organs can be more precisely defined. An understanding of nephron morphology requires knowledge of the physiological or pathological state of the animals, the use of several different techniques concurrently, quantitation of morphological features so defined, and extension of the studies to the molecular level using immunological techniques or x-ray microanalysis.

The functional unit of the kidney is the urinary tubule, which is composed of two segments, the nephron and the collecting system. The nephron, derived from the metanephric blastema, includes the renal corpuscle, S_1, S_2, and S_3 segments of the proximal tubule, the various regions of the thin limb, the medullary ascending thick segment, the cortical ascending thick segment (which includes the macula densa region), and the distal convoluted tubule. The collecting system is derived from the ureteric bud and includes the initial collecting tubule, the collecting tubule in the medullary ray, and the outer and inner medullary collecting duct segments. An intermediate piece, called the connecting tubule, lies between these two parts of the urinary tubule. The connecting tubule segment has been clearly defined only in the rabbit kidney so far (1), but it will probably be shown to exist in other species as well.

Nephrons in a variety of species have been defined as superficial, midcortical, or juxtamedullary on the basis of position of the renal corpuscle in the cortex and anatomy of their postglomerular blood supply (dog [2-4]; rabbit [1]; human [3]; *Psammomys* [5]).

The loop of Henle consists of the pars recta of the proximal tubule, a thin limb segment, and the ascending thick pars recta of the distal tubule. Nephrons are also defined as long-looped or short-looped on the basis of whether their loops turn in the outer or inner medulla. In the human (3) superficial glomeruli generally give rise to short-looped nephrons, juxtamedullary glomeruli give rise to long-looped nephrons, while midcortical glomeruli can give rise to either. In humans there are about seven times more of the short-looped variety of nephron than of the long-looped (6). In certain other species such as the dog and cat, all nephrons turn in the inner medulla and, therefore, are of the long-looped variety (7). In one of these species (the cat), some of the nephrons appear to take on the morphological features characteristic of the short-looped type (1,8).

I. THE NEPHRON

A. Renal Corpuscle

The renal corpuscle is a filtration device responsible for forming an ultrafiltrate of plasma. A double-walled capsule (called Bowman's capsule) surrounds Bowman's space into which an ultrafiltrate of plasma is forced. This capsule consists of flattened parietal cells which form the outer layer, and the elaborately shaped cells of the visceral layer (podocytes) which give rise to secondary processes, called trabeculi, and tertiary processes, called pedicels (or little feet) (Figs. 1 and 2). The podocyte processes line the capillary loops and cause the formation of extensive lateral intercellular channels which provide a large surface area through which the filtrate can move. Changes in podocyte cell shape have been reported by Seiler et al. (9) after the in vivo administration of polycations to rats.

The afferent arteriole to each renal corpuscle enters the corpuscle at the vascular pole and divides to form four to six lobules. These lobules are made up of capillary loops which have a fenestrated endothelium. The capillaries then reunite to form the efferent arteriole which exits in the same region where the afferent arteriole entered. The intraglomerular mesangial cells are located at the hilar or stalk region of the capillary loops, where they occupy a position similar to smooth muscle cells or pericytes seen on other small vessels. Contraction of these cells may affect glomerular permeability. It has been shown that arginine vasopressin and angiotension II cause purified cultures of these cells to contract in vivo (10). These mesangial cells are surrounded by a material known as the mesangial matrix.

The glomerular basement membrane, which lies beneath the podocyte, is composed of a central lamina densa surrounded by two electron-lucent layers, called the lamina rara interna (adjacent to the capillary) and lamina rara externa (adjacent to the podocyte). The basement membrane contains collagenous and noncollagenous glycoproteins and proteoglycans. Several type IV and a type V (AB_2) collagens can be isolated from the glomeruli (11).

Certain other glycoproteins can be identified as well. Fibronectin, a molecule which mediates cell adhesion, was localized to the area surrounding mesangial cells (12). Laminin, another glycoprotein, was found in tubular basement membranes throughout the kidney and in the lamina rara interna and adjacent regions of the lamina densa of the glomerulus (12). Sulfated glycosaminoglycans have been shown to be concentrated in a regular lattice-like network in the glomerular basement membrane as well (13).

Numerous recent studies have shown that molecular size, charge, and hemodynamic conditions determine which of the large molecules presented to the glomerulus are filtered. Changes in these factors alter the way molecules are handled and can lead to the proteinuria seen in various renal diseases.

B. Proximal Tubule

The proximal tubule is the longest nephron segment of those located in the cortex. The lumen of the tubule is widely patent in life due to the effect of blood pressure. The proximal tubule in several species has been divided into three regions, called the S_1, S_2, and S_3 segments. It should be noted, however, that considerable species variation exists, and proximal

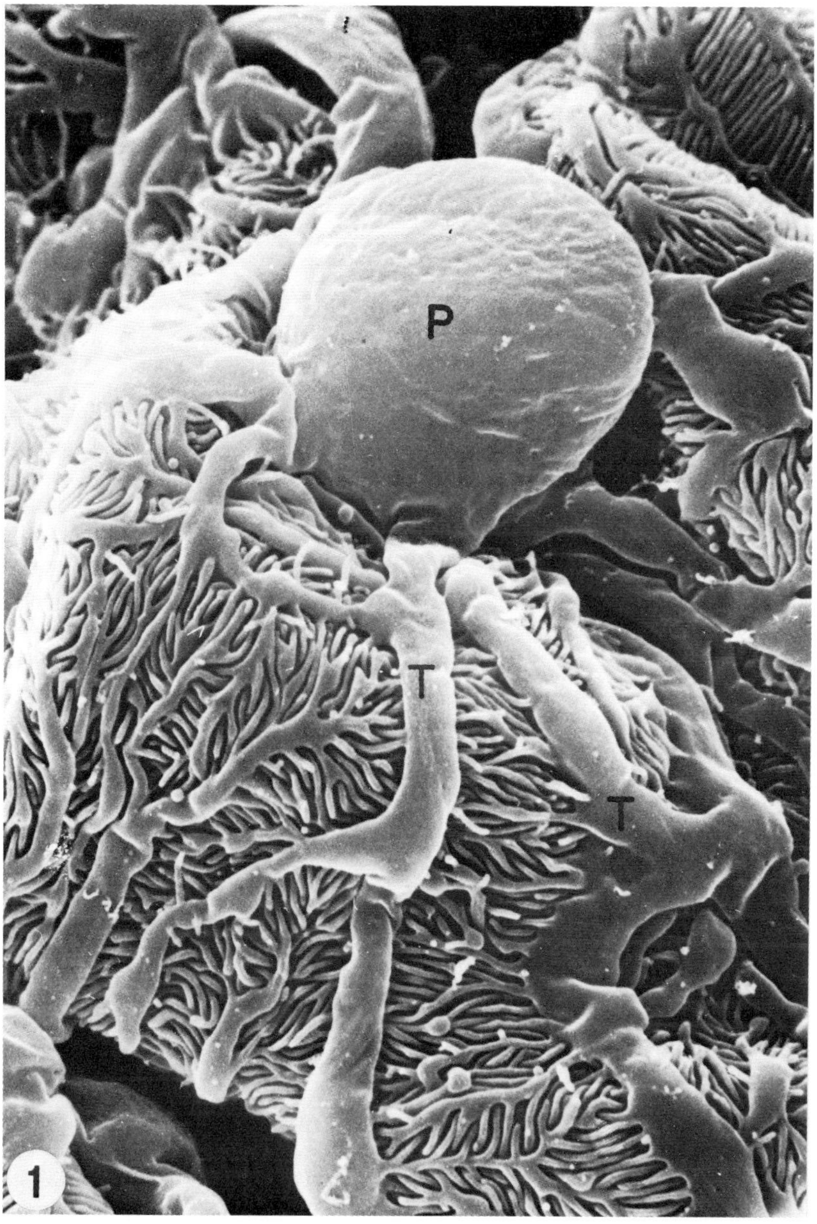

Fig. 1 Scanning electron micrograph showing a portion of the renal corpuscle from the rabbit kidney. Note the podocyte (P) with its long cytoplasmic extensions known as trabeculae (T). These processes or trabeculae give rise to multiple interdigitating pedicels or foot processes (arrows). X 8300.

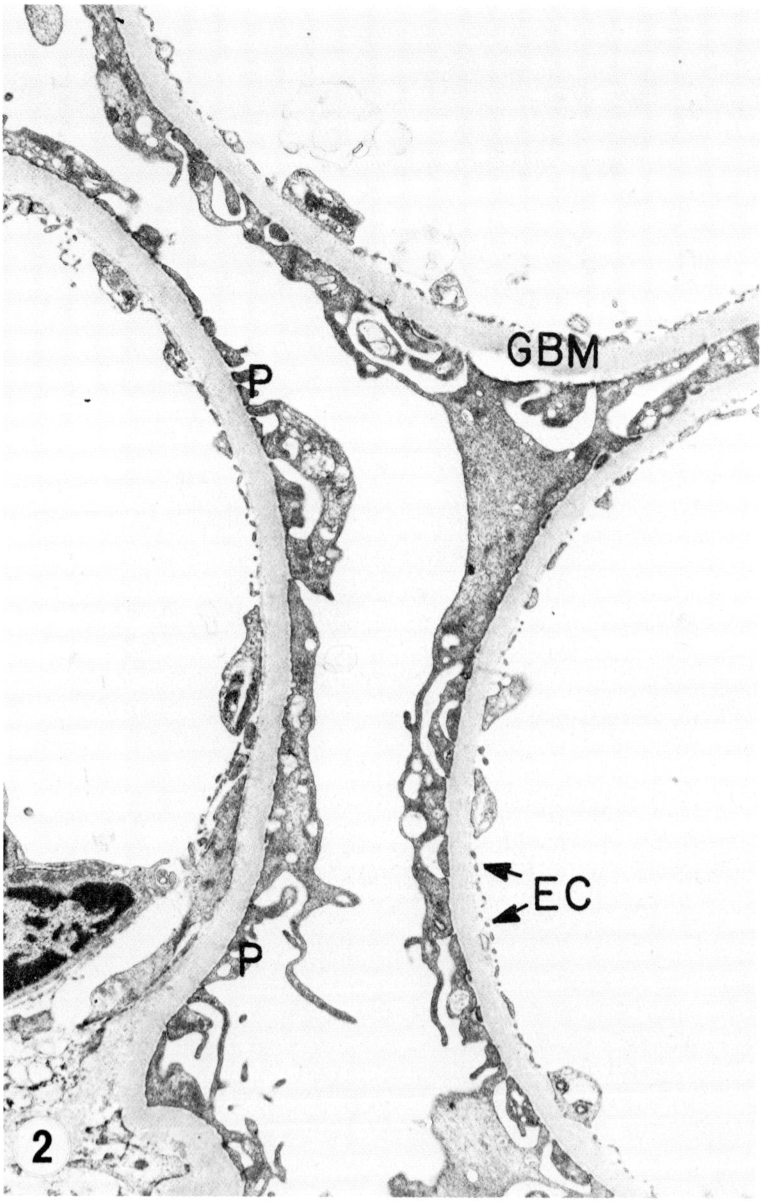

Fig. 2 Transmission electron micrograph showing the glomerular capillary loops from a human kidney. Note the pedicels (P), the glomerular basement membrane (GBM), and the capillary endothelium (EC). × 7400.

tubular structure has not been thoroughly described in humans. The proximal tubule is also divided into the pars convoluta (or convoluted part) and the pars recta (or straight part). The convoluted portion consists of the entire S_1 region and the first part of the S_2 region (Fig. 3 and 4). The pars recta, located in the medullary ray and the outer stripe region of the outer medulla comprises the last part of the S_2 segment and the entire S_3 segment. The pars recta segment comprises the first part of the loop of Henle.

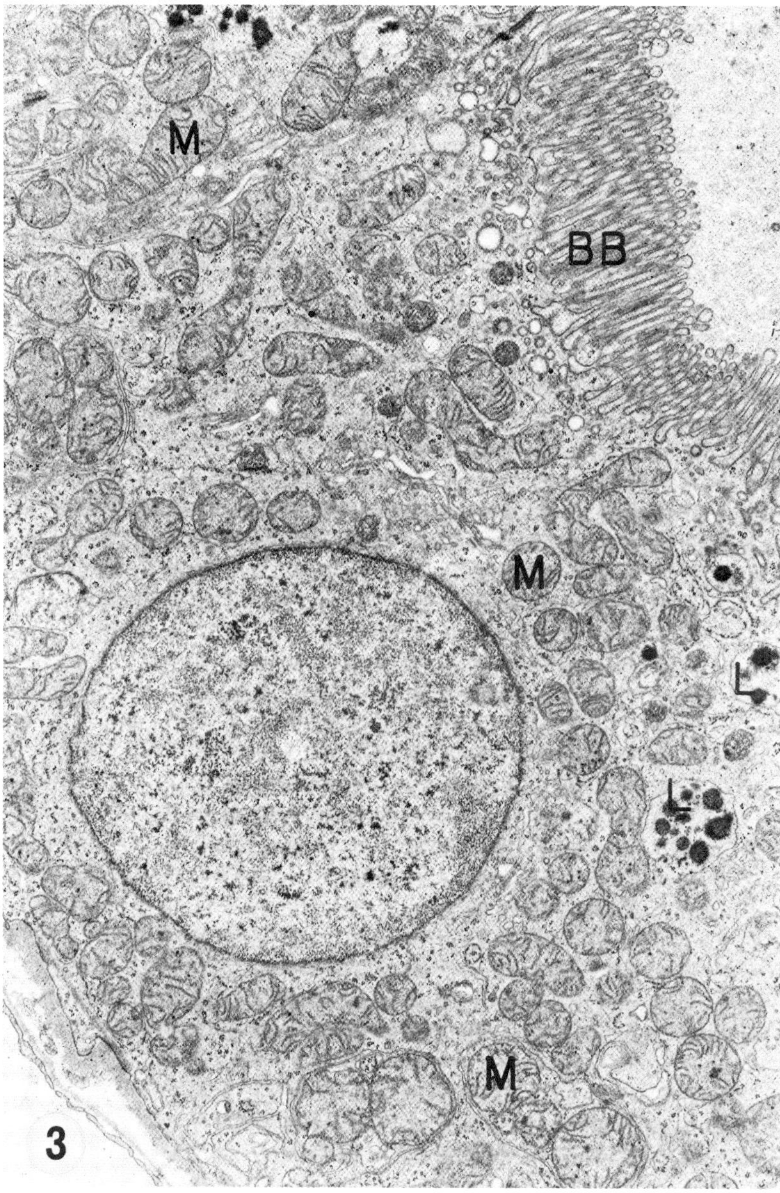

Fig. 3 Transmission electron micrograph showing the proximal convoluted tubule from a human kidney. Note the brush border on the luminal surface (BB), the lysosomes containing dense material (L), and the numerous mitochondria (M). X 7800.

Maunsbach (14) clearly describes the difference in the segments of the rat proximal tubule. In the S_1 segment of the proximal tubule, the cells are tall and are characterized by extensive lateral interdigitating processes which form a system of extensive lateral intercellular channels. These channels appear to play some role in isosmotic sodium chloride transport (see Ch. 2). The cells in this segment contain abundant mitochondria located within the lateral cell processes adjacent to the lateral cell membrane. The mitochondria presu-

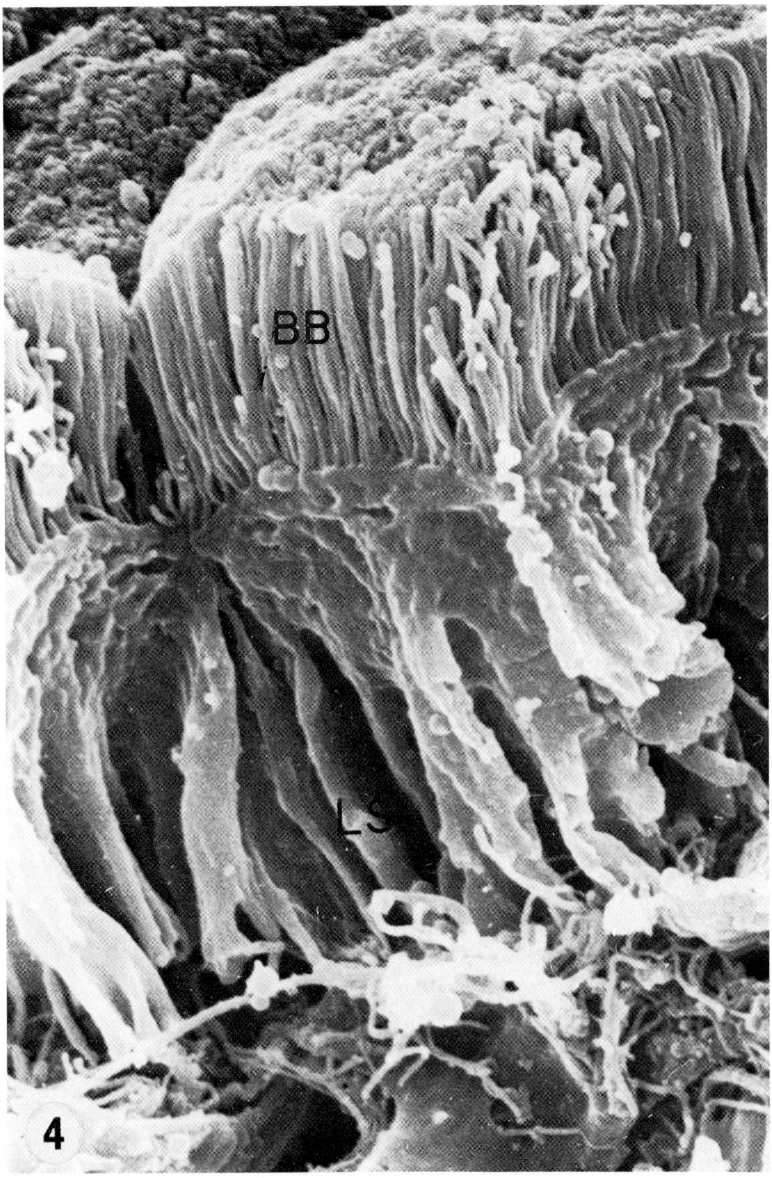

Fig. 4 Scanning electron micrograph showing the proximal convoluted tubule from the rat kidney. Note the brush border (BB) and the extensive lateral intercellular spaces (LS) extending from these cells. X 4700.

mably provide the adenosine triphosphate (ATP) utilized by the sodium-potassium ATPase localized in the lateral cell membranes. These cells possess a prominent microvillus (brush) border which lines the entire apical region of the cells and stains positively with the periodic acid-Schiff's reaction. Each of these microvilli contains a core or bundle of actin filaments. Specific disaccharidases, maltase, alkaline phosphatase, 5'-nucleotidase, and certain ATPases are associated with these microvilli. The increased surface area which is formed by these numerous fingerlike processes presumably has some function with respect to sugar and amino acid reabsorption as well as other absorptive functions. The apical cytoplasm of the cells in the S_1 segment of the proximal convoluted tubule is filled with a prominent endocytic apparatus which consists of apical tubular invaginations, vesicles, and large vacuoles. These cells contain numerous lysosomes which can be either electron dense or electron lucent. The endocytotic apparatus and the numerous cytoplasmic lysosomes are involved in the uptake and subsequent digestion of filtered protein. An overload in this system causes the formation of hyaline droplets in the proximal tubular cells seen in patients with proteinuria.

The cells of the S_2 segment of the proximal tubule perform similar functions and yet a number of fine morphological differences exist between the two segments. Cells from the S_2 region are shorter in height than those of the S_1 segment and these cells have decreased lateral cellular interdigitations. They contain fewer mitochondria. The lysosomes in this segment tend to be relatively electron dense.

The S_1 and S_2 cells of the pars convoluta are held together by shallow tight junctions which can be penetrated by colloidal lanthanum (15,16). The tight junctions and the lateral intercellular spaces form low resistance shunt pathways which are of considerable physiological importance in fluid and electrolyte reabsorption. Desmosomes are only infrequently observed in mammalian proximal tubules. Gap junctions, however, are present along the lateral cell borders (17).

The pars recta (or straight part) of most of the proximal tubules begins in the medullary ray and traverses the outer stripe of the outer medulla. In the case of juxtamedullary nephrons, the pars recta runs directly into and traverses the outer stripe. The pars recta consists of the last part of the S_2 region of the proximal tubule and all of the S_3 segment of the proximal tubule. There appears to be an abrupt transition between the S_2 and S_3 segments. The cells of the S_3 region are shorter in height and less elaborate in shape compared to those of the S_1 and S_2 segments, indicating less involvement with active sodium chloride transport by this segment (Fig. 5). These cells have decreased lateral cellular interdigitations, a less prominent endocytic apparatus and fewer rounder mitochondria. The microvilli lining the apical region of the cells are less well developed in this region in humans. Cells in the S_3 segment also have abundant large microbodies and numerous profiles of smooth-surfaced endoplasmic reticulum. Although the pars recta has been thought to secrete certain organic acids, such as *p*-aminohippuric acid, it has recently been shown that the S_2 region is more active than the S_3 region in this secretory process.

C. Thin Limb of Henle's Loop

Four specific regions of differing morphology are seen in the thin limb of long- and short-looped nephrons (Figs. 6-8). The thin limb structure in the human has not been studied in detail but the cells are generally thicker (Fig. 6). In species which have been well studied (such as rat, mouse, *Psammomys*) a descending thin limb of short-looped nephrons has been identified. These thin limbs generally run within the vascular bundles in the outer medulla (rat [18]; mouse [19]; *Psammomys* [20]). In certain other species, however, they run in the interbundle region (hamster [21]; rabbit [1]; cat [8]). The second region which has been identified is the upper (outer medullary) segment of the thin limb of long-looped nephrons and it traverses the inner stripe region of the outer medulla. The third region is the lower (inner medullary) descending thin limb region of long-looped nephrons which traverses the inner medulla (Fig. 8). Finally, the final region identified is the ascending thin limb of long-looped nephrons (Fig. 8). The morphology of certain regions (the descending

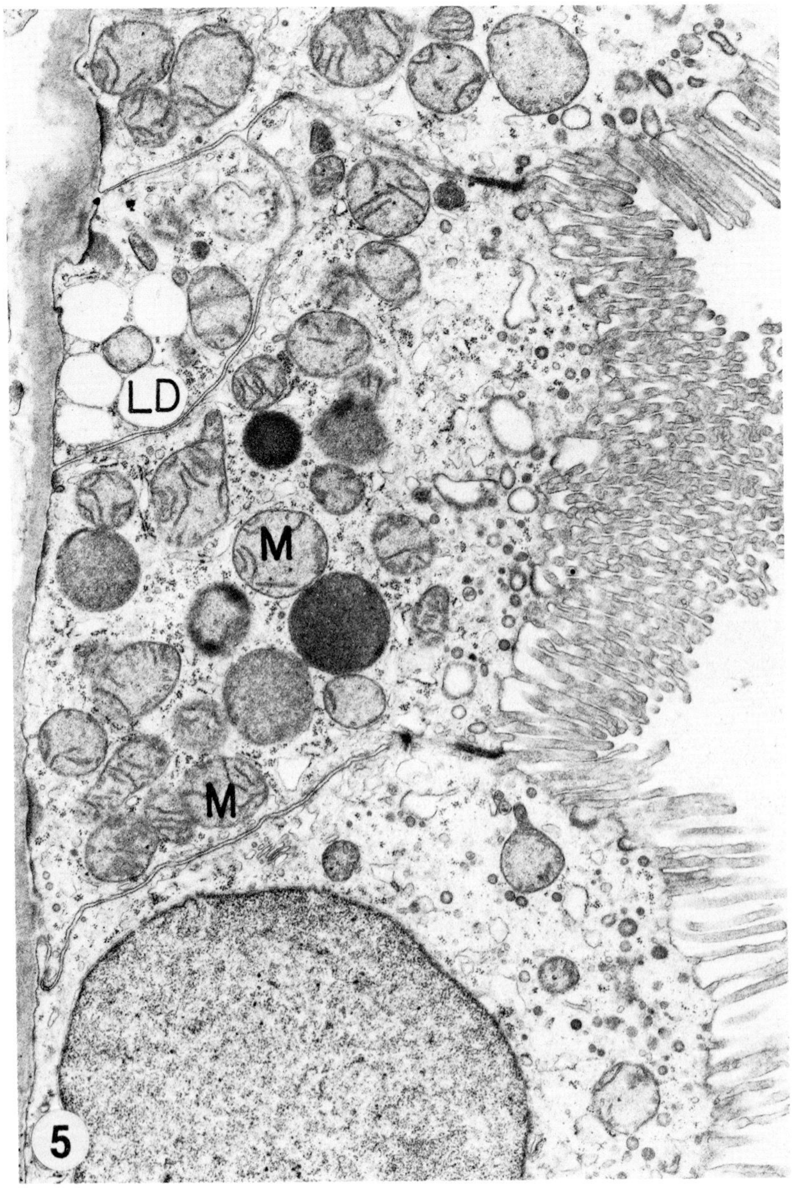

Fig. 5 Transmission electron micrograph of the pars recta segment of the proximal tubule from a human kidney. The cells are much more simplified and box shaped and the mitochondria (M) are fewer in number. A few lipid droplets are seen in the basal aspect of the cell (LD). X 11000.

thin limb of short-looped nephrons and the ascending thin limb of long-looped nephrons) are similar in morphology to the corresponding region in most species studied (1,22). However, the descending regions of long-looped nephrons vary in morphology in different species, being highly specialized in species which can excrete highly concentrated urine.

The descending thin limb of short-looped nephrons has a small luminal diameter and the tubule is generally lined by flat noninterdigitating epithelial cells with few organelles, indi-

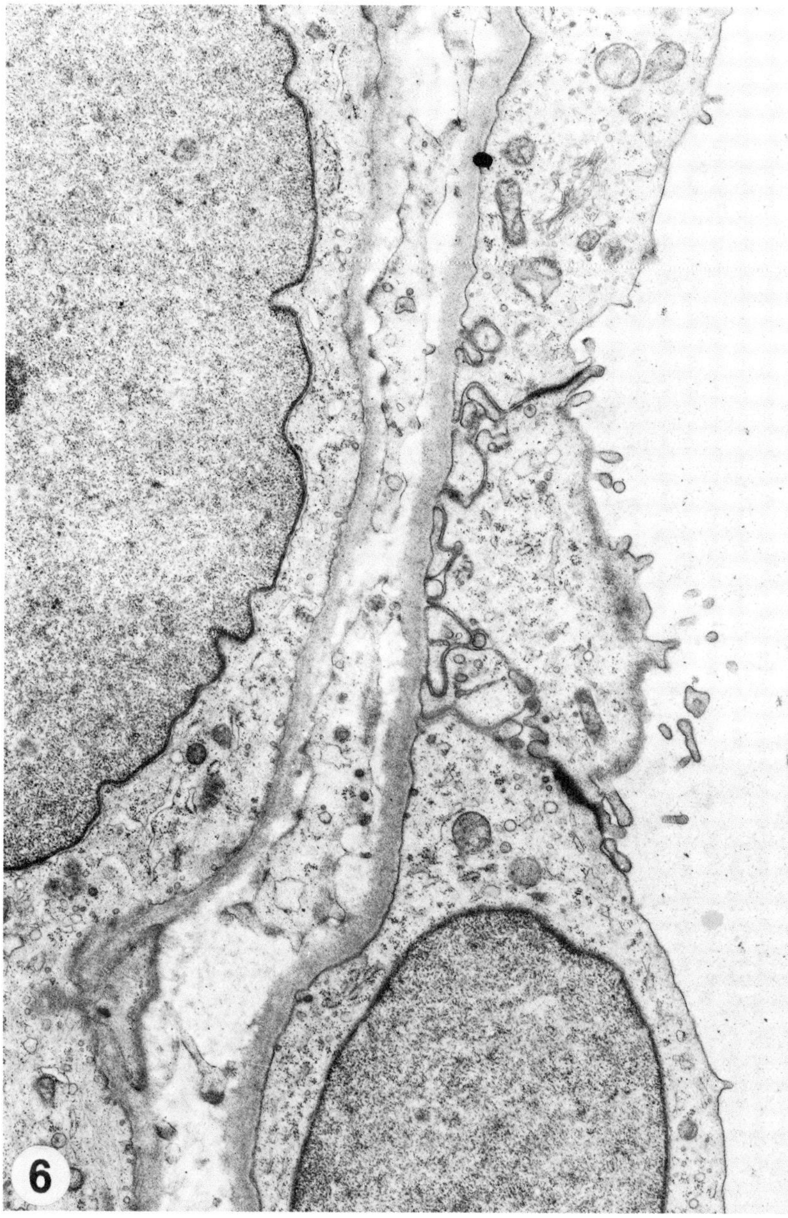

Fig. 6 Transmission electron micrograph of a thin limb of Henle from the human kidney. The cells are very simple in shape and contain few cellular organelles. Since a thorough study of the human thin limb has not been performed the exact region shown here is not possible to identify. X 9700.

cating little machinery for active transport. The cells have a deep tight junction with a high number of junctional fibrils (rabbit [23]; rat [24]), perhaps explaining the low permeability to sodium chloride seen in this segment. Freeze fracture studies of the cell membrane of this segment in the rat showed only a small number of intramembranous particles (24), consistent with the low transepithelial water flux demonstrated for this segment. It, therefore,

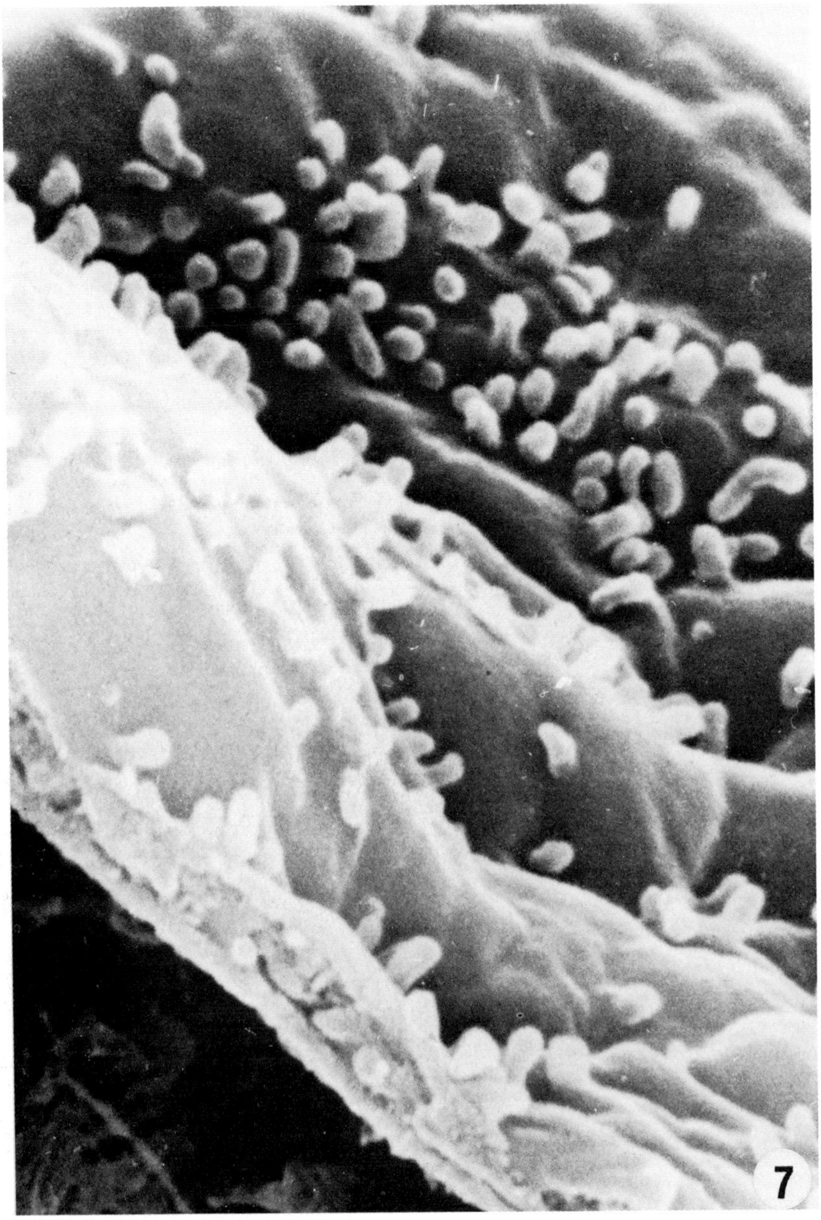

Fig. 7 Scanning electron micrograph showing a thin limb of Henle from a rabbit kidney. This epithelium is extremely thin and has a few scattered microvilli on the luminal surface. X 14400.

has been postulated (20) that recycling of substances such as urea into the lumen of short-looped nephrons from both the ascending venous vasa recta and the pelvic fornix might enhance the medullary accumulation of urea (25).

The morphology of the upper region of the descending thin limb of long-looped nephrons shows considerable morphological variation among species. In species which can excrete a highly concentrated urine such as rat (18,22) and *Psammomys* (26) the epithelium has

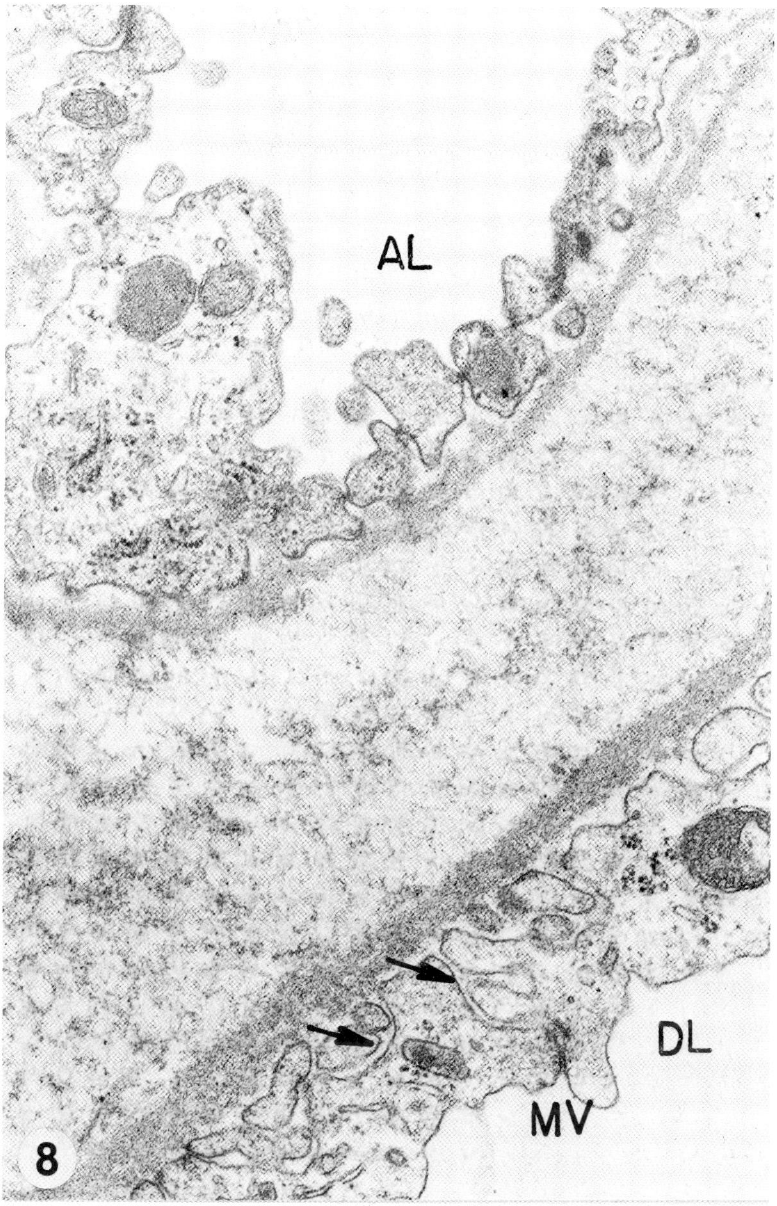

Fig. 8 Transmission electron micrograph showing two types of thin limbs of Henle from a dog kidney. An ascending thin limb of Henle (AL) is shown in the upper portion of the plate. This segment is characterized by numerous cellular profiles, a consequence of the elaborate shape of this region of the tubule. A descending thin limb of Henle (DL) is shown in the lower portion of the micrograph. Note the presence of apical microvilli (MV) and basolateral interdigitations (arrows). X 34000.

numerous mitochondria and microvilli as well as many basal lateral cell projections. In the rabbit (1), however, the epithelium of this region has a simple structure with tight junctions of intermediate lengths. In the rat (24), this upper descending region of the thin limb has a shallow tight junction usually composed of a single fibril which sometimes appears as strands of separated particles. The cells have an extremely complex shape and, therefore, have an elaborate and extensive paracellular pathway. In addition, the cell membranes in the upper descending thin limb have a very high density of intramembranous particles when compared to the other regions of thin limb (24). As the thin limb of the long-looped nephrons descends into the medulla a simpler morphology is seen with respect to cell shape and organelle concentration (Fig. 8). This may relate to the fact that this region does not permit the free passage of sodium chloride across the epithelium. Schwartz et al. (24) have shown that the tight junctions in this region in the rat have a relatively high number of junctional fibrils. The number of intramembranous particles seen is reduced from that found in the outer region of the descending thin limb but is still higher than that seen in the cells of short-looped nephrons.

The ascending thin limb segment of long-looped nephrons (Fig. 8) is similar in all species studied. The epithelium is highly interdigitated and held together by shallow tight junctions. Microvilli are not seen frequently in this region and Schwartz et al. (24) reported a mean of slightly over one junctional fibril in the tight junction. This fibril was continuous and much thicker than that seen in the upper descending portion. As in the descending limb, the elaborate cell shape of this segment creates a large lateral intercellular pathway. However, the cells themselves contain few organelles. The large paracellular pathway might relate to the proposed function of passive efflux of sodium chloride for this region of the thin limb.

D. Distal Tubule

The distal tubule of the mammalian nephron has traditionally been divided into the ascending thick portion of Henle's loop, the macula densa, and the distal convoluted tubule. Recent anatomical and physiological studies suggest that this system of nomenclature is no longer acceptable. The distal tubule is more correctly separated into a medullary ascending thick limb (MAT) (Figs. 9 and 11), a cortical ascending thick limb (CAT) (Fig. 10), and the distal convoluted tubule (DCT) (Fig. 12). According to this scheme, the MAT and the CAT would comprise the thick ascending limb of the loop of Henle and the macula densa would be a specialized region within the CAT segment.

The MAT segment begins at the junction of the inner and outer medulla. It travels through the inner and outer stripes of the outer medulla and eventually enters the cortical medullary rays where it converts to the CAT portion. The epithelium which lines the MAT is composed of a homogeneous population of cells whose height varies from 10-15 μm, according to the species (1,27,28). The luminal surface of these cells is generally smooth, but a few stubby microvilli are present. These cells are joined to one another by relatively shallow tight junctions (0.1-0.2 μm [1]) which have been shown to be freely permeable to colloidal lanthanum (15). Characteristically, there is the extensive interdigitation between these cells, with the cellular processes extending from the basal aspect of the cell toward its apex. The extent to which these processes approach the luminal surface varies with the particular species. The most conspicuous feature of these cells are the long, rod-shaped mitochondria which lie within the cellular processes oriented in an apical-basal direction. As the MAT courses through the outer medulla, it undergoes a gradual decrease in cell height and converts to the CAT in the medullary rays.

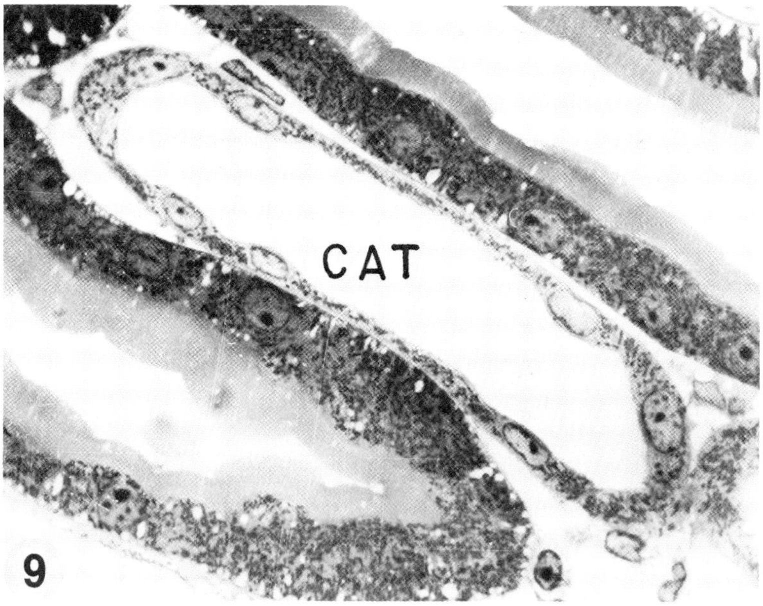

Fig. 9 A light micrograph showing the cortical ascending thick limb of Henle (CAT) from a rat kidney. It is positioned between two S_3 segments of the proximal tubule. Toluidine blue, X 800.

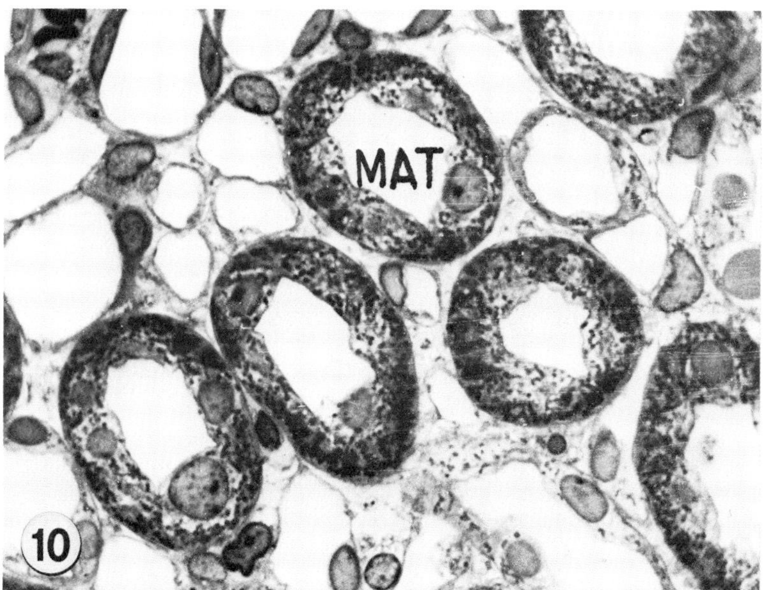

Fig. 10 A light micrograph showing the medullary ascending thick limb of Henle (MAT) from a rat kidney. Compare Figs. 9 and 10 which represent an equivalent magnification to appreciate the difference in cell height between the CAT and MAT segments. Toluidine blue, X 800.

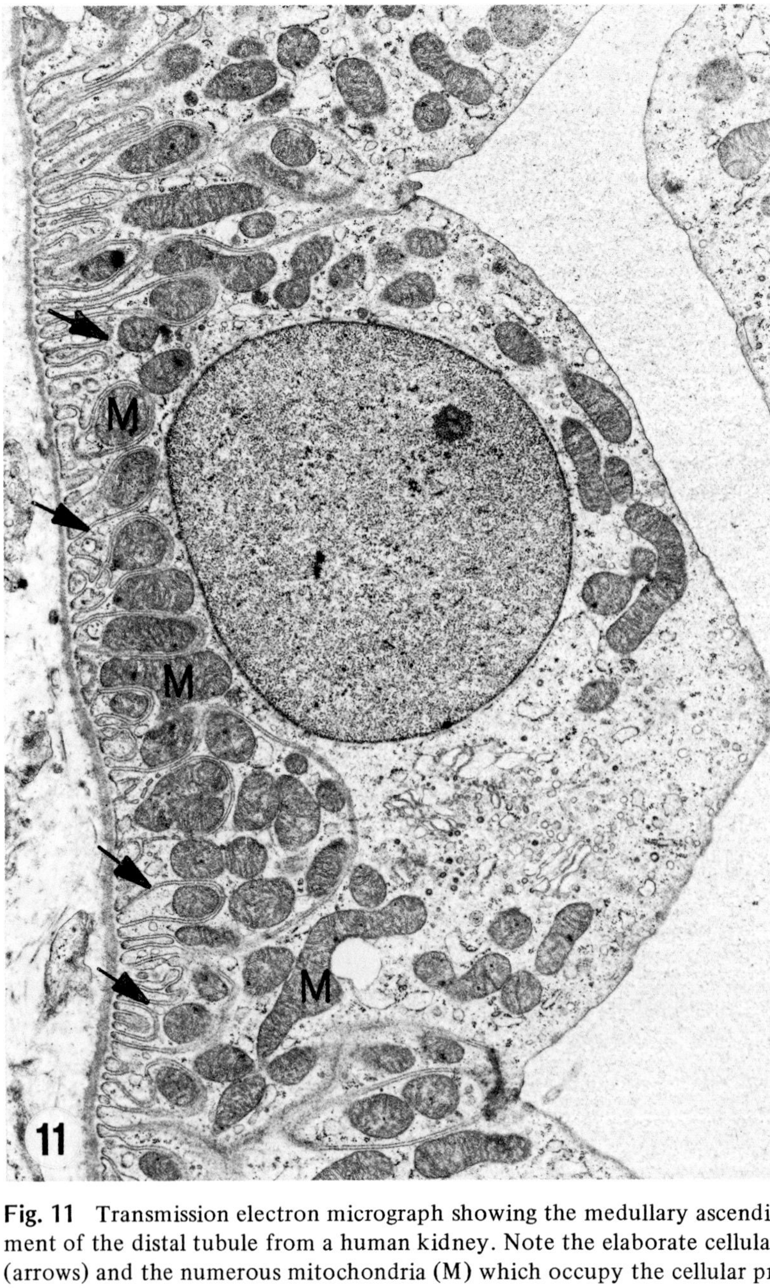

Fig. 11 Transmission electron micrograph showing the medullary ascending thick segment of the distal tubule from a human kidney. Note the elaborate cellular interdigitation (arrows) and the numerous mitochondria (M) which occupy the cellular processes. X 9300.

The CAT, while structurally similar to the MAT, is lower in height and the cells have a more simplified shape. This segment of the distal tubule is the thinnest portion ranging in thickness from 3-6 μm in the rat (28) to as low as 1-2 μm in the rabbit (1). The cells still show extensive interdigitation, but the cellular processes are much less organized. The mitochondria are fewer in number and the nucleus has a flattened appearance because of the marked decrease in cellular height. As the CAT travels through the medullary ray, it approaches its parent glomerulus and gives rise to the specialized plaque of cells known as the

via the connecting tubule into the cortical collecting duct. In the midcortical and juxtamedullary nephrons, the connecting tubule begins a short distance before joining the arcades. The arcades are considered to be connecting tubules. The connecting tubule is composed of two distinct types of cells which include the intercalated cell (see below) and the connecting tubule cell. The connecting tubule cell is somewhat similar to the principal cell which is found throughout the collecting duct system (Fig. 13). These cells have a pale

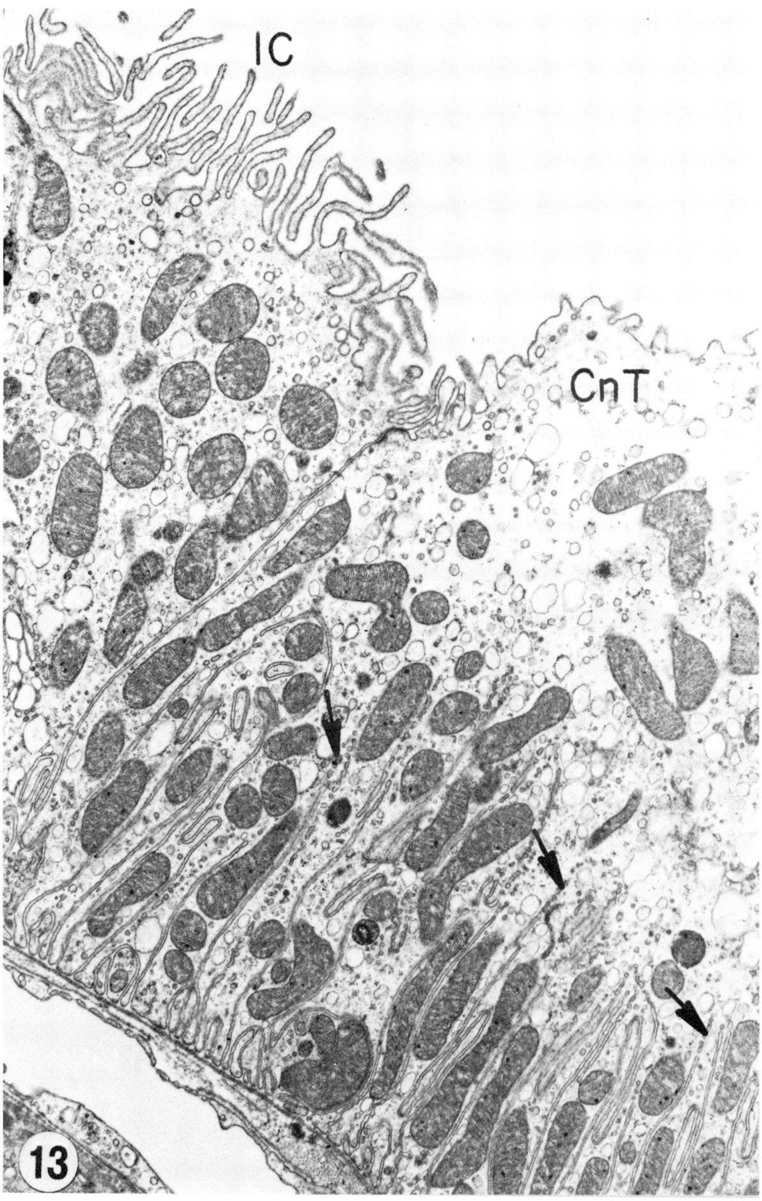

Fig. 13 Transmission electron micrograph showing the connecting tubule from a human kidney. Note the intercalated cell (IC) with its very elaborate luminal surface (microplicae). A connecting tubule cell (CnT) is also apparent and is characterized by numerous true basal infoldings (arrows) which reach to varying distances toward the cell apex. Mitochondria (M) are seen lying between the basal infoldings. X 7300.

cytoplasm, a centrally placed nucleus, and contain mitochondria scattered throughout the cytoplasm. The luminal surface of these cells is generally smooth and the cells are joined together by relatively deep tight junctions. The most significant feature of these cells are the extensive true infoldings of the basal cell membrane. These infoldings penetrate to all regions of the cell and occasionally reach the cell apex (1).

While a clearly defined connecting tubule segment exists for the rabbit kidney, this does not appear to be the case for most other species which have been examined. In the rat (28, 31), the mouse (1), and in man (29,30), the transition from DCT to collecting duct appears to be a gradual transformation. Close examination of the region of transition in the rat and in man (Fig. 13) clearly reveals, however, the presence of connecting tubule cells (Bulger and Dobyan, unpublished observations). The connecting tubule cells of the rat and man generally appear to have much more elaborate basal infoldings than the rabbit. This suggests that a connecting tubule probably also exists for most other species, but it is not as well defined.

The origin of the connecting tubule is still a matter of controversy. Some investigators believe it is derived from the metanephric blastema and, therefore, consider it part of the DCT (6,49). Others hold that it is derived from the ureteric bud and rightfully belongs to the collecting duct system (1). The presence of the intercalated cell in this segment and the close similarity of the connecting tubule cell to the principal cell argue in favor of the ureteric bud origin. It is apparent that detailed studies of this region of transition must be performed for species other than the rabbit before its true significance is understood.

F. Collecting Ducts

The mammalian collecting duct system has been extensively investigated in recent years. It has gained increasing importance as the final regulator of normal fluid and electrolyte balance. The collecting duct system is the primary site of action of ADH and plays a pivotal role in countercurrent exchange and urinary concentration. It is important in sodium and chloride transport and normal acid-base balance and in the control of potassium homeostasis. It has become obvious that the collecting duct system can no longer be envisioned as merely a passive conduit for the elimination of urine.

The mammalian collecting duct system is generally divided into a cortical, medullary, and papillary portion. The collecting duct begins in the cortex where it is continuous with either the connecting tubule of the superficial nephrons or the arcades of the midcortical and juxtamedullary nephrons. The collecting ducts enter the medullary ray and travel through the outer medulla. They begin to fuse after entering the inner medulla and eventually give rise to the large papillary collecting ducts (ducts of Bellini).

Two main types of cells are found throughout the collecting duct system (Figs. 14 and 15). The principal or light cell is the most numerous type and is prevalent along the entire collecting duct tree. These cells have a relatively pale cytoplasm and contain a few oval mitochondria. The cells are joined by a fairly long tight junction consistent with their high electrical resistance. A characteristic feature of the principal cell is the numerous true infoldings of the basal cell membrane. These infoldings are best developed in the cortical portion of the collecting duct and become more simplified in the medullary and papillary regions. The luminal surface of the principal cell is studded with short stubby microvilli. These cells gradually increase in height as the collecting duct travels through the outer medulla (Fig. 15) and reach their greatest height in the papillary region.

The second cell type is the intercalated cell, which is also frequently referred to as the dark cell. These cells are almost exclusively confined to the cortical and outer medullary portions of the collecting duct system. It has been estimated that the intercalated cell

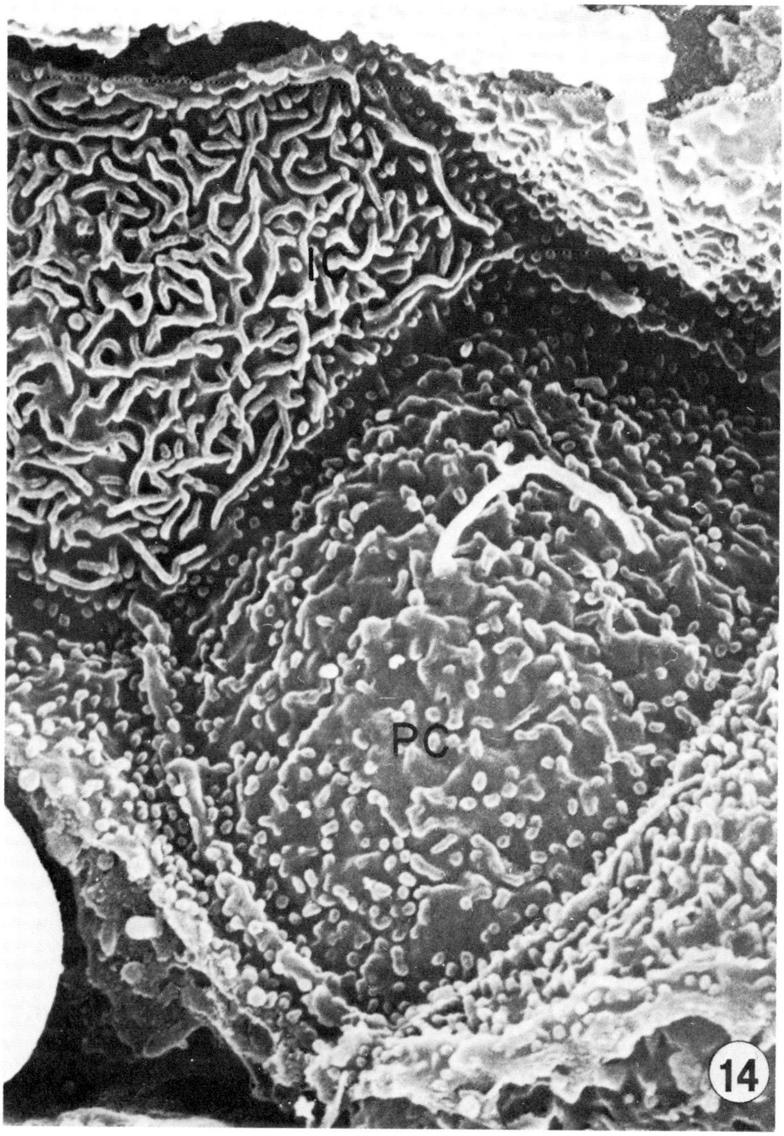

Fig. 14 Scanning electron micrograph showing the two types of cells which are present in the collecting duct system from a rabbit kidney. Note the intercalated cell (IC) with its elaborate luminal surface (microplicae). A principal cell (PC) contains a single cilium and possesses a few stubby microvilli on the luminal surface. X 12000.

accounts for about 33% of the cell population in the cortical collecting duct, about 50% in the outer medullary collecting duct of the rabbit (1), and from 24 to 40% of the cell population in the cortex and 18 to 22% in the outer medulla of the rat kidney (50-52). The intercalated cell is best appreciated for the deep cytoplasmic density which is a consequence of the numerous ribosomes and mitochondria. The luminal surface is covered by microvilli, microplicae (which are ridgelike extensions of the apical cell membrane), or combinations of the two patterns.

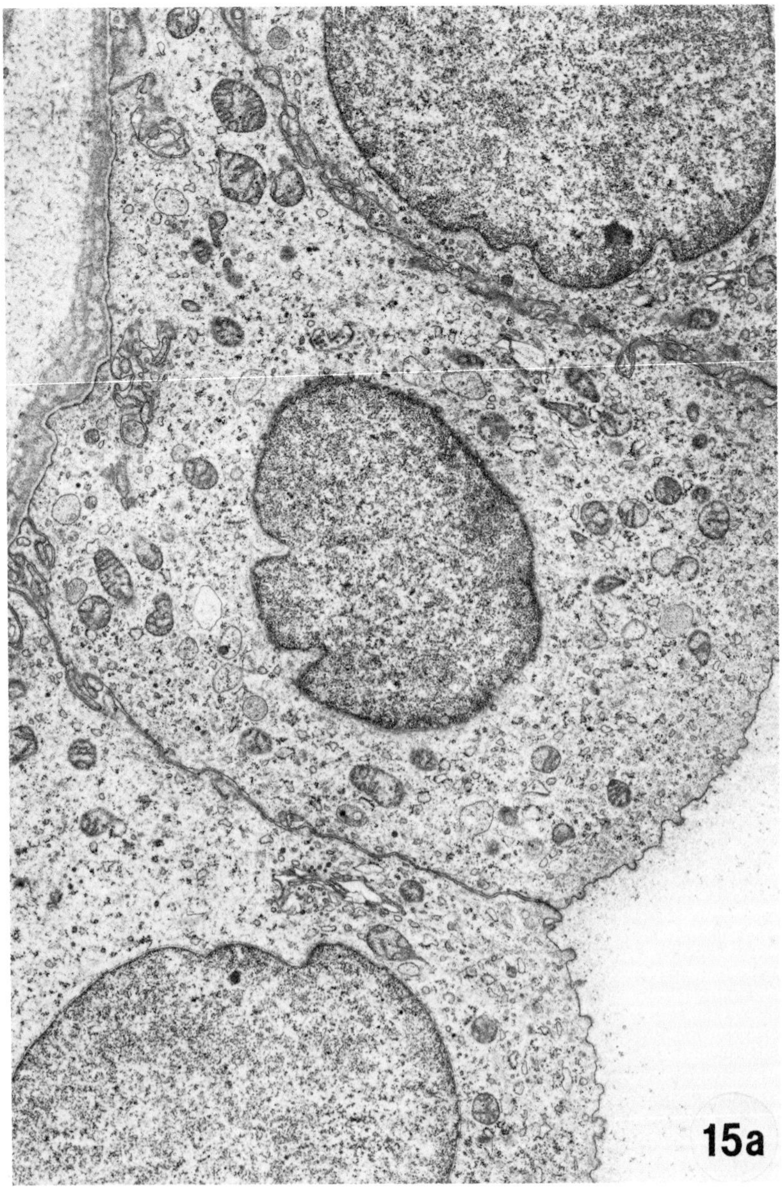

Fig. 15a Transmission electron micrograph showing the inner medullary collecting tubule from a human kidney. These cells are principal cells and have a pale cytoplasm with few cellular organelles such as mitochondria. X 7000.

It has been suggested that more than one type of intercalated cell exists in the mammalian collecting duct. Kaissling and Kriz (1) have described a "black" and "gray" manifestation of the intercalated cell on the basis of differences in cytoplasmic density and cytoplasmic components in the rabbit collecting duct. The gray cell type had a lighter appearance and contained fewer mitochondria and ribosomes. Numerous cytoplasmic vesicles of two main types were almost exclusively characteristic of the gray cell type. These vesicles were either spherical with coated invaginated outer membranes or they presented as flattened vesicles

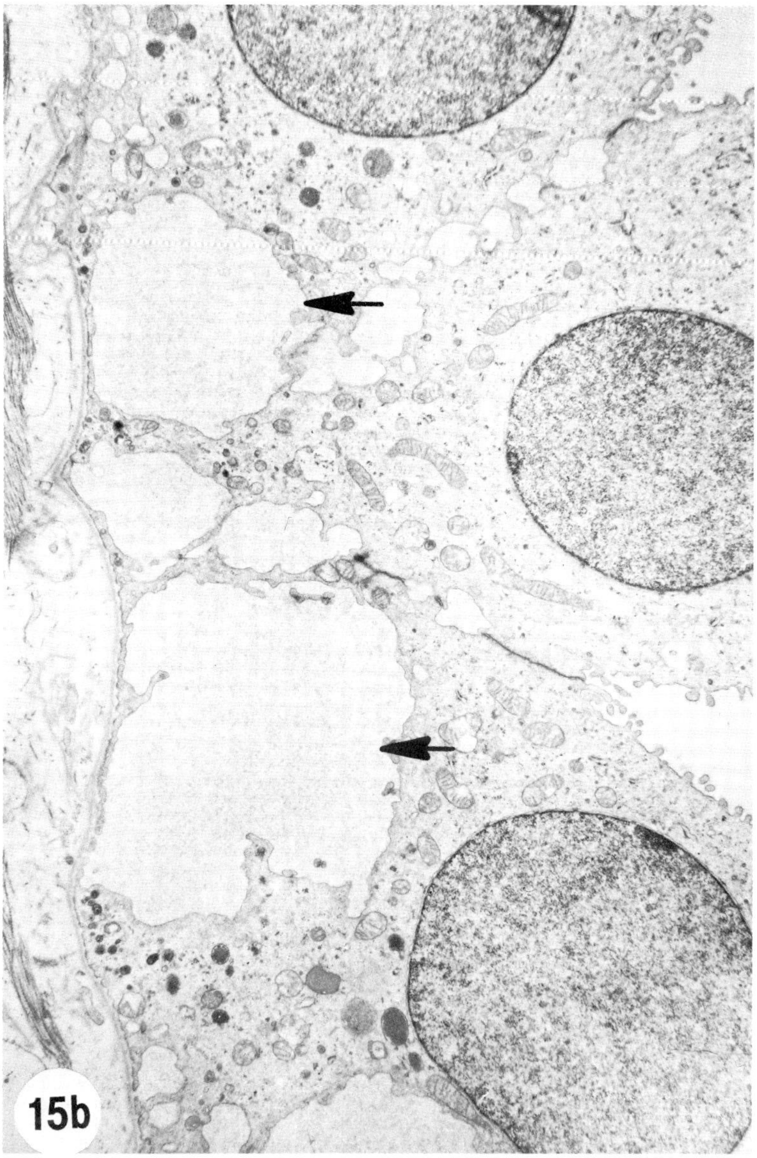

Fig. 15b Transmission electron micrograph showing a medullary collecting tubule of a Brattleboro rat (hereditary diabetes insipitus) after the administration of ADH. Note the large and swollen basal and lateral cell spaces (arrows). X 6000.

which were often piled up in the apical region of the cell. Further evidence supporting two types of intercalated cells came from the freeze-fracture studies of Pricam et al. (53) and Stetson et al. (52). They examined the luminal membrane features as well as the vesicles which are characteristic of the intercalated cell and identified two distinct patterns. Type I cells contained a high density of rod-shaped particles associated with the luminal membrane. Stetson et al. (52) also described a Type II cell which did not possess rod-shaped particles in the luminal membrane, but did contain those particles within the numerous cytoplasmic vesicles. These observations are consistent with the viewpoint that the intercalated cell can exist in several different morphological varieties.

A question which has frequently surfaced in the literature is whether the intercalated cell and the principal cell are two distinct cell types or actually represent the same cell line. This controversy arose after several investigators (54-56) reported an increase in the total number of intercalated cells in response to changes in either acid-base balance or potassium balance. These observations, which relied heavily on scanning electron microscopic observations, suggested that the intercalated cell was actually a functional modification of the principal cell. In the past few years, however, convincing evidence against this theory has emerged suggesting that the intercalated cell represents a distinct and constant cell population which can express differing phenotypic appearances. Hansen and colleagues (50) have quantitated the number of intercalated cells under well-defined conditions of acute respiratory acidosis, acute metabolic alkalosis, chronic metabolic acidosis, and hypo- and hyperkalemia. They found no change in the total number of intercalated cells in any of the physiological conditions studied. Stanton et al. (51) and Stetson et al. (52) also failed to demonstrate any difference in intercalated cell numbers after chronic potassium deprivation, although they did report some structural modifications. These recent studies strongly argue in favor of the intercalated cell as a distinct cell type. It seems plausible that the earlier reports of changes in intercalated cell numbers might have been the result of failure to identify the different varieties which have been recently described.

The collecting duct plays a role in the urinary concentrating mechanism and in controlling the excretion of electrolytes. Recent studies have attempted to ascribe functions to the cell types which line the collecting duct. The principal cell is generally considered to be the site of action of ADH. Several investigators (30,45,57) have shown that the epithelial cells lining the collecting duct swell and the intracellular spaces dilate in response to ADH consistent with bulk water flow across the epithelium (Fig. 15a). Harmanci and co-workers (58, 59) have reported that ADH increases the incidence of intramembrane particle clusters in the luminal membrane of the papillary collecting duct in a dose related fashion. These particle clusters have been related to increased water permeability in other types of epithelium. The principal cell also appears to function in the transport of potassium. Dramatic increases in the basolateral membrane surface density have been reported after potassium adaptation (51,60) or after treatment with agents known to increase potassium secretion along the collecting duct (61). This increase in basolateral surface density might be related to an increase in the number of potassium pump sites which would enhance potassium secretion (60).

The intercalated cell on the other hand may be involved in potassium reabsorption. It has been repeatedly demonstrated that under conditions of potassium deprivation there is enhanced reabsorption of potassium along the nephron. Since changes in intercalated cell structure have been reported after potassium deprivation (50-52,54,55), it seems possible that they may play a role in potassium reabsorption. Finally, several histochemical studies have demonstrated significant carbonic anhydrase activity in the cortical and outer medullary collecting ducts of the human, rat, mouse, and rabbit (62-64). The highest activity was found in the intercalated cell, suggesting a further role in either hydrogen ion secretion or bicarbonate reabsorption.

II. INJURY TO THE KIDNEY

The mammalian nephron is particularly susceptible to a wide variety of pathological agents. The structural integrity of the renal tubule can be compromised in response to ischemic events or nephrotoxic insults. The fact that the kidney received 20-25% of the total cardiac output and yet makes up less than 1% of the total body weight probably accounts for this great sensitivity.

Ischemic or nephrotoxic insults initiate a fairly consistent pattern of cell injury in the kidney. The general pattern of cellular injury has been extensively documented by several investigators (65). After the cell is subjected to an injury, subtle alterations in cellular morphology become apparent. The earliest changes which are identifiable include dilatation of the endoplasmic reticulum and clumping of the nuclear chromatin. As the injury progresses, cell swelling occurs and bleblike extensions of the cell membrane are frequently observed. The mitochondria initially condense and then also begin to undergo swelling. These early changes reflect aberrations in metabolic homeostasis with altered cell-volume regulation. If the insult is removed at this time, either the cells recover completely or they enter into a new but altered steady state. If the insult persists, however, the cells enter a stage of irreversible injury and progress to necrosis (Figs. 16 and 17). Cell swelling will continue until the membranes rupture. The mitochondria undergo high amplitude swelling and contain flocculent matrical densities (Fig. 16). Late in the process of cell injury, the lysosomes lose their structural integrity and begin to release their full complement of hydrolytic enzymes. This signals the beginning of autolysis. Complete disruption of cellular membranes and karyolysis will occur marking the terminal stages of lethal cell injury (Fig. 17).

Since the mammalian nephron contains heterogeneous segments, each with distinct physiological and morphological characteristics, it is not surprising that ischemic or toxic insults affect specific sites along the renal tubule. The proximal tubule (usually the pars

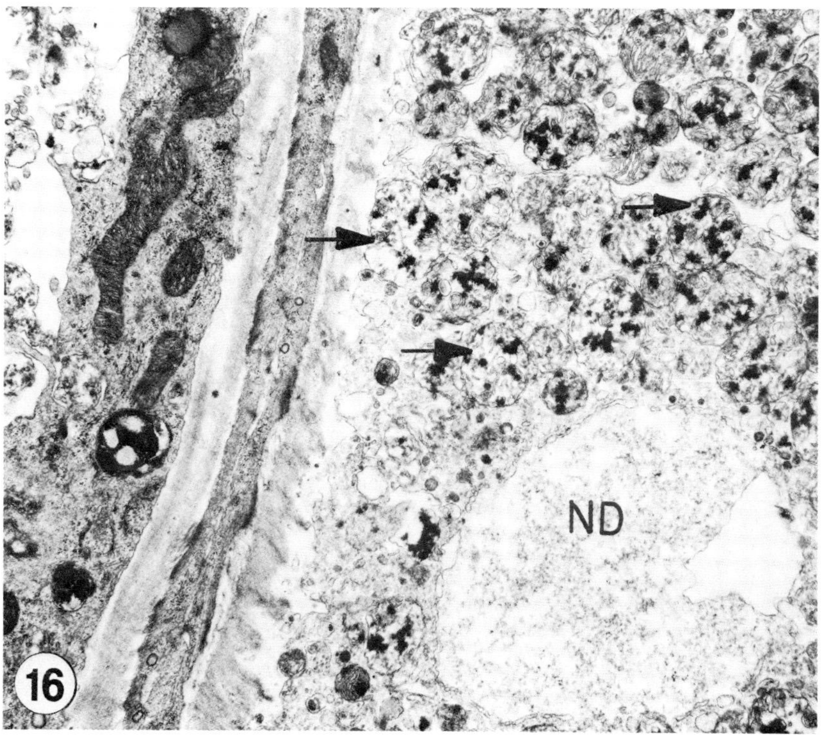

Fig. 16 Transmission electron micrograph from an animal with mercuric chloride-induced acute renal failure showing one proximal tubule containing only necrotic debris (ND) with swollen mitochondria which contain flocculent densities (arrows). The proximal tubule on the left shows an altered tubular cell in the process of relining an injured tubule. X 5600.

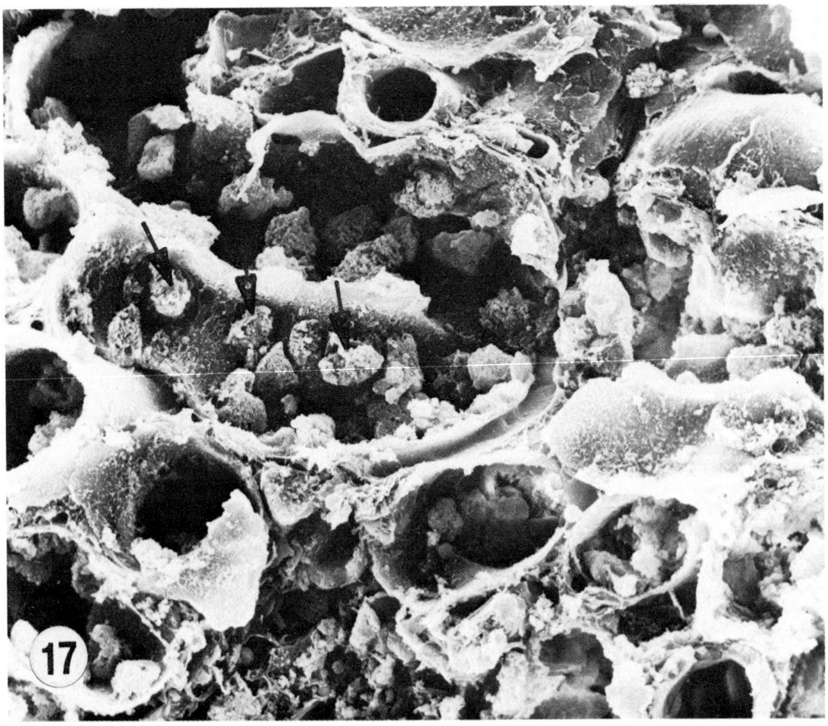

Fig. 17 Scanning electron micrograph of a proximal convoluted tubule containing necrotic cells (arrows) after mercuric chloride-induced acute renal failure. X 600.

recta) is undoubtedly the most sensitive region of the nephron and is vulnerable to both ischemic and toxic insults. This observation has come largely from studies on experimental models of acute renal failure.

Ischemic renal failure is generally produced experimentally by renal artery clamping, the injection of glycerol, or by the intraarterial infusion of norepinephrine. It has been demonstrated that the proximal convoluted tubule is capable of surviving up to 60 min of total renal ischemia induced by renal artery occlusion (66-68). In contrast, the S_3 segment of the proximal tubule located in the outer stripe of the medulla undergoes extensive necrosis with comparable periods of anoxia (69). Venkatachalam et al. (70) used 25 min of renal ischemia and demonstrated a similar site specificity along the proximal tubule. The epithelial cells lining the S_1 and S_2 segments of the proximal tubule suffered a sublethal type of injury which was completely reversible. In contrast, the S_3 cells underwent progressive cell injury and death. Similar findings have also been reported after variable episodes of hypovolemia. Kreisberg et al. (71) and Dobyan et al. (72,73) subjected rats to a transient period of hypovolemia and showed that the pars recta of the proximal tubule situated in the outer stripe region underwent selective necrosis.

The intrarenal infusion of norepinephrine causes immediate vascular shutdown in the kidney and induces a reproducible model of oliguric acute renal failure. Cox et al. (74) and Bulger et al. (32), using a 2-hr infusion, and Cronin et al. (75), using a 40-min infusion, reported widespread tubular necrosis involving all segments of the proximal tubule (Fig. 18). Cox et al. (74) emphasized morphological alterations in the glomerular podocytes, but extensive changes were not seen by Bulger and co-workers (32). The administration of glycerol

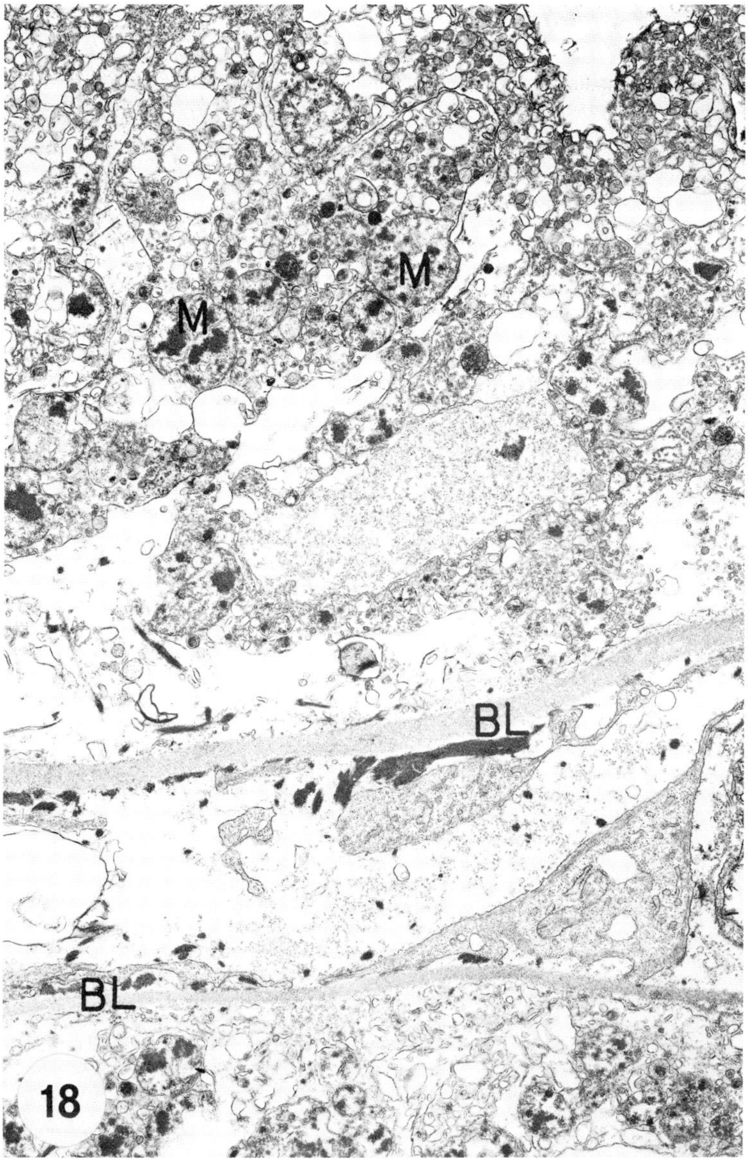

Fig. 18 Transmission electron micrograph showing proximal tubules from the kidney of a dog 24 hr after the intrarenal infusion of norepinephrine. The epithelial cells are completely necrotic and in both tubules only a bare basal lamina remains (BL). Necrotic debris is seen in the lumina of the tubules. Swollen mitochondria with flocculent densities (M) are also apparent. X 8400.

also mimics ischemic acute renal failure by causing volume depletion, hemolysis, and myoglobinemia. The injury induced by this agent is quite similar to other models of vasomotor nephropathy with injury largely confined to the proximal tubule. It is apparent that the proximal tubule responds to alterations in renal hemodynamics in a reproducible and predictable manner.

In addition to ischemic induced renal injury, there are a multitude of chemical agents which exert pronounced effects on the structural integrity of the renal tubule. The majority of nephrotoxic insults are similar to ischemic events with respect to the pattern of injury. The proximal tubule is generally the site along the nephron which is selectively damaged.

Most heavy metals cause widespread acute tubular necrosis of proximal tubules. The administration of mercuric chloride causes selective necrosis of the entire S_3 segment of the proximal tubule (76-79) with higher doses leading to necrosis of S_2 regions as well (76). Uranyl nitrate induces necrosis of the S_2 and S_3 segments (74,80,81). Cis-platinum is a popular chemotherapeutic agent which causes significant impairment in renal function, and when this drug is given to experimental animals it produces selective necrosis of the S_3 segment of the proximal tubule located in the outer stripe of the medulla (64,82-85).

As with other models, the pattern of morphology changes after the necrotic episode to one of tubular regeneration. Cells which are not lethally injured will flatten and spread out to reline the basal lamina of the injured tubule (Fig. 19). Tubules which are in the process of regenerating are low in height, contain numerous free cytoplasmic ribosomes, and possess few cellular organelles. It is interesting to note, however, that cis-platinum seems to have a chronic effect on the renal tubule. Dobyan and co-workers (64) have shown that the administration of cis-platinum to rats induces the formation of cysts. These cysts, which begin as dilatations of the S_3 segment of the proximal tubule, can reach sizes which extend from the outer stripe of the medulla to the subcapsular cortex (Fig. 20).

Agents other than heavy metals have also been shown to cause acute tubular necrosis in experimental animals. The administration of maleic acid to animals is thought to mimic the

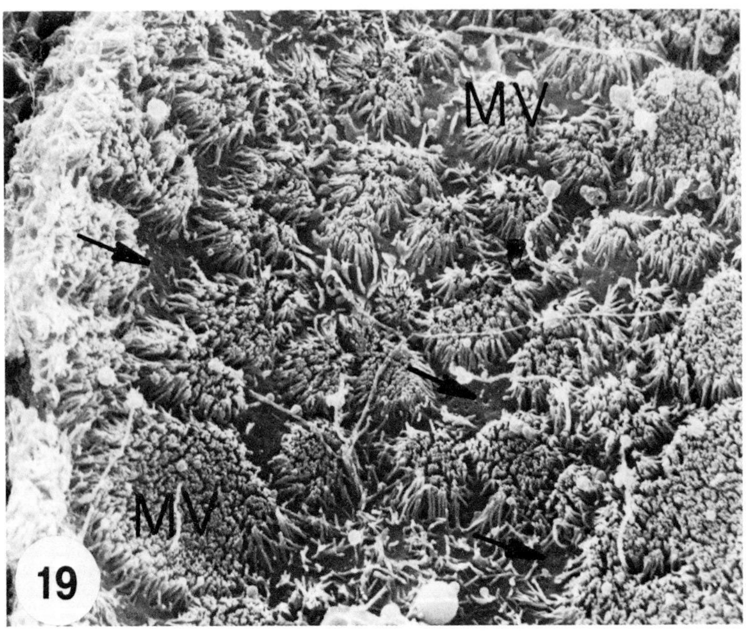

Fig. 19 Scanning electron micrograph showing a proximal tubule of the rat 5 days after the administration of mercuric chloride. This tubule is in the process of regeneration. The tubule is low in height and the luminal surface is studded with clumps of microvilli (MV) of variable lengths. Some areas are devoid of microvilli (arrows). X 2800.

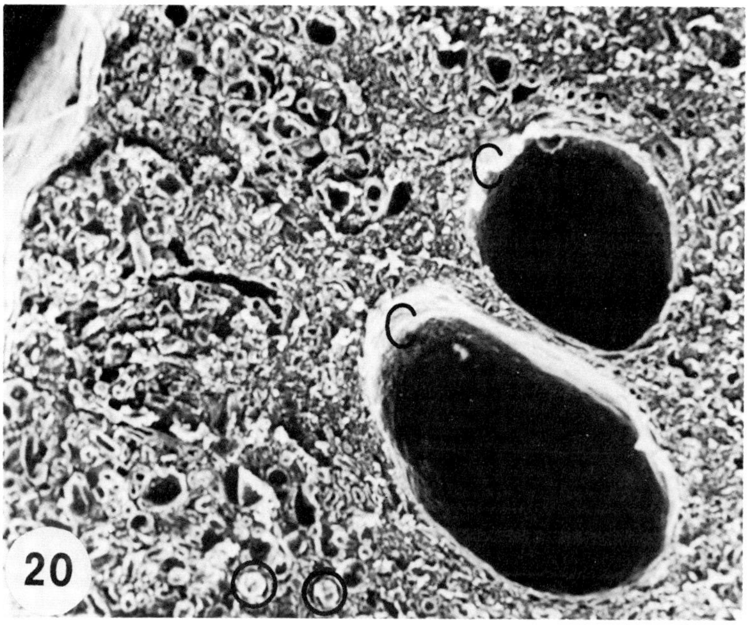

Fig. 20 Scanning electron micrograph showing the cortex of the rat kidney 6 months after a single injection of cis-platinum. Two large cysts (C) can be easily identified in the region of the outer stripe. A renal corpuscle (glomerulus) is encircled to aid in a perception of size. X 470.

physiological effects seen in the Fanconi syndrome (86,87). A recent study by Verani and co-workers (88) has shown that maleic acid causes acute tubular necrosis of the S_2 and S_3 segments of the proximal tubule. Folic acid has been reported to induce changes in the renal tubule, which include tubular dilatation, cast deposition, early cell injury, and frank necrosis (89,90). These same investigators described extensive necrosis of the straight segment of the proximal tubule and ascending thick segment of the distal tubule in the region of the outer medulla. They observed that 4 days after folic acid administration, 91% of the macula densa segments were necrotic.

Nephrotoxicity is one of the major complications of treatment with several classes of antibiotics. The aminoglycosides are frequently associated with antibiotic-associated acute renal failure. Acute tubular necrosis has been reported after the administration of gentamicin, tobramycin, netilmicin, and amikacin (91-95). Most observations regarding aminoglycoside toxicity center on the most nephrotoxic of this group, gentamicin. Gentamicin affects the proximal tubule of both man and experimental animals. The morphological alterations seen include a dramatic increase in the number of large lysosomes which contain large electron-dense myeloid bodies (Fig. 21). This is followed by acute tubular necrosis involving the convoluted portion of the proximal tubule, in particular, the S_2 segment. The injury induced by the aminoglycosides is probably due to a direct toxic effect on the cells of the convoluted tubule. Silverblatt and Kuehn (96), using autoradiography, have shown that labeled gentamicin appears initially over the apical cytoplasm in the region of the endocytotic apparatus and then moves progressively to the cell interior. This suggests that gentamicin is taken up by the proximal tubule cells by the process of endocytosis. In agreement

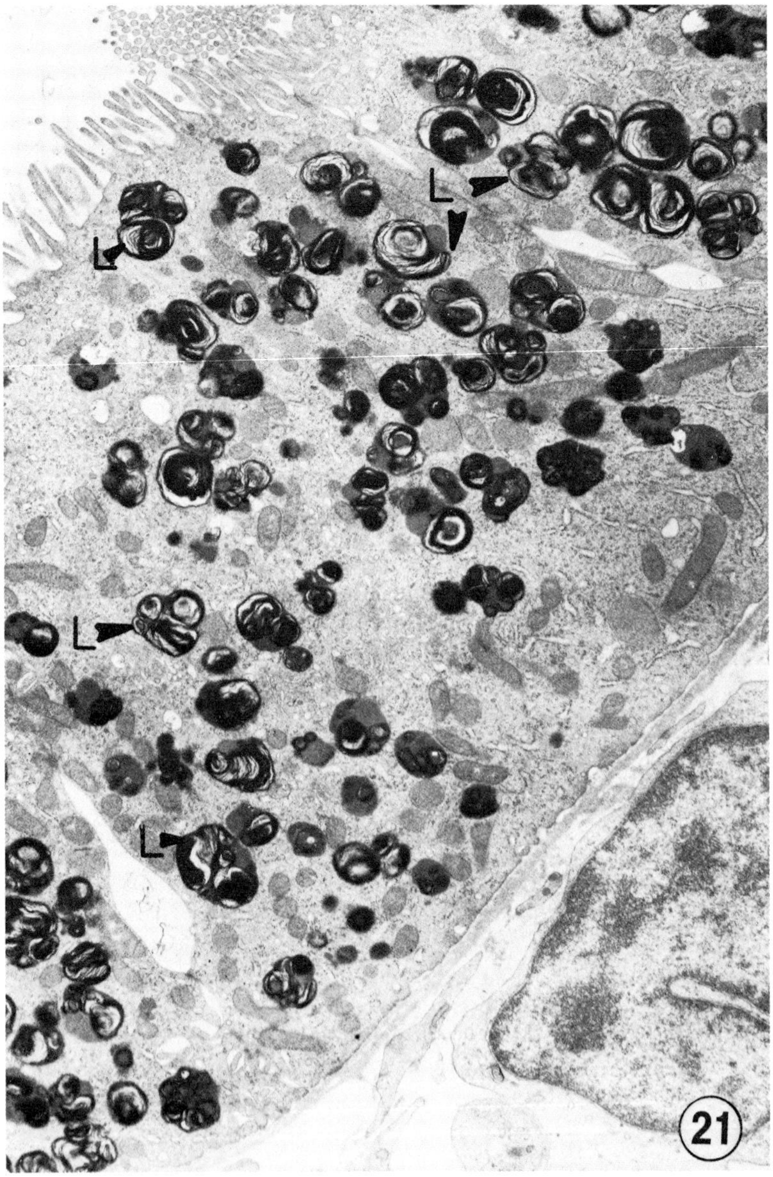

Fig. 21 Transmission electron micrograph showing the proximal tubule from the kidney of a dog receiving repeated injections of the aminoglycoside gentamicin. The most conspicuous feature is the presence of numerous large dense lysosomes (L), which in many instances contain myeloid bodies. X 5000.

with these studies are the observations of Pastoriza-Munoz and co-workers (97) and Sheth et al. (98), who reported that gentamicin is reabsorbed along the proximal convoluted tubule of the rat.

A few of the cephalosporins, in particular cephaloridine, also causes acute tubular necrosis of the proximal tubule, in predominantly the S_2 segment (99). The mechanism of toxicity probably is due to selective uptake of the drug via the organic acid transport system

(100). In this respect, the cytotoxicity of cephaloridine is completely prevented by the administration of probenecid, a drug which inhibits organic anion transport (100,101).

A relationship between the prolonged ingestion of analgesics such as aspirin and phenacetin and renal injury have been reported. The pathological alterations seen along the renal tubule are somewhat unique in that the renal papilla is the primary site of attack. The morphogenesis follows a number of stages from a patchy necrosis to total papillary necrosis (102,103). The necrosis which is localized in the inner medulla and papilla involves the loop of Henle, collecting ducts, capillaries and interstitial cells. Cortical interstitial nephritis has also been described as a consequence of the papillary necrosis (102).

Finally, a number of miscellaneous agents have been examined with respect to their toxic effects on the kidney. For example, lithium salts have been shown to induce pathological alterations in proximal tubules and the collecting ducts (104). The anesthetic methoxyflurane can cause local karyorrhexis, cytoplasmic eosinophilia, and exfoliation of cells in the proximal tubule of experimental animals (105). A detailed review of toxic nephropathy has been recently published by Maher (106).

REFERENCES

1. Kaissling, B.; and Kriz, W. Structural analysis of the rabbit kidney. Adv. Anat. Embryol. Cell Biol. 56:1-123, 1979.
2. Beeuwkes, R., III. Efferent vascular patterns and early vascular-tubular relations in the dog kidney. Am. J. Physiol. 221:1361-1374, 1971.
3. Beeuwkes, R., III. The vascular organization of the kidney. Ann. Rev. Physiol. 42:521-542, 1980.
4. Beeuwkes, R., III. Vascular-tubular relationships in the human kidney. International Symposium on Renal Pathophysiology, edited by Leaf, A., and Giebisch, G. New York, Raven Press, 1980, pp. 155-163.
5. Bankir, L.; Kaissling, B.; de Rouffignac, C.; and Kriz, W. The vascular organization of the kidney of Psammomys obesus. Anat. Embryol. 155:149-190, 1979.
6. Oliver, J. Nephrons and Kidneys. New York, Harper & Row, Hoeber Medical Division, 1968.
7. Sperber, I. Studies on the mammalian kidney. Zool. Bidrag. fran Uppsala 22:249-431, 1944.
8. Kriz, W.; Kaissling, B.; and Pszolla, M. Morphological characterization of the cells in Henle's loop and the distal tubule. In: New Aspects of Renal Function, edited by Vogel, H. G.; and Ullrich, K. J. Amsterdam, Excerpta Medica, 1978, pp. 67-79.
9. Seiler, M. W.; Venkatachalam, M. A.; and Cotran, R. S. Glomerular epithelium: Structural alterations induced by polycations. Science 189:390-393, 1975.
10. Ausiello, D.; Kreisberg, J. I.; Roy, C.; and Karnovsky, M. J. Contraction of cultured rat glomerular cells of apparent mesangial origin after stimulation with angiotensin II and arginine vasopressin. J. Clin. Invest. 65:754-760, 1980.
11. Roll, F. J.; Madri, J. A.; Albert, J.; and Furthmayr, H. Codistribution of collagen type IV and AB2 in the basement membranes and mesangium of the kidney. J. Cell Biol. 85:597-616, 1980.
12. Madri, J. A.; Roll, F. J.; Furthmayr, H.; and Foidart, J. M. Ultrastructural localization of fibronectin and laminin in the basement membranes of the murine kidney. J. Cell Biol. 86:682-687, 1980.
13. Kanwar, Y. S.; and Farquhar, M. G. Anionic sites in the glomerular basement membranes. In vivo and in vitro localization to the laminae rarae by cationic probe. J. Cell Biol. 81:137-153, 1979.
14. Maunsbach, A. V. Observations on the segmentation of the proximal tubule in the rat kidney. Comparison of results from phase-contrast, fluorescence and electron microscopy. J. Ultrastruc. Res. 16:239-258, 1966.

15. Tisher, C. C.; and Yarger, W. F. Lanthanum permeability of the tight junction (zonula occludens) in the renal tubule of the rat. Kidney Int. 3:238-250, 1973.
16. Martinez-Palomo, A.; and Erlij, E. The distribution of lanthanum in tight junctions of the kidney tubule. Pflugers Arch. 343:267, 1973.
17. Silverblatt, F. J.; and Bulger, R. E. Gap junctions occur in vertebrate renal proximal tubule cells. J. Cell Biol. 47:513, 1970.
18. Kriz, W.; Schnermann, J.; and Koepsell, H. The position of short and long loops of Henle in the rat kidney. Z. Anat. Entwickl. Gesch. 138:301-319, 1972.
19. Kriz, W.; and Koepsell, H. The structural organization of the mouse kidney. Z. Anat. Entwickl. Gesch. 144:137-163, 1974.
20. Kaissling, B.; Rouffignac, C. de; Barrett, J. M.; and Kriz, W. The structural organization of the kidney of the desert rodent, Psammomys obesus. Anat. Embryol. 148: 121-143, 1975.
21. Kriz, W.; Barrett, J. M.; and Peter, S. The renal vasculature: Anatomical-functional aspects. Kidney and urinary tract physiology II. Int. Rev. Physiol. 11:1-21, 1976.
22. Schwartz, M. M.; and Venkatachalam, M. A. Structural differences in thin limbs of Henle: Physiological implications. Kidney Int. 6:193-208, 1974.
23. Schiller, A.; Taugner, R.; and Kriz, W. The thin limbs of Henle's loop in the rabbit. A freeze fracture study. Cell Tissue Res. 207:249-265, 1980.
24. Schwartz, M. M.; Karnovsky, M. J.; and Venkatachalam, M. A. Regional membrane specialization in the thin limbs of Henle's loops as seen by freeze-fracture electron microscopy. Kidney Int. 16:577-589, 1979.
25. Stewart, J. Urea handling by the renal countercurrent system: Insights from computer simulation. Pflugers Arch. 356:133-151, 1975.
26. Barrett, J. M.; Kriz, W.; Kaissling, B.; and de Rouffignac, C. The ultrastructure of the nephrons of the desert rodent (Psammomys obesus) kidney: II. Thin limbs of Henle of long-looped nephrons. Am. J. Anat. 151:499-514, 1978.
27. Allen, F.; and Tisher, C. C. Morphology of the ascending thick limb of Henle. Kidney Int. 9:8-22, 1976.
28. Kaissling, B.; Peter, S.; and Kriz, W. The transition of the thick ascending limb of Henle's loop into the distal convoluted tubule in the nephron of the rat kidney. Cell Tissue Res. 182:111-118, 1977.
29. Peter, Karl. Untersuchungen uber Bau Und Entwickelung der Niere, vol. 1. Jena, Verlag von Gustav Fischer, 1909.
30. Tisher, C. C.; Bulger, R. E.; and Valtin, H. Morphology of renal medulla in water diuresis and vasopressin-induced antidiuresis. Am. J. Physiol. 220:87-94, 1971.
31. Crayen, M.; and Thoenes, W. Architektur und cytologische Charakterisierung des distalen Tubulus der Rattenniere. Fortschr. Zool. 23:279-288, 1975.
32. Bulger, R. E.; Cronin, R. E.; and Dobyan, D. C. Glomerular architectural changes after a two-hour infusion of norepinephrine. Am. J. Anat. 159:379-384, 1979.
33. Imbert, M.; Charbardes, D.; Montegut, M.; Glique, A.; and Morel, F. Vasopressin dependent adenylate cyclase in single segments of rabbit kidney tubule. Pflugers Arch. 357:173-186, 1975.
34. Chabardes, D.; Imbert-Teboul, M.; Gagnan-Brunette, M.; and Morel, F. Distribution of adenylate-cyclase-linked hormone receptors in the nephron. In: Endocrinology of Calcium Metabolism, edited by Copp, D. H.; and Talmage, R. V. Amsterdam, Excerpta Medica, 1978, pp. 209-215.
35. Hall, D. A.; and Varney, D. Effect of vasopressin on chloride transport by mouse medullary thick ascending limbs of Henle's loop perfused in vitro. Kidney Int. 16:818 (Abstr.), 1979.
36. Hebert, S. C.; Culpepper, R. M.; and Andreoli, T. E. NaCl transport in mouse medullary thick ascending limbs. I. Functional nephron heterogeneity and ADH-stimulated NaCl cotransport. Am. J. Physiol. 241:F412-F431, 1981.

37. Bourdeau, J. E. L.; and Burg, M. B. Effect of PTH on calcium transport across the cortical thick ascending limb of Henle's loop. Am. J. Physiol. 239:F121-F126, 1980.
38. Suki, W. N.; Rouse, D.; Roland, C. K. N.; and Kokko, J. P. Calcium transport in the thick ascending limb of Henle. Heterogeneity of functions in the medullary and cortical segments. J. Clin. Invest. 66:1004-1009, 1980.
39. Schmidt, U.; and Dubach, U. C. Activity of (Na^+K^+) stimulated adenosine triphosphatase in the rat nephron. Pflugers Arch. 306:219-226, 1969.
40. Guder, W. G.; and Schmidt, U. Sites of enzyme activity along the nephron. Kidney Int. 9:233-243, 1976
41. Schmidt, U.; and Horster, M. Na-K-Activated ATPase: Activity maturation in rabbit nephron segments dissected in vitro. Am. J. Physiol. 233:F55-F60, 1977.
42. Katz, A. I.; Doucet, A.; and Morel, F. Na-K-ATPase activity along the rabbit, rat, and mouse nephron. Am. J. Physiol. 237:F114-F120, 1979.
43. Garg, L. C.; Knepper, M. A.; and Burg, M. B. Mineralocorticoid effects on Na-K-ATPase in individual nephron segments. Am. J. Physiol. 240:F536-F544, 1981.
44. Ernst, S. A. Transport ATPase cytochemistry: ultrastructural localization of potassium-dependent and potassium-independent phosphatase activities in rat kidney cortex. J. Cell Biol. 66:586-608, 1975.
45. Woodhall, P. B.; and Tisher, C. C. Response of the distal tubule and cortical collecting duct to vasopressin in the rat. J. Clin. Invest. 52:3095-3108, 1973.
46. Gross, J. B.; Imai, M.; and Kokko, J. P. A functional comparison of the cortical collecting tubule and the distal convoluted tubule. J. Clin. Invest. 55:1284-1294, 1975.
47. Imai, M. The connecting tubule: A functional subdivision of the rabbit distal nephron segments. Kidney Int. 15:346-356, 1979.
48. Doucet, A.; and Katz, A. I. Mineralocorticoid receptors along the nephron: (^3H) aldosterone binding in rabbit tubules. Am. J. Physiol. 241:F605-F611, 1981.
49. Osathanodh, V.; and Potter, E. L. Development of human kidney as shown by microdissection. III. Formation and interrelationship of collecting tubules and nephrons. Arch. Pathol. Lab. Med. 76:290-302, 1963.
50. Hansen, G. P.; Tisher, C. C.; and Robinson, R. R. Response of the collecting duct to disturbances of acid-base and potassium balance. Kidney Int. 17:326-337, 1980.
51. Stanton, B. A.; Biemesderfer, D.; Wade, J. B.; and Giebisch, G. Structural and functional study of the rat distal nephron: Effects of potassium adaptation and depletion. Kidney Int. 19:36-48, 1981.
52. Stetson, D. L.; Wade, J. B.; and Giebisch, G. Morphologic alterations in the rat medullary collecting duct following potassium depletion. Kidney Int. 17:45-56, 1980.
53. Pricam, C.; Humbert, F.; Perrelet, A.; and Orci, L. A freeze-etch study of the tight junctions of the rat kidney tubules. Lab. Invest. 30:286-291, 1974.
54. Hagege, J.; Gabe, M.; and Richet, G. Scanning of the apical pole of distal tubular cells under differing acid-base conditions. Kidney Int. 5:137-146, 1974.
55. Ordonez, N. G.; and Spargo, B. H. The morphologic relationship of light and dark cells of the collecting tubules in potassium-depleted rats. Am. J. Pathol. 84:317-326, 1976.
56. Evan, A.; Huser, J.; Bengele, H. H.; and Alexander, E. A. The effect of alterations in dietary potassium on collecting system morphology in the rat. Lab. Invest. 42:668-675, 1980.
57. Schafer, J. A.; and Andreoli, T. E. Cellular constraints to diffusion. The effect of antidiuretic hormone on water flows in isolated mammalian collecting tubules. J. Clin. Invest. 51:1264-1278, 1972.
58. Harmanci, M. C.; Kachadorian, W. A.; Valtin, H.; and DiScala, V. A. Antidiuretic hormone-induced intramembranous alterations in mammalian collecting ducts. Am. J. Physiol. 235:F440-443, 1978.
59. Harmanci, M. C.; Stern, P.; Kachadorian, W. A.; and Valtin, H. Vasopressin and collecting duct intramembranous particle clusters: A dose-response relationship. Am. J. Physiol. 239:F560-F564, 1980.

60. Rastegar, A.; Biemesderfer, D.; Kashgarian, M.; and Hayslett, J. P. Changes in membrane surfaces of collecting duct cells in potassium adaptation. Kidney Int. 18:293-301, 1980.
61. Wade, J. B.; O'Neil, R. G.; Pryor, J. L.; and Boulpaep, E. L. Modulation of cell membrane area in renal collecting tubules by corticosteroid hormones. J. Cell. Biol. 81:439-445, 1979.
62. Lonnerholm, G. Histochemical demonstration of carbonic anhydrase activity in the human kidney. Acta Physiol. Scand. 88:455-468, 1973.
63. Lonnerholm, G.; and Riddlestrale, Y. Intracellular distribution of carbonic anhydrase in the rat kidney. Kidney Int. 17:162-174, 1980.
64. Dobyan, D. C.; Hill, D.; Lewis, T.; and Bulger, R. E. Cyst formation in rat kidney induced by cis-platinum administration. Lab. Invest. 45:260-268, 1981.
65. Trump, B. F.; McDowell, E. M.; and Arstila, A. U. Cellular reaction to injury. In: Principles of Pathobiology, edited by Hill, R. B.; and LaVia, M. F. New York, Oxford University Press, 1980, pp. 20-103.
66. Vogt, M. T.; and Farber, E. On the molecular pathology of ischemic renal cell death: Reversible and irreversible cellular and mitochondrial metabolic alterations. Am. J. Pathol. 53:1-26, 1968.
67. Reimer, K. A.; and Jennings, R. B. Alterations in renal cortex following ischemic injury. I. PAH uptake by slices of cortex after ischemia or autolysis. Lab. Invest. 25:176-184, 1971.
68. Glaumann, B.; Glaumann, H.; Berezesky, I. K.; and Trump, B. F. Studies on the pathogenesis of ischemic cell injury. II. Morphological changes of the pars convoluta (P_1 and P_2) of the proximal tubule of the rat kidney made ischemic in vivo. Virchows Arch. (Cell Pathol.) 19:281-302, 1975.
69. Glaumann, B.; and Trump, B. F. Studies on the pathogenesis of ischemic cell injury. III. Morphological changes of the proximal pars recta tubules (P_3) of the rat kidney made ischemic in vivo. Virchows Arch. (Cell Pathol.) 19:303-323, 1975.
70. Venkatachalam, M. A.; Bernard, D. B.; Donohoe, J. F.; and Levinsky, N. G. Ischemic damage and repair in the rat proximal tubule: Differences among the S_1, S_2, and S_3 segments. Kidney Int. 14:31-49, 1978.
71. Kreisberg, J. I.; Bulger, R. E.; Trump, B. F.; and Nagle, R. B. Effects of transient hypotension on the structure and function of the rat kidney. Virchows Arch. (Cell Pathol.) 22:121-133, 1976.
72. Dobyan, D. C.; Nagle, R. B.; and Bulger, R. E. Acute tubular necrosis in the rat kidney following sustained hypotension: Physiologic and morphologic observations. Lab. Invest. 37:411-422, 1977.
73. Dobyan, D. C.; Nagle, R. B.; and Bulger, R. E. Hypovolemic models of acute tubular necrosis in the rat kidney. Virchows Arch. (Cell Pathol.) 25:271-280, 1977.
74. Cox, J. W.; Baehler, R. W.; Sharma, H.; O'Dousio, T.; Osgood, R. W.; Stein, J. H.; and Ferris, T. F. Studies on the mechanism of oliguria in a model of unilateral acute renal failure. J. Clin. Invest. 53:1564-1578, 1974.
75. Cronin, R. E.; DeTorrente, A.; Miller, P. D.; Bulger, R. E.; Burke, T. E.; and Schrier, R. W. Pathogenic mechanisms in early norepinephrine-induced acute renal failure: Functional and histological correlates of protection. Kidney Int. 14:115-125, 1978.
76. Siegel, F. L.; and Bulger, R. E. Scanning and transmission electron microscopy of mercuric chloride-induced acute tubular necrosis in rat kidney. Virchows Arch. (Cell Pathol.) 18:243-262, 1975.
77. Siegel, F. L.; and Bulger, R. E. Scanning and transmission electron microscopy of rat kidney following low dose mercuric chloride administration. Beitr. Pathol. 156:313-342, 1975.

4

Aminoacidurias

JOHN W. FOREMAN and STANTON SEGAL
University of Pennsylvania School of Medicine, Philadelphia, Pennsylvania

I. GENERAL ASPECTS OF AMINO ACID TRANSPORT

One of the major functions of the renal tubule is reclamation of most of the solutes, such as Na^+, K^+, Ca^{2+}, glucose, phosphate, bicarbonate, and amino acids, which are filtered from the renal plasma by the glomerulus. Inherited disorders that affect the transport of individual or all these solutes, when taken as a group, represent a common form of genetic disease. Considered in this chapter are those transport disorders that affect the reabsorption of single or groups of amino acids. Not considered in this chapter are those aminoacidurias which occur from disorders of amino acid metabolism that lead to significant elevations of plasma amino acids which in turn "overflow" into the urine.

A. Mechanisms of Amino Acid Transport

Over the past several decades our concept of the cell membrane and its function has undergone considerable revision. It is clear that the cell membrane is not just an inert lipid barrier separating the cytosol from the extracellular fluid. The cell membrane is a dynamic, fluid structure with a specific organization enabling it to regulate entry and exit of hydrophilic substances, to transmit information from the external environment to the interior of the cell by means of hormone-receptor interactions, and to carry out specific enzymatic processes on both sides of the membrane (1).

The lipid composition of the membrane negates the concept of a simple diffusional model for the translocation of hydrophilic solutes into the cell, since prohibitively high amounts of energy would be required to transport these solutes across the "lipid sea" of the plasma membrane. In addition, simple diffusion would only allow the equilibration of the concentration of solutes within the cell with extracellular fluid; yet, the internal concentration of many solutes, such as amino acids, have been demonstrated to be manyfold greater than the external concentration. This type of transport, termed active, which allows the development of concentration gradients involves the expenditure of energy and specific "carriers," presumably proteins, to mediate the transfer of solutes across the cell membrane. Carriers can also mediate facilitated diffusion which is not energy dependent, but equilibrates substrate concentrations across the cell membrane more rapidly than simple diffusion. A general characteristic of carrier-mediated transport is saturability, which means that the velocity of transport can only increase to a certain maximum with increasing substrate concentrations. Specificity is also a characteristic of carrier-mediated transport in that only a certain substrate or group of substrates with a specific stereoconfiguration and charge can be transported by a single carrier.

The conclusion that membrane carriers are proteins comes from several lines of evidence. First, bacteria as a general model of membrane transport have proteins which bind specific amino acids (2). Mutant bacteria lacking these binding proteins have depressed transport abilities which can be improved by their addition through osmotic shock. Further, the membrane location of these binding proteins was shown with tagged antibodies.

In the renal tubule cell the protein nature of membrane carriers can also be inferred from several experiments. Puromycin, a protein synthesis inhibitor, can after a period of time, lead to impaired amino acid uptake (3). A protein extract from the proximal tubule brush-border membrane can confer some transport characteristics partially resembling that of the brush-border membrane to artificial liposomes (4). Finally, disorders of specific solute transport can be inherited, again implying that proteins are involved in solute transport, since genes code for the synthesis of specific proteins.

B. Techniques of Evaluating Amino Acid Transport

The simplest method of evaluating the transport of an amino acid is to determine its renal clearance. However, this only gives the overall handling of an amino acid by the total nephron population and is essentially a "black box" technique. Studies of this sort have shown that amino acids are virtually completely reabsorbed from the glomerular ultrafiltrate, since less than 2% of the filtered load of most amino acids appears in the final urine. Exceptions to this are glycine in which 5% of the filtered load is excreted and histidine in which 8% is excreted. Clearance studies have shown that aminoacidurias can be divided into three types. The first type occurs when the plasma level and consequently the filtered load of an amino acid are increased beyond the capacity of the kidney to reabsorb it such that an overflow aminoaciduria occurs, as in histidinemia or liver disease. Another type is due to the filtration of amino acids that arise from metabolic defects in intermediary metabolism and for which no carrier or transport system exists such as cystathionine. The third type, which will be discussed in detail later, arises from a specific defect in the ability of the nephron to handle the normal load of a specific amino acid or group of amino acids.

While clearance studies have yielded valuable information indicating that 92-100% of the normal filtered load of amino acids is reabsorbed, the black-box nature of these studies has offered only limited contributions to our understanding of the events at the level of the cell membrane. On the other hand, thin slices of renal cortex incubated in oxygenated buffer have shed much light on the specificity, kinetics, ionic requirements, and other characteristics of amino acid uptake into renal cortical tubule cells. Isolated proximal tubule fragments obtained by a collagenase digestion of these slices has further refined this technique by eliminating architectural concerns due to slice thickness and improving oxygenation of the tissue. A further refinement of in vitro studies of membrane transport has been the isolation of the two membrane species comprising the outer surface of the proximal tubule cell. These two membrane types, the brush-border and basolateral membranes, under certain conditions spontaneously vesiculate, allowing the determination of amino acid uptake across only one membrane type in the absence of significant metabolism.

From studies using these modalities, a model for amino acid uptake has emerged, as shown in Fig. 1. The uptake of most, if not all, amino acids from the tubular lumen across the brush-border membrane is stimulated by influx of sodium which enters the cell because of a favorable electrochemical gradient. This favorable gradient is maintained by the active extrusion of sodium by the enzyme, Na^+-K^+-ATPase, which is located on the basolateral membrane. The transported amino acids can then be either incorporated into protein, metabolized by intracellular enzymes, or transported out of the cell across the basolateral membrane and returned to the blood. Finally, energy is important in maintaining these fluxes to effect net transepithelial transport of amino acids from lumen to blood, although the exact mechanism coupling energy to transepithelial transport is unknown. Amino acid transport is also discussed in Ch. 1.

C. Model of Aminoacidurias

Currently, the exact mechanism leading to any of the aminoacidurias is unknown. There are a number of possible abnormalities which could lead to decreased amino acid uptake,

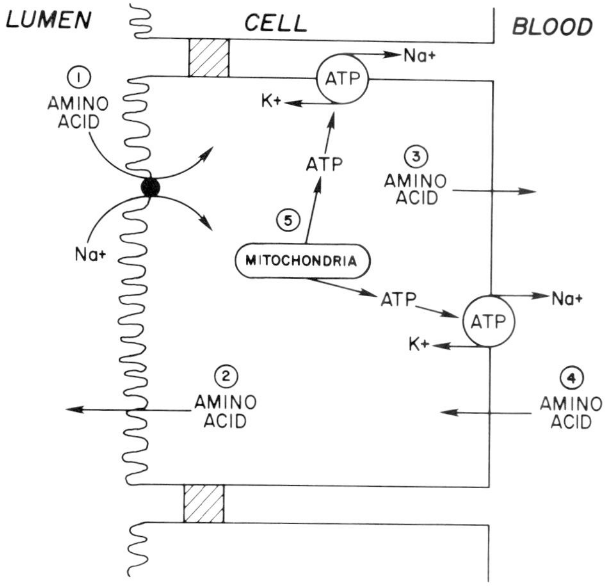

Fig. 1 Model of amino acid transepithelial transport. Amino acids enter the proximal tubule cell from the lumen across the brushborder membrane via specific carriers in conjunction with an ion flux, predominantly the influx of Na^+ down its electrochemical gradient. This electrochemical gradient is maintained by the active extrusion of Na^+ from the cell by Na^+-K^+-ATPase on the basolateral membrane. The transported amino acids then exit the cell at the basolateral membrane again via specific carriers. Amino acids can also enter the cell from the blood across the basolateral membrane and exit across the brush-border membrane. With this arrangement, a defect at any of these sites could lead to increased urine amino acid excretion. There could be a defect in influx across the brush-border membrane (1). The transported amino acid could quickly leak back into the lumen (2). An impairment in the transport across the basolateral membrane (3) or increased uptake from the blood (4) could lead to decreased influx or increased efflux across the brush-border membrane. Finally, a disorder in energy generation or transduction to the membrane could result in an aminoaciduria (5).

as shown in Fig. 1. First, there could be an impairment in amino acid influx from the luminal fluid because of a defective, absent, or abnormally placed carrier in the brush-border membrane. The influx of the amino acid across the brush-border membrane could be normal; but the amino acid quickly backleaks or effluxes into the lumen again. This may be the mechanism of aminoaciduria in the experimental Fanconi syndrome produced by maleic acid (5-6). There could be an impairment in transport out of the cell across the basolateral membrane, leading secondarily to decreased influx. Uptake from blood across the basolateral membrane could be so large that efflux across the brush-border membrane is increased again, analogous to a secretory process. Finally, energy is important in maintaining these fluxes to effect net transepithelial transport of amino acids from lumen to blood, although the exact mechanism coupling energy to transepithelial transport is unknown. Still, a defect in energy generation or transduction to the membrane carriers could lead to aminoaciduria.

D. Normal Amino Acid Excretion

Amino acids in the plasma are freely dialyzable except for tryptophan, which is largely bound to protein, leaving only 10-14% available for ultrafiltration across the glomerular capillary wall. As stated earlier, amino acids are actively transported into the renal tubule cells. This transport takes place predominantly in the proximal convoluted tubule with more than 80% of the normal filtered load of all amino acids, except glycine and histidine, being reabsorbed in the first one-third of the proximal convoluted tubule. With increasing filtered loads, the remaining proximal convoluted and the proximal straight tubule are involved in reabsorption (7). There appears to be little or no uptake in the distal tubule with possibly a small amount in the collecting duct. Recently, using isolated perfused segments of the rabbit nephron, the two transport systems for glycine uptake have been shown to be arranged such that the low-affinity, high-capacity system appears to be in the proximal convoluted tubule and the high-affinity, low-capacity system in the proximal straight (8). This organization would allow the bulk of glycine to be reabsorbed early in the nephron, with the proximal straight segment then able to lower the luminal concentration even further. However, microperfusion studies with histidine have shown a rising K_m with increasing distance down the proximal convoluted tubule (9). Proline reabsorption in the proximal convoluted tubule of the rat also is mediated by multiple transport systems, but without an exact localization of any of these along the tubule (10). Using numerous techniques it appears that most amino acids have multiple transport systems for reabsorption, but the precise spatial arrangement of these systems with respect to distance from the glomerulus is unknown.

Normally, very little amino acid is present in human urine with glycine and histidine accounting for the majority of the α-amino nitrogen excreted. This is because 98% of the filtered amino acids are reabsorbed by the renal tubule after early infancy except for histidine, which is only 92% reabsorbed, and glycine, which is 96% reabsorbed. In the very young infant the percent tubular reabsorption of all amino acids is lower than that of the older child, but this is most evident for glycine, proline, hydroxyproline, serine, alanine, and threonine (11,12). Normal urine amino acid excretion rates for age are shown in Table 1.

II. SPECIFIC DISORDERS OF AMINO ACID TRANSPORT

With these general principles of amino acid transport in mind, the next section deals with specific inherited disorders of renal amino acid handling, listed in Table 2. Not covered in this section but dealt with in Chs. 13 and 14 is the Fanconi syndrome, which has generalized aminoaciduria as one of its manifestations.

Table 1 Urine Amino Acid Excretion in Different Age Groups

	Infants[a] (10 days-7 weeks) (μmol/24 hr)	Children[b] (3-12 years) (μmol/24 hr)	Adults[c,d] (μmol/24 hr)
Taurine	26-257	63-97	78-2349
Aspartic acid		<37	4-57
Threonine	13-100	85-249	54-392
Serine	59-235	155-540	172-772
Glutamine	85-177	140-779	
Asparagine			257-696
Proline	28-96		<87
Glutamic acid	2-10		11-68
Citrulline	Tr		2-43
Glycine	194-787	165-1420	169-1798
Alanine	46-104	102-439	20-797
Valine	12-27	15-51	21-102
½ Cystine	18-28	41-257	67-216
Methionine	1-13	20-95	2-17
Isoleucine	Tr-3	20-56	5-24
Leucine	7-15	21-83	20-62
Tyrosine	22-40	40-168	44-149
Phenylalanine	7-10	24-106	18-103
Ornithine	17-21	<38	5-102
Lysine	39-75	64-642	53-365
Histidine	103-249	306-1285	322-2062
Arginine	Tr-7	<29	2-26

[a]Data from Levy, H. L.; and Mudd, S. H.; Schulman, J. D.; Dreyfus, P. M.; and Abeles, R. H. Am. J. Med. 48:390, 1970.
[b]Data from Carver, M. S.; and Paska, R. Clin. Chim. Acta 6:721, 1961.
[c]Data from Stein, W. H. J. Biol. Chem. 201:75, 1953.
[d]Data from Logan, A.; Schlicke, C. P.; and Manning, G. B. Am. J. Surg. 115:112, 1968.

A. Disorders of Cystine and Dibasic Amino Acids

Classic Cystinuria

Cystine stones in the urinary tract, presumably as a consequence of classic cystinuria, were first described in the early nineteenth century (13-15). Much confusion arose in the early literature because these investigators failed to distinguish between those patients with elevated urinary cystine excretion in concert with the dibasic amino acids, which is classic cystinuria, and those with a generalized aminoaciduria and raised intracellular cystine content, which is cystinosis. In classic cystinuria, the urinary excretion of the amino acids cystine, lysine, ornithine, and arginine markedly exceeds that of normals, but the plasma concentration of all amino acids and the urinary excretion of other amino acids and solutes is normal.

In Vivo Studies

In 1908, Garrod in his famous Croonian lectures (16) introduced the concept that cystinuria was an inborn error of metabolism related to a defect in the catabolic pathway for cystine, although this pathway had yet to be described. Nearly a half century later, Dent and Rose (17) concluded that cystine and the dibasic amino acids share a common renal reabsorptive pathway and that this pathway is defective in cystinuria. They drew these con-

Table 2 Inherited Aminoacidurias

Disease	Clinical findings	Increased urine amino acids	Inheritance
Classic cystinuria	Urolithiasis	Cystine, lysine, ornithine, arginine	Autosomal recessive
Isolated hypercystinuria	None	Cystine	Unknown
Lysinuric protein intolerance	Hyperammonemia, diarrhea, vomiting after protein load	Dibasic amino acids	Autosomal recessive
Hyperdibasicaminoaciduria	Mental retardation	Dibasic amino acids	Unknown
Hyperlysinuria	Mental retardation	Lysine	Unknown
Hartnup disease	Skin rash, cerebellar ataxia, psychiatric disturbances	Neutral amino acids	Autosomal recessive
Methionine malabsorption	White hair, edema, convulsions, acidosis, mental retardation	Methionine, branch-chain amino acids, tyrosine, phenylalanine	Unknown
Histidinuria	Mental retardation	Histidine	Unknown
Iminoglycinuria	None	Glycine, hydroxyproline, proline	Autosomal recessive
Glycinuria	Urolithiasis in some	Glycine	Autosomal recessive
Glucoglycinuria	Glucosuria	Glycine	Autosomal dominant
Dicarboxylic aminoaciduria	? Mental and growth retardation, hypoglycemia in one patient, no findings in another	Glutamic and aspartic acids	Unknown

As with most disorders of amino acid transport, the renal losses of cystine and the dibasic amino acids are probably of negligible nutritional consequence, although as much as several grams of these amino acids can be lost in the adult. In this regard, Colliss et al. (48) reported that the mean height of 44 British patients with cystinuria was statistically less than that of the general population and they attributed this to the renal loss and impaired intestinal absorption of the essential amino acid lysine. However, most if not all of this difference in height could probably be attributed to infections, repeated surgical interventions, and renal insufficiency in these patients. In 64 patients reported by Smith et al. (49), only four patients were below the expected height for age, and three of the four were on the same height percentiles as their unaffected siblings.

A more serious concern is the possible association of cystinuria with central nervous system disorders. Scriver et al. (50) found a higher prevalence of cystinuria is psychiatric patients and Berry (51) observed one positive among 700 mentally retarded children screened for cystinuria. Several reports (52-54) have appeared describing three patients with cystinuria who subsequently developed a spastic paraparesis in the second to fifth decade of life. Careful psychometric testing of 26 homozygous cystinuric patients by Gold et al. (55) failed to reveal any intellectual deficiency when compared to siblings. Smith and Procopis (56) reported a 13-fold higher incidence of heterozygous cystinuria in a mentally deficient population in Australia, but they did not detect any homozygotes. The postulate underlying these studies relating central nervous system dysfunction and cystinuria is that the defective transport system present in the kidney and intestine also appears in the brain. However, studies of cysteine (57), cystine (58,59), and lysine (60) uptake using isolated rat brain synaptosomes and capillaries indicate that the transport systems for these amino acids into the brain are different from those of the kidney and intestine, making this postulate unlikely.

Diagnosis

The diagnosis of cystinuria should be entertained in any patient with a renal calculus. The easiest method for diagnosis is examination of a freshly voided urine for the appearance of the typical flat, hexagonal crystals which are best seen in acidic, concentrated urine (Fig. 5). The best screening procedure is the cyanide-nitroprusside test on urine. Sodium cyanide will reduce cystine to cysteine in urine made alkaline with ammonium hydroxide. The addition of sodium nitroprusside to this will yield a color ranging from pink in normals to violet in homozygotes with cystinuria. A positive reaction is observed with as little as 75-125 mg/g creatinine, which is well below that of homozygotes who excrete more than 250 mg/g creatinine. Some, but not all, heterozygotes will give a weak reaction. A positive reaction will also occur in homocystinuria and acetonuria. Differentiation of cystine and homocystine can be made by a chromatographic method such as paper, thin-layer, or high-voltage electrophoresis. Quantitation of the excretion of cystine and dibasic amino acids is usually done by ion-exchange chromatography. By this method, the upper values of normal in adults are 18, 130, 16, and 22 mg/g creatinine for cystine, lysine, arginine, and ornithine, respectively, while the homozygous cystinuric excretes at least 250 mg/g creatinine of cystine.

From extensive family studies, it has become clear that genetic heterogeneity exists for cystinuria. Harris et al. (61) noted that two distinct genetic mutations appeared to lead to the phenotype of hyperexcretion of cystine and dibasic amino acids. With the demonstration of a gut defect by both in vivo and in vitro methods, Rosenberg et al. (62) were able to distinguish three genotypes of homozygous cystinuria (Table 4). Also, mixed or compound heterozygotes are possible which will yield a urinary excretion pattern similar to the homozygous state. In type I, which is by far the most common, there is an absence of active

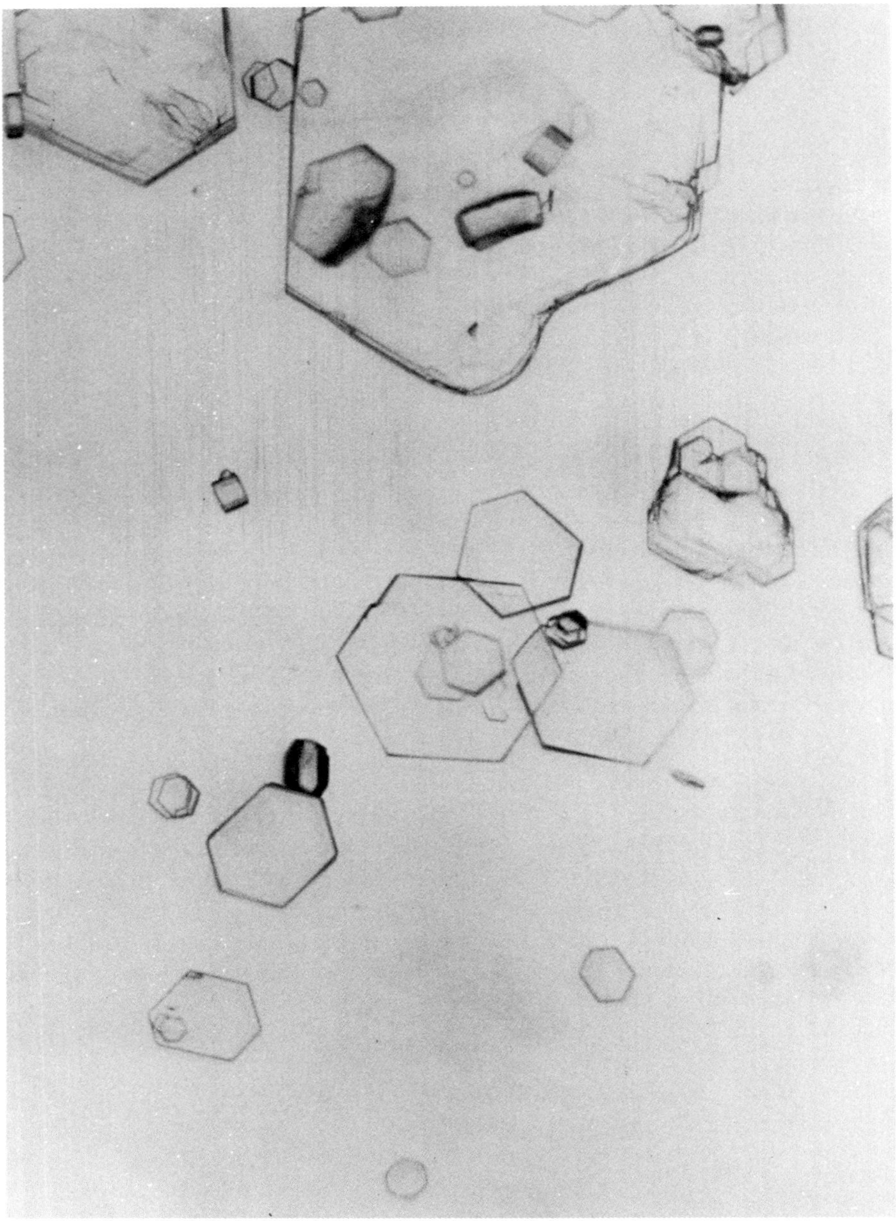

Fig. 5 Cystine crystals as they appear in the urinary sediment.

Table 4 Classification of Cases of Cystinuria

Experimental observations	Type I	Type II	Type III
Intestine:			
In vitro transport	No transport of cystine lysine, or arginine; normal cystine transport	No transport of lysine; markedly reduced cystine transport	Transport of cystine reduced but may be normal; lysine variably reduced
Oral cystine administration	No plasma cystine elevation	No plasma cystine elevation	Slow increase in plasma cystine to normal elevation
Kidney:			
In vitro transport in cortical slices	Reduced lysine transport		Reduced lysine transport
Urinary and amino acid excretion	Increased cystine, lysine, arginine, ornithine excretion	Increased cystine, lysine, arginine, ornithine excretion	Increased cystine, lysine, arginine, ornithine excretion
Urinary amino acid excretion in heterozygotes	Normal	Cystine and lysine above normal	Cystine and lysine above normal

transport of cystine, lysine or arginine by gut mucosa in affected patients and the failure to elevate plasma cystine after an oral cystine load. Heterozygotes of type I have a normal urinary excretion pattern. In type II, lysine uptake is absent and cystine uptake is impaired in gut mucosa with no response to an oral cystine load. Heterozygotes have a modest increase in the excretion of cystine, lysine, arginine, and ornithine, but formation of cystine calculi does not occur. However, there is some evidence that type II heterozygotes have an increased incidence of calcium oxalate stones (63). The elevated urinary cystine excretion may, like uric acid, facilitate calcium oxalate precipitation in an undetermined manner. Type III is characterized by a reduced uptake of cystine and lysine by gut mucosa and slow rise in plasma cystine after an oral load. Heterozygotes also have an increased renal excretion of cystine and dibasic amino acids, albeit less than type II heterozygotes.

Treatment

In a urine with a pH less than 7.5, the upper limit of solubility for cystine is 300 mg/liter. Cystine solubility increases sharply as the pH rises above 7.5, but maintenance of this pH in urine is extremely difficult. A more practical therapeutic maneuver is to increase urine volume. Most cystinuric patients excrete about 0.5-1.0 g of cystine per day. In order to keep the cystine concentration below 300 mg/liter in such patients, an intake of 4 liters or more would be required. Timing of this intake is also important because it is crucial to maintain fluid intake during the night when urine flow is normally slow to prevent supersaturation of this urine with cystine and subsequent crystal formation.

Although rigid adherence to fluid therapy can prevent calculus formation (64), many patients are unable to comply with this regimen or form stones in spite of this. With the introduction of D-penicillamine (β,β-dimethyl cysteine), treatment of patients with recurrent cystine stone formation has changed dramatically (65). Penicillamine can produce a mixed disulfide of penicillamine-cysteine through disulfide exchange. This mixed disulfide is significantly more soluble than cystine. With adequate penicillamine therapy of 1-2 g/day in the adult and 30 mg/kg in the child, cystine excretion can usually be kept below the stone-forming level of 300 mg/liter, preferably below 200 mg/liter. The fall in urinary cystine, however, is not balanced by a rise in the mixed disulfide and there is a fall in plasma cystine, suggesting that the effect of penicillamine on cystine excretion is more complex than just mixed disulfide exchange (66-68).

Unfortunately, penicillamine therapy is often associated with significant side effects. As many as 50% of patients treated with penicillamine will develop fever and a rash and a few of these will also develop arthralgias (66). More serious side effects include the nephrotic syndrome (69-71) and pancytopenia (72). Epidermolysis (73), thrombocytosis (74), and loss of taste (75) have also been reported. Penicillamine also interferes with the action of pyridoxine (76), and supplemental pyridoxine phosphate should be given to patients on penicillamine.

Because of these significant side effects, penicillamine should be restricted to those patients in whom more conservative therapy has failed to prevent stones and should be initiated in a hospital setting to monitor for the possible occurrence of these side effects. Some patients who initially react to penicillamine can later tolerate it when it is reintroduced in slowly increasing doses over 1-2 months.

Other agents have been tried with varying success in patients with cystinuria. *N*-Acetylpenicillamine can form mixed disulfides with cysteine and may be effective in cystinuria (77-79). *N*-Acetylpenicillamine also appears to have fewer side effects than penicillamine, possibly because the amino group is not available for chemical reaction. Mercaptopropionylglycine also has been used with success in some patients (80-84). The amino acid glutamine was reported to dramatically lower urinary cystine excretion after oral administration in two patients (85-87); However, this effect of glutamine on cystine excretion could only be observed after 7 days of administration in one of these two patients (87). Other investigators, however, have not observed any change in cystine excretion with oral glutamine (88,89).

Isolated Hypercystinuria, Lysinuric Protein Intolerance, and Hyperdibasicaminoaciduria

In 1966, Brodehl and his colleagues reported marked cystine excretion with normal dibasic amino acid excretion in a 4-year-old girl and her 2-year-old brother (90). Both parents and another sibling had normal amino acid clearances. Renal stones were not observed in either child. Brodehl named this isolated hypercystinuria to differentiate it from classic cystinuria. The aminoaciduria in these children suggests that cystine is reabsorbed by a second system which is independent of the one shared with the dibasic amino acids. Recent experimental evidence for cystine transport by isolated renal tubules and brush-border membrane vesicles from the rat supports this contention (42-43).

In addition to patients with isolated hypercystinuria, two forms of increased dibasic amino acid excretion without marked cystine excretion have been described. In the first type, which has been termed lysinuric protein intolerance by Perheentupa, patients have been noted to have dibasic aminoaciduria with normal to slightly increased cystine excretion (91-93). These patients also have marked impairment in intestinal dibasic amino acid absorption which may be related to a defect in transport across the basolateral membrane (94). The striking clinical features in these children are vomiting, diarrhea, and lethargy, possibly even coma, after an oral protein load. Leukocytopenia, thrombocytopenia, hepatomegaly, and osteoporosis have also been observed in these patients. Four of 20 patients described by Simell et al. manifested subnormal intelligence (93). Biochemically, these patients develop hyperammonemia with decreased to low normal plasma levels of the dibasic amino acids and massive hyperdibasicaminoaciduria after a protein load. The hyperammonemia can be prevented with the intravenous infusion of arginine, suggesting that it may arise from depletion of the intracellular levels of the urea-cycle intermediates, arginine and ornithine, with the subsequent slowing of this critical pathway for ammonia disposal (91-93). Simell et al. have demonstrated that this impaired uptake of dibasic amino acids by the kidney and intestine in patients with lysinuric protein intolerance also extends to the granulocyte (95) and liver (95,96).

This disorder has been described in several areas of the world, including the United States and Japan, but the highest incidence is in Finland where it occurs once in 60,000-80,000 births (93). Lysinuric protein intolerance is inherited as an autosomal recessive. The most effective treatment appears to be protein restriction to prevent episodic hyperammonemia. The beneficial effects of intravenous arginine and ornithine have led some investigators to try oral supplementation (93,97). This has been helpful in some, but not all, presumably because of variations in absorption of these amino acids in individual patients. Recently, supplemental oral citrulline appears to be the best treatment for lysinuric protein tolerance (98). Citrulline, which is absorbed by an unaffected intestinal transport system, can readily enter the liver where it is converted to arginine and ornithine, correcting the deficiencies of these two amino acids. With this supplementation improved protein tolerance was noted, catch-up growth occurred in seven of nine stunted patients, and liver histology improved in two of four with severe fatty degeneration. Hepatosplenomegaly, osteoporosis, and muscle weakness remained, possibly because of a deficiency of lysine. Supplemental lysine appeared to be of no benefit.

Whelan and Scriver described the second type of hyperdibasicaminoaciduria which presented in 13 members over two generations (99). The urinary excretion of cystine was normal in these patients and they were otherwise asymptomatic. Kihara et al. described a child with mental retardation and hyperdibasicaminoaciduria with normal urinary cystine excretion in an inbred family (100). Both parents excreted increased amounts of dibasic amino acids in contrast to the parents of children with the first type of hyperdibasicamino-aciduria in whom no abnormality in dibasic amino acid excretion can be demonstrated. Also in contrast to patients with the first type of hyperdibasicaminoaciduria, this child did not manifest protein intolerance nor hyperammonemia. It is possible that the patient of Kihara et al. (100) was homozygous for this second type of hyperdibasicaminoaciduria and those of Whelan and Scriver (99) represent heterozygotes.

The patients described by Omura et al. may represent a possible third variation of cystine and dibasic amino acid transport defects (101). They reported a child with markedly increased urinary excretion of lysine with normal excretion of cystine, ornithine, and arginine. Intestinal absorption of lysine was also severely compromised; yet, that of ornithine, arginine, and cystine was normal. This child was profoundly retarded and the authors speculated that a deficiency of the essential amino acid lysine may have been the cause.

B. Disorders of Neutral Amino Acids

Hartnup Disease

In 1956, Baron et al. described four children in a single family with an unusual illness characterized by a pellegralike skin rash, transient cerebellar ataxia, and a defect in the renal reabsorption of neutral amino acids (102). Since then numerous other cases of this disorder have been reported from all over the world (103). Hartnup disease appears to be inherited as an autosomal recessive trait with an incidence of about 1:20,000 (104).

The renal aminoaciduria in Hartnup disease is mainly of neutral amino acids and comprises alanine, serine, threonine, valine, leucine, isoleucine, phenylalanine, tyrosine, tryptophan, histidine, glutamine, and asparagine. The reabsorption of histidine is so low that the clearance of histidine approaches the glomerular filtration rate. The reabsorption of the other neutral amino acids varies between 30 and 60%, which is considerably lower than the normal of over 95%. There is no abnormality in the reabsorption of cystine, dibasic amino acids, dicarboxylic amino acids, glycine, the imino acids, or the β-amino acids. Since this illness is inherited in a simple autosomal recessive fashion, it would appear that the neutral amino acids share a common transport pathway in the kidney. In addition to this common pathway, probably one or more pathways also exist which are specific for each neutral amino acid.

Unlike cystinuria, the excessive renal excretion of the neutral amino acids appear to play only a small role in the pathogenesis of this disorder. Tryptophanuria may contribute to the overall deficiency in nicotinamide, but the major pathogenetic mechanism underlying Hartnup disease is the defect in intestinal absorption of the neutral amino acids in general and tryptophan in particular. Scriver and Shaw (105) have shown that there is a defective intestinal absorption of neutral amino acids by demonstrating an abnormal pattern of amino acids in the stool which is very similar to that of the urine. Milne et al. (106) have further demonstrated this defect in vivo in four ways. First, they showed that unchanged tryptophan could be recovered in stool from Hartnup patients fed large amounts of tryptophan. Secondly, plasma tryptophan rose only slightly after a tryptophan load in Hartnup patients. Thirdly, there was no conversion of orally administered D-tryptophan to indolyl-3-pyruvic by Hartnup patients in contrast to normals. Finally, Hartnup patients excreted abnormally high amounts of tryptophan breakdown products in the urine, which occurred because the unabsorbed tryptophan was metabolized by the gut flora with subsequent absorption and renal excretion of these metabolites. In vitro confirmation of this gut defect came from studies done by Shih and coworkers demonstrating reduced uptake of tryptophan and methionine by gut mucosa from two brothers with Hartnup disease (107). Hartnup patients can absorb oligopeptides containing tryptophan, phenylalanine, and histidine normally and this may be an important way for assimilation of neutral amino acids from the diet in these patients (108,109).

Clinical Aspects

The clinical manifestations of Hartnup disease appear to stem from the malabsorption of tryptophan, leading to nicotinamide deficiency (103). Although the metabolism of tryptophan to nicotinamide and ultimately to nicotinamide adenine nucleotide (NAD) accounts for only a small fraction of the NAD pool, this small deficit appears to be important for the generation of the clinical symptoms of Hartnup disease. Further, Hartnup disease resembles in some respects niacin deficiency, pellegra, which is also thought to lead to a deficiency of NAD. Both diseases are marked by an intermittant, scaly, erythemous rash affecting the face and other exposed body parts which appears to be exacerbated by sunlight, although this has not been convincingly demonstrated.

The other major manifestation is intermittent cerebellar ataxia. This usually appears in concert with worsening of the rash, although it may happen in the absence of a rash, especially after an infection. Typically, when an attack occurs, the patient walks with an unsteady, wide-based gait. Other signs of cerebellar ataxia are often present such as intention tremor, jerky arm movements, and nystagmus. Double vision may also occur. Sensory abnormalities are not found. The onset of the ataxia can be quite abrupt, rapidly reaching a peak. Recovery is gradual, but complete. Some patients have never manifested ataxia, but have had collapsing or fainting attacks which occur without warning. Psychiatric symptoms ranging from mild emotional lability to frank delirium have been evident in a few Hartnup patients. Some patients with Hartnup disease have been mildly retarded, but the original suggestion of progressive mental deterioration is untenable.

These clinical symptoms of Hartnup disease are intermittent and variable. From long-term follow-up of neonatally detected patients, it is clear that many affected individuals never manifest symptoms. Clinically apparent disease can be precipitated by fever, sunlight, sulfonamides, and psychological stress, but always in concert with an inadequate diet. Lessening of clinical expression of the disease with attainment of adulthood also points to some nutrient being in limited supply. During childhood with the stress of growth the supply of this nutrient may be more critical, explaining the improvement in symptoms with aging. Nicotinamide appears to be this nutrient, since clinical improvement follows oral administration of this vitamin. However, it is possible that some or all symptoms could be related to the absorption of a toxin generated by the action of the intestinal flora on the unabsorbed tryptophan and other neutral amino acids.

Diagnosis

The diagnosis should be suspected in any patient with pellegra without a history of niacin or nicotinamide deficiency, especially if the cutaneous and neuropsychiatric manifestations are accompanied by cerebellar signs. The diagnosis can be made by demonstrating excess neutral amino acids in the urine. Hartnup disease can easily be differentiated from the Fanconi syndrome, since the latter has a generalized aminoaciduria not confined to neutral amino acids as well as excess excretion of other urinary solutes such as glucose, phosphate, and bicarbonate.

Treatment

Because of the rarity of Hartnup disease and the transiency of the clinical manifestations, evaluation of various therapeutic modalities is quite difficult. Administration of 40-250 mg of nicotinamide will heal the skin lesions and improve the neurological problems. Undue exposure to sunlight should be avoided, as this probably worsens the rash. Milne has suggested sterilization of the GI tract to minimize the bacterial decarboxylation and thereby reduce the amount of indoles and amines available for absorption (110).

Methionine Malabsorption (Oasthouse Syndrome)

In 1958, Smith and Strang described an infant with white hair, edema, convulsions, and mental retardation who subsequently died at 10 months of age (111). The odor of his urine was distinctly unpleasant, smelling like an oasthouse or dried celery. A urinary ferric chloride test gave a green color and the urine amino acid chromatography had persistently large amounts of methionine, with a smaller increase in the branch chain amino acids as well as phenylalanine and tyrosine. In addition, the urine contained large amounts of α-hydroxybutyric acid. Hooft et al. described a similar 2 year old who also excreted large amounts of α-hydroxybutyric acid in her urine, while her feces contained large amounts of methionine, α-hydroxybutyric acid, and branch-chain ketoacids (112).

Oral methionine loading in the patient described by Hooft et al. (112) led to diarrhea, tachypnea, and marked urinary excretion of α-hydroxybutyric acid (113). Methioninuria was present intermittantly, but most especially after methionine loading (113). In this patient and probably that of Smith and Strang (111), there appeared to be a transport defect in the intestine and kidney that primarily involved methionine. The unabsorbed intestinal methionine was converted to α-hydroxybutyric acid by colonic bacteria which was then absorbed and appeared in the urine. This organic acid may well have given rise to the severe neurological symptoms in these children, since a low methionine diet, with the disappearance of urinary α-hydroxybutyric acid, led to a striking clinical improvement and normalization of the EEG. Further, the malabsorbed methionine probably interfered with branch-chain amino acid absorption with the subsequent generation of their α-ketoacids by colonic bacteria.

Histidinuria

In 1975, Sabater et al. described two mentally retarded male siblings with marked urinary excretion of histidine (114). Further investigation revealed disturbed uptake of histidine both by the intestine and the renal tubule. No other abnormality of amino acid transport was detected. The parents excreted normal amounts of histidine in their urine, but they did exhibit a mild malabsorption of an oral histidine load. From this evidence, there appears to be a transport system specifically for histidine which is defective in these two children.

C. Disorders of Glycine and Imino Acids

Iminoglycinuria

In 1958, Joseph et al. (115) described a patient that had markedly increased amounts of the imino acids proline and hydroxyproline and glycine in his urine and they attributed these biochemical abnormalities to a defect in renal tubular transport of these amino acids. Since then numerous reports of this pattern of aminoaciduria have appeared throughout the world (117-119). Many of the patients initially described suffered from central nervous system (CNS) problems ranging from mental retardation to convulsive disorders in association with this iminoglycinuria. There was concern at first that the CNS disorders were related to the aminoaciduria, but subsequent reports of healthy individuals with iminoglycinuria (120,121) and no apparent illness associated with iminoglycinuria on follow-up of large neonatal screening programs (104,122) have led most investigators to conclude that iminoglycinuria is a benign "experiment of nature."

This experiment of nature points to a common carrier subserving the transport of the amino acids and glycine which is possibly defective in iminoglycinuria. Carrier mediation of proline and hydroxyproline transport by the human kidney was suggested by demonstrations of saturable reabsorption of these amino acids (123,124). A similar pattern of renal handling has also been shown for glycine in the dog (125). In vivo evidence indicating a common carrier mediating the transport of these amino acids is the presence of iminoglycinuria in patients with hyperprolinemia (126). This inhibition of hydroxyproline and glycine reabsorption by proline in the kidney is quite selective, since little or no change occurred in the renal excretion of other amino acids.

Developmental studies have pointed out, however, that more than one system probably mediates tubular reabsorption of glycine and imino acids. Although there is a generalized increase in the urinary excretion of all amino acids in the very immature animal and human, the excretion of glycine and the imino acids is particularly prominent (11,12,127,128). However, by 1 week in the rat and 3-6 months in the human, iminoaciduria disappears, but it is not until 3 weeks of age in the rat and 6-10 months in the human that glycine excretion falls to levels observed in mature individuals. This suggests that separate transport systems, which mature a different rates, exist for glycine and the imino acids in addition to a common system.

In vitro studies using renal cortical slices, isolated tubules, and brush-border membrane vesicles have confirmed this more complex picture of imino acid and glycine transport. The renal cortical slice (37,129-132), the isolated tubule (8,133-135), and the isolated brush-border membrane vesicles (136,137) from the rat have demonstrated that at least two transport systems exist for the uptake of glycine and two transport systems for the uptake of proline. Similar findings have also been observed in renal cortex slices from humans (138, 139). These four systems probably only represent three distinct carriers, since competition studies using renal cortex slices, tubules and brush-border membrane vesicles have shown that at least one separate system exists for the transport of proline and glycine with a single common transport system (130,133,136) (Fig. 6). It is clear from both in vivo (123,140) and in vitro (130,133,134,136) data that the affinity of glycine for this common system is less than proline. From kinetic data, this common system appears to correspond to the high-capacity, low-affinity glycine transport observed in both human and animal kidney

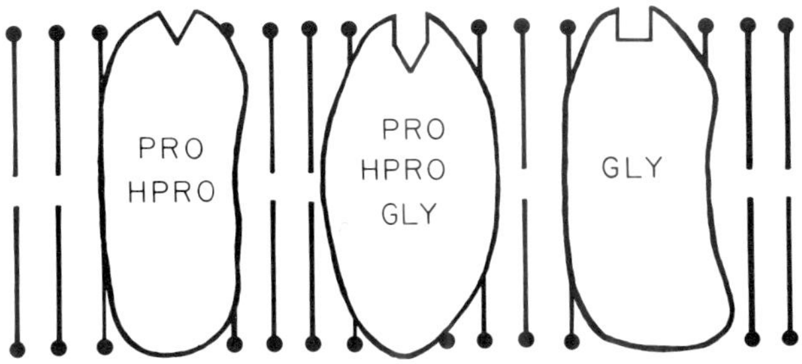

Fig. 6 Schematic drawing of the luminal membrane of the renal proximal tubule cell showing the possible diversity of carrier proteins for glycine (GLY), proline (PRO), and hydroxyproline (HPRO).

cortex (130,133,136,139). The proline transport system that is shared with glycine is not clear. Studies employing renal cortical slices appear to show that glycine and proline interact on the low-affinity proline uptake system (130,131), while studies using isolated renal tubules and brushborder membranes show this interaction occurring on the high-affinity proline uptake system (134,136).

It is fairly certain that this aminoaciduria is inherited as an autosomal recessive trait from the 14 families described with iminoglycinuria. In no report to date has both a parent and a child been described with the mutant phenotype. Levy et al. (104) have reported an incidence of 1:20,000, which indicates that iminoglycinuria is about as common as Hartnup disease but less common than cystinuria.

As in cystinuria, there appear to be several mutant alleles which can give rise to the phenotype of iminoglycinuria. Evidence for this comes from two observations. First, patients from some but not all families have an intestinal transport defect for these amino acids in addition to the renal transport defect (117,141). Secondly, all obligate heterozygotes in some families excrete abnormally high amounts of glycine (120,141-144), but not imino acids, while in other families heterozygotes do not excrete increased amounts of either imino acids or glycine (115-117,145). These differences in families with iminoglycinuria suggest that more than one mutant allele can give rise to this aminoaciduria.

Glycinuria

In 1957, de Vries et al. (146) described a family in whom four females from three successive generations had hyperglycinuria with normal plasma glycine levels and without hyperiminoaciduria. Three of these four women also developed calcium oxalate renal stones, but the relationship to the aminoaciduria remains unclear. Greene et al. (147) described a father and two sons with hyperglycinuria without hyperglycinemia or hyperiminoaciduria. Proline loading in one of the sons demonstrated a normal maximal transport rate for proline, but there was an increase in the splay of the titration curve consistent with an impairment in the binding of proline to the carrier (K_m defect).

It is possible that both of these families contain individuals heterozygous for iminoglycinuria. This would easily explain the apparent dominant nature of transmission. Certainly the family described by Greene et al. (147) appears to be a form of iminoglycinuria.

Kaser et al. (148) described a very different family with hyperglycinuria. Thirteen of 37 members of this family had hyperglycinuria in association with renal glycosuria. Again there was a dominant transmission of the trait. No one was found to have either glycosuria or hyperglycinuria without the other. The defect underlying this combined glucoglycinuria is obscure, but it seems not to affect the combined iminoacid-glycine pathway that is probably responsible for iminoglycinuria.

D. Disorders of Dicarboxylic Amino Acids

Dicarboxylic Aminoaciduria

In 1974, Teijema (149) described a 2-year-old athyreotic acid girl with massive urinary excretion of aspartic and glutamic acid. She also manifested mild hyperprolinemia, hypoglycemia, and mental and growth retardation. The dicarboxylic aminoaciduria was so massive that the excretion rate exceeded filtration, suggesting tubular secretion of these amino acids. The role that the dicarboxylic aminoaciduria played in the hypoglycemia and mental retardation was difficult to ascertain. A second patient described with dicarboxylic aminoaciduria again had such massive excretion of these amino acids that the clearance pattern demonstrated tubular secretion (150). He, however, did not manifest mental retardation, hypoglycemia, or hyperprolinemia.

Both of these children apparently have an isolated abnormality in the handling of dicarboxylic amino acids. The unusual feature of this aminoaciduria is the net secretion of the dicarboxylic amino acids, although net secretion of cystine is observed in many patients with classical cystinuria. Remaining to be defined is whether the origin of this defect lies in impaired reabsorption, increased secretion, or both.

REFERENCES

1. Singer, S. J.; and Nicholson, G. L. The fluid mosaic model of the structure of cell membranes. Science 175:720-732, 1972.
2. Penrose, W. R.; Nichoalds, G. E.; Piperno, J. R.; and Oxender, D. L. Purification and properties of a leucine-binding protein from E. coli. J. Biol. Chem. 243:5921-5928, 1968.
3. Elsas, L. J.; and Rosenberg, L. E. Inhibition of amino acid transport in rat kidney cortex by puromycin. Proc. Natl. Acad. Sci. USA 57:371-378, 1967.
4. Fairclough, P.; Malathi, P.; Preiser, H.; and Crane, R. K. Reconstitution into liposomes of glucose active transport from rabbit renal proximal tubule. Biochim. Biophys. Acta 553:295-306, 1979.
5. Rosenberg, L. E.; and Segal, S. Maleic acid-induced inhibition of amino acid transport in rat kidney. Biochem. J. 92:345-352, 1964.
6. Roth, K. S.; Hwang, S. M.; and Segal, S. Effect of maleic acid on the kinetics of α-methyl-D-glucoside uptake by isolated rat renal tubules. Biochim. Biophys. Acta 426: 675-687, 1976.
7. Stolte, H.; Lustenberger, N.; Weise, M.; Eisenbach, G. M.; and Oelker, H. J. Reabsorption of free amino acids in the single rat nephron. In: Amino Acid Transport and Uric Acid Transport, edited by Silbernagl, S., Lang, F., and Greger, R., Stuttgart, Georg Thieme, 1976, pp. 53-62.
8. Barfuss, D. W.; and Schafer, J. A. Active amino acid absorption by proximal convoluted and proximal straight tubules. Am. J. Physiol. 236:F149-F162, 1979.
9. Lingard, J.; Rumrich, G.; and Young, J. A. Kinetics of L-histidine transport in the proximal convolution of the rat nephron studied using the stationary microperfusion technique. Pflugers Arch. 342:13-28, 1973.
10. Völkl, H.; Silbernagl, S.; and Deetjen, P. Kinetics of L-proline reabsorption in rat kidney by continuous microperfusion. Pflügers Arch. 382:115-121, 1979.
11. Brodehl, J. Postnatal development of tubular amino acid reabsorption. In: Amino Acid Transport and Uric Acid Transport, edited by Silbernagl, S., Lang, F., and Greger, R. Stuttgart, Georg Thieme, 1976, pp. 128-135.
12. Brodehl, J.; and Gellissen, K. Endogenous renal transport of free amino acids in infancy and childhood. Pediatrics 42:395-404, 1968.
13. Wollaston, W. H. On cystic oxide: A new species of urinary calculus. Trans. R. Soc. Lond. 100:223-230, 1810.
14. Stromeyer, L. Oxide cystique. Ann. Chim. Phys. 27:221, 1824.
15. Berzelius, J. J. Calculus urinaries. Traite Chem. 7:424, 1833.
16. Garrod, A. E. Inborn errors of metabolism. Lancet 2, 1908. (Lecture I, p. 1; Lecture II, p. 73; Lecture III, p. 142; Lecture IV, p. 214).
17. Dent, C. E.; and Rose, G. A. Amino acid metabolism in cystinuria. Q. J. Med. 20:205-218, 1951.
18. Robson, E. B.; and Rose, G. A. The effects of intravenous lysine on the renal clearances of cystine, arginine and ornithine in normal subjects, in patients with cystinuria and their relatives. Clin. Sci. 16:75-91, 1957.

19. Lester, F. T.; and Cusworth, D. C. Lysine infusion in cystinuria: Theoretical renal thresholds for lysine. Clin. Sci. 44:99-111, 1973.
20. Kato, T. Renal handling of dibasic amino acids and cystine in cystinuria. Clin. Sci. Molec. Med. 53:9-15, 1977.
21. Webber, W. A.; Brown, J. L.; and Pitts, R. F. Interactions of amino acids in renal tubular transport. Am. J. Physiol. 200:380-386, 1961.
22. Crawhall, J. C.; Scowen, E. F.; Thompson, C. J.; and Watts, R. W. E. The renal clearance of amino acids in cystinuria. J. Clin. Invest. 46:1162-1170, 1967.
23. Segal, S.; and Bovée, K. C. Canine models for human renal transport disorders. In: Models for the Study of Inborn Errors of Metabolism, edited by Hommes, F. A., Elsevier-North Holland, Biomedical Press, 1979, pp. 19-20.
24. Rosenberg, L. E.; Albrecht, I.; and Segal, S. Lysine transport in human kidney: Evidence for two systems. Science 155:1426-1428, 1967.
25. Von Udransky, L.; and Baumann, E. Ueber das Vorkommen von Diaminen, sogenannten Ptomainen, bei Cystinurie. Z. Physiol. Chem. 13:562-594, 1889.
26. Loewy, A.; and Neuberg, C. Über Cystinuria. Z. Physiol. Chem. 43:338-354, 1904.
27. Brand, E.; Cahill, G. H.; and Harris, M. M. Cystinuria II. The metabolism of cysteine, methionine and glutathione. J. Biol. Chem. 109:69-83, 1935.
28. Brand, E.; and Cahill, G. F. Further studies on metabolism of sulfur compounds in cystinuria. Proc. Soc. Exp. Biol. Med. 31:1247, 1934.
29. Milne, M. D.; Asatoor, A. M.; Edwards, K. D. G.; and Loughridge, L. W. The intestinal absorption defect in cystinuria. Gut 2:323-337, 1961.
30. Asatoor, A. M.; Lacey, B. W.; London, D. R.; and Milne, M. D. Amino acid metabolism in cystinuria. Clin. Sci. 23:285-304, 1962.
31. Thier, S.; Fox, M.; Segal, S.; and Rosenberg, L. E. Cystinuria: In vitro demonstration of an intestinal transport defect. Science 143:482-484, 1964.
32. McCarthy, C. F.; Borland, J. L.; Lynch, H. J.; Owens, E. E.; and Tyor, M. P. Defective uptake of basic amino acids and L-cystine by intestinal mucosa of patients with cystinuria. J. Clin. Invest. 43:1518-1524, 1964.
33. Thier, S.; Segal, S.; Fox, M.; Blair, A.; and Rosenberg, L. E. Cystinuria: Defective intestinal transport of dibasic amino acids and cystine. J. Clin. Invest. 44:442-448, 1965.
34. Hellier, M. D.; Perrett, D.; and Holdsworth, C. D. Dipeptide absorption in cystinuria. Br. Med. J. 4:782-783, 1970.
35. Rosenberg, L. E.; Downing, S. J.; and Segal, S. Competitive inhibition of dibasic amino acid transport in rat kidney. J. Biol. Chem. 237:2265-2270, 1962.
36. Schwartzman, L.; Blair, A.; and Segal, S. Exchange diffusion of dibasic amino acids in rat kidney cortex slices. Biochim. Biophys. Acta 135:120-126, 1967.
37. Segal, S.; Schwartzman, L.; Blair, A.; and Bertoli, D. Dibasic amino acid transport by rat kidney cortex slices. Biochim. Biophys. Acta 135:127-135, 1967.
38. Fox, M.; Thier, S.; Rosenberg, L. E.; Kiser, W.; and Segal, S. Evidence against a single renal transport defect in cystinuria. N. Engl. J. Med. 270:556-561, 1964.
39. Segal, S.; and Crawhall, J. C. Characteristics of cystine and cysteine transport in rat kidney cortex slices. Proc. Natl. Acad. Sci. USA 59:231-237, 1968.
40. Segal, S.; and Smith, I. Delineation of separate transport systems in rat-kidney cortex for L-lysine and L-cystine by developmental patterns. Biochem. Biophys. Res. Commun. 35:771-777, 1969.
41. Segal, S.; and Smith, I. Delineation of cystine and cysteine transport systems in rat kidney cortex by development patterns. Proc. Natl. Acad. Sci. USA 63:926-933, 1969.
42. Foreman, J. W.; Hwang, S. M.; and Segal, S. Transport interactions of cystine and dibasic amino acids in isolated rat renal cortical tubules. Metabolism 29:53-61, 1980.
43. Segal, S.; McNamara, P. D.; and Pepe, L. M. Transport interactions of cystine and dibasic amino acids in renal brush border vesicles. Science 197:169-171, 1977.

44. Crawhall, J. C.; and Segal, S. The intracellular ratio of cysteine and cystine in various tissues. Biochem. J. 105:891-896, 1967.
45. Schwartzman, L.; Blair, A.; and Segal, S. A common renal transport system for lysine, ornithine, arginine, and cysteine. Biochem. Biophys. Res. Commun. 23:220-226, 1966.
46. Bostrom, H.; and Hambraeus, L. Cystinuria in Sweden. VII. Clinical, histopathological and medico-sociological aspects of the disease. Acta Med. Scand. (Suppl.) 411:1-128, 1964.
47. Weinberger, A.; Sperling, O.; Rabinovitz, M.; Brosh, S.; Adam, A.; and de Vries, A. High frequency of cystinuria among Jews of Libyan origin. Hum. Hered. 24:568-572, 1974.
48. Colliss, J. E.; Levi, A. J.; and Milne, M. D. Stature and nutrition in cystinuria and Hartnup disease. Br. Med. J. 1:590-592, 1963.
49. Smith, A.; Yu, J. S.; and Brown, D. A. Childhood cystinuria in New South Wales. Arch. Dis. Child. 54:676-681, 1979.
50. Scriver, C. R.; Whelan, D. T.; Clow, C. L.; and Dallaire, L. Cystinuria: Increased prevalence in patients with mental disease, N. Engl. J. Med. 283:783-786, 1970.
51. Berry, H. K. Detection of metabolic disorders among mentally retarded children by means of paper spot tests. Am. J. Ment. Defic. 66:555-560, 1962.
52. Banerji, N. K.; and Miller, J. H. E. Paraplegia associated with cystinuria. J. Neurol. Sci. 12:101-104, 1971.
53. De Meyer, W.; and Gebhard, R. L. Subacute combined degeneration of the spinal cord with cystinuria. Neurology 25:994-997, 1975.
54. Blackburn, C. R. B.; and McLeod, G. CNS lesions in cystinuria. Arch. Neurol. 34:638-639, 1977.
55. Gold, R. J. M.; Dobrinski, M. J.; and Gold, D. P. Cystinuria and mental deficiency. Clin. Genet. 12:329-332, 1977.
56. Smith, A.; and Procopis, P. G. Cystinuria and its relationship to mental retardation. Med. J. Aust. 2:932-933, 1975.
57. Hwang, S. M.; and Segal, S. Developmental and other aspects of [^{35}S] cysteine transport by rat brain synaptosomes. J. Neurochem. 33:1303-1308, 1979.
58. Segal, S.; and Hwang, S. M. L-[^{35}S]Cystine uptake by rat brain synaptosomes. J. Neurochem. 33:697-704, 1979.
59. Hwang, S. M.; Weiss, S. D.; and Segal, S. Uptake of L-[^{35}S] cystine by isolated rat brain capillaries. J. Neurochem. 35:417-424, 1980.
60. Hwang, S. M.; and Segal, S. Developmental and other characteristics of lysine uptake by rat brain synaptosomes. Biochim. Biophys. Acta 557:436-448, 1979.
61. Harris, H.; Mittwoch, U.; Robson, E. B.; and Warren, F. L. Phenotypes and genotypes in cystinuria. Ann. Hum. Genet. 20:57-91, 1955.
62. Rosenberg, L. E.; Downing, S.; Durant, J. L.; and Segal, S. Cystinuria: Biochemical evidence for three genetically distinct diseases. J. Clin. Invest. 45:365-371, 1966.
63. Resnick, M. I.; Goodman, H. O.; and Boyce, W. H. Heterozygous cystinuria and calcium oxalate urolithiasis. J. Urol. 122:52-54, 1979.
64. Dent, C. E.; Friedmann, M.; Green, H.; and Watson, L. C. A. Treatment of cystinuria. Br. Med. J. 1:403-408, 1965.
65. Crawhall, J. C.; Scowen, E. F.; and Watts, R. W. E. Effects of penicillamine on cystinuria. Br. Med. J. 1:585-590, 1963.
66. Bartter, F. C.; Lotz, M.; Thier, S.; Rosenberg, L. E.; and Potts, J. T. Cystinuria: Combined clinical staff conference at the National Institute of Health. Ann. Intern. Med. 62:796-822, 1965.
67. Crawhall, J. C.; and Thompson, C. J. Cystinuria: Effect of D-penicillamine on plasma and urinary cystine concentration. Science 147:1459-1460, 1965.
68. Lotz, M.; and Potts, J. T. Quantitation of the effects of penicillamine therapy in cystinuria. J. Clin. Invest. 43:1293, 1964.

69. Fellers, F. X.; and Shahidi, N. T. The nephrotic syndrome induced by penicillamine therapy. Am. J. Dis. Child. 98:669, 1959.
70. Adams, D. A.; Goldman, R.; Maxwell, M. H.; and Latta, J. H. Nephrotic syndrome associated with penicillamine therapy of Wilson's disease. Am. J. Med. 36:330-336, 1964.
71. Rosenberg, L. E.; and Hayslett, J. P. Nephrotoxic effects of penicillamine in cystinuria. J.A.M.A. 201:698-699, 1967.
72. Corcos, J. M.; Soler-Bechera, J.; Mayer, K.; Freyberg, R. H.; Goldstein, R.; and Jaffe, I. Neutrophilic agranulocytosis during administration of penicillamine. J.A.M.A. 189: 265-268, 1964.
73. Beer, W. E.; and Cooke, K. B. Epidermolysis bullosa induced by penicillamine. Br. J. Dermatol. 79:123-125, 1967.
74. Fawcett, N. P.; Nyhan, W. L.; and Anderson, W. W. Thrombocytosis during treatment of cystinuria with penicillamine therapy. J. Pediatr. 60:976-977, 1966.
75. Keiser, H. R.; Henkiz, R. I.; Bartter, F. C.; and Sjoerdsma, A. Loss of taste during therapy with penicillamine. J.A.M.A. 203:381-383, 1968.
76. Jaffe, I. A.; Altmann, K.; and Merryman, P. The antipyridoxine effect of penicillamine in man. J. Clin. Invest. 43:1869-1873, 1964.
77. Crawhall, J. C.; Purkiss, P.; Watts, R. W. E.; and Young, E. P. The excretion of amino acids by cystinuric patients and their relatives. Ann. Hum. Genet. 33:149-169, 1969.
78. Stokes, G. S.; Potts, J. T.; Lotz, M.; and Bartter, F. C. A new agent in the treatment of cystinuria, N-acetyl-penicillamine. Br. Med. J. 1:284-288, 1968.
79. Stevens, A. D.; and Watts, R. W. E. The treatment of cystinuria with N-acetyl-D-penicillamine, a comparison with the results of D-penicillamine treatment. Q. J. Med. 40: 335-370, 1971.
80. King, J. S. Treatment of cystinuria with α-mercaptopropionylglycine: A preliminary report. Proc. Soc. Exp. Biol. Med. 129:927-932, 1968.
81. Kinoshita, K.; Yachiku, S.; Kotake, T.; Takeuchi, M.; and Sonada, T. Treatment with 2-mercaptopropionylglycine (MPG). Proceedings of the 2nd International Symposium on Thiola. Osaka, Japan. Santen Pharmaceutical Co., Ltd., 1972, p. 50.
82. Sonada, T.; Kinoshita, K.; Kotake, T.; Yachiku, S.; and Takeuchi, M. Effect of thiola on cystinuria. Proceedings of the International Symposium on Thiola. Osaka, Japan. Santen Pharmaceutical Co., Ltd., 1970, p. 231.
83. Nishimura, R.; Ishido, T.; and Takai, S. Studies on cystinuria. Proceedings of the 2nd International Symposium on Thiola. Osaka, Japan. Santen Pharmaceutical Co., Ltd., 1972, p. 47.
84. Hautmann, R.; Terhorst, B.; Stuhlsatz, H. W.; and Lutzeyer, W. Mercaptopropionylglycine: A progress in cystine stone therapy. J. Urol. 117:628-630, 1977.
85. Miyagi, K.; and Nakada, F. Amino acid reabsorption in cystinuria: The effects of monoaminodicarboxylic acids and amido group amino acids with special reference to glutamine. J. Jpn. Soc. Intern. Med. 67:694-702, 1978.
86. Miyagi, K.; Nakada, F.; and Ohshiro, D. Effect of glutamine on cystine excretion in a patient with cystinuria. N. Engl. J. Med. 301:196-198, 1979.
87. Jaeger, P.; and Portman, L. Anticystinuric effect of glutamine and of low sodium diet in cystinuria. Am. Soc. Nephrol. (Abstracts) 33A, 1982.
88. Skovby, F.; Rosenberg, L. E.; and Thier, S. O. No effect of L-glutamine on cystinuria. Letter to the Editor, New Engl. J. Med. 302:236-237, 1980.
89. Van Den Berg, C. J.; Jones, J. D.; and Smith, L. H. Glutamine therapy of cystinuria. Invest. Urol. 18:155-157, 1980.
90. Brodehl, J.; Gellisson, K.; and Kowalewski, S. Isolated cystinuria (without lysine-ornithine-argininuria) in family with hypocalcemia tetany. Klin. Wochenschr. 45:38-40, 1967.
91. Perheentupa, J.; and Visakorpi, J. K. Protein intolerance with deficiency transport of basic amino acids; another inborn error of metabolism. Lancet 2:813-816, 1965.

92. Kekomaki, M.; Visakorpi, J. K.; Perheentupa, J.; and Saxen, L. Familial protein intolerance with deficient transport of basic amino acids; an analysis of 10 patients. Acta Pediatr. Scand. 56:617-630, 1967.
93. Simell, O.; Perheentupa, J.; Rapola, J.; Visakorpi, J.; and Eskelin, L.-E. Lysinuric protein intolerance. Am. J. Med. 59:229-240, 1975.
94. Desjeux, J.-F.; Rajantie, J.; Simell, O.; Dumontier, A.-M.; and Perheentupa, J. Lysine fluxes across the jejunal epithelium in lysinuric protein intolerance. J. Clin. Invest. 65:1382-1387, 1980.
95. Simell, O. Diamino acid transport into granulocytes and liver slices of patients with lysinuric protein intolerance. Pediatr. Res. 9:504-508, 1975.
96. Simell, O.; and Perheentupa, J. Defective metabolic clearance of plasma arginine and ornithine in lysinuric protein intolerance. Metabolism 23:691-701, 1974.
97. Awrich, A. E.; Stackhouse, W. J.; Cantrell, J. E.; Patterson, J. H.; and Rudman, D. Hyperdibasicaminoaciduria, hyperammonemia, and growth retardation: Treatment with arginine, lysine and citrulline. J. Pediatr. 87:731-738, 1975.
98. Rajantie, J.; Simell, O.; Rapola, J.; and Perheentupa, J. Lysinuric protein intolerance: A two year trial of dietary supplementation therapy with citrulline and lysine. J. Pediatr. 97:927-932, 1980.
99. Whelan, D. T.; and Scriver, C. R. Hyperdibasicaminoaciduria: An inherited disorder of amino acid transport. Pediatr. Res. 2:525-539, 1968.
100. Kihara, H.; Valente, M.; Porter, M. T.; and Fluharty, A. L. Hyperdibasicaminoaciduria in a mentally retarded homozygote with a peculiar response to phenothiaxines. Pediatrics 51:223-229, 1973.
101. Omura, K.; Yamanaka, N.; Hijami, S.; Matsuoka, O.; Fujimoto, A.; Issiki, G.; and Tada, K. Lysine malabsorption syndrome: A new type transport defect. Pediatrics 57:102-105, 1976.
102. Baron, D. N.; Dent, C. E.; Harris, H.; Hart, E. W.; and Jepson, J. B. Hereditary pellegra-like skin rash with temporary cerebellar ataxia, constant renal aminoaciduria and other bizarre biochemical features. Lancet 1:421-428, 1956.
103. Jepson, J. B. Hartnup disease. In: The Metabolic Basis of Inherited Disease, 4th ed., edited by Stanbury, J. B., Wyngaarden, J. B., and Fredrickson, D. S. New York, McGraw-Hill, 1978, pp. 1563-1577.
104. Levy, H. L. Genetic screening. In: Progress in Human Genetics, vol. 4, edited by Herns, H., and Hirschorn, K. New York, Plenum Press, 1973, pp. 1-104.
105. Scriver, C. R.; and Shaw, K. N. F. Hartnup disease: An example of genetically determined defective cellular amino acid transport. Can. Med. Assoc. J. 86:232, 1962.
106. Milne, M. D.; Crawford, M. A.; Girao, C. B.; and Loughbridge, L. The metabolic disorder in Hartnup disease. Q. J. Med. 29:407-421, 1960.
107. Shih, V. E.; Bixby, E. M.; Alpers, D. H.; Bartosocas, C. S.; and Thier, S. O. Studies of intestinal transport defect in Hartnup disease. Gastroenterology 61:445-453, 1971.
108. Navab, F.; and Asatoor, A. M. Studies on intestinal absorption of amino acids and a dipeptide in a case of Hartnup disease. Gut 11:373-379, 1970.
109. Asatoor, A. M.; Cheng, B.; Edwards, K. D. G.; Laut, A. F.; Matthews, D. M.; Milne, M. D.; Navab, F.; and Richards, A. J. Intestinal absorption of two dipeptides in Hartnup disease. Gut 11:380-387, 1970.
110. Milne, M. D. Renal tubular dysfunction. In: Diseases of the Kidney, 2nd ed., edited by Strauss, M. B., and Welt, L. G. Boston, Little, Brown, 1972, pp. 1071-1138.
111. Smith, A. J.; and Strang, L. B. An inborn error of metabolism with the urinary excretion of α-hydroxybutyric acid and phenylpyruvic acid. Arch. Dis. Child. 33:109-113, 1958.
112. Hooft, C.; Timmermans, J.; Snoeck, J.; Antener, I.; Oyaert, W.; and Van Den Hende, C. Methionine malabsorption syndrome. Ann. Pediatr. 205:73-84, 1965.
113. Efron, M. L.; and Ampola, M. G. The aminoacidurias. Pediatr. Clin. North Am. 14: 881-903, 1967.

114. Sabater, J.; Ferre, C.; Pulioli, M.; and Maya, A. Histindinuria: A renal and intestinal histidine transport deficiency found in two mentally retarded children. Clin. Genet. 9:117-124, 1976.
115. Joseph, R.; Ribierre, M.; Job, J.-C.; and Girault, M. Maladie familiale associante des convulsions à début très précoce, une albuminorachie et une hyperaminoacidurie. Arch. Fr. Pediatr. 15:374-387, 1958.
116. Tada, K.; Morikawa, T.; Ando, T.; Yoshida, T.; and Mingawa, A. Prolinuria: A new renal tubular defect in transport of proline and glycine. Tohoku J. Exp. Med. 87: 133-143, 1965.
117. Morikawa, T.; Tada, K.; Ando, T.; Yoshida, T.; and Minagawa, A. Prolinuria: Defect in intestinal absorption of imino acids and glycine. Tohoku J. Exp. Med. 90:105-116, 1966.
118. Scriver, C. R.; and Wilson, O. H. Amino acid transport in human kidney: Evidence for genetic control of two types. Science 155:1428-1430, 1967.
119. Scriver, C. R. Familial inimoglycinuria. In: The Metabolic Basis of Inherited Disease, 4th ed., edited by Stanbury, J. B., Wyngaarden, J. B., and Fredrickson, D. S. New York, McGraw-Hill, 1978, pp. 1593-1606.
120. Rosenberg, L. E.; Durant, J. L.; and Elsas, L. J., II. Familial iminoglycinuria: An inborn error of renal tubular transport. N. Engl. J. Med. 278:1407-1413, 1968.
121. Fraser, D. R.; Friedmann, A. I.; Patton, V. M.; Wade, D. N.; and Woolf, L. I. Iminoglycinuria a "harmless' inborn error of metabolism? Humangenetik 6:362-367, 1968.
122. Procopis, P. G.; and Turner, B. Iminoaciduria: A benign renal tubular defect. J. Pediatr. 79:419-422, 1971.
123. Scriver, C. R.; Efron, M. L.; and Schafer, I. A. Renal tubular transport of proline, hydroxyproline and glycine in health and in familial hyperprolinemia. J. Clin. Invest. 43:374-385, 1964.
124. Scriver, C. R.; and Goldman, H. Renal tubular transport of proline, hydroxyproline and glycine. II. Hydroxy-L-proline as substrate and as inhibitor in vivo. J. Clin. Invest. 45:1357-1363, 1966.
125. Pitts, R. F. A renal reabsorptive mechanism in the dog common to glycine and creatinine. Am. J. Physiol. 140:156-168, 1943.
126. Schafer, I. A.; Scriver, C. R.; and Efron, M. L. Familial hyperprolinemia, cerebral dysfunction and renal anomalies occurring in a family with hereditary nephritis and deafness. N. Engl. J. Med. 267:51-60, 1962.
127. Webber, W. A. Amino acid excretion patterns in developing rats. Can. J. Physiol. Pharmacol. 45:867-872, 1967.
128. Blazer-Yost, B.; and Jezyk, P. F. Free amino acids in the plasma and urine of dogs from birth to senescence. Am. J. Vet. Res. 40:832-838, 1979.
129. Rosenberg, L. E.; Blair, A.; and Segal, S. Transport of amino acids by slices of rat-kidney cortex. Biochim. Biophys. Acta 54:479-488, 1961.
130. Mohyuddin, F.; and Scriver, C. R. Amino acid transport in mammalian kidney: Multiple systems for imino acids and glycine in rat kidney. Am. J. Physiol. 219:1-8, 1970.
131. Baerlocher, K. E.; Scriver, C. R.; and Mohyuddin, F. Ontogeny of iminoglycine transport in mammalian kidney. Proc. Natl. Acad. Sci. USA 65:1009-1016, 1970.
132. Segal, S.; Rea, C.; and Smith, I. Separate transport systems for sugars and amino acids in developing rat kidney cortex. Proc. Natl. Acad. Sci. USA 68:372-376, 1971.
133. Hillman, R. E.; Albrecht, I.; and Rosenberg, L. E. Identification and analysis of multiple glycine transport systems in isolated mammalian renal tubules. J. Biol. Chem. 243:5566-5571, 1968.
134. Hillman, R. E.; and Rosenberg, L. E. Amino acid transport by isolated mammalian renal tubules. II. Transport systems for L-proline. J. Biol. Chem. 244:4494-4498, 1969.
135. Roth, K. S.; Hwang, S. M.; London, J. W.; and Segal S. Ontogeny of glycine transport in isolated rat renal tubules. Am. J. Physiol. 233:F241-F246, 1977.

136. McNamara, P.; Ožegović, B.; Pepe, L. M.; and Segal, S. Proline and glycine uptake by renal brushborder membrane vesicles. Proc. Natl. Acad. Sci. USA 73:4521-4525, 1976.
137. McNamara, P.; Pepe, L. M.; and Segal, S. Sodium gradient dependence of proline and glycine uptake in rat renal brushborder membrane vesicles. Biochim. Biophys. Acta 556:151-160, 1979.
138. Holtzapple, P.; Genel, M.; Rea, C.; and Segal, S. Metabolism and uptake of L-proline in human kidney cortex. Pediatr. Res. 7:818-825, 1973.
139. Roth, K. S.; Holtzapple, P.; Genel, M.; and Segal, S. Uptake of glycine by human kidney cortex. Metabolism 28:677-682, 1979.
140. Webber, W. A. Interactions of neutral and acidic amino acids in renal tubular transport. Am. J. Physiol. 202:577-583, 1962.
141. Goodman, S. I.; McIntyre, C. A.; and O'Brien, D. Impaired intestinal transport of proline in a patient with familial iminoaciduria. J. Pediatr. 71:246-249, 1967.
142. Scriver, C. R. Renal tubular transport of proline, hydroxyproline and glycine. III. Genetic basis for more than one mode of transport in human kidney. J. Clin. Invest. 47:823-835, 1968.
143. Whelan, D. T.; and Scriver, C. R. Cystathioninuria and renal iminoglycinuria in a pedigree: A perspective on counseling. N. Engl. J. Med. 278:924-927, 1968.
144. Tancredi, G.; Guazzi, G.; and Auricchio, S. Renal iminoglycinuria without intestinal malabsorption of glycine and imino acids. J. Pediatr. 76:386-392, 1970.
145. Bank, H.; Crispin, M.; Ehrlich, D.; and Szeinberg, A. Iminoglycinuria: A defect of renal tubular transport. Isr. J. Med. Sci. 8:606-612, 1972.
146. de Vries, A.; Kochwa, S.; Lazebnik, J.; Frank, M.; and Djaldetti, M. Glycinuria, a hereditary disorder associated with nephrolithiasis. Am. J. Med. 23:408-415, 1957.
147. Greene, M. L.; Lietman, P. S.; Rosenberg, L. E.; and Seegmiller, J. E. Familial hyperglycemia: New defect in renal tubular transport of glycine and imino acids. Am. J. Med. 54:265-271, 1973.
148. Kaser, H.; Cottier, P.; and Antener, I. Glucoglycinuria, a new familial syndrome. J. Pediatr. 61:386-394, 1962.
149. Teijema, H. L.; Van Gelderen, H. H.; and Gesberts, M. A. H. Laurent de Angulo MSL: Dicarboxylic aminoaciduria: An inborn error of glutamate and aspartate transport with metabolic implications in combination with a hyperprolinemia. Metabolism 23: 115-123, 1974.
150. Melançon, S. B.; Dallaire, L.; Lemieux, B.; Robitaille, P.; and Potier, M. Dicarboxylic aminoaciduria: An inborn error of amino acid conservation. J. Pediatr. 91:422-427, 1977.

5
Glycosurias

SUNG-FENG WEN
University of Wisconsin Center for Health Sciences, Madison, Wisconsin

Glycosuria by definition is a condition in which an increased amount of glucose is excreted in the urine. In the era when glucose was determined by measuring the copper-reducing substances (1,2) the presence of any amount of glucose in the urine was considered as glycosuria, since glucose was thought to be completely absent from the normal urine. With the development of more specific and sensitive enzymatic methods for glucose determination (3,4), a trace amount of glucose is normally detected in the urine and, therefore, glycosuria should now be defined to indicate urinary glucose excretion substantially exceeding the upper limit of normal basal excretion (basal glycosuria).

As urinary glucose excretion is the end result of the renal handling of glucose, it is pertinent to review some aspects of the renal physiology of glucose transport. In this chapter we shall confine our discussion mainly to the transport of D-glucose which is relevant to the clinical glycosurias and the transport of other sugars will be mentioned only in relation to D-glucose transport.

Glucose transport has been widely studied in a number of cell structures, and these can be divided into two major groups (5). The first group is glucose transport in the nonpolarized cells such as erythrocytes. In this group glucose transport demonstrates facilitated diffusion kinetics which is characterized by the lack of sodium dependence, a relative insensitivity to phlorhizin inhibition, and a sensitivity to inhibition by phloretin and cytochalasin B (6,7). The second group includes glucose transport in the polarized cells such as intestinal and renal tubular epithelium. It is characterized by an active transport which is sodium dependent and competitively inhibited by phlorhizin (5,8,9). Intestinal transport of glucose has been extensively investigated because of its easier accessibility due to its size, and it has greatly contributed to the understanding of renal glucose transport owing to the analogy in the membrane structure and the mode of transport (8,10,11). In recent years, however, the direct information on renal tubular mechanisms of glucose transport has become increasingly available with the development of new techniques to study renal tubular transport (5,9, 12-14).

I. PHYSIOLOGY OF RENAL GLUCOSE TRANSPORT

A. Nature of Renal Glucose Reabsorption

Tubular Reabsorptive Capacity for Glucose

Shannon and coworkers (15,16) were the first to study renal glucose transport using the classic clearance techniques to obtain glucose titration curves. In these titration studies, glucose loading is carried out by stepwise increases in the rate of infusion of hypertonic glucose solution to raise plasma glucose concentration as well as the filtered load. As shown in Fig. 1, the progressive rise in the filtered load (FL_G) leads to complete tubular reabsorption of glucose (T_G) until the latter reaches a maximum value (Tm_G). At this point, the tubular reabsorptive capacity for glucose is saturated and no further increase in glucose reabsorption occurs with the increases in the filtered load, resulting in excretion of the excess load into the urine. The curve obtained by plotting T_G against FL_G is called the glucose titration curve. Since the filtered load of glucose is a product of plasma glucose (P_G) and glomerular filtration rate (GFR), and since GFR is usually relatively constant or increases only slightly during glucose loading, it is also customary to plot the glucose titration curve against plasma glucose. Inclusion of urinary glucose excretion (U_GV) in the plot provides the renal threshold for glucose represented by the level of FL_G (or P_G) at which U_GV takes off from the X axis.

The technique of glucose titration was applied and expanded in the evaluation of human renal glucose transport by Smith et al. (17). Normal values of Tm_G determined in human subjects reported by various authors (17-26) are listed in Table 1 (27,28). In both adults and children Tm_G averages in the range of 250-360 mg/min per 1.73 m^2 and Tm_G/GFR averages 2.2-2.8 mg/ml. Tm_G values are similar for adults and children when they are corrected for surface area, but the values in infants are lower due to lower GFR. When Tm_G is factored by GFR, the values become comparable for all groups, indicating that glomerulotubular balance for glucose is maintained at all ages and the lower Tm_G in infants may not be due to tubular immaturity as suggested by some authors (29).

In the actual plotting of the glucose titration curve, a curvilinear transition from complete glucose reabsorption to complete tubular saturation is observed. This curved segment represents a deviation from the theoretical straight lines and is called splay of the glucose titration curve. The beginning of the splay also corresponds to the renal threshold for glu-

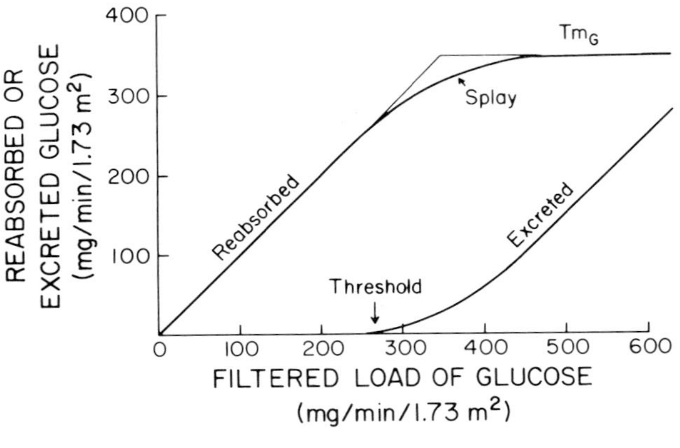

Fig. 1 Glucose titration curve and urinary glucose excretion during glucose loading in normal subjects. Tm_G = tubular maximum for glucose.

Table 1 Normal Values of Tm_G and Tm_G/GFR in Adults, Children, and Infants

Authors	No. of subjects	Tm_G (mg/min per 1.73m^2)	Tm_G/GFR (mg/ml)
Adults			
Smith et al. (17)	35	352 ± 81	2.71 ± 0.45
McPhaul and Simonaitis (18)	16	325 ± 36	2.34 ± 0.21
Letteri and Wesson (19)	19	306 ± 83	2.80 ± 0.10
Elsas and Rosenberg (20)	7	291 ± 27	2.38 ± 0.40
Govaerts and Lambert (21)	45	–	2.41 ± 0.35
Nielsen (22)	3	301 ± 25	2.22 ± 0.30
Children			
Brodehl et al. (23)	16	362 ± 96	2.83 ± 0.47
Stalder (24)	19	304 ± 55	2.22 ± 0.13
Grossmann and Zoellner (25)	65	254 ± 115	–
Infants			
Geckle et al. (26)	10	199 ± 103	2.02 ± 0.39
Brodehl et al. (23)	8	213 ± 71	2.94 ± 0.74

Values are mean ± SD; Tm_G = Tubular maximum for glucose.
Source: Adapted from Refs. 27,28.

cose. Two possible explanations, not mutually exclusive, have been offered to explain the meaning of the splay. One is based on nephron heterogeneity in glucose transport and the other relates to the kinetic function of the carrier-mediated transport process.

According to the theory of nephron heterogeneity, glucose reabsorptive capacity varies from nephron to nephron in that they differ in the level of filtered load of glucose needed to saturate tubular glucose transport. As the glucose titration curve is the composite sum of glucose reabsorption from all nephrons, saturation of some nephrons earlier than others will result in a curvilinear shape of the titration curve before Tm_G for all nephrons is reached. Certain experimental data support such contentions. Oliver et al. (30,31) performed microdissection studies of human and dog nephrons and showed a correlation between structural glomerulotubular balance, expressed as the ratio of glomerular surface to proximal tubule volume (r/R),* and functional glomerulotubular balance for glucose transport derived from the glucose titration curves (17,19). These observations were taken as evidence supporting nephron heterogeneity as the explanation for the splay of the glucose titration curve. Baines (32) also found by micropuncture studies of the rat kidney that the increase in splay following extracellular volume expansion was due to functional nephron heterogeneity in that the glomerulotubular balance of the superficial and deep nephrons was altered in a different manner by volume expansion. A theoretical treatment of renal glucose transport by Burgen (33) led to a similar conclusion in favor of nephron heterogeneity as the cause for the splay.

The alternative explanation for the splay is related to the kinetics of the carrier-mediated glucose transport. Such transport is initiated by a combination of the glucose molecule (G) with a membrane carrier (C) to form a glucose-carrier complex (GC) in a reversible manner:

$$G + C \rightleftarrows GC$$

$$K = \frac{[G] \cdot [C]}{[GC]} \tag{1}$$

$$^*\frac{r}{R} = \frac{\text{(glomerular surface/proximal volume) of a particular nephron}}{\text{mean value (glomerular surface/proximal volume) of all nephrons}}$$

where K is the dissociation constant of the GC complex, [G] is the concentration of glucose in the tubule fluid, and [C] and [GC] are concentrations of free and complexed membrane carrier at the surface of the luminal membrane. From Eq. (1) it can be seen that the affinity of glucose to the carrier is high when K is small and low when K is large. However, since K is probably a finite value, some glucose molecules will escape from binding the carrier and remain unreabsorbed. Thus, glucose reabsorption becomes incomplete even before the transport system is fully saturated, resulting in the formation of splay in the titration curve.

The kinetic explanation of the splay can also be derived from geometrical analysis of the Michaelis-Menten equation which is also applicable to the carrier-mediated transport (34).

We obtain

$$T_G = \frac{Tm_G \cdot TF_G}{TF_G + K_m} \tag{2}$$

Where TF_G denotes mean tubule fluid glucose concentration and K_m is the Michaelis constant. As Tm_G and K_m are constant, Eq. (2) can be rearranged with substitution of X and Y for TF_G and T_G, respectively.

Thus,

$$XY + K_m Y - Tm_G X = 0$$

or

$$(X + K_m)(Y - Tm_G) = -K_m Tm_G \tag{3}$$

Eq. (3) represents a rectangular hyperbola with an asymptote $Y = Tm_G$ (35). As TF_G is roughly proportional to plasma glucose during glucose loading, a similar curve, with a proportional displacement in the direction of X axis, will be obtained when TF_G is replaced by aP_G where a is a constant. Thus, the splay of the titration curve corresponds to the curvilinear portion of the hyperbola.

Although determination of Tm_G by glucose titration is a time-honored method of evaluating renal glucose transport, the existence of Tm_G in vivo in the classic sense has recently been challenged (36-40). A close correlation between GFR and Tm_G has long been recognized (41-44), and an increase in the filtered load through an increase in GFR can further raise Tm_G of the kidney in which tubular glucose transport has already been "saturated," as shown by the prior achievement of Tm_G. Deetjen and Boylan (45) performed in vivo microperfusion studies in the rat proximal tubule and observed that glucose absorption increased with increased perfusion rate with no apparent saturation of glucose transport up to 63×10^{-12} mol/mm per min. Tune and Burg (46), on the other hand, demonstrated Tm_G at 79×10^{-12} mol/mm per min in the isolated rabbit proximal tubule perfused in vitro when the glucose load exceeded 200×10^{-12} mol/min. They attributed the failure of Deetjen and Boylan (45) in demonstrating Tm_G to the submaximal load of glucose employed. However, Stolte et al. (39) were also unable to observe Tm_G during in vivo microperfusion of the rat proximal tubule even though glucose absorption reached 225×10^{-12} mol/mm per min with the glucose load as high as 720×10^{-12} mol/min. Glucose absorption was correlated with fluid absorption over a wide range of glucose concentrations in the perfusate. These different observations between in vivo and in vitro studies are probably related to the lack of glomerulotubular balance in the isolated tubule model owing to the absence of the peritubular capillaries. Bowman and Maack (38) were also unable to show Tm_G in the isolated perfused rat kidney as were von Baeyer et al. (47) in the intact rat kidney in vivo. From these observations it has been suggested that renal glucose transport probably consists of two components: one component is a classic carrier-mediated active transport which is saturable and follows the Michaelis-Menten kinetics; the other is a nonsaturable component which is related to volume absorption (39,40).

Relation to Glomerular Filtration Rate

Dependence of renal glucose transport on GFR has been studied under a number of physiological and experimental conditions (30,32,36,38,41-45). Spontaneous variations in GFR in the same or different animals (36,38,44) and among different nephrons (32) have been shown to correlate with tubular reabsorption of glucose indicating well-maintained glomerulotubular balance under physiological conditions. Similarly, the experimental maneuvers to alter GFR are also associated with proportional changes in Tm_G so that Tm_G/GFR remains relatively constant (41-44).

GFR or flow dependence of renal glucose transport has been interpreted by Barfuss and Schafer (48) in light of a model incorporating interactions between net volume absorption and both saturable and nonsaturable solute absorption. The model includes a saturable, carrier-mediated active transport and a parallel, nonsaturable passive flux. It also incorporates flow dependence of volume absorption and predicts that net glucose transport will be highly flow dependent and will not exhibit a tubular maximum. Although both active and passive components of glucose transport are flow dependent they are related to the luminal glucose concentration rather than the delivery rate of glucose. However, in in vivo microperfusion studies of the rat proximal tubule, Knight et al. (49) observed that the flow dependence of glucose transport was related only to a limited degree to the luminal glucose concentration. Since the passive glucose flux associated with volume absorption could not fully account for the observed flow-dependent increase in glucose absorption, the authors proposed that the flow rate influenced the active component of glucose transport.

GFR dependence of glucose transport should be considered in the context of glomerulotubular balance. As a close relationship between glucose and sodium transport has been well documented (36,50-55), GFR dependence of glucose transport could be the result of the maintenance of glomerulotubular balance for sodium transport in the proximal tubule. The factors which are responsible for the maintenance of glomerulotubular balance have been reviewed elsewhere (56,57). It is of interest to note that glucose as well as amino acids and bicarbonate are among the factors present in the glomerular filtrate which could promote glomerulotubular balance (56-60). Barfuss and Schafer (48) predicted from the flow-dependent model of the nonelectrolyte transport that approximately one-third of ideal glomerulotubular balance could be due to the changes in the delivery rate of solutes such as glucose, amino acids, organic acids, and bicarbonate. However, inconsistent reports have appeared in regard to the effect of glucose on proximal sodium reabsorption. While the presence of luminal glucose has been shown to enhance glucose-dependent sodium transport (60), negative transtubular potential difference (60,62,63,73) and fluid absorption (63-65) of the proximal tubule, others have reported nonsignificant effect on sodium transport (66,67). These conflicting observations suggest that glucose-dependent sodium transport may constitute only a small fraction of total proximal sodium reabsorption (67). If a 1:1 stoichiometric relationship exists between sodium and glucose transport (62), the magnitude of sodium transport that can be affected by glucose transport is indeed small and may not be readily detectable. However, regardless of the role of glucose and other factors involved in proximal sodium transport, GFR dependence of glucose transport appears to be closely related to the glomerulotubular balance of sodium transport (39,40,49).

Sodium Dependence

The relationship between sodium and glucose transport has been extensively investigated in both intestine and kidney (8-11,36,39,50-55). Although Christensen and coworkers (68) had suggested a similar concept, Crane (10) was the first to formulate the sodium-gradient hypothesis to explain the energy source of active sugar transport in the intestine. According to this hypothesis, the transport of glucose from lumen into cell is energized by the concomitant transport of sodium along the sodium gradient. Since sodium and glucose share a common carrier to enter the cell, the energy derived from the preexisting downhill gradient of sodium is utilized to facilitate the uphill movement of glucose across the brush-border membrane. The sodium gradient in turn is produced by an active extrusion of sodium at the basolateral border through the action of Na-K-ATPase. This coupled transport of sodium and glucose, termed cotransport, takes place probably at 1:1 stoichiometric ratio (62) and is electrogenic, carrying a positive charge of sodium ion. More recently, it has been shown that the energy for glucose entry is provided not only by sodium concentration gradient but also by the electrical potential gradient (11,69,70).

In accordance with the concept of sodium-dependent glucose transport, a close correlation between sodium and glucose transport has been observed in a variety of experimental conditions. Thus, Kurtzman et al. (36) varied urinary sodium excretion by extracellular volume expansion and constriction of thoracic vena cava in the dog and showed a correlation of urinary glucose excretion with sodium excretion. Robson et al. (71) also demonstrated a reduction in Tm_G and an increase in the splay of the glucose titration curve in the rat following inhibition of sodium reabsorption by extracellular volume expansion. In micropuncture studies (54,55,72), proximal tubule reabsorption of glucose was inhibited by maneuvers such as volume expansion and administration of acetazolamide which inhibited proximal sodium reabsorption.

Ullrich et al. (53) examined the sodium dependence of active sugar transport in the rat proximal tubule using the technique of simultaneous luminal and capillary microperfusion. They demonstrated that active glucose transport as measured by zero net-flux transtubular concentration difference (Δc) was dependent on the luminal sodium concentration. The effect of sodium on glucose transport was related primarily to an increase in the affinity of glucose to the carrier (a reduction in K_m) without significantly affecting its maximum rate of transport (V_{max}).

More direct support of the sodium-gradient hypothesis is provided by the kinetic studies of glucose transport in the isolated brush-border membrane vesicles (50,51). The accumulation of glucose in the vesicles was stimulated up to 10 times by the presence of sodium gradient which resulted in an "overshoot," as compared to a gradual equilibration with the bathing medium in the absence of the gradient. The movement of sodium-glucose complex into the vesicle was electrogenic and was enhanced by an intravesicular negative potential (14,52). More detailed discussion of the glucose entry step is provided in Ch. 1.

In addition to glucose transport, proximal tubule reabsorption of amino acids and phosphate are also known to derive their energy from the electrochemical gradient of sodium at the brush-border membrane (74-77). In the isolated perfused rabbit proximal tubule, it has been shown that the deletion of glucose or alanine from the perfusate led to enhancement of the transport of phosphate (78). The interaction between glucose and amino acid transport, however, has been more difficult to demonstrate (74,78,79). On the other hand, the maneuvers to reduce sodium-gradient, such as replacement of intraluminal sodium with choline and elimination of potassium from the bath, all reduced absorption of fluid, glucose, and phosphate. That these solutes do not share the common transport carrier is shown by the effect of phlorhizin which inhibits glucose transport but enhances phosphate transport

(78.80.81). It has been postulated that since the transport of all these solutes are dependent on sodium entry at the brush border, their interrelationship is governed by their mutual dependence on the electrochemical gradient of sodium for their transport (11,69,78). As the transport of glucose and amino acids are rheogenic, the alterations in transmembrane potential difference induced by the transport of one solute may influence the rate of entry of the other solutes into the cell. Such electrical coupling has been shown between glucose and alanine transport in the isolated brush-border membrane vesicles of the rat small intestine (69).

Model of Tubular Glucose Transport

The model of glucose entry at the brush-border membrane via sodium-glucose cotransport has been discussed above and is illustrated in Fig. 2. The carrier protein C is bound by both sodium and glucose at the luminal surface and releases them into the cell at the interior surface. Such transport is energized by the sodium concentration gradient and by the intracellular negative potential. The binding of glucose to the carrier is competitively inhibited by phlorhizin. Phlorhizin is a glycoside consisting of a glucose moiety and a phloretin moiety which both bind the carrier at their respective sites. The binding of phlorhizin to the carrier is competitively inhibited by D-glucose but not by L-glucose (82). The sugar binding sites of the carrier demonstrate stereochemical and configurational specificity, although some variations in the structural requirements have been reported by different authors (5,14,53, 83,84). The major requirements may include D-pyranose ring, a methyl or hydroxymethyl group at C_5, and a hydroxyl group at C_2 (53,84). Thus, Ullrich (14,53) showed that L-glucose, D-mannose, 2-deoxy-D-glucose, and D-fructose were not actively transported by the rat proximal tubule. A deviation from the D-glucose configuration at C_3 (3-*O*-methyl-D-glucose) or C_4 (D-galactose) allowed active transport at a reduced rate, whereas the absence of a hydroxyl group at C_3 (3-deoxy-D-glucose) abolished the transport. Deviations at C_1 or C_6 did not significantly alter the magnitude of active transport. Others, however, have shown slightly different structural requirements based on different experimental models (5,83-85).

Glucose transport at the basolateral membrane is less well understood than that at the brush-border membrane as isolation of the pure basolateral membrane is technically more difficult (50). Such information is also derived from the studies using multiple indicator dilution (5,86,87), kidney slices (83), and teased tubules (88). Glucose exit from cell to

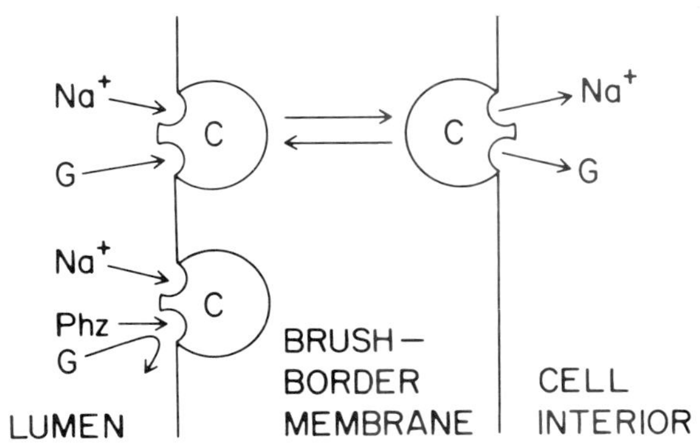

Fig. 2 Model for glucose entry at the brush border. C = carrier; G = glucose; Phz = phlorhizin.

peritubular capillaries is most likely passive, as intracellular glucose concentration has been shown to exceed that of the surrounding medium (46). However, because of the relatively low permeability of glucose across the membrane, a carrier-mediated transport in the form of facilitated diffusion has been suggested (5,88). The available data from in vivo (86,87) and in vitro studies (50,88) also indicate a stereospecific transport which is sodium independent and is inhibitable by phloretin and cytochalasin B and less by phlorhizin. Thus, glucose transport at the basolateral membrane mimicks that of nonpolarized cells (6,7).

In addition to an active glucose transport from lumen to blood, there is also a passive transport pathway for glucose across the proximal tubule. The passive component of glucose transport has been examined by inhibition of the active transport with phlorhizin (89, 90) or by evaluation of the passive permeation of L-glucose (91). Passive backleak of glucose is relatively small under normal conditions (89,90) and varies in degree among different species (92). The passive component becomes more significant when plasma glucose concentration is increased (89,90). As a steep glucose concentration gradient normally exists along the proximal tubule, the leaked load can significantly contribute to the luminal glucose concentration and further add to the active glucose reabsorption (92). The contribution of the passive transport to the overall handling of glucose by the renal tubule is probably greater when the permeability of the proximal tubule is increased by certain experimental conditions (55,93-95). Such an increase in permeability has been shown following administration of maleic acid (93,95) and when intratubular pressure is increased by maneuvers such as saline infusion (94). Therefore, the observed reduction in net glucose reabsorption under these conditions may be due, in part, to increased backleak of glucose (55,95).

With consideration of the factors discussed above, a model of proximal glucose transport can be summarized as in Fig. 3. The net transport of glucose is the sum of two independent fluxes. One is an active, carrier-mediated transport which is saturable and sodium dependent. This component derives its energy from the electrochemical gradient of sodium at the brush-border membrane and is the major pathway for glucose transport from lumen to blood. The second component is a passive leak pathway which is dependent on tubular permeability and transepithelial glucose concentration gradient. Its contribution to the net glucose transport is most significant when the plasma glucose concentration is raised or when tubular permeability is increased by experimental maneuvers. The cellular site of the leak pathway for glucose is unknown, but it could be the paracellular channel as this has been shown to be the case with glycine (96). Both active and passive components of glucose transport are thought to be flow dependent (48) and this may be related to the alterations in luminal glucose concentration (48) and volume reabsorption (39,40).

Renal Glucose Metabolism

A detailed discussion of renal glucose metabolism is beyond the scope of this chapter and only certain pertinent features will be summarized. An excellent review of the subject is available elsewhere (97).

Although the kidney is known to participate in both production and utilization of glucose, neither addition nor uptake of glucose by the kidney is demonstrable when glucose concentrations in the renal artery and vein are measured (98-100). This is because of the canceling effect of simultaneous production and utilization of glucose as well as the high rate of renal blood flow. When the isolated rat kidney is perfused with a solution containing glucose as the sole substrate considerable glucose utilization can be shown (101). In the intact dog kidney, production and utilization of glucose are similar in magnitude and account for less than 1% of the renal glucose load during both metabolic acidosis and alkalosis

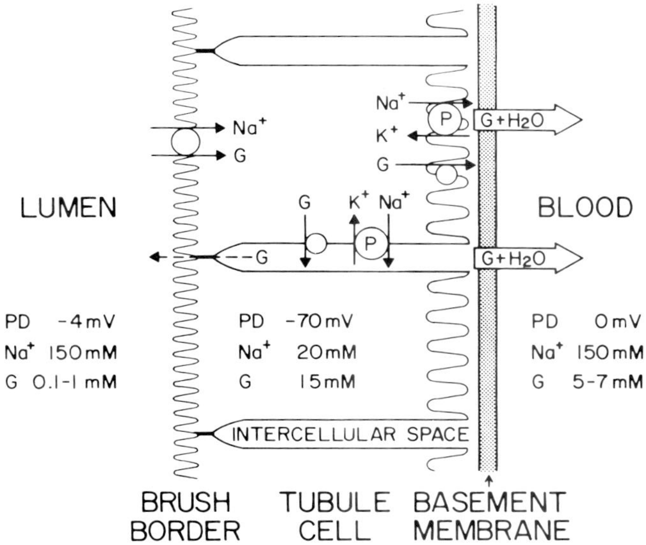

Fig. 3 Model for glucose transport across proximal tubular epithelium. Glucose enters the cell at the brush border through a cotransport system with sodium utilizing its favorable electrochemical gradient. Na-K-ATPase at the basolateral membrane actively extrudes Na^+ to create the electrochemical gradient. Glucose exit at the basolateral membrane is probably also carrier mediated in the form of facilitated diffusion along a favorable glucose gradient. Glucose and other solutes with accompanying water are then taken up by the peritubular capillary through the effect of Starling's forces. Under certain conditions, glucose may also leak back into the tubule lumen probably via the intercellular channel. P = pump; PD = potential difference; G = glucose.

(102). About two-thirds of the glucose utilized by the isolated rat kidney has been shown to be converted to CO_2 (103). In the renal medulla, glucose is converted to lactate through anaerobic glycolysis.

Net addition of glucose to the renal venous blood can be demonstrated in hepatectomized animals (104), in patients with respiratory acidosis (105), and during prolonged starvation (106). The contribution of the kidney to the total gluconeogenesis ranges from 26% in the normal rats to 47-55% in the state of fasting, metabolic acidosis, or diabetes (107). The renal capacity for gluconeogenesis exceeds that of the liver when compared in unit gram of tissue. Renal gluconeogenesis is regulated by intracellular pH and the enzyme phosphenol-pyruvate carboxykynase (PEPCK) appears to play a major role in mediating renal production of glucose during acidosis (108-112).

Since glucose is metabolized in the kidney, it was thought that renal glucose transport may also involve phosphorylation–dephosphorylation processes in the glucose metabolism (113-114). Glucose is phosphorylated by hexokinase (nonspecific alkaline phosphatase) and ATP within the tubule cell and this phosphorylation step was thought to enhance tubular glucose uptake across the luminal membrane by removing free glucose and creating a concentration gradient favorable for glucose entry. The second step in glucose transport was the hydrolysis of glucose-6-phosphate which was presumed to occur at a site further away from the luminal membrane and thus to yield a high glucose concentration toward the peritubular membrane, favoring glucose exit from the cell. However, several observations provided evidence against phosphorylation as a required step in the renal glucose transport. Dinitrophenol, which uncouples aerobic phosphorylation, did not block glucose reabsorption when given to an intact animal (115); phlorhizin, which nearly completely inhibited glucose transport, did not inhibit alkaline phosphatase in the proximal convoluted tubule (116). Although phlorhizin in high dosage was shown to inhibit oxidative metabolism (117), its competitive inhibition of active glucose transport was demonstrated at a very low dose in the absence of any effect on metabolism (5). A glycosuric dose of phlorhizin did not alter the rate of disappearance of injected ^{32}P-labeled inorganic phosphate from the plasma, suggesting normal synthesis of glucose esters (118). In patients with glycogen storage disease in whom glucose-6-phosphatase was lacking, glycosuria was not present (119).

Although renal glucose transport may not significantly involve metabolic processes, renal glucose metabolism does provide energy for sodium transport (120). It is well known that renal sodium reabsorption accounts for most, if not all, of the energy consumption by the kidney and 20-30 meq of sodium is estimated to be reabsorbed per mmole of oxygen utilized in ATP formation (121-122). Under normal conditions about 95% of the ATP produced in the kidney is derived from aerobic oxidative metabolism and only 5% is provided by anaerobic metabolism, including medullary glycolysis (123,124). Of the aerobic pathways approximately 13% is derived from oxidation of glucose to CO_2 (125), while other substrates such as lactate, glutamate, free fatty acids, and citrate provide the remainder of energy (97). Thus, glucose is one of the important energy sources for active sodium reabsorption.

In summary, glucose is most likely transported across the proximal tubule cell in the form of intact molecules without undergoing metabolic processes. Although glucose utilization and production occur in the kidney, they constitute less than 1% of the total renal glucose load and neither addition nor extraction of glucose by the kidney is demonstrable under most conditions. However, renal glucose metabolism can significantly influence sodium transport, since glucose is one of the energy sources for active sodium reabsorption.

B. Site of Renal Glucose Transport

Proximal Tubule

The pioneer micropuncture studies in amphibians and mammals by Walker et al. (126,127) showed that glucose is filtered by the glomerulus and the glucose concentration in the glomerular filtrate is the same as that in the blood. In the proximal convoluted tubule, glucose is reabsorbed against an increasing glucose gradient resulting from an active reabsorption and little glucose remains in the tubule fluid of the late proximal segment. In more recent years, with the use of specific enzymatic methods for glucose determination in the tubule fluid, the profile of glucose reabsorption in the proximal tubule has been more clearly defined (55,72,128-130). The major portion of the filtered glucose is reabsorbed in the early segment of the proximal tubule and 90-98% is reabsorbed at the end of the accessible segment of the proximal convoluted tubule (72,128-130). Variation in the extent of proximal reabsorption is probably related to the difference in species and sex of the animals used for micropuncture. Frohnert et al. (129) showed that while about 98% of the filtered glucose was reabsorbed in the proximal tubule of the male rats, proximal glucose reabsorption in the female rats was less complete. In the dog, proximal glucose reabsorption was about 90% of the filtered load, which was also less than that in the rat, probably reflecting less complete fluid reabsorption (55,72). Proximal glucose reabsorption is readily inhibited by maneuvers which also inhibit proximal sodium reabsorption such as saline infusion (55, 72) or administration of acetazolamide (54). While inhibition by these maneuvers is nonspecific and partial, phlorhizin completely abolishes proximal glucose reabsorption, indicating its specific action on the active transport (126,127,130,131).

McKeown et al. (132) compared glucose transport in the early and late segments of the isolated rabbit proximal tubule from the cortical and juxtamedullary nephrons. They found that the early proximal segment had a greater capacity to absorb glucose than the late segment but there were no significant differences between the cortical and juxtamedullary nephrons. Tune and Burg (46) showed the Tm_G in the proximal convoluted segment was some 13 times that of the straight segment in the isolated perfused rabbit tubule. In vivo microperfusion of the rat kidney by von Baeyer (133) also demonstrated a limited glucose transport capacity in the short loop of Henle, which may largely represent the proximal straight tubule. Barfuss and Schafer (91) also found lower glucose transport capacity and lower glucose permeability of the rabbit proximal straight segment than those of the proximal convoluted segment. They concluded that the high transport capacity with moderate leak in the early proximal tubule allows the establishment of a steep glucose gradient which is maintained by a system of low transport capacity with low leak in the late proximal segment.

Other Nephron Sites

Although the proximal tubule site of glucose reabsorption is well established, glucose transport in other nephron segments has not been clarified. Micropuncture studies in the proximal and distal tubules of the dog showed that inhibition of proximal glucose reabsorption is usually associated with an increase in glucose reabsorption in the segment between the late proximal tubule and the distal tubule (designated as intermediate segment for brevity) (72, 134,173). This segment appears to play an important role in the regulation of urinary glucose excretion, since glycosuria was prevented by glucose reabsorption at this site (72,173). Significant glucose absorption in the intermediate segment (or short loop of Henle) has also been shown in the rat by microinjection (85,267,291,292) and microperfusion techniques (133,293). The anatomical location of glucose transport in the intermediate segment remains unknown. Although the proximal straight segment could be largely responsible, the possible participation in glucose reabsorption by the loop of Henle cannot be completely excluded.

Micropuncture studies in the rat by Frohnert et al. (129) demonstrated no glucose reabsorption in the distal tubule, but a significant difference in fractional delivery of glucose was observed between the late distal tubule and the final urine. Although glucose reabsorption in the collecting duct may be suggested from such findings, the possible nephron heterogeneity between the superficial and deep nephrons renders such a conclusion highly speculative. Glucose reabsorption in the distal nephron segments was also evaluated by intratubular microinjections of labeled glucose in the distal tubule. While virtually complete recovery of the radioactivity in the urine was reported in male rats, indicating no glucose absorption (85,291,292), significant glucose absorption in the distal nephron segments was observed in female rats (267). In micropuncture studies of the renal papilla and the superficial nephrons in female rats (134), no significant glucose reabsorption was observed in the distal tubule or the collecting duct. On the other hand, mean tubule fluid to plasma (TF/P) glucose ratios at the bend of Henle's loop was much higher than the values in the distal tubule or the collecting duct. As TF/P inulin ratios, which estimate fluid reabsorption, were unchanged or increased in the latter distal segments, it is likely that some glucose reabsorption occurred at a site distal to the bend of the loop. The possible distal glucose reabsorptive sites, therefore, include the ascending loop of Henle and the cortical collecting tubule. However, the magnitude of glucose reabsorption at these sites is apparently small and unlike the intermediate segment their significance in the overall handling of glucose by the nephron remains unclear.

II. GLYCOSURIAS

A. Basal Glycosuria

In the era when glucose was measured by the determination of reducing substances (1,2) no glucose could normally be detected in the urine. However, these methods overestimate blood glucose and underestimate urine glucose concentrations (135). As normal urine contains less than 15 mg/dl of glucose (136), it also shows a negative reaction with the reagent strips which require a greater than 40 mg/dl concentration for a positive reaction. Quantitative enzymatic methods using glucose oxidase (3) or hexokinase-glucose-6-phosphate dehydrogenase (4) allow a more accurate determination of glucose in both blood and urine (135); The basal excretion of trace amounts of glucose in normal urine measured by these methods averages 75 mg/24 hr with a range of 15-135 mg/24 hr or 300 nmol/min with a range of 60-540 nmol/min (136-141). A higher normal range of 132-316 mg/24 hr per 1.73 m^2 was reported by Elsas and Rosenberg (20). There is a diurnal variation of basal glucose excretion which is higher in the afternoon and evening and is only minimally affected by the urine flow rate (136,139).

The existence of basal glycosuria poses a problem in the definition of the renal threshold for glucose. The renal threshold for glucose is originally defined as the plasma glucose concentration above which the filtered glucose escapes tubular reabsorption and appears in the urine. During glucose titration studies this can be calculated by the ratio of tubular glucose reabsorption to GFR (T_G/GFR) when glucose first appears in the urine (142). Since the filtered load of glucose is completely reabsorbed below the threshold (i.e., $P_G \cdot \text{GFR} = T_G$), T_G/GFR provides the plasma glucose concentration at the threshold. The normal threshold has been reported to be in the range of 140-190 mg/dl (142). With the presence of basal glycosuria it becomes more difficult to define what degree of urinary glucose excretion constitutes frank glycosuria. Various criteria have appeared in the literature, including the values greater than 10 mg/hr (240 mg/24 hr) (140), 500 mg/24 hr (143), 1 mg/min (1440 mg/24 hr) (20), etc. Elsas and Rosenberg (20) proposed a minimal threshold ($Fmin_G$), which is defined as the filtered load of glucose at which 1 mg/min of glucose is excreted in the urine. They obtained a normal mean of 224 ± 41 mg/min per 1.73 m^2 (or a mean P_G of 189 ± 44 mg/dl), which is slightly higher than the range reported by Smith (142).

B. Hyperglycemic Glycosurias

Diabetes Mellitus and Other Related Metabolic Disorders

Glycosuria in diabetes mellitus and other disorders of abnormal carbohydrate metabolism is caused by hyperglycemia, with the filtered load of glucose exceeding the renal threshold. However, urinary excretion of glucose does not always correlate quantitatively with the degree of hyperglycemia, since both lowered (144,145) and elevated (146) renal thresholds for glucose are seen in some diabetic patients. As the sodium dependence of glucose transport is well established, the variations in the renal threshold for glucose in diabetic patients should also be interpreted in light of its relationship to sodium excretion. Thus, those patients undergoing natriuresis which involves a reduction in proximal sodium reabsorption are expected to show a lowered renal threshold; whereas sodium-retaining patients, including those with congestive heart failure or diabetic nephropathy, should have an elevated threshold. Therefore, the past practice of using glycosuria as a guide for diabetic control is apparently less than satisfactory.

Iatrogenic Glycosuria

Intravenous infusion of 5% dextrose in water (containing 5000 mg/dl glucose) is a frequent cause of hyperglycemia and glycosuria when given at a rate exceeding the rate of utilization. In addition, the size of extracellular volume and the state of renal excretion of sodium can also influence the degree of glycosuria. In profoundly diuretic states such as diabeter insipidus, postobstructive diuresis, or the diruretic phase of acute renal failure, infusion of 5% dextrose in water or saline to replace the urinary loss of volume frequently leads to glycosuria and osmotic diuresis which may perpetuate or aggravate the preexisting diuresis. Glycosuria in these conditions can be heavy and at times may be the major cause for massive diuresis. In extreme cases, development of hyperglycemic coma has been reported following a 5% dextrose infusion for fluid replacement in children with postoperative diabetes insipidus (147). To prevent glycosuria and osmotic diuresis as well as hyperglycemia, 2.5 or 3% dextrose solution has been successfully used without the danger of hemolysis (148).

C. Unclassified Glycosuria

There are a group of patients in whom the mechanism of glycosuria is unknown or poorly defined. Marble (149) refers to these conditions as unclassified glycosuria. They include a number of endocrine diseases such as hyperthyroidism, hyperpituitarism, and hyperadrenocorticism, and intracranial diseases such as brain tumors, cerebral hemorrhage, and head injury. Alimentary glycosurua follows ingestion of a large amount of carbohydrate and a variety of other acute and chronic conditions, including infection, malignant neoplasms, and hepatic and renal diseases, are also listed under the category of unclassified glycosuria. In many of these conditions hyperglycemia could be the cause of glycosuria, but this is poorly documented probably due to its intermittent nature. In some of the other cases of unclassified glycosuria renal glycosuria may be the underlying mechanism, but further documentation is needed to clarify the possible causes of glycosuria in these conditions.

D. Renal Glycosurias

History and Definition of Renal Glycosuria

Renal glycosuria denotes excessive urinary excretion of glucose in the absence of hyperglycemia and therefore is a result of defective tubular reabsorption of glucose. As the quantity of urinary glucose excretion varies widely among patients with renal glycosuria and especially because of the presence of basal glycosuria in normal subjects, some difficulties have been encountered in the quantitative definition of renal glycosuria. Further, this has been complicated by the existence of intermittent and persistent varieties of renal glycosuria and has been the subject of controversy with respect to the criteria for the diagnosis of renal glycosuria.

Renal glycosuria was first reported by Klemperer in 1896 (150). He described a case of glycosuria in which its detection had been preceded by a renal disease. He initially called it diabetes renalis, but later he suggested the term nephrogenous glycosuria. As the earlier experimental study of von Mehring in 1886 (cited in Ref. 150) had demonstrated glycosuria without hyperglycemia following injection of phlorhizin, Klemberer theorized that the glycosuria was independent of carbohydrate intake, but was caused by the leakage of the kidney as a result of renal disease similar to that induced by phlorhizin. Bönninger in 1907 (151) described a patient with glycosuria in whom the clinical features were similar to diabetes renalis but no preexisting renal disease was detected. He pointed out the benign nature of the disease with no transition into diabetes mellitus. Salomon in 1914 (152) proposed the term diabetes innocens to stress the favorable course and to be differentiated from diabetes mellitus. Rosenfeld in 1916 (153) suggested the name diabetes innocuus, and in 1917 Jacobsen (cited in Ref. 154) called it renal diabetes or renal glycosuria. Objecting to the term renal diabetes, Goto in 1918 (155) named it alimentary renal glycosuria. Umber and Rosenberg in 1924 (156) inferred that the condition was neither renal nor diabetic and suggested the name glycosuria innocens. Holst in 1926 (157) used the term benign glycosuria, and Hjärne in 1927 (154) preferred the term orthoglycemic glycosuria. In these early reports on renal glycosuria the diagnosis was made largely on detection of a positive urinary sugar reaction in the absence of the manifestations of diabetes mellitus.

Hjärne's extensive study of 19 cases in a Swedish family included those with intermittent glycosuria which developed in the postprandial period or during the course of a glucose tolerance test (154). Lawrence (158) also used a criterion of diagnosing renal glycosuria in any patient who developed glycosuria at any time during an otherwise normal glucose tolerance test. Lawrence studied Royal Air Force inductees in whom glycosuria was found by a preliminary test. During glucose tolerance tests he found 65% of the 800 inductees to have renal glycosuria (158). Since glycosuria is not an infrequent association with otherwise normal glucose tolerance tests (20,159,160), Lawrence's criterion (158) grossly overdiagnoses renal glycosuria in the clinical setting. In contrast, Marble (149,161) adopted very stringent criteria and restricted the diagnosis of renal glycosuria to conditions in which the renal threshold is extremely low, as indicated by the presence of glucose in all specimens of urine examined, including those after an overnight fast. In addition, normal carbohydrate metabolism should be confirmed by a glucose tolerance test and other forms of melituria (such as pentosuria, fructosuria, galactosuria, lactosuria, sucrosuria, and maltosuria) must be excluded.

Although Marble's rigid criteria undoubtedly reassures the accuracy of the diagnosis of renal glycosuria and has greatly contributed to the understanding of the genetic transmission of the glucose transport defect (162), many milder cases with intermittent renal glycosuria will be excluded. As random testing of urine for glucose may not provide adequate quantitative information, a determination of 24-hr urinary glucose excretion should be obtained. Owing to the presence of basal glycosuria and the wide range of normal values of urinary glucose excretion (136-141,143), a clear cut-off point for renal glycosuria is difficult to define and is inevitably arbitrary. Elsas and Rosenberg (143) proposed that a 24-hr urinary glucose excretion of greater than 500 mg/1.73 m^2 (on a diet of about 30 cal/kg with 50% carbohydrate) should be considered glycosuric.

Pathophysiology of Renal Glycosuria

The classic demonstration of renal glycosuria is to perform a glucose titration study to document a lowered renal threshold for glucose. According to the pattern of glucose titration curves, two types of renal glycosuria are generally identified, as shown in Fig. 4. In type A glycosuria there is a lowering of both the threshold and Tm_G; in type B, the threshold is lowered by an exaggerated splay but Tm_G is normal (163,164,170). As has been discussed previously, the splay of the glucose titration curve is explained by either a functional nephron heterogeneity or the kinetics of the carrier-mediated transport. According to the theory of nephron heterogeneity by Reubi (163,170), the increase in the splay of type B renal glycosuria indicates an exaggeration of the heterogeneity with regard to glomerulotubular balance for glucose in that a greater number of nephrons show defective glucose reabsorption relative

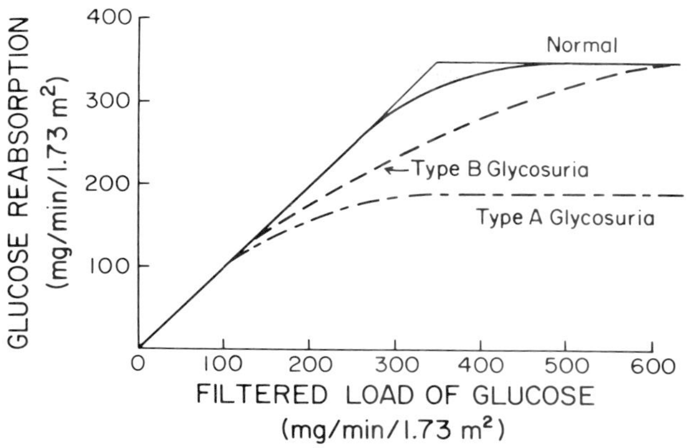

Fig. 4 Glucose titration curves for normal subjects and patients with type A and type B renal glycosuria.

to the filtered load, while other nephrons maintain normal or supernormal glomerulotubular balance. In type A renal glycosuria on the other hand, the glucose transport defect exists in most or all of the nephrons.

The kinetic interpretation of renal glycosuria was provided by Woolf et al. (165). Based on a theoretical model of the carrier-mediated transport system, they calculated and plotted glucose titration curves by varying the amount of carrier substance (E) and the affinity of glucose for the carrier (K_m). When E was given only one-half of the normal value the curve resembled that of type A renal glycosuria. When E was normal but K_m was raised (that is, the affinity was reduced), the curve resembled that of type B renal glycosuria. Thus, in type A renal glycosuria glucose-binding sites of the tubule are reduced, while in type B the affinity of glucose to the carrier is reduced but the number of binding sites remains normal.

Although the use of glucose titration curves to classify renal glycosuria into type A and type B categories provides valuable quantitative information and have greatly contributed to the genetic analysis, existence of different clinical types of renal glycosuria have been questioned (27,166,167). Examination of Tm_G and Tm_G/GFR values of the patients with renal glycosuria (Table 2) reveals that there is a gradual transition from low to high values among these patients without clear separation into two groups. Moreover, Reubi (169,170) observed in a case of renal glycosuria due to ferricyanide poisoning that a type A pattern was demonstrated in the early stage, but it progressively transformed into type B patterns in the late and recovery stages (Fig. 5). Reubi interpreted these observations to indicate a transition from uniformly impaired glucose transport in all nephrons in the early stage to an uneven recovery among the nephrons in the later stages. The observations also suggest that type A and type B renal glycosurias may not be separate entities but merely the manifestations of differing severity of the glucose transport defect. Thus, increased splay of the glucose titration curve determines the appearance of recognizable glycosuria in mild disease as in type B glycosuria, whereas reduced maximum reabsorptive rate is the determinant of the magnitude of glycosuria in type A glycosuria. The report of a pedigree in which both type A and type B renal glycosuria occurred in the same family (20) may also indicate that these two types represent different degrees of glycosuria and not necessarily a coincidence of two different mutant genes inherited. Moreover, the demonstration of increased splay in type A renal glycosuria by McPhaul and Simonaitis (18) also suggests that such abnormality is not limited to type B renal glycosuria.

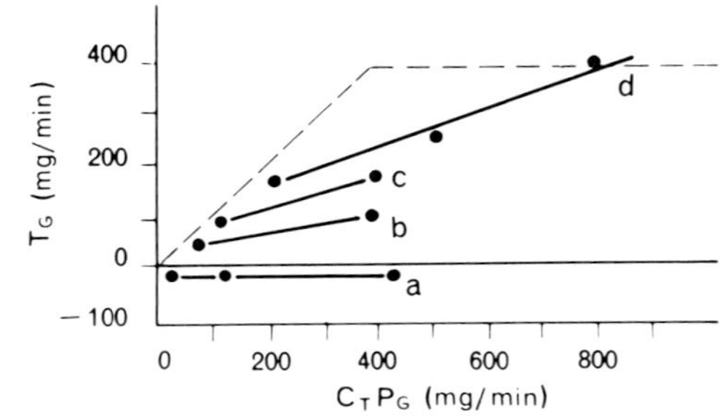

Fig. 5 Transition from type A to type B renal glycosuria caused by potassium ferricyanide poisoning. T_G = tubular glucose reabsorption; C_T = thiosulfate clearance (GFR); P_G = plasma glucose concentration; a = 6 days after poisoning; b = 14 days; c = 19 days; d = 28 days. (From Ref. 170).

With all the usefulness of glucose titration studies in evaluating renal glycosuria, there is an artifactual component inherent in the technique. Glucose titration requires infusion of large quantities of hypertonic glucose solution which leads to extracellular volume expansion, osmotic diuresis, and release of insulin, all of which inhibit proximal sodium and glucose reabsorption (55,72,171-174). As volume expansion is known to reduce Tm_G and increase splay of the glucose titration curve (71), lack of standardization of the volume of fluid infused during glucose loading may also influence the pattern of the titration curve. Such alterations in glucose transport by glucose loading may explain in part the "fatigue" of glucose reabsorption during glucose titration studies reported in some patients with renal glycosuria (175,176).

Certain information on the mechanism of renal glycosuria can also be obtained from the evaluation of renal glucose transport without glucose loading. In micropuncture studies in the dog, proximal tubule glucose reabsorption was inhibited by extracellular volume expansion (55,72) and administration of low-dose maleic acid (55) or acetazolamide (54). Despite a reduction in proximal glucose reabsorption, these maneuvers failed to induce glycosuria owing to a compensatory reabsorption of glucose at a further distal site. Only when high-dose maleic acid was administered did significant glycosuria occur even though the proximal effect was comparable to that of the other maneuvers (55). It follows, therefore, that inhi-

Table 2 Distribution of Tm_G Values Among Patients with Type A and Type B Renal Glycosuria

Renal glycosuria	Tm_G range (mg/min)	No. of patients	Tm_G/GFR range (mg/ml)	No. of patients
Type A	21-100	5	0.11-0.60	2
	101-150	8	0.61-1.00	6
	151-200	8	1.01-1.40	5
	201-250	8	1.41-1.80	13
Type B	251-300	7	1.81-2.20	8
	301-350	6	2.21-2.60	6
	351-400	1	2.61-3.00	3

Source: Data from Refs. 22,164,168,170,193,194,277,278.

bition of glucose transport at both proximal and distal sites is necessary for glycosuria to develop. Subsequent distal tubule micropuncture studies indicated that the distal site of glucose transport was the intermediate segment which includes the proximal straight segment and the loop of Henle (72,173).

Administration of maleic acid is known to cause experimental Fanconi syndrome (177, 178,181, Ch. 12). Maleic acid inhibits some metabolic enzymes including Na-K-ATPase (179, 180) and such metabolic effect can lead to inhibition of active transport of sodium at the basolateral membrane and consequently a reduction in electrochemical gradient of sodium at the luminal membrane. Since the entry step of glucose and other solutes at the luminal membrane is dependent on sodium gradient, transport of these solutes becomes defective. Another theory on the mechanism of transport defects in the Fanconi syndrome has been proposed by Bergeron et al. (95). They studied the transport of amino acids, glucose, and phosphate in maleate-induced Fanconi syndrome in the rat by microinjection, stop-flow, and microperfusion techniques. Bergeron et al. observed that the efflux of molecules from the tubule cells was increased throughout the proximal and distal tubule suggesting enhanced cell membrane permeability (95). Maesaka and McCaffery (93) also demonstrated tubular leakage of lissamine green and inulin from the proximal or distal segments in maleic acid-treated rats. These observations suggest that the glycosuria induced by maleic acid and probably that of the human Fanconi syndrome are caused by an increased permeability of the proximal and distal tubule membrane with leakage of solutes, including glucose. As the entry of labeled solutes into the proximal tubule cell was unaltered and fully compensates for the increased efflux, Bergeron et al. (95) proposed that the tubular dysfunction in the Fanconi syndrome is primarily determined by tubular leakage at distal sites. Micropuncture observations in the dog showing a significant distal effect of maleic acid on glucose transport, albeit the evidence is indirect, is also consistent with their proposal (55). The mechanism of glycosuria in this model is in contrast to that of phlorhizin-induced glycosuria in which sodium-glucose cotransport at the brush-border membrane is specifically inhibited. The mechanism of the isolated renal glycosuria encountered in the clinical setting is probably more analogous to the latter model, but the precise information on the glucose transport defect is not available. The possibilities include an alteration in the affinity of glucose to the carrier or a reduction in the number of glucose carriers, or both.

Primary Renal Glycosuria (Familial Renal Glycosuria; Benign Glycosuria)

Primary renal glycosuria is an inherited defect in renal tubular reabsorption of glucose. It is an isolated renal glycosuria not associated with any other tubular dysfunction, and although it is usually a life-long abnormality, no progressive alteration in renal function or systemic metabolism is encountered.

Incidence

The condition is usually detected in the second decade. but it may be seen at any age ranging from 4 weeks to 60 years (149,160). Both sexes are equally affected. The true incidence of the disease is unknown because of the difficulty in defining the diagnostic criteria for renal glycosuria, as discussed in Sect. II.D. With the use of the stringent criteria developed by Marble (149,161), renal glycosuria is uncommon. Only 85 out of 50,000 cases (0.17%) of melituria at the Joslin Clinic in Boston were found to have renal glycosuria. Crombie (182) reported an incidence of 0.29% and Harkness (183) 0.63% using less rigid criteria. If we assume that 3% of the general population has melituria, the incidence of renal glycosuria will be 1:20,000 by Marble's criteria (149,161).

Heredity

The familial occurrence of renal glycosuria has long been recognized. Hjärne in 1927 (154) reported 19 cases of orthoglycemic glycosuria in several generations of a Swedish family and made an extensive review of the literature on the subject. These cases included those with intermittent glycosuria who spilled glucose in the urine only in the postprandial period or after a glucose load. As parent to offspring transmission was seen with about 50% of the offspring being affected from an affected parent, Hjärne concluded that the mode of inheritance was consistent with an autosomal dominant character and this view was held and supported by most other authors at the time (184-187). In 1964, Khachadurian and Khachadurian (162) performed quantitative evaluations of renal glycosuria in six cases out of three families, and provided evidence for an autosomal recessive inheritance. By determination of 24-hr urinary glucose excretion, they observed that although mild intermittent glycosuria appeared in successive generations, heavy persistent glycosuria did not. They further observed that parents of persons with heavy persistent glycosuria showed either intermittent glycosuria or no glycosuria. They suggested that heavily glycosuric patients were homozygous, whereas mild, intermittently glycosuric parents were heterozygous for the affected gene. They also proposed to use the terms renal glycosuria and renal glycosuria trait to describe the homozygous and heterozygous individuals, respectively.

As quantitative evaluation of glycosuria is important in differentiating homozygous from heterozygous individuals, Elsas, Rosenberg, and coworkers (20,188) performed glucose titration studies in three pedigrees to reevaluate the mode of genetic transmission (Fig. 6). In pedigree Holm the proband (III-1) had severe type A renal glycosuria, whereas both parents (II-1 and II-2) and one in each set of grandparents (I-2 and I-3) had mild type A renal glycosuria. The pattern of inheritance was that of an autosomal recessive trait in that only the proband with severe glycosuria was a homozygote and the affected parents and grandparents with mild glycosuria were heterozygotes. Similarly, in pedigree Hol two sons with severe type A renal glycosuria were homozygotes, and the remaining two sons and the mother with milder forms of renal glycosuria were heterozygotes. The son II-4 showed a titration curve of type B renal glycosuria which prompted the authors to speculate that the father who could not be studied might have had type B renal glycosuria. While such a coincidence of type A and type B renal glycosuria occurring in the same family is possible, an alternative explanation is that type B renal glycosuria could be merely a manifestation of a mild form of type A renal glycosuria rather than representing a genetically different type (see the preceding section). In pedigree Cov both children had mild type A renal glycosuria with both parents showing normal titration curves. In this family the children were homozygous with overt manifestation of glycosuria, while the parents were thought to be heterozygous with their abnormality being so mild that it could not be demonstrated by glucose titration. These observations of Elsas, Rosenberg, and co-workers (20, 188) further established the autosomal recessive character of inheritance in primary renal glycosuria. Unlike glucose-galactose malabsorption, primary renal glycosuria is not associated with an intestinal defect in glucose transport (20), suggesting different mutant genes for these two disorders (189).

Pathology

In primary renal glycosuria a structural basis for the functional defect has not been clearly shown. Although Grote and Heilmann (190) earlier reported the renal histological picture in a patient with a lowered renal threshold for glucose, the case was complicated by diabetes mellitus, gastric carcinoma, and pneumonia. The first histological description of the kidney in a patient with primary renal glycosuria, therefore, was made by Monasterio (191). Based

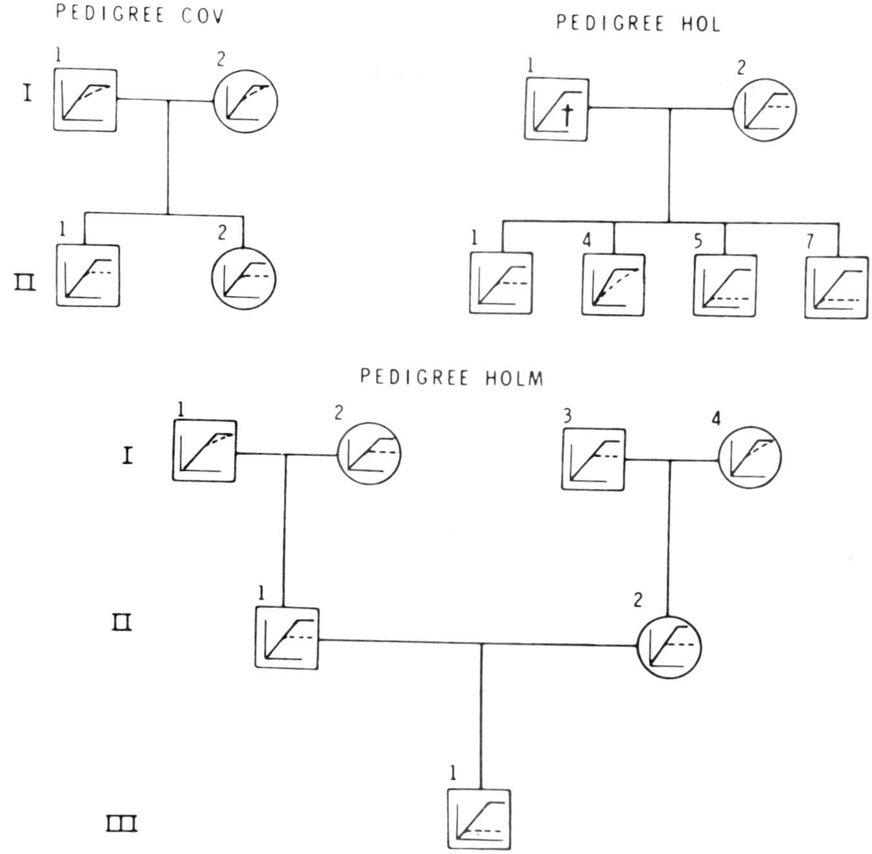

Fig. 6 Patterns of inheritance in three families with renal glycosuria. For explanation of symbols, see text. (From Ref. 188.)

on the examination of a specimen obtained by surgery, the author observed a diffuse flattening of the proximal tubule epithelium which on occasion was so striking as to result in an ectasia of the tubule lumen. Monasterio et al. (192) later followed 15 patients with renal glycosuria in three of whom needle biopsy of the kidney was obtained. The histological findings were similar to but less pronounced than the earlier report by Monasterio (192). The latter author proposed the term glycosuric tubular dysplasia to describe the renal lesion. Subsequently, Monasterio et al. (193) again reported two male patients with renal glycosuria in whom a large specimen of renal tissue was obtained by surgery for light and electron microscopic examinations as well as for microdissection. Both patients had normal glucose tolerance curves and excreted 27-100 g and 6-51 g of glucose per day, respectively. Fifty complete nephrons from each patient were microdissected for the measurement of glomerular surface and proximal tubule length and volume. The ratios of the glomerular parameters to tubular dimensions (r/R) were similar to the normal subjects and, therefore, the structural equivalent of glomerulotubular imbalance could not be demonstrated. The histological examinations, however, revealed abnormalities confined to the proximal tubule, including vacuolization, accumulation of periodic acid-Schiff-positive material and dissolution of the finer cytoplasmic elements of the brush border and the mitochondrial apparatus. These lesions were thought to be nonspecific but reversible, accounting for the benign nature of renal glycosuria.

The findings of Monasterio (191-193) were not confirmed by most other authors (194-196). Leonardi et al. (194) studied five cases of renal glycosuria from two families and in three of them needle biopsies of the kidney were obtained. No structural abnormalities were found, including normal alkaline phosphatase activity in the brush-border membrane of the proximal tubule. Electron microscopic examination also did not detect alterations in the fine structures of the proximal tubule cells, which would be considered typical of renal glycosuria. Freeman and Roberts (195) also reported electron microscopic findings of five renal biopsies from patients with renal glycosuria. Two showed no abnormalities and three had slight thickening of the tubular basement membrane which was nonspecific. Other authors also reported similar negative findings (196). Although Monasterio (193) argued that needle biopsy of the kidney may be subject to a sampling error and abnormal findings are more likely to be observed from larger surgical specimens, the question of any detectable structural alterations in primary renal glycosuria remains unresolved. As the tubular defect in glucose transport may involve only the biochemical alterations in the carrier protein for glucose, such subtle abnormalities may not be demonstrable morphologically. The minor and nonspecific tubular pathology shown by some authors may not necessarily be related to the selective tubular defect in glucose transport. An analogous condition is seen in glucose-galactose malabsorption in which the small intestinal mucosa with severe glucose transport defect showed no morphological abnormalities (195).

Clinical Features

The patients with primary renal glycosuria are mostly asymptomatic and the detection of glycosuria by a routine urinalysis is the usual event leading to the diagnosis. Despite considerable glycosuria in many of these patients, polyuria and polydipsia, the frequent symptoms of diabetes mellitus, are usually absent. The degree of glycosuria varies widely, ranging from less than 1 g to over 100 g/24 hr, with the majority excreting 5-30 g/24 hr. While the majority of patients diagnosed according to Marble's criteria should have persistent glycosuria, other patients may have only intermittent glycosuria probably representing the heterozygotes (162).

The diagnosis of primary renal glycosuria should be based on a 24-hr urinary glucose excretion of greater than 500 mg on a diet containing 30 cal/kg of which about 50% is carbohydrate (143). Diabetes mellitus should be excluded by obtaining fasting and postprandial blood glucose and, if necessary, by a glucose tolerance test. Other causes of renal tubular dysfunction should be excluded by determination of renal clearances of phosphate, amino acids, uric acid, and bicarbonate and by testing urinary acidification. Increased rates of urinary lactate excretion have been reported in primary renal glycosuria (198), but the significance of this observation is unknown. One should also rule out other known causes of renal glycosuria such as pregnancy and chronic renal failure. A positive family history is useful in supporting the familial nature of the disease, and evaluation of other family members should provide further information on the pattern of genetic transmission. A glucose titration study is a valuable research tool in providing quantitative information on renal glycosuria, but it is not required in establishing the diagnosis.

Transition of primary renal glycosuria into diabetes mellitus has been reported by some authors (159,199). However, these cases probably represent coexistence of both conditions in the same individuals rather than a causal relationship between the two conditions. Moreover, a low renal threshold for glucose is also seen frequently in diabetic patients (144,145), and these cases may account for some of the reports on the apparent transition from renal glycosuria to diabetes mellitus.

The clinical course of primary renal glycosuria is invariably benign with no deterioration in renal function or metabolic state throughout life. Although the degree of renal glycosuria may vary from time to time, it usually remains stable over many decades without progression, and the patient's general condition of health also remains unaltered. As expected from the benign nature of the abnormality, no treatment is indicated in this condition. In patients with heavy glycosuria, however, prolonged fasting should be avoided to prevent hypoglycemia and ketosis. The most important diagnostic implication of primary renal glycosuria is in its differentiation from diabetes mellitus so that the unnecessary and often dangerous insulin and other hypoglycemic treatments can be avoided.

Glucose-Galactose Malabsorption

A syndrome of malabsorption of monosaccharides glucose and galactose was first reported in 1962 almost simultaneously by Swedish (200,201) and French authors (202). Since then over 20 cases have been reported (203). The clinical features are characteristic. Shortly after birth the affected children develop severe watery diarrhea, dehydration, and failure to thrive on an ordinary diet containing carbohydrate. The stools are acidic and show high contents of glucose and galactose. The diarrhea is more or less continuous and severe as long as the diet contains any carbohydrate of which glucose and galactose are the major constituents. Little or no rise in blood levels of these hexoses occurs after ingestion of food. The diarrhea promptly subsides when dietary carbohydrate is replaced by fructose. Sucrose is also better tolerated than other dissacharides because one of its monosaccharide component is fructose. The recognition of this disorder is important, since the child may die from dehydration and malnutrition.

The intestinal defect is caused by the absence of active transport of glucose and galactose in the jejunum most likely involving the step of hexose uptake at the brush border (197, 204,205). No structural abnormalities in the intestinal mucosa have been observed (197, 204). Fructose and xylose are transported by the intestine through mechanisms different from that of glucose and galactose, and therefore their absorption is unaffected in this disorder (205). Accumulation of amino acids and the Na-K-ATPase activity in the intestinal biopsy specimens and intestinal sodium transport are also normal (197). Although phlorhizin normally inhibits intestinal glucose uptake, no effect is observed in the affected patients (197). Three adult cases of glucose-galactose malabsorption have also been reported (207,208). The disorder is inherited as an autosomal recessive trait (209), with the heterozygotes exhibiting an intermediate defect in the rate of intestinal glucose uptake (205).

In the majority of patients with glucose-galactose malabsorption, a mild defect in renal glucose reabsorption has been demonstrated (176,197,200,205,210,211). The 24-hr urinary glucose excretion is usually in the range of 0.4-1.0 g and glucose titration studies show a reduced threshold with normal or only slightly reduced Tm_G (type B renal glycosuria) (197, 210,212). Liu et al. (176), however, reported a patient with severe depression of Tm_G which was associated with a "fatigue" of glucose reabsorption and a low GFR. The defect in renal glucose reabsorption is most regularly seen in homozygotes (197,205). The occurrence of an analogous defect in glucose transport in both intestine and renal tubule suggests that the disorder is caused by mutation of a gene locus shared by both systems. Similar inborn errors of amino acid transport involving both renal tubule and intestine have been reported in cystinuria, Hartnup disease, and iminoglycinuria (213-215). As a complete defect in intestinal glucose transport is associated with a partial defect in renal glucose transport in glucose-galactose malabsorption, the kidney probably contains a glucose transport system which is not shared by the intestine (205) and a defect in such a transport system is seen in primary renal glycosuria. In glucose-galactose malabsorption the expression of the defect in glucose transport is probably confined to intestine and kidney, since the intravenous glucose tolerance test is normal (216) and red cell glucose transport is also intact (217).

Renal Glycosuria in the Fanconi Syndrome

The Fanconi syndrome is the generalized dysfunction of the proximal tubule leading to excessive urinary losses of a number of solutes which are normally reabsorbed in this segment. These solutes include glucose, amino acids, phosphate, urate, and bicarbonate. As a detailed description of the syndrome is covered in Chs. 13 and 14, only some pertinent aspects related to glycosuria will be discussed here.

Renal glycosuria is one of the cardinal symptoms of the Fanconi syndrome and was first described by de Toni (218) in connection with this syndrome. The degree of glycosuria varies from mild to severe and the renal threshold for glucose is also reduced to a variable degree. The pattern of glucose titration curves in the Fanconi syndrome has not been adequately investigated because of the potential hypokalemic effect of glucose loading (219-221). In the few cases studied, Tm_G was either low or normal (222-224). However, glucose loading tended to be submaximal in these studies and a further rise in Tm_G with greater glucose loading could not be excluded in some of the patients showing low Tm_G (222-225). Occasionally, Tm_G declined with prolonged glucose loading (225) probably due to the "fatigue" caused by extracellular volume expansion.

The nature of tubular defects in the Fanconi syndrome remains unknown. One theory postulates that the first step of glucose uptake by the brush-border membrane is intact (294) and the defect is in the inability to maintain the steep glucose gradient after glucose reabsorption owing to an increase in tubule membrane permeability. Such an increase in membrane permeability has been shown in the experimental model of the Fanconi syndrome induced by maleic acid (93,95), leading to the leakage of a number of solutes, including glucose. Another theory is that active sodium extrusion at the basolateral membrane is reduced due to a defective Na-K-ATPase (179,180), resulting in the lowering of a sodium gradient at the luminal membrane and reduced entry of sodium-dependent solutes into the tubule cell. It is also possible that the mechanism of tubular dysfunction is different depending on the underlying etiology of the Fanconi syndrome. Thus, sodium-dependent glucose transport into the brush-border membrane vesicles in the maleic acid-induced model was shown to be intact (294), whereas that in the anhydro-4-epitetracycline-induced model was reduced (295).

The Fanconi syndrome develops in a variety of diseases with or without specific etiology. The primary Fanconi syndrome usually occurs sporadically, but hereditary incidence of the syndrome has also been reported. The secondary Fanconi syndrome includes those with inborn errors of metabolism and those with acquired diseases. Among the inborn errors of metabolism are cystinosis, glycogenosis, Lowe's syndrome, galactosemia, fructose intolerance, tyrosinemia, and Wilson's disease. In acquired diseases, multiple myeloma, nephrotic syndrome, transplanted kidney, and intoxications with heavy metals, maleic acid, lysol, and outdated tetracycline are associated with the Fanconi syndrome (222).

In glycogen storage disease most patients do not develop the Fanconi syndrome (226, 227). In a small number of patients who do develop the Fanconi syndrome, renal glucose reabsorption is most severely affected and the term renal glucose-losing syndrome has been proposed by Brodehl (222) to distinguish it from other forms of the Fanconi syndrome with milder glycosuria. Fellers et al. (228) called it pseudophlorhizin diabetes because the severity of glycosuria mimicked that caused by phlorhizin. It appears to occur in a special type of glycogenosis, which is separate from any other known types, including type I with hepatic glucose-6-phosphatase deficiency (222). The glycogen storage involves both liver and kidney. Since the first description by Fanconi and Bickel in 1949 (221), more than 10 cases of glycogenosis associated with the Fanconi syndrome have been reported mostly in the European literature (221,222,224,228-232). All cases have been small children with their ages ranging from 1 to 6 years and the first symptoms of the Fanconi syndrome have been observed at as early as 1½ months of age (229). The major features include hepatic accumulation of glycogen (greater than 8 g/100 g wet tissue) and severe Fanconi syndrome. Aminoaciduria is generalized and massive, and phosphaturia is also severe, leading to rickets, osteoporosis, and growth retardation. Moderate to severe acidosis also develops. However, the most prominent feature is the profound degree of glycosuria with 24-hr urinary glucose excretion, averaging 189 g/1.73 m^2 (range 74-240 g/1.73 m^2). The massive glycosuria is associated with normoglycemia and, on occasion, hypoglycemia. One case reported by Brodehl et al. (222) had fractional glucose reabsorption of only 30% of the filtered load. Glucose and galactose tolerance are also impaired and ketonemia and ketonuria are frequent. Although the tubular dysfunction is severe, only mild histological changes in the kidney are described (222). Some accumulation of glycogen is shown in the proximal tubule and the ascending loop of Henle, but it is less prominent than that of type I glycogenosis. With electron microscopy, giant mitochondria are seen in the proximal tubule cells and triple-layered mitochondrial crystals are displaced and found beside the membrane. The treatment of this disorder is mainly symptomatic, including frequent protein-enriched feedings for hypoglycemia and fluid and alkaline administration during acute decompensation caused by infections or surgery. The long-term prognosis appears good, since renal function with regard to GFR remains unaltered and tubular dysfunction tends to improve with age.

Renal Glycosuria Associated with Other Specific Tubular Defects

A few specific defects in amino acid and phosphate transport are associated with renal glycosuria and these rare combinations of specific tubular defects should be differentiated from the Fanconi syndrome in which generalized tubular dysfunction is the main feature. Careful scrutiny is required in the cases of the incomplete Fanconi syndrome in which at least one of the cardinal features of the syndrome is not present. For example, certain cases with combined glycosuria and aminoaciduria should be classified as the incomplete Fanconi syndrome because of the generalized nature of aminoaciduria (233,234).

In glucoglycinuria renal glycosuria is associated with glycinuria but without other forms of aminoaciduria. Käser et al. (235,236) reported a 9-year-old boy with cystic fibrosis who was found to have renal glycosuria and glycinuria. The patient had normal urea and creatinine clearances and daily urinary glucose excretion was in the range of 2-4 g. A glucose titration study showed a reduced renal threshold at 70 mg/dl but the Tm_G was normal indicating a type B renal glycosuria. The 24-hr urinary glycine excretion was 194-300 mg, occasionally rising to 600-700 mg (normal: 83-114 mg). The excretion patterns of other amino acids were essentially normal. Examination of the patient's relatives revealed combined renal glycosuria and glycinuria in 13 out of 45 apparently healthy individuals. Neither of the two tubular defects occurred alone in these relatives and it was suggested that the disorder is inherited as an autosomel dominant trait. No other families of glucoglycinuria have been reported. These rare cases of glucoglycinuria must be differentiated from those of isolated glycinuria (237,238), iminoglycinuria (215,239), and generalized aminoacidurias with prominent glycinuria (240).

Renal glycosuria is also associated with familial hypophosphatemia (or phosphate diabetes) (241,242). Dent (241) reported four adult cases of familial hypophosphatemia with osteomalacia in whom the tubular defects in phosphate and glucose transport appeared to coexist. However, only one of them had pronounced renal glycosuria (above 0.5%), and the other three had mild and intermittent glycosuria. Magid et al. (242) also reported a 16-year-old boy with hypophosphatemic rickets and renal glycosuria. The 24-hr urinary glucose excretion was 9.47 g and Tm_G was marginally suppressed at 286 mg/min per 1.73 m^2. Aminoaciduria was absent. Although the patient's mother also had hypophosphatemic osteomalacia with phosphate reabsorptive defect, she had no glycosuria. Some of the earlier reports on similar cases of hypophosphatemic rickets or osteomalacia were associated with renal glycosuria (243-245), but they could not be differentiated from the Fanconi syndrome in the absence of information on urinary amino acid excretion. Others (246) reported the absence of generalized aminoaciduria but glycosuria was mild and intermittent.

A third syndrome of combined tubular defects involving the transport of glucose, phosphate, and glycine has been reported by Scriver et al. (247). They reported a 16-year-old boy who developed rickets at the age of 9 and later was found to have severe hypophosphatemia caused by impairment in renal conservation of phosphate. The defect in phosphate transport was so severe that net tubular secretion of phosphate was demonstrated on several occasions. Urinary excretion of glycine was increased with glycine clearance of 6.5-16.7 ml/min and fractional glycine reabsorption of 72-91% (normal >93%). Urinary excretion of glycyl-proline was also increased. A glucose titration study showed a reduced renal threshold at 78 mg/dl and Tm_G was markedly depressed. The inhibited transport of glycine, glucose, and phosphate appeared to be noncompetitive in nature, since infusion of one of these solutes did not alter urinary excretion of the others and infusion of L-proline, the competitive inhibitor of glycine transport, showed normal responses. Brodehl (222) reported another patient with hypophosphatemic rickets associated with renal glycosuria and glycinuria. This patient had renal glycosuria since the age of 4 and urinary glucose excretion ranged 10-40 g/24 hr at the age of 17. The renal threshold for glucose was low at 70 mg/dl, but Tm_G was not determined. Glycine clearance was 11.6 ml/min per 1.73 m^2 and fractional glycine reabsorption was 89.4%. Excretion of other amino acids was normal.

Glycosuria in Pregnancy

Renal glycosuria occurs frequently during pregnancy and represents an important diagnostic problem with regard to the differentiation from gestational diabetes mellitus. Since the first observation of renal glycosuria in pregnancy by Blot in 1856 (248), a wide range of incidence has been reported in the literature (140,141,249,250). The incidence varies from less than 2% (249) to 88% (140) depending on the criteria of renal glycosuria, the analytic methods for glucose used, gestational age, and time, duration, and frequency of urinary glucose determination. Using conventional reagent strips for glycosuria screening in random urine samples, Chen et al. (249) observed a 1.7% incidence of renal glycosuria in a large population of pregnancies collected over 6 years. Soler and Malins (140) on the other hand reported that urinary glucose excretion above the normal rate of 10 mg/hr occurred in 88% of women during pregnancy when the determinations were made over a 2-hr period. Glycosuria was slight during fasting and increased after meals. Lind and Hytten (141) made serial studies of 24-hr urinary glucose excretion in 30 pregnant women from the tenth to fortieth gestational weeks and again postpartum. In 26 women (87%), the 24-hr urinary glucose excretion was greater than the nonpregnant upper limit of 140 mg with 12 (40%) excreting less than 500 mg, four (13%) in the range of 500-1000 mg, and 10 (33%) more than 1000 mg.

Urinary glucose excretion increases within 4 weeks of gestation reaching a near-peak value at 8-11 weeks (251,252). Thereafter, it either continues to rise to peak in the early third trimester or remains unchanged throughout the pregnancy (141). The glycosuria is frequently intermittent and conspicuously variable from day to day and during the course of the day (140,141). The increased urinary glucose excretion reverts to normal within a week after delivery (141).

Davison and Hytten (253) examined renal glucose reabsorption following intravenous glucose infusion in glycosuric and nonglycosuric pregnant women during gestation and again at 8-10 weeks postpartum. Throughout pregnancy, in both groups, the renal reabsorption of glucose was less effective than in the nonpregnant state. Of interest was the observation that the glycosuric group exhibited less efficient glucose reabsorption for the given levels of filtered load than the nonglycosuric group not only during pregnancy but also postpartum when the women were no longer glycosuric. Davison and Hytten (253) concluded that pregnancy imposes some specific change in the glucose reabsorptive capacity and that women who develop glycosuria in pregnancy may, in addition, have preexisting inefficiency in glucose reabsorption or an element of tubular damage. In this connection, Davison and coworkers (252) showed that pregnant women with a well-documented history of urinary tract infection preceding the pregnancy had significantly higher rates of urinary glucose excretion than those with a negative history.

The cause of renal glycosuria in pregnancy has not been clearly defined. Two potential effects of pregnancy on renal glucose transport have been considered. One is the greatly increased GFR during pregnancy which raises the filtered load of glucose to the level that exceeds the normal tubular reabsorptive capacity. The other is an inhibitory effect of pregnancy on tubular glucose reabsorption through some unidentified mechanism.

It has long been known that remarkable hemodynamic alterations occur in pregnancy with a 30-50% increase in GFR (254,255). Christensen (256) performed glucose titration studies in pregnant women and found that Tm_G was not significantly different from the nonpregnant controls while the renal threshold was lower. The lowered renal threshold was thought to be due to the increase in GFR. Welsh and Sims (257) also performed glucose titration studies in 29 pregnant women, 13 with glycosuria. Tm_G for the glycosuric women was 310 ± 18 mg/min, which was significantly lower than the 378 ± 20 mg/min for the nonglycosuric pregnant women, or 366 ± 16 mg/min for the nonpregnant women. As Tm_G should normally increase with an increase in GFR (41-43), the absence of such an increase in Tm_G in the nonglycosuric pregnant women indicates that the tubular glucose reabsorptive capacity was also lower than that of the nonpregnant control. The glycosuric pregnant women, therefore, had far lower Tm_G for a given filtered load of glucose than the control. Such relationship between Tm_G and GFR is illustrated in Fig. 7, in which the regression lines for the three groups are plotted. It can be noted that for a given GFR, Tm_G was clearly lower for the normal pregnant group than the control group and lowest for the glycosuric pregnant group. The slope of regression lines was not significantly different for the three groups, indicating a constant relationship between Tm_G and GFR. Recent glucose titration studies in glycosuric pregnant women by Drexel and Seiler (258) also confirmed the markedly reduced Tm_G consistent with type A renal glycosuria.

The underlying mechanism of reduced tubular glucose reabsorption in pregnancy is unknown. Although the pregnant kidney is known to be able to reabsorb sodium avidly (259, 265,296), the presence of extracellular volume expansion during pregnancy may well alter the glomerulotubular balance of the proximal nephron. The increased clearances of uric acid (252,260) and amino acids (261) in addition to that of glucose, also suggest a generalized impairment of proximal tubular function. However, the filtration fraction, which determines the peritubular capillary physical forces (262), has been reported to be increased (259,263), decreased (252), or unchanged (264). Moreover, in micropuncture studies of the pregnant rat, Alexander et al. (259) could not demonstrate significant alterations in

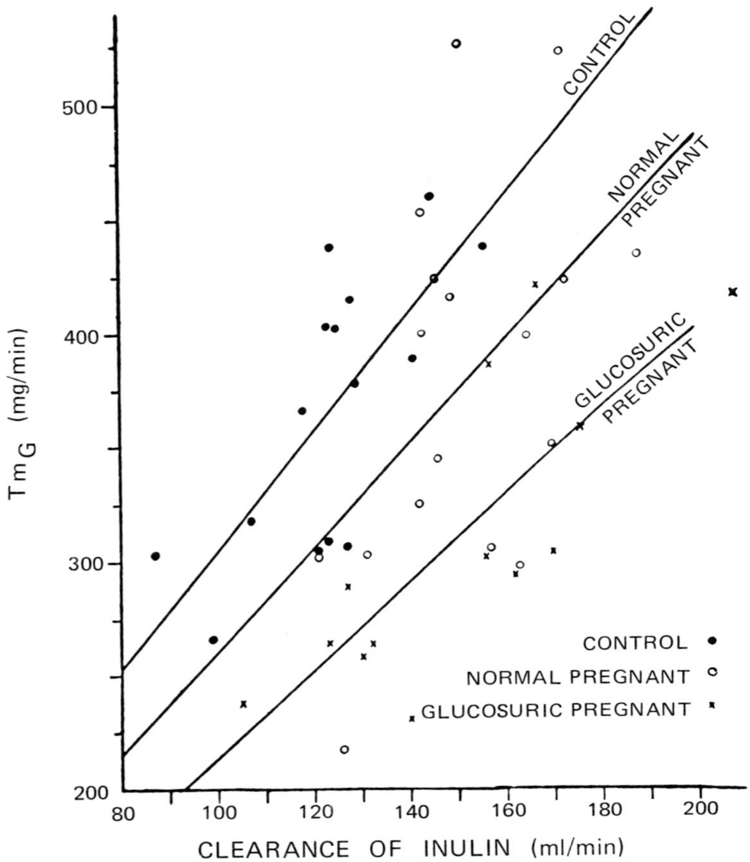

Fig. 7 Regression lines of tubular maximum for glucose (Tm_G) plotted against GFR in control, normal-pregnant and glycosuric-pregnant women. (From Ref. 257.)

proximal glomerulotubular balance, while Garland and Green (297) showed reduced fractional proximal fluid reabsorption only in late pregnancy. Bishop and Green (266) were also unable to show altered glomerulotubular balance for sodium in the proximal tubule and suggested that a distal segment was responsible for the glycosuria of pregnancy (267). In addition to the hemodynamic alterations in pregnancy, other possible factors for renal glycosuria include a number of hormones, especially sex hormones, which are increased during pregnancy and decline rapidly after delivery (265,268). Whether these hormones exert any effect on renal glucose transport remains to be elucidated.

Renal Glucose Spillage in Chronic Renal Failure and Nephrotic Syndrome

As chronic renal disease progresses, the functioning nephron population diminishes and the remaining nephrons undergo adaptation in order to maintain homeostasis of electrolytes and nonelectrolytes (269). As a result, excretion of these solutes per nephron is greatly enhanced. Thus, fractional sodium reabsorption in the proximal tubule and in some distal segments is reduced in chronic renal failure (270) by certain as yet unidentified factors (271). As glucose transport is closely related to sodium transport, one would expect that fractional glucose reabsorption is also reduced in chronic renal failure. Indeed, Rieselbach et al. (272)

observed that the splay of glucose titration curves was increased in patients with chronic renal failure when GFR was less than 15 ml/min, indicating a reduced renal threshold for glucose. In patients with GFR less than 10 ml/min there was a marked exaggeration of the splay, while in those with GFR greater than 15 ml/min the splay was similar to the normal group. The increase in splay was thought to be due to an increase in nephron heterogeneity of chronic renal disease (273) or an alteration in the kinetics of glucose transport. Regardless of the mechanism, the increase in splay is related to the uremic environment, since the unilateral pyelonephritic kidney in the rat exhibited exaggerated splay only in the uremic state following contralateral nephrectomy (274).

Similar observations were made by McPhaul and Simonaitis (18) in glomerulonephritic patients. However, lowered renal threshold for glucose and increased splay of the glucose titration curve were found in much wider range of GFR than that reported by Rieselbach et al. (272). As the majority of patients reported by McPhaul and Simonaitis (18) had heavy proteinuria in excess of 3.5 g/24 hr, the presence of nephrotic syndrome could also have contributed to the development of abnormal glucose titration curve at higher GFR levels (see below).

The relationship of the exaggerated splay to renal adaptation in chronic renal failure was examined by Schmidt and Danovitch (275) in dogs with experimentally induced renal insufficiency. They found that Tm_G was reduced and the splay was markedly exaggerated when the animals were on a constant salt intake of 85 mmol/day (CSI). These animals were undergoing sodium adaptation with fractional sodium excretion (FE_{Na}) of 4.56-8.14%. When these animals were placed on a diet with proportional reduction of sodium intake according to the level of GFR (PRS) FE_{Na} was 0.38-0.72%, indicating no sodium adaptation, and Tm_G/GFR rose significantly with reversion of the splay to normal. When PRS dogs were fed a CSI diet just prior to the study, Tm_G/GFR and the splay remained essentially similar to those of PRS dogs despite an increase in FE_{Na} to 3.13%. Thus, the abnormal splay of glucose titration curves in chronic renal failure is related to the long-term adaptation in sodium transport but not directly to the concurrent sodium excretion.

The site of altered glucose transport in the nephron was examined by micropuncture in the remnant kidney model of the dog (72). Although uremic dogs showed increased single nephron GFR and reduced fractional reabsorption of sodium and glucose in the proximal tubule, no glycosuria was detected owing to an increase in glucose reabsorption in the intermediate segment (between the late proximal tubule and the distal tubule) (Fig. 8). Following extracellular volume expansion there was a further reduction in proximal sodium and glucose reabsorption. The ensuing increase in the delivery of glucose to the intermediate segment exceeded the reabsorptive capacity of this segment and resulted in glycosuria. This was in marked contrast to the control group in which the increased glucose delivery of volume expansion was fully compensated by reabsorption in the intermediate segment and no glycosuria developed. It appears, therefore, that both the proximal tubule and the intermediate segment play an important role in the regulation of urinary glucose excretion in the uremic state.

The spillage of glucose in patients with chronic renal failure is usually mild and not clinically significant. However, it may occasionally cause confusion with diabetes mellitus, especially because carbohydrate tolerance is also impaired in the uremic state (276).

In nephrotic syndrome features of tubular dysfunction including glycosuria, aminoaciduria, phosphaturia, renal potassium wasting, and hyperchloremic acidosis have been described (279-283). These features represent nonspecific tubular dysfunction and therefore are similar to those of the Fanconi syndrome. The commonest manifestations are aminoaciduria and glycosuria (284). As the filtered protein is reabsorbed into the proximal tubule

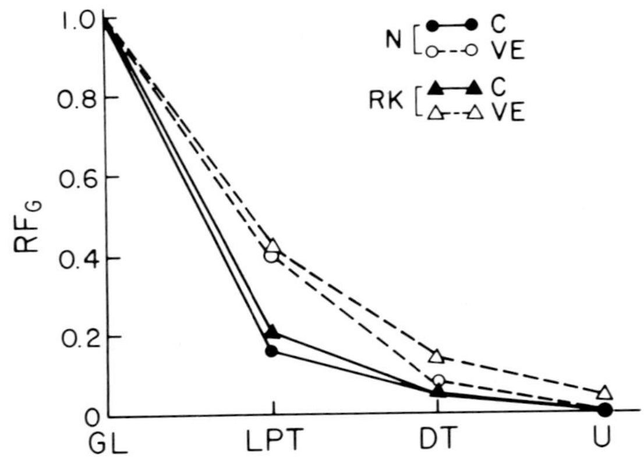

Fig. 8 Remaining fractions of filtered glucose (RF_G) at nephron sites in normal (N) and uremic remnant-kidney (RK) dogs before (C) and after extracellular volume expansion (VE). GL = glomerulus; LPT = late proximal tubule; DT = distal tubule; U = final urine. (From Ref. 72.)

epithelium through endocytosis and catabolized in the lysosomes (285,286), it is thought that tubular damage occurs in the process resulting in tubular dysfunction. Another mechanism which may lead to tubular dysfunction in nephrotic syndrome is related to hypoalbuminemia. Despite the well-known picture of renal retention of sodium in nephrotic syndrome it has been shown that proximal reabsorption of sodium is reduced probably as the result of decreased plasma oncotic pressure in the peritubular capillaries, reducing the uptake of proximal reabsorbate (287,288). The enhanced overall reabsorption of sodium, therefore, appears to be a function of the distal nephron segments (288). Since the transport of glucose and other solutes in the proximal tubule are sodium dependent, defective glucose reabsorption may result from a low oncotic pressure in the peritubular capillaries in nephrotic syndrome. The demonstration of enhanced proximal glucose reabsorption following hyperoncotic albumin infusion to raise peritubular oncotic pressure is also supportive of such a mechanism (289). Usberti et al. (290) performed glucose titration studies in patients with nephrotic syndrome in whom there was moderate impairment of renal function. They reported that the splay of the glucose titration curve was increased but Tm_G/GFR was unchanged in nephrotic patients as compared with nonnephrotic patients. Their findings were similar to those of McPhaul and Simonaitis (18) in that glycosuria was observed at higher levels of GFR than those reported by Rieselbach et al. (272). In the studies of Usberti et al. (290) a significant correlation was found between glucose reabsorption per 100 ml GFR and serum albumin as well as between splay point, which is a measure of renal threshold, and serum albumin or GFR. Thus, glycosuria may develop in patients with nephrotic syndrome or chronic renal failure, conditions that frequently coexist in the same individual.

REFERENCES

1. Folin, O.; and Wu, H. A system of blood analysis. J. Biol. Chem. 38:81-110, 1919.
2. Somogyi, M. Determination of blood sugar. J. Biol. Chem. 160:69-73, 1945.
3. Middleton, J. E.; and Griffith, W. J. Rapid colorimetric micro-method for estimating glucose in blood and C.S.F. using glucose oxidase. Br. Med. J. 2:1525-1527, 1957.

4. Peterson, J. I.; and Young, D. S. Evaluation of the hexokinase/glucose-6-phosphate dehydrogenase method of determination of glucose in urine. Anal. Biochem. 23:301-316, 1968.
5. Silverman, M. Glucose transport in the kidney. Biochim. Biophys. Acta 457:303-351, 1976.
6. Kotyk, A. Mechanisms of nonelectrolyte transport. Biochim. Biophys. Acta 300:183-210, 1973.
7. Lieb, W. R.; and Stein, W. D. Carrier and non-carrier models for sugar transport in the human red blood cell. Biochim. Biophys. Acta 265:187-207, 1972.
8. Schultz, S. G.; and Curran, P. F. Coupled transport of sodium and organic solutes. Physiol. Rev. 50:637-718, 1970.
9. Ullrich, K. J. Sugar, amino acid, and Na^+ cotransport in the proximal tubule. Ann. Rev. Physiol. 41:181-195, 1979.
10. Crane, R. K. Hypothesis of the mechanism of intestinal active transport of sugars. Fed. Proc. 21:891-895, 1962.
11. Schultz, S. G. Sodium-coupled solute transport by the small intestine; a status report. Am. J. Physiol. 233:E249-E254, 1977.
12. Morel, F.; and de Rouffignac, C. Kidney. Ann. Rev. Physiol. 35:17-54, 1973.
13. Mudge, G. H.; Berndt, N. O.; and Valtin, H. Tubular transport of urea, glucose, phosphate, uric acid, sulfate, and thiosulfate. In: Handbook of Physiology: Renal Physiology, edited by Orloff, J., and Berliner, R. W. Washington, D.C., American Physiological Society, 1973, pp. 587-652.
14. Ullrich, K. J. Renal tubular mechanisms of organic solute transport. Kidney Int. 9: 134-148, 1976.
15. Shannon, J. A.; and Fisher, S. The renal tubular reabsorption of glucose in the normal dog. Am. J. Physiol. 122:765-774, 1938.
16. Shannon, J. A.; Farber, S.; and Troast, L. The measurement of glucose Tm in the normal dog. Am. J. Physiol. 133:752-761, 1941.
17. Smith, H. W.; Goldring, W.; Chasis, H.; Ranges, H. A.; and Bradley, S. E. The application of saturation methods to the study of glomerular and tubular function in the human kidney. J. Mt. Sinai Hosp. 10:59-108, 1943.
18. McPhaul, J. J.; and Simonaitis, J. J. Observations on the mechanisms of glycosuria during glucose loads in normal and nondiabetic subjects. J. Clin. Invest. 47:702-711, 1968.
19. Letteri, J. M.; and Wesson, L. G. Glucose titration curves as an estimate of intrarenal distribution of glomerular filtrate in patients with congestive heart failure. J. Lab. Clin. Med. 65:387-405, 1965.
20. Elsas, L. J.; and Rosenberg, L. E. Familial renal glycosuria: A genetic reappraisal of hexose transport by kidney and intestine. J. Clin. Invest. 48:1845-1854, 1969.
21. Govaerts, P.; and Lambert, P. P. Pathogenie du diabete renal. Acta Clin. Belg. 4:341-370, 1949.
22. Nielsen, A. L. On the mechanism of glycosuria. Acta Med. Scand. 130: 219-231, 1948.
23. Brodehl, J.; Franken, A.; and Gellissen, K. Maximal Tubular reabsorption of glucose in infants and children. Acta Paediatr. Scand. 61:413-420, 1972.
24. Stalder, G. Funktionen des Tubulusepithels. Mod. Probl. Paediatr. 6:22-56, 1960.
25. Grossmann, P.; and Zoellner, K. Bestimmung der Funkionsfähigkeit des proximalen Tubulus mit Hilfe von Glukose und p-Aminohippursäure bei kindern. Acta Biol. Med. Germ. 20:413-419, 1968.
26. Gekle, D.; Janovsky, M.; Slechtova, R.; and Martinek, J. Einfluss der glomerulären Filtrationsrate auf die tubuläre Glucosereabsorption bei Kindern. Klin. Wochenschr. 45: 416-419, 1967.
27. Brodehl, J. Renal glycosuria. In: Pediatric Kidney Disease, edited by Edelmann, C. M., Jr., Boston, Little, Brown, 1978, pp. 1036-1047.
28. DeFronzo, R. A.; and Thier, S. O. Inherited disorder of renal tubule function. In: The Kidney, 2nd ed., edited by Brenner, B. M., and Rector, F. C. Jr. Philadelphia, Saunders, 1981, 1816-1871.

29. Tudvad, F. Sugar reabsorption in prematures and full-term babies. Scand. J. Clin. Lab. Invest. 1:218-283, 1949.
30. Oliver, J.; and MacDowell, M. The structural and functional aspects of the handling of glucose by the nephrons and the kidney and their correlation by means of structural-functional equivalents. J. Clin. Invest. 40:1093-1112, 1961.
31. Bradley, S. E.; Laragh, J. H.; Wheeler, H. O.; MacDowell, M.; and Oliver, J. Correlation of structure and function in the handling of glucose by the nephrons of the canine kidney. J. Clin. Invest. 40:1113-1131, 1961.
32. Baines, A. D. Effect of extracellular fluid volume expansion on maximum glucose reabsorption rate and glomerular tubular balance in single rat nephron. J. Clin. Invest. 50: 2414-2425, 1971.
33. Burgen, A. S. V. A theoretical treatment of glucose reabsorption in the kidney. Can. J. Biochem. 34:466-474, 1956.
34. Koushanpour, E. Biochemical basis of tubular transport. In: *Renal Physiology: Principles and Functions*. Philadelphia, Saunders, 1976, pp. 121-149.
35. Thomas, G. B., Jr. The hyperbola. In: *Calculus and Analytic Geometry*. 4th ed. Reading, Massachusetts, Addison-Wesley, 1968, 344-352.
36. Kurtzman, N. A.; White, M. G.; Rogers, P. W.; and Flynn, J. J., III. Relationship of sodium reabsorption and glomerular filtration rate to renal glucose reabsorption. J. Clin. Invest. 51:127-133, 1972.
37. Kurtzman, N. A.; and Pillay, V. K. G. Renal reabsorption of glucose in health and disease. Arch. Intern. Med. 131:901-904, 1973.
38. Bowman, R. H.; and Maack, T. Glucose transport by the isolated perfused rat kidney. Am. J. Physiol. 222:1499-1504, 1972.
39. Stolte, H.; Hare, D.; and Boylan, J. W. D-glucose and fluid reabsorption in the proximal surface tubule of the rat kidney. Pflügers Arch. 334:193-206, 1972.
40. Hare, D.; and Stolte, H. Rat proximal tubule D-glucose transport as a function of concentration, flow and radius. Pflügers Arch. 334:207-221, 1972.
41. Handley, C. A.; and Moyer, J. H. Significance of the GFR/Tm_G ratio. Am. J. Physiol. 180:151-155, 1955.
42. Kwang, T. F.; and Bennett, C. M. Relationship between glomerular filtration rate and maximum tubular reabsorptive rate of glucose. Kidney Int. 5:23-29, 1974.
43. Schultze, R. G.; and Berger, H. The influence of GFR and saline expansion on Tm_G of the dog kidney. Kidney Int. 3:291-297, 1973.
44. Van Liew, J. B.; Deetjen, P.; and Boylan, J. W. Glucose reabsorption in the rat kidney: Dependence on glomerular filtration. Pflügers Arch. 295:232-244, 1967.
45. Deetjen, P.; and Boylan, J. W. Glocuse reabsorption in the rat kidney. Microperfusion studies. Pflügers Arch. 299:19-29, 1968.
46. Tune, B. M.; and Burg, M. B. Glucose transport by proximal renal tubules. Am. J. Physiol. 221:580-585, 1971.
47. von Baeyer, H.; Haeberle, D. A.; Van Liew, J. B.; and Hare, D. Glomerular tubular balance of renal D-glucose transport during hyperglycemia. Pflügers Arch. 384:39-47, 1980.
48. Barfuss, D. W.; and Schafer, J. A. Flow dependence of nonelectrolyte absorption in the nephron. Am. J. Physiol. 236:F163-174, 1979.
49. Knight, T. F.; Senekjian, H. O.; Sansom, S. C.; Weinman, E. J. Proximal tubule glucose efflux in the rat as a function of delivered load. Am. J. Physiol. 238:F499-F503, 1980.
50. Kinne, R.; Murer, H.; Kinne-Saffran, E.; Thees, M.; and Sachs, G. Sugar transport by renal plasma membrane vesicles: Characterization of the system in the brush border microvilli and basal lateral plasma membranes. J. Membr. Biol. 21:375-395, 1975.
51. Aronson, P. S.; and Sacktor, B. The Na^+ gradient-dependent transport of D-glucose in renal brush border membranes. J. Biol. Chem. 250:6032-6039, 1975.

52. Murer, H.; and Hopfer, U. Demonstration of electrogenic Na^+-dependent D-glucose transport in intestinal brush border membranes. Proc. Natl. Acad. Sci. 71:484-488, 1974.
53. Ullrich, K. J.; Rumrich, G.; and Klöss, S. Specificity and sodium dependence of the active sugar transport in the proximal convolution of the rat kidney. Pflügers Arch. 351:35-48, 1974.
54. Wen, S. F.; Boynar, J. W., Jr.; and Stoll, R. W. Effects of diuretics on renal glucose transport in the dog. Clin. Sci. Mol. Med. 54:481-488, 1978.
55. Wen, S. F. Micropuncture studies of glucose transport in the dog: Mechanism of renal glycosuria. Am. J. Physiol. 231:468-475, 1976.
56. Lassiter, W. E. Disorders of sodium metabolism. In: *Strauss and Welt's Diseases of the Kidney*, 3rd ed., edited by Earley, L. E., and Gottschalk, C. W., Boston, Little, Brown, 1979, pp. 1507-1541.
57. Gertz, K. H.; and Boylan, J. W. Glomerular-tubular balance. In: *Handbook of Physiology: Renal Physiology*, edited by Orloff, J., and Berliner, R. W., American Physiological Society, Washington, D.C., 1973, pp. 763-790.
58. Bartoli, E.; and Earley, L. E. Importance of utrafilterable plasma factors in maintaining tubular reabsorption. Kidney Int. 3:142-150, 1973.
59. Bartoli, E.; Conger, J. D.; and Earley, L. E. Effect of intraluminal flow on proximal tubular reabsorption. J. Clin. Invest. 52:843-849, 1973.
60. Kokko, J. P. Proximal tubule potential difference. Dependence on glucose, HCO_3^- and amino acids. J. Clin. Invest. 52:1362-1367, 1973.
61. Hilden, S. A.; and Sacktor, B. D-Glucose-dependent sodium transport in renal brush border membrane vesicles. J. Biol. Chem. 254:7090-7096, 1979.
62. Frömter, E.; and Luer, K. Electrical studies on sugar transport kinetics of rat proximal tubule. Pflügers Arch. 343:R47, 1973.
63. Burg, M. B.; Patlak, C. S.; Green, N.; and Villey, D. Organic solutes in fluid absorption by renal proximal convoluted tubules. Am. J. Physiol. 231:627-637, 1976.
64. Weinman, E. J.; Suki, W. N.; and Eknoyan, G. D-Glucose enhancement of water reabsorption in the proximal tubule of the rat kidney. Am. J. Physiol. 231:777-780, 1976.
65. Imai, M.; Seldin, D. W.; and Kokko, J. P. Effect of perfusion rate on the fluxes of water, sodium, chloride and urea across the proximal convoluted tubule. Kidney Int. 11:18-27, 1977.
66. Green, R.; and Giebisch, G. Ionic requirements of proximal tubular sodium transport. I. Bicarbonate and chloride. Am. J. Physiol. 229:1205-1215, 1975.
67. Bishop, J. H. V.; Green, R.; and Thomas, S. Effects of glucose on water and sodium reabsorption in the proximal convoluted tubule of the rat kidney. J. Physiol. 275:481-493, 1978.
68. Riggs, T. R.; Walker, L. M.; and Christensen, H. N. Potassium migration and amino acid transport. J. Biol. Chem. 233:1479-1484, 1958.
69. Murer, H.; Sigrist-Nelson, K.; and Hopfer, U. On the mechanism of sugar and amino acid interaction in intestinal transport. J. Biol. Chem. 250:7392-7396, 1975.
70. Sacktor, B.; and Beck, J. C. Na^+-Electrochemical potential-mediated transport of D-glucose in renal brush border membrane vesicles. Curr. Probl. Clin. Biochem. 8:159-169, 1977.
71. Robson, A. M.; Srivastava, P. L.; and Bricker, N. S. The influence of saline loading on renal glucose reabsorption in the rat. J. Clin. Invest. 47:329-335, 1968.
72. Wen, S. F.; and Stoll, R. W. Effect of volume expansion on renal glucose transport in normal and uremic dogs. Am. J. Physiol. 236:F567-F574, 1979.
73. Maruyama, T.; and Hoshi, T. The effect of D-glucose on the electrical potential profile across the proximal tubule of the newt kidney. Biochim. Biophys. Acta 282:214-225, 1972.

74. Ullrich, K. J.; Rumrich, G.; Klöss, S. Sodium dependence of the amino acid transport in the proximal convolution of the rat kidney. Pflugers Arch. 351:49-60, 1974.
75. Evers, J.; Murer, H.; and Kinne, R. Phenylalanine uptake in isolated renal brush border vesicles. Biochim. Biophys. Acta 426:598-615, 1976.
76. Hammerman, M. R.; and Sacktor, B. Transport of amino acids in renal brush-border membrane vesicles. Uptake of L-proline. J. Biol. Chem. 252:591-595, 1977.
77. Hoffman, N.; Thees, M.; and Kinne, R. Phosphate transport by isolated renal brush border vesicles. Pflügers Arch. 362:147-156, 1976.
78. Dennis, V. W.; and Brazy, P. C. Sodium, phosphate, glucose, bicarbonate, and alanine interactions in the isolated proximal tubule of the rabbit kidney. J. Clin. Invest. 62: 387-397, 1978.
79. Fass, S. J.; Hammerman, M. R.; and Sacktor, B. Transport of amino acids in renal brush border membrane vesicles. Uptake of the neutral amino acid L-alanine. J. Biol. Chem. 252:583-590, 1977.
80. Cohen, J. J.; Berglund, F.; and Lotspeich, W. D. Inter-relationship during renal tubular reabsorption in the dog among several anions showing a sensitivity to glucose and phlorizin. Am. J. Physiol. 189:331-338, 1957.
81. Pitts, R. F.; and Alexander, R. S. The renal reabsorption mechanism for inorganic phosphate in normal and acidotic dogs. Am. J. Physiol. 142:648-662, 1944.
82. Frasch, W.; Frohnert, P. P.; Bode, F.; Baumann, K.; and Kinne, R. Competitive inhibition of phlorhizin binding by D-glucose and the influence of sodium: A study on isolated brush border membrane of rat kidney. Pflügers Arch. 320:265-284, 1970.
83. Kleinzeller, A.; McAvoy, E. M.; and McKibbin, R. D. Active renal hexose transport. Structural requirements. Biochim. Biophys. Acta 600:513-529, 1980.
84. Crane, R. K. Intestinal absorption of sugars. Physiol. Rev. 40:789-825, 1960.
85. Knight, T.; Sansom, S.; and Weinman, E. J. Renal tubular absorption of D-glucose, 3-0-methyl-D-glucose, and 2-deoxy-D-glucose. Am. J. Physiol. 233:F274-F277, 1977.
86. Silverman, M.; Aganon, M.A.; and Chinard, F. P. D-Glucose interactions with renal tubule cell surfaces. Am. J. Physiol. 218-735-742, 1970.
87. Silverman, M. The chemical and steric determinants governing sugar interactions with renal tubular membranes. Biochim. Biophys. Acta 332:248-262, 1974.
88. Kleinzeller, A.; and McAvoy, E. M. Sugar transport across the peritubular face of renal cells of the flounder. J. Gen. Physiol. 62:169-184, 1973.
89. Loeschke, K.; Baumann, K.; Renschler, H.; and Ullrich, K. J. Differenzierung zwischen aktiver und passiver Komponente des D-Glucosetransports am proximalen Konvolut der Rattenniere. Pflügers Arch. 305:118-138, 1969.
90. von Baeyer, H.; von Conta, C.; Haeberle, D.; and Deetjen, P. Determination of transport constants for glucose in the proximal tubule of the rat kidney. Pflügers Arch. 343:273-286, 1973.
91. Barfuss, D. W.; and Schafer, J. A. Differences in active and passive glucose transport along the proximal nephron. Am. J. Physiol. 241:F322-F332, 1981.
92. Warnock, D. G.; Patlak, C. S.; and Burg, M. B. Contribution of leaked load to solute transport by renal tubules. Am. J. Physiol. 234:F480-F484, 1978.
93. Maesaka, J. K.; and McCaffery, M. Evidence for renal tubular leakage in maleic acid-induced Fanconi syndrome. Am. J. Physiol. 239:F507-F513, 1980.
94. Lorentz, W. B.; Jr.; Lassiter, W. E.; and Gottschalk, C. W. Renal tubular permeability during increased intrarenal pressure. J. Clin. Invest. 51:484-492, 1972.
95. Bergeron, M.; Dubord, L.; and Hausser, C. Membrane permeability as a cause of transport defects in experimental Fanconi syndrome. A new hypothesis. J. Clin. Invest. 57: 1181-1189, 1976.
96. Barfuss, D. W.; Mays, J. M.; and Schafer, J. A. Peritubular uptake and transepithelial transport of glycine in isolated proximal tubules. Am. J. Physiol. 238:F324-F333, 1980.

97. Cohen, J. J.; and Kamm, D. E. Renal metabolism: Relation to renal function. In: The Kidney, edited by Brenner, B. M., and Rector, F. C. Jr. Philadelphia, Saunders, 1981, pp. 144-248.
98. Dies, F.; Herrera, J.; Matos, M.; Avelar, E.; and Ramos, G. Substrate uptake by dog kidney in vivo. Am. J. Physiol. 218:405-410, 1970.
99. Chinard, F. P.; Taylor, W. R.; Nolan, M. F.; and Enns, T. Renal handling of glucose in dogs. Am. J. Physiol. 196:535-544, 1959.
100. Bollman, J. L.; and Grindlay, J. H. Measurements of renal gluconeogenesis. Am. J. Physiol. 170:38-44, 1952.
101. Bowman, R. H. Gluconeogenesis in the isolated perfused rat kidney. J. Biol. Chem. 245:1604-1612, 1970.
102. Costello, J.; Scott, J. M.; Wilson, P.; and Bourke, E. Glucose utilization and production by the dog kidney in vivo in metabolic acidosis and alkalosis. J. Clin. Invest. 52: 608-611, 1973.
103. Gregg, C. M.; Cohen, J. J.; Black, A. J.; Espeland, M. A.; and Feldstein, M. L. Effects of glucose and insulin on metabolism and function of the perfused rat kidney. Am. J. Physiol. 235:F52-F-61, 1978.
104. Reinecke, R. M. The kidney as a source of glucose in the eviscerated rat. Am. J. Physiol. 140:276-285, 1943.
105. Aber, G. M.; Morris, L. O.; and Housley, E. Gluconeogenesis by the human kidney. Nature 212:1589-1590, 1966.
106. Owen, O. E.; Felig, P.; Morgan, A. P.; Wahren, J.; and Cahill, G. F., Jr. Liver and kidney metabolism during prolonged starvation. J. Clin. Invest. 48:574-583, 1969.
107. Kida, K.; Nakajo, S.; Kamiya, F.; Toyama, Y.; Nishio, T.; and Nakagawa, H. Renal net glucose release in vivo and its contribution to blood glucose in rats. J. Clin. Invest. 62:721-726, 1978.
108. Dawson, A. G. Contribution of pH-sensitive metabolic processes to pH homeostasis in isolated rat kidney tubules. Biochim. Biophys. Acta 499:85-98, 1977.
109. Kamm, D. E.; and Cahill, G. F., Jr. Effects of acid-base status on renal and hepatic gluconeogenesis in diabetes and fasting. Am. J. Physiol. 216:1207-1212, 1969.
110. Alleyne, G. A. O.; and Scullard, G. H. Renal metabolic response to acid-base changes. I. Enzymatic control of ammoniagenesis in the rat. J. Clin. Invest. 48:364-370, 1969.
111. Iynedjian, P. B.; Ballard, F. J.; and Hanson, R. W. The regulation of phosphoenolpyruvate carboxykinase (GTP) synthesis in rat kidney cortex. The role of acid-base balance and glucocorticoids. J. Biol. Chem. 250:5596-5603, 1975.
112. Kamm, D. E.; and Strope, G. L. Renal cortical and hepatic phosphoenolpyruvate carboxykinase in the diabetic rat. Effect of acid-base status. Metabolism 23:1073-1079, 1974.
113. Taggart, J. V. Mechanisms of renal tubular transport. Am. J. Med. 24:774-784, 1958.
114. Pitts, R. F. Tubular reabsorption. In: Physiology of the Kidney and Body Fluids, 3rd ed., Chicago, Year Book, 1974, pp. 71-98.
115. Mudge, G. H., and Taggart, J. V. Effect of 2,4-dinitrophenol on renal transport mechanisms in the dog. Am. J. Physiol. 161:173-180, 1950.
116. Kritzler, R. A.; and Gutman, A. B. Alkaline phosphatase activity of the proximal convoluted tubules and the mechanism of phlorizin glycosuria. Am. J. Physiol. 134:94-101, 1941.
117. Lotspeich, W. D.; and Keller, D. M. A study of some effects of phlorizin on the metabolism of kidney tissue in vitro. J. Biol. Chem. 222:843-853, 1956.
118. Dratz, A. F.; and Handler, P. Renal phosphate and carbohydrate metabolism studied with the aid of radiophosphorus. J. Biol. Chem. 197:419-431, 1952.
119. Cori, G. T. Glycogen structure and enzyme deficiencies in glycogen storage disease. Harvey Lect. 48:145-171, 1954.
120. Ross, B. D.; Epstein, F. H.; and Leak, A. Sodium reabsorption in the perfused rat kidney. Am. J. Physiol. 225:1165-1171, 1973.

121. Cohen, J. J.; and Barac-Nieto, M. Renal metabolism of substrates in relation to renal function. In: *Handbook of Physiology*: *Renal Physiology*, edited by Orloff, J.; and Berliner, R. W., Washington, D. C., American Physiological Society, 1973, pp. 909-927.
122. Knox, F. G.; Fleming, J. S.; and Rennie, D. W. Effect of osmotic diuresis on sodium reabsorption and oxygen consumption of the kidney. Am. J. Physiol. 210:751-759, 1966.
123. Pitts, R. F.; and Stone, W. J. Renal metabolism of alanine. J. Clin. Invest. 46:530-538, 1967.
124. Randall, H. M., Jr.; and Cohen, J. J. Anaerobic CO_2 production by dog kidney in vitro. Am. J. Physiol. 211:493-505, 1966.
125. Garza-Quintero, B.; Cohen, J. J.; Brand, P. H.; and Kook, Y. J. Steady-state glucose oxidation by dog kidney in vivo: Relation to Na^+ reabsorption. Am. J. Physiol. 228: 549-555, 1975.
126. Walker, A. M.; and Hudson, C. L. The reabsorption of glucose from the renal tubules in amphibia and the action of phlorizin upon it. Am. J. Physiol. 188:130-143, 1937.
127. Walker, A. M.; Bott, P. A.; Oliver, J.; and MacDowell, M. C. The collection and analysis of fluid from single nephrons of the mammalian kidney. Am. J. Physiol. 134: 580-595, 1941.
128. Rohde, R.; and Deetjen, P. Die Glucoseresorption in der Rattenniere. Mikropunktionsanalysen der tubulären Glucosekonzentration bei freiem Fluss. Pflügers Arch. 302: 219-232, 1968.
129. Frohnert, P. P.; Höhmann, B.; Zwiebel, R.; and Baumann, K. Free-flow micropuncture studies of glucose transport in the rat nephron. Pflügers Arch. 315:66-85, 1970.
130. Bishop, J. H. V.; Green, R.; and Thomas, S. Free-flow reabsorption of glucose, sodium, osmoles and water in the rat proximal convoluted tubule. J. Physiol. 288: 331-351, 1979.
131. Wen, S. F. Effect of phlorhizin on renal glucose and phosphate transport in the dog. Clin. Sci. 57:367-374, 1979.
132. McKeown, J. W.; Brazy, P. C.; and Dennis, V. W. Intrarenal heterogeneity for fluid, phosphate, and glucose absorption in the rabbit. Am. J. Physiol. 237:F312-F318, 1979.
133. von Baeyer, H. Glucose transport in the short loop of Henle of the rat kidney. Pflügers Arch. 359:317-323, 1975.
134. McSherry, N. R.; and Wen, S. F. Segmental analysis of renal glucose transport in young female rats. J. Physiol. 356:9-19, 1984.
135. Davison, J. M.; and Cheyne, G. A. Renal reabsorption of glucose. Lancet 1:787-788, 1972.
136. Keller, D. M. Glucose excretion in man and dog. Nephron 5:43-66, 1968.
137. Fine, J. Glucose content of normal urine. Br. Med. J. 1:1209-1214, 1965.
138. Froesch, E. R.; and Renold, A. E. Specific enzymatic determination of glucose in blood and urine using glucose oxidase. Diabetes 5:1-6, 1956.
139. Schubert, G. E.; Schuster, H. P.; and Baum, P. Physiologische Glucosurie bei verschiedenen Diuresezuständen. Klin. Wochenschr. 42:619-622, 1964.
140. Soler, N. G.; and Malins, J. M. Prevalence of glucosuria in normal pregnancy. A. quantitative study. Lancet 1:619-621, 1971.
141. Lind, T.; and Hytten, F. E. The excretion of glucose during normal pregnancy. J. Obstet. Gynaecol. Br. Common. 79:961-965, 1972.
142. Smith, H. W. Clearances involving active tubular reabsorption. In: The Kidney. New York, Oxford University Press, 1951, pp. 81-142.
143. Elsas, L. J., II; Rosenberg, L. E. Renal glycosuria. In: Strauss and Welt's Disease of the Kidney, 3rd ed., edited by Earley, L. E., and Gottschalk, C. W., Boston, Little, Brown, 1979, pp. 1021-1028.

144. Nelson, A. R.; Perkoff, G. T.; and Tyler, F. H. Renal glucosuria in pre-existing diabetes. Arch. Intern. Med. 113:649-654, 1964.
145. Robertson, J. A.; and Gray, C. H. Mechanism of lowered renal threshold for glucose in diabetes. Lancet 2:12-15, 1953.
146. Grant, J. L. Elevated glucose threshold in Kimmelstiel-Wilson syndrome. N. Engl. J. Med. 251:302-304, 1954.
147. Freidenberg, G. R.; Kosnik, E. J.; and Sotos, J. F. Hyperglycemic coma after suprasellar surgery. N. Engl. J. Med. 303:863-865, 1980.
148. Andreoli, T. E.; and Schafer, J. A. Nephrogenic diabetes insipidus. In: *The Metabolic Basis of Inherited Disease*, 4th ed., edited by Stanbury, J. B., Wyngaarden, J. B., and Fredrickson, D. S. New York, McGraw-Hill, 1978, pp. 1634-1659.
149. Marble, A. Nondiabetic melituria. In: *Joslin's Diabetes Mellitus*, 11th ed. edited by Marble, A., White, P., Bradley, R. F., and Krall, L. P. Philadelphia, Lea & Febiger, 1971, pp. 818-829.
150. Klemperer, G. Über regulatorische Glykosurie und renalen Diabetes. Berl. Klin. Wochenschr. 33:571, 1896.
151. Bönninger, M. Beitrag zur Frage des Nierendiabetes. Dtsch. Med. Wochenschr. 34: 780-783, 1908.
152. Salomon, H. Über den Diabetes innocens der Jugendlichen, zugleich ein Beitrag zur Frage des renalen Diabetes. Dtsch. Med. Wochenschr. 40:217-221, 1914.
153. Rosenfeld, D. Über Diabetes innocuus. Berl. Klin. Wochenschr. 53:1093, 1916.
154. Hjärne, U. A study of orthoglycaemic glycosuria with particular reference to its hereditability. Acta Med. Scand. 67:422-571, 1927.
155. Goto, K. Alimentary renal glycosuria. Arch. Intern. Med. 22:96-113, 1918.
156. Umber, F.; and Rosenberg, M. Zur Diagnose und Prognose der Glycosuria innocens. Z. Klin. Med. 100:655-674, 1924.
157. Holst, J. E. The occurrence of benign glycosuria in diabetes mellitus. Arch. Int. Med. 38:279-291, 1926.
158. Lawrence, R. D. Symptomless glycosurias: Differentiation by sugar tolerance test. Med. Clin. North Am. 31:289-297, 1947.
159. Drucker, W. D.; Fitch, R. F.; and Gaston, J. H. Diabetes mellitus and pre-existing renal glycosuria. Arch. Intern. Med. 110:199-204, 1962.
160. Horowitz, L.; and Schwarzer, S. Renal glycosuria: Occurrence in two siblings and a review of the literature. J. Pediatr. 47:634-639, 1955.
161. Marble, A.; Joslin, E. P.; Dublin, L. I.; and Marks, H. H. Studies in diabetes mellitus. VII. Non-diabetic glycosuria. Am. J. Med. Sci. 197:533-556, 1939.
162. Khachadurian, A. K.; and Khachadurian, L. A. The inheritance of renal glycosuria. Am. J. Hum. Genet. 16:189-194, 1964.
163. Reubi, F. C. Glucose titration in renal glycosuria. In: *Ciba Foundation Symposium on the Kidney*. Boston, Little, Brown, 1954.
164. Bradley, S. E.; Bradley, G. P.; Tyson, C. J.; Curry, J. J.; and Blake, W. C. Renal function in renal diseases. Am. J. Med. 9:766-798, 1950.
165. Woolf, L. I.; Goodwin, B. L.; and Phelps, C. E. Tm-Limited renal tubular reabsorption and the genetics of renal glycosuria. J. Theoret. Biol. 11:10-21, 1966.
166. Taggart, J. V. Combined clinics on disorders of renal tubular function. Am. J. Med. 20:448-461, 1956.
167. Krane, S. M. Renal glycosuria. In: The Metabolic Basis of Inherited Disease, 4th ed., edited by Stanbury, J. B., Wyngaarden, J. B., and Fredrickson, D. S. New York, McGraw-Hill, 1978, pp. 1607-1617.
168. Froesch, E. R.; Winegrad, A. I.; and Renold, A. E. Die tubuläre Nierenfunction bei verscheidenen Formen des renalen Diabetes Mellitus. Helv. Med. Acta 24:548-555. 1957.
169. Reubi, F. C.; and Wüthrich, F. Glycosurie rénale massive consécutive a l'ingestion de ferricyanure de potassium. Acta Clin. Belg. 10:198-208, 1955.

170. Reubi, F. C. Tubular syndromes. In: Clearance Tests in Clinical Medicine, Springfield, Illinois, Charles C Thomas, 1963, pp. 157-173.
171. Seely, J. F.; and Dirks, J. H. Micropuncture study of hypertonic mannitol diuresis in the proximal and distal tubule of the dog kidney. J. Clin. Invest. 48:2330-2340, 1969.
172. DeFronzo, R. A., Goldberg, M., and Agus, Z. S. The effects of glucose and insulin on renal electrolyte transport. J. Clin. Invest. 58:89-90, 1976.
173. Wen, S. F.; Boynar, J. W., Jr.; and Stoll, R. W. Mechanism of glycosuria during volume expansion superimposed on subthreshold glucose loading. J. Lab. Clin. Med. 101:708-716, 1983.
174. Wen, S. F.; and McSherry, N. R. Renal glucose transport during endogenous hyperglycemia. Internatl. Congr. Nephrol. (Abstracts) 8:39, 1981.
175. Chaptal, J.; Benezech, C.; Jean, R.; Campo, C.; and Dejeanne, M. G. Etude sur le diabete renal chez l'enfant: Exploration biologique de deux cas; Discussion nosologique. Arch. Fr. Pediatr. 11:273-280, 1954.
176. Liu, H. Y.; Anderson, G. J.; Tsao, M. U.; Moore, B. F.; and Giday, Z. Tm glucose in a case of congenital intestinal and renal malabsorption of monosaccharides. Pediatr. Res. 1:386-394, 1967.
177. Berliner, R. W.; Kennedy, T. J.; and Hilton, J. G. Effect of maleic acid on renal function. Proc. Soc. Exp. Biol. Med. 75:791-794, 1950.
178. Harrison, H. H.; and Harrison, H. C. Experimental production of renal glycosuria, phosphaturia and aminoaciduria by injection of maleic acid. Science 120:606-608, 1954.
179. Angielski, S.; and Rougulski, J. Effect of maleic acid on the kidney. I. Oxidation of Krebs cycle intermediates by various tissues of maleate-intoxicated rats. Acta Biochim. Pol. 9:357-365, 1962.
180. Kramer, H. J.; and Gonick, H. C. Experimental Fanconi syndrome. I. Effect of maleic acid on renal cortical Na-K-ATPase activity and ATP levels. J. Lab. Clin. Med. 76: 799-808, 1970.
181. Kramer, H. J.; and Gonick, H. C. Effect of maleic acid on sodium-linked tubular transport in experimental Fanconi syndrome. Nephron 10:306-319, 1973.
182. Crombie, D. L. Incidence of glycosuria and diabetes. Proc. R. Soc. Med. 55:205-207, 1961.
183. Harkness, J. Prevalence of glycosuria and diabetes mellitus. A comprehensive survey in an urban community. Br. Med. J. 1:1503-1507, 1962.
184. Brown, M. S.; and Polshuck, R. Familial renal glycosuria, J. Lab. Clin. Med. 20:605-608, 1935.
185. Fischer, A. F. Intermittent and continuous renal glycosuria. Am. J. Dis. Child. 50: 166-177, 1935.
186. Babson, S. G. Renal glycosuria. A hereditary and clinical study of one family. J. Pediatr. 17:781-790, 1940.
187. Parkes-Weber, F. A glycosuric family without hyperglycemia. Lancet 2:71-72, 1931.
188. Elsas, L. J.; Busse, D.; and Rosenberg, L. E. Autosomal recessive inheritance of renal glycosuria. Metabolism 20:968-975, 1971.
189. Scriver, C. R.; Chesney, R. W.; and McInnes, R. R. Genetic aspects of renal tubular transport: Diversity and topology of carriers. Kidney Int. 9:149-171, 1976.
190. Grote, L. R.; and Heilmann, P. Ein anatomischer Befund bei renalen Diabetes. Zentralbl. Allg. Pathol. 64:65-70, 1935.
191. Monasterio, G. Histologischer und physio-pathologischer Beitrag zur Pathogenese des Diabetes Renalis. Klin. Wochenschr. 18:538-541, 1939.
192. Monasterio, G.; Muiesan, G.; Pardelli, G.; Marinozzi, V.; and Bosman, C. Diabetes renale o tubulodisplasia glicosurica. Minerva Nefrol. 10:42-66, 1963.
193. Monasterio, G.; Oliver, J.; Muiesan, G.; Pardelli, G.; Marinozzi, V.; and MacDowell, M. Renal diabetes as a congenital tubular dysplasia. Am. J. Med. 37:44-61, 1964.

194. Leonardi, P.; Ruol, A.; and Munari, R. Morphological aspects of renal glycosuria. Am. J. Med. Sci. 239:721-727, 1960.
195. Freeman, J. A.; and Roberts, K. E. A fine structural study of renal glycosuria. Exp. Mol. Pathol. 2:83-92, 1963.
196. Reubi, F. Nierenkrankheiten. Bern and Stuttgart, Hans Huber, 1961.
197. Meeuwisse, G. W.; and Dahlquist, A. Glucose-galactose malabsorption: A study with biopsy of the small intestinal mucosa. Acta Paediatr. Scand. 57:273-280, 1968.
198. Anderson, J.; and Mazza, R. Pyruvate and lactate excretion in patients with diabetes mellitus and benign glycosuria. Lancet 2:270-272, 1963.
199. Ackerman, I. P.; Fajans, S. S.; and Conn, J. W. The development of diabetes mellitus in patients with non-diabetic glycosuria. Clin. Res. 6:251, 1958.
200. Lindquist, B.; and Meeuwisse, G. W. Chronic diarrhea caused by monosaccharide malabsorption. Acta Paediatr. Scand. 51:674-685, 1962.
201. Lindquist, B.; Meeuwisse, G. W.; and Melin, K. Glucose-galactose malabsorption. Lancet 2:666, 1962.
202. Laplane, R.; Polonovski, C.; Etienne, M.; Debray, P.; Lods, J.-C.; and Pissarro, B. L'intolérance aux sucres a transfert intestinal actif: Ses rapports avec l'intolérance au lactose et le syndrome coeliaque. Arch. Fr. Pediatr. 19:895-944, 1962.
203. Gray, G. M. Intestinal disaccharidase deficiency and glucose-galactose malabsorption. In: The Metabolic Basis of Inherited Disease, 4th ed., edited by Stanbury, J. B., Wyngaarden, J. B. and Fredrickson, D. S. New York, McGraw-Hill, 1978, pp. 1526-1536.
204. Schneider, A. J.; Kinter, W. B.; and Stirling, C. E. Glucose-galactose malabsorption. Report of a case with autoradiographic studies of a mucosal biopsy. N. Engl. J. Med. 274:305-312, 1966.
205. Elsas, L. J.; Hillman, R. E.; Patterson, J. H.; and Rosenberg, L. E. Renal and intestinal hexose transport in familial glucose-galactose malabsorption. J. Clin. Invest. 49:576-585, 1970.
206. Meeuwisse, G. W.; and Melin, K. Glucose-galactose malabsorption. A clinical study of 6 cases. Acta Paediatr. Scand. (Suppl.) 188:3-18, 1969.
207. Phillips, S. F.; and McGill, D. S. Glucose-galactose malabsorption in an adult: Perfusion studies of sugar, electrolyte, and water transport. Am. J. Digest. Dis. 18:1017-1014, 1973.
208. Hughes, W. S.; Senior, J. R. The glucose-galactose malabsorption syndrome in a 23-year-old woman. Gastroenterology 68:142-145, 1975.
209. Melin, K.; and Meeuwisse, G. W. Glucose-galactose malabsorption. A genetic study. Acta Paediatr. Scand. (Suppl.) 188:19-24, 1969.
210. Meeuwisse, G. W. Glucose-galactose malabsorption: Studies on renal glycosuria. Helv. Paediatr. Acta 25:13-24, 1970.
211. Eggermont, E.; and Loeb, H. Glucose-galactose malabsorption. Lancet 2:343-344, 1966.
212. Abraham, J. M.; Levin, B.; Oberholzer, V. G.; and Russell, A. Glucose-galactose malabsorption. Arch. Dis. Child. 42:592-597, 1967.
213. Rosenberg, L. E.; Downing, S.; Durant, J.; and Segal, S. Cystinuria: Biochemical evidence for three genetically distinct diseases. J. Clin. Invest. 45:365-371, 1966.
214. Jepson, J. Hartnup disease. In: The Metabolic Basis of Inherited Disease, 4th ed., edited by Stanbury, J. B., Wyngaarden, J. B., and Fredrickson, D. S. New York, McGraw-Hill, 1978, pp. 1563-1577.
215. Morikawa, T.; Tada, K.; Ando, T.; Yoshida, T.; Yokoyama, Y.; and Arakawa, T. Prolinuria: Defect in intestinal absorption of imino acids and glycine. Tohoku J. Exp. Med. 90:105-116, 1966.
216. Meeuwisse, G. W.; and Lindquist, B. Glucose-galactose malabsorption. Studies on the intermediate carbohydrate metabolism. Acta Paediatr. Scand. 59:74-79, 1970.
217. Meeuwisse, G. W. Glucose-galactose malabsorption. A study on the transfer of glucose across the red cell membrane. Scand. J. Clin. Lab. Invest. 25:145-149, 1970.

218. de Toni, G. Remarks on the relations between renal rickets (renal dwarfism) and renal diabetes. Acta Paediatr. 16:479-484, 1933.
219. Bickel, H.; and Hickmans, E. M. Part 7: Some biochemical aspects of Lignac-Fanconi disease. Acta Paediatr. (Suppl.) 90:137-170, 1952.
220. Debré, R.; Marie, J.; Cléret, F.; and Messimy, R. Rachitisme tardif coexistant avec une néphrite chronique et une glycosurie. Arch. Med. Enf. 37:597-606, 1934.
221. Fanconi, G.; and Bickel, H. Die chronische Aminoacidurie (Aminosäurendiabetes oder nephrotischglukosurischer Zwergwuchs) bei der Glykogenose und der Cystinkrankheit. Helv. Paediatr. Acta 4:359-396, 1949.
222. Brodehl, J. The Fanconi syndrome. In: Pediatric Kidney Disease, edited by Edelmann, C. M. Jr. Boston, Little, Brown, 1978, pp. 955-987.
223. Bradley, S. E. Disorders of renal tubular function. Am. J. Med. 20:457-461, 1956.
224. Bauer, B. Debré-De-Toni-Fanconi-Syndrom mit Glykogenose der Leber. Klin. Wochenschr. 46:317-328, 1968.
225. Reem, G. H.; Isaacs, M.; and Vanamee, P. Renal transport of urate, phosphate and glucose in Fanconi syndrome. J. Clin. Endocrinol. Metab. 27:1141-1150, 1967.
226. Howell, R. R. The glycogen storage disease. In: The Metabolic Basis of Inherited Disease, 4th ed., edited by Stanbury, J. B., Wyngaarden, J. B., and Fredrickson, D. S. New York, McGraw-Hill, 1978, pp. 137-159.
227. Moses, S. W.; and Gutman, A. Inborn errors of glycogen metabolism. Adv. Pediatr. 19:95-169, 1972.
228. Fellers, F. X.; Piedrahita, V.; and Galan, E. M. Pseudo-phlorhizin diabetes (abstract). Pediatr. Res. 1:304, 1967.
229. Garty, R.; Cooper, M.; and Tabachnik, E. The Fanconi syndrome associated with hepatic glycogenosis and abnormal metabolism of galactose. J. Pediatr. 85:821-823, 1974.
230. Lambert, F.; and Mayer, H. Glykogenose der Leber mit Galaktoseverwertungsstörung und schwerem Fanconi-Syndrom. Z. Kinderheilkd. 98:133-145, 1967.
231. Odievre, M. Glycogénose hepato-rénale avec tubulopathie complex. Rev. Int. Hepatol. 26:1-70, 1966.
232. Rotthauwe, H. W.; Fichsel, H.; Heldt, H. W.; Kirten, E.; Reim, M.; Schmidt, E.; and Wesemann, W. Glykogenose der Leber mit Aminoacidurie und Glukosurie. Klin. Wochenschr. 41:818-825, 1963.
233. Halvorsen, S.; and Aas, K. Renal tubular defects in fibrous dysplasia of the bones: Reports of two cases. Acta Paediatr. Scand. 50:297-303, 1961.
234. Luder, J.; and Sheldon, W. Familial tubular absorption defect of glucose and amino acids. Arch. Dis. Child. 30:160-164, 1955.
235. Käser, H.; Cottier, P.; and Antener, I. Glucoglycinuria, a new familial syndrome. J. Pediatr. 61:386-394, 1962.
236. Käser, H.; Cottier, P.; and Antener, I. Die Glukoglycinurie, ein neues familiäre Syndrom. Helv. Paediatr. Acta 16:586-608, 1961.
237. DeVries, A.; Kochwa, S.; Lazebnik, J.; Frank, M.; and Djaldetti, M. Glycinuria, a hereditary disorder associated with nephrolithiasis. Am. J. Med. 23:408-415, 1957.
238. Greene, M. L.; Lietman, P. S.; Rosenberg, L. E.; and Seegmiller, J. E. Familial hyperglycinuria: New defect in renal tubular transport of glycine and imino acids. Am. J. Med. 54:265-271, 1973.
239. Joseph, R.; Ribierre, M.; Job, J. C.; and Girault, M. Maladie familiale associante des convulsions a début tres précoce une hyperalbuminoarchie et une hyperaminoacidurie. Arch. Fr. Pediatr. 15:374-387, 1958.
240. Brodehl, J. Renal hyperaminoaciduria. In: Pediatric Kidney Disease, edited by Edelmann, C. M. Boston, Little, Brown, 1978, pp. 1047-1079.
241. Dent, C. E. Rickets and osteomalacia from renal tubule defects. J. Bone Joint Surg. 34B:266-274, 1952.

242. Magid, G. J.; Maloney, J. R.; Sirota, J. H.; and Schwab, E. A. Familial hypophosphatemia: Studies on its pathogenesis in an affected mother and son. Ann. Intern. Med. 64:1009-1027, 1966.
243. Cook, W. T.; Barelay, J. A.; Govan, A. D. T.; and Nagley, L. Osteoporosis associated with low serum phosphorus and renal glycosuria. Arch. Intern. Med. 80:147-164, 1947.
244. Milkman, L. A. Multiple spontaneous idiopathic symmetrical fractures. Am. J. Roentgenol. 32:622-634, 1934.
245. Hunter, D. Studies in calcium and phosphorus metabolism in generalized disease of bones. Proc. R. Soc. Med. 28:1619-1644, 1935.
246. Burnett, C. H.; Dent, C. E.; Harper, C.; and Warland, B. J. Vitamin D-resistant rickets: Analysis of twenty-four pedigrees with hereditary and sporadic cases. Am. J. Med. 36:222-232, 1964.
247. Scriver, C. R.; Goldbloom, R. B.; and Roy, C. Hypophosphatemic rickets with renal hyperglycinuria, renal glycosuria and glycylprolinuria. Pediatrics 34:357-371, 1964.
248. Blot, H. De la glycosurie physiologique chez les femmes en couches, les nourrices et un certain nombre de femmes enceintes. Gaz. Hop. Civils Milit. 29:482-484, 1856.
249. Chen, W. W.; Sese, L.; Tantakasen, P.; and Tricomi, V. Pregnancy associated with renal glucosuria. Obstet. Gynecol. 47:37-40, 1976.
250. Fine, J. Glycosuria of pregnancy. Br. Med. J. 1:205-210, 1967.
251. Davison, J. M. Changes in renal function and other aspects of homeostasis in early pregnancy (abstract). J. Obstet. Gynaecol. Br. Common. 81:1003, 1974.
252. Davison, J. M.; and Dunlop, W. Renal hemodynamics and tubular function in normal human pregnancy. Kidney Int. 18:152-161, 1980.
253. Davison, J. M.; and Hytten, F. E. The effects of pregnancy on the renal handling of glucose. Br. J. Obstet. Gynaecol. 82:374-381, 1975.
254. Sims, E. A. H.; and Krantz, K. E. Serial studies of renal function during pregnancy and the puerperium in normal women. J. Clin. Invest. 37:1764-1774, 1958.
255. Davison, J. M.; and Hytten, F. E. Glomerular filtration during and after pregnancy. J. Obstet. Gynaecol. Br. Common. 81:588-595, 1974.
256. Christensen, P. J. Tubular reabsorption of glucose during pregnancy. Scand. J. Clin. Lab. Invest. 10:364-373, 1958.
257. Welsh, G. W.; and Sims, E. A. H. The mechanism of renal glycosuria in pregnancy. Diabetes 9:363-369, 1960.
258. Drexel, H.; and Sailer, S. Kinetics of glucose handling in renal glycosuria during pregnancy. Klin. Wochenschr. 58:1299-1306, 1980.
259. Alexander, E. A.; Churchill, S.; Bengele, H. H. Renal hemodynamics and volume homeostasis during pregnancy. Kidney Int. 18:173-178, 1980.
260. Semple, P. F.; Carswell, W.; and Boyle, J. A. Serial studies of the renal clearance of urate and inulin during pregnancy and after the puerperium in normal women. Clin. Sci. Mol. Med. 47:559-565, 1974.
261. Hytten, F. E.; and Cheyne, G. A. The aminoaciduria of pregnancy. J. Obstet. Gynaecol. Br. Common. 79:424-432, 1972.
262. Lewy, J. E.; and Windhager, E. E. Peritubular control of proximal tubular fluid reabsorption in the kidney. Am. J. Physiol. 214:943-954, 1968.
263. Davison, J. M.; and Lindheimer, M. D. Changes in renal haemodynamics and kidney weight during pregnancy in the unanesthetized rat. J. Physiol. 301:129-136, 1979.
264. Baylis, C. The mechanism of the increase in the glomerular filtration rate in the twelve-day pregnant rat. J. Physiol. 305:405-414, 1980.
265. Lindheimer, M. O.; and Katz, A. I. The renal response to pregnancy. In: The Kidney, 2nd ed., edited by Brenner, B. M., and Rector, F. C. Jr. Philadelphia, Saunders, 1981, pp. 1762-1815.
266. Bishop, J. H. V.; and Green, R. Effects of pregnancy on glucose reabsorption by the proximal convoluted tubule in the rat. J. Physiol. 319:271-285, 1981.

267. Bishop, J. H. V.; and Green, R. Glucose handling by distal portions of the nephron during pregnancy in the rat. J. Physiol. 336:131-142, 1983.
268. Carpenter, C. W. Urinary estrogen excretion in the puerperium. Am. J. Obster. Gynecol. 99:303-307, 1967.
269. Bricker, N. S.; Klahr, S.; Lubowitz, H.; and Rieselbach, R. E. Renal function in chronic renal disease. Medicine 44:263-288, 1965.
270. Wen, S. F.; Wong, N. L. M.; Evanson, R. L.; Lockhart, E. A.; and Dirks, J. H. Micropuncture studies of sodium transport in the remnant kidney of the dog. The effect of graded volume expansion. J. Clin. Invest. 52:386-397, 1973.
271. Bricker, N. S. The control of sodium excretion with normal and reduced nephron population. The pre-eminence of third factor. Am. J. Med. 43:313-321, 1967.
272. Rieselbach, R. E.; Shankel, S. W.; Slatopolsky, E.; Lubowitz, H.; and Bricker, N. S. Glucose titration studies in patients with chronic progressive renal disease. J. Clin. Invest. 46:157-163, 1967.
273. Rocha, A.; Marcondes, M.; and Malnic, G. Micropuncture study in rats with experimental glomerulonephritis. Kidney Int. 3:14-23, 1973.
274. Shankel, S. W.; Robson, A. M.; and Bricker, N. S. On the mechanism of splay in the glucose titration curve in advanced experimental renal disease in the rat. J. Clin. Invest. 46:164-172, 1967.
275. Schmidt, R. W.; and Danovitch, G. M. Glucose reabsorption in experimental renal insufficiency: Effects of proportional reduction of sodium intake. Kidney Int. 16:590-599, 1979.
276. DeFronzo, R. A.; Andres, R.; Edgar, P.; and Walker, W. G. Carbohydrate metabolism in uremia: A review. Medicine 52:468-481, 1973.
277. Lambert, P. P. A study of the mechanism by which toxic tubular damage changes the renal threshold. In: Ciba Foundation Symposium on the Kidney. Boston, Little, Brown, 1954.
278. Robertson, J. A.; and Gray, C. H. Renal function tests in renal glycosuria including observations during pregnancy. Lancet 2:15-16, 1953.
279. Stanbury, S. W.; and Macauley, D. Defects of renal tubular function in the nephrotic syndrome. Q. J. Med. 26:7-30, 1957.
280. Stickler, G. B.; Hayles, A. B.; Power, M. H.; and Ulrich, J. A. Renal tubular dysfunction complicating the nephrotic syndrome. Pediatrics 26:75-85, 1960.
281. Stickler, G. B.; Rosevear, J. W.; and Ulrich, J. A. Renal tubular dysfunction complicating the nephrotic syndrome: The disturbance in calcium and phosphorus metabolism. Proc. Mayo Clin. 37:376-388, 1962.
282. Bouissou, F.; Barthe, Ph.; and Pierragi, M. Th. Severe idiopathic nephrotic syndrome with tubular dysfunction (report of nine pediatric cases). Clin. Nephrol. 14:135-141, 1980.
283. McVicar, M.; Exeni, R.; and Susin, M. Nephrotic syndrome and multiple tubular defects in children: An early sign of focal segmental glomerulosclerosis. J. Pediatr. 97: 918-922, 1980.
284. Woolf, L. I.; and Giles, H. McC. Urinary excretion of amino acids and sugar in the nephrotic syndrome. Acta Paediatr. 45:489-500, 1956.
285. Maunsbach, A. B. Albumin absorption by renal proximal tubule cells. Nature 212: 546-547, 1966.
286. Strauss, W. Cytochemical observations on the relationship between lysosomes and phagosomes in kidney and liver by combined staining for acid phosphatase and intravenously injected horseradish peroxidase. J. Cell Biol. 20:497-507, 1964.
287. Grausz, H.; Lieberman, R.; and Earley, L. E. Effect of plasma albumin on sodium reabsorption in patients with nephrotic syndrome. Kidney Int. 1:47-54, 1972.
288. Bernard, D. B.; Alexander, E. A.; Couser, W. G.; and Levinsky, N. G. Renal sodium retention during volume expansion in experimental nephrotic syndrome. Kidney Int. 14:478-485, 1978.

289. Kawamura, J.; Mazumdar, D. C.; and Lubowitz, H. Effect of albumin infusion on renal glucose reabsorption in the rat. Am. J. Physiol. 232:F286-F290, 1977.
290. Usberti, M.; Federico, S.; Cianciaruso, B.; Costanzo, R.; Russo, D.; and Andreucci, V. E. Relationship between serum albumin concentration and tubular reabsorption of glucose in renal disease. Kidney Int. 18:546-551, 1979.
291. Kramp, R. A.; and Lorentz, W. B. Glucose transport in chronically altered rat nephrons. Am. J. Physiol. 243:F393-F403, 1982.
292. Boonjarern, S.; Mehta, P. K.; Laski, M. E.; Earnest, W. R.; and Kurtzman, N. A. Effect of furosemide on renal handling of glucose in the rat. Am. J. Physiol. 232:F438-F442, 1977.
293. Bishop, J. H. V.; and Green, R. Glucose transport by short loops of Henle in the rat. J. Physiol. 320:127-138, 1981.
294. Silverman, M. The mechanism of maleic acid nephropathy: Investigations using brush border membrane vesicles. Membr. Biochem. 4:63-69, 1981.
295. Yanase, M.; Orita, Y.; Okada, N.; Nakanishi, T.; Horio, M.; Ando, A.; and Abe, H. Decreased Na^+-gradient-dependent D-glucose transport in brush-border membrane vesicles from rabbits with experimental Fanconi syndrome. Biochim. Biophys. Acta 733:95-101, 1983.
296. Atherton, J. C.; and Pirie, S. C. The effect of pregnancy on glomerular filtration rate and salt and water reabsorption in the rat. J. Physiol. 319:153-164, 1981.
297. Garland, H. O.; and Green, R. Micropuncture study of changes in glomerular filtration and ion and water handling by the rat kidney during pregnancy. J. Physiol. 329: 389-409, 1982.

6
Phosphaturic Syndromes

RUSSELL W. CHESNEY
University of Wisconsin Center for Health Sciences, Madison, Wisconsin

I. THE INORGANIC ANION PHOSPHATE AND ITS BIOLOGICAL ROLE

Phosphorus is the second most abundant mineral element in the human body, and fully 75% of total body phosphorus is found in bone. Since elemental phosphorus is unstable, virtually all molecules of this element are in the form of the inorganic anion, phosphate or PO_4 (1). Phosphates are found throughout the body as: (1) a component of organic compounds—adenosine triphosphate (ATP), diphosphate (ADP), and monophosphate (AMP) and other nucleotides, creatinine phosphate, DNA, RNA, acylphosphates, and phosphorylated glycolytic compounds; (2) phospholipids, which are important membrane constituents; (3) phosphoproteins; and (4) a component of hydroxyapatite (Ca_{10} $[PO_4]_6[OH]_2$), octocalcium phosphate, and amorphous calcium phosphate, all of which comprise bone mineral (2).

Finally, there is a fairly substantial pool of inorganic phosphate that circulates in the blood, is found in all cells (particularly in muscle), is localized in particular subcellular fractions (such as the mitochondria and nucleus), and is absolutely required for all phosphorylation steps. The high-energy phosphate bond is not only essential for life, but it also can only derive from the inorganic phosphate pool within a given cell. The third phosphate joined to ADP by an ester linkage can only arise from inorganic phosphate and cannot arise from other organic phosphorylated compounds.

Since phosphate is such an important chemical in living organisms, the importance of physiological mechanisms to maintain phosphate concentrations within various pools and intracellular sites cannot be overestimated. Factors regulating the intestinal absorption of phosphate are relatively unimportant in phosphate homeostasis. Clearly, the renal transepithelial transport and reclamation of phosphate is the major mechanism for maintaining body stores of this compound (1,4).

II. RENAL REGULATION OF PHOSPHATE HOMEOSTASIS

A. General Considerations

Before discussing those syndromes that have excessive renal phosphate wasting as a common feature, we will briefly review the major intrarenal mechanisms for the efficient reabsorption and excretion of phosphate. At the outset, it is important to recognize that the most essential regulators of renal phosphate handling are the dietary intake of phosphate and the circulating level of metabolically active parathyroid hormone (PTH) (5). In states of excessive phosphate ingestion, urinary phosphate excretion will increase, in part since greater phosphate absorption from the intestine will cause a fall in the ionized fraction of calcium which in turn will stimulate immunoreactive parathyroid hormone (iPTH) (1,5). With decreased dietary intake, the renal tubular reabsorption of phosphate will rise dramatically (6). In the phosphate depletion syndrome, the urine will be essentially free of phosphate (7).

Phosphate in blood exists in one of two forms: $Na_2{}^{2+}HPO_4{}^{2-}$ or $Na^+H_2PO_4{}^-$. Since the pKa_2 of the phosphoric acid buffering system is roughly 6.8, at pH 7.4 fully 80% is present as $Na_2{}^{2+}HPO_4{}^{2-}$ (3). The concentration of phosphate in the glomerular ultrafiltrate is approximately 90% of that in plasma, with the other 10% remaining in the blood as calcium-phosphate microcrystals that are poorly filtered (8).

B. Renal Tubular Sites of Transport

The site in the tubule where most phosphate is reabsorbed is the proximal convoluted tubule with a further large fraction being reclaimed from the pars recta (9) (see Chs. 2 and 3). In intact animals, about 70% of the filtered load is reabsorbed in the convoluted proximal tubule vs. 80% in the thyroparathyroidectomized (TPTX) animal. Reabsorption in the pars recta accounts for another 15% in TPTX animals (10). There is a terminal phosphate reabsorption, accounting for approximately 5-15% of the filtered load, and reaccumulation at this locus may be of great importance in terms of the regulation of phosphate excretion (9). Certainly, fractional delivery of phosphate to the distal tubule is higher than in ureteral urine, regardless of the parathyroid status of the animal. Current evidence would suggest that the arcades connecting the collecting duct to the distal tubule are the most likely sites for terminal phosphate reabsorption (11). Nonetheless, there may be more avid reabsorption in deep nephrons that are inaccessible to conventional micropuncture techniques (10). Furthermore, discrepancies between animal species and techniques used do not provide a clear mechanism of terminal nephron reabsorption. Deep nephrons have longer arcades, and the cells lining this portion of the nephron demonstrate PTH-sensitive adenylate cyclase activity. The importance of this terminal nephron site can best be seen in the chronic TPTX animal, where 10% of the filtered load reaches this segment, but only 2% of the load is found in the urine.

C. Mechanisms of Transport

The mechanism of transport is much clearer in the proximal tubule and to a certain extent in the pars recta. Since the uptake of phosphate occurs against both an electrical and a chemical gradient, the transepithelial transport of phosphate is active. The active component is clearly located at the brush border or luminal membrane, since movement across the antiluminal or basal-lateral membrane could be passive by electrochemical criteria; i.e., the inside of the tubular cell is negative, and there is a high intracellular phosphate concentration (10). As with many other organic solutes, including glucose and amino acids, the energy for the active brush-border membrane uptake of phosphate comes from sodium going down its electrochemical gradient (12) (see Chs. 1 and 2). Phosphate transfer occurs as a result of a secondary active transport process with the energy utilized to extrude sodium from the cell at the basal-lateral membrane by means of Na-K-ATPase. The agents which block Na-K-ATPase activity, including ouabain or the removal of potassium, block phosphate reabsorption (13).

Two factors which strongly influence proximal tubule handling are PTH and volume expansion (14). Saline expansion results in a marked reduction in proximal tubule phosphate reabsorption, as shown by micropuncture studies. Phosphaturia is evident if these expanded animals have intact parathyroids, but is absent in TPTX animals. One hypothesis is that saline loading results in a dilution of ionized calcium that in turn causes PTH secretion which blocks proximal phosphate reabsorption. With the infusion of calcium along with saline expansion, the phosphaturic response is blocked (15). Volume expansion also influences the $TmPO_4$ as it does Tm-glucose and the fractional excretion of sodium, perhaps via the natriuretic third factor effect (see Ch. 8, Sect. IV), but again it is difficult to exclude the role of PTH on the reduced $TmPO_4$ found (10,15). Complete saturation of the transport system in the brush-border membrane is dependent on the sodium concentration, the affinity of the transporter for sodium, the ambient medium pH, and luminal phosphate content (10). The half-maximal saturation concentration (K_m) is 0.7 mmol in the proximal tubule and 0.2 mmol in the pars recta in rats (10). Hence, affinity for phosphate is actually greater in the pars recta. The low K_m value found in this latter nephron locale permits the reaccumulation of phosphate at low intraluminal concentrations (10).

Since the volume of the proximal tubule far exceeds the pars recta, more phosphate is transported in the proximal tubule (16). Nonetheless, the pars recta is important in the reclamation of phosphate in the volume-loaded state, particularly in the absence of PTH (10,13,14). Transfer of phosphate out of this segment may account for the high plasma values of phosphate found in PTH-deficient states, such as idiopathic or postsurgical hypoparathyroidism or pseudohypoparathyroidism (17).

Distal or terminal nephron transport is important in the virtually complete extraction of this anion after phosphate depletion or after parathyroidectomy (13,14).

D. Secretion by the Tubule

Turning from the net reabsorption of this anion, we will discuss the controversial issue as to whether net secretion of phosphate may sometimes be found (18). It is easy to demonstrate phosphate secretion in the kidneys of lower vertebrates, including snakes, fish, frogs, alligators, and birds. The acute elevation of plasma phosphate concentration will result in CPO_4/GFR values greater than 2. The administration of PTH will augment this net secretion.

The net secretion of phosphate in mammalian species and in man is difficult to demonstrate unequivocally (19). It can sometimes be seen after the acute infusion of phosphate and some marker of clearance such as inulin. Using the technique of microperfusion in dogs and rats, with care to remove all contaminated samples, no evidence for peritubular to luminal influx of phosphate was found. Thus, it appears that phosphate transport in the proximal tubule is basically a unidirectional event with reabsorption unopposed by backflux (20). Conclusive evidence for net secretion in the distal nephron and cortical collecting tubule is absent, and studies purporting to show terminal nephron secretion can just as easily be explained by the influence of deep nephron contribution to the terminal nephron ultrafiltrate. Clearly, definitive proof for tubule secretion of phosphate, in quantities exceeding net reabsorption, does not currently exist (14,18,19).

III. FACTORS ALTERING PHOSPHATE TRANSPORT BY THE NEPHRON

A variety of endogenous agents alter the net reabsorption of phosphate and are important in both the physiological regulation of phosphate homeostasis and in the pathophysiological mechanisms found in certain phosphaturic and phosphate-retaining conditions (1,5,10, 13). An entire spectrum of ions and hormones influences renal phosphate handling: PTH, calcitonin, vitamin D metabolites, cortisol, thyroxine, angiotensin, growth hormone, magnesium, calcium, lithium, bicarbonate, glucose, amino acids, and phosphate itself.

A. Parathyroid Hormone

Of these agents, PTH clearly exerts the greatest influence. PTH appears to act in several nephron segments, including the proximal tubule, the pars recta, and the terminal nephron, i.e., all nephron locations capable of phosphate reabsorption (21). Parathyroid hormone appears to block the maximal transport of phosphate at the level of the brush-border membrane (22). As is widely recognized, PTH binds to its receptor on the antiluminal or peritubular membrane which leads to increased activity of the adenylate cyclase system (hormone receptor, N-protein or coupling protein, and adenylate cyclase) and, accordingly, to increased intracellular levels of cyclic AMP (cAMP) (23-25). This cyclic AMP in turn appears to enhance the activity of a luminal membrane protein kinase (26) which phosphorylates luminal membrane proteins (27). It is also possible, although unproven, that cAMP results in increased concentrations of calcium and phosphate within the cell which blocks further transepithelial phosphate transport (28) or that cAMP makes tubular membranes "leaky," especially at the lateral intracellular spaces, thus permitting the backleak of phosphate and other ions (29). These two intriguing hypotheses need further experimental proof.

There are three clear lines of evidence supporting the contention that PTH action is mediated via cAMP: (1) tissue levels of cAMP rise shortly after PTH administration, followed by a rapid urinary excretion of this cyclic nucleotide (30); (2) PTH-sensitive adenylate cyclase is located in those nephron sites where phosphate is being reabsorbed (31); (3) the addition of cAMP or its more soluble analog, dibutyryl cAMP, to the bathing medium will completely simulate the physiological actions of PTH, including decreased phosphate transport (21). As discussed later, if the generation of cAMP is blocked for any reason, phosphaturia will not follow PTH administration. The best examples of this are seen in hypercalcemia and in pseudohypoparathyroidism type I (25,32). Of interest, in the phosphate depletion syndrome (see below), both PTH-induced or exogenously administered cAMP will not invoke phosphaturia (33,34). Thus, there is "blunting" of the phosphaturic effect of this hormone despite the presence of the "second messenger."

The influence of PTH on the tubule may also act by two additional mechanisms: inhibition of sodium and fluid reabsorption (35), and inhibition of phosphate reabsorption by tubular fluid alkalinization (36). The former hypothesis may be relevant in terms of proximal tubular phosphate reabsorption, since the delivery of sodium and phosphate to the distal nephron is increased (35). However, in the terminal nephron, virtually all of this sodium is reabsorbed, and even more phosphate is excreted. Thus, this hypothesis is clearly not relevant in the terminal nephron. Urinary alkalinization, on the other hand, would favor the formation of divalent phosphate (HPO_4^{2-}) which is more highly charged and thus less capable of transmembrane movement (13,21). Lang (10) makes the point that tubular fluid alkalinization under other experimental circumstances may actually enhance phosphate reabsorption and that inhibition of protein secretion by chemical agents such as sulfonated stilbenes may not alter phosphate handling (37). These other hypotheses do not seem to explain PTH-induced phosphaturia as clearly as does the adenylate-cyclase-cAMP theory.

Perhaps, the most convincing evidence that cAMP directly influences phosphate transport following phsophorylation comes from studies in PTH-treated rats where Na^+-dependent phosphate transport was inhibited, but glucose, sodium, and mannitol uptake were unaffected. Intravenous infusion of dibutyryl cAMP 1 hr prior to sacrifice also decreased brush-border membrane phosphate uptake. Both PTH and cAMP were ineffective when added directly in vitro to brush-border membrane vesicles isolated from normal rats (38). Accordingly, some prior interaction between PTH and/or cAMP and the membrane is needed, and only Na-dependent phosphate transport is affected.

B. Calcitonin

Calcitonin (CTC) is a hormone that also demonstrates a phosphaturic effect even though plasma phosphate concentrations are sometimes reduced (39). In intact animals, this phosphaturia and hypophosphatemia could be secondary to hypocalcemia from the hormone and a consequent augmentation of PTH secretion. However, CTC will lower serum phosphate even in TPTX animals. Calcitonin does block phosphate reabsorption regardless of serum calcium level, GFR, or the prevailing phosphate concentration in serum, thereby implying a direct tubular effect. Calcitonin receptors are found in tubules (40), and some authors have found increased cAMP secretion (41). Various species differences in relation to the renal tubular response to CTC have been found, making a cogent hypothesis for its action difficult to formulate (39). At present, it remains uncertain whether CTC has specific actions in terms of phosphate reabsorption or whether its effect is the consequence of its action on other ions such as calcium.

C. Vitamin D

At present, it is not established whether vitamin D and its two major circulating metabolites—25(OH)D (25-hydroxyvitamin D) and $1,25(OH)_2D$ (1,25-dihydroxyvitamin D)—directly influence phosphate transport. Experimental studies have demonstrated both an increase (42) and a decrease (43) in phosphate excretion after introduction of vitamin D analogs. Vitamin D metabolism proceeds normally with the formation of $1,25(OH)_2D$ in the presence of PTH, and in the absence of this hormone, the levels of $1,25(OH)_2D$ are reduced (44). Furthermore, both PTH and vitamin D metabolites influence calcium absorption from the gut and release from bone (44). Therefore, it is difficult to discount changes in serum or, more importantly, tubular calcium values as being of equal importance in assessing the renal phosphaturic effects of vitamin D metabolites. Phosphate clearance is increased in hypoparathyroid man following correction of hypocalcemia (45). On the other hand, the acute intra-arterial infusion of calcium will enhance phosphate reabsorption (46).

Clearly, the effect of vitamin D analogs on phosphate excretion depends on prior vitamin D status and the level of urinary cAMP (47). The chronic administration of $1,25(OH)_2D$ to TPTX rats results in decreased urinary phosphate excretion (48); this effect is probably related to the calcemic effect of this metabolite, much as was found in the studies of Eisenberg (45) in hypoparathyroid man.

Another factor that can govern the response of the tubule to either PTH, vitamin D, or calcium level is the adaptive mechanism that responds to the dietary intake of phosphate (49,50). With reduced dietary intake of phosphate (the phosphate-depleted state), little of this anion is excreted in the urine, and the phosphaturic response to PTH is blunted (51). This adaptive response is expressed at the brush-border membrane where greater accumulation by vesicles is evident (52,53).

Phosphate-depleted rats that are given $1,25(OH)_2D$ chronically have a return of phosphaturia with a loss of this adaptive response; this effect is again seen at the brush border membrane (52,55). Further, these changes may be related to the regulation of renal phosphate transport by either serum or intracellular calcium concentrations. Even after phosphate loading of TPTX animals, which normally leads to phosphaturia, if the predictable drop in serum calcium is prevented by calcium infusion, the decline in $TmPO_4$ is not as great (56). Finally, by using the calcium ionophore A23187, which shifts extracellular calcium into the cell, it can be shown that the phosphaturia of phosphate loading is related to hypocalcemia and reduced intracellular calcium content (57).

D. Glucose

Both glucose and galactose infusion will augment phosphate excretion. Many parallels have been noted between glucose and phosphate transport, since both are taken up more avidly in early proximal tubules, both have saturation kinetics and the transport of each is sodium dependent (58). The kinetics of renal tubular phosphate reabsorption in vivo reveal that glucose inhibits in a competitive fashion (59). Dextrose infusion sufficient to induce glucosuria will depress phosphate reabsorption by 20%, possibly suggesting some sharing of transport pathways. However, the use of the inhibitor phloridzin neatly distinguishes each transport site because glucose reabsorption is blocked while phosphate reaccumulation is actually enhanced (60). This glucose effect is shared by galactose and fructose, and these sugars inhibit phosphate reabsorption in man (61). Maleic acid, a known mitochondrial poison (particularly of succinylcoenzyme A) will augment both hexose and phosphate excretion (62). In addition, ouabain and other cardiac glycosides which block Na-K-ATPase activity will inhibit both glucose and phosphate transport (63). It is also clear that brush-border membrane vesicle uptake of both glucose and phosphate is sodium dependent (64). The remarkable set of parallelisms is not dependent on the action of insulin, since the renal transport of both compounds occurs independently of the hormonal action of insulin (65).

In the phosphate-depleted state the Tm-glucose falls, as further evidence of a common mechanism. When PTH is given to dogs the Tm-glucose rises, while phosphaturia ensues (66). Most authors conclude that there is no direct proof that glucose and phosphate actually share carriers, but that both compounds compete for a common energy source (58,67).

E. Amino Acids

Amino acids, like glucose and phosphate, are also avidly reabsorbed in the early proximal tubule (67). Again, amino acid reabsorption is sodium dependent (67,68), and the accumulation of many amino acids by brush-border membrane vesicles is dependent on a sodium gradient (69). An interaction of phosphate and amino acids has been shown, both after infusion and in cortex slice experiments in vitro (70). As is the situation in the interaction between glucose and phosphate, amino acids most probably compete for a common energy source intended for renal tubular epithelial transport processes.

F. Other Hormones

A large number of hormones influence the renal handling of phosphate, including PTH, CTC, growth hormone, vasopressin, thyroxine, glucagon, insulin, glucocorticoids, estrogens, and catecholamines (39). The scope of this chapter does not permit a detailed discussion of hormonal action on phosphate transport. Clearly, several of these hormones have greater clinical relevance and will be further discussed.

Growth Hormone

Growth hormone has an antiphosphaturic action, and the plasma phosphate of acromegalic subjects is higher than normal (71). A hypophosphaturic action of growth hormone is noted 3 hr after a dose in rats (72), and both GFR and $TmPO_4$/GFR are increased after human growth hormone administration (73). The mechanism of this action of growth hormone is not established, although it may involve enhanced sodium reabsorption, insulin release, or an increase in the synthesis of $1,25(OH)_2D$ (39). Growth hormone does not appear to play a role in the renal adaptive mechanisms in phosphate depletion (74).

Glucocorticoids

Low circulating phosphate concentrations and hyperphosphaturia are commonly found in adrenocortical hyperfunction (75). This effect is not related to mineralocorticoid activity (76). The increased clearance of phosphate is independent of PTH secretion, since it has been found in hyperparathyroidism (77).

G. Other Compounds

The administration of lithium (Li) will blunt the phosphaturic effect of PTH (78). Not only does Li block the adenylate cyclase-cAMP system in the renal tubule, but the infusion of cAMP in the presence of Li fails to evoke a phosphaturic response. It has been previously mentioned that phosphate reabsorption is highly dependent on the presence of active sodium transport. Therefore, it is possible that Li replaces sodium and blocks transport. Certainly, the replacement of intraluminal sodium by stepwise increases in choline will progressively reduce phosphate reabsorption (79).

Virtually all diuretics will induce phosphaturia, including osmotic agents, mercurial diuretics, acetazolamide, thiazides, and loop diuretics (80). None of the potassium-sparing agents will block phosphate reabsorption. Of the other diuretics, carbonic anhydrase inhibitors are the most potent. These agents block bicarbonate reabsorption and cause an alkaline urine which favors formation of the more polar and less permeable phosphate anion, HPO_4^{2-}, rather than $H_2PO_4^-$ (81). However, this mechanism is unlikely to cause phosphaturia, since acetazolamide leads to a fall in proximal tubular pH (80). The acetazolamide effect is dependent on the presence of bicarbonate in the urine (82) and is not dependent on the presence of PTH (83). Nonetheless, acetazolamide will affect the adenylate cyclase system and augment the formation of cAMP in studies in rats (84). Ethacrynic acid and furosemide, which do not alter cAMP levels, do augment phosphate excretion.

Some anatomic manipulations will alter the renal handling of phosphate. After the relief of unilateral ureteral obstruction, hypophosphaturia is found on the previously obstructed side in comparison to the normal kidney (85). The fractional excretion of water and sodium is increased in the obstructed side, providing evidence for a dissociation between the renal handling of sodium and phosphate in this condition. Although extracellular volume expansion and the infusion of PTH in dogs will enhance phosphate excretion, a blunting of this response is evident in the obstructed kidney (86). This hypophosphaturia may be related to enhanced uptake by the proximal tubule and decreased sodium (and water) reaccumulation at a distal site.

On the other hand, compensatory phosphaturia is found after unilateral nephrectomy in rats (87). This increase in the fractional excretion of phosphate occurs despite thyroparathyroidectomy and under constant PTH infusion, indicating that secondary hyperparathyroidism after nephrectomy is not essential to compensatory phosphaturia.

IV. TECHNIQUES USED IN EVALUATING RENAL TUBULAR PHOSPHATE TRANSPORT

Although it would seem that one could assess the renal excretion of phosphate by measuring the clearance of phosphate—$C_{PO_4} = U_{PO_4}V/PO_{4\,(serum)}$—this technique is dependent on both GFR and the circulating serum phosphate concentration. Several methods have been devised, including the phosphate clearance/creatinine clearance ratio (C_{PO_4}/C_{Cr}), the percent tubular reabsorption of phosphate (%TRP) (88), the phosphate excretion index

(PEI), and the index of phosphate excretion (89). Each of these techniques has a wide range of normal values, and there is overlap between healthy subjects and individuals with disorders of phosphate metabolism (90). Several approaches have been taken to best determine the renal threshold concentration for phosphate.

The direct method of determining the reabsorption of phosphate is to infuse inorganic phosphate via an intravenous line so that the plasma level rises linearly. The excretion rate can then be estimated at various times after infusion, and a renal threshold can be found by extrapolation. This technique allows one to determine the interrelationship between the theoretical renal threshold, the GFR, and the tubular maximum for phosphate ($TmPO_4$) (91-93). However, the limit or threshold phosphate concentration can be derived from knowledge of phosphate excretion, serum phosphate, and the GFR under steady-state conditions. Bijvoet (89,92) has shown that the greater the serum phosphate value in comparison to the phosphate threshold value, the greater will be the fraction of the filtered load.

Using the methods established by Bijvoet (89,92), one can estimate the relationship between the fraction of the filtered load that is filtered and the ratio of the phosphate threshold to the prevailing plasma phosphate. First, one needs to know the ratio of the phosphate clearance to creatinine clearance (C_{PO_4}/C_{Cr}). This ratio is obtained from simultaneous measurements of phosphate and creatine in plasma and urine:

$$C_{PO_4}/C_{Cr} = \frac{\text{Urine }(PO_4) \times \text{Volume} \times \text{Plasma }(Cr)}{\text{Plasma }(PO_4) \times \text{Urine }(Cr) \times \text{Volume}}$$

$$= \frac{U_{PO_4} \times P_{Cr}}{U_{Cr} \times P_{PO_4}}$$

One can use a single urine sample obtained after the first morning void (8-10 A.M.) and ignore urine volume. From the C_{PO_4}/C_{Cr} one can determine the percent tubular reabsorption of phosphate (%TRP) = 1 - (C_{PO_4}/C_{Cr}). Using the complex calculations derived from infusion studies (91-93), it was found that the $TmPO_4$/GFR = TRP $\times$ plasma (PO_4). These calculations have been simplified by a nomogram which will derive the renal threshold concentration for phosphate from the plasma phosphate concentration and the C_{PO_4}/C_{Cr} or the TRP (94) (Fig. 1). This nomogram is useful in the discussion of the phosphaturic syndromes to follow.

The excretion of phosphate has a circadian variation and is lowest during the morning, reaching its highest level between 6 P.M. and midnight (95). This circadian rhythm can be reversed by nighttime feeding (96). This observation is important in individuals fed by parenteral alimentation methods, since they are often fed during the night. Other factors, such as cortisol secretion and muscle activity, may also govern the circadian variability of excretion. The dietary intake of phosphate regulates the amount excreted each day and, in the phosphate depletion syndrome, urinary phosphate concentrations are negligible (7,97). Following the feeding of phosphate, its renal excretion rapidly increases, probably related to the higher filtered load rather than to PTH secretion (98).

There are numerous indices of renal phosphate handling that can be utilized (Table 1). Each of these techniques has distinct shortcomings, particularly when plasma phosphate levels are rapidly changing. When phosphate intake is normal and the GFR does not vary greatly, a fasting plasma phosphate will indicate whether hyperreabsorption or hyperex-

Table 1 Variables Which Influence the Tubular Reabsorption of Phosphate

Variable	Symbol	Calculation	Dimensions	Average	Range
Plasma phosphate	PO_4		mass/vol; mg/100 dl	3.2	2.3-4.4
Glomerular filtration rate	GFR		vol/time; ml/min	100	80-120
Filtered load	LPO_4	$(PO_4) \times GFR$	mass/time; mg/min	3.2	
Urinary excretion rate	UPO_4		mass/time, mg/min	0.36	0.14-0.57
Tubular reabsorption rate	TPO_4	$LPO_4 - UPO_4 V$	mass/time, mg/min	2.84	
Maximum tubular reabsorption rate	Tm	a	mass/time; mg/min	3.2	
Limit or threshold phosphate concentration	$TmPO_4/GFR$	See Fig. 1	mass/vol; mg/100 dl	3.2	2.5-4.2
Phosphate clearance	CPO_4	$UPO_4 V/(PO_4)$	vol/time, ml/min	12	
Phosphate/creatinine clearance	CPO_4/C_{Cr}	$UPO_4 V/LPO_4$	No dimension	0.12	
Fractional reabsorption of filtered load	TRP	$TPO_4/LPO_4 = 1 - UPO_4 V/LPO_4$	No dimension	0.88	
Phosphate excretion index	PEI	b	Dimension?		±0.09
Index of phosphate excretion	IPE	c	mass/vol, mg/100 dl		±0.50

[a] Relationship between PO_4 excretion rate and plasma PO_4 concentration.
[b] $PEI = CPO_4/C_{Cr} - 0.055(PO_4) + 0.07$; (PO_4) is expressed in mg/100 dl.
[c] $IPE = UPO_4 V/GFR - (PO_4 - 2.5)/2$; (PO_4) is expressed in mg/100 dl.
Source: Ref. 89.

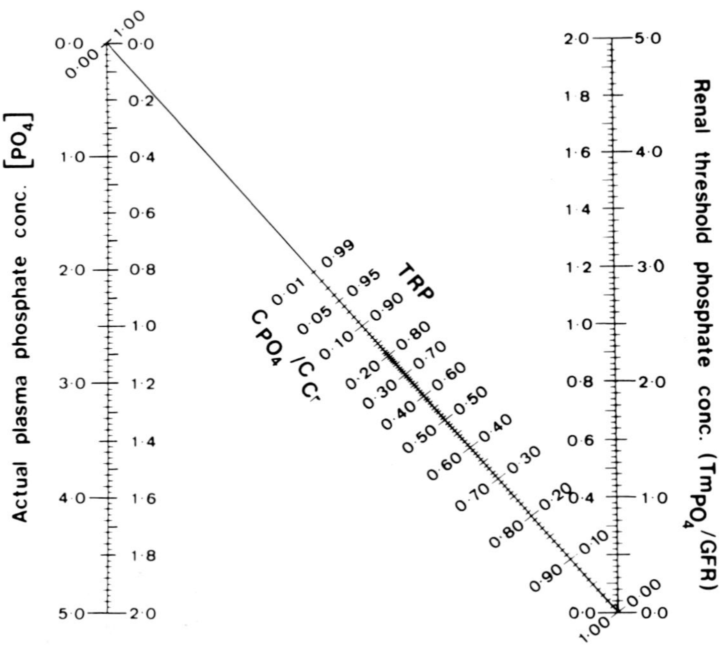

Fig. 1 Nomogram for the derivation of the renal threshold concentration for phosphate. (From Ref. 94.)

creation is present. Nonetheless, determination of the $TmPO_4/GFR$ will indicate the renal threshold. This method is greatly simplified by use of the nomogram in Fig. 1. When phosphate excretion is examined in children it must be recalled that plasma phosphate values are higher (1) and that the normal values for $TmPO_4/GFR$ are also higher (99), with a mean value of 4.97 ± 0.61 mg/dl (SE). Finally, as shown in hypoparathyroid individuals, one can examine the $TmPO_4/GFR$ rather than phosphate excretion after PTH infusion (17). Probably the easiest means of assessing the causes of abnormal plasma phosphate values is by an examination of the $TmPO_4/GFR$ ratio.

V. PHOSPHATURIC SYNDROMES

A. Primary Hypophosphatemic Rickets (X-Linked Hypophosphatemic Rickets)

Primary hypophosphatemic rickets represents the most prevalent form of rickets seen in North America and Western Europe (100). This disorder is characterized by an increased renal clearance of phosphate, despite moderate hypophosphatemia, normocalcemia, short stature, and hypomineralization of the growth plate of bone which is not corrected by doses of vitamin D that ordinarily cure vitamin D deficiency (100,101). The characteristic bone lesion in hypophosphatemic rickets involves hypomineralization, both at the epiphyseal cartilage and at the endosteal bone surface (102-104). Vitamin D therapy will improve the radiological appearance of the epiphyseal lesion, but fails to heal the osteomalacic lesion at the endosteal surface.

Several names for this disorder are in common usage in the literature, so that the reader must be aware of the different terms. The prominent names are: vitamin D-resistant rickets, familial vitamin D-resistant rickets with hypophosphatemia, X-linked hypophosphatemic rickets, familial X-linked hypophosphatemic rickets, familial hypophosphatemic rickets, primary hypophosphatemic rickets, renal phosphate diabetes, familial hypophosphatemia, and renal hypophosphatemic rickets (105). The term primary hypophosphatemic rickets seems preferable, since the role of hypophosphatemia on the bone disease is emphasized and since not all cases are familial or have an X-linked inheritance pattern.

Biochemical Abnormality and Pathophysiology

The universal biochemical abnormality is hypophosphatemia with a moderate but sustained reduction in serum phosphate values to 1.0-2.5 mg/dl (0.13-0.34 mM/liter). Just as serum phosphate values are higher during childhood, these values are higher in affected children than in adults with the condition (106). Serum calcium values are usually in the low normal range (9.0-9.3 mg/dl), and alkaline phosphatase activity is moderately increased. Urinary calcium excretion is low and phosphate excretion is very high, particularly in view of the prevailing serum phosphate concentration (107). Since hyperphosphaturia is evident despite hypophosphatemia, the $TmPO_4/GFR$ is reduced and usually is below 1.8 mg/dl (102-104, 108). The fecal concentration of both calcium and phosphate is elevated (109). The values for iPTH are normal in untreated patients but rise after oral phosphate treatment (110). Some patients have been described who clearly have secondary hyperparathyroidism and glandular hyperplasia (111,112). Renal tubular glucose and amino acid excretion are not features of this entity.

The pathogenesis of primary hypophosphatemic rickets is not fully established. Basically, two opposing theories are espoused to explain the phosphaturia in the face of hypophosphatemia:

1. That a renal tubular defect in the reabsorption of phosphate, presumably related to a missing or abnormal transport protein, accounts for decreased reclamation of this anion
2. That a defect in vitamin D metabolism results in decreased intestinal calcium and phosphate absorption, secondary hyperparathyroidism, and resultant phosphaturia.

Since iPTH values are normal in untreated patients, the reduced reabsorption of phosphate in this second hypothesis relies on a "hypersensitivity of the renal tubule to the phosphaturic action of PTH" (107,113). Intricate clinical research studies have been performed to establish which of these theories is correct, but to date the available data could be interpreted as favoring either theory. Moreover, all studies involving the infusion of calcium to patients fail to account for the influence of this divalent cation on intrarenal blood flow and phosphate handling at the level of the renal tubule.

In the first hypothesis, the renal lesion exists at the level of the renal tubule, most likely at the renal brush-border membrane (114). The main support for this theory comes from the fact that patients do not have hypercalcemia, do not have increased iPTH levels, do not have hypercalcuria, and do not have the hyperexcretion of amino acids, bicarbonate, uric acid, glucose, and cAMP expected if the tubule were hyperresponsive to the physiological action of PTH (67,115-117). The recent description of a patient with X-linked hypophosphatemia and hypoparathyroidism occurring coincidentally tends to favor this hypothesis (119). This patient, with no detectable circulating PTH, had renal phosphaturia after serum calcium levels had been normalized by therapy with $1,25(OH)_2D_3$, indicating that hypophosphatemia and hyperphosphaturia can prevail without circulating PTH. Nonetheless, an elevation of serum calcium (and presumably of renal tubular cell calcium) values was needed before phosphaturia was evident.

A comparable defect in intestinal phosphate transport has been postulated; it is based on the initial findings of Albright et al. (109). Impaired phosphate absorption is found in infusion studies (120) and in gut biopsy specimens (121), but others have failed to confirm this finding (122,123). More recently, Walton (124), using a triple lumen tube, described impaired jejunal phosphate absorption along with the defect in calcium absorption reported in 1937 by Albright et al. (109). Scriver (115) has made the point that calcium malabsorption could be the consequence of higher intestinal phosphate concentrations after microcrystal formation.

In the second hypothesis, PTH plays a pivotal role in hyperphosphaturia. Increased phosphate excretion following stimulation of the tubule by PTH could reduce %TRP and the $TmPO_4/GFR$ (1) and the increase of these indices after the induction of hypercalcemia (125,126). Hahn et al. (107) found that iPTH (C-terminal) concentrations in untreated patients were mildly elevated to 11.4 ng/ml (vs. 5.1 ng/ml in controls), and that urinary cAMP excretion was twice normal. The infusion of PTH both lowered $TmPO_4/GFR$ and increased cAMP; the infusion of ionic calcium suppressed PTH release, cAMP urinary excretion, and phosphaturia. Short et al. (127) found normal iPTH values and urinary cAMP excretion rates, but their diet contained a lower phosphate content than that provided in the study of Hahn et al. (107). When the patients in Short's study (127) received enough intravenous calcium to raise the serum value to 13-15 mg/dl the %TRP rose and urinary cAMP excretion rates fell. Exogenous PTH led to an exaggerated phosphaturic response. Scriver (115,116) has argued that calcium infusion could not only suppress PTH secretion but also influence phosphate handling directly, as previously shown by the studies of Lavender and Pullman (128).

In at least two patients with X-linked hypophosphatemia, the renal tubular phosphate leak was unaltered by subtotal parathyroidectomy, but not all the functioning glandular tissue was removed (112,129). In another patient, a renal transplant did not alter hyperphosphaturia (130). Nonetheless, the donated kidney came from an HLA-identical sibling in whom pretransplant phosphate levels were unavailable. Following donation of the kidney, the donor had a serum phosphate of 3.2 mg/dl and a $TmPO_4/GFR$ of 2.3 mg/dl, the latter value being subnormal.

Two conclusions are possible from these contradictory findings. First, there is considerable heterogeneity in this condition which accounts for normal PTH values and tubular responsiveness to PTH in some patients and not in others. Alternatively, this condition may involve a variety of confounding factors that ultimately results in renal hyperphosphaturia. Certainly, the changes in vitamin D metabolism evident in these patients appears to be another variable in the pathogenesis of this condition.

Albright et al. (109) originally postulated that a defect in vitamin D metabolism would be found. The circulating values for 25(OH)D appear to be completely normal in untreated patients (131,132). The values of $1,25(OH)_2D$ are less certain but appear to be "normal" or just subnormal in untreated patients (102,103,133) and reduced in patients treated with vitamin D_2 (134-136). With dietary phosphate deprivation, the values for $1,25(OH)_2D$ actually fall in patients, whereas they rise in normal controls (137). Certainly, in view of their hypophosphatemia, the low normal or subnormal values of calcitriol found in these patients indicate a relative reduction of calcitriol synthesis. Until vitamin D turnover rates are examined, it is not clear whether this relative calcitriol deficiency represents a lower synthetic rate of this metabolite. When the concentrations of $24,25(OH)_2D$ are examined, they are either normal (134) or slightly reduced (136). In conclusion, the main abnormality in vitamin D metabolism appears to be an apparent reduction in the circulating values of $1,25(OH)_2D$ that is relevant only because of hypophosphatemia, which should stimulate greater production of $1,25(OH)_2D$. Obviously, turnover studies of vitamin D metabolites will be informative in these patients.

An important animal model of X-linked hypophosphatemia has been found in an inborn strain of laboratory mice, the Hyp/Y mouse (138). These animals have an X-linked form of rickets with hypophosphatemia and short stature. Since both human and murine disease are inherited on the X-chromosome, and since there is preservation of genes coded on the X-chromosome among mammals, this mouse model may be comparable to the human disease. The Hyp/Y mouse demonstrates diminished intestinal uptake of phosphate and calcium (139) and decreased proximal tubular reabsorption of phosphate (140), with normal terminal nephron accumulation and decreased bone ash (138). It is known that sodium-dependent, azide-inhibitable phosphate transport by brush-border membrane vesicles is impaired in Hyp/Y or male mice (114). Accumulation by female hemizygotes is also impaired but not to the same extent. When mice are fed a phosphate-depleted diet, brush-border vesicle uptake rate will increase by 200%, indicating that the renal epithelium in these mice adapts to an altered dietary intake (141). As in human disease, serum PTH values are normal and PTH infusion does not alter renal tubular phosphate handling (142). Moreover, after acute TPTX and phosphate loading a renal tubular phosphate leak is still found.

The levels of vitamin D metabolites in these mice are normal (143), but are low in view of the hypophosphatemia. After phosphate deprivation, the serum levels of $1,25(OH)_2D$ rise in normal mice, but they either do not change or actually fall in Hyp/Y mice (144), as was noted in man (137). Treatment with oral phosphate will improve bone mineralization (138). Therapy with $1,25(OH)_2D$ will improve intestinal calcium transport, but it does not influence gut transport of phosphate (139). Although both 1α-(OH)D (a synthetic analog) and $1,25(OH)_2D$ will increase urinary phosphate conservation and improve rachitic bone morphology, only the synthetic analog will improve phosphate homeostasis by raising plasma values (145). Future studies with this animal model will undoubtedly assist our understanding of phosphate homeostasis and proper treatment regimens in the human disease, but the disease in the mouse seems to be a more homogeneous one than found in man.

At present, a simple unified theory of the pathogenesis of primary hypophosphatemic rickets in man is not possible. At least six major problems must be resolved:

1. Is the defect in brush border membrane vesicle transport found in the mouse analogous to disease in humans?
2. Is the renal handling of phosphate altered by normal circulating concentrations of PTH without any other hormone effects?
3. Do the normal or subnormal circulating values for $1,25(OH)_2D$ found in patients truly indicate relative deficiency because of the hypophosphatemia that prevails?
4. Does calcium infusion result in an appreciable alteration of phosphate handling in this condition, so that studies using this approach to suppress endogenous PTH secretion should be viewed with caution?
5. Is calcium homeostasis of importance in setting the $TmPO_4/GFR$ as suggested in the patient described by Lyles et al. (119)?
6. Does the paradoxical fall in serum $1,25(OH)_2D$ values after dietary phosphate deprivation indicate an important defect in vitamin D metabolism?

Until these questions are reasonably answered, one must view any unified hypothesis with caution.

Clinical Features and Diagnosis

The smooth bowing of the lower limbs which is characteristic of primary hypophosphatemic rickets usually appears at the onset of walking or at approximately 12 months of age. When weight-bearing begins (105) (Fig. 2) growth retardation and bowing are mainly confined to the lower limbs, and one may see pelvic deformities, coxa vara, genu valgum, and smooth bowing. Early craniostenosis is frequent and usually leads to a protuberant forehead and an enlarged bridge of the nose; this feature is more evident in males (109). In contrast to patients with vitamin D deficiency, these patients do not have enamel hypoplasia of the teeth but do have defective dentin formation. A histological examination of the teeth will demonstrate interglobular dentine, which is felt to be characteristic of the disorder (119,146).

Patients have all the radiological signs of rickets (Fig. 3) with coarse trabeculation, most notably at the distal ends of long bones. Two distinct features can be noted–rickets in the region of the epiphysis and metaphysis and a widened bone shaft with a loose reticular pattern to bone trabeculae. In the untreated state, evidence of hyperparathyroidism is not found, and Looser-Milkman striae are almost never found. Children appear to be undermineralized

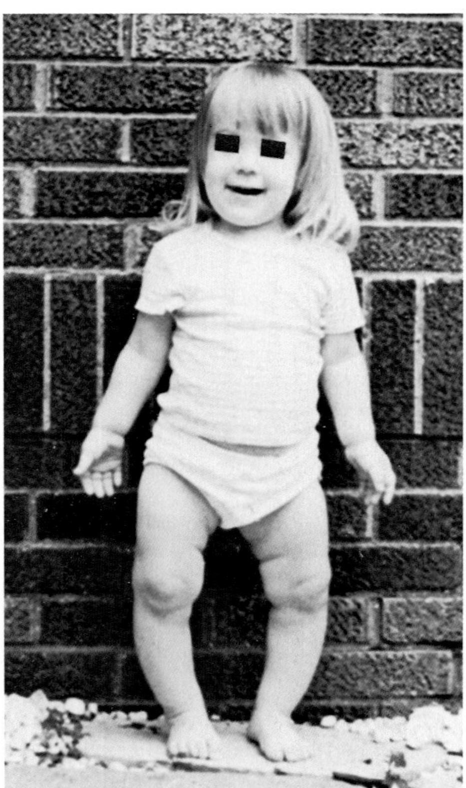

Fig. 2 The typical patient with X-linked hypophosphatemic rickets prior to the onset of vitamin D and phosphate therapy.

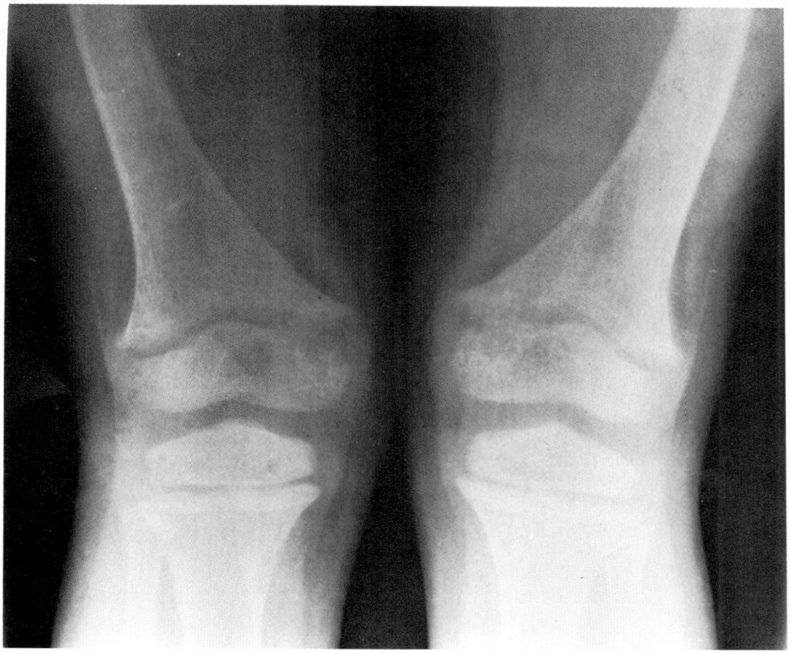

Fig. 3 Roentgenograms of the knees of a girl with X-linked hypophosphatemic rickets. Note the metaphyseal widening and the fraying at the ends of the metaphyses as well as the coarse and thickened trabecular bone at the distal end of the femur and proximal tibia.

(134,147), but young adults may have supranormal bone tissue, osteosclerosis, and increased bone calcium, as determined by in vivo neutron activation analysis (148). Histological examination of bone reveals two typical lesions—the hypomineralization of cartilage at the growth plate and the undermineralized osteoid at endosteal bone surfaces (103). One may also see abnormal deposition of bone minerals, irregular cement lines, abnormal orientation of collagen fibers, and increased low-density bone around osteocytic lacunae (149,150).

Male patients with hypophosphatemic rickets will always manifest disease, but females are variably affected. In X-linked disease, by definition, females are heterozygotes and males are hemizygotes. Untreated females may have mild fasting hypophosphatemia and mild bowing and be of normal height. Untreated patients remain short, and an adult height of 140-155 cm is typical (151). In adult life, patients show evidence of degenerative joint disease with severe pains and other rheumatic manifestations (152). These joint manifestations are frequently prominent, may affect job opportunities, and possibly indicate the need for lifelong therapy.

The inheritance pattern of hypophosphatemic rickets is usually X-linked (153). Other inheritance patterns, including autosomal dominant (154), autosomal recessive (155), and sporadic (156), have rarely been reported. Clearly, however, the predominant mode of inheritance is X-linked dominant. This pattern was perceived long after the description of the disease (151), probably since simple D-deficiency rickets was far more common (153). As Scriver states (153), "The inherited forms (of rickets), previously submerged, merely became more prominent as the flood of rickets of environmental origin abated." In addition, other inheritance patterns are more common in diseases to be discussed later.

Therapy

Treatment of hypophosphatemic rickets with immense daily doses of vitamin D will improve the radiological appearance of the epiphyseal lesion. This form of therapy, often requiring doses of 150,000 U (3333 μg) of vitamin D per day, does not prevent the continuing deformity of the lower limbs, prevent recurrence of deformity after surgical correction, or restore a normal growth pattern (151,154). The risk-benefit ratio of vitamin D alone is very high, with frequent toxocity, including hypercalcemia, hypercalciuria, nephrocalcinosis, and renal damage, as evidenced by a fall in endogenous creatinine clearance (151,157).

Although early studies indicated disappointing results using phosphate supplements (158, 159), when the frequent and large doses of phosphate that could achieve positive phosphate balance were used (160,161) healing of rickets occurred. Long-term studies of the daily provision of 1-4 g of inorganic phosphate given every 4-5 hr indicate that both healing of rickets and increased growth velocity will ensue (154,162-164). Catch-up growth is possible and, if phosphate is started early in life, reasonable height can be achieved and maintained (1, 153,154). Following an oral phosphate dose, the serum value for this anion peaks in 90-120 min and returns to pretherapy values in 4 hr (162). As anticipated, oral phosphate loading will increase PTH secretion which can actually cause hyperparathyroid bone disease. Vitamin D_2 in moderately high doses along with oral calcium can be used to prevent this side effect of phosphate therapy (165).

Trials with 25(OH)D and supplemental phosphate have not corrected the bone lesion in this form of rickets and do not appear to offer any substantial advantage, since this form of therapy does not completely heal the bone lesion (166,167).

Patients have been given short-term trials of $1,25(OH)_2D$ therapy. This therapy leads to improved intestinal calcium absorption and causes a transient rise in serum phosphate values. Nonetheless, in these trials, lasting up to 2 weeks, no healing of bone disease was noted (168-170), and this form of therapy clearly does not correct the renal tubular phosphate leak.

More recently, trials with long-term $1,25(OH)_2D$ have indicated that this form of therapy is the most effective means of dealing with this disorder (102,103,171-176). Therapy with $1,25(OH)_2D$ (approximately 65 ng/kg body wt per day) appears to improve both calcium and phosphate balance, increase bone mineralization, and possibly increase linear growth rate. Both the rachitic lesion at the growth plate and the mineralization defect at the endosteal surface are corrected, which cannot be shown for any other form of treatment (102, 103,171). No improvement in the renal tubular phosphate leak is found (103,171,176) and the $TmPO_4/GFR$ is either unchanged or may actually fall (Table 2). Where vitamin D_2 and phosphate treatment fails to correct the defect in bone mineral content, therapy with this more active metabolite will correct this defect (176). Further trials will demonstrate whether $1,25(OH)_2D$ given over decades will prevent the degenerative joint disease that is so prevalent in adult hypophosphatemic subjects.

B. Hypophosphatemic Nonrachitic Bone Disease

Sometimes patients with renal hypophosphatemia may demonstrate short stature and bowing without clearcut radiological evidence of rickets. Scriver (177,178) has chosen to use another term to identify such patients–hypophosphatemic nonrachitic bone disease (HMBD). This disorder may be either sporadic or autosomal dominant, with the latter mode of inheritance being the typical one (178,179). These patients have femoral bowing, elbow flexion contractures, increased bone density, and coarse trabeculae on radiological examination.

The fractional renal excretion of phosphate is normal in the fasting hypophosphatemic state in HMBD, whereas it is massively increased at an equivalent plasma phosphate level in

Table 2 Urine Phosphate (PO_4) Excretion[a]

Vitamin D_2 and oral phosphate therapy							
P_{Cr} (mg/dl)	PPO_4 (mg/dl)	U_{Cr} (mg/dl)	UPO_4 (mg/dl)	PO_4/Cr	PO_4/24 hr	%TRP	$TmPO_4$/GFR
0.47 ± 0.03 n = 13	2.6 ± 0.18 n = 13	54.6 ± 3.2 n = 13	94.1 ± 7.4 n = 13	1.93 ± 0.24 n = 13	569.9 ± 102 n = 13	67.00 ± 4.55 n = 13	1.99 ± .24 n = 13

Calcitriol and oral phosphate therapy							
P_{Cr} (mg/dl)	PPO_4 (mg/dl)	U_{Cr} (mg/dl)	UPO_4 (mg/dl)	PO_4/Cr	PO_4/24 hr	%TRP	$TmPO_4$/GFR
0.49 ± 0.02 n = 28	3.3[b] ± 0.08 n = 28	74.4 ± 7.3 n = 28	245.0[b] ± 16.6 n = 28	3.74[b] ± 0.30 n = 28	1656.0[b] ± 160 n = 28	47.00[b] ± 3.37 n = 28	1.53[b] ± 0.12 n = 28

[a]Values are the mean ± SE.
[b]Different from values on vitamin D_2, $p < 0.01$.

primary hypophosphatemia (Fig. 4). Urinary phosphate and cAMP excretion is increased by the infusion of PTH extract in contrast to the findings in primary hypophosphatemia. Plasma iPTH values and $1,25(OH)_2D$ levels are completely normal (135). Accordingly, the renal tubular phosphate leak is milder. As Scriver states (178), "The most simple explanation for the different phenotypes is that independent gene products, each responsible for a different aspect of phosphate homeostasis, are affected by the two mutations."

Treatment with $1,25(OH)_2D$ therapy alone, at doses of 1 μg daily, appeared to raise the prevailing serum phosphate value, improve the tubular reabsorption of phosphate, significantly raise the $TmPO_4$/GFR, and heal the osteomalacia of endosteal trabecular bone (178). This form of disease is not common, but should be sought by physicians caring for hypophosphatemic patients.

C. Vitamin D-Deficiency Rickets

Once widely common, vitamin D-deficiency rickets was related to air pollution from the large factory wastes of the industrial revolution in the temperate zones of North America and Western Europe (100). In the late eighteenth and nineteenth centuries, the smoke-choked air of urban centers prevented the ultraviolet rays of sunlight striking the skin of the inhabitants of these cities. 7-Dehydrocholesterol, contained in the skin, did not undergo conversion to pre-vitamin D_3 and vitamin D_3 (44). Rickets became an epidemic disorder that was only cured after vitamin D was discovered by Mellanby and after Steenbock and Hess independently discovered that ultraviolet irradiation of ergosterol could provide a readily available source of vitamin D in the diet (180). Vitamin D supplements are now universally used in milk products in the temperate zones of modern industrialized nations.

Hypophosphatemia and hyperphosphaturia in vitamin D-deficiency rickets is the consequence of secondary hyperparathyroidism (115). The sequence of events is vitamin D deficiency followed by a fall in plasma ionized calcium as intestinal calcium absorption declines

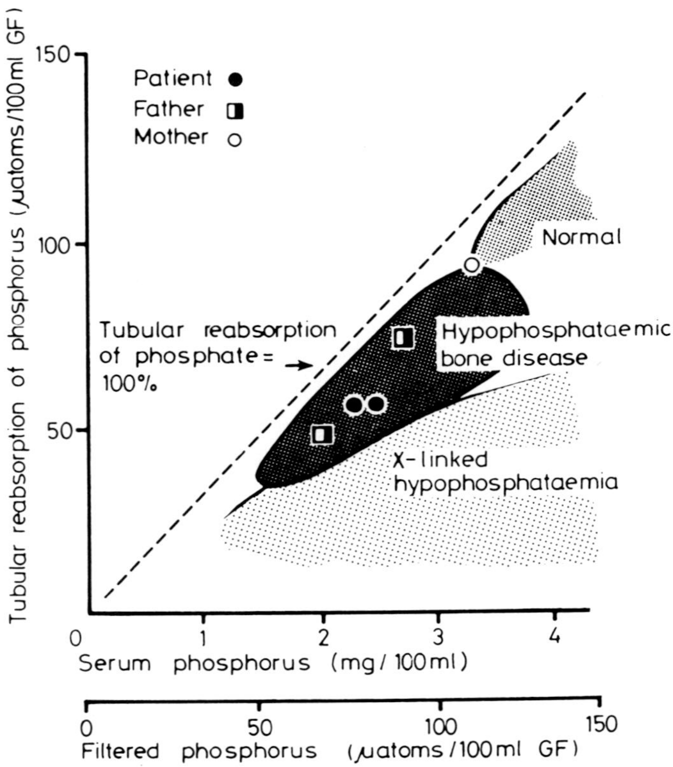

Fig. 4 The relationship between the tubular reabsorption of phosphorus and the serum concentration of phosphate in the members of a family with hypophosphatemic bone disease. Also shown are the patterns of phosphate excretion in X-linked hypophosphatemia and in normal individuals. (From Ref. 178.)

(stage I rickets). The reduction of ionized calcium leads to a rise in iPTH secretion, which causes a normalization of serum calcium and a fall in serum phosphate (stage II rickets) (1, 115). The serum value for calcium rises, since bone resorption is enhanced by the local action of PTH on osteoclast activation; PTH results in phosphaturia and a fall in $TmPO_4$/GFR by mechanisms previously discussed. In stage III rickets, the final stage, the biochemical features are hypocalcemia, hypophosphatemia, phosphaturia, and aminoaciduria. This aminoaciduria is possibly caused by excessive calcitonin secretion or renal tubular cell calcium deficiency rather than by hyperparathyroidism per se (181,182). Thyroparathyroidectomy will block the phosphaturia of vitamin D deficiency in experimental animals (rats) as evidence of the central role of iPTH in the phosphate leak of D deficiency (183).

When circulating vitamin D metabolite concentrations are measured, the values for 25-(OH)D and 24,25$(OH)_2$D are always low (184-188) and those for 1,25$(OH)_2$D are either low (185) or in the normal range (184,187,188). The values for 25(OH)D are low, since this is the major circulating metabolite (20-60 ng/ml) in plasma. The serum values for 24,25$(OH)_2$D are reduced, since three factors—25(OH)D deficiency, hypocalcemia, and hypophosphatemia—will inhibit the activity of the 24-hydroxylase enzyme system (189). The values for 1,25$(OH)_2$D in plasma should probably not be considered normal, since these subjects are hypocalcemic and hypophosphatemic and have elevated iPTH values, all known stimuli of the synthesis of this metabolite (188). It is likely that under these circumstances the values for $1,25(OH)_2D$ should actually be supranormal. In general, the values for 25(OH)D are 0-5 ng/ml. For $24,25(OH)_2D$, they are not detectable (vs. 1.5-4.0 ng/ml normally). For $1,25(OH)_2D$, the values are 25-50 pg/ml (vs. 20-60 pg/ml normally) (188). Because of these differences, it is probably best to term this disorder 25(OH)D deficiency.

Currently, six groups appear to be at risk for 25(OH)D deficiency: premature infants, vegetarian Asiatics living in Europe, strict vegetarians and their offspring, the elderly, patients receiving long-term anticonvulsant therapy, and patients with gastrointestinal malabsorption of vitamin D (189,190). The rickets of prematurity is seen at about 12 weeks of age in rapidly growing infants whose bone growth demands large amounts of calcium and phosphate. Most infants affected have been fed low phosphate formulas, such as human breast milk or soy-protein milk (190). The values for 25(OH)D in sera are low (191-193), but increasing the phosphate content of the diet appears to improve this condition (194). Asiatics living in large European urban areas eating a "vegan diet" have a high incidence of osteomalacia (184,185,195), and treatment of these individuals with vitamin D_3 (75 μg daily) will heal bone disease, correct hyperphosphaturia, and cause $1,25(OH)_2D$ values to rise to greater than 120 pg/ml (185). Serum $24,25(OH)_2D$ values will become normal only after 25(OH)D values do.

An epidemic of rickets has been described among black children living in cities on the East Coast of the United States whose parents belong to religious sects that require dietary restriction and a distinctive dress of all members (196). The children are breast-fed for several years and eat only a vegetarian diet. Their mothers wear dark robes exposing only the forehead and eyes. This combination of poor calcium, phosphate, and vitamin D intake in conjunction with scant exposure to sunlight leads to rickets in these children. Rickets in the elderly is related to the same group of features: inadequate dietary sources of minerals and vitamin D and poor sunshine exposure. Another pathogenic factor in the aged is the very low circulating values for $1,25(OH)_2D$ found in patients in the sixth decade and beyond (197).

A final group at particular risk are nonambulatory patients treated with anticonvulsants. Since 1968 it has been appreciated that some patients with epilepsy receiving phenytoin and phenobarbital develop hypophosphatemia and phosphaturia along with elevated serum alkaline phosphatase activity (198-202). These drugs appear to enhance the conversion of 25-(OH)D to inactive products outside the normal vitamin D metabolic pathway (199). Since patients have calcium malabsorption, 25(OH)D deficiency, and elevated iPTH concentrations, it could be anticipated that $1,25(OH)_2D$ levels would be normal. The levels are quite normal in man (188,203), and the activity of 1α-hydroxylase is increased in chickens (204).

Therapy of D-deficiency hypophosphatemia is straightforward: Replace vitamin D in doses large enough to correct intestinal calcium absorption and reduce iPTH secretion to raise the serum phosphate level (188,202,205). Usually, daily doses of 10-30 μg (400-1200 U) are sufficient. Obviously, if patients would also drink vitamin D-fortified milk, which contains calcium and phosphate, the healing of rickets would be accelerated.

D. Vitamin D-Dependency Rickets

This autosomal recessive disorder was initially described by Fraser and Salter (206) and by Prader et al. (207) and is now known as autosomal recessive vitamin D-dependent rickets (ARVDDR). This disorder presents earlier than any other form of rickets, at 12 weeks of life (Table 3), with hypocalcemia, irritability, convulsions, and a bulging fontanelle (208). These children demonstrate the classic radiological features of rickets, aminoaciduria, phos-

Table 3 Clinical Features of the Forms of Rickets in Which Vitamin D Is Important

	Vitamin D-deficiency rickets	Primary hypophosphatemic rickets	Vitamin D-dependency rickets	Vitamin D-dependency rickets not responsive to calcitriol
Bone disease	Rickets Bowing	Rickets Bowing	Rickets Bowing	Rickets Bowing
Muscle weakness	Yes	No	Yes	Yes
Age of onset	9-12 months	12-18 months	3-6 months	3-6 months
Serum calcium level	↓	Normal or slightly ↓	↓	↓
Serum phosphate level	↓	↓	↓	↓
Serum alkaline phosphatase	↑	↑	↑	↑
Serum immunoreactive PTH level	↑	Normal or minimal ↑	↑	↑
Increased aminoaciduria	Yes	No	Yes	Yes
$TmPO_4$ at endogenous (PO_4)	↓	↓	↓	↓
Urinary phosphate at:				
Endogenous levels	↑	↑	↑	↑
Loaded levels	↑	↑	↑	↑
Intestinal calcium absorption	↓	↓ or normal	↓	↓
Genetics	None	X-linked dominant Autosomal dominant Autosomal recessive	Autosomal recessive	Autosomal recessive: often in offspring of consanguineous mating between first cousins; Alopecia, common
Response to 10 μg vitamin D_3/day	Curative	None	None	None
Response to 2 μg $1,25(OH)_2D_3$/day	Curative	None	Curative	None
Response to 1 mg vitamin D_3/day	Curative Hypercalcemia	Rickets partially healed Hypophosphatemia persists	Curative	Bone disease partially healed hypophosphatemia corrected
Oral phosphate supplementation		Heals rickets increased growth		

phaturia, and hypophosphatemia with very high iPTH values. Severe tooth enamel hypoplasia is found and indicates hypocalcemia in early life (209). The finding that 100,000 U or more is required to correct the plasma mineral abnormalities and the rickets suggests a defect in vitamin D metabolism. Small doses of 1,25$(OH)_2$D or its 1α-hydroxy analog will reverse all the features of this disorder (208,210,211). Moreover, when plasma values of 1,25$(OH)_2$D have been measured, they are markedly reduced, averaging 6-9 pg/ml (208,212).

The diagnosis of this condition can be established by several features: hypocalcemia and hypophosphatemia at an early age, enamel hypoplasia, very low 1,25$(OH)_2$D concentrations despite adequate vitamin D intake or even high-dose therapy, and the finding of siblings with this condition whose parents are normal (208,209). This condition is far more rare than either vitamin D deficiency or primary hypophosphatemia.

The therapy of this condition is specifically the 1α-hydroxylated vitamin D metabolites. Daily therapy at 1-3 μg will cure the disease in most cases (208-210,213), but the curative doses of 1,25$(OH)_2$D may vary, indicating some heterogeneity in this condition (213). Obviously, the dose needed to initially heal rickets and reverse hyperphosphaturia and iPTH secretion is higher than the maintenance dose of 1,25$(OH)_2$D (208,213).

What is currently unclear is the precise intracellular location of the defect in 1,25$(OH)_2$D synthesis. There could be a defect in 25(OH)D transport across cell membranes, a defect in 25(OH)D binding in renal tubular epithelium, a transport defect at the mitochondrial membranes, or a variety of abnormalities in the 25(OH)D-1α-hydroxylase enzyme per se. As with any inborn error of vitamin metabolism, one may have defective apoenzyme, deficient apoenzyme, or abnormalities of the various components of the enzyme, which include an iron-sulfur protein and a flavoprotein (214). With the development of methods aimed at measuring the 1α-hydroxylase activity in mammalian kidney, it may become possible to delineate the defect (215). Studies in a Hanoverian pig strain with an animal model of ARVDDR may also offer clues to the nature of this enzyme defect (216).

E. Vitamin D-Dependent Rickets Not Responsive to 1,25$(OH)_2$D (Vitamin D-Dependent Rickets Type II)

In rare instances, patients with vitamin D-dependent rickets have been identified who fail to respond to high-dose vitamin D_2 or physiological doses of 1,25$(OH)_2$D that ordinarily cure ARVDDR (217-223). The circulating values of 1,25$(OH)_2$D in these patients are greater than 150 pg/ml (or more than five times normal), and therapy with 1,25$(OH)_2$D may raise these values to more than 300 pg/ml without any regression of the biochemical and radiological symptoms. Bell (224,225) has suggested what appears to be a refractoriness of target organs to 1,25$(OH)_2$D and uses the term vitamin D-dependent rickets type II.

Secondary hyperparathyroidism is evident from measurement of serum values, bone histological demonstration of osteitis fibrosa, augmented urinary cAMP excretion, and aminoaciduria (218,226). The elevated plasma concentrations of 1,25$(OH)_2$D are related to this hyperparathyroidism; the even higher values after vitamin D administration are also most likely related to iPTH action. Since vitamin D therapy will normally suppress the synthesis of (or at least the plasma values for) 1,25$(OH)_2$D (227), the even higher values of 1,25-$(OH)_2$D after vitamin D therapy indirectly imply a defect in the binding of this active metabolite. Two other lines of evidence suggest a receptor defect. First, intestinal ^{47}Ca absorption is impaired, despite the high 1,25$(OH)_2$D concentrations (219,223,226). Second, the binding of radiolabeled 1,25$(OH)_2$D to the nuclear receptors of cultured skin fibroblasts is reduced in these patients as compared to controls (Fig. 5) (228).

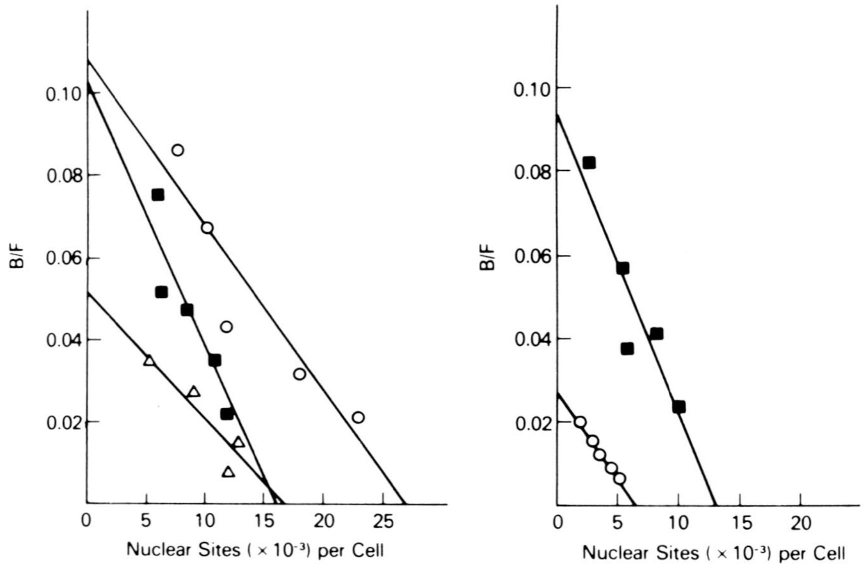

Fig. 5a The nuclear uptake of tritiated (^{3}H-1,25$(OH)_2D_3$) by the skin fibroblast cultured from normal subjects. Shown in the figure is the ratio of bound to free hormone (B/F) and the number of nuclear binding sites X 10^{-3} per cell. Symbols represent individual patients.

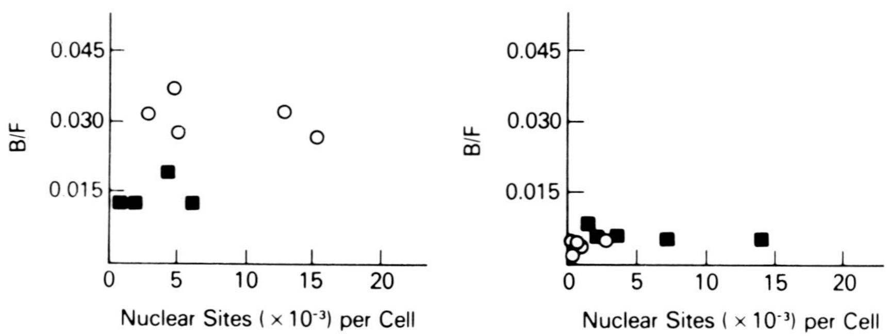

Fig. 5b The nuclear uptake of tritiated 1,25$(OH)_2D_3$ by skin fibroblast cultured from patients with type II vitamin D-dependent rickets. In this figure, no specific binding was detectable in numerous passages of these cells (From Ref. 228.)

An important subset of this syndrome has, in addition, alopecia totalis and short stature as prominent features (217,220-223) (Fig. 6). This form of type II vitamin D-dependent rickets is familial, and affected children are often the products of consanguineous mating between first cousins. Sibling pairs have all the common biochemical and histological features of vitamin D-dependent rickets.

Treatment of this form of rickets is difficult, and doses of 1,25$(OH)_2$D between 5 and 40 μg daily may be necessary. In one unusual patient who was receiving 17.5 mg of vitamin D_2 each day, the serum 25(OH)D concentration was only 18 ng/ml, and the value for 1,25-$(OH)_2$D was 21.2 ng/ml (21,200 pg/ml) (226). A dose of 20-50 μg of 25(OH)D corrected the osteomalacia and hypophosphatemia for reasons that are unclear. Another patient appeared to respond to oral 24,25$(OH)_2$D treatment (222).

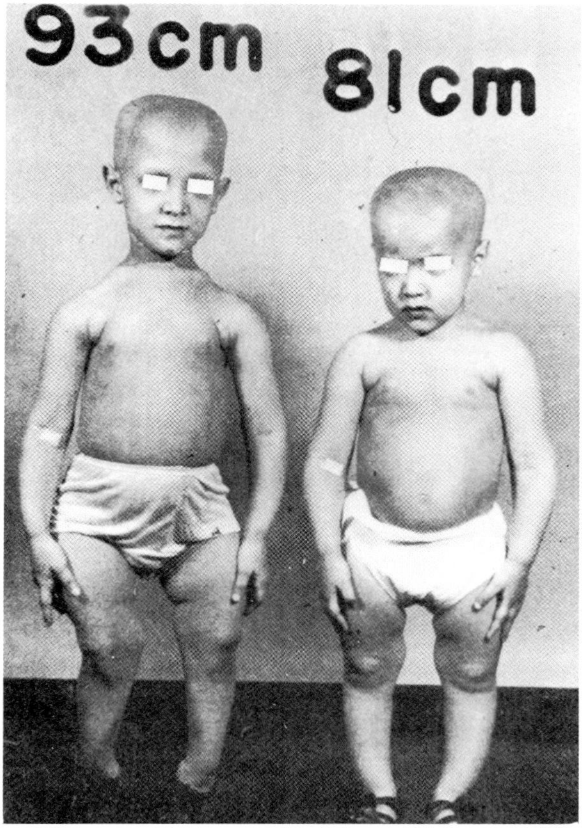

Fig. 6 The typical phenotype features of two boys with type II vitamin D-resistant rickets and alopeica. The boy on the left is 93 cm tall, the one on the right 81 cm. (From Ref. 220.)

Several of these patients have become pregnant and delivered normal offspring (225,229). Cord blood values for 1,25$(OH)_2$D are excessively high, and transient mild hypercalcemia is found. None of the offspring are affected, since these children are heterozygotes.

F. Oncogenous Rickets with Phosphaturia

Another condition with hypophosphatemia and osteomalacia and for which there is less evidence for an abnormality in vitamin D metabolism is oncogenous rickets (230). Hyperphosphaturia with rickets or endosteal osteomalacia has been described in approximately 30 patients with tumors of soft tissue or bone or with a hereditary syndrome involving dysplasia of mesenchymal tissue, such as polyostotic fibrous dysplasia, neurofibromatosis, or the epidermal nevus syndrome (231,232). These patients have primary hyperphosphaturia not related to elevated iPTH values and have normocalcemia, normal renal function, and no evidence of generalized aminoaciduria. A clinical resemblance between these patients and patients with adult sporadic hypophosphatemic osteomalacia is apparent (233,234), since both groups demonstrate marked bone pain, muscle weakness, Looser-Milkman zones, malaise, and a decline in stature from the collapse of vertebral bodies. Finally, both groups often have hyperglycinuria as an isolated aminoaciduria.

Table 4 Tumor Types Associated With Hypophosphatemic Osteomalacia (Oncogenous Rickets)

Author	Tumor type	Site	Surgical cure
McCance	Degenerating osteoid tumor	Femur	Yes
Hague	Malignant neurolemmoma	Axilla	No
Prader	Reparative giant cell granuloma	Rib	Yes
Dent	Degenerative osteoid tissue	Thigh	Yes
Yoshikawa	Cavernous hemangioma	Thigh	Yes
Castleman	Giant cell tumor	Femur	Yes
Balsan	Dense fibrous bony tissue	Calvarium	Yes
Salassa	Benign sclerosing hemangioma	Groin	Yes
Salassa	Benign sclerosing hemangioma	Thigh	Yes
Evans	Hemangiopericytoma	Femur	Partial
Stanbury	Malignant mesenchymoma	Fibula	No
Stanbury	Malignant mesenchymoma	Lower leg	No
Olefsky	Ossifying mesenchymal tumor	Pharynx	Yes
Pollack	Nonossifying fibroma	Radius	Yes
Wyman	Malignant pleomorphic tumor	Tibia	Yes
Drezner	Giant cell tumor	Iliac wing	Yes
Daniels	Multiple sclerosing hemangioma	Skull, ribs, pelvis	No
Moser	Ossifying mesenchymal tumor	Toe	Yes
Willhoite	Ossifying mesenchymal tumor	Ulna	Yes
Luiovitz	Hemangiopericytoma	Malleolus	Yes
Luiovitz	Hemangiopericytoma	Knee	No
Peacock	Benign chondroblastoma	Not reported	Not reported
Fukumoto	Benign osteoblastoma	Tibia	Yes
Nortman	Mesenchymoma	Nasal	No
Dent	Not identified	Nasal antrum	Yes
Dent	Not identified	Nasal antrum	Yes
Dent	Not identified	Rectus abdominus sheath	Yes
Parker	Giant cell tumor	Distal radius	Yes

Source: Adapted from Simpson, D.P.; Wen, S.E.; and Chesney, R.W. Fluid and electrolyte abnormalities of malignancy. In: Cancer and the Kidney, edited by Frei, E., III; and Reisselbach, R.H. Philadelphia, Lea & Febiger, 1981.

Some as yet uncharacterized substance within the tumor directly causes hyperphosphaturia (230,233). Approximately 75% of the cases reported have regression of the hypophosphatemic osteomalacia by surgical excision of the tumor. In metastatic tumors, complete removal of tumor is impossible, and phosphate wasting continues (235-237) (Table 4). Histological classification of these tumors has been clouded by the plethora of names given, and the basic tumor type is an ossifying mesenchymal tumor of bone or soft tissue (237), found to be made up of osteoclasts, osteoid, collagen, cartilage, or vascular elements. After successful tumor excision, hypophosphatemia and hyperphosphaturia return to normal.

In four recently described cases (patients #16,23,24, and 28 in Table 4), there is a defect in vitamin D metabolism with normal 25(OH)D values and very reduced $1,25(OH)_2D$ values (238-241). These patients differ from the bulk of patients with oncogenous rickets in that they have generalized aminoaciduria (238,239,241) and elevated iPTH values (238,241) as well as glucosuria. Therapy with $1,25(OH)_2D$ at 2.5-3.0 μg daily improved calcium and phosphate balance and led to bone healing in two of the children (239,240). After tumor excision, serum $1,25(OH)_2D$ values rose into the normal range.

That a failure of the conversion of 25(OH)D to 1,25$(OH)_2$D by the kidney is at the heart of this disorder seems unlikely for several reasons. The hypocalcemia, aminoaciduria, and elevated iPTH values of vitamin D deficiency are unusual in patients with these tumors (115, 230). Secondly, homogenates of the tumor infused into laboratory animals cause renal tubular phosphate wasting (242), suggesting a direct local action of the tumor. As Parker et al. (238) suggest, "The rapid correction of phosphorus excretion that we found postoperatively would be consistent with a (tumoral) phosphaturic substance in addition to the altered metabolism of vitamin D."

Removal of tumor is the best form of therapy, but oral phosphate supplements may help alleviate bone pain and myopathy. Oral 1,25$(OH)_2$D therapy can be given if surgery must be postponed.

G. Adult Sporadic Hypophosphatemic Osteomalacia

Patients who develop hypophosphatemic osteomalacia between the ages of 15 and 60 are said to have the syndrome of adult sporadic hypophosphatemic osteomalacia (244,245). The typical patient has onset at ages 20-35 or after 50 years, and there is no previous history of rickets, short stature, bone pain, or bone disease. The typical patient manifests profound bone pain, myopathy, Looser-Milkman zones, and collapsed "codfish" vertebrae (246). The spine is particularly affected, and compression fractures result in considerable loss of height. As noted previously, hyperglycinuria is common, and glucosuria may also be found.

Patients are normocalcemic and have serum phosphate values in the range of 2.0-2.5 mg/dl (0.5-0.7 mmol/liter), with a mild elevation of serum alkaline phosphatase activity (247). The $TmPO_4$/GFR is reduced and, as in nonrachitic hypophosphatemic bone disease, normal urinary phosphate excretion values are evident at the endogenous levels of phosphate. Marked hyperphosphaturia (>1500 mg/24 hr) is found after phosphate loading (244,248).

The pathogenesis of this disorder is uncertain, but neither hyperparathyroidism or excessive calcitonin secretion are found (249). Subtotal parathyroidectomy does not change the hyperphosphaturia and hypophosphatemia (250,251). Nonetheless, several cases of parathyroid adenomas have been found in patients with adult sporadic hypophosphatemic osteomalacia (244,250,251), presumably related to reduced intestinal calcium absorption and negative calcium balance with years of hyperplasia of the glands leading to adenoma formation. No evidence for a defect in vitamin D metabolism is found, since exogenous 1,25$(OH)_2$D therapy will improve intestinal ^{47}Ca absorption and increase urinary calcium and phosphate excretion, but it does not affect hypophosphatemia and bone mineralization (252). The plasma values for 25(OH)D, 24,25$(OH)_2$D, and 1,25$(OH)_2$D are in the normal range, and even after raising both 25(OH)D and 1,25$(OH)_2$D values by treatment, hypophosphatemia is unchanged (249). These findings suggest a PTH-independent and vitamin D-independent renal phosphate leak. It is possible that some of these patients have occult mesenchymal tumors capable of elaborating a phosphaturic substance; clearly, the presence of tumor should be sought. Nonetheless, the pathogenesis of the phosphate leak and of the glycine leak remains uncertain.

The diagnosis of this condition is made by the history of pains in muscle, bones, joints, or "the princess-on-the-pea syndrome" (247), or by malaise and numbness. Radiological abnormalities are fairly distinctive, with markedly diminished bone density, reduced cortical thickness, and after years codfish vertebrae, kyphosis, scoliosis, and angulation of bones (248). The symptoms are so much like the phosphate depletion syndrome (7) that a careful inquiry regarding the use of aluminum hydroxide-containing antacids should be obtained.

Treatment with vitamin D and oral phosphate supplements will improve all symptoms (244,245,247-249,252). Either 1α-hydroxy analogs (1-2 μg/day), 25(OH)D (50-100 μg/day), or vitamin D_2 (100,000-300,000 U/day) are used and result in increased ^{47}Ca absorption and improved calcium and phosphate balance. Both radiological and histological evidence of bone healing can be found, but with rare exceptions (253), phosphate and vitamin D must be given for life. Because of the overlap in findings between these patients and those with oncogenous rickets a thorough search for a tumor is needed.

REFERENCES

1. Harrison, H. E.; and Harrison, H. C. Disorders of Calcium and Phosphate Metabolism in Childhood and Adolescence, Philadelphia, Saunders, 1979, pp. 53-84.
2. Raisz, L. G. Bone metabolism and calcium regulation. In: Metabolic Bone Disease, vol. 1, edited by Avioli, L. V., and Karne, S. M. New York, Acadmic Press, 1977, pp. 1-49.
3. Lenninger, A. L. Catabolism and the generation of phosphate-bond energy in biochemistry: The molecular basis of cell structure and function. In: Biochemistry, New York, Worth, 1970, pp. 267-481.
4. Massry, S. G.; and Fleisch, H. The Renal Handling of Phosphate. New York, Plenum Press, 1980.
5. Massry, S. G.; Friedler, R. M.; and Coburn, J. W. Excretion of phosphate and calcium: Physiology of their renal handling and relation to clinical medicine. Arch. Intern. Med. 131:828-859, 1973.
6. Trohler, U.; Bonjour, J. P.; and Fleisch, H. Inorganic phosphate homeostasis: Renal adaptation to the dietary intake of phosphate in intact and thyroparathyroidectomized rats. J. Clin. Invest. 54:264-273, 1976.
7. Lotz, M.; Zisman, E.; and Bartter, F. C. Evidence for a phosphorus-depletion syndrome in man. N. Engl. J. Med. 278:409-415, 1968.
8. Harris, C. A.; Sutton, R. A. L.; and Dirks, J. H. Effects of hypercalcemia on calcium and phosphate ultrafilterability and tubular reabsorption in the rat. Am. J. Physiol. 233: F201-F206, 1977.
9. Amiel, C. Sites of renal tubular reabsorption of phosphate. In: The Renal Handling of Phosphate, edited by Massry, S. G., and Fleisch, H. New York, Plenum Press, 1980, pp. 39-55.
10. Lang, F. Renal handling of calcium and phosphate. Klin. Wochenschr. 58:985-1003, 1980.
11. Poujeol, P.; Corman, B.; Touvay, C.; and de Rouffignac, C. Phosphate reabsorption in rat nephron terminal segments: Intrarenal heterogeneity and strain differences. Pflugers Arch. 371:39-44, 1977.
12. Hoffmann, N.; Thees, M.; and Kinne, R. Phosphate transport by isolated renal brush border vesicles. Pflugers Arch. 362:147-156, 1976.
13. Dennis, V. W.; Stead, W. W.; and Myers, J. L. Renal handling of phosphate and calcium. Ann. Rev. Physiol. 41:257-271, 1979.
14. Knox, F. G.; Osswald, H.; Marchand, G. R.; Spielman, W. S.; Haas, J. A.; Berndt, T.; and Youngberg, S. P. Phosphate transport along the tubule. Am. J. Physiol. 233:F261-F268, 1977.
15. Gradowska, L.; Caglar, S.; Rutherford, E.; Harter, H.; and Slatopolsky, E. On the mechanism of the phosphaturia of extracellular fluid volume expansion in the dog. Kidney Int. 3:230-237, 1973.
16. Dennis, V. W.; Woodhall, P. B.; and Robinson, R. R. Characteristics of phosphate transport in isolated proximal tubule. Am. J. Physiol. 231:797-785, 1976.
17. Drezner, M.; Neelon, F. A.; and Lebovitz, H. W. Pseudohypoparathyroidism type II: A possible defect in the reception of the cyclic-AMP signal. N. Engl. J. Med. 389:1056-1060, 1973.

18. Schneider, E. G.; Hanson, R. C.; Childers, J. W.; Fitzgerald, E. M.; and Gleason, S. D. Is phosphate secreted by the kidney? In: The Renal Handling of Phosphate, edited by Massry, S. G., and Fleisch, H. New York, Plenum Press, 1980, pp. 59-78.
19. Knox, F. G.; Schneider, E. G.; Willis, L. R.; Strandhoy, J. W.; and Ott, C. E. Site and control of phosphate reabsorption by the kidney. Kidney Int. 3:347-353, 1973.
20. Greger, R. F.; Lang, F. C.; Knox, F. G.; and Lechene, C. R. Absence of significant secretory flux of phosphate in the proximal convoluted tubule. Am. J. Physiol. 232:F235-F238, 1977.
21. Lau, K.; Goldfarb, S.; and Goldberg, M. The effects of parathyroid hormone on renal phosphate handling. In: The Renal Handling of Phosphate, edited by Massry, S. G., and Fleisch, H. New York, Plenum Press, 1980, pp. 115-135.
22. Kinne, R.; Berner, W.; Hoffmann, H.; and Murer, H. Phosphate transport by isolated renal and intestinal plasma membranes. Adv. Exp. Med. Biol. 81:265-277, 1977.
23. Aurbach, G. D.; and Heath, D. Parathyroid hormone and calcitonin regulation of renal function. Kidney Int. 6:331-345, 1974.
24. Chase, L. R.; and Aurbach, G. D. Parathyroid function and the renal excretion of 3',5' adenylic acid. Proc. Natl. Acad. Sci, USA 58:518-525, 1967.
25. Chase, L. R.; and Aurbach, G. D. Renal adenyl cyclase: Anatomically separate sites for parathyroid hormone and vasopressin. Science 159:545-547, 1968.
26. Kinne, R.; Shlatz, L. J.; Kinne-Saffnan, E.; and Schwartz, I. L. Distribution of membrane-bound cyclic AMP-dependent protein kinase in plasma membranes of cells of the kidney cortex. J. Membr. Biol. 24:145-159, 1975.
27. Shlatz, L. J.; Schwartz, I. L.; Kinne-Saffran, E.; and Kinne, R. Distribution of parathyroid hormone-stimulated adenylate cyclase in plasma membranes of cells of the kidney cortex. J. Membr. Biol. 24:131-144, 1975.
28. Rasmussen, H.; Pechet, M.; and Fast, D. Effect of dibutyryl cyclic adenosine 3',5'-monophosphate, theophylline and other nucleotides upon calcium and phosphate metabolism. J. Clin. Invest. 47:1843-1850, 1968.
29. Lorentz, W. B., Jr. Effect of parathyroid hormone on renal tubular permeability. Am. J. Physiol. 231:1401-1407, 1976.
30. Kaminsky, N. I.; Broadus, A. E.; Hardman, J. G.; Jones, D. L., Jr.; Ball, J. H.; Sutherland, E. W.; and Liddle, G. W. Effects of parathyroid hormone on plasma and urinary adenosine 3'5'-monophosphate in man. J. Clin. Invest. 49:2387-2395, 1970.
31. Chabardes, D.; Imbert, M.; and Morel, F. Localization of PTH action sites along the rabbit nephron. In: Phosphate Metabolism in Kidney and Bone, International Workshop, edited by Avioli, L. V., Bordier, P., Fleisch, H., Massry, S., and Slatopolsky, E. Paris, Nouvelle Imprimerie, 1975, pp. 123-132.
32. Popovtzer, M. M.; Flis, R. S.; Mahandru, S. S.; and Blum, M. Effect of the divalent cation Ionophore (A23187) on renal handling of phosphorus. Kidney Int. 12:164-171, 1977.
33. Steele, T. H. Renal resistance to parathyroid hormone during phosphorus deprivation. J. Clin. Invest. 58:1461-1464, 1976.
34. Harter, H. R.; Mercado, A. M.; Rutherford, W. E.; Rodriguez, H.; Slatopolsky, E.; and Klahr, S. Effects of phosphate depletion and parathyroid hormone on renal glucose reabsorption. Am. J. Physiol. 227:1422-1427, 1974.
35. Agus, Z. S.; Puschett, J. B.; Senesky, D.; and Goldberg, M. Mode of action of parathyroid hormone and cyclic adenosine 3'5'-monophosphate on renal tubular phosphate reabsorption in the dog. J. Clin. Invest. 50:617-626, 1971.
36. Arruda, J. A. L.; Nascimento, L.; Westenfelder, C.; and Kurtzman, N. A. Effect of parathyroid hormone on urinary acidification. Am. J. Physiol. 232:F423-F429, 1977.
37. Ullrich, K. J. Mechanisms of cellular and subcellular transport of phosphate. In: Proceedings of the 3rd International Workshop of Phosphate. Madrid, 1977, pp. 3-10.

38. Hirsch, P. F.; and Munson, P. L. Thyrocalcitonin. Physiol. Rev. 49:548-622, 1969.
39. Ritz, E.; Kreusser, W.; and Bommer, J. Effects of hormones other than parathyroid hormones on renal handling of phosphate. In: The Renal Handling of Phosphate, edited by Massry, S. G., and Fleisch, H. New York, Plenum Press, 1980, pp. 137-196.
40. Marx, S. J.; and Aurbach, G. D. Renal receptors for calcitonin: Coordinate occurence with calcitonin-activated adenylate cyclase. Endocrinology 97:448-453, 1975.
41. Kurokawa, K.; Nagata, N.; Sasaki, M.; and Nakane, K. Effects of calcitonin on the concentration of cyclic adenosine 3'5'-monophosphate in rat kidney in vivo and in vitro. Endocrinology 94:1514-1518, 1974.
42. Levine, B. S.; Brautbar, N.; and Coburn, J. W. Does vitamin D affect the renal handling of calcium and phosphorus? Miner. Electrolyte Metab. 1:295-302, 1978.
43. Popovtzer, M. M.; and Robinette, J. B. Effect of 25(OH)-vitamin D_3 on urinary excretion of cyclic adenosine monophosphate. Am. J. Physiol. 229:907-910, 1975.
44. DeLuca, H. F. The vitamin D system in the regulation of calcium and phosphorus metabolism. W.O. Atwater Memorial Lecture, Nutrit, Rev. 37:161-193, 1979.
45. Eisenberg, E. Effects of serum calcium level and parathyroid extract on phosphate and calcium excretion in hypoparathyroid patients. J. Clin. Invest. 44:942-945, 1965.
46. Lavender, A. R.; and Pullman, T. N. Changes in inorganic phosphate excretion induced by renal arterial infusion of calcium. Am. J. Physiol. 205:1025-1032, 1963.
47. Puschett, J. B.; and Kuhrman, M. S. Renal tubular effects of 1,25-dihydroxyvitamin D_3: Interactions with vasopressin and parathyroid hormone in the vitamin D-depleted rat. J. Lab. Clin. Med. 92:895-903, 1978.
48. Bonjour, J. P.; and Fleisch, H. Calcium supply and renal handling of phosphate. Miner. Electrolyte Metab. 3:261-267, 1980.
49. Trohler, U.; Bonjour, J. P.; and Fleisch, H. Inorganic phosphate homeostasis: Renal adaptation to the dietary intake in intact and thyroparathyroidectomized rats. J. Clin. Invest. 57:264-273, 1976.
50. Steele, T. H.; and DeLuca, H. F. Influence of dietary phosphorus on renal phosphate reabsorption in the parathyroidectomized rat. J. Clin. Invest. 57:867-874, 1976.
51. Bonjour, J. P.; Trohler, U.; Preston, C.; and Fleisch, H. Parathyroid hormone and renal handling of Pi: Effect of dietary Pi and diphosphonates. Am. J. Physiol. 234:F497-F505, 1978.
52. Stoll, R.; Kinne, R.; and Murer, H. Effect of dietary phosphate intake on phsophate transport by isolated rat renal brush-border vesicles. Biochem. J. 180:465-470, 1979.
53. Bonjour, J. P.; Preston, C.; and Fleisch, H. Effect of 1,25-dihydroxyvitamin D_3 on the renal handling of Pi in thyroparathyroidectomized rats. J. Clin. Invest. 60:1419-1428, 1977.
54. Gloor, H. J.; Bonjour, J. P.; Caverzasio, J.; and Fleisch, H. Resistance to the phosphaturic and calcaemic actions of parathyroid hormone during phosphate depletion. J. Clin. Invest. 63:371-377, 1979.
55. Agus, Z. S.; Wasserstein, A.; and Goldfarb, S. PTH, calcitonin, cyclic nucleotides and the kidney. Ann. Rev. Physiol. 43:583-595, 1981.
56. Frick, A.; and Dursasin, I. Maximal reabsorptive capacity for inorganic phosphate (Tm_{Pi}) in the absence of parathyroid hormone in the rat: Decrease of the Tm_{Pi} during prolonged administration of phosphate and the role of calcium. Pflugers Arch. 377:9-14, 1978.
57. Oberleithner, H.; Lang, F.; Greger, R.; and Sporer, H. Influence of calcium and ionophore 23187 on tubular phosphate reabsorption. Pflugers Arch. 379:37-41, 1979.
58. Ginsburg, J. N. Effect of glucose and free fatty acid on phosphate transport in dog kidney. Am. J. Physiol. 222:1153-1160, 1972.
59. Pitts, R. F.; and Alexander, R. S. The renal reabsorptive mechanism for inorganic phosphate in normal and acidotic dogs. Am. J. Physiol. 142:648-666, 1944.

60. Cohen, J. J.; Berglund, E.; and Lotspeich, W. D. Renal tubular reabsorption of acetoacetate, inorganic sulfate and inorganic phosphate in the dog as affected by glucose and phloridzin. Am. J. Physiol. 184:91-96, 1956.
61. Segal, S.; Thier, S.; Fox, M.; and Rosenberg, L. Inhibitory effect of sugars on amino acid accumulation by slices of rat kidney cortex. Biochim. Biophys. Acta 65:567-568, 1962.
62. Harrison, H. E.; and Harrison, H. C. Experimental production of renal glycosuria, phosphaturia and aminoaciduria by injection of maleic acid. Science 120:606-608, 1954.
63. Csaky, T. Z.; Prachnamboli, K.; Eiseman, B.; and Ho, P. M. The effect of digitalis on the renal tubular transport of glucose in normal and heartless dogs. J. Pharmacol. Exp. Ther. 150:275-284, 1964.
64. Evers, C.; Murer, H.; and Kinne, R. Effect of parathyrin on the transport properties of isolated renal brush border vesicles. Biochem. J. 172:49-56, 1978.
65. DeFronzo, R. A.; Goldberg, N.; and Agus, Z. S. The effects of glucose and insulin on renal electrolyte transport. J. Clin. Invest. 58:83-90, 1975.
66. Harter, H. R.; Mercado, A.; Rutherford, W. E.; Rodriguez, H.; Slatopolsky, E.; and Klahr, S. Effects of phosphate depletion and parathyroid hormone on renal glucose reabsorption. Am. J. Physiol. 227:1422-1427, 1974.
67. Scriver, C. R.; Chesney, R. W.; and McInnes, R. R. Genetic aspects of renal tubular transport diversity and topology of carriers. Kidney Int. 9:149-171, 1976.
68. Curran, P. F. Active transport of amino acids and sugars. Arch. Int. Med. 129:258-269, 1972.
69. Rozen, R.; Tenenhouse, H. S.; and Scriver, C. R. Taurine transport in renal brush-border membrane vesicles. Biochem. J. 180:245-248, 1979.
70. Drummond, K. N.; and Michael, A. F. Specificity of the inhibition of tubular phosphate reabsorption by certain amino acids. Nature 201:1333-1334, 1964.
71. Reifenstein, E. C.; Kinsell, L. W.; and Albright, F. Observations on the use of the serum phosphorus level as an index of pituitary growth hormone activity; The effect of estrogen therapy in acromegaly. Endocrinology 39:71A, 1946.
72. Durand, D.; Prelot, M.; and Raoul, Y. Effets precoces de l'hormone de croissance sur les phosphates seriques et urinaires du rat. Experientia 32:120-122, 1976.
73. Corvilain, J.; and Abramow, M. Some effects of human growth hormone on renal hemodynamics and on tubular phosphate transport in man. J. Clin. Invest. 41:1230-1235, 1962.
74. Lee, D. B. N.; Brautbar, N.; Walling, M. W.; Silis, V.; Carlson, H. E.; Grindeland, R. E.; Coburn, J. W.; and Kleeman, C. R. Role of growth hormone in experimental phosphorus deprivation in the rat. Calcif. Tissue Int. 32:105-112, 1980.
75. Gallagher, J. C.; and Wilkinson, R. The effect of ethinyloestradiol on calcium and phosphorus metabolism of post-menopausal women with primary hyperparathyroidism. Clin. Sci. 45:785-802, 1973.
76. Anderson, J.; and Forster, J. B. Effect of cortisone on urinary phosphate excretion in man. Clin. Sci. 18:437-439, 1959.
77. Goldsmith, R. S.; Siemsen, A. W.; Mason, A. D., Jr.; and Forland, M. Primary role of plasma hydrocortisone concentration in the regulation of the normal forenoon pattern of urinary phosphate excretion. J. Clin. Endocrinol. 25:1649-1659, 1965.
78. Arruda, J. A. L.; Richardson, J. M.; Wolfson, J. A.; Nascimento, L.; Rademacher, D. R.; and Kurtzman, N. A. Lithium administration and phosphate excretion. Am. J. Physiol. 231:1140-1146, 1976.
79. Dennis, V. W.; Stead, W. W.; and Myers, J. L. Renal handling of phosphate and calcium. Ann. Rev. Physiol. 41:257-271, 1979.
80. Martinez-Maldonado, M.; and Eknoyan, G. Role of extracellular fluid volume expansion and diuretics in renal handling of phosphate. In: The Renal Handling of Phosphate, edited by Massry, S. G., and Fleisch, H. New York, Plenum Press, 1980, pp. 265-286.

81. Puschett, J. B.; and Goldberg, M. The relationship between the renal handling of phosphate and bicarbonate in man. J. Lab. Clin. Med. 73:965-969, 1969.
82. Besarab, A.; Silva, P.; Ross, B.; and Epstein, F. Bicarbonate and sodium reabsorption by the isolated perfused kidney. Am. J. Physiol. 228:1525-1530, 1975.
83. Beck, L. H.; and Goldberg, M. Effects of acetazolamide and parathyroidectomy on renal transport of sodium, calcium and phosphate. Am. J. Physiol. 224:1136-1142, 1973.
84. Rodriguez, H. J.; Walls, J.; Yates, J.; and Klahr, S. Effect of acetazolamide on the urinary excretion of cyclic AMP and on the activity of renal adenyl cyclase. J. Clin. Invest. 53:122-130, 1974.
85. Better, O. S.; Tuma, S.; Kedar, S.; and Chaimowitz, C. Enhanced tubular reabsorption of phosphate: Following relief of unilateral ureteral obstruction in man. Arch. Intern. Med. 135:245-248, 1975.
86. Chamiovitz, C.; Dickmeyer, J.; Friedler, R. M.; Kurokawa, K.; and Massry, S. G. Studies on mechanism of hypophosphaturia after relief of unilateral ureteral obstruction. Nephron 19:333-341, 1977.
87. Lehne, C.; and Coe, F. L. Compensatory phosphaturia after unilateral nephrectomy in the rat. Am. J. Physiol. 231:1625-1629, 1976.
88. Nordin, B. E. C.; and Fraser, R. Assessment of urinary phosphate excretion. Lancet 1:947-950, 1960.
89. Bijvoet, O. L. M. Indices for the measurement of the renal handling of phosphate. In: The Renal Handling of Phosphate, edited by Massry, S. G., and Fleisch, H. New York, Plenum Press, 1980, pp. 1-38.
90. Anonymous. Plasma-phosphate and tubular reabsorption of phosphate. Lancet 1:820-821, 1970.
91. Anderson, J.; and Parsons, V. The tubular maximal resorptive rate for inorganic phosphate in normal subjects. Clin. Sci. 25:431-441, 1963.
92. Bijvoet, O. L. M. Relation of plasma phosphate concentration to renal tubular absorption of phosphate. Clin. Sci. 37:23-36, 1969.
93. Stamp, T. C. B.; and Stacey, T. E. Evaluation of theoretical renal phosphorus threshold as an index of renal phosphorus handling. Clin. Sci. 39:505-516, 1970.
94. Walton, R. J.; and Bijvoet, O. L. M. Nomogram for the derivation of renal threshold phosphate concentration. Lancet 2:309-311, 1975.
95. Wesson, L. G. Electrolyte excretion in relation to diurnal cycles of renal function. Medicine 43:547-592, 1964.
96. Dossetor, J. B.; Gorman, H. M.; and Beck, J. C. The diurnal rhythm of urinary electrolyte excretion. I. Observations in normal subjects. Metabolism 12:1083-1099, 1963.
97. Robertson, W. G. Urinary excretion. In: Calcium, Phosphate and Magnesium Metabolism, edited by Nordin, B. E. C., London, Churchill Livingstone, 1976, pp. 113-161.
98. Goldman, R.; and Bassett, S. H. Renal regulation of phosphorus excretion. J. Clin. Endocrinol. 18:981-990, 1958.
99. Corvilain, J. Growth and renal control of plasma phosphate. J. Clin. Endocrinol. 16: 1507-1521, 1956.
100. Fraser, D.; and Scriver, C. R. Familial forms of vitamin D-resistant rickets revisited: X-linked hypophosphatemia and autosomal recessive vitamin D dependency. Am. J. Clin. Nutr. 29:1315-1329, 1976.
101. Williams, T. F.; Winters, R. W.; and Burnett, C. H. Familial (hereditary) vitamin D-resistant rickets with hypophosphatemia. In: The Metabolic Basis of Inherited Disease, edited by Stanbury, J. B., Wyngaarden, J. B., and Fredrickson, D. S. New York, McGraw-Hill, 1972, pp. 1465-1485.
102. Drezner, M. K.; Lyles, K. W.; Haussler, M. R.; and Harrelson, J. M. Evaluation of a role for 1,25-dihydroxyvitamin D_3 in the pathogenesis and treatment of X-linked hypophosphatemic rickets and osteomalacia. J. Clin. Invest. 66:1020-1032, 1980.

103. Glorieux, F. H.; Marie, P. J.; Pettilor, J. M.; and Delvin, E. E. Bone response to phosphate salts, ergocalciferol and calcitriol in hypophosphatemic vitamin D-resistant rickets. N. Engl. J. Med. 303:1023-1031, 1980.
104. Costa, T.; Marie, P. J.; Scriver, C. R.; Cole, D. E. C.; Reade, T. M.; Nogrady, B.; Glorieux, F. H.; and Delvin, E. E. X-linked hypophosphatemia: Effect of calcitriol on renal handling of phosphate, serum phosphate and bone mineralization. J. Clin. Endocrinol. Metab. 52:463-472, 1981.
105. Chesney, R. W. Tubular defects in phosphate reabsorption in clinical medicine. In: The Renal Handling of Phosphate, edited by Massry, S. G., and Fleisch, H. New York, Plenum Press, 1980, pp. 321-366.
106. Stickler, G. B.; Beabout, J. W.; and Riggs, B. L. Vitamin D-resistant rickets: Clinical experience with 41 typical familial hypophosphatemic patients and 2 atypical non-familial cases. Mayo Clin. Proc. 45:197-218, 1970.
107. Hahn, T. J.; Scharp, C. R.; Halstead, L. R.; Haddad, J. G.; Karl, D. M.; and Avioli, L. V. Parathyroid hormone status and renal responsiveness in familial hypophosphatemic rickets. J. Clin. Endocrinol. Metab. 41:926-937, 1975.
108. Chesney, R. W.; Mazess, R. B.; Rose, P.; Hamstra, A. J.; Deluca, H. F.; and Breed, A. L. Long-term influence of calcitriol and supplemental phosphate in X-linked hypophosphatemic rickets. Pediatrics 71:559-567, 1983.
109. Albright, F.; Butler, A. M.; and Bloomberg, E. Rickets resistant to vitamin D therapy. Am. J. Dis. Child. 54:529-547, 1937.
110. Arnaud, C ; Glorieux, F.; and Scriver, C. R. Serum parathyroid hormone in X-linked hypophosphatemia. Science 173:845-847, 1971.
111. Kleerekoper, M.; Coffey, R.; Greco, T.; Nichols, S.; Cooke, N.; Murphy, W.; and Avioli, L. V. Hypercalcemic hyperparathyroidism in hypophosphatemic rickets. J. Clin. Endocrinol. Metab. 45:86-94, 1977.
112. Tarwalkar, Y B.; Musgrave, J. E.; Buist, N. R. M.; Campbell, R. A.; and Campbell, J. R. Vitamin D-resistant rickets and parathyroid adenomas: Renal transport of phosphate. Am. J. Dis. Child. 128:704-708, 1974.
113. Glorieux, F.; and Scriver, C. R. Loss of a parathyroid hormone-sensitive component of phosphate transport in X-linked hypophosphatemia. Science 175:997-999, 1972.
114. Tenenhouse, H. S.; Scriver, C. R.; McInnes, R. R.; and Florieux, F. H. Renal handling of phosphate in vivo and in vitro by the X-linked hypophosphatemic male mouse (Hyp/Y): Evidence for a defect in the brush-border membrane. Kidney Int. 14:236-244, 1978.
115. Scriver, C. R. Rickets and the pathogenesis of impaired tubular transport of phosphate and other solutes. Am. J. Med. 57:43-49, 1974.
116. Scriver, C. R. Transepithelial transport of phosphate: Perspectives from man and mouse. In: Pediatric Diseases Related to Calcium, edited by DeLuca, H. F., and Anast, C. S. New york, Elsevier, 1980, pp. 165-178.
117. Glorieux, F. H.; and Scriver, C. R. Transport, metabolism and clinical use of inorganic phosphate in X-linked hypophosphatemia. In: The Clinical Aspects of Metabolic Bone Disease, edited by Frame, B., Parfitt, A. M., and Duncan, H. Amsterdam, Excerpta Medica ICS, 1973, pp. 421-426.
118. Glorieux, F. H.; and Scriver, C. R. Parathyroid hormone secretion in X-linked hypophosphatemia. N. Engl. J. Med. 290:1329-1330, 1974.
119. Lyles, K. W.; McNamara, C. R.; and Drezner, M. K. Coincidence of hypoparathyroidism and X-linked hypophosphatemic rickets: An experiment of nature illuminating the physiological factors which regulate the renal tubular defect. Calcif. Tissue Int. 33:309A, 1981.
120. Condon, J. R.; Nassim, J. R.; and Rutter, A. Pathogenesis of rickets and osteomalacia in familial hypophosphatemia. Arch. Dis. Child. 46:269-272, 1971.

121. Short, E. M.; Binder, H. J.; and Rosenberg, L. E. Familial hypophosphatemic rickets: Defective transport of inorganic phosphate by intestinal mucosa. Science 179:700-702, 1973.
122. Gerbaux-Balsan, S. L'absorption intestinale du phosphore dans le rachitisme vitamine-resistant hypophosphatemique herditaire: Effets de fortes surcharges de phosphore et des regimes tres pauvres en calcium. Rev. Fr. Etud. Clin. Biol. 10:65-72, 1965.
123. Glorieux, F. H.; Morin, C. L.; Travers, R.; Delvin, E. E.; and Porier, R. Intestinal phosphate transport in familial hypophosphatemia. Pediatr. Res. 10:691-696, 1976.
124. Walton, J. Familial hypophosphatemic rickets: A delineation of its subdivisions and pathogenesis. Clin. Pediatr. 15:1007-1012, 1976.
125. Falls, W. F., Jr.; Carter, N. W.; Rector, F. W.; and Seldin, D. W. Familial vitamin D-resistant rickets: Study of six cases with evaluation of the pathogenic role of secondary hyperparathyroidism. Ann. Intern. Med. 68:553-560, 1968.
126. Field, M. J.; and Reiss, E. Vitamin D-resistant rickets: The effect of calcium infusion on phosphate reabsorption. J. Clin. Invest. 39:1807-1812, 1960.
127. Short, E.; Morris, R. C., Jr.; and Spencer, M. Exaggerated phosphaturic response to circulating parathyroid hormone in patients with familial X-linked hypophosphatemic rickets. J. Clin. Invest. 58:152-163, 1976.
128. Lavender, A. R.; and Pullman, T. N. Changes in inorganic phosphate excretion induced by the renal arterial infusion of calcium. Am. J. Physiol. 205:1025-1032, 1963.
129. Glorieux, F. H.; Scriver, C. R.; Reade, T. M.; Goldman, H.; and Roseborough, A. Use of phosphate and vitamin D to prevent dwarfism and rickets in X-linked hypophosphatemia. N. Engl. J. Med. 287:481-487, 1972.
130. Morgan, J. M.; Hawley, W. L.; Chenoweth, A. I.; Retan, W. J.; and Diethelm, A. G. Renal transplantation in hypophosphatemia with vitamin D-resistant rickets. Arch. Intern. Med. 134:549-552, 1974.
131. Haddad, J. G., Jr.; Chyu, K. J.; Hahn, T. J.; and Stamp, T. C. B. Serum concentrations of 25-hydroxyvitamin D in sex-linked hypophosphatemic vitamin D-resistant rickets. J. Lab. Clin. Med. 81:22-27, 1973.
132. Balsan, S.; and Garabedian, M. 25-Hydroxycholecalciferol: A comparative study in deficiency rickets and different types of resistant rickets. J. Clin. Invest. 51:749-759, 1972.
133. Delvin, E. E.; and Glorieux, F. H. Serum 1,25-dihydroxyvitamin D concentration in hypophosphatemic vitamin D-resistant rickets. Calcif. Tissue Int. 33:173-175, 1981.
134. Chesney, R. W.; Mazess, R. B.; Rose, P.; Hamstra, A. J.; and DeLuca, H. F. Supranormal 25-hydroxyvitamin D and subnormal 1,25-dihydroxyvitamin D. Am. J. Dis. Child. 134:140-143, 1980.
135. Scriver, C. R.; Reade, T. M.; DeLuca, H. F.; and Hamstra, A. J. Serum 1,25-dihydroxyvitamin D levels in normal subjects and in patients with hereditary rickets or bone disease. N. Engl. J. Med. 299:976-979, 1978.
136. Posen, S. Personal communication.
137. Insogna, K.; Stewart, A.; and Gertner, J. Impaired response to acute phosphorus deprivation in sex-linked hypophosphatemic rickets. Calcif. Tissue Int. 33:315A, 1981.
138. Eicher, E. M.; Southard, J. L.; Scriver, C. R.; and Glorieux, F. H. Hypophosphatemia: Mouse model for human familial hypophosphatemic (vitamin D-resistant) rickets. Proc. Natl. Acad. Sci. USA 73:4667-4671, 1976.
139. O'Doherty, P. J. A.; DeLuca, H. F.; and Eicher, E. M. Intestinal calcium and phosphate transport in genetic hypophosphatemic mice. Biochem. Biophys. Res. Comm. 71:617-621, 1976.
140. Giasson, S. D.; Brunetti, M. G.; Danan, G.; Vigneault, N.; and Carriere, S. Micropuncture study of renal phosphorus transport in hypophosphatemic vitamin D-resistant rickets mice. Pflugers Arch. 371:33-38, 1977.

141. Tenenhouse, H. S.; and Scriver, C. R. Renal adaptation to phosphate deprivation in the Hyp mouse with X-linked hypophosphatemia. Can. J. Biochem. 57:938-944, 1979.
142. Cowgill, L. D.; Goldfarb, S.; Lau, K.; Slatopolsky, E.; Agus, Z. S. Evidence for an intrinsic renal tubular defect in mice with genetic hypophosphatemic rickets. J. Clin. Invest. 63:1023-1210, 1979.
143. Meyer, R. A., Jr.; Gray, R. W.; and Meyer, M. H. Abnormal vitamin D metabolism in the X-linked hypophosphatemic mouse. Endocrinology 107:1577-1581, 1980.
144. Meyer, R. A., Jr.; Gray, R. W.; Kiebzak, G. M.; Mish, P. M. Altered vitamin D, cyclic nucleotide and trace mineral metabolism in the X-linked hypophosphatemic mouse. In: Phosphate and Minerals in Health and Disease, edited by Massry, S. G. New York, Plenum Press, 1980, pp. 351-354.
145. Beamer, W. G.; Wilson, M. C.; and DeLuca, H. F. Successful treatment of genetically hypophosphatemic mice by 1α-hydroxyvitamin D_3 but not 1,25-dihydroxyvitamin D_3. Endocrinology 106:1949-1955, 1980.
146. Gorlin, R. Thoma's Oral Pathology, St. Louis, C. V. Mosby, 1970, p. 117.
147. Chesney, R. W.; Mazess, R. B.; Rose, P.; and Jax, D. K. Bone mineral status measured by direct photon absorptiometry in childhood renal disease. Pediatrics 60:864-872, 1977.
148. Harrison, J. E.; Cumming, W. A.; Fornasier, V.; Fraser, D.; Kooh, S. W.; and McNeill, K. G. Increased bone mineral content in young adults with familial hypophosphatemic vitamin D refractory rickets. Metabolism 25:33-40, 1976.
149. Parfitt, A. M. Hypophosphatemic vitamin D refractory rickets and osteomalacia. Orthop. Clin. North Am. 3:653-680, 1972.
150. Witmer, G.; and Balsan, S. Biopsie osseuse dans quatre cas de rachitisme vitamine D-resistant idiopathique. Pathol. Biol. 16:421-429, 1968.
151. Winters, R. W.; Graham, J. B.; Williams, T. F.; McFalls, V. W.; and Burnett, C. H. A genetic study of familial hypophosphatemia and vitamin D-resistant rickets with a review of the literature. Medicine 37:97-142, 1958.
152. Moser, C. R.; and Fessel, W. J. Rheumatic manifestations of hypophosphatemia. Arch. Intern. Med. 134:674-678, 1974.
153. Scriver, C. R. The William Allan Memorial Award Address: On phosphate transport and genetic screening, "Understanding Backward–Living Forward" in human genetics. Am. J. Hum. Genet. 31:243-263, 1979.
154. Harrison, H. E.; Harrison, H. C.; Lifshitz, F.; and Johnson, A. D. Growth disturbance in hereditary hypophosphatemia. Am. J. Dis. Child. 112:290-297, 1966.
155. Stamp, T. C. B.; and Baker, L. R. I. Recessive hypophosphatemic rickets and possible aetiology of the "vitamin-D resistant" syndrome. Arch. Dis. Child. 51:360-365, 1976.
156. Kistler, H. J.; Bonetti, A.; Frey, P.; and Fischer, J. A. Sproadische hypophosphatemische vitamin-D-resistente Osteomalazie (Phosphatdiabetes) im Erwachsenenalter and Hyperparathyreoidismus. Schweiz. Med. Wochenschr. 106:1855-1862, 1976.
157. Stickler, G. B.; Jowsey, J.; and Bianco, A. J., Jr. Possible detrimental effect of large doses of vitamin D in familial hypophosphatemic vitamin D-resistant rickets. J. Pediatr. 79:68-71, 1971.
158. Frame, B.; Smith, R. W., Jr.; Fleming, J. L.; and Hanson, G. Oral phosphates in vitamin D-refractory rickets and osteomalacia. Am. J. Dis. Child. 106:147-153, 1963.
159. Stickler, G. B.; Hayles, A. B.; and Roserear, J. W. Familial hypophosphatemic vitamin D-resistant rickets. Am. J. Dis. Child. 110:664-667, 1965.
160. Gerbeaux-Balsan, S. L'absorption intestinale du phosphore dans le rachitisme vitamine-resistant hypophosphatemique hereditaire. Effets de fortes surcharges de phosphore et des regimes tres pauvres en calcium. Rev. Fr. Etud. Clin. Biol. 10:65-72, 1965.
161. West, C. D.; Blanton, J. C.; Silverman, F. N.; and Holland, N. H. Use of phosphate salts as an adjunct to vitamin D in the treatment of hypophosphatemic vitamin D-refractory rickets. J. Pediatr. 64:469-477, 1964.

162. Glorieux, F. H.; Scriver, C. R.; Reade, T. M.; Goldman, H.; and Roseborough, A. Use of phosphate and vitamin D to prevent dwarfism and rickets in X-linked hypophosphatemia. N. Engl. J. Med. 287:481-487, 1972.
163. McEnery, P. T.; Silverman, F. N.; and West, C. D. Acceleration of growth with combined vitamin D-phosphate therapy of hypophosphatemic resistant rickets. J. Pediatr. 80:763-774, 1972.
164. Evans, G. A.; Arulanantham, K.; and Gage, J. R. Primary hypophosphatemic rickets: Effect of oral phosphate and vitamin D on growth and surgical treatment. J. Bone joint Surg. 62A:1130-1138, 1980.
165. Teitelbaum, S. L.; Rosenberg, E. M.; Bates, M.; and Avioli, L. V. The effects of phosphate and vitamin D therapy on osteopenic, hypophosphatemic osteomalacia of childhood. Clin. Orthop. Relat. Res. 116:38-47, 1976.
166. Puschett, J. B.; Genel, M.; Rastegar, A.; Anast, C.; DeLuca, H. F.; and Friedman, A. Long-term therapy of vitamin D-resistant rickets with 25-hydroxycholecalciferol. Clin. Pharmacol. Ther. 17:202-211, 1975.
167. Cohanin, M.; DeLuca, H. F.; and Yendt, E. Effects of prolonged treatment with 25-hydroxyvitamin D in hypophosphatemic (vitamin D refractory) rickets and osteomalacia. John Hopkins Med. J. 131:118-132, 1972.
168. Glorieux, F. H.; Scriver, C. R.; Holick, M. F.; and DeLuca, H. F. X-linked hypophosphatemic rickets: Inadequate therapeutic response to 1,25-dihydroxycholecalciferol. Lancet 2:287-289, 1973.
169. Brickman, A. S.; Coburn, J. W.; Kurokawa, K.; Bethune, J. E.; Harrison, H. E.; and Norman, A. W. Actions of 1,25-dihydroxycholecalciferol in patients with hypophosphatemic vitamin D-resistant rickets. N. Engl. J. Med. 289:495-498, 1973.
170. Russell, R. G. G.; Smith, R.; Preston, C.; Walton, R. J.; Woods, C. G.; Henderson, R. G.; and Norman, A. W. The effect of 1,25-dihydroxycholecalciferol on renal tubular reabsorption of phosphate intestinal absorption of calcium and bone histology in hypophosphatemic renal tubular rickets. Clin. Sci. Mol. Med. 48:177-186, 1975.
171. Costa, T.; Marie, P. J.; Scriver, C. R.; Cole, D. E. C.; Reade, T. M.; Nogrady, B.; Glorieux, F. H.; Delvin, E. E. X-linked hypophosphatemia: Effect of calcitriol on renal handling of phosphate, serum phosphate and bone mineralization. J. Clin. Endocrinol. Metab. 52:463-472, 1981.
172. Hirschman, G. H.; DeLuca, H. F.; Chan, J. C. M. Hypophosphatemic vitamin D-resistant rickets: Metabolic balance studies in a child receiving 1,25-dihydroxyvitamin D_3, phosphate and ascorbic acid. Pediatrics 61:451-457, 1978.
173. Chan, J. C. M.; Lovinger, R. D.; and Mamunes, P. Renal hypophosphatemic rickets: Growth acceleration after long-term treatment with 1,25-dihydroxyvitamin D_3. Pediatrics 66:445-454, 1980.
174. Rasmussen, H.; Pechet, M.; Anast, C.; Maxure, A.; Gertner, J.; Broadus, A. E. Long-term treatment of familial hypophosphatemic rickets with oral phosphate and 1α-hydroxyvitamin D. J. Pediatr. 99:26-34, 1981.
175. Peacock, M.; Heyburn, P. J.; and Aaron, J. E. Treatment of vitamin D-resistant hypophosphatemic osteomalacia with 1α-hydroxyvitamin D_3. Calcif. Tissue Res. (Suppl.) 22:55-62, 1977.
176. Chesney, R. W.; Mazess, R. B.; Rose, P.; Hamstra, A. J.; DeLuca, H. F.; and Breed, A. L. Long-term influence of calcitriol (1,25$(OH)_2$-Vitamin D) and supplemental phosphate in X-linked hypophosphatemic rickets. Calcif. Tissue Int. 33:307, 1981.
177. Scriver, C. R.; MacDonald, W.; Reade, T. M.; Glorieux, F. H.; and Nogrady, B. Hypophosphatemic nonrachitic bone disease: An entity distinct from X-linked hypophosphatemia in the renal defect, bone involvement and inheritance. Am. J. Med. Genet. 1:101-117, 1977.
178. Scriver, C. R.; Reade, T.; Halal, F.; Costa, T.; and Cole, D. E. C. Autosomal hypophosphatemic bone disease responds to 1,25$(OH)_2$ D_3. Arch. Dis. Child. 56:203-207, 1981.

179. Frymoyer, J. W.; and Hodgkin, W. Adult-onset vitamin D-resistant hypophosphatemic osteomalacia. J. Bone Jt. Surg. 59A:101, 1977.
180. Chesney, R. W. Modified vitamin D compounds in the treatment of certain bone diseases. In: Nutritional Pharmacology, edited by Spiller, G. A. New York, Liss, 1981, pp. 147-202.
181. McInness, R. R.; and Scriver, C. R. Effect of calciotropic hormones and cyclic nucleotides on aminoaciduria and phosphaturia. Pediatr. Res. 14:218-223, 1980.
182. Phillips, M. E.; Havard, J.; and O'Herud, B. Aminoaciduria in chronic renal failure—Its relationship to vitamin D and parathyroid status. Am. J. Clin. Nutr. 33:1541-1545, 1980.
183. Grose, J. H.; and Scriver, C. R. Parathyroid-dependent phosphatemia and aminoaciduria in the vitamin D-deficient rat. Am. J. Physiol. 214:370-377, 1968.
184. Eastwood, J. B.; de Wardner, H. E.; Gray, R. W.; and Lemann, J. L., Jr. Normal plasma-1,25$(OH)_2$-vitamin D concentrations in nutritional osteomalacia. Lancet 1:465-466, 1979.
185. Papapoulos, S. E.; Clemens, T. L.; Fraher, L. J.; Gleed, J.; and O'Riordan, J. L. H. Metabolites of vitamin D in human vitamin D deficiency: Effect of vitamin D_3 or 1,25-dihydroxycholecalciferol. Lancet 2:612-615, 1980.
186. Nguyen, T. M.; Guillozo, H.; Garabedian, M.; Mallet, E.; and Balsan, S. Serum concentrations of 24,25-dihydroxyvitamin D in normal children and in children with rickets. Pediatr. Res. 13:973-976, 1979.
187. Rasmussen, H.; Baron, R.; Broadus, A.; DeFronzo, R.; Lang, R.; and Horst, R. 1,25-$(OH)_2 D_3$ is not the only metabolite involved in the pathogenesis of osteomalacia. Am. J. Med. 69:360-368, 1980.
188. Chesney, R. W.; Zimmerman, J.; Hamstra, A.; DeLuca, H. F.; and Mazess, R. B. Vitamin D metabolite concentrations in vitamin D deficiency: Are calcitriol levels normal? Am. J. Dis. Child. 135:1025-1028, 1981.
189. Tanaka, Y.; Lorenc, R. S.; and DeLuca, H. F. The role of 1,25-dihydroxyvitamin D_3 and parathyroid hormone in the regulation of chick renal 25-hydroxyvitamin D_3-24-hydroxylase. Arch. Biochem. Biophys. 171:521-526, 1975.
190. Chesney, R. W. Current clinical applications of vitamin D metabolite research. In: Clinical Orthopaedics and Related Research, edited by Urist, M. R. Philadelphia, Lippincott, 16:285-314, 1981.
191. Hoff, N.; Haddad, J. G.; Teitelbaum, S.; McAlister, W.; and Hillman, L. S. Serum concentrations of 25-hydroxyvitamin D in rickets of extreme prematurity. J. Pediatr. 94: 460-466, 1979.
192. Rowe, J. C.; Wood, D. H.; Rowe, D. W.; and Raisz, L. G. Nutritional hypophosphatemic rickets in a premature infant fed breast milk. N. Engl. J. Med. 300:293-305, 1979.
193. Steichen, J. J.; Ho, M.; Hug, G.; and Tsang, R. C. Elevated serum 1,25$(OH)_2$-vitamin D concentrations in rickets of prematurity. Pediatr. Res. 14:581, 1980.
194. Fleischman, A. F.; Perl, H.; and Skolnick, L. Rickets in the small premature—A preventable disorder. Pediatr. Res. 14:571, 1980.
195. Haddad, J. G.; and Stamp, T. C. Circulating 25-hydroxyvitamin D in man. Am. J. Med. 57:57-62, 1974.
196. Bachrach, S. An outbreak of vitamin D-deficiency rickets in a susceptible population. Pediatrics 64:871-877, 1979.
197. Riggs, B. L.; Gallagher, J. C.; DeLuca, H. F.; Edis, A. J.; Lambert, P. W.; and Arnaud, C. D. A syndrome of osteoporosis, increased serum immunoreactive parathyroid hormone and inappropriately low serum 1,25-dihydroxyvitamin D. Mayo Clin. Proc. 53: 701-706, 1978.
198. Kruse, R. Osteopathien bei autiepileptischer langzeit therapie (Vorlaufige Mitteilung), Monatsschr. Kinderheilkd. 116:378-384, 1968.

199. Hahn, T. J.; Birge, S. J.; Scharp, C. R.; and Avioli, L. V. Phenobarbital-induced alterations in vitamin D metabolism. J. Clin. Invest. 51:741-748, 1972.
200. Hahn, T. J.; Hendin, B. A.; Scharp, C. R.; and Haddad, J. G. Serum 25-hydroxycholecalciferol levels and bone mass in children on chronic anticonvulsant therapy. N. Engl. J. Med. 292:550-554, 1975.
201. Tolman, K. G.; Jubiz, W.; Sannella, J. J.; Madsen, J. A.; Belsey, R. E.; Goldsmith, R. S.; and Freston, J. W. Osteomalacia associated with anticonvulsant drug therapy in mentally retarded children. Pediatrics 56:45-51, 1975.
202. Borgstedt, A. D.; Bryson, M. G.; Young, L. W.; and Forbes, G. F. Long-term administration of anti-epileptic drugs and the development of rickets. J. Pediatr. 81:9-15, 1972.
203. Jubiz, W.; Haussler, M. R.; McCain, T. A.; and Tolman, K. G. Plasma 1,25-dihydroxyvitamin D levels in patients receiving anticonvulsant drugs. J. Clin. Endocrinol. Metab. 44:617-623, 1977.
204. Levison, J. C.; Kent, G. N.; Worth, G. K.; and Retallack, R. Anticonvulsant induced increase in 25-hydroxyvitamin D_3-1α-hydroxylase. Endocrinology 101:1898-1901, 1977.
205. Dunnigan, M. G.; McIntosh, W. B.; Sutherland, G. R.; Gardee, R.; Glekin, B.; Ford, J. A.; and Robertson, I. Policy for prevention of Asian rickets in Britain: Preliminary assessment of Glasgow rickets compaign. Br. Med. J. 282:357-360, 1981.
206. Fraser, D.; and Salter, R. B. The diagnosis and management of the various types of rickets. Pediatr. Clin. North Am., May, 417-441, 1958.
207. Von Prader, A.; Illig, R.; and Heierli, E. Eine besondere form der primaren vitamin D resistenten rachitis mit hypocalcamie und autosomal dominantem erbgang: die hereditare pseudo-mangelrachitis. Helv. Pediatr. Acta 16:452-468, 1961.
208. Delvin, E. E.; Glorieux, F. H.; Marie, P. J.; and Pettifor, J. M. Vitamin D dependency: Replacement therapy with calcitriol. J. Pediatr. 99:26-34, 1981.
209. Arnaud, C.; Maijer, R.; Reade, T.; Scriver, C. R.; and Whelan, D. T. Vitamin D dependency: An inherited post-natal syndrome with secondary hyperparathyroidism. Pediatrics 46:871-880, 1970.
210. Fraser, D.; Kooh, S. W.; Kind, H. P.; Holick, M. F.; Tanaka, Y.; and DeLuca, H. F. Pathogenesis of hereditary vitamin D-dependent rickets: An inborn error of vitamin D metabolism involving defective conversion of 25-hydroxyvitamin D to 1α,25-dihydroxyvitamin D. N. Engl. J. Med. 289:817-822, 1973.
211. Reade, T. M.; Scriver, C. R.; Glorieux, F. H.; Nogrady, B.; Delvin, E.; Poirier, R.; Holick, M. F.; and DeLuca, H. F. Response to crystalline 1α-hydroxyvitamin D_3 in vitamin D dependency. Pediatr. Res. 9:593-599, 1975.
212. Scriver, C. R.; Reade, T. M.; DeLuca, H. F.; and Hamstra, A. J. Serum 1,25-dihydroxyvitamin D levels in normal subjects and patients with hereditary rickets or bone disease. N. Engl. J. Med. 299:976-979, 1978.
213. Balsan, S. Vitamin D metabolites in pediatric pharmacology. In: Pediatric Diseases Related to Calcium, edited by DeLuca, H. F., and Anast, C. S. New York, Elsevier, 1980, pp. 241-256.
214. Pedersen, J. I.; Ghazarian, J. G.; Orme-Johnson, W.; and DeLuca, H. F. Isolation of chick renal mitochondrial ferredoxin active in the 25-hydroxyvitamin D_3-1α-hydroxylase system. J. Biol. Chem. 251:3933-3941, 1976.
215. Tanaka, Y.; and DeLuca, H. F. Measurement of chick kidney 25-hydroxyvitamin D_3-1α-hydroxylase without use of radioactive substrate. Anal. Biochem. 110:102-107, 1981.
216. Brandis, M.; Murer, H.; Stange, G.; Kamran, D.; and Harmeyer, J. Phosphate transport in renal tubular brush border vesicles in a pig strain of vitamin D-dependent rickets. Pediatr. Res. 14:988, 1980.

217. Balsan, S.; Garabedian, M.; Sorgniard, R.; Holick, M.; and DeLuca, H. F. 1,25-Dihydroxyvitamin D_3 and 1α-hydroxyvitamin D_3 in children: Biologic therapeutic effects in nutritional rickets and different types of vitamin D resistance. Pediatr. Res. 9:586-593, 1975.
218. Brooks, M. H.; Bell, N. H.; Love, L.; Stern, P. H.; Orfei, E.; Queener, S. H.; Hamstra, A. J.; and DeLuca, H. F. Vitamin D-dependent rickets type II: Resistance of target organs to 1,25-dihydroxyvitamin D. N. Engl. J. Med. 298:996-999, 1978.
219. Marx, S. J.; Speigel, A. M.; Brown, E. M.; Gardner, D. G.; Downs, R. W., Jr.; Attie, M.; Hamstra, A. J.; and DeLuca, H. F. A familial syndrome of decrease in sensitivity to 1,25-dihydroxyvitamin D. J. Clin. Endocrinol. Metab. 47:1303-1310, 1978.
220. Rosen, J. F.; Fleischman, A. R.; Finberg, L.; Hamstra, A.; and DeLuca, H. F. Rickets with alopecia: An inborn error of vitamin D metabolism. J. Pediatr. 94:729-735, 1979.
221. Sockalosky, J. J.; Ulstrom, R. A.; DeLuca, H. F.; and Brown, D. M. Vitamin D-resistant rickets: End-organ unresponsiveness to $1,25(OH)_2 D_3$. J. Pediatr. 96:701-703, 1980.
222. Liberman, U. A.; Halabe, A.; Samuel, R.; Kauli, R.; Edelstein, S.; Weisman, Y.; Papapoulos, S. E.; Fraker, L. J.; Clemens, T. L.; and O'Riordan, J. L. H. End-organ resistance to 1,25-dihydroxycholecalciferol. Lancet 1:504-507, 1980.
223. Tsuchuya, T.; Matsuo, N.; Cho, H.; Kumagai, M.; Yasaka, A.; Suda, T.; Orimo, H.; and Shiraki, M. An unusual form of vitamin D-dependent rickets in a child: Alopecia and marked end-organ hyposensitivity to biologically active vitamin D. J. Clin. Endocrinol. Metab. 51:685-690, 1980.
224. Bell, N. H. Hypercalcemic and hypocalcemic disorders. Diagnosis and treatment. Nephron 23:147-151, 1979.
225. Bell, N. H. Vitamin D-dependent rickets type II. Calcif. Tissue Int. 31:89-91, 1980.
226. Zerwekh, J. E.; Glass, K.; Jowsey, J.; and Pak, C. Y. C. A unique form of osteomalacia associated with end-organ refraction to 1,25-dihydroxyvitamin D and apparent defective synthesis of 25-hydroxyvitamin D. J. Clin. Endocrinol. Metab. 49:171-175, 1979.
227. Stern, P. H.; de Olazabal, J.; and Bell, N. H. Evidence for abnormal regulation of circulating 1α,25-dihydroxyvitamin D in patients with sarcoidosis and normal calcium metabolism. J. Clin. Invest. 66:852-855, 1980.
228. Eil, C.; Liberman, U. A.; Rosen, J. F.; and Marx, S. J. A cellular defect in hereditary vitamin D-dependent rickets type II: Defective nuclear uptake of 1,25-dihydroxyvitamin D in cultured skin fibroblasts. N. Engl. J. Med. 304:1588-1591, 1981.
229. Marx, S. J.; Swart, E. G., Jr.; Hamstra, A. J.; and DeLuca, H. F. Normal intrauterine development of the fetus of a woman receiving extraordinarily high doses of 1,25-dihydroxyvitamin D_3. J. Clin. Endocrinol. Metab. 51:1138-1142, 1980.
230. Harrison, H. E. Oncogenous rickets: Possible elaboration by a tumor of a humoral substance inhibiting tubular reabsorption of phosphate. Pediatrics 52:432-434, 1973.
231. Aschenberg, L. C.; Solomon, L. M.; Zeis, P. M.; Justice, P. M.; and Rosenthal, I. M. Vitamin D-resistant rickets associated with the epidermal nevus syndrome: Demonstration of a phosphaturic substance in the dermal lesions. J. Pediatr. 91:56-60, 1977.
232. Prader, A.; Illig, R.; Uelinger, E.; and Stadler, G. Rachitis infolge knoch or tumors. Helv. Pediatr. Acta 14:554-565, 1959.
233. Chesney, R. W. Tubular defects in phosphate reabsorption in clinical medicine. In: The Renal Handling of Phosphate, edited by Massry, S. G., and Fleisch, H. New York, Plenum Press, 1980, p. 336.
234. Daniels, R. A.; and Weisenfeld, I. Tumorous phosphaturic osteomalacia: Report of a case associated with multiple hemangiomas of bone. Am. J. Med. 67:155-159, 1979.
235. Wyman, A. L.; Paradinas, F. J.; and Daly, J. R. Hypophosphatemic osteomalacia associated with a malignant tumor of the tibia: Report of a case. J. Clin. Pathol. 30:328-335, 1977.

236. Olefsky, J.; Kempson, R.; Jones, H.; and Reaven, G. Tertiary hyperparathyroidism and apparent "cure" of vitamin D-resistant rickets after removal of an ossifying fibroma of bone. N. Engl. J. Med. 286:740-745, 1972.
237. Chesney, R. W.; Simpson, D. P.; and Wen, S. F. Effects of tumor on fluid and electrolytes. In: Cancer and the Kidney, edited by Frei, E., III, and Reisselbach, R. H. Philadelphia, Lea & Febiger, 1982, pp. 534-593.
238. Parker, M. S.; Klein, I.; Haussler, M. R.; and Mintz, D. H. Tumor-induced osteomalacia: Evidence of a surgically correctable alteration in vitamin D metabolism. JAMA 245:492-493, 1981.
239. Drezner, M. K.; and Feinglos, M. N. Osteomalacia due to 1α,25-dihydroxycholecalciferol deficiency. J. Clin. Invest. 60:1046-1053, 1977.
240. Nortman, D. F.; Coburn, J. W.; Brautbar, N.; Sherrard, D. J.; Haussler, M. R.; Singer, F. R.; Brickman, A. S.; and Barton, R. T. Treatment of mesenchymal tumor-associated osteomalacia with 1,25$(OH)_2D_3$: Report of a case. In: Vitamin D: Basic Research and Its Clinical Application, edited by Schaefer, K., and Norman, A. W. Berlin, Walter deGruyter, 1979, pp. 1167-1168.
241. Fukumoto, Y.; Tauri, S.; Tsukiyama, K.; Ichihara, K.; Moriwaki, K.; Nonaka, K.; Mizushima, T.; Kobayashi, Y.; Dokoh, S.; Funkunaga, M.; and Morita, R. Tumor-induced vitamin D-resistant hypophosphatemic osteomalacia associated with proximal renal tubular dysfunction and 1,25-dihydroxyvitamin D deficiency. J. Clin. Endocrinol. Metab. 49:873-878, 1979.
242. Chesney, R. W. Metabolic bone disease. Pediatr. in Rev. 5:227-237, 1984.
243. Pollack, J. A.; Schiller, A. L.; and Crawford, J. D. Rickets and myopathy cured by removal of a non-ossifying fibroma of bone. Pediatrics 52:364-371, 1973.
244. Dent, C. E.; and Stamp, T. C. B. Hypophosphatemic osteomalacia presenting in adults. Q. J. Med. 40:303-329, 1971.
245. Offerman, G.; von Herrath, D.; and Delling, G. Idiopathische hypophosphatamische Osteomalagie. Dtsch. Med. Wochenschr. 101:1684-1689, 1976.
246. Segar, W. E.; Iber, F. L.; and Kyle, L. H. Osteomalacia of unknown etiology. N. Engl. J. Med. 254:1011-1017, 1956.
247. Lundberg, E.; Bergengren, H.; and Lindqvist, B. Mild phosphate diabetes in adults. Acta Med. Scand. 204:93-96, 1978.
248. Teitelbaum, S. L.; Rosenberg, E. M.; Bates, M.; and Avioli, L. V. The effects of phosphate and vitamin D therapy on osteopenic, hypophosphatemic osteomalacia of childhood. Clin. Orthop. 116:38-47, 1976.
249. Ulmann, A.; Bouchard, P.; Garabedian, M.; Bourdeau, A.; Witmer-Cournot, G.; Lacour, B.; Balsan, S.; and Funck-Brentano, J. L. Plasma vitamin D metabolites in a patient with sporadic hypophosphatemic osteomalacia (adult-onset type). Eur. J. Clin. Invest. 10:369-372, 1980.
250. Glanville, H. J.; and Bloom, R. Case of renal tubular osteomalacia (Dent type 2) with later development of autonomous parathyroid tumors. Br. Med. J. 2:26-29, 1965.
251. Thomas, W. C., Jr.; and Fry, R. M. Parathyroid adenomas in chronic rickets. Am. J. Med. 49:404-407, 1970.
252. Offermann, G.; Delling, G.; and Haussler, M. R. 1,25-Dihydroxycholecalciferol in hypophosphataemic osteomalacia presenting in adults. Acta Endocrinol. 88:408-416, 1978.
253. Dent, C. E.; and Friedman, M. Hypophosphatemic osteomalacia with complete recovery. Br. Med. J. 1:1676-1679, 1964.

7

Abnormalities of Uric Acid Transport

HARRY O. SENEKJIAN,* THOMAS F. KNIGHT,† and EDWARD J. WEINMAN‡
Veterans Administration Medical Center and Baylor College of Medicine, Houston, Texas

I. URATE METABOLISM

The body pool of urate represents a balance between urate production and urate excretion. Input into the urate pool derives in large measure from the catabolism of endogenously produced nucleic acids. Only 20% of the pool arises from the dietary intake of purines (1). The elimination of urate from the body is mainly by renal excretion. Gastrointestinal excretion by intestinal uricolysis accounts for less than one-third of the total production rate of urate per day in normal man (1, 2). The factors which control nucleic acid production and its breakdown into urate have recently been reviewed in detail and will not be considered further (3-5). The factors which modulate the rate of intestinal uricolysis have not been extensively studied. Indeed, most of the investigative effort has been directed toward examination of the mechanisms which subserve the excretion of urate by the kidneys.

The renal handling of urate has been studied to a variable degree in man and a variety of laboratory animals using clearance, tissue slice, in vivo micropuncture, and in vitro microperfusion techniques. In addition, preliminary data on the transport of urate in isolated membrane vesicles have recently become available (see Ch. 1). In most species examined, urate undergoes filtration and net tubular reabsorption and/or tubular secretion. In some animals and in humans, the evidence would suggest that there is bidirectional transport of urate across the renal tubular cells. It has also been demonstrated that in some species the renal cells themselves are capable of de novo production of urate (6). The importance of the contribution of urate production by the kidneys, however, is unknown at the present time.

Animal experiments have been performed in an attempt to understand the mechanisms which modulate the transport of urate in the kidney, with the ultimate goal of translating animal studies to the understanding of the biology of man. Several major experimental diffi-

Current affiliations:
*University of Utah, Salt Lake City, Utah
†University of Nebraska College of Medicine, Omaha, Nebraska
‡University of Texas School of Medicine at Houston, Houston, Texas

culties, however, have precluded the adaptation of a unified model of the handling of urate by the human kidney from animal studies. First, in many mammals, excluding man, urate is catabolized to allantoin. As a consequence, the plasma concentration of urate is considerably lower than that of man. Second, there exists marked species variability in the relative contributions of the absorptive and secretory fluxes of urate to urate excretion. In some animals net reabsorption of filtered urate is normally present, while in other species net secretion of urate is observed. Third, in animals, as compared to man, there are differing sensitivities to drugs which affect the rates of urate transport. Finally, the relative specificities of the organic acid secretory system in the renal tubules for urate and other organic anions differ in different species. A review of the similarities and differences between various experimental animals has recently been published (7,8). It remains problematic, therefore, whether or not a clear model of urate handling by the kidney in man can be developed at the present time, due to the fact that there is marked variability between species and that studies in man are, by necessity, indirect. The animal experiments, however, have provided direct insights which are appropriate for the species under study and may be applicable to man.

Urate is freely filtered at the glomerulus and protein binding determined by both in vitro and in vivo techniques is felt to be less than 10% (9,10). It had been suggested, based on some in vitro studies, that plasma binding of urate may be considerably higher than that noted above and that the action of some uricosuric drugs may depend upon their ability to displace urate bound to protein (11-13). These studies have not been confirmed, and it is now accepted by most investigators that the binding of urate to plasma proteins is not an important variable (10).

The renal handling of urate has been extensively studied in the rat. In this species, only 10-30% of the urate filtered at the glomerulus is excreted in the urine, indicating that there is net reabsorption of urate (9,14-17). Free-flow micropuncture studies have shown that the proximal convoluted tubule is the major nephron site of urate reabsorption (9,14,15, 18,19). The reabsorption of filtered urate also occurs, albeit to a lesser extent, at a nephron site between the proximal and distal tubule (14,19). This latter flux is believed to represent the contribution of the proximal straight tubule. There is no evidence for the transport of urate in the distal convoluted tubule or in the collecting duct system (18,20). Evidence to date would indicate that internephronal heterogeneity for urate transport does not seem to exist in the rat (18).

In the proximal convoluted tubule, the tubular fluid to plasma concentration of urate is less than one, a finding which suggests that the tubular absorption of urate is an active transport mechanism (18). More detailed studies have shown that in the rat proximal tubule the absorption of urate can occur in the absence of a favorable electrochemical gradient; that is, urate absorption is an active transport process (21). The absorptive flux demonstrates first-order saturation kinetics, and estimates of the K_m and V_{max} have been published (22). The absorptive flux can be inhibited by probenecid and some diuretic agents (16,23). The absorption of urate, however, is not intimately linked to that of sodium (9,16,17,21). Expansion of the extracellular fluid volume inhibits the absorptive flux of urate, while volume depletion enhances the tubular absorption of urate (17,19,20). The mechanism of these responses involves alteration of the specific mechanism for absorption and perhaps alterations in the flow rate of urine along the proximal tubule induced by changes in the extracellular fluid volume (24). Changes in the flow rate could conceivably result in changes in the mean intraluminal concentration of urate and thus alter the absorptive flux of urate independent of changes in sodium absorption.

In the proximal tubule of the rat, there is also a secretory mechanism which transports urate from the peritubular capillary blood into the lumen (21,25,26). The secretory flux, too, follows first-order saturation kinetics, and the K_m and V_{max} have been determined (25). The secretory flux is inhibitable by probenecid, other organic acids, some diuretic agents and pyrazinamide (16,27,28). In the rat, the plasma concentration of urate is well below the K_m for both the absorptive and secretory transport systems. In response to an exogenous load of urate, there is an increase in the clearance of urate, presumably reflecting the increased contribution of urate secreted from the capillary blood into the lumen (15). In addition to the facilitated transport systems noted above, urate can also diffuse in and out of the lumen of the tubule by passive diffusion along concentration gradients (21). Solvent drag, however, does not significantly influence net urate transport (22).

In contrast to the rat, the fractional excretion of urate in the rabbit is close to or in some experimental circumstances, in excess of the filtered load (29,30). The demonstration of a clearance of urate greater than the filtered load is evidence for net urate secretion. Studies on isolated brush-border vesicles of the rabbit had suggested the possibility of an active transport mechanism for the absorption of urate (31). Studies in isolated in vitro perfused segments of the rabbit proximal tubule, however, have not indicated the presence of an active absorptive mechanism (32,33). As in the rat, in the rabbit some urate absorption can occur by passive diffusion, presumably by a paracellular pathway (32). The superficial proximal tubules of the rabbit are capable of net secretion of urate (32,33). Recent evidence suggests that the juxtamedullary proximal tubules have a lower capacity for urate secretion than do superficial cortical proximal tubules, and that nephron heterogeneity for the transport of urate exists in this species (34). The secretory process in the superficial proximal tubules is an active transport mechanism and the K_m and V_{max} have been determined (32, 33). Some studies have suggested that the relationship between urate and its carrier in the rabbit is allosteric (33). The secretory flux of urate is inhibitable by probenecid (33). Isolated tubule and tissue slice studies have demonstrated that the cell concentration of urate exceeds that of the surrounding media, evidence indicating that active uptake occurs across the antiluminal border of the cell (35,36). The mechanism subserving the movement of urate from the cell into the lumen, however, has not been elucidated, and both passive and/or facilitated mechanisms may be operative.

In the mongrel dog, the fractional excretion of urate is less than 100%, indicating net reabsorption of filtered urate in this species (37). Evidence for both active absorption and secretion of urate has been presented (38,39). A recent set of studies has provided some insights into the mechanism of absorption in this species. The uptake of urate into brush-border membrane vesicles is energized, not by a sodium gradient as is the case for glucose, but rather by a proton gradient (40). Additional studies have suggested that the uptake of urate across the luminal membrane is mediated by an anion exchange mechanism where other anions are exchanged for urate (41). The applicability of these findings to other species, however, remains to be determined. For example, good evidence exists for the presence of an anion exchange mechanism in the brush-border vesicles of the rabbit, yet facilitated urate absorption has not been unequivocally demonstrated in this species (32,33,42).

The discussion of the transport of urate in the rat, rabbit, and dog highlight some of the differences between species and the difficulties of adapting a unified model. In addition, significant differences in the renal handling of urate exist between the species already discussed and between the snake, chicken, monkey, and mini-pig (7,8). In some but not all species, *p*-aminohippurate inhibits the flux of urate (7). The response to diuretic agents, pyrazinamide and, possibly, other drugs differs between species as well. Thus, the presence in some species, of absorptive and secretory mechanisms existing simultaneously, the experimental difficulties in examining single unidirectional fluxes, the lack of truly specific inhibitors of only a single flux, and the presence of significant passive diffusion, have made the formulation of a single model of urate transport by the renal tubular cells difficult, if not impossible.

In man, the methods of study are more indirect. The fractional excretion of urate in normal man is less than 10% of the filtered load (43). A tubular maximum for absorption has been reported in some studies (44). Under some experimental conditions, and in some clinical disorders in man, the clearance of urate has been shown to exceed the filtered load, a finding demonstrating the presence of a secretory mechanism (45-47). Attempts to quantitate the contribution of the absorptive and secretory mechanisms to the overall renal excretion of urate in man have proven to be particularly difficult and, in some respects, confusing. Studies of this type in man have involved the use of pyrazinamide, a drug which is believed to be a relatively specific inhibitor of urate secretion (48,49). This drug, however, may have activity on both the secretory and reabsorptive processes, and its specificity is not supported by animal studies (28,50). Nonetheless, a large number of studies employing pyrazinamide have been performed in man. Following the administration of pyrazinamide to man, the clearance and fractional excretion of urate is decreased (48,49). If it is assumed that urate secretion is nearly totally inhibited and the absorptive flux is unaltered, the results suggest that nearly 98% of the filtered load of urate is absorbed and that 2% escapes into the urine (49). The 2% that escapes reabsorption accounts for 20% of the urinary excretion of urate. By extrapolation, then, 80% of the urinary excretion of urate derives from tubular secretion. Under some experimental circumstances, the results obtained with pyrazinamide suggest that the tubular secretion of urate is quite large and that some of the secreted urate is back reabsorbed at a nephron site distal to the secretory site (the so-called postsecretory reabsorptive site) (51). Thus, the following sequence of events has been postulated: filtered urate is reabsorbed; urate secretion occurs at a site further along the nephron; and some of the secreted urate is back reabsorbed at the postsecretory reabsorptive site (Fig. 1). It is

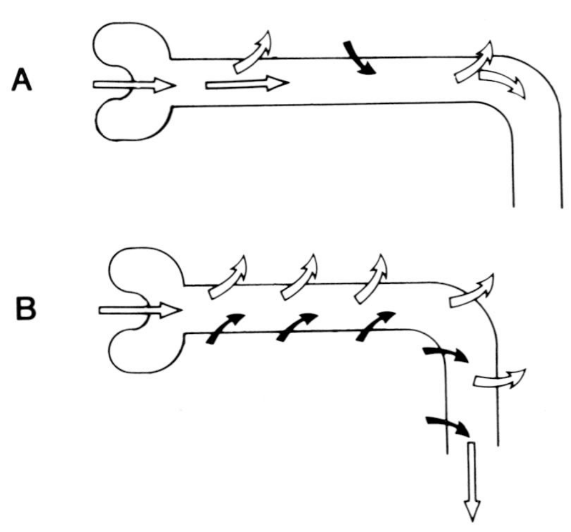

Fig. 1 Current concepts of the handling of urate by the proximal tubule. In the classic sequence of events (A), filtered urate is reabsorbed, followed by secretion at a site further along the nephron; finally, some of the secreted urate is back reabsorbed at the postsecretory reabsorptive site. In (B), secretion and reabsorption occur simultaneously along the length of the proximal convoluted and proximal straight tubules.

Table 1 Renal Tubular Abnormalities of Uric Acid Transport

- I. Hereditary disorders
  - A. Gouty arthritis and hyperuricemia
    1. Overproduction of uric acid
    2. Defective renal excretion of uric acid
  - B. Hyperuricemia due to increased renal tubular reabsorption
  - C. Hypouricemia due to isolated renal tubular defect (Dalmatian dog mutation)
  - D. Hypouricemia due to generalized renal tubular defect
    1. Fanconi syndrome
    2. Wilson's disease
    3. Sickle cell anemia
- II. Acquired disorders
  - A. Systemic diseases
    1. Retained organic acids–ketoacidosis, lactic acidosis
    2. Congestive heart failure
    3. Malignancy
    4. Syndrome of inappropriate ADH
    5. Normal pregnancy
    6. Preeclampsia and eclampsia
  - B. Drug-induced disorders
    1. Chronic administration of diuretics
    2. Salicylates
    3. X-ray contrast agents
    4. Glyceryl guaiacolate
    5. Probenecid
    6. Sulfinpyrazone
  - C. Toxic agents
    1. Lead (saturnine gout)
    2. Beryllium

recognized, however, that such an axial nephronal assymetry may not have any true anatomical basis and that secretion and reabsorption may occur across the same nephron segments. While the latter is demonstrable in some animals, no clear evidence favoring the axial arrangement of absorptive, secretory, and postsecretory reabsorptive sites is available (21, 22,25). Nonetheless, schema for understanding renal tubular disorders of urate transport and the effect of pharmacological agents on the excretion of urate have been formulated based on this axial model. Despite the limitations of this model, the use of such schema provides a tool for remembering and categorizing certain disease states and sites of action of drugs (52).

With respect to man, the apparent absorptive and secretory mechanisms for urate transport are probably located in the proximal tubule. Both mechanisms can be inhibited by other organic acids, but the sensitivity for inhibition of the secretory system appears to be greater than that of the absorptive system. This fact is suggested by the so-called paradoxical response to drugs such as salicylates. In low doses, salicylate administration results in a rise in the plasma concentration of urate and a decrease in the urinary excretion of urate (53). In higher doses, the drug is uricosuric (53). It has been postulated that salicylates in low doses inhibit the secretory flux relatively more than the absorptive flux. In higher doses, both secretion and absorption are inhibited, and the net result is an increase in the urinary excretion of urate and a fall in the plasma concentration of urate. This paradoxical response has been noted with a number of drugs, and is evident in some animal studies (28,54).

It becomes apparent from the above considerations that disorders of tubular function, especially those involving the proximal convoluted tubule, may result in an altered metabolism of urate. Depending upon which transport system is most affected, hyperuricemia or hypouricemia may ensue. These alterations may occur as congenital or acquired defects and/or in response to drugs or toxins (Table 1). The transport of urate may be altered as a direct consequence of the disease condition or exposure, or as an indirect consequence of alteration in extracellular fluid volume, the generation of other organic acids which compete with urate for transport, or alterations in the tubular flow rate or tubular fluid composition. It is not presently possible in all cases to define precisely the nature of the defects due to the limitations of the currently available experimental methods.

In the following discussion, we have attempted to categorize the available literature on the abnormalities in the renal tubular transport of urate in clinical conditions in which the abnormalities in the renal handling of urate are a major manifestation of the disease process. We note, again, that some of these studies are difficult to evaluate, based on the factors just discussed.

II. HEREDITARY DISORDERS OF URIC ACID TRANSPORT

A. Isolated Defects of Uric Acid Transport

Gouty Arthritis and Hyperuricemia

Gouty arthritis is the most common and most extensively studied clinical disorder of abnormal urate metabolism. The prevalence of gouty arthritis has been estimated to be as high as 3% (55). Attacks of gouty arthritis are almost always associated with hyperuricemia and a correlation between the plasma level of uric acid and the risk of developing acute arthritis was suggested by the findings of the Framingham study (55). In that study of over 5000 individuals, the prevalence of gouty arthritis was 90% in patients with plasma concentrations of urate greater than four standard deviations (SDs) above normal. The normal serum level of uric acid (as measured colorimetrically by a modification of the Folin method) was 5.21 ± 1.11 (SD) mg/dl in men and 4.00 ± 0.94 mg/dl in women (55,56). Similar results were obtained in a study of serum uric acid in England and Scotland (57). Others, however, using an automated chemical analysis system, determined that the serum uric acid level was 6.1 ± 1.1 and 4.8 ± 1.3 mg/dl in normal men and women, respectively (58). Thus, there is variability among series as to the true "normal" serum level of uric acid. The definition of hyperuricemia may also be based on its solubility characteristics. Thus, at physiological pH, serum containing uric acid in a concentration greater than 8.0 mg/dl (measured colorimetrically) in men is considered supersaturated (59). This corresponds to a level greater than two standard deviations above the mean for most published studies. The definition of hyperuricemia, however, is still arbitrary and is based upon evaluation of the specific population under study and the method of determination.

As noted earlier, the metabolism of urate involves de novo production of urate from nucleic acids and excretion predominantly by the kidneys (1,2). Based on measured de novo production rates of urate, patients with primary gout may be subdivided into those who overproduce urate and those whose production rate is normal. This latter group are considered to have a defect in urate excretion. These two types of hyperuricemic patients can be differentiated by determining the 24-hour urinary excretion of urate. On a purine-free diet, normal humans excrete less than 600 mg/24 hr (60). Hyperuricemic humans who excrete greater than 600 mg/24 hr are considered to be overproducers of urate, and account for approximately 20% of a population of patients with gouty arthritis. Eighty percent of hyperuricemic patients excrete normal amounts of urate in the urine and are considered to have a renal defect in urate transport. The clinical syndromes of urate overproduction have been discussed in a number of recent reviews, and will not be discussed further (4,61,62).

The nature of the renal defect leading to hyperuricemia and gout has been the subject of extensive investigation. The possibility that gout may be caused by a specific impairment in the renal excretion of uric acid was first suggested by Garrod in 1848 (63). In 1957, however, Gutman and Yu published the results of a series of studies performed on patients with gouty arthritis (64). No abnormalities in renal function or in the renal handling of urate were found, and they concluded that no renal defect in urate handling existed in these patients. Nugent and Tyler reported results of clearance experiments in patients with gout and in nongouty subjects, and found no differences in the renal clearance of urate between these two groups under control conditions (65). The plasma level of urate, however, was significantly higher in the patients with gout (9.2 mg/dl) as compared to controls (5.6 mg/dl). When the normal subjects were fed RNA, so as to increase their plasma level of urate to a level similar to that of the gouty subjects, the renal clearance of urate was greater in the normal than in the gouty subjects, implying a defect in the renal excretion of urate in the latter group. Although overproduction was also possible, they argued against this mechanism as being a major factor in the genesis of gout, since most gouty patients do not excrete increased amounts of urate and many gouty patients have normal uric acid pools. These findings were supported by later studies of Lathem and Rodnan (66).

Using an analogous experimental design, Yu et al. increased the plasma concentration of urate in gouty and nongouty subjects by feeding RNA or by the intravenous infusion of uric acid (67). No discernible differences in the clearance of urate by the kidneys was observed. Moreover, pyrazinamide suppressed urinary excretion of urate equally in both groups of subjects, suggesting that there was no defect in the renal secretion of urate. This study was followed by another study of gouty and nongouty subjects utilizing the pyrazinamide (PZA) suppression test, which again demonstrated no defect in the renal handling of urate in gouty subjects (68).

In 1962 Seegmiller et al. performed experiments in which the plasma concentration of urate was increased by feeding RNA to normal subjects and to patients with gout (69). The subjects with gout were subdivided into those individuals with normal rates of production of urate (presumed underexcretors) and those with overproduction of urate. The fractional excretion of urate in the normoproducers was significantly lower than that of the overproducers and of the normal subjects who received RNA. These findings suggested a defect in the excretion of urate in the normoproducers. A major criticism of this study, however, was that plasma concentrations of urate were not entirely comparable in the two subgroups of gouty patients (70).

Rieselbach et al. (71) extended the approach utilized by Seegmiller and colleagues (69). Urate metabolism was studied in 15 men with gouty arthritis and compared with a group of normals. The turnover rate of urate was determined using 2-^{14}C urate. Of the 15 gouty patients studied, nine were found to be overproducers of urate and six were normoproducers. The urinary excretion of urate correlated well with the turnover data. The administration of pyrazinamide resulted in similar fractional rates of excretion of urate in the two groups of patients, implying that both groups have similar renal reabsorptive capacities for urate. Urate secretion, however, was quite different. At any given plasma concentration of urate, the overproducers of urate had higher rates of secretion of urate than the normoproducers.

In an attempt to settle the issue of whether a renal abnormality in urate handling exists in gouty patients, Simkin critically analyzed the data from the above-mentioned studies (Fig. 2)

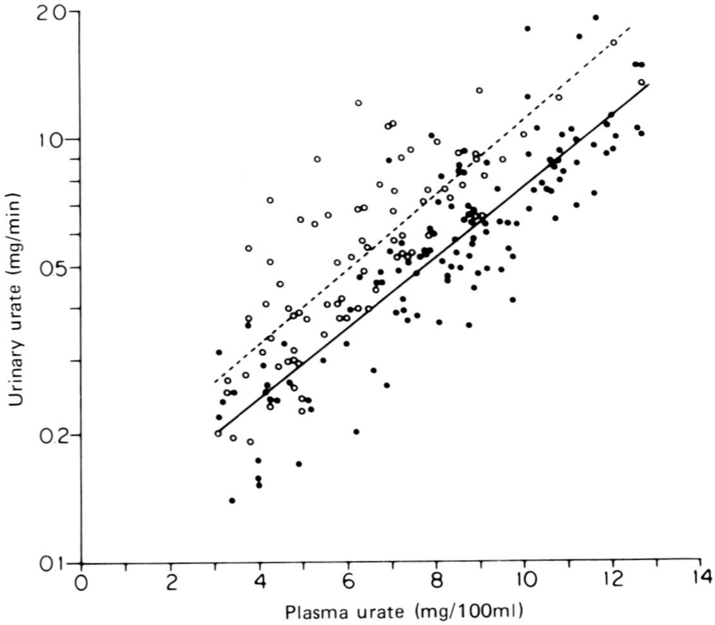

Fig. 2 Uric acid excretion at varying plasma concentrations of urate in normals and gouty subjects. The slopes of the regression lines through normal (open circles) and gouty (closed circles) patients are not significantly different from each other. (From Simkin, P. A. Arthritis and Rheum. 22:99, 1979.)

(72). The urinary excretion rate of uric acid was compared with the plasma level of urate in 73 gouty subjects and 36 normals. The cumulative data fit regression lines that had parallel slopes but different intercepts. It was deduced that at any plasma concentration of urate, gouty individuals will excrete only 71% as much urate as normals. Said in another way, the plasma concentration of urate in gouty individuals must be 1.7 mg/dl higher than normals to achieve the same rate of urate excretion.

In summary, it would seem that gout is a disease of multiple metabolic defects. A subset of patients can be identified who overproduce urate and have abnormally high rates of excretion of urate by the kidneys. As compared to normal controls, the rates of absorption and secretion of urate are appropriate to the plasma concentrations of urate. In another group of patients, a defect in the renal excretion of urate exists, with or without coexistent abnormalities in the rate of production. Based on the results of the pyrazinamide suppression test, the renal defect would seem to be one of an inadequate rate of secretion of urate in the face of an elevation in the plasma concentration of urate. The tubular reabsorptive mechanisms, however, would seem to be intact.

An association between gout, hyperuricemia, and polycystic and medullary cystic disease of the kidney has been described (73-75). Renal function in some of these cases was well preserved, and the hyperuricemia was apparently due to undersecretion of uric acid. Further studies of patients with these defects will be required, however, to ascertain whether the defect is due to specific tubular transport abnormalities or to a decreased rate of excretion due to the decrease in the glomerular filtration rate.

Hyperuricemia Due to Increased Renal Tubular Reabsorption

Two families have been described with hyperuricemia of no discernible secondary cause and normal glomerular filtration rates (76). The endogenous rate of production of urate was normal as determined by the rate of ^{14}C glycine incorporation into urate. The fractional excretion rate of urate was less than 5.5%. Tubular secretion and reabsorption of uric acid were assessed following the administration of probenecid and pyrazinamide. The results were interpreted to indicate an enhanced rate of urate absorption and a normal rate of secretion. As stated previously, such studies must be interpreted with caution, especially since the drugs used affect the renal tubular transport of each other in addition to their effects on urate transport. Nonetheless, if these studies are confirmed, they would represent the first description of primary hyperuricemia due to enhanced tubular reabsorption rather than defective secretion of urate.

Hypouricemia Due to Isolated Renal Tubular Defect

The Tecumseh study (77) of 6000 normal persons identified 1% of that population as having a serum concentration of urate less than 2.0 mg/dl, a finding that has since been confirmed by others (78). Investigation of persons with hypouricemia has revealed either a decreased rate of production of urate or increased rate of urinary excretion of urate. Decreased production of uric acid may be due to a deficiency of the enzyme xanthine oxidase (xanthinuria), following the administration of allopurinol, or in severe liver disease. Increased renal excretion of urate may be due to hereditary or acquired disorders of renal tubular function or the administration of uricosuric drugs.

The first report of hypouricemia due to a specific renal absorptive defect appeared in 1950 (45). The patient described had a serum concentration of urate which ranged between 0.2 and 0.6 mg/dl and a fractional rate of excretion of 150%. No other studies of renal tubular function were included in the report. Three additional reports have described other patients with hypouricemia and fractional rates of excretion of urate greater than 100% (47,79,80). In the patient described by Khachadurian and Arslanian (47), no tubular defects other than that of urate transport were found. Simkin et al. (79) administered pyrazinamide, salicylate, or probenecid to a patient with hypouricemia and a fractional rate of urate excretion greater than 100%. All three drugs reduced the fractional rate of excretion to approximately 100%, indicating defective reabsorption of urate as the causative defect. This defect has been termed the Dalmatian dog mutation in man, in analogy to the finding in the Dalmatian coach hound (46). The Dalmatian, in contrast to other strains of dog, has an inherited defect in tubular absorption of urate. Whereas the defect in urate transport in Dalmatians seems to be generalized and the defect for urate transport is also found in their red blood cells, humans with hypouricemia seem to have the defect localized to the renal tubules (81).

A number of additional studies have been published describing patients with hypouricemia (82-91) due to increased renal excretion of uric acid. By contrast to the patients described above, all of these individuals had hypouricemia, but the fractional rate of excretion of urate, although elevated, was less than 100%. Utilizing the pharmacological probes pyrazinamide and probenecid, it would seem that the basic defect in all the reported cases is that of impaired reabsorption of urate rather than increased tubular secretion. Some authors have attempted to localize the defect to the pre- or postsecretory reabsorptive site (86,87), but as noted previously the results of studies using pharmacological probes must be interpreted with caution.

A familial occurrence of defective tubular reabsorption of urate has been noted in a number of kindred studies. The inheritance pattern appears to be an autosomal recessive trait (82,83,88,90). Although the condition would seem to be benign, a number of associated abnormalities have been described, including uric acid lithiasis, calcium oxalate lithiasis, bone disease, and hypercalciuria (80,82,84,90). The hypercalciuria has been attributed to increased intestinal absorption of calcium, although a coexistent renal tubular defect for calcium absorption is also possible.

B. Hypouricemia Due to Renal Defect: Generalized Disorders

The Fanconi Syndrome (92,93)

Hyperuricosuria and hypouricemia are well recognized features of the Fanconi syndrome. Studies with pyrazinamide and probenecid (92) have demonstrated that there is a defect in the reabsorption of urate. The rates of secretion of urate appear to be normal (92).

Wilson's Disease (94-96)

Wilson's disease is associated with multiple renal tubular absorptive defects, including defects in the transport of urate. Hyperuricosuria has been described by a number of authors. Low plasmic uric acid concentrations and fractional excretion rates in excess of 20-30% of the filtered load are frequently seen. The defect, based on pharmacological studies, appears to be one of defective tubular reabsorption of urate. Of interest, treatment with penicillamine in some cases has returned the pattern of urate excretion toward normal (97,98).

Sickle Cell Anemia (99,100)

The most common abnormality of uric acid metabolism described in sickle cell disease is hyperuricemia. In a study of 20 cases of hemoglobin S disease (either SS or SC), nine had hyperuricemia, but only one patient had gout (99). The proposed mechanism of the hyperuricemia was an increased rate of production due to increased turnover of nucleic acids. The renal handling of urate was studied in seven young adults with sickle cell anemia, uric acid overproduction, and normouricemia (100). Urate clearance in these subjects was increased compared to normals, as was the fractional rate of excretion of urate. Administration of pyrazinamide resulted in a quantitatively greater suppression of urate excretion than in normals. These findings were interpreted to indicate that patients with sickle cell anemia are hypersecretors of uric acid. The increase in the rate of secretion of urate thus serves to maintain the plasma concentration of urate at normal levels and prevent the development of gout.

III. ACQUIRED DISORDERS OF URIC ACID TRANSPORT

A. Uric Acid Abnormalities Associated with Systemic Diseases

A number of systemic diseases may be associated with changes in the transport of urate in the kidney which result in either hyperuricemia or hypouricemia. Although specific transport abnormalities are present in some of the conditions to be described, the majority are the consequence of either retention of other organic anions, drug administration, or alteration in the volume of extracellular fluid. Frequently more than one factor is present. Hyperuricemia may be seen in conditions marked by increased production or retention of other organic acids (101,102). These organic acids compete with urate for the tubular secretory site in the kidney. Diabetic ketoacidosis, ketoacidosis associated with fasting, and lactic acidosis may all be accompanied by an elevation in the serum concentration of urate (103, 104). These forms of hyperuricemia rarely result in urate deposition or specific clinical signs. The hyperuricemia is usually transient and disappears when the underlying abnormality is corrected. In addition to the decreased secretory flux of urate in such clinical conditions, it is quite likely that the reabsorptive flux of urate is also enhanced due to the coexisting decrease in the extracellular fluid volume.

Hyperuricemia is a common finding in patients with congestive heart failure. In this situation, the primary defect is likely to be an enhanced rate of absorption of urate. It has been demonstrated both in animals and man that depletion of the extracellular fluid volume and a decrease in the effective blood volume is associated with an increased rate of tubular absorption of urate (20,105). The mechanism responsible for the increased absorptive flux may be related to slower rates of flow of tubular fluid in the proximal convoluted tubule (24). A decreased rate of urate secretion may also exist consequent to lactic or keto acid generation.

Malignant diseases are most commonly associated with hyperuricemia secondary to increased production of urate. However, a small percentage of patients with malignant diseases may have hypouricemia due to abnormalities in renal tubular reabsorption of urate. In a study of 53 patients with serum urate concentrations less than 2 mg/dl, nine patients, or 17%, were noted to have malignant disease (78). Four of these patients were studied in detail and were found to have increased fractional excretion of urate, without evidence of other defects in tubular absorptive function. Hypouricemia has been reported in patients with carcinoma of the lung, acute myeloblastic leukemia, and Hodgkin's disease (106,107). In one case of Hodgkin's disease, hypouricemia was noted to parallel disease activity (107). The mechanisms responsible for the increased excretion of urate in these disorders, however, have not been fully elucidated. It is possible that there are substances produced by these tumors that directly interfere with urate transport.

In addition to a possible direct effect of malignancy on the absorptive mechanism for urate, increased rates of excretion of urate regularly accompany the syndrome of inappropriate secretion of antidiuretic hormone (SIADH) seen with some malignant diseases. Only one of 17 patients with SIADH studied by Beck had a serum concentration of uric acid in excess of 4.0 mg/dl (108). Clearance studies demonstrated an increased fractional rate of excretion of urate in three of these patients studied in greater detail. Restriction of water, which normalized the serum concentration of sodium, returned the fractional rate of excretion of urate to normal. It was suggested that the hypervolemia that accompanies SIADH was responsible for the increased clearance of urate (108). Antidiuretic hormone itself is unlikely to participate directly in this phenomenon, since ADH, if it has any direct effect on the transport of urate, enhances urate absorption across various epithelial tissues (109, 110). Serum urate concentrations less than 4.0 mg/dl are so commonly seen with SIADH that it has been recommended as a useful laboratory test to separate SIADH from other causes of hyponatremia. In the study of Beck, no patient with hyponatremia caused by other mechanisms had a serum concentration of urate of less than 5 mg/dl (108).

Normal pregnancy results in an increase in urate excretion, most likely reflecting the expanded extracellular fluid volume (111). Preeclampsia and eclampsia are associated with a fall in the fractional rate of excretion of urate. The exact mechanism responsible for this decreased excretion of urate has not been clearly defined, but may be related to the decreased extracellular fluid volume as compared to normal pregnancy or the retention of organic acids (112). The change in the serum concentration of urate in pregnancy has been used as a biochemical marker of preeclampsia in pregnant women.

Other diseases that have been causally associated with abnormalities in renal urate transport include cirrhosis, essential hypertension, and renovascular hypertention (113-115);

B. Drug-Induced Disorders of Urate Transport

Drugs may also cause disorders of urate transport by the kidney. Hyperuricemia or hypouricemia may result, depending on whether the secretory or reabsorptive system for urate is affected.

The chronic administration of diuretics is the most common drug-related cause of hyperuricemia (116). The primary effect of these agents on urate transport is secondary to the diuretic-induced changes in the extracellular fluid volume and the influence of the state of hydration on urate reabsorption in the proximal convoluted tubule (17). In addition, since diuretics are organic acids, they may inhibit the secretory flux of urate by competing for the common organic acid secretory system. Studies in man and in the rat, however, would suggest that the prime cause of diuretic induced hyperuricemia is depletion of the extracellular fluid volume (17,117).

The second most common cause of drug-induced hyperuricemia is the administration of salicylates in low doses (53). Administration of acetylsalicylate at a dose of 1.2 g for 4 days led to an increase in the plasma concentration of urate of 1.0-1.8 mg/dl in males and 1.0 mg/dl in females. Yu and Gutman found that the maximal antiuricosuric effect of salicylates occurred at a plasma salicylate concentration of 5 mg/dl (53). It has been proposed that salicylates in low doses inhibit the renal tubular secretion of uric acid. Other pharmacological agents are less commonly associated with hyperuricemia, but they should be kept in mind in the evaluation of patients with elevated blood levels of uric acid.

Pharmacological agents may also be associated with hypouricemia due to increased renal excretion of urate. The most common cause of hypouricemia in hospitalized patients is drug administration. Ramsdell and Kelly found that drugs could be implicated as the cause of hypouricemia in two-thirds of the patients they studied (78). The three most commonly associated agents were salicylates (in high doses and plasma salicylate concentration greater than 10 mg/dl), x-ray contrast agents, and glyceryl guaiacolate. In addition, both probenecid and sulfinpyrazone induce an increased rate of urate excretion in the urine. In patients with hyperuricemia, the administration of either probenecid or sulfinpyrazone reduces the plasma concentration of urate toward normal. However, both drugs have been used in clinical circumstances not directly related to hyperuricemia. When administered to patients who initially have normal plasma concentrations of urate hypouricemia may be induced.

Studies performed in patients receiving radiocontrast agents have demonstrated that the administration of these agents results in marked uricosuria (118). Based on the ability of pyrazinamide to abolish the uricosuria, it has been suggested that these agents enhance secretion of uric acid (119). It is possible, however, that these agents may also interfere with the postsecretory reabsorption of uric acid. The orally administered cholecystographic dyes iopanoic acid (Telepaque) and calcium ipodate (Oragrafin) appear to be the most potent uricosuric dyes and their effects may be evident for up to 7 days after administration (119).

Glyceryl guaiacolate (Robitussin) has been shown to increase the fractional excretion of urate (120). Presumably, this is the result of inhibition of urate reabsorption.

C. Disorders of Urate Transport Secondary to Toxic Agents

Hyperuricemia may be seen in patients with chronic lead intoxication, so-called saturnine gout. It has been proposed that the mechanism responsible for the hyperuricemia seen with lead intoxication involves enhanced urate reabsorption. Emmerson examined patients with lead intoxication using the pyrazinamide suppression test and found that urate secretion was within the range seen in normals (121).

Chronic beryllium intoxication may also be associated with hyperuricemia in 40% of cases (122). Renal clearance studies have shown a decrease in the fractional excretion of urate in these patients. The authors (122) suggested that this was due to decreased secretion of urate, either by a direct interference with cellular metabolism or by an indirect effect of an unidentified organic acid which interfered with urate excretion.

IV. CLINICAL CONSEQUENCES OF ABNORMALITIES OF URATE TRANSPORT

Regardless of the pathophysiology, there are only a limited number of clinical expressions of disordered urate metabolism. Urate itself is not toxic to tissue. The major clinical expressions of these diseases are related to the precipitation of urate, and include the development of gouty arthritis and/or the formation of kidney stones. A relationship between the serum concentration of uric acid and the development of gouty arthritis was suggested from the results of the Framingham study (55). It has become clear, however, that other factors in addition to hyperuricemia contribute to the development of attacks of gouty arthritis (123). Moreover, the data of the Framingham study showing a relationship between attacks of arthritis and the serum concentration of uric acid are rather limited. The relationship between the serum concentration of urate and the development of uric acid nephrolithiasis in published studies is weak or nonexistent (124,125). This is perhaps not surprising, since the critical variable is likely to be the urine concentration of uric acid. Most studies, however, report only the absolute rates of urate excretion, a value which may or may not correlate with the incidence of stones. It is also likely that other factors, such as the urine pH, may influence the incidence of stones (126). Nonetheless, hyperuricemia when associated with increased rates of excretion of urate, volume depletion, and/or acidic urine, or renal tubular defects of absorption and hyperuricosuria is a clinical circumstance which favors the crystallization of uric acid and the formation of kidney stones.

In addition to arthritis and nephrolithiasis, abnormalities in urate metabolism have been implicated in other disease conditions. Hyperuricosuria, with or without hyperuricemia, is often observed in patients with calcium oxalate kidney stones. In one series of 460 calcium stone-forming patients, 25% were identified as having hyperuricosuria alone or hyperuricosuria as well as hypercalciuria (127). The mechanism of the hyperuricosuria is unclear. It has been shown that these patients ingest excessive amounts of purine-rich foods in their diet (128). In addition, a number of these stone-formers have also been shown to be overproducers of uric acid (127,129). The existence of a subgroup of patients with hyperuricosuria due to increased fractional excretion of uric acid is possible, but has not yet been documented (130). Uric acid and/or sodium urate appear to provide a nidus for the crystallization of calcium oxalate or alter the physicochemical properties of calcium and oxalate in solution (129,131,132). In some patients, the coexistence of several renal tubular absorptive defects may result in nephrolithiasis, and therapy directed toward reduction of the urinary concentration of uric acid may reduce the incidence of calcium oxalate stones (129).

Chronic hyperuricemia and/or hyperuricosuria has been postulated to result in gouty nephropathy, a slowly progressive form of renal insufficiency (133-135). The pathological findings include interstitial nephritis with or without arteriosclerotic changes in the glomeruli, blood vessels, and renal interstitium. These findings are nonspecific and their relationship to the abnormalities in urate metabolism are unclear. In addition, in a series of 20 patients with asymptomatic hyperuricemia, 63% were found to have one or more renal functional abnormalities (136). These included abnormal urine sediments, submaximal urine concentrating ability, proteinuria, and diminished titratable acid excretion. Only 10% of the patients, however, had abnormal glomerular filtration rates. The most recent evidence would indicate that hyperuricemia per se, in the absence of stones, does not lead to a decline in renal function above and beyond that predicted to occur by aging alone (137,138). If significant decrements in renal function occur in such patients, it can often be ascribed to coexisting renal disease or a toxic nephropathy such as that seen in lead intoxication (138, 139). Finally, the changes in renal function over time in hyperuricemic individuals is similar whether or not pharmacological therapy is administered to treat the hyperuricemia (137, 138). At the present time, then, it appears unlikely that gouty nephropathy is a distinct clinical entity.

Hyperuricemia has been noted in some, but not all, clinical studies to be a risk factor for the development of arteriosclerosis and cardiovascular disease (140-142). These relationships are difficult to discern from the available literature and are complicated by the association of hyperuricemia with hypertension, obesity, glucose intolerance, and diuretic administration (123). While no definitive statement about the relationship between urate and arteriosclerosis can be made, it would appear that hyperuricemia is not a major risk factor or at best only a minor risk factor. Moreover, there is no evidence to date to indicate that hypouricemic therapy is of any value in reducing the risk of cardiovascular disease.

Therapy for patients with abnormalities in urate metabolism has recently been reviewed (59,143). Patients with acute alterations in the serum concentration of urate, such as those associated with alterations in the extracellular fluid volume or the generation of other organic acids, rarely manifest clinically recognized sequelae of the hyperuricemia. Therapy is directed only toward the primary disease process. This statement, however, does not necessarily apply to patients with cancer undergoing chemotherapy or radiation therapy when the risk of uric acid-induced acute renal failure is a possible complication, or in patients with extreme obesity, especially during periods of weight reduction using starvation regimens (104). Patients with chronic hyperuricemia without documented episodes of gouty arthritis or uric acid kidney stones probably should not receive pharmacological agents to reduce the serum concentration of urate (144). Patients with attacks of gouty arthritis, in addition to anti-inflammatory medication, can and should be treated with specific therapy directed toward reducing the serum concentration of uric acid. In like manner, patients with uric acid stones or calcium oxalate stones with coexisting hyperuricosuria should receive hypouricemic therapy. In theory, the choice of therapy depends on whether overproduction or underexcretion of uric acid is the cause of hyperuricemia. Drugs used to treat hyperuricemia include uricosuric agents that block the renal tubular reabsorption of uric acid (probenecid, sulfinpyrazone) or agents that inhibit the production of uric acid by blocking the enzyme xanthine oxidase (allopurinol). Patients who are found to be overproducers of uric acid, as well as patients with renal disease (especially those with uric acid nephrolithiasis or urate nephropathy) should be treated with allopurinol. Patients who are underexcretors of uric acid may be treated with a uricosuric agent if renal function is relatively normal. Treatment with a uricosuric agent results in an increase in renal uric acid excretion with the risk of developing renal calculi. Thus, the choice between these two forms of therapy must be made on an individual basis, and careful follow-up of serum and urinary levels of uric acid must be obtained.

ACKNOWLEDGMENT

The authors wish to acknowledge the secretarial assistance of Polly Dunham.

REFERENCES

1. Sorensen, L. B. Degradation of uric acid in man. Metabolism 8:687-703, 1959.
2. Sorensen, L. B. The elimination of uric acid in man. Scand. J. Clin. Lab. Invest. 12 (Suppl. 54):35-46, 1960.
3. Kelley, W. Pathophysiology of purine metabolism in man. Enzyme 18:161-175, 1974.
4. Wyngaarden, J. B. Metabolic defects of primary hyperuricemia and gout. Am. J. Med. 56:651-664, 1974.
5. Seegmiller, J. E. Intermediary purine metabolism and its regulation. In: Gout and Uric Acid Metabolism, edited by Talbott, J. H., and Yu, T.-F. New York, Stratton Intercontinental Medical Book, 1976, pp. 39-57.
6. Chin, T. Y.; Cacini, W.; Zmuda, M. J.; and Quebbemann, A. J. Quantification of renal uric acid synthesis in the rat. Am. J. Physiol. 238:F481-F487, 1980.
7. Weiner, I. M. Urate transport in the nephron. Am. J. Physiol. 237:F85-F92, 1979.
8. Roch-Ramel, F.; and Weiner, I. M. Renal excretion of urate: Factors determining the action of drugs. Kidney Int. 18:665-676, 1980.
9. Roch-Ramel, F.; Diezi-Chomety, F.; DeRougemont, D.; Tellier, M.; Widmer, J.; and Peters, G. Renal excretion of uric acid in the rat: A micropuncture and microperfusion study, Am. J. Physiol. 230:768-776, 1976.
10. Kovarsky, J.; Holmes, E. W.; and Kelley, W. N. Absence of significant urate binding to human serum proteins. J. Lab. Clin. Med. 93:85-91, 1979.
11. Campion, D. S.; Bluestone, R.; and Klinenberg, J. R. Uric acid: Characterization of its interaction with human serum albumin. J. Clin. Invest. 52:2383-2386, 1973.
12. Campion, D. S.; Bluestone, R.; and Klinenberg, J. R. Displacement by uricosuric agents of sodium urate bound to human serum albumin. Biochem. Pharmacol. 23:1653-1657, 1974.
13. Schlosstein, L. H.; Kippen, I.; Whitehouse, M. W.; Bluestone, R.; Paulus, H. E.; and Klinenberg, J. R. Studies with some novel uricosuric agents and their metabolites: Correlation between clinical activity and drug-induced displacement of urate from its albumin binding sites. J. Lab. Clin. Med. 82:412-418, 1973.
14. Senekjian, H. O.; Knight, T. F.; and Weinman, E. J. Micropuncture study of the renal handling of [6-^{14}C]-urate in the rat. Miner. Electrolyte Metab. 2:155-160, 1979.
15. DeRougemont, D.; Henchoz, M.; and Roch-Ramel, F. Renal urate excretion at various plasma concentrations in the rat: A free-flow micropuncture study. Am. J. Physiol. 231:387-392, 1976.
16. Weinman, E. J.; Knight, T. F.; McKenzie, R.; and Eknoyan, G. Dissociation of urate from sodium transport in the rat proximal tubule. Kidney Int. 10:295-300, 1976.
17. Weinman, E. J.; Steplock, D.; Suki, W. N.; and Eknoyan, G. Urate reabsorption in proximal convoluted tubule of the rat kidney. Am. J. Physiol. 231:509-515, 1976.
18. Frommer, J. P.; Sheth, A. U.; Senekjian, H. O.; Babino, H.; and Weinman, E. J. Free-flow micropuncture study of renal urate transport in the Munich-Wistar rat. Miner. Electrolyte Metab. 7:324-330, 1982.
19. Roch-Ramel, F.; Granges, F.; Roth, L.; Widmer, J.; and Weiner, I. M. Renal handling of urate by non-diuretic and diuretic rats. Renal Physiol. 2:122-129, 1979-80.
20. Weinman, E. J.; Eknoyan, G.; and Suki, W. N. The influence of the extracellular fluid volume on the tubular reabsorption of uric acid. J. Clin. Invest. 55:283-291, 1975.
21. Weinman, E. J.; Senekjian, H. O.; Sansom, S. C.; Steplock, D.; Sheth, A.; and Knight, T. F. Evidence for active and passive urate transport in the rat proximal tubule. Am. J. Physiol. 240:F90-F93, 1981.
22. Sansom, S. C.; Senekjian, H. O.; Knight, T. F.; Babino, H.; Steplock, D.; and Weinman, E. J. Determination of the apparent transport constants for urate absorption in the rat proximal tubule. Am. J. Physiol. 240:F406-F410, 1981.

23. Knight, T. F.; Senekjian, H. O.; Sansom, S. C.; and Weinman, E. J. The effect of intraluminal D-glucose and probenecid on urate absorption in the rat proximal tubule. Am. J. Physiol. 236:F526-F529, 1979.
24. Senekjian, H. O.; Knight, T. F.; Sansom, S.; and Weinman, E. J. Effect of flow rate and the extracellular fluid volume on proximal urate and water absorption. Kidney Int. 17: 155-161, 1980.
25. Weinman, E. J.; Sansom, S. C.; Steplock, D.; Sheth, A.; Knight, T. F.; and Senekjian, H. O. The secretion of urate in the proximal convoluted tubule of the rat. Am. J. Physiol. 239:F383-F387, 1980.
26. Kramp, R. A.; and Lenoir, R. H. Characteristics of urate influx in the rat nephron. Am. J. Physiol. 229:1654-1661, 1975.
27. Frankfurt, S. J.; and Weinman, E. J. The effect of probenecid on urate transport in the rat kidney. Proc. Soc. Exp. Biol. Med. 155:554-557, 1977.
28. Frankfurt, S. J.; and Weinman, E. J. Pyrazinoic acid and urate transport in the rat. Proc. Soc. Exp. Biol. Med. 159:16-20, 1978.
29. Roch-Ramel, F.; DeRougemont, D.; Peters, G.; and Weiner, I. M. Micropuncture study of urate excretion by the kidney of the rat, the Cebus monkey and the rabbit. In: Amino Acid Transport and Uric Acid Transport, edited by Silbernagel, S., Lang, F., and Greger, R. Stuttgart, George Thieme, 1976, pp. 188-191.
30. Poulsen, H.; and Praetorius, E. Tubular excretion of uric acid in rabbits. Acta Pharmacol. Toxicol. 10:371-378, 1954.
31. Boumendil-Podevin, E. F.; Podevin, R. A.; and Priol, C. Uric acid transport in brush border membrane vesicles isolated from rabbit kidney. Am. J. Physiol. 236:F519-F525, 1979.
32. Senekjian, H. O.; Knight, T. F.; and Weinman, E. J. Urate transport by the isolated perfused S_2 segment of the rabbit. Am. J. Physiol. 240:F530-F535, 1981.
33. Shimomura, A.; Chonko, A.; Tanner, R.; Edwards, R.; and Grantham, J. The nature of urate transport in isolated rabbit proximal tubules. Am. J. Physiol. 241:F565-F578, 1981.
34. Weber, J. L.; Kokko, J. P.; Jacobson, H. R. Heterogeneity of uric acid transport in proximal tubules. Am. Soc. Nephrol. Abstr.:154A, 1980.
35. Plaats, M. M.; and Mudge, G. H. Accumulation of uric acid by slices of kidney cortex. Am. J. Physiol. 200:387-391, 1961.
36. Kippen, I.; Nakata, N.; and Klinenberg, J. R. Uptake of uric acid by separated renal tubules of the rabbit. I. Characteristics of transport. J. Pharmacol. Exp. Ther. 201: 218-225, 1977.
37. Roch-Ramel, F.; Wong, L. N. M.; and Dirks, J. H. Renal excretion of urate in mongrel and Dalmatian dogs: A micropuncture study. Am. J. Physiol. 231:326-331, 1976.
38. Yu, T. F.; Berger, L.; Kupfer, S.; and Gutman, A. B. Tubular secretion of urate in the dog. Am. J. Physiol. 199:1199-1204, 1960.
39. Nolan, R. P.; and Foulkes, E. C. Studies on renal urate secretion in the dog. J. Pharmacol. Exp. Ther. 179:429-437, 1971.
40. Blomstedt, J. W.; and Aronson, P. S. pH Gradient-stimulated transport of urate and p-aminohippurate in dog renal microvillus membrane vesicles. J. Clin. Invest. 65:931-934, 1980.
41. Kahn, A. M.; and Aronson, P. S. Cl-Coupled urate transport in dog renal cortical microvillus membrane vesicles (Abstr.). Fed. Proc. 40:463, 1981.
42. Warnock, D. G.; and Yee, V. J. Chloride uptake by brush border membrane vesicles isolated from rabbit renal cortex. J. Clin. Invest. 67:103-115, 1981.
43. Steele, T. H.; and Boner, G. Origins of the uricosuric response. J. Clin. Invest. 52:1368-1375, 1973.
44. Berliner, J. W.; Hilton, J. G.; Yu, T. F.; and Kennedy, T. J., Jr. The renal mechanism for urate excretion in man. J. Clin. Invest. 29:396-401, 1950.

45. Praetorius, E.; and Kirk, J. E. Hypouricemia: With evidence for tubular elimination of uric acid. J. Lab. Clin. Med. 35:865-868, 1950.
46. Green, M. L.; Marcus, R.; Aurbach, G. D.; Kazam, E. S.; and Seegmiller, J. E. Hypouricemia due to isolated renal tubular defect: Dalmatian dog mutation in man. Am. J. Med. 53:361-367, 1972.
47. Khachadurian, A. K.; and Arslanian, M. J. Hypouricemia due to renal uricosuria. Ann. Intern. Med. 78:547-550, 1973.
48. Yu, T.-F.; Berger, L.; Stone, D. J.; Wolfe, J.; and Gutman, A. B. Effect of pyrazinamide and pyrazinoic acid on urate clearance and other discrete renal functions. Proc. Soc. Exp. Biol. Med. 96:264-267, 1957.
49. Steele, T. G.; and Rieselbach, R. E. The renal mechanism for urate homeostasis in normal man. Am. J. Med. 43:868-875, 1967.
50. Fanelli, G. M. Jr.; Bohn, D. L.; and Reilly, S. S. Renal urate transport in the chimpanzee. Am. J. Physiol. 220:613-620, 1971.
51. Diamond, H. S.; and Paolino, J. S. Evidence for a postsecretory reabsorptive site for uric acid in man. J. Clin. Invest. 52:1491-1499, 1973.
52. Steele, T. H. Renal excretion of uric acid. Arthritis Rheum. 18(Suppl.):793-804, 1975.
53. Yu, T. F.; and Gutman, A. B. Study of the paradoxical effects of salicylates in low, intermediate, and high dosages on the renal mechanism of excretion of urate in man. J. Clin. Invest. 38:1298-1315, 1959.
54. Yu, T. F.; and Gutman, A. B. Paradoxical retention of uric acid by uricosuric drugs in low dosage. Proc. Soc. Exp. Biol. Med. 90:542-547, 1955.
55. Hall, A. P.; Barry, P. E.; Dawber, T. R.; and McNamara, P. M. Epidemiology of gout and hyperuricemia: A long-term population study. Am. J. Med. 42:27-37, 1967.
56. Jacobson, B. M. The uric acid in the serum of gouty and non-gouty individuals. Determination by Folin's recent method and its significance in the diagnosis of gout. Ann. Int. Med. 11:1277-1295, 1937.
57. Sturge, R. A.; Scott, J. T.; Kennedy, A. C.; Hart, D. P.; and Buchanan, W. W. Serum uric acid in England and Scotland. Ann. Rheum. Dis. 36:420-427, 1977.
58. Drum, D. E.; Goldman, P. A.; and Jankowski, C. B. Elevation of serum uric acid as a clue to alcohol abuse. Arch. Int. Med. 141:477-479, 1981.
59. Simkin, P. A. Management of gout. Ann. Intern. Med. 90:812-816, 1979.
60. Seegmiller, J. E.; Grayzel, A. I.; Laster, L.; and Liddle, L. Uric acid production in gout. J. Clin. Invest. 40:1304-1314, 1961.
61. Boss, G. R.; and Seegmiller, J. E. Hyperuricemia and gout: Classification, complications and management; N. Engl. J. Med. 300:1459-1468, 1979.
62. Smyth, C. J. Disorders associated with hyperuricemia. Arthritis Rheum. 18(Suppl.): 713-719, 1975.
63. Garrod, A. B. Observations on certain pathological conditions of blood and urine in gout, rheumatism in Bright's disease. Tr. M-Chir. Soc. 31:83-98, 1848.
64. Gutman, A. B.; and Yu, T. F. Renal function in gout. With a commentary on the renal regulation of urate excretion, and the role of the kidney in the pathogenesis of gout. Am. J. Med. 23:600-622, 1957.
65. Nugent, C. A.; and Tyler, F. H. The renal excretion of uric acid in patients with gout and in non-gouty subjects. J. Clin. Invest. 38:1890-1898, 1959.
66. Lathem, W.; and Rodnan, G. P. Impairment of uric acid excretion in gout. J. Clin. Invest. 41:1955-1963, 1962.
67. Yu, T. F.; Berger, L.; and Gutman, A. B. Renal function in gout. II. Effect of uric acid loading on renal excretion of uric acid. Am. J. Med. 33:829-844, 1962.
68. Gutman, A. B.; Yu, T. F.; and Berger, L. Renal function in gout. III. Estimation of tubular secretion and reabsorption of uric acid by use of pyrazinamide (pyrazinoic acid). Am. J. Med. 47:575-592, 1969.
69. Seegmiller, J. E.; Grayzel, A. I.; Howell, R. R.; and Plato, C. The renal excretion of uric acid in gout. J. Clin. Invest. 41:1094-1098, 1962.

70. Rieselbach, R. E.; and Steele, T. H. Influence of the kidney upon urate homeostasis in health and disease. Am. J. Med. 56:665-675, 1974.
71. Rieselbach, R. E.; Sorensen, L. B.; Shelp, W. D.; and Steele, T. H. Diminished renal urate secretion per nephron as a basis for primary gout. Ann. Intern. Med. 73:359-366, 1970.
72. Simkin, P. A. Uric acid excretion in patients with gout. Arthritis Rheum. 22:98-99, 1979.
73. Newcombe, D. S. Gouty arthritis and polycystic kidney disease. Ann. Intern. Med. 79: 605-606, 1973.
74. Martinez-Maldonado, M. Polycystic kidney disease and hyperuricemia. Ann. Intern. Med. 80:116, 1974.
75. Thompson, G. R.; Weiss, J. J.; Goldman, R. T.; and Rigg, G. A. Familial occurrence of hyperuricemia, gout and medullary cystic disease. Arch. Intern. Med. 138:1614-1617, 1978.
76. Stapleton, F. B.; and Nyhan, W. L. Increased renal tubular reabsorption of uric acid in familial hyperuricemia (Abstr.). Clin. Res. 27:824A, 1979.
77. Mikkelsen, W. M.; Dodge, H. J.; and Valkenburg, H. The distribution of serum uric acid values in a population unselected as to gout or hyperuricemia: Tecumseh, Michigan, 1959-1960. Am. J. Med. 39:242-251, 1965.
78. Ramsdell, C.; and Kelley, W. N. The clinical significance of hypouricemia. Ann. Intern. Med. 78:239-242, 1973.
79. Simkin, P. A.; Skeith, M. D.; and Healey, L. A. Suppression of uric acid secretion in a patient with renal hypouricemia. Isr. J. Med. Sci. 9:1113, 1973.
80. Hedley, J. M.; and Phillips, P. J. Familial hypouricaemia associated with renal tubular uricosuria and uric acid calculi: Case report. J. Clin. Pathol. 33:971-972, 1980.
81. Sperling, O.; Boer, P.; Weinberger, A.; and DeVries, A. Transport into erythrocytes and absorption of uric acid in hereditary renal hypouricemia. Biomedicine 23:157-159, 1975.
82. Sperling, O.; Weinberger, A.; Oliver, I.; Lieberman, U. A.; and DeVries, A. Hypouricemia, hypercalciuria and decreased bone density: A hereditary syndrome. Ann. Intern. Med. 80:482-487, 1974.
83. Akaoka, I.; Nishizawa, T.; Yano, E.; Takeuchi, A.; Nishida, Y.; Yoshimura, T.; and Horiuchi, Y. Familial hypouricemia due to renal tubular defect of urate transport. Ann. Clin. Res. 7:318-324, 1975.
84. Akaoka, I.; Nishizawa, T.; Yano, E.; Kamatani, N.; Nishida, Y.; and Sasaki, S. Renal urate excretion in five cases of hypouricemia with an isolated renal defect of urate transport. J. Rheum. 4:86-94, 1977.
85. Benjamin, D.; Sperling, O.; Weinberger, A.; Pinkhas, J.; and DeVries, A. Familial hypouricemia due to isolated renal tubular defect. Nephron 18:220-225, 1977.
86. Benjamin, D.; Sperling, O.; Weinberger, A.; and Pinkhas, J. Familial hypouricemia due to isolated renal tubular abnormality. Biomedicine 29:54-56, 1978.
87. Sperling, O.; Weinberger, A.; Benjamin, D.; Pinkhas, J.; and DeVries, A. Hereditary renal hypouricemia: Heterogeneity of tubular abnormality. Monogr. Hum. Genet. 10: 122-126, 1978.
88. Frank, M.; Many, M.; and Sperling, O. Familial renal hypouricemia: Two additional cases with uric acid lithiasis. Br. J. Urol. 51:88-91, 1979.
89. Barrientos, A.; Perez-Diaz, V.; Diaz-Gonzalez, R.; and Rodicio, J. L. Hypouricemia by defect in the tubular reabsorption. Arch. Intern. Med. 139:787-789, 1979.
90. DeVries, A.; and Sperling, O. Inborn hypouricemia due to isolated renal tubular defect. Biomedicine 30:75-80, 1973.
91. Fujiwara, Y.; Takamitsu, Y.; Ueda, N.; Orita, Y.; and Abe, H. Hypouricemia due to an isolated defect in renal tubular urate reabsorption. Clin. Nephrol. 13:44-48, 1980.
92. Meisel, A. D.; and Diamond, H. S. Hyperuricosuria in the Fanconi syndrome. Am. J. Med. Sci. 273:109-115, 1977.

93. Wallis, L. A.; and Engle, R. L. The adult Fanconi syndrome. II. Review of eighteen cases. Am. J. Med. 22:13-23, 1957.
94. Bishop, C.; Zimdahl, W. T.; and Talbott, J. H. Uric acid in two patients with Wilson's disease. Proc. Soc. Exp. Biol. Med. 86:440-441, 1954.
95. Mahoney, J. P.; Sandberg, A. A.; Gubler, C. J.; Cartwright, G. E.; and Wintrobe, M. M. Uric acid metabolism in hepatolenticular degeneration. Proc. Soc. Exp. Biol. Med. 88:427-430, 1975.
96. Wilson, D. M.; and Goldstein, N. P. Renal urate excretion in patients with Wilson's disease. Kidney Int. 4:331-336, 1973.
97. Leu, M. L.; Strickland, G. T.; and Gutman, R. A. Renal function in Wilson's disease: Response to penicillamine therapy. Am. J. Med. Sci. 260:381-398, 1970.
98. Sorensen, L. B.; and Kappas, A. The effect of penicillamine therapy on uric acid metabolism in Wilson's disease. Trans. Assoc. Am. Physicians 79:157-162, 1966.
99. Gold, M. S.; Williams, J. C.; Spivack, M.; and Grann, V. Sickle cell anemia and hyperuricemia. J.A.M.A. 206:1572-1573, 1968.
100. Diamond, H. S.; Meisel, A.; Sharon, E.; Holden, D.; and Cacatian, A. Hyperuricosuria and increased tubular secretion of urate in sickle cell anemia. Am. J. Med. 59:796-802, 1975.
101. Goldfinger, S.; Klinenberg, J. R.; and Seegmiller, J. E. Renal retention of uric acid induced by infusion of beta-hydroxybutyrate and acetoacetate. N. Engl. J. Med. 272:351-355, 1965.
102. Yu, T. F.; Sirota, J. H.; Berger, L.; Halpern, M.; and Gutman, A. B. Effect of sodium lactate infusion on urate clearance in man. Proc. Soc. Exp. Biol. Med. 96:809-813, 1957.
103. Padova, J.; and Bendersky, G. Hyperuricemia in diabetic ketoacidosis. N. Engl. J. Med. 267:530-534, 1962.
104. Shapiro, J. R.; Klinenberg, J. R.; Peck, W.; Goldfinger, S. E.; and Seegmiller, J. E. Hyperuricemia associated with obesity and intensified by caloric restriction. Arthritis Rheum. 7:343, 1964.
105. Steele, T. H. Evidence for altered renal urate reabsorption during changes in volume of the extracellular fluid. J. Lab. Clin. Med. 74:288-299, 1969.
106. Dwosh, I. L.; Roncari, D. A. K.; Marliss, E.; and Fox, I. H. Hypouricemia in disease: A study of different mechanisms. J. Lab. Clin. Med. 90:153-161, 1977.
107. Bennett, J. S.; Bond, J.; Singer, I.; and Gottlieb, A. J. Hypouricemia in Hodgkin's disease. Ann. Intern. Med. 76:751-756, 1972.
108. Beck, L. H. Hypouricemia in the syndrome of inappropriate secretion of antidiuretic hormone. N. Engl. J. Med. 301:528-530, 1979.
109. Levine, S. D.; Franki, N.; Einhorn, R.; and Hays, R. M. Vasopressin stimulated movement of drugs and uric acid across the toad urinary bladder. Kidney Int. 9:30-35, 1976.
110. Meisel, A.; and Diamond, H. Effect of vasopressin on uric acid excretion: Evidence for distal nephron reabsorption of urate in man. Clin. Sci. Molec. Med. 51:33-40, 1976.
111. Hill, L. M. Metabolism of uric acid in normal and toxemic pregnancy. Mayo Clinic Proc. 53:743-751, 1978.
112. Handler, J. S. The role of lactic acid in the reduced excretion of uric acid in toxemia of pregnancy. J. Clin. Invest. 39:1526-1532, 1960.
113. Matz, R.; Christodoulou, J.; Vianna, N.; and Ruwitch, J. Renal tubular dysfunction associated with alcoholism and liver disease. N.Y. State J. Med. 69:1312-1314, 1969.
114. Cannon, P. J.; Stason, W. B.; Demartini, F. E.; Sommar, S. C.; and Laragh, J. H. Hyperuricemia in primary and renal hypertension. N. Engl. J. Med. 275:457-464, 1966.
115. Simon, N. M.; Smucker, J. E.; O'Conor, V. J. Sr.; and delGreco, F. Differential uric acid excretion in essential and renal hypertension. Circulation 39:121-125, 1969.

116. Demartini, F. E.; Wheaton, E. A.; Healey, L. A.; and Laragh, J. H. Effect of chlorothiazide on the renal excretion of uric acid. Am. J. Med. 32:572-577, 1961.
117. Suki, W. N.; Hull, A. R.; Rector, F. C. Jr.; and Seldin, D. W. Mechanism of the effect of thiazide diuretics on calcium and uric acid (Abstr.). J. Clin. Invest. 46:1121, 1967.
118. Mudge, G. H. Uricosuric action of cholecystographic agents. A possible factor in nephrotoxicity. N. Engl. J. Med. 284:929-933, 1971.
119. Postlewaite, A. E.; and Kelley, W. N. Uricosuric effect of radiocontrast agents. A study in man of four commonly used preparations Ann. Intern. Med. 74:845-852, 1971.
120. Ramsdell, C. M.; Postlewaite, A. E.; and Kelley, W. N. Uricosuric effects of glyceryl guaiacolate. J. Rheumatol. 1:114-116, 1974.
121. Emmerson, B. T.; Mirosch, W.; and Douglas, J. B. The relative contributions of tubular reabsorption and secretion to urate excretion in lead nephropathy. Aust. N.Z. J. Med. 1:353-362, 1971.
122. Kelley, W. N.; Goldfinger, S. E.; and Hardy, H. L. Hyperuricemia in chronic beryllium disease. Ann. Intern. Med. 70:977-983, 1969.
123. Fessel, W. J.; Siegelaub, A. B.; and Johnson, E. S. Correlates and consequences of asymptomatic hyperuricemia. Arch. Intern. Med. 132:44-54, 1973.
124. Gutman, A. B.; and Yu, T. F. Uric acid nephrolithiasis in gout. Ann. Intern. Med. 67: 756-779, 1968.
125. Yu, T.; and Gutman, A. B. Uric acid nephrolithiasis in gout. Ann. Intern. Med. 67: 1133-1148, 1967.
126. Sperling, O.; DeVries, A.; and Kedem, O. Studies on the etiology of uric acid lithiasis. IV. Urinary non-dialyzable substances in idiopathic uric acid lithiasis. J. Urol. 94: 286-292, 1965.
127. Coe, F. L. Hyperuricosuric calcium oxalate nephrolithiasis. Kidney Int. 13:418-426, 1978.
128. Kavalich, A. G.; Moran, E.; Coe, F. L. Dietary purine consumption by hyperuricosuric calcium oxalate kidney stone formers and normal subjects. J. Chronic Dis. 29:745-760, 1976.
129. Coe, F. L.; and Kavalich, A. G. Hypercalciuria and hyperuricosuria in patients with calcium nephrolithiasis. N. Engl. J. Med. 291:1344-1350, 1974.
130. Broadus, A. E.; and Thier, S. O. Metabolic basis of renal-stone disease. N. Engl. J. Med. 300:839-845, 1979.
131. Coe, F. L.; Lawton, R. L.; Goldstein, R. B.; and Tembe, V. Sodium urate accelerates precipitation of calcium oxalate in vitro. Proc. Soc. Exp. Biol. Med. 149:926-929, 1975.
132. Prien, E. L.; and Prien, E. L., Jr. Composition and structure of urinary stone. Am. J. Med. 45:654-672, 1978.
133. Talbott, J. H.; and Terplan, K. L. The kidney in gout. Medicine (Baltimore) 39:405-467, 1960.
134. Fineberg, S. K.; and Altschul, A. The nephropathy of gout. Ann. Intern. Med. 44: 1182-1194, 1956.
135. Gonick, H. C.; Rubin, M. E.; Gleason, I. O.; and Sommers, S. C. The renal lesion in gout. Ann. Intern. Med. 62:667-674, 1965.
136. Fessel, W. J. Renal outcomes of gout and hyperuricemia. Am. J. Med. 67:74-82, 1979.
137. Berger, L.; and Yu, T. F. Renal function in gout. Am. J. Med. 59:605-613, 1975.
138. Batuman, V.; Maesaka, J. K.; Haddad, B.; Tepper, E.; Landy, E.; and Wedeen, R. P. The role of lead in gout nephropathy. N. Engl. J. Med. 304:520-523, 1981.
139. Meyers, A. R.; Epstein, F. H.; Dodge, H. J.; and Mikkelsen, W. M. Relationship of serum uric acid to risk factors in coronary heart disease. Am. J. Med. 45:520-528, 1968.

140. Fessel, W. J. High uric acid as an indicator of cardiovascular disease. Am. J. Med. 68: 401-404, 1980.
141. Coronary Drug Project Research Group. Serum uric acid: Its association with other risk factors and with mortality in coronary heart disease. J. Chronic Dis. 56:557-569, 1976.
142. Boss, G. R.; and Seegmiller, J. E. Hyperuricemia and gout. N. Engl. J. Med. 300:1459-1468, 1979.
143. Duffy, W. B.; Senekjian, H. O.; Knight, T. F.; and Weinman, E. J. Management of asymptomatic hyperuricemia. J.A.M.A. 246:2215-2216, 1981.

8

Isolated Proximal (Type 2) Renal Tubular Acidosis

CHESTER M. EDELMANN, JR.
Albert Einstein College of Medicine of Yeshiva University, New York, New York

The renal defect in proximal (or type 2) renal tubular acidosis (RTA) is characterized by: (1) the urinary excretion of a large fraction of the filtered load of bicarbonate when the concentration of bicarbonate in plasma is within the range of normal, (2) the excretion of an acid, bicarbonate-free urine when the concentration of bicarbonate in plasma is below the patient's renal threshold, and (3) a normal capacity to reduce urinary pH to minimally low levels and to excrete titratable acid and ammonium (1-7).

When type 2 RTA occurs in an isolated form, without other abnormalities in renal function and without an identifiable etiology, it is referred to as idiopathic, primary, or isolated type 2 RTA (1-3). Secondary type 2 RTA occurs as part of the idiopathic renal Fanconi syndrome (2,8-10) and is encountered in a number of metabolic disturbances, including cystinosis (2,11), Wilson's disease (12,13), hereditary intolerance to fructose (14,15), tyrosinemia (16), Lowe's syndrome (17-19), and both vitamin D deficiency (20) and vitamin D dependency (21). It has been reported in association with the nephrotic syndrome (22), and following renal transplantation (23-25) and renal vascular accidents (26); it occurs secondary to a number of drugs and toxins, including outdated tetracycline (27), methyl-3-chromone (28), and valproic acid (29); and it has been reported in a variety of other conditions, including Leigh's syndrome (30), osteopetrosis (31,32), tetralogy of Fallot (33), and hyperparathyroidism (34,35). Isolated type 2 RTA, described and characterized by Rodriguez-Soriano and associates (1,2), is the subject of this chapter. Type 2 RTA as a feature of Fanconi syndrome is discussed in Ch. 14.

I. CLINICAL FEATURES

All patients who have been reported with nonfamilial isolated type 2 RTA have been within the pediatric age group. Most are diagnosed before 18 months of age (1-3,36-40) (Table 1). The great majority are males, in contrast to the female preponderance in patients with type 1 RTA. The presenting symptom is growth failure (failure to thrive), with length falling farther below the third percentile as time progresses. A striking feature, which remains unexplained, is persistent vomiting, which occurs almost uniformly in early infancy.

Table 1 Clinical and Laboratory Characteristics of Isolated Type 1 and Type 2 Renal Tubular Acidosis in Children

	Type 1	Type 2
Mode of presentation	Growth failure; rarely rickets, nephrocalcinosis, nephrolithiasis	Growth failure
Age of presentation	Occasionally infancy; often early childhood or later	Usually infancy
Familial occurrence	Occasional	Rare
Sex predilection, F:M	4:1	1:4
Associated complications	Nephrocalcinosis, nephrolithiasis, urinary concentrating defect, rickets, hypokalemia	None
Urinalysis	Usually normal	Usually normal
Urinary pH	Above 6, regardless of level of plasma bicarbonate	4.5-7.8, depending on level of plasma bicarbonate
Serum chemistries	Hyperchloremic metabolic acidosis; hypokalemia	Hyperchloremic metabolic acidosis
Renal bicarbonate threshold	Normal	Low
Maximal rates of excretion of titratable acid and ammonium in urine	Impaired	Normal
Glomerular filtration rate	Normal to low	Normal
Hypercalciuria	Present	Absent
Ratio of urinary: plasma PCO_2	Below normal	Not adequately evaluated; probably normal
Hydrogen ion balance	Positive	Normal (zero)
Persistence of defect	Permanent	Transient

Although most cases are sporadic (41), familial occurrence of type 2 RTA has been reported. In the family described by Brenes et al. (42) nine members were affected, including five females and four males, ranging in age from 2 to 27 years. The series reported by Rodriguez-Soriano et al. (2) included two boys, first cousins, whose mothers were sisters. Winsnes et al. (43) reported two brothers with type 2 RTA; these boys also had mental retardation, nystagmus, corneal opacities, cataracts, glaucoma, and enamel defects of the permanent teeth, and probably should be considered as having secondary type 2 RTA. The two brothers described by Guibaud and associates (31) had persistent type 2 RTA and osteopetrosis. It is interesting in this regard that the brother and sister reported by Bourke et al. (44) also had osteopetrosis, but they had renal abnormalities characteristic of type 1 RTA. In neither report could a relationship between RTA and osteopetrosis be established.

In most patients, physical examination reveals only growth failure. If acutely ill when initially seen, patients may give evidence of dehydration and poor nutrition. Urinalysis reveals no abnormalities. Renal function is normal, except for the abnormality in reabsorption of bicarbonate. Children with type 2 RTA and systemic abnormalities may represent variants or secondary forms of the disease. For example, Donckerwolcke et al. (37,38) reported a 20-month-old girl with type 2 RTA, bilateral band keratopathy, and psychomoter retardation.

The patient described by Graziani et al. (40) is difficult to classify. This 4-year-old girl presented with rickets, failure to thrive (height below third percentile), metabolic acidosis, and a moderately elevated BUN. Urinary concentrating ability was normal, and a urinary pH of 4.6 was observed following an arginine load. The bicarbonate threshold was 17 mmol/liter. Aminoaciduria and glucosuria were absent. Thus, except for the presence of bone disease, which did not respond to large doses of vitamin D, she appeared to have type 2 RTA. She was treated with low doses of sodium bicarbonate, inadequate to correct metabolic acidosis, and resumed a normal pattern of growth. Her rickets healed, and after 3 years of treatment she was able to maintain normal acid-base balance without therapy. In many ways this patient is similar to the 44-year-old woman reported by York and Yendt (45) who presented with osteomalacia and isolated renal loss of bicarbonate, although neither vitamin D deficiency nor hyperparathyroidism was excluded. The bone disease healed with treatment with vitamin D and sodium bicarbonate.

In patients with isolated type 2 RTA, during periods of uncorrected metabolic acidosis dehydration and volume contraction may result in a temporary decrease in glomerular filtration rate. With rehydration, this rapidly returns to normal. Except for hyperchloremic acidosis, serum electrolytes, including calcium, inorganic phosphate, and potassium, are within normal limits (1-3). The finding of aminoaciduria, phosphaturia, glucosuria, and uricosuria, which are characteristic of the Fanconi syndrome, exclude the diagnosis of isolated type 2 RTA. The complications of type 1 RTA, including bone disease, nephrocalcinosis, urolithiasis, hypokalemia, and a defect in urinary concentration, are uniformly absent in isolated type 2 RTA (1-5). This may be explained by their ability to maintain hydrogen ion balance, as discussed in the next section.

II. PATHOPHYSIOLOGY

A. Bicarbonate Reabsorption

Untreated patients demonstrate hyperchloremic metabolic acidosis, usually of moderate severity. The urinary pH, as in normal subjects, ranges from mildly acid to neutral. Bicarbonate titration studies have revealed levels of the renal bicarbonate threshold between 15 and 20 meq/liter (2,5,10,31,32,36,37,39,40,42,43); except for the depressed threshold, however, the titration curve has a normal configuration (Fig. 1). During metabolic acidosis, or in response to ammonium chloride or arginine infusion, urinary pH falls to levels comparable to those seen in normal subjects, and the rates of excretion of titratable acid and ammonium also are within the range of normal (46,47). When patients are treated and their serum bicarbonate concentration is raised to normal levels, a brisk bicarbonaturia is observed, equal to 15-20% or more of the filtered load (2).

The magnitude of the bicarbonate loss observed in some patients with type 2 RTA had led to the conclusion that the abnormality resides in the proximal tubule, since the rate of excretion of bicarbonate in urine appears to exceed the usual total rate of delivery to the distal portion of the nephron. These observations, however, do not exclude the possibility of a combined proximal and distal defect. Nevertheless, the unimpaired ability to acidify the urine and to excrete titratable acid and ammonium suggest that distal acidification mechanisms are intact. Other distal functions, such as the renal concentrating capacity and the ability to excrete a load of potassium, also are unimpaired, adding credence to the argument that the defect is limited to the proximal nephron.

In contrast to patients with the Fanconi syndrome, other proximal functions are normal: aminoaciduria, glucosuria, phosphaturia, uricosuria, and cation wastage are not observed.

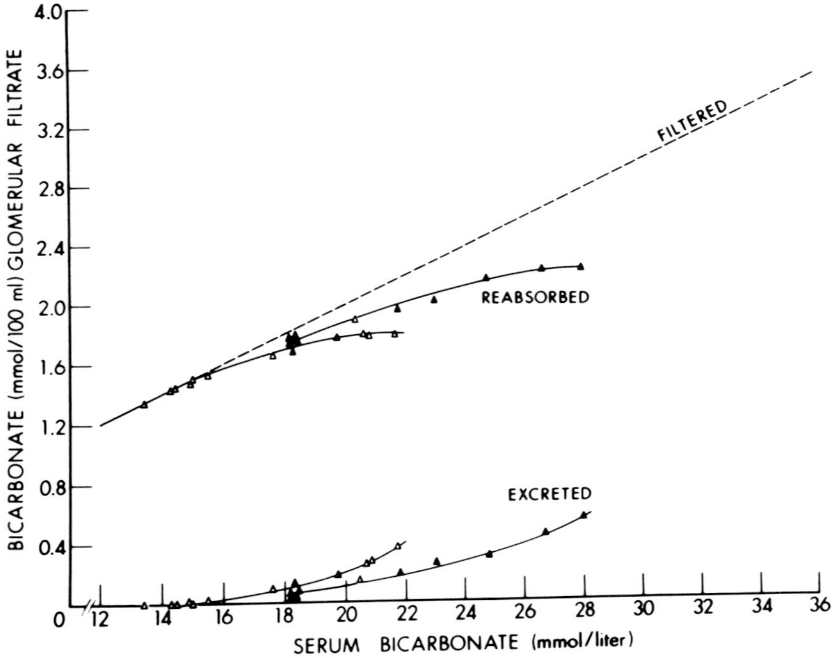

Fig. 1 Bicarbonate titration curves in two children with isolated type 2 renal tubular acidosis. (From Ref. 2.)

Rodriguez-Soriano (10) examined the renal handling of sodium and water in children with either type 1 or type 2 RTA using clearance techniques to estimate rates of proximal reabsorption and distal delivery. Those with type 2 RTA demonstrated decreased proximal reabsorption of sodium and water, coinciding with the presumed site of decreased reabsorption of bicarbonate. All but one of the patients with type 2 RTA had the Fanconi syndrome, however, and the one exception was a child with metachromatic leukodystrophy and aminoaciduria in addition to acidosis. The relevance of these studies to patients with isolated type 2 RTA, therefore, is uncertain.

Patients with isolated type 2 RTA exhibit many of the same functional characteristics as subjects given carbonic anhydrase inhibitors (48-52), suggesting that a deficiency in carbonic anhydrase activity might underlie their disease. Matsuda et al. (53) reported three children with RTA and skeletal demineralization following long-term anticonvulsant therapy that included acetazolamide. They concluded that the rickets resulted from the same mechanism that has been reported in other children on long-term anticonvulsant therapy (interference with vitamin D metabolism) and that the RTA was due to acetazolamide. In two of these children in whom acetazolamide could be discontinued, the acidosis and rickets resolved following treatment with phosphate and high doses of vitamin D.

Rodriguez-Soriano et al. (1) administered acetazolamide to two children with isolated type 2 RTA during the course of a bicarbonate titration study. A marked increase in the rate of urinary excretion of bicarbonate and a decrease in the rate of reabsorption were observed. This study demonstrated the presence of inhibitable renal carbonic anhydrase activity, but it could not exclude the possibility of a proximal deficiency or absence, with normal carbonic anhydrase activity in the distal tubular epithelium. It is also worth noting that a marked increase in urinary excretion of bicarbonate has been noted following administration of acetazolamide to patients with type 1 RTA (54,55).

In the patient with type 2 RTA reported by Donckerwolcke et al. (37) essentially no response was observed following the administration of acetazolamide at doses as high as 25 mg/kg and with serum bicarbonate levels as high as 35 meq/liter. It is of interest that this patient had a limitation in urinary concentrating capacity, suggesting an associated defect in distal nephron function. She also had bilateral band keratopathy, possibly removing her from the category of isolated type 2 RTA. In the two brothers with type 2 RTA reported by Winsnes et al. (43), a high dose of acetazolamide lowered the tubular bicarbonate reabsorption substantially. These children also had abnormalities other than type 2 RTA, as mentioned above. In the woman with type 2 RTA and osteomalacia reported by York and Yendt (45), a subnormal response was noted following the administration of acetazolamide. In contrast, the brothers with type 2 RTA and osteopetrosis studied by Guibaud et al. (31) had a vigorous response to acetazolamide. The pattern of response obviously has been quite variable, probably reflecting pathophysiological variations in the patients studied.

Shapira et al. (56) reported a family with an enzymatically inactive red cell carbonic anhydrase B and RTA. They postulated that a renal tubular defect similar to that observed in the red cell might explain the occurrence of RTA. It is of interest that these patients had type 1 RTA, suggesting the possibility of an abnormality in carbonic anhydrase limited to the distal nephron. Two children reported by Kondo et al. (57) also had type 1 RTA in association with an inactive form of erythrocyte carbonic anhydrase B.

The data thus are inconclusive, and the basic defect in type 2 RTA remains unknown. It is tempting to speculate that at least in some patients a deficiency in proximal tubular carbonic anhydrase is the major factor. It is not possible, of course, to exclude a defect in the carbonic anhydrase nondependent reabsorption of bicarbonate, if such a mechanism is in fact present in the human.

B. Hydrogen Ion Balance

One of the striking features of isolated type 2 RTA is that despite persistent metabolic acidosis, bone disease is not observed. Metabolic bone disease occurs in type 2 RTA associated with the Fanconi syndrome and is ameliorated by administration of vitamin D (58). It has been suggested that a defect in vitamin D metabolism might contribute also to the rickets that occurs in patients with type 1 RTA (see Ch. 1). Studies of vitamin D metabolism in patients with isolated type 2 RTA have not been reported. Whether or not metabolic acidosis per se affects vitamin D metabolism is controversial (59,60).

It is generally accepted that one of the major factors causing the bone disease in patients with type 1 RTA is acidemia, alkaline salts of bone serving as buffers for retained hydrogen ion (51,61-63) (see Ch. 11). Normal subjects given large acid loads by Lemann and coworkers (51,63) went into positive hydrogen ion balance and demonstrated an increase in their rate of urinary excretion of calcium, suggesting buffering of the retained H^+ by bone. In patients with type 1 RTA, hypercalciuria, in combination with a high urinary pH and low concentration of citrate (64,70), leads to nephrocalcinosis and nephrolithiasis.* It has been suggested that patients with type 2 RTA do not have hypercalciuria because the increased delivery of bicarbonate to the distal nephron enhances calcium reabsorption in that segment. Indeed, Sutton et al. (72) have shown in dogs a direct relationship between the concentration

*It is worth noting the comment by Wrong and Feest (71), however, that the great majority of their patients have *not* had hypercalciuria. (Also, see Ch. 11.)

of bicarbonate in distal tubular fluid and the rate of calcium reabsorption at that site. This, of course, cannot explain the absence of hypercalciuria in untreated patients with type 2 RTA, in whom bicarbonaturia is absent. It has been presumed, although of course it cannot be known for certain, that in the untreated state the fractional reabsorption of bicarbonate in the proximal tubule is normal, the load of filtered bicarbonate during metabolic acidosis being within the proximal tubular reabsorptive capacity. Only with treatment and restoration of normal levels of bicarbonate in plasma is the proximal tubular capacity overwhelmed, with markedly increased distal delivery and urinary excretion. Increased distal delivery of bicarbonate during treatment, however, may account for the decrease in urinary excretion of calcium that has been noted in children with isolated type 2 RTA following correction of acidosis (1,2).

In patients with isolated type 2 RTA, urine can be acidified and the rate of excretion of net acid is normal. These features along with the absence of hypercalciuria, bone disease, nephrolithiasis, and nephrocalcinosis led us to hypothesize (2) that they are able to maintain hydrogen ion balance, in contrast to patients with type 1 RTA or chronic renal insufficiency (58). If this formulation is correct, patients with isolated type 2 RTA would have no need to utilize bone as a source of buffer. This hypothesis was tested by Lemann et al. (73), who studied two members of a family with isolated type 2 RTA. The 19-year-old proband and his 23-year-old brother were observed during stable acidosis, with serum bicarbonate levels of 12.4 and 19.1 meq/liter, respectively. As predicted, they were found to be in hydrogen ion balance, and neither subject demonstrated hypercalciuria. Similar studies have not been done in children, but presumably the absence of hypercalciuria and bone disease can be explained in a similar fashion.

It is also pertinent that in the study of Lemann and associates (51) of the mechanism by which chronic metabolic acidosis augments urinary calcium excretion, six normal subjects given ammonium chloride more than doubled their urinary rate of excretion of calcium during acidosis, interpreted as reflecting the buffering effect on bone of retained hydrogen ion, whereas three subjects rendered acidotic by administration of acetazolamide had no statistically significant change in urinary calcium excretion.

C. Impairment of Growth

An intriguing question, which remains unanswered is why children with isolated type 2 RTA fail to grow normally. The answer would seem to be that acidemia per se interferes with normal growth mechanisms (74). Several interesting studies have been reported. Weber and associates (75) examined the possibility that chronic metabolic acidosis might interfere with the metabolism of vitamin D or cause secondary hyperparathyroidism, with negative results. McSherry (7) has shown blunted release of growth hormone in children with RTA stimulated with arginine and L-dopa infusion, with a normal response following correction of acidosis. In other studies in children with RTA, effects of acidosis on collagen synthesis were demonstrated (7). It appears likely that acidosis has multiple metabolic effects, and further studies of the type cited will be necessary to fully elucidate the nature of the disturbance.

Maren and associates (76) treated adult beagles with large doses of acetazolamide for periods lasting as long as 16 months. Despite persistent, severe metabolic acidosis, the dogs remained healthy and some showed evidence of growth. A group of puppies started on treatment with acetazolamide at the time of weaning were described as growing normally, although a control group not receiving acetazolamide was not available for comparison. In addition, the dose of acetazolamide used was much smaller than that given to the adult animals, and only a slight degree of acidosis was produced: average values of blood pH and bicarbonate were

7.28 and 19.2 meq/liter, respectively. In another experiment, 4-week-old rats were given sufficient acetazolamide to produce severe acidosis. Growth slowed markedly, but is was noted that there was a striking decrease in food intake, and, therefore, the effects of acidosis and inadequate nutrition could not be separated.

Cooke and associates (74) studied 30-day-old rats made acidotic with ammonium chloride or acetazolamide. All animals were compared to pair-fed controls. Uninephrectomized animals given ammonium chloride developed a slight degree of acidosis and demonstrated slowing of growth. Those given both ammonium chloride and acetazolamide had a marked decrease in their rate of growth. Rats treated with acetazolamide alone, however, with blood pH averaging 7.13, had a weight gain indistinguishable from their controls! This observation remains unexplained and, to my knowledge, unconfirmed.

Since children with isolated type 2 RTA represent the only instance in which chronic metabolic acidemia occurs as an isolated abnormality and, presumably, in the absence of a positive hydrogen ion balance, the disease provides a unique opportunity to explore the effect of acidemia on growth.

III. RENAL HISTOLOGY

Based on the few patients with isolated type 2 RTA that have been studied, renal histology appears to be unremarkable. In the two patients with isolated type 2 RTA biopsied by Rodriguez-Soriano and associates (1), renal histology was interpreted as normal. One of the brothers with type 2 RTA reported by Winsnes et al. (43) died following head trauma. At autopsy "the glomeruli appeared normal. In the proximal tubular epithelium cells, vacuolization and increased fat content was observed" (43). Histological data in other patients with isolated type 2 RTA are not available.

IV. DIAGNOSIS

The diagnosis of isolated type 2 RTA usually is not difficult. The problem almost always presents in a child with failure to thrive, in whom persistent and otherwise unexplained hyperchloremic metabolic acidosis has been demonstrated. Nonrenal causes of acidemia must be excluded. Renal insufficiency is readily excluded by measurement of serum concentrations of urea or creatinine or performance of renal clearances.

In the absence of an identifiable cause of acidosis, and with normal or near normal renal function, the diagnosis of RTA is suggested. Several random urines should be examined, preferably using early morning specimens. The finding of a urine pH of 5.5 or below excludes the diagnosis of type 1 RTA. If low levels of urinary pH are not recorded, despite acidemia, an acid-loading test should be performed. The short ammonium chloride loading test is simple to do and provides all the needed information (3,46,47,77).

Untreated subjects with RTA, similar to normal individuals, have levels of serum bicarbonate in the vicinity of their renal threshold. Depression of the resting serum bicarbonate concentration by several millimoles results, therefore, in a serum level well below the threshold and stimulates formation of maximally acid urine. During the ammonium chloride loading test, therefore, if an approriately low level of urinary pH is not observed, the diagnosis of type 1 RTA is established (Fig. 2). On the other hand, a fall in urinary pH to 5.5 or less suggests the diagnosis of type 2 RTA (Fig. 3). An exception to this may be patients who are able to acidify the urine well below pH 5.5, but appear to have a limitation in the rate of secretion of H^+ in the distal nephron, as suggested by a subnormal increase in urinary PCO_2 during bicarbonate loading (78) (see Ch. 9).

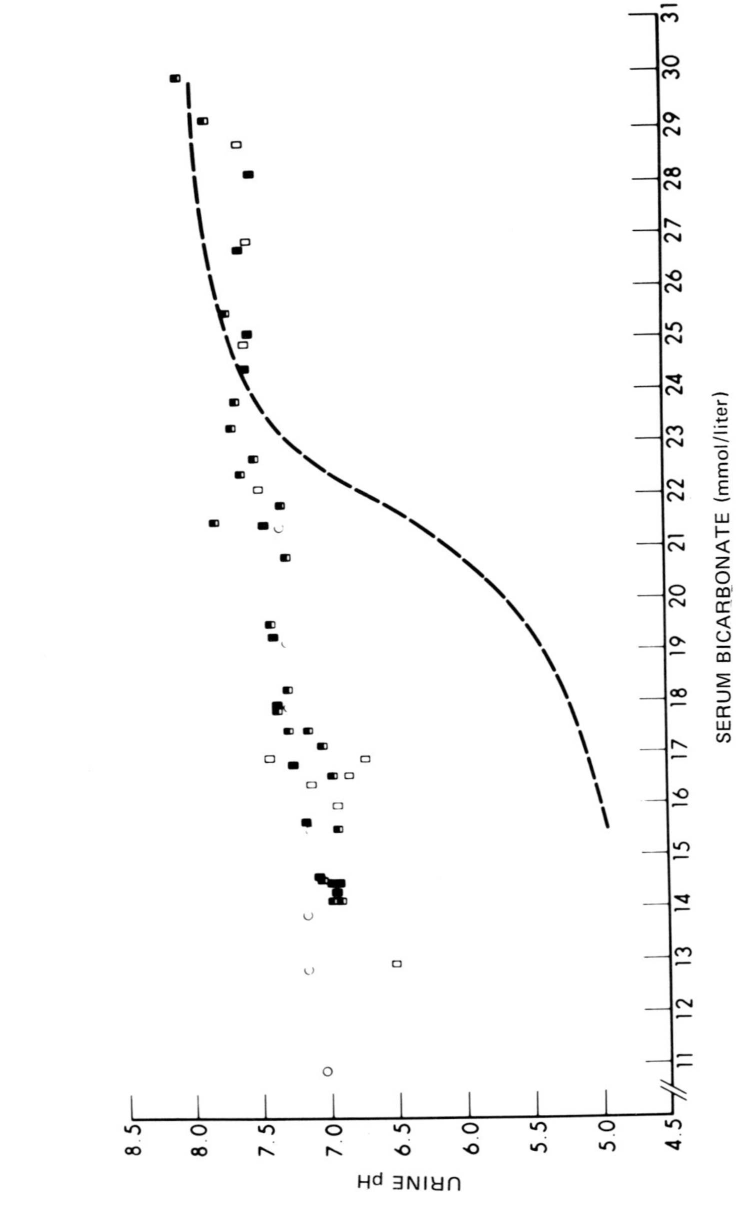

Fig. 2 Data from normal infants (broken line) and from infants and children with type 1 renal tubular acidosis. In the subjects with RTA, minimal decreases in urinary pH are observed, despite marked reduction in the concentration of bicarbonate in serum. (From Ref. 3.)

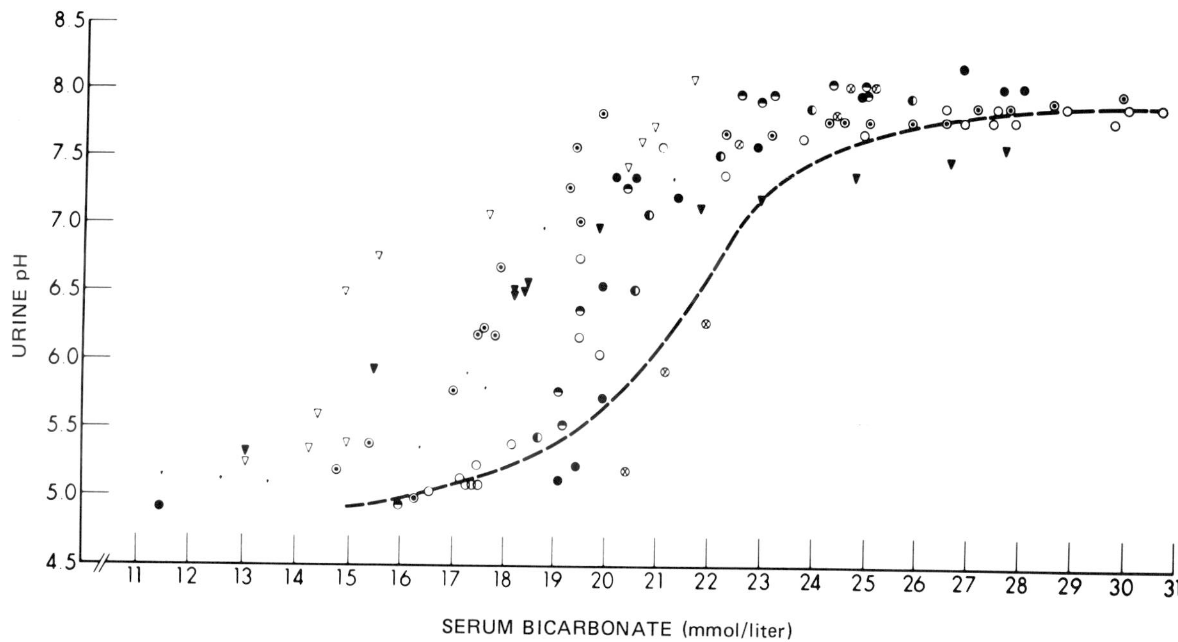

Fig. 3 Data from normal infants and from infants and children with type 2 renal tubular acidosis. All subjects achieved comparably low values of urinary pH, either spontaneously or during ammonium chloride acidosis. All those with type 2 RTA had renal thresholds for bicarbonate below the level of normal, reflected by a displacement of their response curves to the left. (From Ref. 3.)

The diagnosis of type 2 RTA can be confirmed by the performance of a bicarbonate titration test (36,47,79), although that difficult procedure usually is not needed. The level of the threshold can be determined easily in any clinical unit, as described in the following. The patient is given sufficient alkali over the course of several days to bring the serum bicarbonate concentration well into the normal range. Treatment is then discontinued, permitting the serum concentration to fall steadily toward pretreatment levels. Paired samples of blood and urine are examined once or twice daily. The serum bicarbonate concentration that is associated with a fall in urinary pH from 6.5 to 7.0 down to 5.5-6.0 identifies the level of the threshold. Values of the threshold below normal (see Table 2) establish the diagnosis of type 2 RTA.

With the diagnosis of type 2 RTA, secondary forms of the disease must be excluded. Appropriate examinations should be done to rule out other proximal tubular abnormalities, such as glucosuria, aminoaciduria, and phosphaturia. The various diseases and abnormalities associated with type 2 RTA, discussed above, should be considered. In the absence of an identifiable etiology and with the exclusion of other proximal tubular defects, the diagnosis of isolated type 2 RTA is established.

McSherry et al. (80) described infants with type 1 RTA who, in contrast to older children and adults, excreted large amounts of bicarbonate in the urine when plasma levels were brought within the range of normal. Similar cases have been reported by Leumann and Steinmann (81) and Rodriguez-Soriano and associates (82) (Fig. 4). These infants do not have a unique form of RTA; their bicarbonate wasting is the consequence of severe type 1 RTA in infants with immature renal function, in whom the fractional delivery of bicarbonate out of the proximal nephron (a characteristic of the immature kidney) overwhelms the distal reabsorptive capacity, resulting in a large bicarbonate leak. Similar to patients with type 2 RTA, their therapeutic requirement for maintenance of normal levels of bicarbonate in plasma is much greater than the typical patient with distal RTA. With age, as the kidney matures, the dosage requirement for bicarbonate progressively decreases, although the type 1 RTA remains as a permanent defect. This special characteristic of infants with type 1 RTA, if not fully appreciated, can lead to confusion in establishing the correct diagnosis.

So-called type 4 RTA is also of the distal type, and includes a variety of disorders in which the common factor is either aldosterone deficiency or reduced tubular responsiveness to aldosterone, resulting in hyperkalemia (83, Ch. 10). McSherry (7) has described subtypes of type 4 RTA, subtype 5 being designated the early childhood type, characterized by hyperchloremic acidosis, hyperkalemia, and aciduria. She has encountered 13 children with this disorder with equal frequency in girls and boys, and frequent familial occurence. Although the disorder is transient, and has features similar to those found in patients with isolated type 2 RTA, a striking difference in the latter group of patients is the preponderance of males and the absence of hyperkalemia. McSherry's patients (7) are described as having reduced

Table 2 Normal Serum Bicarbonate Concentrations

Age group	Renal bicarbonate threshold (meq/L)	Reference
Adults	24-26	79
Children	22-25	36
Birth to 1 year	21-22	47
Low-birth-weight infants	15-20	102

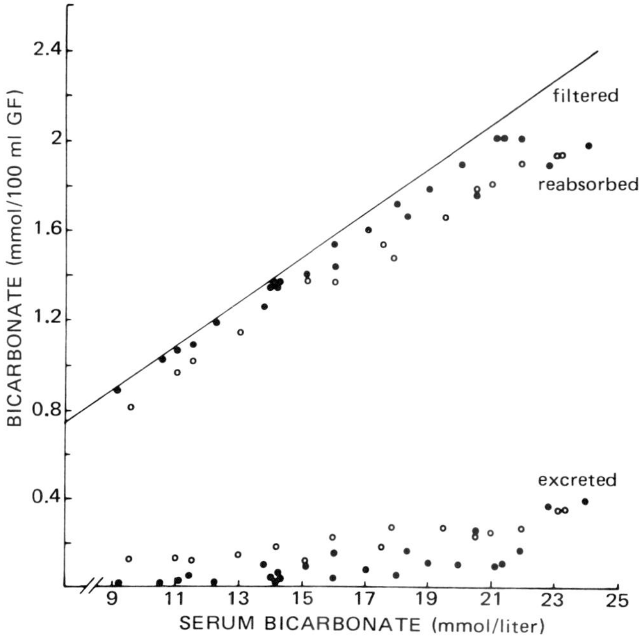

Fig. 4 Bicarbonate titration data in three infants with type 1 renal tubular acidosis and bicarbonate wasting. (From Ref. 82.)

secretion of hydrogen ion and potassium, evidencing impaired distal nephron function. Neither of these features has been characteristic of the patients with isolated type 1 RTA described by us or by others.

V. TREATMENT

Patients with type 2 RTA excrete 15% or more of filtered bicarbonate when serum bicarbonate concentrations are brought within the range of normal. The magnitude of this bicarbonate loss can be appreciated from the following example. A 6-month-old child has an absolute rate of glomerular filtration of 15-20 ml/min. With a serum bicarbonate concentration of 21 meq/liter, 450-600 meq of bicarbonate are filtered each 24 hr. If 15% is excreted in the urine, the daily loss of bicarbonate will be 70-90 meq, or approximately 10-15 meq/kg body weight. The *minimum* starting dose of alkali in patients with type 2 RTA, therefore, is approximately 10 meq/kg per 24 hr, with adjustment in dose as necessary to maintain a serum concentration well within the range of normal.

For this purpose, sodium bicarbonate, sodium lactate, sodium citrate, or other organic salts of sodium can be used. Since sodium bicarbonate is inexpensive and readily available, we have used it almost exclusively, with good results. Infants and small children can be given sodium bicarbonate powder, purchased as baking soda, mixed with jelly, pudding, or chocolate syrup. One measuring teaspoon of baking soda weighs approximately 3.7 g and contains 44 meq of bicarbonate.

It might be anticipated that while on therapy, flooding the distal nephron with sodium bicarbonate would enhance the exchange of sodium for potassium and result in excessive urinary losses of this ion and consequent hypokalemia. This had not been our experience, however, and children with isolated type 2 RTA, ingesting normal diets, have not required potassium supplementation. This, of course, is in striking contrast to patients with type 2 RTA as part of the Fanconi syndrome, who regularly demonstrate hypokalemia and require potassium supplementation, with or without treatment for correction of acidosis. As discussed in the following section, the use of hydrochlorothiazide in children with type 2 RTA also mandates potassium supplementation.

Hydrochlorothiazide was first described in the treatment of RTA by Rampini et al. (9). A patient with the idiopathic Fanconi syndrome so treated had correction of acidosis, return of urinary calcium to normal, and resolution of severe rickets. However, another patient of theirs with cystinosis failed to respond (9). In the patient with isolated type 2 RTA reported by Donckerwolcke (38) a dose of bicarbonate of 22 meq/kg failed to current acidosis, which was then easily controlled when hydrochlorothiazide was given. This produced severe hypokalemia, which was not fully corrected despite large supplemental doses of potassium. Callis et al. (11) successfully corrected the acidosis in two children with cystinosis, noting that the rate of excretion of urinary calcium also returned to normal and that there was a marked increase in tubular reabsorption of filtered phosphate.

That the beneficial effect of hydrochlorothiazide is produced by inducing a mild degree of plasma volume contraction, which enhances reabsorption in the proximal tubule, is supported by the studies of Oetliker and Rossi (18) in two children with Lowe's syndrome. They demonstrated a clear effect of extracellular volume on tubular reabsorption of bicarbonate. Conversely, Broyer and associates (36) noted that when they infused bicarbonate at high rates in children with type 2 RTA, they lowered the bicarbonate threshold. In two patients with Leigh's syndrome and type 2 RTA, Gruskin and co-workers (30) found that administration of larger and larger doses of bicarbonate, in an attempt to bring serum levels up to normal, led to a progressive *decrease* in tubular reabsorption.

It would seem appropriate, therefore, to employ hydrochlorothiazide in any patient requiring such large doses of sodium bicarbonate to make correction of acidosis impossible or impractical. It must be recognized, however, that when hydrochlorothiazide is used, potassium supplementation is necessary. The starting dose of hydrochlorothiazide is 1.5-2 mg/kg per day, with a smaller dose once acidosis is corrected.

Therapeutic efforts are directed toward maintenance of a normal plasma concentration of bicarbonate throughout the 24-hr period. Thus, the first dose of alkali is given on arising in the morning, the last dose just before going to sleep at night. As a consequence of bringing the plasma bicarbonate concentration within the range of normal, and thus well above the patient's threshold, the urinary bicarbonate wastage probably leads to a rapid decline in the plasma concentration between each dose, particularly during the night. Theoretically, the use of a diuretic to reduce the bicarbonate leak might minimize these fluctuations in plasma bicarbonate. This possibility, however, has not been tested. Moreover, with treatment as described, growth is normalized, suggesting that the day and night variations in serum bicarbonate concentration may not be important (5).

Long-term therapy with sodium bicarbonate or other alkalizing salts does not appear to have any untoward effects. Nevertheless, Nishi and associates (84) have reported a case of copper deficiency occurring in a child with isolated type 2 RTA fed a low copper-containing formula. They proposed that alkali therapy inhibited copper absorption.

VI. PROGNOSIS

In most if not all patients with isolated type 2 RTA, an accelerated rate of growth accompanies correction of acidosis. Children regain normal percentiles, and, although long-term follow-up data are limited, their ultimate height appears to be unaffected by the initial period of stunting (5). After 1 or more years of treatment, therapy can be withdrawn and children continue to maintain normal values of blood pH and bicarbonate and to grow normally. The family reported by Brenes et al. (42) represents an exception to this rule, since as adults they demonstrated short stature and continued to be acidemic. Interestingly, these authors (42) concluded that since their adult patients were asymptomatic and growth potential was lacking, treatment would serve no useful purpose.

VII. RELATIONSHIP OF ISOLATED TYPE 2 RTA TO LIGHTWOOD'S SYNDROME

In 1935, at the annual meeting of the British Paediatric Association, Lightwood (85) reported a group of six infants with a clinical course characterized by anorexia, constipation, vomiting, and failure to thrive. Physical examination revealed wasting and hypotonia. In some, blood urea levels were elevated. The infants all died between the ages of 5 and 11 months from intercurrent infection. An unexpected finding at autopsy was nephrocalcinosis. In 1936, Butler et al. (86) described four similar infants, with the additional characteristics of unexplained episodes of dehydration and metabolic acidosis. All died, despite attempts at therapy; at autopsy, all had nephrocalcinosis. The similarity of these cases to those reported by Lightwood (85) was noted, but no explanation for the acidosis could be found. Lightwood and coworkers (87) described another infant in 1936, in a report with the intriguing title "Persistent acidosis in an infant: Cause not yet ascertained."

Hartmann described a 4-month-old infant with persistent acidosis, similar to the patients reported by Lightwood and others, and was the first to implicate the kidney as the site of the defect (88). He demonstrated "a persistent excretion of $BHCO_3$ into the urine as the only clearly evident expression of renal insufficiency, which led to chronic severe acidosis and which necessitated the continued oral administration of relatively enormous doses of alkali."

The first adult reported with RTA was a 29-year-old woman with recurrent episodes of urolithiasis. She had metabolic acidosis, and it was noted that her minimum urinary pH following ammonium chloride was 6.3. With a combination of sodium citrate-citric acid, her acidosis was fully corrected (89).

Albright and associates (90) further clarified the difference between the acidosis associated with *glomerular insufficiency* (chronic progressive renal disease and azotemia) from that associated with *tubular insufficiency* (with normal overall renal function). They reported six new cases of RTA and concluded that renal tubular insufficiency decreased the ability to make ammonia and to excrete an acid urine. This in turn led to a demand for calcium as a base, dissolving calcium salts from the bones, and leading to hypercalciuria. They clearly differentiated the bone disease they observed in their patients with tubular insufficiency from so-called renal rickets associated with uremia. They also commented that "the tubular acidosis associated with the Fanconi syndrome is entirely different from the tubular acidosis discussed. . . ." in their paper, the first (unrecognized) distinction between type 1 and type 2 RTA. The prescient statement preceding their discussion of tubular acidosis that "this section, in the authors' opinion, constitutes the most important part of this paper," reveals the wisdom and perspicacity of these investigators.

For a period of time, the infants and children reported with RTA seemed to be indistinguishable from the adults with that condition. However, following the diagnosis of large numbers of infants with RTA in England, Scotland, and Wales, and the recognition that their abnormality was transient, it was generally accepted that Lightwood's disease represented an infantile, transient form of RTA, in contrast to Albright's disease, or the adult-type, permanent disorder.

In the decade from 1945 to 1955 more than 100 cases of Lightwood's syndrome were reported from Great Britain; major series included those of Lightwood et al. (91), Carré and associates (92), Doxiadis (93), Latner and Burnard (94), and Buchanan and Komrower (95). As quickly as Lightwood's syndrome appeared, it as rapidly declined. Lightwood and Butler (96) surveyed seven university centers in England, Scotland, and Wales for the period 1950 through 1959. The rapid appearance and disappearance of infantile RTA suggested the possibility that an environmental agent might have played an important etiological role. Factors that were considered included the excessive amounts of vitamin D to be found at that time in many of the foods fed to infants, the presence of mercury in teething powders, and the recent introduction of sulfonamide as an antimicrobial agent. None of these, however, provided a satisfactory answer. The decline in Lightwood's syndrome preceded the decrease in the vitamin D content of baby food. Few infants had been treated with sulfonamide or had been given mercury-containing teething powder. Moreover, with respect to the latter, Williams et al. (97) had carefully studied 22 infants with pink disease; none was either acidotic or hypokalemic.

Apart from its etiology, what was the nature of the disturbance in infants with Lightwood's syndrome? It was assumed for many years that these infants had a gradient-type RTA, i.e., inability to acidify their urine appropriately (91), as demonstrated in adults by Albright and associates (90). This, however, was never adequately assessed.

It is of interest that most infants reported with Lightwood's syndrome were boys. With appropriate treatment and correction of acidosis, normal patterns of growth were resumed, and treatment could be discontinued entirely after a year or two. In several reports in which dosage requirements were given, it can be calculated that infants needed as much as 150 meq of alkali per day to maintain correction of acidosis. In the majority of infants, nephrocalcinosis, urolithiasis, rickets, hypokalemia, and concentrating defects were absent. It was noted, moreover, that infants who had nephrocalcinosis at the time of diagnosis usually failed to recover; many of these infants also had urinary concentrating defects.

It is apparent that the characteristics of most infants with Lightwood's syndrome suggest type 2 rather than type 1 RTA, although as discussed above, the need for large doses of alkali does not distinguish between type 2 RTA and infantile type 1 RTA with bicarbonate wasting. However, patients described in the latter category have had permanent disease, even though their dosage requirement decreases with age (80-82).

The data of Latner and Burnard (94) are of pathophysiological interest. They studied the response of six infants (all male) with Lightwood's syndrome to the infusion of neutral sodium phosphate. All infants reduced their urinary pH to 5.09-5.80, in comparison to preinfusion values of 6.27-6.91. These findings speak against the diagnosis of type 1 RTA, since patients with that condition who have been studied did not lower their urinary pH following administration of neutral phosphate to levels below 6.0 (54,98).

Latner and Burnard (94) also noted a marked increase in urinary PCO_2 following phosphate infusion, a finding which also might be taken to rule against the diagnosis of type 1 RTA (99). However, Reynolds (98) infused neutral phosphate into three adults with type 1 RTA and observed the urinary PCO_2 to increase to as high as 191 torr. Since there is uncertainty concerning the significance of the failure of most patients with type 1 RTA to increase urinary PCO_2 during an alkaline diuresis to the same levels as normals (100,101), the data of Latner and Burnard (94) remain inconclusive (see also Ch. 9).

Thus, the nature of Lightwood's syndrome, as well as its mysterious appearance and disappearance in Great Britain, remains unknown. Most of its features and particularly its transient nature suggest isolated type 2 RTA, but this cannot be stated with certainty. What is clear, however, is that the terms *infantile* and *adult* RTA are misleading and should be abandoned. Type 1 RTA in the infant, child, or adult is a permanent defect and appears to have similar pathophysiological characteristics. Type 2 RTA is encountered in all age groups, although to date the transient form of isolated type 2 RTA has been limited to infants.

REFERENCES

1. Rodriguez-Soriano, J.; Boichis, H.; Stark, H.; and Edelmann, C. M., Jr. Proximal renal tubular acidosis. A defect in bicarbonate reabsorption with normal urinary acidification. Pediatr. Res. 1:81-98, 1967.
2. Rodriguez-Soriano, J.; Boichis, H.; Edelmann, C. M., Jr. Bicarbonate reabsorption and hydrogen ion excretion in children with renal tubular acidosis. J. Pediatr. 71:802-813, 1967.
3. Rodriguez-Soriano, J.; and Edelmann, C. M., Jr. Renal tubular acidosis. Ann. Rev. Med. 20:363-382, 1969.
4. Morris, R. C., Jr.; Sebastian, A.; and McSherry, E. Renal acidosis. Kidney Int. 1:322-340, 1972.
5. Nash, M. A.; Torrado, A. D.; Greifer, I.; Spitzer, A.; and Edelmann, C. M., Jr. Renal tubular acidosis in infants and children. Clinical course, response to treatment and prognosis. J. Pediatr. 80:738-748, 1972.
6. Rodriguez-Soriano, J. Renal tubular acidosis. In: Pediatric Nephrology—*Proceedings of the 5th International Pediatric Nephrology Symposium*, edited by Gruskin, A. B., and Norman, M. E. Boston, Martinus Nijhoff, 1981, pp. 28-36.
7. McSherry, E. Renal tubular acidosis in childhood. Kidney Int. 20:799-809, 1981.
8. Tegelaers, W. H. H.; and Tiddens, H. W. Nephrotic-glucosuric-aminoaciduric dwarfism and electrolyte metabolism. Helv. Paediatr. Acta 10:269-278, 1955.
9. Rampini, S.; Fanconi, A.; Illig, R.; and Prader, A. Effect of hydrochlorothiazide on proximal renal tubular acidosis in a patient with idiopathic "deToni-Debré-Fanconi syndrome." Helv. Paediatr. Acta 23:13-21, 1968.
10. Rodriguez-Soriano, J.; Vallo, A.; Castillo, G.; and Oliverso, R. Renal handling of water and sodium in children with proximal and distal renal tubular acidosis. Nephron 25:193-198, 1980.
11. Callis, L.; Castelló, F.; Fortuny, G.; Vallo, A.; and Ballabriga, A. Effect of hydrochlorothiazide on rickets and on renal tubular acidosis in two patients with cystinosis. Helv. Paediatr. Acta 25:602-619, 1970.
12. Morgan, H. G.; Stewart, W. K.; Lowe, K. G.; Stowers, J. M.; and Johnstone, J. H. Wilson's disease and the Fanconi syndrome. Q. J. Med. 31:361-384, 1962.
13. Wilson, D. M.; and Goldstein, N. P. Bicarbonate excretion in Wilson's disease (hepatolenticular degeneration). Mayo Clin. Proc. 49:394-400, 1974.
14. Morris, R. C., Jr. An experimental renal acidification defect in patients with hereditary fructose intolerance. I. Its resemblance to renal tubular acidosis. J. Clin. Invest. 47:1389-1398, 1968.
15. Morris, R. C., Jr. An experimental renal acidification defect in patients with hereditary fructose intolerance. II. Its distinction from classic renal tubular acidosis; its resemblance to the renal acidification defect associated with the Fanconi syndrome of children with cystinosis. J. Clin. Invest. 47:1648-1663, 1968.
16. Gentz, J.; Jagenburg, R.; and Zetterström, R. Tyrosinemia. An inborn error of tyrosine metabolism with cirrhosis of the liver and multiple renal tubular defects (deToni-Debré-Fanconi syndrome). J. Pediatr. 66:670-696, 1965.
17. Lamy, M.; Frézal, J.; Rey, J.; and Larsen, C. Étude métabolique du syndrome de Lowe, Rev. Fr. Etud. Clin. Biol. 7:271-283, 1962.

18. Oetliker, O.; and Rossi, E. The influence of extracellular fluid volume on the renal bicarbonate threshold. A study of two children with Lowe's syndrome. Pediatr. Res. 3: 140-148, 1969.
19. Matsuda, I.; Takeda, T.; Sugai, M.; and Matsuura, N. Oculocerebro-renal syndrome in a child with a normal urinary acidification and a defect in bicarbonate reabsorption. Am. J. Dis. Child. 117:205-212, 1969.
20. Guignard, J. P.; and Torrado, A. Proximal renal tubular acidosis in vitamin D deficiency rickets. Acta Paediatr. Scand. 62:543-546, 1973.
21. Stoop, J. W.; Schraagen, M. J. C.; and Tiddens, H. A. W. M. Pseudo vitamin D deficiency rickets. Acta Paediatr. Scand. 56:607-616, 1967.
22. Stickler, G. B.; Rosevear, J. W.; and Ulrich, J. A. Renal tubular dysfunction complicating the nephrotic syndrome: The disturbance in calcium and phosphorus metabolism. Mayo Clin. Proc. 37:376-387, 1962.
23. Massry, S. G.; Preuss, H. G.; Maher, J. F.; and Schreiner, G. E. Renal tubular acidosis after kidney homotransplantation. Studies on mechanism. Am. J. Med. 42:284-292, 1967.
24. Wilson, D. R.; and Siddiqui, A. A. Renal tubular acidosis after kidney transplantation. Natural history and significance. Ann. Intern. Med. 79:352-361, 1973.
25. Vertuno, L. L.; Preuss, H. G.; Argy, W. P., Jr.; and Schreiner, G. E. Fanconi syndrome following homotransplantation. Arch. Intern. Med. 133:302-305, 1974.
26. Stark, H.; and Geiger, R. Renal tubular dysfunction following vascular accidents of the kidneys in the newborn period. J. Pediatr. 83:933-940, 1973.
27. Wegienka, L. C.; and Weller, J. M. Renal tubular acidosis caused by degraded tetracycline. Arch. Intern. Med. 114:232-235, 1964.
28. Otten, J.; and Vis, H. L. Acute reversible renal tubular dysfunction following intoxication with methyl-3-chromone. J. Pediatr. 73:422-425, 1968.
29. Lenoir, G. R.; Pèrignon, J.-L.; Gubler, M-C.; and Broyer, M. Valproic acid: A possible cause of proximal tubular renal syndrome. J. Pediatr. 96:503-504, 1981.
30. Gruskin, A. B.; Patel, M. S.; Linshaw, M.; Ettenger, R.; Huff, D.; and Grover, W. Renal function studies and kidney pyruvate carboxylase in subacute necrotizing encephalomyelopathy (Leigh's syndrome). Pediatr. Res. 7:832-841, 1973.
31. Guibaud, P.; Larbre, M.; Freycon, M. T.; and Genoud, J. Ostéopétrose et acidose rénale tubularie. Deux cas de cette association dans une fratrie. Arch. Fr. Pediatr. 29:269-286, 1972.
32. Vainsel, M.; Fondu, P.; Cadranel, S.; Rocmans, C.; and Gepts, W. Osteopetrosis associated with proximal and distal tubular acidosis. Acta Paediatr. Scand. 61:429-434, 1972.
33. Rodriguez-Soriano, J.; Vallo, A.; Chouza, M.; and Castillo, G. Proximal renal tubular acidosis in tetralogy of Fallot. Acta Paediatr. Scand. 64:671-674, 1975.
34. Siddiqui, A. A.; and Wilson, D. R. Primary hyperparathyroidism and proximal renal tubular acidosis: Report of two cases. Can. Med. Assoc. J. 106:654-659, 1972.
35. Muldowney, F. P.; Carroll, D. V.; Donohoe, J. F.; and Freaney, R. Correction of renal bicarbonate wastage by parathyroidectomy. Implications in acid-base homeostasis. Q. J. Med. 40:487-498, 1971.
36. Broyer, M.; Proesmans, W.; and Royer, P. La titration des bicarbonates chez l'enfant normal et au cours de diverses néphropathies. Rev. Fr. Etudes Clin. Biol. 14:556-568, 1969.
37. Donckerwolcke, R. A.; Van Stekelenburg, G. J.; and Tiddens, H. A. A case of bicarbonate-losing renal tubular acidosis with defective carboanhydrase activity. Arch. Dis. Child. 45:769-773, 1970.
38. Donckerwolcke, R. A.; Van Stekelenburg, G. J.; and Tiddens, H. A. Therapy of bicarbonate-losing renal tubular acidosis. Arch. Dis. Child. 45:774-779, 1970.
39. Schoeneman, M.; Lifshitz, F.; and Diaz-Bensussen, S. The transport of bicarbonate by the small intestine of a patient with proximal renal tubular acidosis. Pediatr. Res. 8: 735-739, 1974.

40. Graziani, G.; DeVecchi, A.; and Rosti, D. Primary proximal renal tubular acidosis. A therapeutic approach and long-term follow-up. Helv. Paediatr. Acta 31:427-434, 1976.
41. Scriver, C. R.; Chesney, R. W.; and McInnes, R. R. Genetic aspects of renal tubular transport: Diversity and topology of carriers. Kidney Int. 9:149-171, 1976.
42. Brenes, L. G.; Brenes, J. N.; and Hernandez, M. M. Familial proximal renal tubular acidosis. A distinct clinical entity. Am. J. Med. 63:244-252, 1977.
43. Winsnes, A.; Monn, E.; Stokke, O.; and Feyling, T. Congential, persistent proximal type renal tubular acidosis in two brothers. Acta Paediatr. Scand. 68:861-868, 1979.
44. Bourke, E.; Delaney, V. B.; Mosawi, M.; Reavey, P.; and Weston, M. Renal tubular acidosis and osteopetrosis in siblings. Nephron 28:268-272, 1981.
45. York, S. E.; and Yendt, E. R. Osteomalacia associated with renal bicarbonate loss. Can. Med. Assoc. J. 94:1329-1342, 1966.
46. Edelmann, C. M., Jr.; Biochis, H.; Rodriguez-Soriano, J.; and Stark, H. The renal response of children to acute ammonium chloride acidosis. Pediatr. Res. 1:452-460, 1967.
47. Edelmann, C. M., Jr.; Rodriguez-Soriano, J.; Boichis, H.; Gruskin, A. B.; and Acosta, M. Bicarbonate reabsorption and hydrogen ion excretion in normal infants. J. Clin. Invest. 46:1309-1317, 1967.
48. Nadell, J. The effects of the carbonic anhydrase inhibitor "6063" on electrolyes and acid-base balance in two normal subjects and two patients with respiratory acidosis. J. Clin. Invest. 32:622-629, 1953.
49. Leaf, A.; Schwartz, W. B.; and Relman, A. S. Oral administration of a potent carbonic anhydrase inhibitor ("Diamox"). N. Engl. J. Med. 250:759-764, 1954.
50. Seldin, D. W.; Portwood, R. M.; Rector, F. C., Jr.; and Cade, R. Characteristics of renal bicarbonate reabsorption in man. J. Clin. Invest. 38:1663-1671, 1959.
51. Lemann, J., Jr.; Litzow, J. R.; Lennon, E. J.; and Kelly, O. A. Studies of the mechanism by which chronic metabolic acidosis augments urinary calcium excretion in man. J. Clin. Invest. 46:1318-1328, 1967.
52. White, M. G.; and Asch, M. J. Acid base effects of topical mafenide acetate in the burned patient. N. Engl. J. Med. 284:1281-1286, 1971.
53. Matsuda, I.; Takekoshi, Y.; Shida, N.; Fujieda, K.; Nagai, B.; Arashima, S.; Anakura, M.; and Oka, Y. Renal tubular acidosis and skeletal demineralization in patients on long-term anticonvulsant therapy. J. Pediatr. 87:202-205, 1975.
54. Frick, P. G.; Rubini, M. E.; and Meroney, W. H. Recurrent nephrolithiasis associated with an unusual tubular defect and hyperchloremic acidosis. Am. J. Med. 25:590-599, 1958.
55. Webster, G. D.; Huth, E. J.; Elkinton, J. R.; and McCance, R. A. The renal excretion of hydrogen ion in renal tubular acidosis: II. Quantitative response to the carbonic anhydrase inhibitor, acetazolamide. Am. J. Med. 29:576-585, 1960.
56. Shapira, E.; Ben-Yoseph, Y.; Eyal, F. G.; and Russell, A. Enzymatically inactive red cell carbonic anhydrase B in a family with renal tubular acidosis. J. Clin. Invest. 53:59-63, 1974.
57. Kondo, T.; Taniguchi, N.; Taniguchi, K.; Matsuda, I.; and Murao, M. Inactive form of erythrocyte carbonic anhydrase B in patients with primary renal tubular acidosis. J. Clin. Invest. 62:610-617, 1978.
58. Brenner, R. J.; Spring, D. B.; Sebastian, A.; McSherry, E. M.; Genant, H. K.; Palubinskas, A. J.; and Morris, R. C., Jr. Incidence of radiographically evident bone disease, nephrocalcinosis, and nephrolithiasis in various types of renal tubular acidosis. N. Engl. J. Med. 307:217-222, 1982.
59. Kawashima, H.; Kraut, J. A.; and Kurokawa, K. Metabolic acidosis suppresses 25-hydroxyvitamin D_3-1α-hydroxylase in the rat kidney. Distinct site and mechanism of action. J. Clin. Invest. 70:135-140, 1982.
60. Kraut, J. A.; Gordon, E.; Horst, R. L.; Ransom, J. C.; Slatopolsky, E.; Coburn, J. W.; and Kurokawa, K. Effect of chronic metabolic acidosis on vitamin D metabolism in man. Kidney Int. 23:103, 1983.

61. Goodman, A. D.; Lemann, J., Jr.; and Lennon, E. J. Production, excretion and net balance of fixed acid in patients with renal acidosis. J. Clin. Invest. 44:495-506, 1965.
62. Lemann, J., Jr.; Lennon, E. J.; Goodman, A. D.; Litzow, J. R.; and Relman, A. S. The net balance of acid in subjects given large loads of acid or alkali. J. Clin. Invest. 44:507-517, 1965.
63. Lemann, J., Jr.; Litzow, R.; and Lennon, E. J. The effects of chronic acid loads in normal man. Further evidence for the participation of bone mineral in the defenses against chronic metabolic acidosis. J. Clin. Invest. 45:1608-1614, 1966.
64. Fourman, P.; and Robinson, J. R. Diminished urinary excretion of citrate during deficiencies of potassium in man. Lancet 2:656-657, 1953.
65. Harrison, H. E. Mechanisms of action of vitamin D. Pediatrics 14:285-295, 1954.
66. Harrison, H. E.; Chisolm, J. J., Jr.; and Harrison, H. C. Congential tubular acidosis (abstr.). A.M.A. J. Dis. Child. 96:588, 1958.
67. Bauld, W. S.; MacDonald, S. A.; and Hill, M. C. Effect of renal tubular acidosis on calcium excretion. Br. J. Urol. 30:285-291, 1958.
68. Dedmon, R. E.; and Wrong, O. The excretion of organic anion in renal tubular acidosis with particular reference to citrate. Clin. Sci. 22:19-32, 1962.
69. Morrissey, J. F.; Ochoa, M., Jr.; Lotspeich, W. D.; and Waterhouse, C. Citrate excretion in renal tubular acidosis. Ann. Intern. Med. 58:159-166, 1963.
70. Nordin, B. E. C.; and Smith, D. A. Citric acid excretion in renal stone disease and in renal tubular acidosis. Br. J. Urol. 35:438-444, 1963.
71. Wrong, O. M.; and Feest, T. G. Renal tubular acidosis. N. Engl. J. Med. 304:1548, 1981.
72. Sutton, R. A. L.; Wong, N. L. M.; and Dirks, J. H. Effects of metabolic ecidosis and alkalosis on sodium and calcium transport in the dog kidney. Kidney Int. 15:520-533, 1979.
73. Lemann, J., Jr.; Wilz, D. R.; and Brenes, L. G. Acid, calcium, and phosphorus balances in proximal renal tubular acidosis (abstr.). Kidney Int. 10:560, 1976.
74. Cooke, R. E.; Boyden, D. G.; and Haller, E. The relationship of acidosis and growth retardation. J. Pediatr. 57:326-337, 1960.
75. Weber, H. P.; Gray, R. W.; Dominguez, J. H.; and Lemann, J., Jr. The lack of effect of chronic metabolic acidosis on 25-OH-vitamin D metabolism and serum parathyroid hormone in humans. J. Clin. Endocrinol. Metab. 43:1047-1055, 1976.
76. Maren, T. H.; Mayer, E.; and Wadsworth, B. C. Carbonic anhydrase inhibition. I: The pharmacology of Diamox 2-acetylamino-1,3,4-thiadiazole-5-sulfonamide. Bull. Johns Hopkins Hosp. 95:199-243, 1954.
77. Wrong, O.; and Davies, H. E. F. The excretion of acid in renal disease. Q. J. Med. 28: 259-313, 1959.
78. Batlle, D.; Grupp, M.; Gavira, M.; and Kurtzman, N. A. Distal renal tubular acidosis with intact capacity to lower urinary pH. Am. J. Med. 72:751-758, 1982.
79. Pitts, R. F.; Ayer, J. L.; and Schiess, W. The renal regulation of acid-base balance in man. III. The reabsorption and excretion of bicarbonate. J. Clin. Invest. 28:35-44, 1949.
80. McSherry, E.; Sebastian, A.; and Morris, R. C., Jr. Renal tubular acidosis in infants: The several kinds, including bicarbonate-wasting, classic renal tubular acidosis. J. Clin. Invest. 51:499-514, 1972.
81. Leumann, E. P.; and Steinmann, B. Persistent and transient distal renal tubular acidosis with bicarbonate wasting. Pediatr. Res. 9:767-773, 1975.
82. Rodriguez-Soriano, J.; Vallo, A.; and Garcia-Fuentes, M. Distal renal tubular acidosis in infancy: A bicarbonate losing state. J. Pediatr. 86:524-532, 1975.
83. Sebastian, A.; McSherry, E.; and Morris, R. C., Jr. Metabolic acidosis with special reference to the renal acidoses. In: The Kidney, edited by Brenner, B. M., and Rector, F. C. Philadelphia, Saunders, 1976, pp. 615-660.
84. Nishi, Y.; Kittaka, E.; Fukuda, K.; Hatano, S.; and Usui, T. Copper deficiency associated with alkali therapy in a patient with renal tubular acidosis. J. Pediatr. 98:81-83, 1981.

85. Lightwood, R. Calcium infarction of kidneys in infants, Br. Paed. Assoc. Proc. (abstr.), Arch. Dis. Child. 10:205, 1935.
86. Butler, A. M.; Wilson, J. L.; and Farber, S. Dehydration and acidosis with calcification at renal tubules. J. Pediatr. 8:489-499, 1936.
87. Lightwood, R.; Maclagan, N. F.; and Williams, J. G. Persistent acidosis in an infant: Cause not yet ascertained. Proc. R. Soc. Med. 29:1431-1433, 1936.
88. Hartmann, A. F. Clinical studies in acidosis and alkalosis; use and abuse of alkali in states of bicarbonate deficiency due to renal acidosis and sulfanilamide alkalosis. Ann. Intern. Med. 13:940-956, 1939.
89. Baines, G. H.; Barclay, J. A.; and Cooke, W. T. Nephrocalcinosis associated with hyperchloraemia and low plasma-bicarbonate. Q. J. Med. 14:113-123, 1945.
90. Albright, F.; Burnett, C. H.; Parson, W.; Reifenstein, E. C., Jr.; and Roos, A. Osteomalacia and late rickets. The various etiologies met in the United States with emphasis on that resulting from a specific form of renal acidosis, the therapeutic indications for each etiological subgroup, and the relationship between osteomalacia and Milkman's syndrome. Medicine 25:399-479, 1946.
91. Lightwood, R.; Payne, W. W.; and Black, J. A. Infantile renal acidosis. Pediatrics 12: 628-644, 1953.
92. Carré, I. J.; Wood, B. S. B.; and Smallwood, W. C. Idiopathic renal acidosis in infancy. Arch. Dis. Child. 29:326-333, 1954.
93. Doxiadis, S. A. Idiopathic renal acidosis in infancy. Arch. Dis. Child. 27:409-427, 1954.
94. Latner, A. L.; and Burnard, E. D. Idiopathic hyperchloraemic renal acidosis in infants (nephrocalcinosis infantum): Observations on the site and nature of the lesion. Q. J. Med. 19:285-301, 1950.
95. Buchanan, E. U.; and Komrower, G. M. The prognosis of idiopathic renal acidosis in infancy with observations on urine acidification and ammonia production in children. Arch. Dis. Child. 33:532-535, 1958.
96. Lightwood, R.; and Butler, N. Decline in primary infantile renal acidosis: Aetiological implications. Br. Med. J. 1:855-857, 1963.
97. Williams, H.; MacDonald, W. B.; and Callow, V. Pink disease. Its relation to adrenal function and the value of salt and desoxycorticosterone treatment. Med. J. Aust. 1: 363-365, 1951.
98. Reynolds, T. B. Observations on the pathogenesis of renal tubular acidosis. Am. J. Med. 25:503-515, 1958.
99. Halperin, M. L.; Goldstein, M. B.; Haig, A.; Johnson, M. D.; and Stinebaugh, B. J. Studies on the pathogenesis of type 1 (distal) renal tubular acidosis as revealed by urine PCO_2 tensions. J. Clin. Invest. 53:669-677, 1974.
100. Maren, T. H. Carbon dioxide equilibria in the kidney: The problems of elevated carbon dioxide tension, delayed dehydration, and disequilibrium pH. Kidney Int. 14: 395-405, 1978.
101. DuBose, T. D., Jr. Hydrogen ion secretion by the collecting duct as a determinant of the urine to blood PCO_2 gradient in alkaline urine. J. Clin. Invest. 69:145-156, 1982.
102. Schwartz, G. J.; Haycock, G. B.; Edelmann, C. M., Jr.; and Spitzer, A. Late metabolic acidosis: A reassessment of the definition. J. Pediatr. 95:102-107, 1979.

9

The Defect in Distal (Type 1) Renal Tubular Acidosis

DANIEL C. BATLLE
University of Illinois College of Medicine and West Side Veterans Administration Hospital, Chicago, Illinois

NEIL A. KURTZMAN*
University of Illinois College of Medicine, Chicago, Illinois

I. THE DEFECT IN DISTAL RENAL TUBULAR ACIDOSIS

The first cases of renal tubular acidosis (RTA) were described in children suffering from nephrocalcinosis and acidosis in 1935 by Lightwood (1) and 1936 by Butler et al. (2). The classic studies of Albright and colleagues (3) characterized the clinical features of the syndrome, documented its association with rickets or osteomalacia, and pointed out the basic defect in tubular function. Although this disorder seemed to be relatively rare at first, appearing with other disturbances of renal tubular transport that were genetically determined in some cases (4-7), the syndrome rapidly achieved great interest among students of pathophysiology because it was a model of disease in which the biochemical and molecular basis of its pathogenesis could be approached.

More than a decade after the first cases were reported, studies of urinary acidification in patients with RTA, generalized renal disease, and normal subjects (8-17) established two general types of RTA. In one, the urine pH could be lowered below 5.5 if systemic acidemia was of sufficient severity. At normal or higher values of plasma bicarbonate, however, these patients wasted large amounts of bicarbonate into the urine. A second group of patients was delineated in whom the urine pH could not be lowered below 5.5, regardless of the degree of acidemia present. Subsequently, the former disorder has been termed proximal (or type 2) RTA, since bicarbonate reabsorption is predominantly a function of the proximal tubule. The latter disorder is usually referred to as distal (or type 1), classic RTA, since development of the steep urine to plasma pH gradient is a function of the distal nephron. Patients with both types of RTA differed from patients with acidosis of chronic renal failure in whom the ability to lower urine pH during acidemia was maintained and bicarbonate wasting at normal plasma bicarbonate concentrations was rarely observed.

The exact defect causing classic RTA has interested nephrologists for many years (18-29). The prevailing view, proposed by Seldin and Wilson (27), and Rector (28) was that

**Current affiliation*: Texas Tech University Health Sciences Center, Lubbock, Texas

distal RTA was the result of an inability to maintain a steep pH gradient across the distal nephron. Seldin and Wilson (27) concluded that hydrogen ion secretion was not impaired in patients with type 1 RTA largely because maximal reabsorptive capacity for bicarbonate (a phenomenon which mainly reflects proximal acidification) during bicarbonate loading was either normal or increased in these patients. Since hydrogen ion secretion mediates bicarbonate reabsorption, they suggested that hydrogen ion secretion in the distal nephron was intact. Since the urine could not be acidified and hydrogen ion secretion seemed to be intact, a backleak of acid in the distal nephron was suggested as the likely mechanism responsible for impaired distal acidification.

Halperin and colleagues (29) reasoned that the reverse took place in patients with type 1 RTA. Based on the assumption that the ability to raise the urinary carbon dioxide tension greatly in excess of that of blood during bicarbonate loading reflected hydrogen ion secretion, and because this ability was markedly impaired in patients with distal RTA, they concluded that hydrogen ion secretion was impaired and that this impairment was responsible for the defect in type 1 RTA (29). The secretion of hydrogen ions into the distal nephron lumen containing bicarbonate results in the formation of carbonic acid. The delayed dehydration of this acid then results in a rise in urinary PCO_2. There is no reason why a "leaky" tubule would not exhibit backleak of carbonic acid under conditions of bicarbonate loading (30). This backleak of carbonic acid would prevent the urinary PCO_2 from rising, even though hydrogen ion secretory capacity was intact. Hence, a low urinary PCO_2 during bicarbonate loading in itself does not necessarily exclude acid backleak as a mechanism responsible for type 1 RTA. Acid backleak should also result in failure to lower urinary pH maximally.

Because acid backleak cannot be clearly differentiated from failure to secrete hydrogen ions by the measurement of either the urinary PCO_2 during bicarbonate loading or urinary pH during acidosis we have examined the pathogenesis of type 1 RTA by the systematic use of sodium sulfate and neutral phosphate infusion (31-42). Using these tools in animals with experimental distal acidification defects (31-33) as well as by studies in acidifying membranes (i.e., the turtle bladder) (43-46) several types of distal acidification defects have been postulated. Recent studies in humans have further expanded our understanding of the pathogenesis of type 1 RTA (35-41). A form of hyperkalemic type 1 RTA associated with impaired urinary potassium secretion and aldosterone unresponsiveness has been recently characterized (37,41). These studies emphasize the importance of renal potassium handling and its interrelationship with hydrogen ion secretion in the pathogenesis of certain types of type 1 RTA. In this chapter we will discuss the pathogenesis of type 1 RTA in an attempt to correlate experimental models of impaired distal urinary acidification and human type 1 RTA.

II. DISTAL URINARY ACIDIFICATION

The distal nephron performs three functions relative to urinary acidification. It reclaims the relatively small amount of bicarbonate that exits from the proximal nephron. In general, this does not amount to much more than 10% of the filtered bicarbonate. It also titrates urinary buffer. Divalent basic phosphate is converted to the acid monovalent form. It should be emphasized that some of this titration of phosphate takes place in the proximal tubule. Ammonia formed in tubular cells diffuses into the lumen of the distal nephron where hydrogen ion secretion converts it to nondiffusible ammonium. Hydrogen ion secretion and titration of urinary buffers result in the lowering of urine pH to the minimal values commonly observed. During acidemia urine pH may fall as low as 4.5.

Much of our recent knowledge concerning the mechanism of distal urinary acidification results from the study of the acidification process in vitro using either the toad or turtle bladder

(43-58). These membranes are capable of developing large pH gradients and in almost all regards appear analogous to the distal nephron of the mammalian kidney. The best available evidence suggests that proton translocation in the isolated bladder epithelium (50) and possibly in the distal nephron (most importantly in the collecting tubule) results from a specific hydrogen ion pump. The pump represents the active component of acidification (51). It is influenced by electrochemical gradient such that lowering mucosal pH by about 3 pH units brings hydrogen ion secretion to zero. Establishing an electrical gradient of 180 mV lumen positive also stops hydrogen ion secretion (52). Hydrogen ion secretion may be further abolished by the combination of an electrical or chemical gradient; 1 pH unit is equivalent to about 58 mV. The passive component of acidification consists of the backleak of acid from the mucosal to the serosal surface (53). The distal nephron and the turtle or toad bladders are very "tight" epithelia; thus, the passive component under ordinary circumstances is very small and can usually be ignored (54). However, it is likely that the distal nephron is not as tight an epithelium as the bladder; the passive component, therefore, may be significant.

The secretion of protons is influenced by the availability of hydrogen ion (53). The removal of hydrogen ion from water liberates hydroxyl which is buffered by CO_2 and converted to bicarbonate (55,56). Bicarbonate thus formed is then removed from the cell. Therefore, there are two critical steps regulating the formation and removal of bicarbonate. Inhibition of either of these two factors will increase cell pH and decrease the availability of protons (53,55,56). The first of these factors is carbonic anhydrase activity. Carbonic anhydrase catalyzes the reaction:

$$CO_2 + OH^- = HCO_3$$

Accordingly, the inhibition of proton transport by carbonic anhydrase inhibiting drugs is the result of decreased buffering of hydroxyl within the cell.

The positive serosal potential difference (PD) permits negatively charged bicarbonate to leave the cell passively. This exit step for bicarbonate is in some way dependent upon the presence of a specific protein in the serosal membrane. The importance of this protein for bicarbonate exit has been definitely demonstrated in erythrocytes. Disulfonic stilbenes (e.g., SITS) irreversibly bind to this protein, an effect that decreases the rate of bicarbonate exit from the cell (57,58). Accordingly, SITS inhibits acidification not by a direct effect on the pump but by increasing intracellular pH.

Both the bladder and the mammalian collecting tubule have the capacity to secrete bicarbonate (54,59,60). Net acidification, therefore, is the rate of proton secretion minus bicarbonate secretion. However, it is not currently known whether bicarbonate secretion plays a significant role in acidification in the distal nephron.

III. FACTORS INFLUENCING DISTAL ACIDIFICATION

A. Blood pH

Wide fluctuations of pH from normal markedly influence the rate of distal acidification. For example, respiratory alkalosis markedly inhibits this process (61,62). To what extent this inhibition is also the result of hypocapnia, independent of altered pH, is not clearly known. We have recently demonstrated that rats recovering from hypoxemia-induced respiratory alkalosis have reduced distal hydrogen secretion (63). Chronic alkali loading also is associated with a reduced rate of distal hydrogen ion secretion (63). Hence, exposure to an alkalemic environment results in depression of distal urinary acidification. This adaptive response may be mediated by small changes in intracellular pH.

The extent to which minimal alterations in blood pH influence distal acidification has not yet been totally established. Undetectable changes in blood pH may be the mechanism that modulates the response to altered dietary acid content. The rabbit, for example, under usual circumstances consumes a diet with a high alkaline ash content. Administration of an acid ash diet to rabbit, however, results in the elaboration of an acid urine (64). Blood pH is maintained at a normal level. The stimulus that tells the rabbit distal nephron to excrete acid when the diet is altered may be a very small change in blood pH. Alternatively, intracellular pH may be the one dominant determinant in modulating the kidney's response to differing acid loads.

B. Sodium Transport and Potential Difference

The rate of active hydrogen ion secretion is exquisitely sensitive to alterations in transepithelial electrical gradient (46,65). Under ordinary circumstances, the tubular lumen is negative to the peritubular space, favoring secretion of positively charged ions and thereby stimulating urine acidification. The main determinant of this PD is sodium transport.

Sodium reabsorption is a function of sodium delivery to the distal nephron, the level of mineralocorticoid activity, and the nature of the accompanying anion. To the extent that anion composition is constant, the PD is a function of distal sodium delivery and mineralocorticoid activity. If distal sodium delivery is increased by infusing sodium with an impermeant anion, a greater negative PD will develop, thereby increasing proton secretion (36, 46,66).

C. Aldosterone

In addition to its effect on sodium reabsorption, aldosterone influences urinary acidification through several other mechanisms (44,67-69). The conductance of acidifying membranes for protons is increased when aldosterone is added to the serosal media (44). Aldosterone also affects acid-base balance indirectly by its effect on potassium balance. Potassium depletion stimulates and potassium excess inhibits ammonia synthesis (70). Furthermore, aldosterone itself may increase ammonia synthesis. The effect of aldosterone on urinary acidification is discussed in more detail in Ch. 10.

D. Potassium

Alterations in potassium homeostasis in the absence of other stimuli to aldosterone release influence acidification, in our view, solely by modulating the rate of ammonia synthesis or aldosterone formation and release. Potassium depletion accompanied by aldosterone excess greatly increases acid excretion.

IV. EVALUATION OF DISTAL ACIDIFICATION

A. Minimal Urine pH and Acid Excretion During Metabolic Acidosis

Measurement of urine pH is the first step in assessing the integrity of distal urinary acidification. If systemic acidosis is present the urine pH should be below 5.5. The finding of a urine pH below 5.5 suggests appropriate urinary acidification and, by conventional definition, excludes type 1 RTA. If the patient is acidotic, there is no need to perform an ammonium chloride loading test. Mild acidosis is sufficient to evaluate urinary acidification and there is no need to induce severe acidosis. It should be noted, however, that systematic studies in patients with type 1 RTA evaluating the effect of progressively lowering blood pH on urine pH are not currently available. Our approach to patients in whom type 1 RTA is suspected and the urine pH is low (i.e., below 5.5) during acidosis is to measure urine PCO_2 during bicarbonate loading. This maneuver can uncover a defect in the rate of distal H^+ secretion if urine PCO_2 does not increase normally (39,40). A urine pH below 5.5 can be found in patients with type 2 RTA and is also characteristic of patients with acidosis due to selective aldosterone deficiency (35,37,41,71). Patients with a proximal defect in bicarbonate reabsorption can lower the urine pH below 5.5 when the serum bicarbonate concentration falls to very low levels, i.e., to a level of serum bicarbonate where reabsorption of the filtered bicarbonate is complete and bicarbonate excretion ceases. In addition, these patients are able to increase urinary PCO_2 during bicarbonate loading.

The urine pH should be measured (by a pH meter) from freshly voided urine in the morning and collected in mineral oil. Urine pH is influenced by the patient's position and urine flow. Since in the recumbent position the urine pH may increase, it is preferable to ask the patient to void in the upright position. If systemic acidosis is not present at the time of study, NH_4Cl can be given orally in a dose of 0.1 g/kg of body weight daily for 3-5 days. A 24-hr urine collection for measurement of acid excretion can be started on the third day of NH_4Cl administration as described by Elkinton et al. (10). Alternatively, a single dose of the same amount of NH_4Cl may be given; urine is then collected hourly from 2 to 8 hr after the NH_4Cl ingestion (9). In our experience, the 3-day test gives more reliable results and we prefer it because it allows time for a maximal increase in ammonium excretion. The urine pH in normal subjects falls below 5.5 (usually below 5.0) by the first day and remains low thereafter. The finding of a urinary pH above 5.5 in the face of acidosis is the most specific (but not the most sensitive) criteria for the diagnosis of type 1 RTA (see below).

The amount of secreted H^+ excreted in the urine bound to ammonia is measured as ammonium excretion. Titratable acidity is the amount of H^+ bound to HPO_4^- and to a lesser extent, to other weak acids such as creatinine and uric acid. The sum of titratable acid and ammonium excretion minus the trivial amount of bicarbonate excreted normally equals net acid excretion. Net acid excretion represents the net amount of HCO_3 added to the blood via tubular regeneration. Both ammonium excretion and titratable acidity are decreased in renal insufficiency. Thus, it is important to compare acid excretion between patients and controls with similar glomerular filtration rate (GFR).

An alternative acidifying agent is calcium chloride (2 meq/kg of body weight orally). This substance gives results similar to NH_4Cl and can be used in patients who cannot tolerate ammonium chloride (i.e., nausea and vomiting) or in patients with liver insufficiency in whom ammonium chloride is contraindicated (72).

B. Renal Handling of Bicarbonate

In patients with type 1 RTA, bicarbonate reabsorption is incomplete at low plasma levels of bicarbonate, but increases normally with increasing plasma bicarbonate concentration. Thus, maximal bicarbonate reabsorption is normal or slightly increased in type 1 RTA, probably as a result of volume contraction and/or hypokalemia.

An easy method to evaluate the renal handling of bicarbonate consists of calculating the fraction of filtered bicarbonate excreted in the urine at normal plasma bicarbonate levels. Fractional excretion of bicarbonate is greater than 15% in patients with type 2 RTA (73). In type 1 RTA, fractional excretion of bicarbonate is usually less than 5%, since the amount of bicarbonate delivered to the defective distal nephron is small (73). Fractional bicarbonate excretion is calculated by dividing bicarbonate clearance by GFR.

C. Sodium Sulfate Infusion

Normal subjects are able to lower the urine pH maximally when distal sodium reabsorption is avid and distal Na delivery is adequate. The first requirement can be accomplished by placing the subject on a low salt diet (i.e., 20 meq Na daily for 3 days) which in turn stimulates aldosterone release and thereby enhances the capacity for distal Na reabsorption (12,15). Distal Na delivery is then promoted by the acute administration of a salt of a poorly reabsorbable anion such as sodium sulfate (500 ml of 4% Na_2SO_4 infused over 60 min). Sodium sulfate infusion can also be performed after the administration of 9-fluorohydrocortisone (1 mg orally 12 hr preceding Na_2SO_4 infusion), which ensures avid Na reabsorption. This maneuver obviates the need for prior salt restriction, since it ensures that sufficient mineralocorticoid activity is present (36-38).

The Na_2SO_4 test properly performed results in a fall of urine pH below 5.5 (usually below 5.0) regardless of whether systemic acidosis is present It should be pointed out that urine collections should continue for 2-3 hr after Na_2SO_4 infusion is discontinued because some subjects have a late response. Patients with chronic renal insufficiency also respond normally to Na_2SO_4 despite their inability to retain salt maximally (15). Another agent that can be used to evaluate sodium-dependent distal acidification is furosemide (74), which results in a fall in urine pH comparable to that elicited by Na_2SO_4 infusion.

D. Urinary PCO_2 as an Index of Distal Acidification

Normally, after alkalinization of the urine with sodium bicarbonate loading, the PCO_2 of urine reaches a value considerably higher than that of blood (29,76-80). Secreted hydrogen ion reacts with bicarbonate to form carbonic acid. The dehydration of carbonic acid to CO_2 and H_2O proceeds slowly, since carbonic anhydrase is not present in the lumen of the distal nephron. This delay in carbonic acid dehydration allows the development of a high PCO_2 as the tubular urine reaches the terminal nephron where the surface to volume relationship is unfavorable for CO_2 diffusion. The infusion of carbonic anhydrase dissipates the high urine to blood (U-B) PCO_2 normally seen in alkaline urine (80). This observation has been interpreted to indicate that the U-B PCO_2 gradient was the direct result of proton secretion (80). Subjects with impaired distal acidification invariably fail to raise the urinary PCO_2 substantially above that of blood (29,39,40). Normally, the U-B PCO_2 gradient rises markedly after maximal alkalinization of the urine (urine pH of 7.8 or higher), provided that urine bicarbonate concentration is sufficiently high (i.e., above 100 meq/l). Impaired concentrating capacity also may prevent the rise in urine PCO_2 during bicarbonate loading despite adequate distal H^+ secretion (76). This lack of increase in U-B PCO_2 results from insufficient availability of bicarbonate. A concentrating defect can impair the achievement of sufficiently high urinary concentrations of bicarbonate and thereby prevent a normal rise in urine PCO_2 (39,75).

The various factors that affect urinary PCO_2 generation need to be considered. We studied several animal models of impaired urinary acidification as well as the factors that influence PCO_2 generation in the urine. A number of important regulatory events emerged from these studies. A tight correlation exists between urinary PCO_2 and urinary bicarbonate concentration (33,39,40,75). The concentration of bicarbonate in the urine, per se, could influence urine PCO_2 through its "ampholyte" effect (75,77). According to this formulation, bicarbonate combines with bicarbonate to form carbonic acid and carbonate, a CO_2-generating effect unrelated to urinary acidification. Recently, Stinebaugh and associates (78) have argued that such an effect of bicarbonate concentration can generate CO_2 only if bicarbonate is added to urine as opposed to elevation of bicarbonate concentration secondary to water abstraction. If this argument is correct, urinary PCO_2 can be elevated as a consequence of the ampholyte effect only by bicarbonate secretion. As has been mentioned, there is some evidence to suggest that bicarbonate is secreted in the mammalian collecting tubule. However, whether bicarbonate secretion contributes in any demonstrable amount to urinary PCO_2 generation is not known.

Because of the correlation between urinary bicarbonate concentration and PCO_2, it was postulated that at least part of the CO_2 tension in highly alkaline urine resulted from the concentration of the urine rather than from its acidification (75). That there is a contribution attributable to acidification, however, can clearly be demonstrated by observing the urinary PCO_2 at high levels of urine bicarbonate concentration. At such levels the urine PCO_2 in subjects with impaired distal acidification is significantly lower than in normal subjects (39). Patients with impaired distal urinary acidification (39,40) commonly elaborate urine with pH values in excess of 8.0 (a value seldom seen in normal subjects during bicarbonate loading). [Note: The use of the U-B PCO_2 as a marker of distal acidification has recently been questioned (81).]

A critical dependence of urine PCO_2 on urinary phosphate concentration exists when the pH of the urine is close to the pK of the phosphate buffer system (i.e., 6.8) (33-36,38-40,79). In highly alkaline urine (pH greater than 7.8) phosphate concentration plays no role in generation of urine PCO_2 (33). At a urine pH close to 6.8, the urine bicarbonate concentration is low and concentrating capacity plays no role in the ability of the kidney to generate a high urine PCO_2. Accordingly, the effect of phosphate infusion on urinary PCO_2 of patients with a urine pH at or near 6.8 is a pure test of urinary acidification (35,36,39,40). This test is performed by infusing neutral sodium phosphate (0.6 mmol/kg of body weight diluted in 180 ml of normal saline) slowly at a constant rate of 1-2 ml/min. This maneuver usually results in a two- to threefold increase in plasma phosphate concentration (35,36,39). Urinary phosphate concentration must increase above 20 mmol in two or three successive urine collections at 2-4 hr after beginning the phosphate infusion. Under these conditions, U-B PCO_2 rises markedly in normal subjects and patients with renal insufficiency (35,36,39).

The response to phosphate buffer infusion on urine PCO_2 can be employed to assess the mechanism responsible for impaired distal acidification (35,36,38-41). For example, if type 1 RTA were the result of impaired distal proton secretion, the urine PCO_2 should not increase normally in response to phosphate loading at a urine pH of 6.8, since phosphate loading tests proton secretory ability (35,36). If, however, the cause of type 1 RTA were a backleak of acid, then the response to phosphate administration as regards urine PCO_2 might well be normal, inasmuch as proton secretion would be intact; the secreted proton would be bound to phosphate buffer and probably be much less diffusible than in the absence of such a buffer. Thus, a backleak defect might respond normally to phosphate administration.

V. EXPERIMENTAL DEFECTS IN DISTAL URINARY ACIDIFICATION

A. Amphotericin

The antifungal antibiotic amphotericin B may cause type 1 RTA in humans (25). The effect of this agent on urinary acidification has been studied in the rat (83,84). Experimental animals develop incomplete type 1 RTA following exposure to this drug. The mechanism whereby this agent might interfere with urinary acidification has been elucidated using the turtle bladder as an experimental model (43). This membrane secretes protons in a fashion analogous to the distal nephron of mammals and is markedly affected by exposure to amphotericin. Amphotericin causes no defect in proton secretion or the ability to generate large pH gradients when added to a turtle bladder preparation (43). What it does is to markedly increase the permeability of this membrane to acid (43). Secreted acid back diffuses resulting in a decrease in net acidification. Thus, by inference, type 1 RTA seen in patients exposed to amphotericin could be attributed to an increase in the permeability of the distal nephron to acid (i.e., acid backleak). This mechanism, however, has not been characterized in experimental animals or patients receiving this drug. One could predict that urinary pH would fall and U-B PCO_2 would rise normally in response to sodium sulfate and sodium phosphate, respectively (34,36).

B. Lithium

Animals treated with lithium chloride develop hyperchloremic metabolic acidosis (32,85). Proximal bicarbonate reabsorption as assessed by bicarbonate titration is normal (32). The urine pH during systemic acidosis, however, is inappropriately high (32,85). The U-B PCO_2 gradient during bicarbonate loading is low even when corrected for urinary bicarbonate concentration. Thus, lithium administration in large doses quite clearly causes overt type 1 RTA. The response of U-B PCO_2 to phosphate loading and the urine pH in response to sodium sulfate loading is normal (32,33). That is to say, these animals which are not able to lower urine pH during systemic acidosis are able to lower urine pH normally during sodium sulfate administration. As a result of these observations it was postulated (32,33) that lithium caused a type of acidification defect analogous to that just described for amphotericin; i.e., that the permeability of the distal nephron for acid was increased.

To further examine this issue additional studies in the turtle bladder were performed (45). These studies did not support the backleak hypothesis because the addition of lithium to the mucosal side of this membrane had no effect on proton secretion under short circuit conditions and failed to demonstrate a backleak of acid (45). In addition there was no enhancement of bicarbonate secretion in the lithium-treated bladder (45). The turtle bladder generates a lumen-negative potential difference by reabsorbing far more sodium than it secretes protons. This negative potential difference in and of itself favors proton secretion. To examine proton secretion in this preparation, independent of any effect of sodium reabsorption, the bladder potential difference can be reduced to zero (short circuited) by the passage of an electrical current in the appropriate direction. Accordingly, to study the possibility that lithium might have an effect on hydrogen ion secretion indirectly by affecting sodium reabsorption, the effect of lithium on the bladder must be studied under open circuit conditions; i.e., sodium reabsorption must be allowed to generate a mucosal-negative potential difference.

In experiments using the open-circuited bladder, Arruda et al. (45) observed that lithium reduced the normal lumen negative potential difference to a value that was close to zero. This reduction in the favorable electrical gradient for proton secretion markedly reduced the rate of hydrogen ion secretion. Restoration of the potential difference restored the rates of hydrogen ion secretion to control values despite the fact that lithium was still present in the mucosal solution (45). Therefore, lithium impairs urinary acidification by reducing hydrogen ion secretion as a consequence of the impairment of the favorable electrical gradient for proton transport (i.e., lithium induces a voltage dependent type of acidification defect). The observation in vivo that sodium sulfate and sodium phosphate administration to lithium-treated animals produced a normal acidifying response can be explained as the consequence of enhanced distal delivery of sodium which in turn increases sodium reabsorption by displacing lithium, and thereby regenerates the luminal-negative potential difference. This mechanism is likely responsible for the distal acidification defect observed in patients receiving chronic lithium therapy (39). Patients, however, have incomplete type 1 RTA, so that metabolic acidosis is rarely seen (see Sect. VI.H, Rate-Dependent Type 1 RTA).

C. Amiloride

Amiloride administration to dogs causes hyperkalemic metabolic acidosis (86). When this diuretic is given to rats an incomplete (nonacidotic) form of type 1 RTA develops (46). Rats so treated are unable to raise the U-B PCO_2 gradient (46). Furthermore, they are unable to lower the urine pH normally when challenged with acid and respond abnormally to the acidifying effects of either sodium phosphate or sodium administration (46). This response closely resembles that seen in the postobstructive kidney described below. However, amiloride causes an acidification pattern identical to that seen with lithium in the turtle bladder (46). in open circuit conditions amiloride-treated bladders demonstrate decreased hydrogen ion secretion which is totally reversed by the restoration of the potential difference, even in the continued presence of the diuretic (46). The difference in response to amiloride and lithium in vivo is likely the consequence of a persistent and irreversible blockade of distal sodium transport secondary to the continued presence of amiloride. By blocking the cellular channels for sodium reabsorption, amiloride prevents increased distal delivery of this cation from having its normal effect on distal voltage. That is to say, amiloride induces an irreversible distal acidification defect (as long as it is present).

Amiloride-induced hyperkalemia is the totally predictable result of a decrease in distal potential difference. Lithium does not cause hyperkalemia, possibly because it impairs potassium reabsorption in more proximal portions of the nephron. In fact, the overall effect of lithium on renal potassium excretion is to increase it (unpublished observations).

D. Urinary Tract Obstruction

It has long been recognized that urinary tract obstruction interferes with urinary acidification (87-91). We further studied this issue by examining the acidification defect induced by unilateral ureteral obstruction for 24 hr (31). The postobstructive kidney was unable to raise the U-B PCO_2 gradient in response to either bicarbonate or phosphate loading. In addition, the acidifying response to sodium sulfate administration was markedly abnormal (31). The urine pH was inappropriately high during ammonium chloride-induced metabolic acidosis. While this defect in acidification was initially attributed to a secretory failure of the proton pump (31), the above-mentioned effect of amiloride and our observations in patients with obstructive uropathy (37) suggested an alternative explanation. The failure to secrete acid and potassium normally in the postobstructive kidney could be the consequence of a primary impairment in sodium reabsorption (37). The failure of sodium reabsorption would reduce the favorable gradient for potassium and proton translocation and, thus, reduce potassium secretion and distal urinary acidification (37,66).

E. Aldosterone Deficiency

Deficiency of aldosterone also results in a form of type 1 RTA. Aldosterone affects distal urinary acidification through at least two mechanisms: it increases the rate of proton secretion and helps establish the lumen-negative potential difference normally seen in the distal nephron. This latter effect is secondary to its action on sodium reabsorption. Because the force of the proton pump is not believed to be influenced by aldosterone (44), one would predict that the ability to lower urine pH in response to acidosis in the absence of this hormone would be intact. This, indeed, is the case. Since deficiency of aldosterone should slow the rate of proton transport, one might predict the U-B PCO_2 gradient would be depressed in the absence of this hormone. Such, however, is not the case (67). Aldosterone-deficient subjects are able to raise the U-B PCO_2 during either bicarbonate or phosphate loading in a fashion indistinguishable from normal (36,67). This intact ability to raise the urinary U-B PCO_2 in the absence of aldosterone suggests that this hormone does not regulate the rate of distal proton secretion to a major extent. The acidosis that develops in patients with aldosterone deficiency is related to hyperkalemia and decreased ammonium excretion (see below).

VI. CLASSIFICATION AND CHARACTERIZATION OF THE DEFECT CAUSING TYPE 1 RTA

The following classification of type 1 RTA is based on our current understanding of the mechanisms regulating acidification of the urine by the distal nephron. Some of the mechanisms delineated below are represented by well-defined clinical syndromes. Others represent clinical pictures still evolving, while several are purely theoretical.

A. Pure Proton Secretory Defect

The pure proton secretory defect results from failure of the proton pump. Since the proton pump is defective, urine pH can not be maximally lowered regardless of the intensity of the

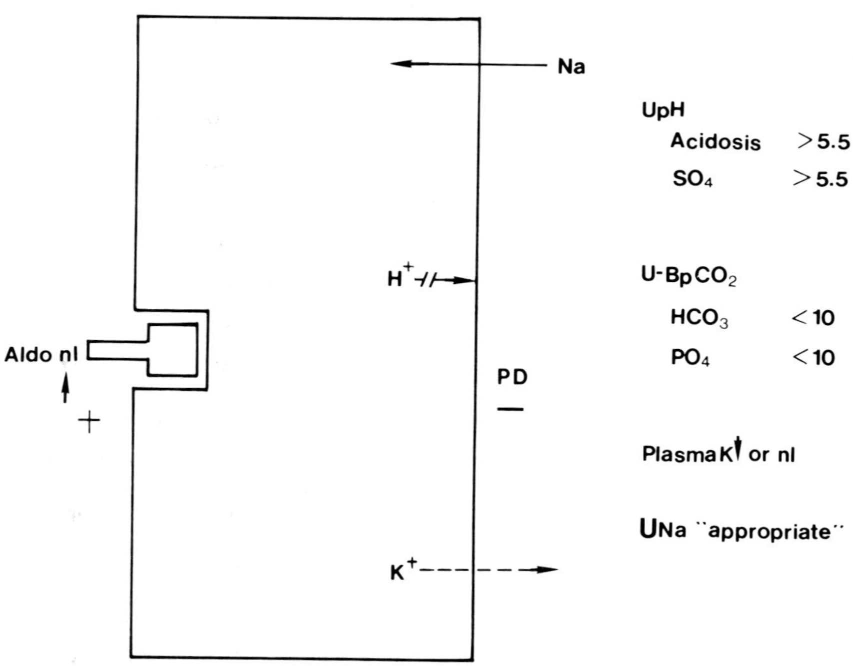

Fig. 1 Depicts the features of a defect in distal acidification as a consequence of impaired hydrogen ion secretion (i.e., proton pump failure). Potassium excretion is not impaired in such a defect and may be high, leading to hypokalemia (see text).

stimulus. Therefore, as outlined in Fig. 1, the urine pH will be greater than 5.5 both during systemic acidosis or following the administration of sodium sulfate (35,36). The U-B PCO_2 will likewise be depressed both during bicarbonate and phosphate loading (35,36). This failure to respond to phosphate or bicarbonate is the result of inability to secrete protons normally under any circumstances. This failure to lower urine pH and to increase urinary PCO_2 normally contrasts markedly with some of the derangements to be described below. In addition, urine sodium concentration will be roughly appropriate for the state of volume and dietary sodium intake. Likewise potassium homeostasis will be maintained. Similarly, aldosterone is regulated appropriately for the state of volume and potassium homeostasis.

This mechanism has been shown to be operative in patients with various causes of acquired type 1 RTA (35,36). It is currently unknown whether the hereditary form of type 1 RTA associated with hypokalemia and nephrocalcinosis results from this mechanism. As recently summarized (42) a few patients with nephrocalcinosis responded to sodium sulfate infusion by lowering urinary pH below 5.5, whereas others did not (22,23,36). Some of the patients in whom sodium sulfate resulted in lowering of urine pH had an incomplete form of type 1 RTA (23). We think that a normal response to sodium sulfate in this setting is also consistent with a mild secretory defect (unpublished observations). As of this writing, however, systematic studies evaluating the response to phosphate and sulfate loading in patients with hereditary type 1 RTA are not available. It is conceivable that there may be more than one type of distal acidification defect underlying the various causes of hereditary type 1 RTA(24).

Patients with type 1 RTA have been shown to waste small amounts of salt in the urine (92). This salt wastage tendency may be the result of tubular damage secondary to nephrocalcinosis rather than an inherent part of the tubular defect. The hypokalemia often seen in these patients is likely the result of intact potassium secretory capacity in the face of high levels of aldosterone, secondary to variable degrees of volume contraction and an increase in distal delivery of sodium with poorly reabsorbable anions (93). The intact capacity to secrete potassium in the face of this defect is emphasized by the response of these patients to sodium sulfate (35,36). This maneuver markedly increases potassium excretion, while failing to maximally acidify the urine (35,36), strongly suggesting that the distal nephron's capacity to generate a negative potential difference is intact. Hence, impaired Na reabsorption is not likely to be the primary event leading to decreased distal acidification in these patients (36).

B. Backleak of Acid

Acid backleak results from an increase in the permeability to acid in the distal nephron. The only well-defined example of a defect in distal urinary acidification secondary to this mechanism results from the administration of amphotericin B. This antibiotic is well known to cause type 1 RTA in humans (25). Unfortunately, the response of amphotericin-treated patients with type 1 RTA to the infusion of sulfate, phosphate, or bicarbonate has not been studied. Therefore, the formulation to be presented regarding this defect is to a large extent theoretical (Fig. 2).

The urine pH in patients with amphotericin-induced type 1 RTA is inappropriately high (25). We believe that these patients, if infused with sodium sulfate, would lower the urine pH. If distal nephron permeability is increased in this disorder, it is our feeling that sulfate will still be poorly reabsorbed. The reabsorption of sodium under this circumstance will generate a negative electrical potential difference, retarding the backleak of protons even in the face of a "leaky" distal nephron.

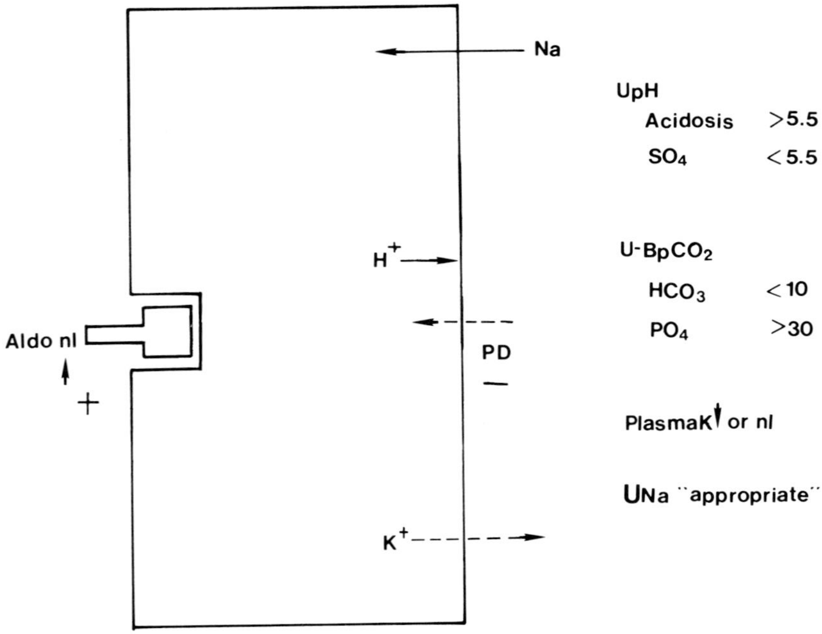

Fig. 2 Depicts the features of a distal acidification defect resulting from backleak (broken line) of acid (H^+ or carbonic acid) in the face of unimpaired hydrogen ion secretion. Hypokalemia develops as a result of increased tubular permeability for potassium.

Urine to blood PCO_2 during bicarbonate loading also has not been measured in patients with amphotericin-induced type 1 RTA, although the acute infusion of this antibiotic results in an inability to raise the urine PCO_2 normally during bicarbonate loading in rats (84). The failure to raise urine PCO_2 normally would occur if a leaky distal nephron allowed increased back diffusion of carbonic acid. If the proton pump is intact hydrogen ions will be secreted normally even in the presence of amphotericin. During bicarbonate loading, the secretion of protons will result in the formation of carbonic acid. If carbonic acid back diffuses in increased amounts, a low urinary PCO_2 will result. The infusion of phosphate should in our opinion result in a normal elevation of U-B PCO_2. Phosphate is much less diffussable than is carbonic acid. The secretion of protons in the presence of large amounts of urinary phosphate would result in titration of the alkaline form of phosphate to its acid counterpart. Acid phosphate would not back diffuse as rapidly as carbonic acid and would appear in the terminal nephron, where it can donate a proton to bicarbonate, leading to the generation of a high urine PCO_2. Since sodium transport is not reduced by the presence of amphotericin, the exchange of sodium for potassium would be accelerated, explaining why these patients develop an exaggerated kaliuresis and hypokalemia.

C. Voltage-Dependent

In order to generate a negative intratubular potential difference in the distal nephron, sodium must be reabsorbed. Failure to reabsorb sodium in this nephron segment as the result of an intrinsic tubular defect will result in a decrease in the potential difference. Since proton secretion is stimulated by the presence of a negative luminal potential difference, the rate of distal acidification will decrease in proportion to the decrease in sodium transport.

This would be the case even if the hydrogen pump were totally intact. In addition to the effect of this defect on acidification, potassium secretion will fall markedly for the same reason. Since potassium secretion is largely passive, the effect of this defect may be more pronounced on potassium excretion than on acidification. Thus, it is common to find patients who likely have this defect whose major clinical manifestation is hyperkalemia rather than metabolic acidosis.

Obviously, a defect in sodium transport will be reflected by an inability to conserve sodium normally. Since relatively small amounts of sodium are reabsorbed in the more distal portions of the nephron, this defect may be manifested only when the patient is placed on a very low sodium diet. Occassionally one may observe patients with more profound sodium wastage (41). Since this defect is the result of a failure in tubular function rather than a deficiency of aldosterone, these patients should have normal or even increased levels of plasma aldosterone (37). Typically, these patients do not lower urine pH normally during systemic acidosis (37), or during sodium sulfate infusion (37). Occassionally, however, patients with this defect respond normally to sodium sulfate (36). Such patients likely have a defect in sodium transport that can be overcome by delivering large amounts of sodium to the distal nephron and should also respond normally to phosphate infusion (36) (Fig. 3). Those patients who are unresponsive to sodium sulfate are also unresponsive to phosphate (36). All patients with this defect would be expected to have an abnormally low urine PCO_2 during bicarbonate loading (36).

Clinical examples of this form of hyperkalemic type 1 RTA are obstructive uropathy and certain forms of interstitial nephritis such as is seen in patients with hemoglobinopathies S

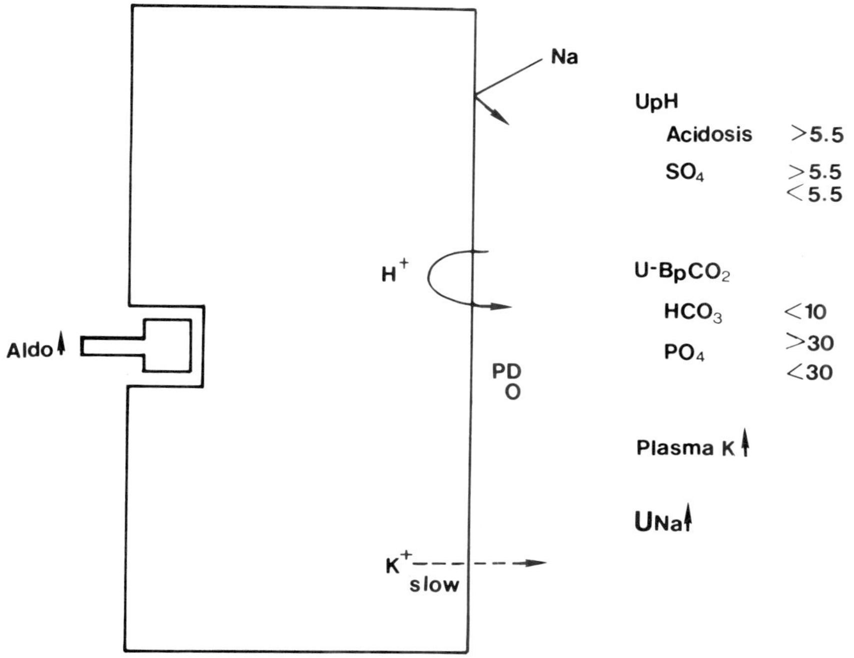

Fig. 3 Depicts the features of decreased H^+ and K^+ secretion as consequence of failure to establish a normal potential difference (PD). This results from a primary impairment in sodium reabsorption (see text).

(36,37,46). Some of these patients may have selective aldosterone deficiency combined with voltage dependent type 1 RTA (37,94).

D. Aldosterone Deficiency

Over the past few years the syndrome of isolated hypoaldosteronism has become a well-recognized clinical entity (71,94-98), a common feature of which is hyperchloremic metabolic acidosis. It is well accepted that the defect in urinary acidification seen in these patients does not result from impaired proximal bicarbonate reabsorption. For this reason and since aldosterone exerts its tubular effect in the collecting tubule, the hyperchloremic acidosis has been attributed to a defect in the distal nephron. This type of defect is called by some workers type 4 RTA (71) (see Ch. 10). In our view this term lacks precision, since patients with both aldosterone deficiency and aldosterone resistance have many common features (94). For this reason we favor the terms aldosterone deficiency or aldosterone resistance, since they both describe the primary defect involved and indicate the appropriate therapy.

As shown in Fig. 4 patients with aldosterone deficiency acidify the urine in a fashion very similar to that observed in normal subjects. Urine pH is appropriately acid both during systemic acidosis (71,94,95) and during sulfate loading (36). Urine PCO_2 is normal both during bicarbonate (67) and phosphate loading (36). The reason why the absence of aldosterone does not impair urinary acidification, as assessed by these tests, but does result in systemic acidosis is not totally clear. It may relate to an effect of aldosterone on urinary

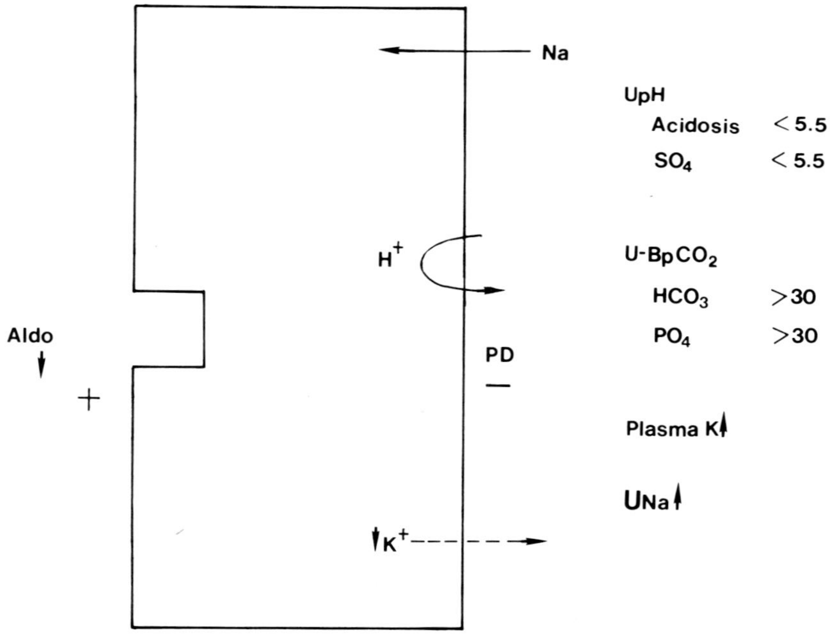

Fig. 4 Depicts the features of aldosterone deficiency. Observe that H^+ secretion is not impaired, but potassium excretion is decreased. Na reabsorption may be decreased but not to the extent of interfering with the achievement of a substantial PD. Ammonium excretion is decreased (see text).

ammonia formation (68,71,94). On the other hand, experimental animals with aldosterone deficiency are able to increase urinary ammonium excretion normally, at least acutely (67). An additional factor not present in adrenalactomized animals may be the presence of renal insufficiency. Almost all patients with this disorder have a moderate reduction in glomerular filtration rate (71,95-97). The combination of reduced GFR and aldosterone deficiency may be decisive in the generation of the acidosis (94). Studies of experimental animals with aldosterone deficiency have been limited to those with intact renal function.

Potassium homeostasis is clearly abnormal in selective aldosterone deficiency. Aldosterone concentrations in the blood are decreased in relation to the volume status and the serum potassium concentration. This is a critical feature which distinguishes aldosterone deficiency from aldosterone resistance (see below). In all other regards the two syndromes are similar. An additional factor which may decrease urinary ammonium excretion is hyperkalemia (98). The effects of hyperkalemia and aldosterone deficiency on decreased ammonia production may be additive.

E. Aldosterone Resistance

As shown in Fig. 5, aldosterone resistance is indistinguishable from aldosterone deficiency except that blood aldosterone concentration is normal or elevated in the former. Aldosterone resistance may be differentiated from the hyperkalemic acidosis due to voltage-dependent defect by the failure of patients with the latter disorder to lower urine pH during acidosis.

The best known example of this disorder is the form of pseudohypoaldosteronism described in children (99-103). Interestingly, one of the major manifestations of this disorder

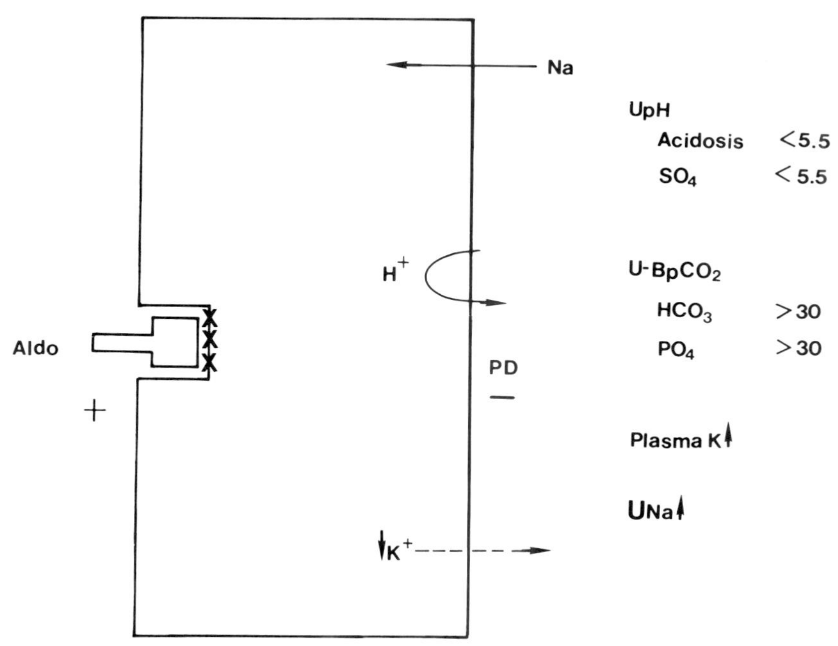

Fig. 5 Depicts the features associated with aldosterone resistance. The features of this defect are similar to those seen in aldosterone deficiency except that plasma aldosterone concentration is increased.

is sodium wastage, well in excess of that seen in patients with selective aldosterone deficiency. In adults, however, a distinctive form of hyperkalemic hyperchloremic acidosis associated with normal or increased plasma aldosterone levels, and all the urinary features of aldosterone resistance except salt wastage, has been described (104-107). In one of these patients mineralocorticoid administration failed to increase potassium excretion even when coupled with intravenous infusion of sodium chloride (107). The infusion of sodium sulfate, however, resulted in a normally large increase in urinary potassium excretion. The basic cause of the defect could be an inability to generate a negative potential difference in the lumen of the distal nephron as a result of increased permeability of the distal nephron to chloride (i.e., "chloride shunt") (107). As shown in Fig. 6, this defect should be associated with a normal acidification response to systemic acidosis or sulfate administration. It is also likely that these patients would raise urinary PCO_2 normally if infused with either bicarbonate or phosphate.

In this regard, the syndrome resembles that form of voltage-dependent type 1 RTA which responds normally to phosphate and sulfate administration (36). It differs from that syndrome in that patients with a chloride shunt are able to lower the urine pH normally in response to systemic acidosis. Furthermore, patients with a chloride shunt have no tendency to waste sodium, whereas sodium wastage is a feature of voltage-dependent type 1 RTA. As a result of enhanced NaCl reabsorption these patients may develop hypertension and suppression of plasma renin activity (107).

F. Increased Bicarbonate Secretion

There is evidence that both anuran membranes and mammalian collecting tubules may secrete bicarbonate, as discussed above. The magnitude of this process and the role which it

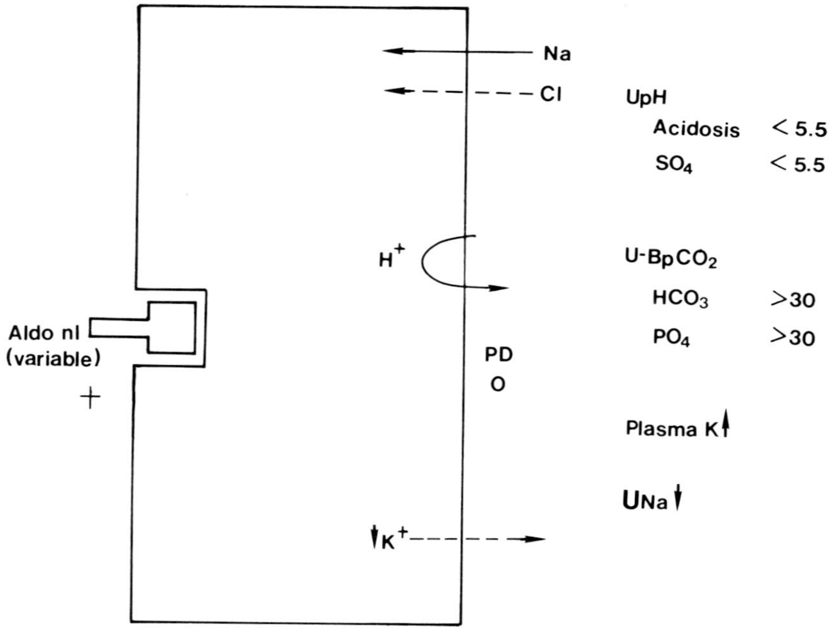

Fig. 6 Depicts the features associated with enhanced Cl reabsorption (chloride shunt) causing a decrease in PD and, thus, a decrease in potassium excretion. The rate of H^+ secretion is also probably decreased. These patients, however, can lower urinary pH during acidosis.

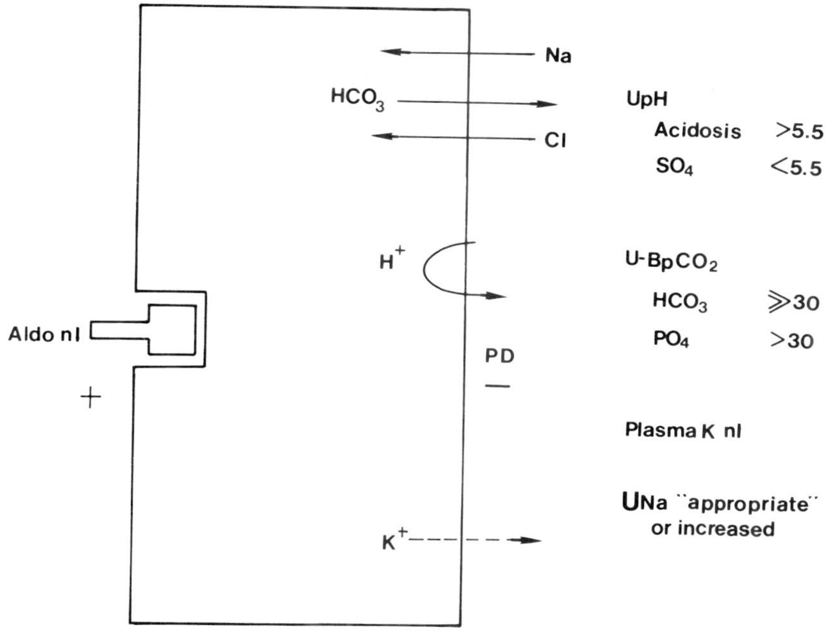

Fig. 7 Depicts the theoretical features associated with a distal acidification defect resulting from bicarbonate secretion. Urine-blood (U-B) PCO_2 during bicarbonate loading should be normal or even increased as a result of bicarbonate secretion. This defect is purely theoretical (see text).

plays in urinary acidification is imperfectly understood. It is within the realm of possibility that an increase in bicarbonate secretion could result in type 1 RTA. We must emphasize, however, that there is no experimental or clinical example of such a defect. We feel the characteristic feature of this defect, if it exists, would be an enhanced capacity to raise the urine PCO_2 during bicarbonate loading (Fig. 7). This is the only form of type 1 RTA that should have this characteristic. Increased ability to raise urinary PCO_2 would be due to increased amounts of bicarbonate in tubular urine stimulating carbonic acid and CO_2 generation. The mechanism is identical to that observed if one adds sodium bicarbonate to a beaker of water. The failure to lower urine pH normally during systemic acidosis would simply be the result of bicarbonate wastage. The effect of sulfate administration is problematic, though we think the response could be normal.

G. Defect in Hydroxyl Disposal

The secretion of a proton into the tubular lumen results in the liberation of hydroxyl from water. Under ordinary conditions this hydroxyl is titrated within the cell by CO_2 to bicarbonate, a reaction catalyzed by carbonic anhydrase. Bicarbonate once formed is removed from the cell and returned to the blood. Thus, a deficiency in this enzyme might result in a decrease in proximal as well as distal urinary acidification. One family with congenital carbonic anhydrase deficiency and RTA has been described (108). It is not clear, however, whether these patients had type 1 RTA in addition to type 2 RTA.

An inability to extrude bicarbonate from the cell would also retard urinary acidification. Experimentally, substances such as SITS reduce urinary acidification by interfering with the exit step for bicarbonate, but no clinical example of such a defect is known.

H. Rate-Dependent Type 1 RTA

All the defects in distal urinary acidification characterized by an inability to lower urine pH normally during acidemia might be thought of as examples of an inability to maintain a sharp pH gradient between tubular urine and blood. Most of the mechanisms previously discussed might result in a failure to maintain a steep pH gradient. As described above, an inability to secrete protons will result in such a defect as will an increase in backleak of acid or a voltage dependent defect. Another mechanism, however, that might result in impaired distal urinary acidification is a decrease in the rate of urinary acidification which is insufficient to prevent the generation of a steep pH gradient (40). This defect could represent a separate category in itself or an early manifestation of other forms of type 1 RTA. We recently described a group of patients with impaired distal urinary acidification as deduced from the inability to raise urine PCO_2 during bicarbonate loading who were able to lower urine pH normally during systemic acidosis (39,40). These patients also raised urine PCO_2 normally in response to phosphate administration (39,40). Our explanation for this defect is that the rate of proton secretion was reduced, but not to the point where it prevented the lowering of the urine pH during acidemia (40).

Based on these observations we proposed that the most sensitive index of the rate of distal urinary acidification is the urine PCO_2 during bicarbonate loading (39,40). A possible explanation for this observation is that bicarbonate loading raises the blood pH. When blood pH is elevated the stimulus to distal urinary acidification might be reduced. If there is a subtle defect in the rate of urinary acidification, bicarbonate loading would offer the setting most likely to disclose the defect. On the other hand, during systemic acidosis the fall in blood pH

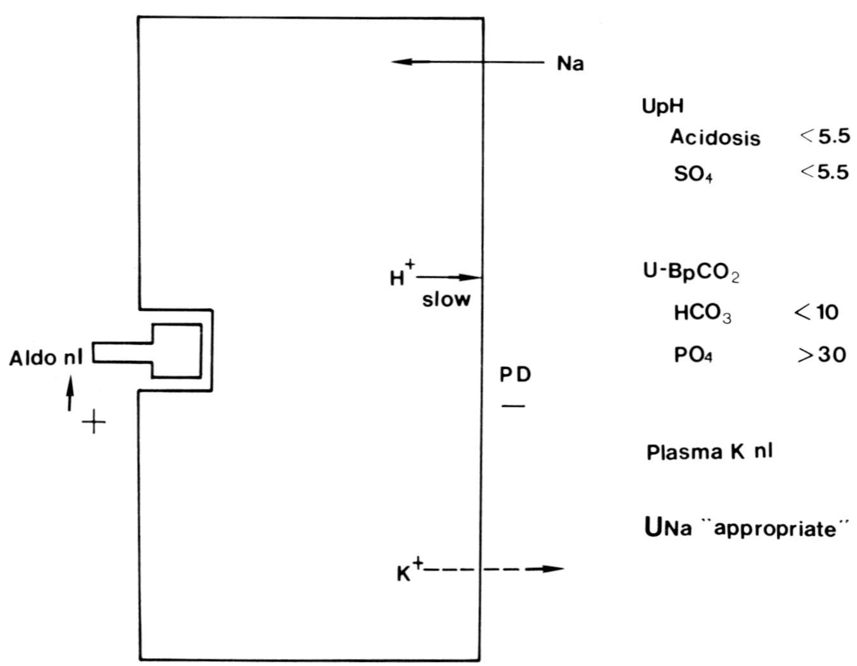

Fig. 8 Depicts the features of a rate-dependent defect in distal acidification. Observe that only the U-B PCO_2 during bicarbonate loading is abnormal (see text).

Table 1 Classification of Type 1 RTA According to Abnormal Mechanism of Distal Acidification and Associated Features

	Example	Plasma K	K excretion (baseline)	U-B PCO_2 during $NaHCO_3$ infusion	U-B PCO_2 during phosphate infusion	Na_2SO_4 urine pH	Na_2SO_4 K excretion	Plasma ↓ aldosterone
A. Failure to lower urine pH during acidosis								
I. Isolated secretory defect for H^+	Renal transplant chronic rejection	Normal or low	Normal or increased	Low	Low	> 5.5	Normal or increased	Normal or increased
II. Acid backleak	Amphotericin B	Normal or low	Normal or increased	Low	Normal	< 5.5	Normal or increased	Normal or increased
III. Voltage-dependent defect								
a. Severe impairment of distal Na transport	Obstructive uropathy, SS hemoglobinopathy	Increased	Decreased	Low	Low	> 5.5	Decreased	Normal or[c] increased
b. Mild impairment of distal Na transport or delivery[a]	SC hemoglobinopathy	Increased	Decreased	Low	Normal	< 5.5	Normal	Normal or increased
B. Preserved ability to lower urine pH during acidosis								
IV. Rate-dependent defect in H^+ secretion[a]	Li therapy, analgesic-induced interstitial nephritis	Normal	Normal	Low	Normal	< 5.5	Normal	Normal
V. Selective aldosterone deficiency	Diabetic nephropathy	Increased	Decreased	Normal	Normal	< 5.5	Subnormal	Decreased
VI. Aldosterone resistance	Pseudohypoaldosteronism of infancy, Cl shunt[b]	Increased	Decreased	Normal	Normal	< 5.5	Subnormal	Increased[c]

[a]A rate-dependent defect may result from various mechanisms (i.e., a mild or partial secretory defect or from a mild voltage-dependent defect).
[b]Important differences exist between aldosterone resistance associated with pseudohypoaldosteronism and a chloride shunt–type of tubular dysfunction. The former is associated with salt wastage, whereas the latter is associated with volume expansion and hypertension.
[c]In patients with a voltage-dependent defect and in those with aldosterone resistance, plasma aldosterone should be increased in response to hyperkalemia. The absence of increased plasma aldosterone suggest that selective aldosterone deficiency is also present.
Source: Adapted from Ref. 42.

presents a major stimulus to urinary acidification which may override the expression of a mild defect. Further supporting this notion is the observation that all but one of the patients we have seen with this type of disorder have not had spontaneous acidosis (39,40). This defect is consistently present in persons receiving chronic lithium therapy in whom metabolic acidosis is not present (39). Interestingly, we have observed one patient with interstitial nephritis due to analgesic abuse and persistent hyperchloremic metabolic acidosis who was unable to raise the urine PCO_2 normally during bicarbonate loading but who consistently lowered the urine pH to below 5.3 (40). Hence, although a rate-dependent defect is likely to occur in subjects with mildly impaired distal acidification, it can also occur in subjects with hyperchloremic acidosis. Until more patients with hyperchloremic acidosis associated with this peculiar pattern of urinary acidification are described it seems reasonable to consider that a rate-dependent defect is the early expression of most kinds of distal acidification defects. According to this view, the definition of incomplete type 1 RTA should be expanded to include patients in whom the only detectable abnormality in urinary acidification is a low U-B PCO_2 gradient during $NaHCO_3$ loading (39,40) (see Fig. 8).

REFERENCES

1. Lightwood, R. Communication No. 1. Arch. Dis. Child. 10:205-206, 1935.
2. Butler, A. M.; Wilson, J. L.; and Farber, S. Dehydration and acidosis with calcification of the renal tubules. J. Pediatr. 8:489-499, 1936.
3. Albright, F.; Burnett, C. H.; Parson, W.; Reifenstein, E. C., Jr.; and Roos, A. Osteomalacia and late rickets. The various etiologies met in the United States with emphasis on that resulting from a specific form of renal acidosis, the therapeutic indications for each etiological subgroup, and the relationship between osteomalacia and Milkman's syndrome. Medicine 25:399-479, 1946.
4. Latner, A. L.; and Burnard, E. D. Idiopathic hyperchloraemic renal acidosis of infants. (Nephrocalcinosis infantorum.) Observations on the site and nature of the lesion. Q. J. Med. 19:285-301, 1950.
5. Jackson, W. P. U.; and Linder, G. C. Innate functional defects of the renal tubules, with particular reference to the Fanconi syndrome. Cases with retinitis pigmentosa. Q. J. Med. 22:133-156, 1953.
6. Mudge, G. H. Clinical patterns of tubular dysfunction. Am. J. Med. 24:785-804, 1958.
7. Huth, E. J.; Webster, G. D., Jr.; and Elkinton, J. R. The renal excretion of hydrogen ion in renal tubular acidosis. III. An attempt to detect latent cases in a family; comments on nosology, genetics and etiology of the primary disease. Am. J. Med. 29:586-598, 1960.
8. Smith, L. H., Jr.; and Schreiner, G. E. Studies on renal hyperchloremic acidosis. J. Lab. Clin. Med. 43:347-358, 1954.
9. Wrong, O.; and Davies, H. E. F. The excretion of acid in renal diseases. Q. J. Med. 28: 259-313, 1959.
10. Elkinton, J. R.; Huth, E. J.; Webster, G. D., Jr.; and McCance, R. A. The renal excretion of hydrogen ion in renal tubular acidosis. Am. J. Med. 29:554-575, 1960.
11. Wrong, O. Urinary hydrogen ion excretion. J. Clin. Pathol. 18:520-526, 1965.
12. Schwartz, W. B.; Jenson, R. L.; and Relman, A. S. Acidification of the urine and increased ammonia excretion without change in acid-base equilibrium: Sodium reabsorption as a stimulus to the acidifying process. J. Clin. Invest. 34:673-680, 1955.
13. Steinmetz, P. R.; Eisenger, R. P.; and Lowenstein, J. The excretion of acid in unilateral renal disease in man. J. Clin. Invest. 44:582-591, 1965.
14. Steinmetz, P. R.; and Bank, N. Effects of acute increases in the excretion of solute and water on renal acid excretion in man. J. Clin. Invest. 42:1142-1149, 1963.

15. Seldin, D. W.; Colman, A. J.; Carter, N.; and Rector, F. C., Jr. The effect of Na_2SO_4 on urinary acidification in chronic renal disease. J. Lab. Clin. Med. 69:893-903, 1967.
16. Rodriguez-Soriano, J. R.; Biochis, M.; and Edelman, C. M., Jr. Bicarbonate reabsorption and hydrogen ion excretion in children with renal tubular acidosis. J. Pediatr. 71:802-813, 1967.
17. Morris, R. C., Jr. Renal tubular acidosis. Mechanisms, classification and implications. New Engl. J. Med. 281:1405-1413, 1969.
18. Reynolds, T. B. Observations on the pathogenesis of renal tubular acidosis. Am. J. Med. 25:503-515, 1958.
19. Frick, P. G.; Rubini, M. E.; and Meroney, W. H. Recurrent nephrolithiasis associated with an unusual tubular defect and hyperchloremic acidosis. Am. J. Med. 25:590-599, 1958.
20. Seldin, D. W.; Rector, F. C., Jr.; Portwood, R.; and Carter, N. Pathogenesis of hyperchloremic acidosis in renal tubular acidosis. Geneva, Proceedings of the 1st International Congress of Nephrology, 1960, pp. 725-728.
21. Royer, P.; Lestradet, H.; Nordmann, R.; Mathiel, H.; and Rodriguez-Soriano, J. Etudes sur quatre cas d'acidose tubulaire chronique idiopathique avec hypocitraturie. Sem. Hop. Paris, 38:808-829, 1962.
22. Tannen, R. L.; Falls, W. F.; and Brackett, N. C. Incomplete renal tubular acidosis: Some clinical and physiological features. Nephron 15:111-113, 1975.
23. Buckalew, V. M., Jr.; McCurdy, D. K.; Ludwig, G. D.; Chaykin, L. B.; and Elkinton, J. R. Incomplete renal tubular acidosis, physiologic studies in three patients with a defect in lowering urine pH. Am. J. Med. 45:32-42, 1968.
24. Buckalew, V. M., Jr.; Purvis, M. L.; Shulman, M. G.; Herndon, N. C.; and Rudman, D. Hereditary renal tubular acidosis. Medicine 53:229-254, 1974.
25. McCurdy, D. K., Frederic, M.; and Elkinton, J. R. Renal tubular acidosis due to amphotericin B. N. Engl. J. Med. 276:124-130, 1968.
26. Gyory, A. Z.; and Edwards, K. D. G. Effect of mersalyl, ethacrynic acid and sodium sulfate infusion on urinary acidification in hereditary renal tubular acidosis. Med. J. Aust. 2:940-945, 1971.
27. Seldin, D. W.; and Wilson, J. D. Renal tubular acidosis. In: The Metabolic Basis of Inherited Disease, 3rd ed., edited by Stanbury, J. B., Wyngarden, J. B., and Frederickson, D. New York, McGraw-Hill, 1972, pp. 1548-1566.
28. Rector, F. C., Jr. Acidification of the urine. In: Renal Physiology, edited by Orloff, J., and Berliner, R. W. Baltimore, Williams & Wilkins, 1973, pp. 431-454.
29. Halperin, M. L.; Goldstein, M. B.; Haig, A.; Johnson, M. D.; and Stinebaugh, B. J. Studies on the pathogenesis of type 1 (distal) renal tubular acidosis as revealed by the urinary PCO_2 tensions. J. Clin. Invest. 53:669-677, 1974.
30. Sebastian, A.; McSherry, E.; and Morris, R. C., Jr. On the mechanism of the inappropriately low urinary carbon dioxide tension (U-B PCO_2) in classic (type 1) renal tubular acidosis (RTA). Clin. Res. 22:544A, 1974.
31. Thirakomen, K.; Kozlov, N.; Arruda, J. A. L.; and Kurtzman, N. A. Renal hydrogen ion secretion following the release of unilateral ureteral obstruction. Am. J. Physiol. 231: 1233-1239, 1976.
32. Nascimento, L.; Rademacher, D.; Hamburger, R.; Arruda, J. A. L.; and Kurtzman, N. A. On the mechanism of lithium-induced renal tubular acidosis. J. Lab. Clin. Med. 89: 445-462, 1977.
33. Arruda, J. A. L.; Nascimento, L.; Kumar, S.; Sodhi, B.; and Kurtzman, N. A. Factors influencing the formation of urinary carbon dioxide tension. Kidney Int. 11:307-317, 1977.
34. Arruda, J. A. L.; and Kurtzman, N. A. Mechanism and classification of deranged distal urinary acidification. Am. J. Physiol. 8:F515-F523, 1980.

35. Batlle, D. C.; Moses, M. F.; Manaligod, J.; Arruda, J. A. L.; and Kurtzman, N. A. The pathogenesis of hyperchloremic metabolic acidosis associated with renal transplantation. Am. J. Med. 70:786-796, 1981.
36. Batlle, D. C.; Sehy, J. T.; Roseman, M. K.; Arruda, J. A. L.; and Kurtzman, N. A. Clinical and pathophysiologic spectrum of acquired distal renal tubular acidosis. Kidney Int. 20:389-396, 1981.
37. Batlle, D. C.; Arruda, J. A. L.; and Kurtzman, N. A. Hyperkalemic distal renal tubular acidosis associated with obstructive uropathy. N. Engl. J. Med. 304:373-380, 1981.
38. Batlle, D. C.; and Arruda, J. A. L. The renal tubular acidosis syndromes. Miner. Electrolyte Metab. 5:83-99, 1981.
39. Batlle, D. C.; Gaviria, M.; Grupp, M.; Arruda, J. A. L.; Wynn, J.; and Kurtzman, N. A. Distal nephron function in patients receiving chronic lithium therapy. Kidney Int. 21: 477-485, 1982.
40. Batlle, D. C.; Grupp, M.; Gaviria, M.; and Kurtzman, N. A. Distal renal tubular acidosis with intact ability to lower urine pH. Am. J. Med. 72:751-758, 1982.
41. Batlle, D. C.; Itsarayoungyuen, K.; Arruda, J. A. L.; and Kurtzman, N. A. Hyperkalemic hyperchloremic metabolic acidosis in patients with sickle cell hemoglobin. Am. J. Med. 72:188-192, 1982.
42. Batlle, D. C.; and Kurtzman, N. A. Distal renal tubular acidosis. Pathogenesis and classification. Am. J. Kidney Dis. 1:328-344, 1982.
43. Steinmetz, P. R.; and Lawson, W. J. Defect in urinary acidification induced in vitro by amphotericin B. J. Clin. Invest. 49:596-601, 1970.
44. Al-Awqati, G.; Norby, L. H.; Mueller, A.; and Steinmetz, P. R. Characteristics of stimulation of H^+ transport by aldosterone in turtle urinary bladder. J. Clin. Invest. 58: 351-358, 1976.
45. Arruda, J. A. L.; Dytko, G.; Mola, R.; and Kurtzman, N. A. On the mechanism of lithium-induced distal renal tubular acidosis: Studies in the turtle bladder. Kidney Int. 17: 196-204, 1980.
46. Arruda, J. A. L.; Subbarayudu, K.; Kytko, G.; Mola, R.; and Kurtzman, N. A. Voltage dependent distal acidification defect induced by amiloride. J. Lab. Clin. Med. 95:407-416, 1980.
47. Steinmetz, P. R.; Omachi, R. S.; and Frazier, H. S. Independence of hydrogen ion secretion and transport of other electrolytes in turtle bladder. J. Clin. Invest. 46:1541-1548, 1967.
48. Steinmetz, P. R. Acid-base relations in epithelium of turtle bladder; site of active step in acidification and role of metabolic CO_2. J. Clin. Invest. 48:1258-1265, 1969.
49. Steinmetz, P. R.; and Lawson, L. R. Effect of luminal pH on ion permeability and flows of Na^+ and H^+ in turtle bladder. Am. J. Physiol. 220:1573-1580, 1971.
50. Dixon, T. E.; and Al-Awqati, Q. Urinary acidification in turtle bladder is due to a reversible proton-translocating ATPase. Proc. Natl. Acad. Sci. USA 76:3135-3138, 1979.
51. Beauwens, R.; and Al-Awqati, Q. Active H^+ transport in the turtle urinary bladder. J. Gen. Physiol. 68:421-439, 1976.
52. Al-Awqati, Q.; Meuller, A.; and Steinmetz, P. R. Transport of H^+ against electrochemical gradients in turtle urinary bladder. Am. J. Physiol. 233:F502-F508, 1977.
53. Steinmetz, P. R. Cellular mechanisms of urinary acidification. Physiol. Rev. 54:890-956, 1974.
54. Leslie, B. R.; Schwartz, J. H.; and Steinmetz, P. F. Coupling between Cl absorption and HCO_3 secretion in turtle urinary bladder. Am. J. Physiol. 225:610-617, 1973.
55. Schwartz, J. H.; Finn, J. T.; Vaughan, G.; and Steinmetz, P. R. Distribution of metabolic CO_2 and the transported ion species in acidification by turtle bladder. Am. J. Physiol. 226:283-289, 1974.
56. Schwartz, J. H.; Rosen, S.; and Steinmetz, P. R. Carbonic anhydrase function and the epithelial organization of H^+ secretion in turtle urinary bladder. J. Clin. Invest. 51:2653-2662, 1972.

57. Cohen, L. H.; Mueller, A.; and Steinmetz, P. R. Inhibition of the HCO_3 exit step in urinary acidification by a disulfonic stilbene. J. Clin. Invest. 61:981-986, 1978.
58. Husted, R. F.; Cohen, L. H.; and Steinmetz, P. R. Pathways for bicarbonate transfer across the serosal membrane of turtle urinary bladder: Studies with a disulfonic stilbene. J. Membr. Biol. 47:27-37, 1979.
59. McKinney, T. D.; and Burg, M. B. Bicarbonate absorption by rabbit cortical collecting tubules in vitro. Am. J. Physiol. 234:F141-F145, 1978.
60. McKinney, T. D.; and Burg, M. B. Bicarbonate secretion by rabbit cortical collecting tubules in vitro. J. Clin. Invest. 61:1421-1427, 1978.
61. Giammarco, R. A., Goldstein, M. B.; Halperin, M. L.; and Stinebaugh, B. J. Effect of hyperventilation on distal nephron hydrogen ion secretion. J. Clin. Invest. 58:77-82, 1976.
62. Sehy, J. T.; Roseman M. K.; Arruda, J. A. L.; and Kurtzman, N. A. Characterization of distal hydrogen ion secretion in acute respiratory alkalosis. Am. J. Physiol. 235: F203-F208, 1978.
63. Batlle, D. C.; Itsarayoungyuen, K.; Downer, M.; Foley, R.; Arruda, J. A. L.; and Kurtzman, N. A. Suppression of distal urinary acidification after recovery from chronic hypocapnia. Am. J. Physiol. 245:F433-F442, 1983.
64. Cruz-Soto, M.; Batlle, D. C.; Sabatini, S.; Arruda, J. A. L.; and Kurtzman, N. A. Distal acidification in the rabbit: Role of diet and blood pH. Am. J. Physiol. 12:F364-F371, 1982.
65. Ziegler, T. W.; Fanestil, D. D.; and Ludens, J. H. Influence of transepithelial potential difference on acidification in the toad urinary bladder. Kidney Int. 10:279-286, 1976.
66. Kurtzman, N. A. "Short-circuit" distal renal tubular acidosis. J. Lab. Clin. Med. 95: 633-636, 1980.
67. DiTella, P. J.; Sodhi, B.; McCreary, J.; Arruda, J. A. L.; and Kurtzman, N. A. Mechanism of the metabolic acidosis of selective mineralocorticoid deficiency. Kidney Int. 14: 466-477, 1978.
68. Hulter, H. N.; Ilnicki, L. P.; Harbottle, J. A.; and Sebastian, A. Impaired renal H^+ secretion and NH_3 production in mineralocorticoid-deficient glucocorticoid-replete dogs. Am. J. Physiol. 232:F136-F146, 1977.
69. Hulter, H. N.; Sebastian, A.; Sigala, J. F.; Light, J. H.; Glynn, R. D.; Schambelan, M.; and Biglieri, E. G. Pathogenesis of renal hyperchloremic acidosis resulting from dietary potassium restriction in the dog: Role of aldosterone. Am. J. Physiol. 238:F79-F91, 1980.
70. Tannen, R. L. Relationship of renal ammonia production and potassium homeostasis. Kidney Int. 11:453-465, 1977.
71. Sebastian, A.; Schambelan, M.; Lindenfeld, S.; and Morris, R. C., Jr. Amelioration of metabolic acidosis with fluorocortisone therapy in hyporeninemic hypoaldosteronism. N. Engl. J. Med. 297:576-589, 1977.
72. Oster, J. R.; Hotchkiss, J. L., Carbon, M.; and Vaamonde, C. A short duration renal acidification test using calcium chloride. Nephron 14:281-292, 1975.
73. Sebastian, A.; McSherry, E.; and Morris, R. C., Jr. Metabolic acidosis with special reference to renal acidosis. In: The Kidney, vol. II, edited by Brenner, B., and Rector, F. C. Philadelphia, Saunders, 1976, pp. 615-660.
74. Batlle, D. C. Furosemide as a tool to evaluate cortical collecting duct function. Clin. Research 32:800A, 1984.
75. Arruda, J. A. L.; Nascimento, L.; Mehta, P. K.; Rademacher, D. R.; Sehy, J. T.; Westenfelder, C.; and Kurtzman, N. A. The critical importance of urinary concentrating ability in the generation of urinary carbon dioxide tension. J. Clin. Invest. 60:922-935, 1977.
76. Kurtzman, N. A.; and Arruda, J. A. L. Physiologic significance of urinary carbon dioxide tension. Miner. Electrolyte Metab. 1:241-246, 1978.

77. Maren, T. H. Carbon dioxide equilibria in the kidney: The problems of elevated carbon dioxide tension, delayed dehydration, and disequilibrium pH. Kidney Int. 14:395-405, 1978.
78. Stinebaugh, B. J.; Esquenazi, R.; Schloeder, F. X.; Suki, W. N.; Goldstein, M. B.; and Halperin, M. L. Control of the urine-blood PCO_2 gradient in alkaline urine. Kidney Int. 17:31-39, 1980.
79. Stinebaugh, B. J.; Schloeder, F. X.; Gharafry, E.; Suki, W. N.; Goldstein, M. B.; and Halperin, M. L. Mechanism by which neutral phosphate infusion elevates urine PCO_2. J. Lab. Clin. Med. 89:946-958, 1977.
80. Ochwadt, B. K., and Pitts, R. F. Effect of intravenous infusion of carbonic anhydrase on carbon dioxide tension of alkaline urine. Am. J. Physiol. 185:426-429, 1956.
81. Batlle, D. C. Delta urine PCO_2 rather than U-B PCO_2 as an index of distal acidification. Semin. Nephrol. 2:189-190, 1982.
82. Dubose, T. D., Jr. Hydrogen ion secretion by the collecting duct as a determinant of the U-B PCO_2 gradient in alkaline urine. J. Clin. Invest. 69:145-156, 1982.
83. Roscoe, J. M.; Goldstein, M. B.; Halperin, M. L.; Schloeder, F. X.; and Stinebaugh, B. J. Amphotericin-induced urine acidification defect in rats. J. Lab. Clin. Med. 89:463-470, 1977.
84. Julka, N. K.; Arruda, J. A. L.; and Kurtzman, N. A. The mechanism of amphotericin-induced distal acidification defect in rats. Clin. Sci. 56:555-562, 1979.
85. Roscoe, M.; Goldstein, M. B.; Halperin, J. L.; Wilson, D. R.; and Stinebaugh, B. J. Lithium-induced impairment of urine acidification. Kidney Int. 9:344-350, 1976.
86. Hulter, H. N.; Ilnicki, L. P.; Licht, J. H.; and Sebastian, A. On the mechanism of diminished urinary carbon dioxide tension caused by amiloride. Kidney Int. 21:8-13, 1982.
87. Ericsson, N. O.; Winberg, J.; and Zetterstrom, R. Renal function in infantile obstructive uropathy. Acta Paediatr. 44:444-459, 1955.
88. Earley, L. E. Extreme polyuria in obstructive uropathy: Report of a case of "water-losing nephritis" in an infant, with a discussion of polyuria. N. Engl. J. Med. 255:600-605, 1956.
89. Berlyne, G. M. Distal tubular function in chronic hydronephrosis. Q. J. Med. 30:339-355, 1961.
90. Walls, J.; Buerkert, J.; Purkerson, M. L.; and Klahr, S. Nature of the acidifying defect after relief of ureteral obstruction. Kidney Int. 7:304-316, 1975.
91. Harris, R. H.; and Yarger, W. E. Renal function after release of unilateral ureteral obstruction in rats. Am. J. Physiol. 227:806-815, 1974.
92. Sebastian, A.; McSherry, E.; and Morris, R. C., Jr. Impaired renal conservation of sodium and chloride during sustained correction of systemic acidosis in patients with type 1, classic renal tubular acidosis. J. Clin. Invest. 58:454-469, 1976.
93. Sebastian, A.; McSherry, E.; and Morris, R. C., Jr. Renal potassium wasting in renal tubular acidosis. Its occurrence in types 1 and 2 despite sustained correction of systemic acidosis. J. Clin. Invest. 50:667-678, 1971.
94. Batlle, D. C. Hyperkalemic hyperchloremic metabolic acidosis associated with selective aldosterone deficiency and distal renal tubular acidosis. Semin. Nephrol. 1:260-273, 1981.
95. Perez, G. O.; Oster, J. R.; and Vaamonde, C. A. Renal acidosis and renal potassium handling in selective hypoaldosteronism. Am. J. Med. 57:809-816, 1974.
96. Shambelan, M.; Sebastian, A.; and Biglieri, E. G. Prevalance, pathogenesis, and functional significance of aldosterone deficiency in hyperkalemic patients with chronic renal insufficiency. Kidney Int. 17:89-101, 1980.
97. Arruda, J. A. L.; Batlle, D. C.; Sehy, J. T.; Roseman, M.; Baranowski, R. L.; and Kurtzman, N. A. Hyperkalemia in renal insufficiency: Role of aldosterone deficiency and tubular unresponsiveness to aldosterone. Am. J. Nephrol. 1:160-167, 1981.

98. Szylman, P.; Better, O. S.; Chaimowitz, C.; and Rosler, A. Role of hyperkalemia in the metabolic acidosis of isolated hypoaldosteronism. N. Engl. J. Med. 294:361-365, 1976.
99. Thorn, G. W.; Koepj, G. F.; and Clinton, M., Jr. Renal failure simulating adrenocortical insufficiency. N. Engl. J. Med. 231:76-85, 1944.
100. Cheek, D. B.; and Perry, J. W. A salt-wasting syndrome in infancy. Arch. Dis. in Child. 33:252-256, 1958.
101. Donnel, G. N.; Litman, N.; and Roldan, M. Pseudohypo-adrenalocorticism. Renal sodium loss, hyponatremia, and hyperkalemia due to a renal tubular insensitivity to mineralocorticoids. Am. J. Dis. Child. 97:813-828, 1959.
102. Stanbury, S. W.; and Mahler, R. F. Salt-wasting renal disease. Metabolic observations on a patient with "salt-losing nephritis." Q. J. Med. 28:425-447, 1959.
103. Walker, W. G.; Jost, L. J.; Johnson, J. R.; and Kowarski, A. Metabolic observations on salt wasting in a patient with renal disease. Am. J. Med. 39:505-519, 1965.
104. Arnold, J. E.; and Healy, J. K. Hyperkalemia, hypertension and systemic acidosis without renal failure associated with a tubular defect in potassium excretion. Am. J. Med. 47:461-472, 1969.
105. Gordon, R. D.; Geddes, R. A.; Oawsey, C. G. K.; and O'Halloran, M. W. Hypertension and severe hyperkalemia associated with suppression of renin and aldosterone and completely reversed by dietary sodium restriction. Aust. Ann. Med. 4:287-294, 1970.
106. Spitzer, A.; Edelmann, C. M., Jr.; Goldberg, L. D.; and Henneman, P. H. Short stature, hyperkalemia and acidosis: A defect in renal transport of potassium. Kidney Int. 3: 251-257, 1973.
107. Schambelan, M.; Sebastian, A.; and Rector, F. C., Jr. Mineralocorticoid resistant renal hyperkalemia without salt wasting (type II pseudohypoaldosteronism). Role of increased renal chloride reabsorption. Kidney Int. 19:716-727, 1981.
108. Shapira, E.; Gen-Yoseph, F. G. E.; and Russel, A. Enzymatically inactive red cell carbonic anhydrase in a family with renal tubular acidosis. J. Clin. Invest. 53:59-63, 1974.

10

Hyperkalemic Renal Tubular Acidosis

ANTHONY SEBASTIAN, MORRIS SCHAMBELAN, HENRY N. HULTER, TERRY MAHER,* IRA KURTZ,† EDWARD G. BIGLIERI, FLOYD C. RECTOR, JR., and R. CURTIS MORRIS, JR.
University of California at San Francisco, San Francisco, California

I. INTRODUCTION

Metabolic acidosis is commonly associated with hyperkalemia in chronic diseases of the kidney that result in diffuse histologically evident parenchymal damage and reduced glomerular filtration rate (1). Usually acidosis is proportional in severity to the degree of glomerular insufficiency (2-5), whereas hyperkalemia may be only minimal even in patients with far advanced glomerular insufficiency (6-9). In patients selected because of severe hyperkalemia (serum potassium concentration > 5.5 meq/liter), the most common diagnoses of the underlying renal disease are tubulointerstitial nephritis and diabetic nephropathy (5,10-12), and in these patients a characteristic pattern of renal tubular dysfunction has been delineated (13-15): Renal bicarbonate reabsorption is reduced at normal plasma bicarbonate concentration (sustained by alkali therapy), but the magnitude of the reduction (<15%) is not sufficient to indicate impaired bicarbonate reabsorption in the proximal tubule (13-15). The ability of the kidney to establish steep hydrogen ion concentration gradients between blood and urine during spontaneously occurring acidosis appears unimpaired (10,11,13-15). Despite highly acidic urine during acidosis, renal net acid excretion is subnormal, due in part to reduced urinary excretion of ammonium, which in turn appears to be due in part to reversible suppression of renal ammoniagenesis caused by hyperkalemia (10). This impairment in renal ammoniagenesis is evident even in patients with only minimal reduction in glomerular filtration rate. Renal clearance of potassium is greatly reduced, and serum potassium concentrations increase strikingly in response to increased dietary potassium (5). Proximal tubular dysfunction evidenced by hyperaminoaciduria, glucosuria, or increased renal clearance of phosphate has not been described. The tubular dysfunction in these patients is physiologically distinguishable from that in patients with other recognized syndromes of renal tubular acidosis (RTA), and the resulting syndrome of hyperkalemic RTA has been given the designation type 4 RTA (10,15-18).

Current affiliation
*Nephrology Medical Group Inc., San Pablo, California
†University of California at Los Angeles, Los Angeles, California

Table 1 Clinical Spectrum of Hyperkalemic Renal Tubular Acidosis

- Aldosterone Deficiency
  - Combined deficiency of aldosterone and adrenal glucocorticoid hormones
    - Addison's disease (24)
    - Bilateral adrenalectomy (24,25)
    - Inherited impairment of steroidogenesis: 21-hydroxylase deficiency (26-29)
  - Aldosterone deficiency without glucocorticoid deficiency
    - Inherited impairment of aldosterone biosynthesis: corticosterone methyl oxidase deficiency (30-36)
    - Chronic heparin administration (37)
    - Secondary to deficient renin secretion (5,13,24,38-45)
      - Chronic diffuse histologically evident renal parenchymal disease and reduced glomerular filtration rate
        - Diabetic nephropathy
        - Tubulointerstitial nephritis
        - Obstructive uropathy
        - Renal transplantation
      - Indomethacin administration (46-48)
    - Inhibition of formation of angiotension II: administration of converting enzyme inhibitors (49)
    - Acquired adrenal insensitivity to angiotensin II (50)
    - Chronic idiopathic hypoaldosteronism in adults and children (51-56)
- Pseudohypoaldosteronism (attenuated renal response to aldosterone with secondary hyperreninemia and hyperaldosteronism)
  - Classic pseudohypoaldosteronism of infancy (type 1 pseudohypoaldosteronism) (30, 57-81)
  - Chronic tubulointerstitial disease with glomerular insufficiency and salt-wasting nephritis (82-84)
  - Drugs: spironolactone, amiloride, triamterene
  - Abnormally increased levels of endogenous aldosterone antagonists (e.g., progesterone): 21-hydroxylase deficiency (85,86)
- Aldosterone Deficiency + Attenuated Renal Response to Aldosterone
  - Inherited impairment of steroidogenesis causal of aldosterone deficiency and increased levels of endogenous aldosterone antagonists
    - 21-hydroxylase deficiency (congenital adrenal hyperplasia) (85,86)
  - Selective ion transport defect of the renal tubule causal of renal resistance to the kaliuretic and acid excretory effects of mineralocorticoid and causal of impaired renin secretion (type 2 pseudohypoaldosteronism) (87-96)
  - Chronic diffuse histologically evident renal parenchymal disease and reduced glomerular filtration rate
    - Associated deficient renin secretion (10,13,24,38-42,97)
    - Renin status uncertain (98)
  - Obstructive uropathy with deficient renin secretion (43)
  - Renal transplantation with deficient renin secretion (99)
  - Lupus nephritis with deficient renin secretion (100)
- Uncertain Pathophysiology
  - Chronic pyelonephritis (11,101)
  - Lupus nephritis (102)
  - Renal transplantation (103)
  - Acute glomerulonephritis (104)
  - Renal amyloidosis (105)

The physiological characteristics of the renal tubular dysfunction in patients with type 4 RTA are those that would be predicted to occur as a result of deficiency of aldosterone (16, 18-20). In the initial group of patients in whom the syndrome of type 4 RTA was characterized, severe aldosterone deficiency unassociated with glucocorticoid deficiency was found in association with chronic renal parenchymal disease (10,14). Subsequently, it has become evident that the syndrome of type 4 RTA can occur in a wide variety of clinical disorders that cause aldosterone deficiency even in the absence of primary renal disease (Table 1) (18, 21-23).

Type 4 RTA also occurs in a wide variety of clinical disorders of both renal and extrarenal origin in which the secretion rates and plasma concentrations of aldosterone are not distinctly subnormal as judged by comparison of the values of these parameters with those in normal subjects ingesting similar amounts of sodium and potassium (Table 1). Nevertheless, aldosterone deficiency is likely to be present in many of those disorders inasmuch as the observed values of plasma and urine aldosterone concentrations are subnormal by comparison with those observed in normal subjects rendered hyperkalemic and acidotic by administration of exogenous potassium and acid loads (106-111). Since a physiologically appropriate increment in aldosterone secretion in response to hyperkalemia and acidemia may be an important determinant in the renal defense mechanism that limits the severity of the electrolyte and acid-base disturbances, such "relative" aldosterone deficiency might be a major determinant of hyperkalemia and RTA in these patients. Presently there are no well-established criteria for determining the physiological appropriateness of aldosterone levels in relation to the degree and duration of hyperkalemia and metabolic acidosis, and this circumstance precludes dismissal of aldosterone deficiency as a major pathogenetic factor in many patients with type 4 RTA in whom aldosterone levels are not unequivocally subnormal.

In some clinical disorders in which type 4 RTA occurs, there appears to be "end-organ resistance" to the renal action of aldosterone as evidenced by the persistence of hyperkalemia and RTA despite the presence of exceedingly high levels of endogenous aldosterone or as evidenced by the lack of therapeutic response to chronic administration of large amounts of exogenous mineralocorticoid steroid. Such end-organ resistance may be either of a specific nature, as that resulting from the presence of steroid antagonists to aldosterone receptor-binding or from defects of the aldosterone receptor itself; or the resistance may be of a nonspecific nature, as that resulting from diffuse renal parenchymal damage or from transport dysfunctions that preclude the final expression of the aldosterone effector mechanism.

Some investigators reserve the designation type 4 RTA for those patients with the syndrome of type 4 RTA who have unequivocal aldosterone deficiency. For reasons that will become apparent from the discussion in the following sections, we prefer to employ this designation in all patients with hyperkalemic RTA who manifest the syndrome of type 4 RTA as defined in the first paragraph of this section, whether aldosterone deficiency is present or absent, or the status of aldosterone activity and renal responsiveness is known.

II. ROLE OF ALDOSTERONE IN RENAL ACIDIFICATION

A. Effect of Hypermineralocorticoidism on Renal and Systemic Acid-Base Homeostasis in Humans

In normal humans, the administration of mineralocorticoid hormones that possess minimal glucocorticoid activity results in augmentation of renal hydrogen ion secretion (112-118). Acute administration of aldosterone in large amounts to normal subjects results within hours in a decrease in urine pH (114-117) and an increase in net acid excretion (114,115,117,118).

Chronic administration of large amounts of aldosterone results in a sustained increase in plasma bicarbonate concentration and blood pH indicative of the development of metabolic alkalosis (119). Whereas the degree of metabolic alkalosis is relatively slight, it can be calculated that the continued reabsorption by the kidney of the associated increased filtered bicarbonate load requires a sustained increase in net rate of renal hydrogen ion secretion exceeding 250 meq/day, which is four to five times more hydrogen ion secreted than that normally excreted in the urine as net acid. Chronic administration of mineralocorticoid hormones results in the development of metabolic alkalosis also in dogs (120,121), and it has been demonstrated in this species that the renal acid-excretory and systemic alkalosis-producing effect of mineralocorticoid administration is markedly augmented by preexisting restriction of dietary intake of potassium (121).

B. Effect of Aldosterone Deficiency on Renal and Systemic Acid-Base Homeostasis

Studies in Dogs

The effect of aldosterone deficiency on the renal acidification process has been extensively studied in adrenalectomized dogs maintained postoperatively on physiological replacement doses of glucocorticoid and mineralocorticoid hormones (19,122). When the administration of mineralocorticoid hormones is discontinued net acid excretion decreases, and hyperkalemia and hyperchloremic acidosis occur (Fig. 1). The reduction in net acid excretion is accounted for largely by a reduction in urine ammonium excretion, which in turn appears to be due to diminished renal production of ammonia, since it occurs in the absence of an increase in urine pH or a decrease in urine flow.

Among the factors that might diminish renal production of ammonia in the mineralocorticoid-deficient dog, potassium retention and hyperkalemia were suggested by the finding that the excretion rates of ammonium varied inversely with the degree of hyperkalemia. The relationship between these two parameters was further investigated in studies in which restriction of potassium in the diet precluded the occurrence of potassium retention and hyperkalemia when the administration of mineralocorticoid hormones was discontinued (19). In these dogs maintained normokalemic, the cumulative reduction in ammonium excretion was significantly less than that which occurred in the dogs that became hyperkalemic, even though the pH of the urine was significantly greater in the normokalemic dogs. Thus, the production of ammonia was suppressed to a lesser extent when hyperkalemia was prevented. Indeed, ammonia production might not have decreased at all, since the reduction in urinary ammonium excretion was a consequence, at least in part, of the increase in urine pH that occurred when mineralocorticoid hormones were withheld. These results permit the conclusion, therefore, that potassium retention contributes to the reduction in renal production of ammonia in mineralocorticoid deficiency. This conclusion is in accord with observations of Tannen that suggest that the administration of exogenous potassium loads can suppress the production of ammonia by the mammalian kidney (123) and with the observation of Szylman et al. (97) in a patient with isolated aldosterone deficiency that correction of hyperkalemia increased ammonium excretion without a decrease in urine pH.

The results of the cited studies in adrenalectomized dogs indicate also that aldosterone deficiency impairs the rate capacity of the distal nephron to secrete H^+, but it does not impair its ability to generate normally steep lumen to blood H^+ concentration gradients (19, 122). When luminal buffer concentration is low, as when renal production and urine excretion of ammonia are greatly reduced by hyperkalemia, the urine pH in mineralocorticoid-

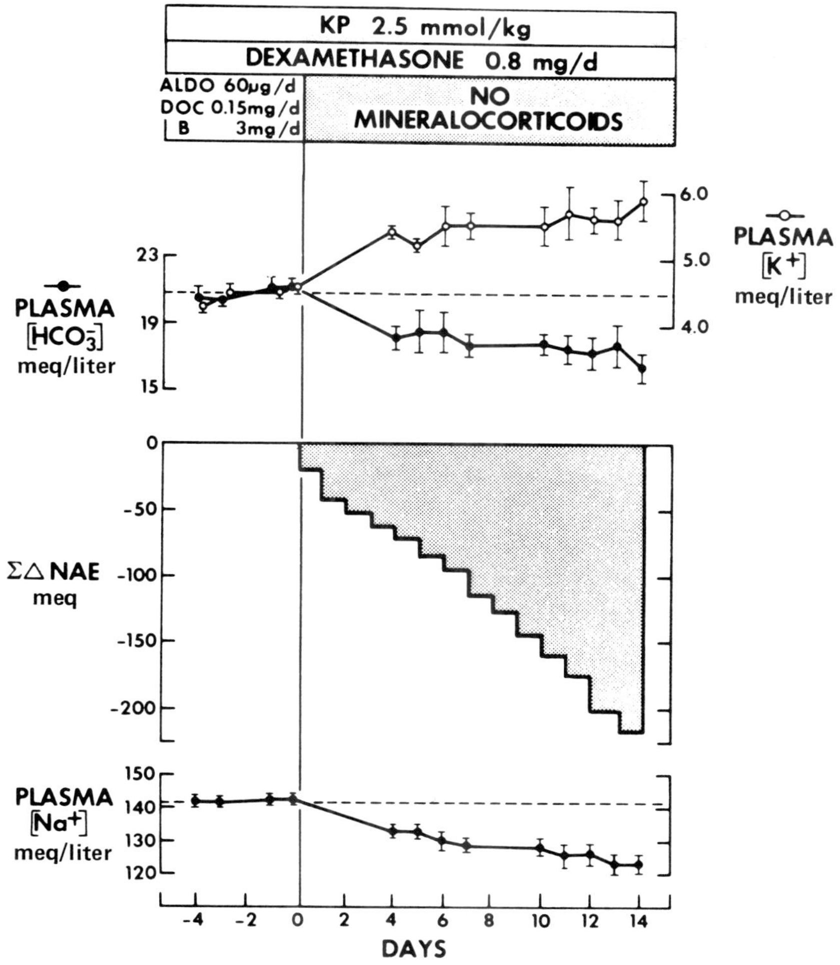

Fig. 1 Effect of mineralocorticoid discontinuation on plasma and urinary acid-base and electrolyte composition in adrenalectomized dogs maintained on dexamethasone without direct effort to maintain normal sodium balance or to prevent development of hyperkalemia. (From Refs. 19,122.)

deficient dogs is not different from that in mineralcorticoid-replete dogs in whom similar degrees of metabolic acidosis have been induced by exogenous acid feeding (Fig. 2). However, when the amount of luminal buffer is increased, reflected by an increase in urine ammonium excretion, the urine pH increases to a substantially greater degree in mineralocorticoid-deficient dogs than in mineralocorticoid-replete dogs, indicating in the former group that the secretion of H^+ increases at a blunted rate (Fig. 2).

Studies in Turtle Bladders

The above findings in the dog are consistent with the results of in vitro studies in turtle bladders. Turtle bladders are H^+-secreting epithelia that resemble the mammalian collecting tubules and ducts (in contradistinction to earlier nephron segments) with respect to embryo-

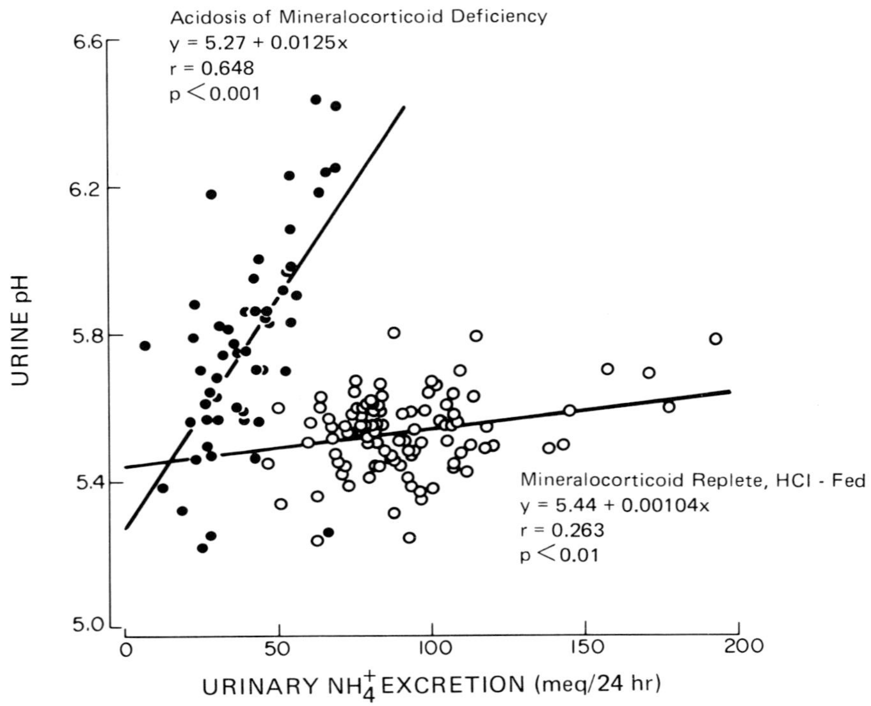

Fig. 2 Daily urine pH as a function of daily urinary ammonium excretion in mineralocorticoid-deficient glucocorticoid-replete adrenalectomized dogs (n = 5) and in mineralocorticoid-replete hydrochloric acid-fed dogs (n = 8) during steady-state metabolic acidosis. Consequent to hyperkalemia-induced suppression of renal ammoniagenesis in mineralocorticoid deficiency, a reduced availability of ammonia for diffusion into tubular fluid appears to reduce intraluminal buffering of secreted hydrogen ion and thereby reduce intraluminal (and urine) pH even though the rate capacity of the hydrogen ion transport mechanism has been dampened simultaneously. Thus, during the period of mineralocorticoid deficiency, the pH of urine varied directly with the excretion rate of ammonium, which in turn varied inversely with plasma potassium concentration (not shown). If, during chronic metabolic acidosis, the rate of ammonia production determines both urine pH and the rate of urine ammonium excretion, the value of urine pH for any given rate of ammonium excretion can be taken as an index of the hydrogen ion secretory capacity in the distalmost segments of the nephron, assuming that the excretion rate of nonammonia buffer is constant. Hence, in the mineralocorticoid-deficient dog, it can be inferred that hydrogen ion secretory capacity of the distal nephron is subnormal, since over a wide range of urine ammonium excretion rates urine pH was greater than in similarly acidotic acid-fed mineralocorticoid-replete dogs. The slope of the relationship between urine pH and urine ammonium excretion is an index of the rate capacity of the hydrogen ion transport mechanism of the distal nephron, and appears to be subnormal in mineralocorticoid deficiency; the y-intercept at x = 0 (i.e., the value of urine pH at zero ammonium excretion) is an index of the hydrogen ion concentration gradient-generating ability of the transport mechanism, and appears to be intact in mineralocorticoid deficiency. (From Ref. 19.)

logical origin, structure, and function (124-130). In these epithelia, the H^+ secretory mechanism is electrogenic (i.e., it is capable of transporting a net positive charge into the lumen), and it is not dependent on Na^+ resorption, although the rate of H^+ secretion may be influenced by the rate of Na^+ resorption. Secretion of H^+ occurs even under conditions in which Na^+ transport is prevented and no favorable transepithelial electrical potential difference is permitted to develop. Under these conditions, the rate of H^+ secretion decreases in response to an increase in the transepithelial H^+ concentration gradient against which H^+ is secreted; when the concentration of H^+ in the mucosal fluid is approximately 1000 times greater (i.e., 3 pH units less) than that in the serosal fluid, the net rate of H^+ secretion is reduced to zero (Fig. 3). This reflects cessation of unidirectional H^+ secretion from cell to lumen; backleak of H^+ from the mucosal fluid into the cell or serosal fluid is negligible. The magnitude of the transepithelial H^+ concentration gradient required to nullify net H^+ secretion is an index of the "driving force" (protonmotive force) of the H^+ secretory pump. Aldosterone deficiency decreases the rate of H^+ secretion when the transepithelial H^+ concentration gradient is nonlimiting for H^+ secretion but does not affect the protonmotive force of the H^+ secretory pump (130) (Fig. 3).

A characteristic of electrogenic H^+ secretion is dependence of the secretory rate on the transepithelial electrical potential difference (131). The net rate of H^+ secretion is modulated by the transepithelial electrical potential difference, which ordinarily is determined in part by the net rate of sodium resorption. In the absence of a transepithelial H^+ concentration gradient, H^+ secretion can be nullified by an unfavorable transepithelial electrical gradient (lumen-positive) that is energetically equivalent to the H^+ concentration gradient that nullifies H^+ secretion in the absence of an electrical gradient (129). Aldosterone stimulation of H^+ secretion is at least in part due to the increased lumen-negative electrical potential that results from aldosterone stimulation of active sodium reabsorption.

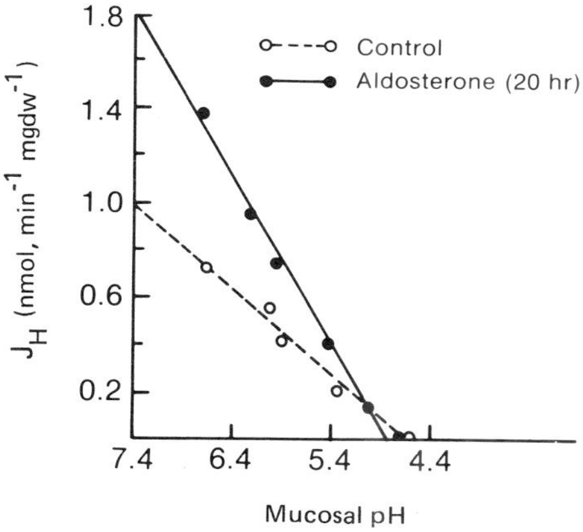

Fig. 3 The relationship of H^+ secretion (J_H) to the applied pH gradient (against which H^+ is secreted) in ouabain-treated freshwater turtle (*Pseudemys scripta*) bladders studied under short-circuit conditions in both control (unfilled circles, freshly pithed) and aldosterone-treated (filled circles, 20 hr) hemibladders. Aldosterone increased the rate of H^+ secretion at nonlimiting H^+ concentration gradients (increased slope), but it did not alter the applied H^+ gradient at which net H^+ secretion ceases (the proton motive force of the pump). (From Ref. 183.)

Studies in Rabbit Isolated Perfused Renal Tubules

Recent studies of acidification of luminal fluid by the rabbit cortical collecting tubule perfused in vitro indicate that the physiological characteristics of the H^+ secretory mechanism in the mammalian distal nephron are similar to those defined in the urinary bladder of the toad and turtle (132,133). The data support the existence of a distinct acidification mechanism that is both active and electrogenic, and stimulated by the magnitude of the sodium-dependent lumen-negative potential. Electrogenic H^+ secretion is stimulated by pretreatment of the animals with mineralocorticoid hormone (132). Mineralocorticoid hormone stimulation of H^+ secretion in the rabbit cortical collecting tubule is in part due to stimulation of active sodium reabsorption, since in the presence of luminal sodium mineralocorticoid hormone administration is associated with a large and significant increase in lumen-negative electrical potential, and in part due to a more direct effect on the proton secretory mechanism, since in the absence of luminal sodium mineralocorticoid hormone administra-

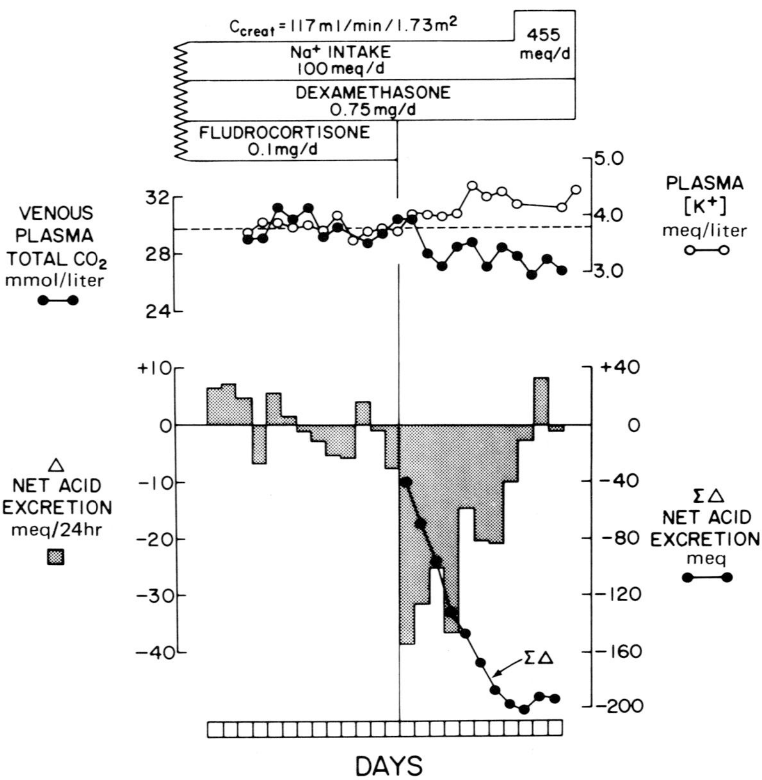

Fig. 4 Representative study of the effect of discontinuation of mineralocorticoid replacement therapy in an adrenalectomized patient without apparent intrinsic renal disease. The dashed line in the upper panel represents the mean control value of both plasma total carbon dioxide and potassium concentration (P_K). Values of Δ net acid excretion (ΔNAE) represent the difference between the daily net acid and the mean control values. Values of $\Sigma\Delta$ net acid excretion ($\Sigma\Delta$NAE) represent the accumulated sum of the daily values of Δ net acid excretion during the period of mineralocorticoid discontinuation. (From Ref. 25.)

tion results in a large and significant increase in lumen-positive electrical potential attributable to H^+ secretion (132).

In outer medullary collecting tubules, unlike the circumstance in cortical collecting tubules, mineralocorticoid hormone does not stimulate Na^+ reabsorption, nor does it alter the transtubular electrical potential difference, which is oriented lumen-positive in the collecting tubules that are located in the inner stripe of the outer medulla (134). The lumen-positive potential results from electrogenic H^+ secretion, which occurs despite the absence of Na^+ reabsorption, but is accompanied by Cl^- secretion at nearly identical rates (135-137). Mineralocorticoid hormone stimulates H^+ secretion in this nephron segment. Adrenalectomy reduces the rate of H^+ secretion, aldosterone replacement restores the rate, which suggests that normal levels of aldosterone secretion maintain the normal rate of H^+ secretion in this nephron segment (138). The intrinsic H^+ secretory capacity of this nephron segment exceeds that of the cortical collecting tubule and approaches 25% of that of the proximal convoluted tubule (135). Thus, mineralocorticoid hormone-stimulated H^+ secretion in the outer medullary collecting tubule may be the major determinant of distal nephron H^+ secretion rates in the mammalian kidney under ordinary physiological conditions, and in physiological and pathological states of altered mineralocorticoid levels. Morphological evidence has been ad-

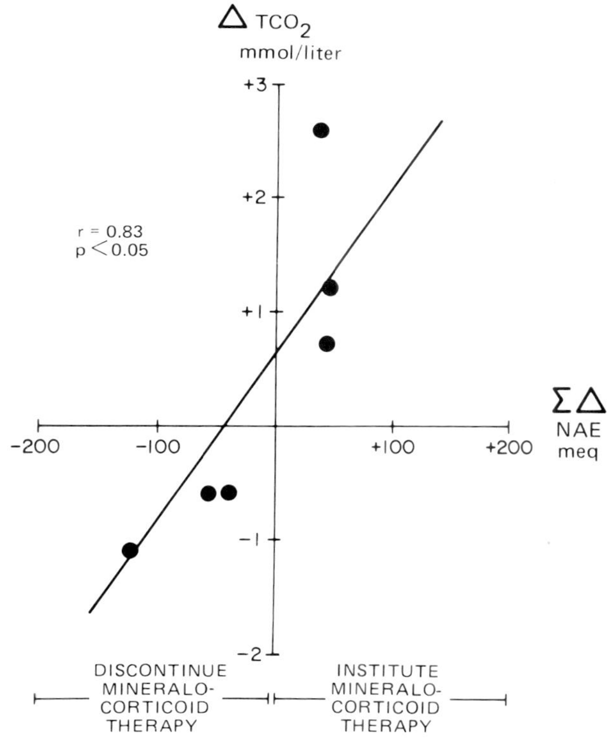

Fig. 5 Relationship between change in plasma carbon dioxide content and the cumulative change in urinary net acid excretion ($\Sigma\Delta$NAE, meq) following the first 5 days of discontinuation or initiation of mineralocorticoid replacement therapy in six adrenalectomized patients without apparent intrinsic renal disease. In one patient the duration of study was only 3 days. (From Ref. 25.)

duced in the rat that H^+ secretion in the outer medullary collecting duct is mediated by secretory pumps located in the luminal membrane of mitochondria-rich cells in this segment (139).

Studies in Humans

Studies similar to those in adrenalectomized dogs have been performed in adrenalectomized humans to investigate the renal and systemic acid-base consequences of mineralocorticoid deficiency in the absence of both glucocorticoid deficiency and renal disease (25) (Fig. 4). Glucocorticoid replacement was provided with dexamethasone, mineralocorticoid replacement with fludrocortisone or aldosterone. Following a control period, mineralocorticoid replacement was either discontinued or initiated. Net acid excretion and plasma total CO_2 decreased in each patient in whom mineralocorticoid was discontinued and increased in each patient in whom mineralocorticoid was initiated. The changes in plasma total CO_2 correlated with the changes in net acid excretion (Fig. 5) and the changes in net acid excretion correlated positively with the changes in sodium balance (Fig. 6) and negatively with the changes in potassium balance and plasma potassium concentration (Fig. 7). The magnitude of the cumulative reduction in net acid excretion correlated also with the basal rate of net acid excretion, hence presumably with the basal rate of endogenous acid production.

These findings provide the first evidence that renal acidification in humans is under stimulation by mineralocorticoid at levels of mineralocorticoid not exceeding those prevailing in normal subjects ingesting typical acid-producing diets of normal sodium and potassium content. The extent to which the tonic stimulation of renal acidification is mediated by a

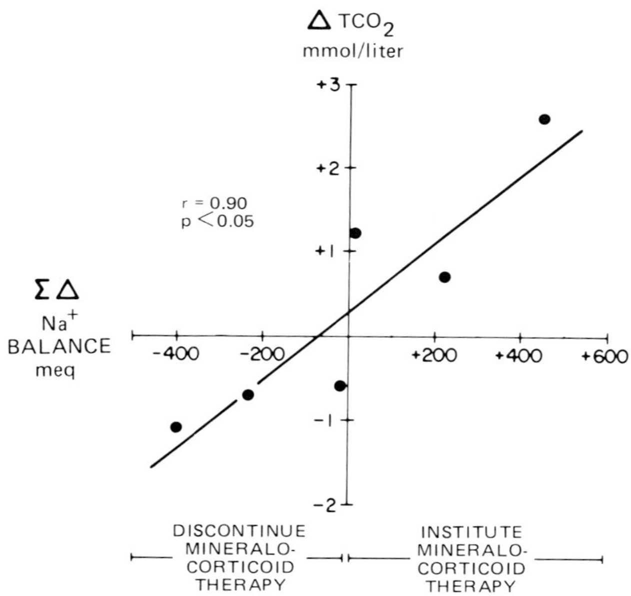

Fig. 6 Relationship between change in plasma carbone dioxide content and the cumulative change in sodium balance ($\Sigma\Delta$ Na^+ balance, meq) following the first 5 days of discontinuation or initiation of mineralocorticoid replacement therapy in six adrenalectomized patients without apparent intrinsic renal disease. The changes in sodium balance were calculated from the changes in urinary sodium excretion relative to intake. In one patient the duration of study was only 3 days. (From Ref. 25.)

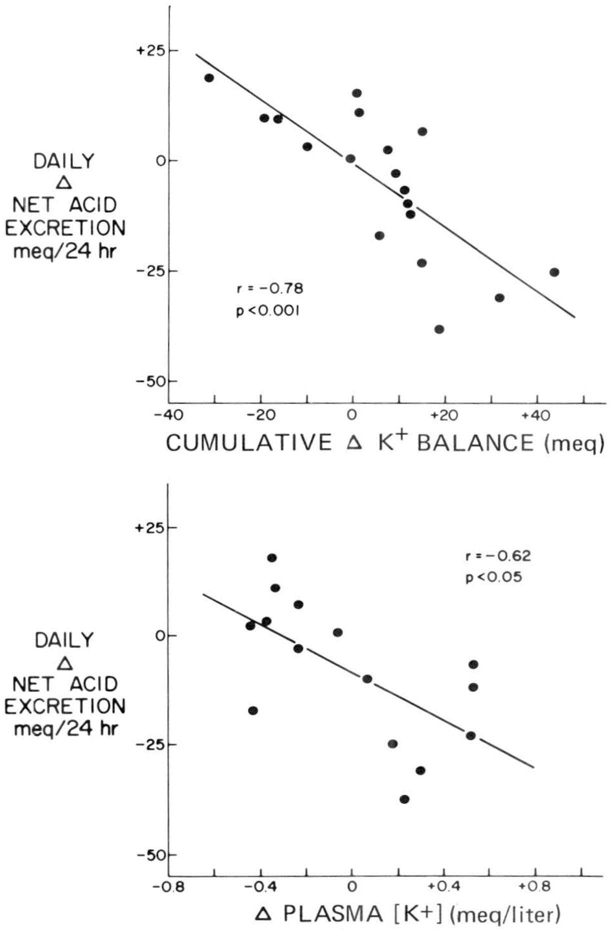

Fig. 7 Relationship between daily Δ net acid excretion (ΔNAE) and the cumulative change in potassium balance (upper panel) and the change in plasma potassium concentration (lower panel) following discontinuation or institution of mineralocorticoid replacement therapy (days 1-3) in six adrenalectomized patient without apparent intrinsic renal disease. Values of Δ excretion, balance, and concentration represent the difference between the daily values of excretion, balance, and concentration, respectively, and the corresponding mean control values. The changes in potassium balance were calculated from the changes in urinary potassium excretion relative to intake; values of cumulative Δ potassium balance represent the accumulated sum of the daily values of Δ potassium balance during the period of mineralocorticoid discontinuation.

direct effect of mineralocorticoid on renal H^+ transport or by an indirect effect dependent on stimulation of renal sodium and/or potassium transport was not determined. Nevertheless, the findings implicate mineralocorticoid deficiency in humans as a significant renal acidosis-producing condition not dependent on the presence of renal disease or glucocorticoid deficiency.

Table 2 Possible Mechanisms Whereby Aldosterone Stimulates Collecting Duct Hydrogen Ion Secretion

1. Increased lumen pH secondary to stimulation of cellular production of NH_3
2. Increased lumen electronegativity secondary to stimulation of Na^+ reabsorption
3. Increased production and utilization of metabolic energy for H^+ secretion
4. Increased conductance (or decreased resistance) of proton transport through H^+ secretory pump pathway
5. Increased numbers of H^+ secretory pumps

C. Cellular Mechanisms Whereby Aldosterone Stimulates Acidification

Possible mechanisms whereby aldosterone stimulates hydrogen ion secretion are outlined in Table 2. These possible mechanisms are not mutually exclusive and their postulation is based on current knowledge of the molecular mechanisms related to aldosterone action and renal acidification.

III. HYPERKALEMIC RTA IN PATIENTS WITH HISTOLOGICALLY EVIDENT DIFFUSE RENAL PARENCHYMAL DISEASE: ROLE OF ALDOSTERONE

A. Prevalence of Aldosterone Deficiency in Patients with Chronic Renal Insufficiency

To investigate the prevalence of aldosterone deficiency in hyperkalemic patients with diffuse renal parenchymal disease and chronic renal insufficiency, Schambelan et al. measured plasma and urine aldosterone levels in 31 such patients who had creatinine clearances ranging from 10 to 56 ml/min per 1.73 m^2 and serum potassium concentrations ranging from 6.0 to 8.7 meq/liter when dietary potassium was unrestricted at the time of initial diagnosis (5). None of the patients had cortisol deficiency. Urine aldosterone excretion ranged from 0.8 to 10.9 μg/24 hr when the subjects were in a steady state while ingesting a constant diet containing 108-128 meq sodium and 30-64 meq potassium (Fig. 8). Under similar conditions in 29 normal subjects, urine aldosterone ranged from 4.2 to 15.6 μg/24 hr. By comparison with these values in normal subjects, 14 of the 31 patients had frank hypoaldosteronism. However, aldosterone excretion rates in patients with chronic hyperkalemia should be compared with values observed in normal subjects who also have chronic hyperkalemia, inasmuch as hyperkalemia per se ordinarily stimulates aldosterone secretion (106-109). But no such data are available in normal subjects with chronic experimental hyperkalemia. Therefore, in the patients with chronic renal insufficiency, aldosterone levels were evaluated by comparing the ratio of urine aldosterone excretion to the serum potassium concentration ($U_{aldo}V/S_K$) with the ratio observed in the normal subjects studied (Fig. 9). In 23 of the 31 patients, $U_{aldo}V/S_K$ was distinctly subnormal, and these patients were diagnosed as having hypoaldosteronism and designated subgroup A. In the remaining eight patients, $U_{aldo}V/S_K$ was within the range observed in normal subjects, and these patients were designated subgroup B. Since the values of $U_{aldo}V/S_K$ in normal subjects who have chronic hyperkalemia are not known, the possibility could not be excluded that the patients in subgroup B also had hypoaldosteronism, but relatively less severe compared to that in subgroup A. Further evidence of hypoaldosteronism in subgroup B is the finding that normokalemic patients with chronic renal insufficiency characteristically have substantially higher concentrations of

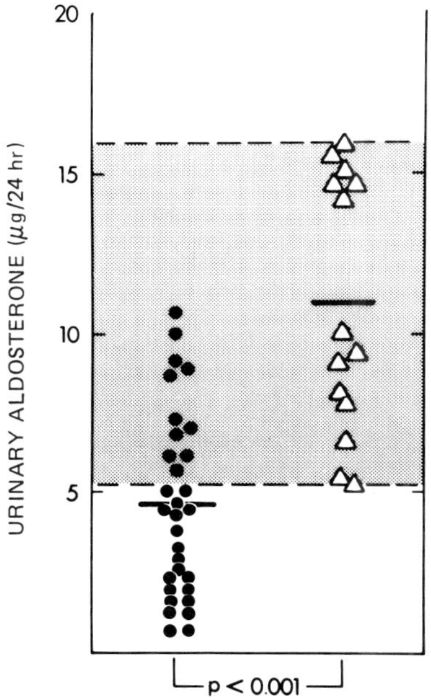

Fig. 8 Values of urinary aldosterone excretion in patients with hyperkalemia and chronic renal insufficiency (filled circles) and in normal subjects (unfilled triangles). Shaded area delimits the range of values in normal subjects. (From Ref. 5.)

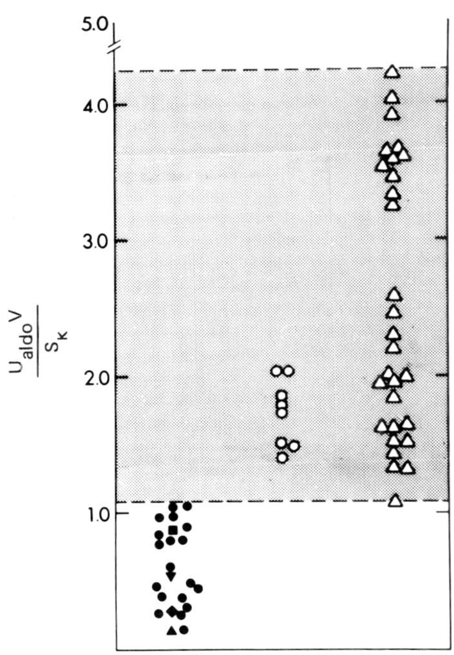

Fig. 9 Values for the ratio of urinary excretion of aldosterone-18-glucuronide to serum potassium concentration ($U_{aldo}V/S_K$) in patients with hyperkalemia and chronic renal insufficiency (filled symbols and unfilled circles) and in normal subjects (unfilled triangles). Two subgroups of patients are identified: 23 patients (filled symbols) in whom values of this ratio are below the range in normal subjects (shaded area) and eight patients (unfilled circles) in whom the value of this ratio fell within the normal range. (From Ref. 5.)

plasma aldosterone than were observed in the patients in subgroup B (6,7,9). The results of the study by Schambelan et al. (5) indicate that hypoaldosteronism occurs commonly in patients with chronic renal insufficiency who have hyperkalemia.

B. Functional Significance of Aldosterone Deficiency in the Pathogenesis of Hyperkalemia in Patients with Chronic Renal Insufficiency

The results of the study by Schambelan et al. (5) also indicated clearly that aldosterone deficiency contributed to the pathogenesis of hyperkalemia in patients with chronic renal insufficiency. In both subgroups A and B, a significant positive correlation was observed between the serum potassium concentration and the steady-state urinary excretion rate of potassium (Fig. 10). Urinary potassium excretion in the steady state is presumed to reflect net dietary load of potassium (diet minus stool potassium). A significantly greater degree of hyperkalemia was observed in the patients with hypoaldosteronism (subgroup A) than in those without overt hypoaldosteronism (subgroup B) in relation to the net dietary load of potassium (Fig. 10). It is conceivable that the presence of hyperkalemia in subgroup B, albeit of lesser severity than in subgroup A, is related to the relative degree of hypoaldosteronism in these patients. Viewed in another way, these data indicate that renal clearance of potassium is impaired in hyperkalemic patients with chronic renal insufficiency, and that the magnitude of this impairment is related to the extent to which aldosterone secretion is subnormal.

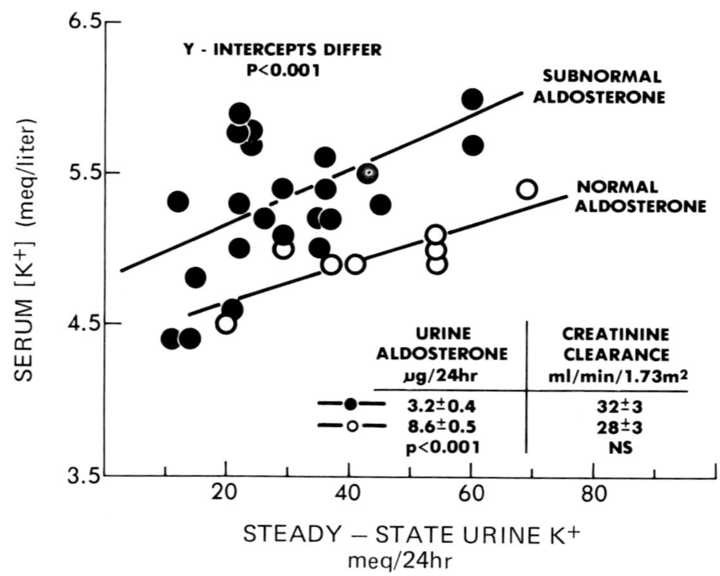

Fig. 10 Relationship between serum potassium concentration and urinary potassium excretion in patients with isolated hypoaldosteronism (subgroup A) (filled circles) and patients with chronic renal insufficiency without hypoaldosteronism (subgroup B, unfilled circles). As indicated by regression lines, a significant positive correlation between these variables was observed both in the patients in subgroup A ($y = 0.020x + 4.72$; $r = 0.56$; $p<0.01$) and in those in subgroup B ($y = 0.013x + 4.38$; $r = 0.83$; $p<0.01$). The y intercept was significantly greater ($p<0.001$) in the patients in subgroup A than it was in those in subgroup B, but the slopes did not differ significantly in the two groups (analysis of covariance).

C. Renal and Systemic Acid-Base Response to Mineralocorticoid Replacement Therapy in Patients with Chronic Renal Insufficiency

The role of aldosterone deficiency in the pathogenesis of metabolic acidosis in patients with diffuse renal parenchymal disease and reduced glomerular filtration rate (GFR) has been investigated in studies in which the potent mineralocorticoid fludrocortisone was administered to patients with hyperkalemic RTA and hypoaldosteronism in the setting of chronic tubulo-interstitial nephritis (10). Administration of physiological amounts of fludrocortisone in some cases resulted in large increases in net acid excretion of sufficient magnitude to substantially ameliorate the degree of systemic acidosis. In the patients in whom glomerular filtration rate was not markedly subnormal (i.e., GFR >30 ml/min), the increase in net acid excretion was due almost entirely to an increase in urinary ammonium excretion. In the patients in whom glomerular filtration rate (and presumably also renal mass) was more markedly reduced, the contribution of urine ammonium excretion to the increase in net acid excretion was less; increased titratable acid excretion contributed substantially. Analysis of the changes in urine pH and ammonium excretion indicated that administration of exogenous mineralocorticoid both augmented renal ammonia production and stimulated renal hydrogen ion secretion. The augmentation of ammonia production appeared to be due to the correction of hyperkalemia, but a more direct effect of mineralocorticoid on renal ammonia-genesis cannot be excluded. The findings in this investigation and the interpretation of the findings are described more fully in the following sections.

The results obtained in the study of one patient are summarized in Fig. 11, which depicts the renal and systemic acid-base effects of chronic administration of a physiological replacement dose of fludrocortisone (0.10-0.15 mg/day) in a patient with chronic tubulo-interstitial renal disease (creatinine clearance 13 ml/min per 1.73 m^2) and hyporeninemic hypoaldosteronism. Fludrocortisone administration was associated with a reduction in urine pH, an increase in net acid excretion, and a substantial amelioration of systemic acidosis and hyperkalemia. The observed reduction in urine pH during fludrocortisone administration suggests that even though the urine was highly acidic in the pretreatment period, acidification was impaired owing to aldosterone deficiency, and that mineralocorticoid replacement ameliorates the impairment by stimulation of H^+ secretion. Presumably the pretreatment values of urine pH would have been considerably higher than those observed had the pretreatment rate of renal ammonia production not been limited in this patient owing to a marked reduction in renal mass.

In other patients with type 4 RTA and chronic renal insufficiency and hypoaldosteronism, administration of physiological amounts of fludrocortisone has had little or no effect on acid-base balance, but administration of "superphysiological" amounts resulted in a substantial increase in net acid excretion and amelioration of systemic acidosis (10). The requirement for superphysiological amounts of exogenous mineralocorticoid raises the possibility that in addition to deficiency of aldosterone, the kidney may be hyporesponsive to the action of aldosterone in some patients. This circumstance might not be specific for patients with chronic renal insufficiency who have hyperkalemic RTA. Chronic renal disease may in some way limit the renal response to aldosterone, since the secretion rate and plasma concentration of aldosterone is commonly supernormal in patients with chronic renal insufficiency (6,7,9). Thus, failure to correct metabolic acidosis might reflect failure to administer hormone in a amount appropriate for the degree of renal insufficiency. This possibility is suggested by the finding of Daughaday and Rendleman (140) in an adrenalectomized patient with pyelonephritis that the amount of exogenous mineralocorticoid hormone required to maintain correction of acidosis and hyperkalemia increased greatly as the renal disease

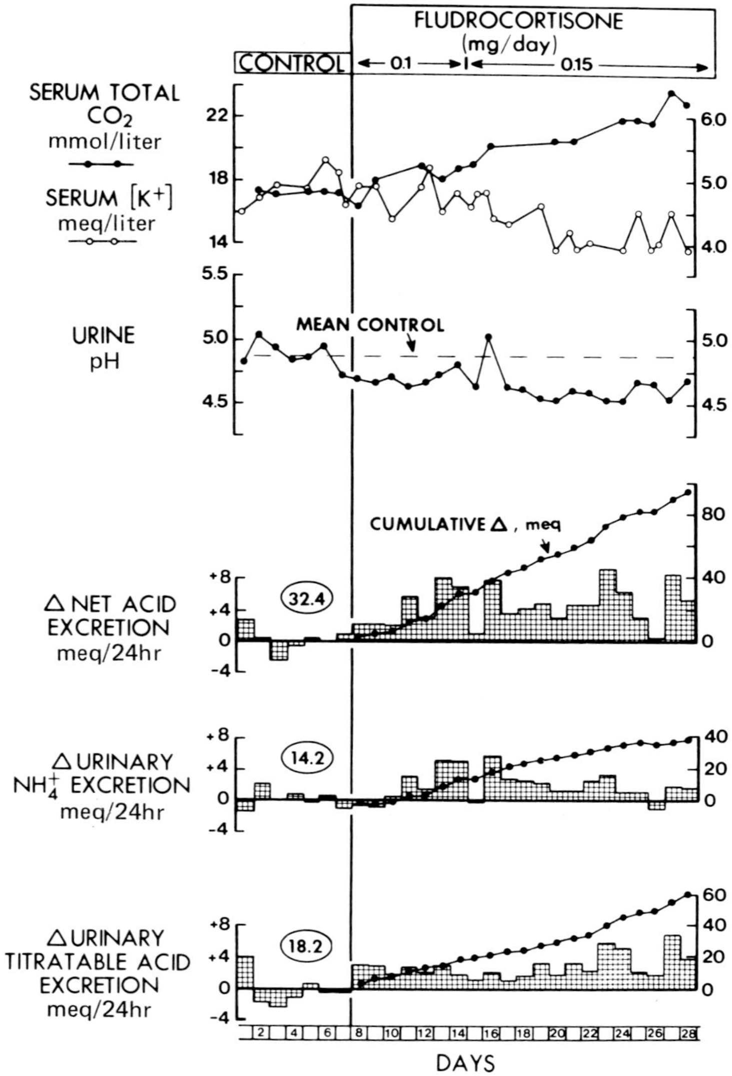

Fig. 11 Effect of orally administered fludrocortisone on serum carbon dioxide content and potassium concentration, urine pH and urinary titratable acid, and ammonium and net acid excretion in a patient with hyporeninemic hypoaldosteronism and chronic renal insufficiency (creatinine clearance 13 ml/min per 1.73 m^2). Systemic acidosis had not previously been treated. The severity of hyperkalemia had been mitigated before the study was initiated by the provision of a low-normal dietary intake of potassium. In the three bottom panels, the hatched bars represent the difference between the measured values of acid excretion and the mean value before therapy; the magnitude of these differences is indicated by the scale on the left-hand side of the panel. For reference, the mean control value is designated by the numerals within the ellipse. The accumulated values of the daily differences are shown by the solid circles and are indicated by the scale on the right-hand side of the panel. The observed reduction in urine pH during fludrocortisone administration suggests that even though the urine was highly acidic in the pretreatment period, acidification was impaired owing to aldosterone deficiency, and that mineralocorticoid replacement ameliorates the impairment by stimulation of H^+ secretion. Presumably the pretreatment values of urine pH would have been considerably higher had the pretreatment rate of renal ammonia production not been limited in this patient owing to a marked reduction in renal mass. (From Ref. 10.)

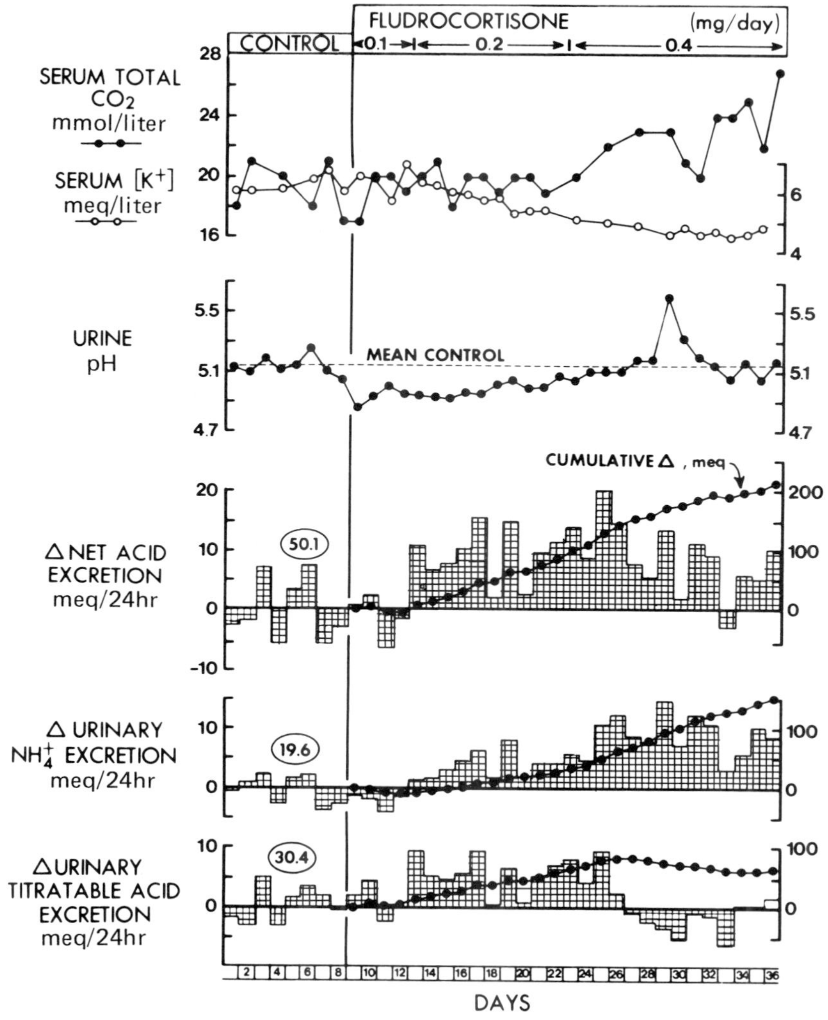

Fig. 12 Effect of fludrocortisone on serum carbon dioxide content and potassium concentration, urine pH and urinary titratable acid, and ammonium and net acid excretion in a patient with hyporeninemic hypoaldosteronism and chronic renal insufficiency (creatinine clearance, 36 ml/min per 1.73 m^2). Systemic acidosis had not previously been treated. In the three bottom panels, the hatched bars represent the difference between the measured value of acid excretion and the mean value before therapy; the magnitude of these differences is indicated by the scale on the left-hand side of the panel. For reference, the mean control value is designated by the numerals within the ellipse. The accumulated values of the daily differences are shown by the solid circles and are indicated by the scale on the right-hand side of the panel. (From Ref. 10.)

progressed. Failure to correct acidosis in some cases might also reflect an inadequate duration of hormone administration to achieve the requisite cumulative acid-excretory effect given that the number of functioning nephrons is greatly reduced (10). Superphysiological amounts of exogenous mineralocorticoid may be appropriate replacement therapy for patients with aldosterone deficiency and reduced numbers of functioning nephrons.

In patients with type 4 RTA and hypoaldosteronism in whom glomerular filtration rate is not markedly reduced (i.e., creatinine clearance >30 ml/min), the increase in net acid excretion observed during mineralocorticoid therapy is accounted for predominantly by increased urine ammonium excretion (Fig. 12). Urine pH decreased when mineralocorticoid therapy was initiated, but with continued therapy it increased in parallel with the observed increase in urine ammonium excretion (Figs. 12 and 13). These findings suggest that the rate of renal production of ammonia increased during mineralocorticoid therapy. A primary increase in ammonia production would result in an increase in the amount of ammonia diffusing into the tubular lumen, which would both augment the excretion of ammonium and, by increasing the amount of luminal buffer, raise urine pH. Urine ammonium excretion correlated inversely with serum potassium concentration (Fig. 13) and did not decrease on discontinuation of mineralocorticoid therapy if hyperkalemia was prevented from recurring by reduction of dietary potassium intake; titratable acid and net acid excretion decreased, however (Fig. 14). Thus, in patients with hypoaldosteronism and chronic renal insufficiency, administration

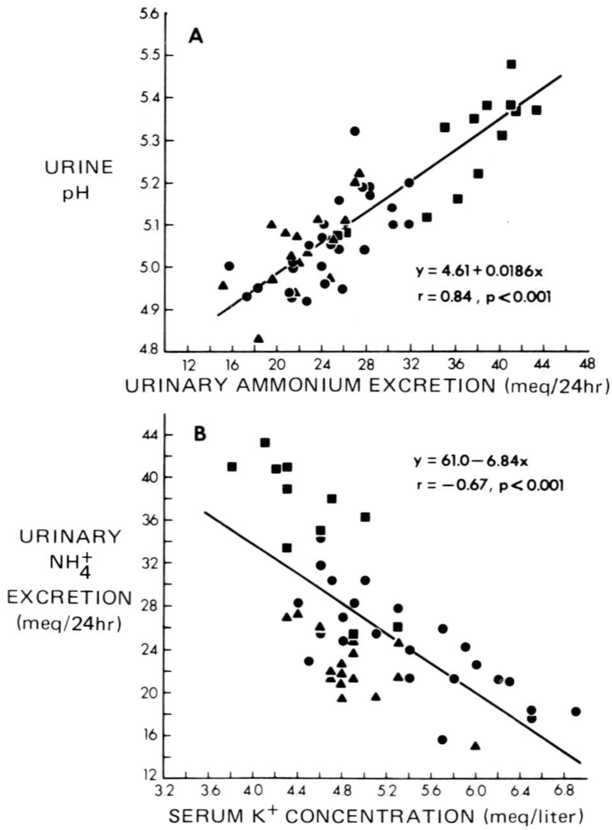

Fig. 13 Relation between (A) urine pH and urinary ammonium excretion and (B) urinary ammonium excretion and serum potassium concentration during oral administration of fludrocortisone therapy in patients with hyporeninemic hypoaldosteronism without far advanced chronic renal insufficiency (creatinine clearance, 35-44 ml/min per 1.73 m^2). (From Ref. 10.)

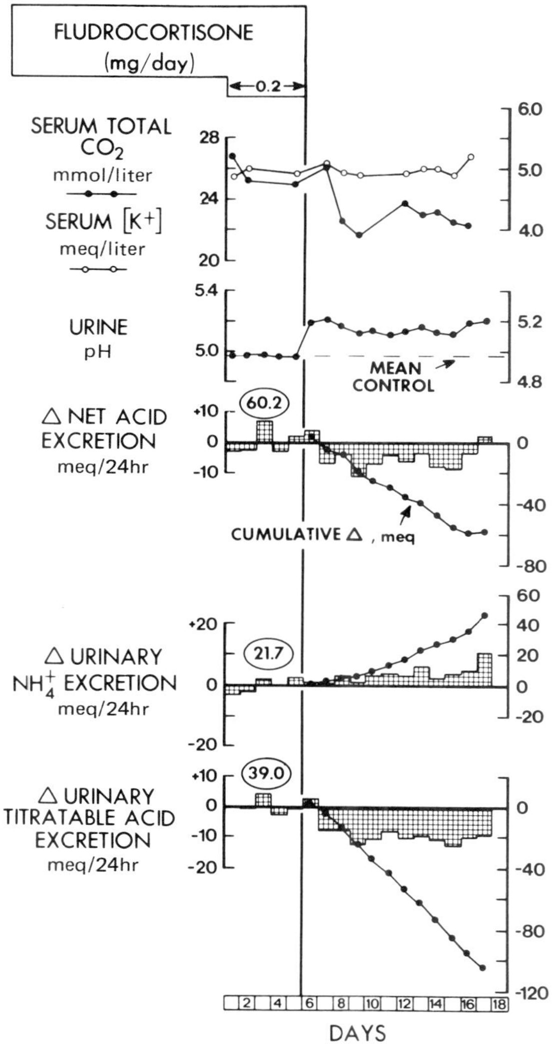

Fig. 14 Effect of discontinuation of fludrocortisone on serum carbon dioxide content and potassium concentration, urine pH and urinary titratable acid, and ammonium and net acid excretion in a patient with hyporeninemic hypoaldosteronism and chronic renal insufficiency (creatinine clearance, 35 ml/min per 1.73 m^2). In this study dietary intake of potassium was reduced when therapy was discontinued; the serum potassium concentration remained constant. The rate of urinary ammonium excretion did not decrease when therapy was discontinued, despite a sustained increase in urine pH. (From Ref. 10.)

of mineralocorticoid can augment both renal H^+ secretion and, by correction of hyperkalemia, renal ammonia production.

The results depicted in Fig. 15 provide additional evidence that in patients with type 4 RTA and hypoaldosteronism mineralocorticoid replacement therapy stimulates renal hydrogen ion secretion independently of its effect (direct or indirect) to stimulate renal ammonia production. This figure shows the relationship between urine pH and urine ammonium

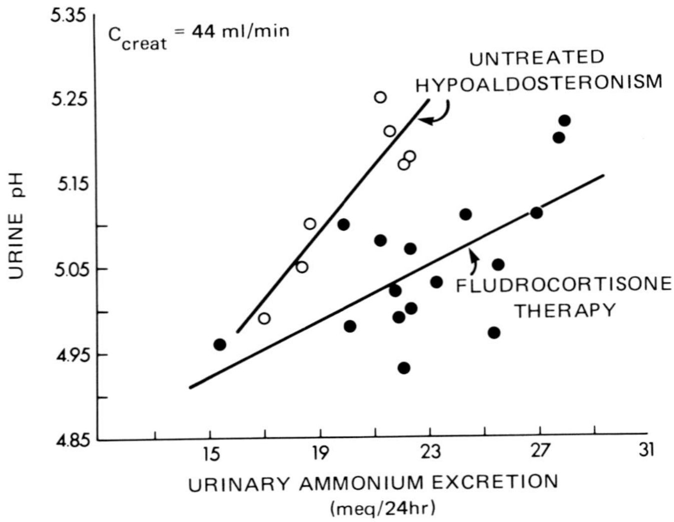

Fig. 15 Relationship between daily urine pH and urine ammonium excretion in a patient with type 4 RTA and hypoaldosteronism studied prior to (unfilled circles) and after (filled circles) initiation of chronic fludrocortisone therapy. Under both conditions urine ammonium excretion varied inversely with serum potassium concentration (data not shown). Prior to initiation of fludrocortisone therapy serum potassium concentration increased progressively in response to an increase in dietary potassium intake; urine ammonium excretion and urine pH decreased. After initiation of chronic fludrocortisone therapy, while dietary potassium intake was maintained constant, serum potassium concentration decreased progressively from supernormal to normal levels; urine ammonium excretion and urine pH increased. The parallel relationship between urine pH and ammonium excretion in both cases reflects the buffering effect of ammonia diffusion into tubular fluid; the amount of ammonia available for diffusion is modulated by potassium balance. Since during fludrocortisone therapy urine pH is lower in relation to urine ammonia content, it may be inferred that fludrocortisone in some way increases the capacity of the distal nephron to secrete hydrogen ion. When urine ammonium excretion approaches zero, however, the reduced availability of luminal buffer obviates the need for mineralocorticoid stimulation of distal nephron hydrogen ion secretory capacity for acidification of the urine, suggesting that the blood to urine hydrogen ion concentration gradient-generating ability of the collecting duct is unaffected by mineralocorticoid deficiency.

excretion prior to initiation of fludrocortisone therapy (unfilled circles) and during the period of fludrocortisone therapy (filled circles). During the pretreatment period, the relationship between these two variables was dictated by a decreasing rate of ammonium excretion that was associated with an increase in plasma potassium concentration, a non-steady-state condition caused by renal potassium retention. During the treatment period, the relationship between these two variables was dictated by an increasing rate of ammonium excretion that was associated with a decreasing plasma potassium concentration, a consequence of fludrocortisone-stimulated renal potassium excretion. Since during both periods urine pH correlated positively with urine ammonium excretion, it may be inferred that the changes in urine pH reflected to a considerable extent the effect of corresponding changes in the rate of renal production of ammonia and the consequent changes in the availability of ammonia for diffusion into the urine. As shown in the figure, considerably smaller changes in urine pH occurred during the fludrocortisone treatment period than during the pretreatment period despite changes in the rate of renal production of ammonia that resulted in a similar range of urine ammonium excretion rates in the two periods. That is, the slope of the relation between urine pH and urine ammonium excretion is considerably lower during fludrocortisone therapy than it is during the pretreatment period. Since urine pH is lower in relation to urine buffer (ammonia) content during fludrocortisone therapy, it may be inferred that fludrocortisone in some way increases the capacity of the distal nephron to titrate luminal buffers. As previously discussed in relation to the studies depicted in Fig. 2, the slope of the positive correlation between urine pH and urine ammonium excretion can be taken as an index of the hydrogen ion secretory capacity of the distal nephron, and the value of urine pH at very low or near zero urine ammonium excretion rates can be taken as an index of the hydrogen ion concentration-gradient-generating ability of the distal nephron. Thus, as in dogs and turtles, mineralocorticoid appears to increase the rate capacity of the distal nephron for hydrogen ion secretion when luminal buffer availability is not limiting, but does not affect the hydrogen ion concentration-gradient-generating ability when luminal buffer availability is near zero.

D. Renal and Systemic Acid-Base Response to Correction of Hyperkalemia by Dietary Potassium Restriction in Patients with Chronic Renal Insufficiency

To what extent does hyperkalemia per se contribute to the pathogenesis of metabolic acidosis in patients with chronic renal insufficiency? The effect of acute or chronic hyperkalemia on renal acid-base homeostasis in man and other mammals is incompletely understood. Hyperkalemia is a potential renal acidosis-producing factor, inasmuch as potassium loading suppresses renal production of ammonia (123) and diminishes bicarbonate reabsorptive capacity during bicarbonate loading (141). But the effect on renal bicarbonate reabsorption at normal or subnormal plasma bicarbonate concentrations has not been evaluated. Acute potassium chloride loading in nonbicarbonate-loaded rats results in a suppression of bicarbonate reabsorption in the proximal tubule, but the influence of attendant extracellular fluid volume expansion was not excluded, and net renal bicarbonate reabsorption was not measured (142). Long-term potassium loading in dogs reportedly has no significant effect on net acid excretion or plasma bicarbonate concentration in some studies (143), and results in hyperkalemic renal tubular acidosis in others (144). In the experimental model of hyperkalemic RTA induced by administration of amiloride (see below) neither the magnitude of reduction in net acid excretion nor the degree of metabolic acidosis was influenced when hyperkalemia was prevented from occurring by appropriate adjustment of dietary potassium intake on initiation of amiloride administration (145).

To investigate the specific role of hyperkalemia in the pathogenesis of metabolic acidosis in chronic renal insufficiency, chronic balance studies were performed wherein hyperkalemia was corrected solely by restriction of dietary potassium in three patients with moderate chronic renal insufficiency (C_{creat}36, 44, 58 ml/min per 1.73 m^2) (146). Reduction of potassium intake was effected by equimolar substitution of sodium for potassium in the electrolyte supplement to a whole-food diet of intrinsic low potassium content. This maneuver resulted in correction of hyperkalemia and a significant and sustained amelioration of metabolic acidosis (Figs. 16 and 17). Net acid excretion increased following the reduction of potassium intake, but the increase was transient and of insufficient magnitude to fully account for the magnitude of the observed increment in plasma bicarbonate concentration, suggesting the contribution of an extrarenal mechanism of bicarbonate input to the extra-

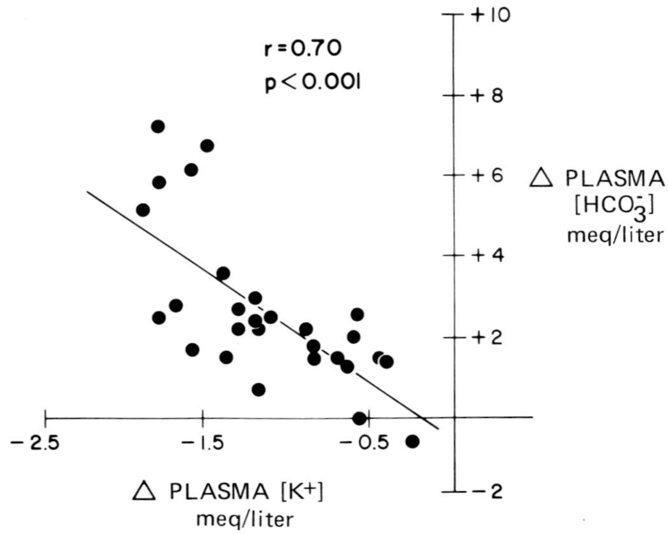

Fig. 16 Relation between the change in plasma bicarbonate concentration and the change in plasma potassium concentration in response to dietary potassium restriction in three patients with hyperkalemia, metabolic acidosis, and chronic renal insufficiency. Δ plasma $[HCO_3^-]$ is calculated as the difference between the value observed during dietary K^+ restriction and the mean control value; Δ plasma $[K^+]$ is calculated in a similar manner. In one patient, data are for serum potassium.

cellular compartment (Fig. 17). Evidence for such an extrarenal mechanism was obtained only during the transition period, when plasma potassium concentration was decreasing. During sustained normokalemia, the increased plasma bicarbonate concentration was maintained entirely as a consequence of a sustained increase in total renal hydrogen ion secretion inasmuch as the attendant increased filtered bicarbonate load was reabsorbed completely without a reduction in net acid excretion from control values (Fig. 18). These results thus indicate that at least in some patients with moderate chronic renal insufficiency, metabolic acidosis can be ameliorated by restriction of dietary potassium without administration of medication or change in diet anion. Amelioration of acidosis is initiated by both extrarenal and renal mechanisms and is sustained by an increase in the set-point at which the kidney regulates plasma bicarbonate.

It is possible that in these studies of dietary potassium restriction a limitation was imposed on the magnitude of the increase in set-point of renal regulation of plasma bicarbonate concentration owing to suppression of aldosterone secretion by the adrenal glands in response to potassium restriction (106,147-149). Urine aldosterone excretion decreased during potassium restriction, presumably secondary to the observed reduction in plasma renin activity and plasma potassium concentration. Plasma renin activity and potassium concentration are the two major regulators of aldosterone secretion (108). It is reasonable to postulate that the acidosis-ameliorating effect of potassium restriction was limited by the observed reduction in aldosterone, since it is known that in subjects without renal disease the prevailing level of mineralocorticoid provides a tonic stimulation of renal acid excretion required to maintain normal plasma acid-base composition (25). Furthermore, it is known that in such patients with chronic renal insufficiency mineralocorticoid deficiency can lead to a reduction

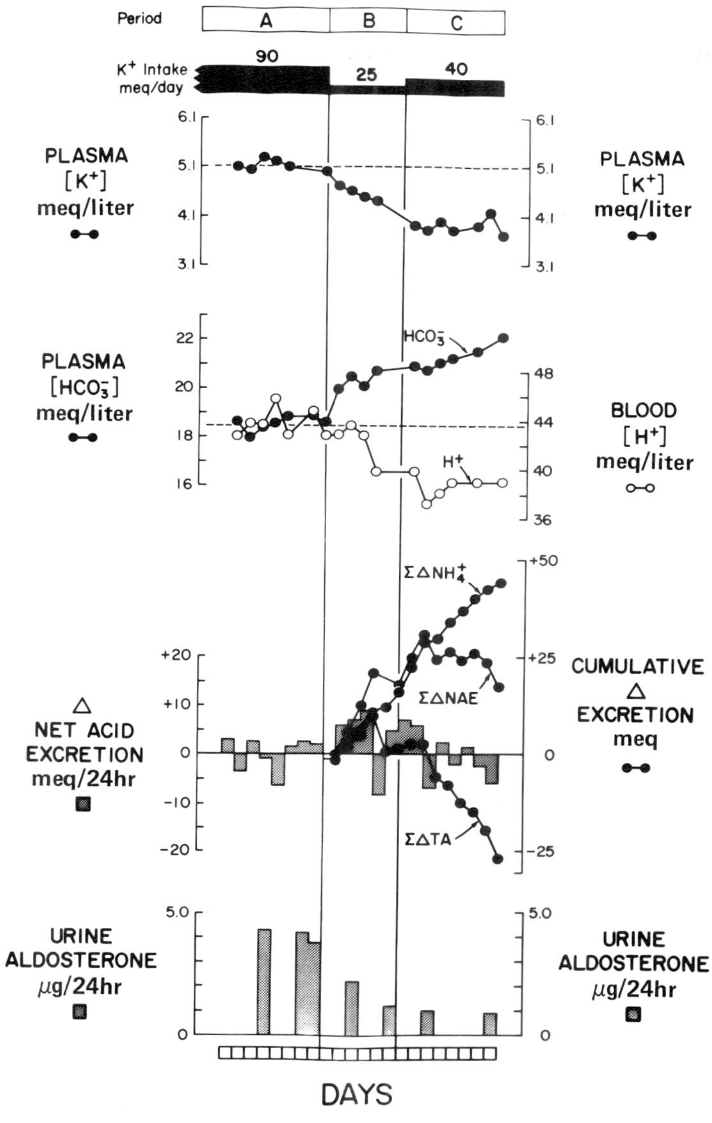

Fig. 17 Effect of restriction and partial replenishment of dietary potassium on plasma potassium concentration, plasma bicarbonate and blood hydrogen ion concentrations, and the urine excretion of ammonium, titratable acid, net acid, and aldosterone in a patient with hyperkalemia, metabolic acidosis, and chronic renal insufficiency (creatinine clearance 36 ml/min per 1.73 m^2). In the middle panel, the horizontal line labeled zero represents the mean value of net acid excretion obtained in the control period (period A), and the shaded bars represent the difference between the daily value and the mean control value of net acid excretion. The magnitude of these daily differences is indicated by the scale on the left side of the panel. The accumulated daily differences in urine excretion of net acid, ammonium, and titratable acid are depicted by the filled circles and quantified by the scale on the right side of the panel.

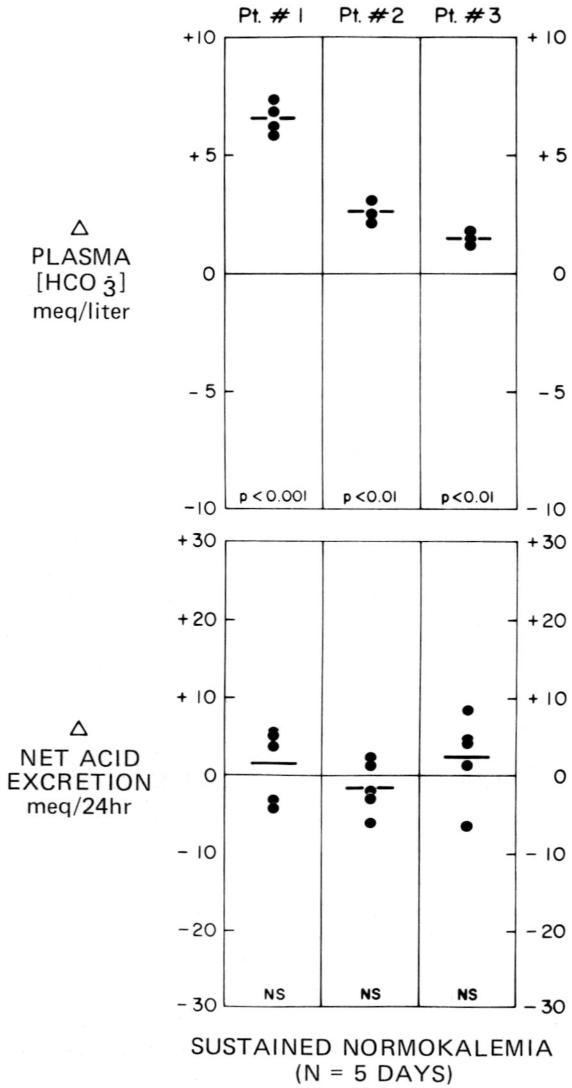

Fig. 18 Magnitude of the change from the mean control value in plasma bicarbonate concentration and daily net acid excretion during the last 5 days of a period of sustained normokalemia induced by dietary potassium restriction in three patients with hyperkalemia, metabolic acidosis, and chronic renal insufficiency.

in net acid excretion and development of metabolic acidosis independent of changes in plasma potassium concentration (10) (Fig. 14). However, reduced levels of aldosterone during potassium restriction might be offset by potentiated renal action of aldosterone mediated by reduction in body potassium stores, since it is known that the acid excretory response to administered mineralocorticoid can be greatly augmented by dietary potassium restriction (121). The interrelation between plasma potassium concentration and circulating aldosterone levels with respect to regulation of renal acidification requires further investigation both in healthy subjects and in patients with chronic renal insufficiency who have spontaneous disturbances in potassium and aldosterone metabolism.

E. Incidence of Metabolic Acidosis in Patients with Hypoaldosteronism and Chronic Renal Insufficiency

It is widely held that metabolic acidosis is not an invariable accompaniment of hypoaldosteronism in patients with chronic renal disease (20,150), and that it occurs only in about 50% of cases in some series (150). The possibility can be considered that metabolic acidosis is an invariable accompaniment of hypoaldosteronism but is not always discerned. The range of values of plasma bicarbonate concentration and blood pH in normal subjects is sufficiently broad that a substantial degree of metabolic acidosis might be present, yet the values of plasma bicarbonate concentration and blood pH are not below the lower limits of the normal range (151). Furthermore, the lower limits of the normal range for plasma bicarbonate concentration and blood pH differ among normal individuals depending on the set-point at which blood carbon dioxide is regulated by the respiratory system in response to factors other than blood acidity (151). Hence, in patients with hypoaldosteronism in whom plasma bicarbonate concentration and blood pH fall within the broad range of values in normal subjects, these values might be distinctly subnormal when consideration is made for the effect of PCO_2. This possibility is supported by observations in adrenalectomized patients in whom hypoaldosteronism is induced experimentally by withholding mineralocorticoid replacement therapy (25). In these patients, metabolic acidosis occurs without reduction in plasma bicarbonate concentration or blood pH to values below the lower limits of the broad range of values for the normal population. The occurrence of more severe degrees of metabolic acidosis in patients with hypoaldosteronism and chronic renal disease may reflect amplification of the renal acidification dysfunction by additional factors (e.g., the intake level of sodium and consequent amount of sodium delivery to the distal nephron; intake level of potassium and degree of hyperkalemia; the number of residual functioning nephrons) (10,15,21).

F. Therapeutic Alternatives in Patients with Type 4 RTA and Chronic Renal Parenchymal Disease

Treatment of patients with type 4 RTA and chronic renal insufficiency with mineralocorticoid may not always be indicated, however. Some patients are hypertensive and have measured increases in extracellular fluid volume and total exchangeable sodium content (12,42). Treatment with mineralocorticoid in these patients, by increasing renal tubular reabsorption of sodium chloride, might exacerbate the degree of hypertension and lead to other deleterious consequences of extracellular fluid volume expansion. In one patient studied in our laboratory, the occurrence of hypertension 2 years after initiating fludrocortisone therapy necessitated its discontinuation. Patients with hyporeninemic hypoaldosteronism in the older age groups may have limited cardiac reserve. In such patients, the combination of a fixed level of circulating (exogenous) mineralocorticoid hormone and unrestricted salt intake and physical activity might lead to congestive heart failure.

Alternative therapeutic measures that can be considered in patients with hyporeninemic hypoaldosteronism and type 4 renal tubular acidosis include restriction of dietary potassium, administration of potassium-binding resins, and sodium bicarbonate, or loop diuretics, or both. Despite impairment in renal bicarbonate resorption, administration of 1.5-2.0 meq/kg of sodium bicarbonate per day may be sufficient to sustain correction of acidosis, since glomerular filtration rate is usually reduced. Correction of acidosis usually mitigates the severity of hyperkalemia. Often, the serum potassium concentration can be maintained at less than 5.0 meq/liter with combined alkali therapy and modest dietary potassium restriction. The severity of hyperkalemia and acidosis can be mitigated by oral administration of potassium-binding resins (97), but many patients find the medication unpalatable.

Chronic administration of the chloruretic agent furosemide can also ameliorate acidosis and hyperkalemia in patients with type 4 RTA (152). Chronic administration of furosemide is known to result in an increase in net acid and potassium excretion in dogs, and causes persisting hypokalemic metabolic alkalosis. Furosemide is known to inhibit active chloride reabsorption in the loop of Henle, an effect that results in saluresis and secondary hyperaldosteronism (153). The kaliuretic and acid excretory response can be attributed to increased secretion of potassium and hydrogen ion in the distal nephron secondary to the combined effect of increased distal delivery of sodium and increased circulating levels of aldosterone. More recently, it has been demonstrated in dogs that the acid excretory response to furosemide administration can occur under experimental conditions in which salt depletion and hyperaldosteronism are prevented from occurring (154). These studies raise the possibility that furosemide more directly stimulates renal hydrogen ion secretion (154). In patients with type 4 RTA, the magnitude of the acid excretory response to furosemide correlates with the prevailing levels of endogenous aldosterone (152). Patients with the most marked degrees of hypoaldosteronism have only a minimal response despite several weeks of therapy. Coadministration of mineralocorticoid hormone (fludrocortisone) greatly potentiates the ameliorative effect of furosemide in these patients.

IV. HYPERKALEMIC RTA IN PATIENTS WITHOUT HISTOLOGICALLY EVIDENT DIFFUSE RENAL PARENCHYMAL DISEASE: ROLE OF ALDOSTERONE

In a wide spectrum of clinical disorders, chronic renal hyperkalemia and type 4 RTA occur in the absence of diffuse renal parenchymal disease and reduced glomerular filtration rate (Table 1). In some of these conditions, such as Addison's disease or corticosterone methyl oxidase deficiency, renal hyperkalemia and type 4 RTA can be attributed to a deficiency of aldosterone and can be corrected by administration of exogenous mineralocorticoid hormone in physiological replacement doses. In other conditions, aldosterone deficiency is not clearly present, and hyperkalemia and acidosis persist despite administration of even superphysiological doses of mineralocorticoids. In the absence of histologically evident diffuse renal parenchymal disease, such mineralocorticoid resistant renal hyperkalemia and acidosis occurs in two distinctly different clinical syndromes: (1) classic pseudohypoaldosteronism of infancy, characterized by renal salt wasting and hypotension (30,57-81), and (2) a syndrome of chronic mineralocorticoid-resistant hyperkalemia and acidosis unaccompanied by renal salt wasting or hypotension, and frequently associated with hypertension (87-96). These two syndromes have been designated as type 1 and 2 pseudohypohypoaldosteronism, respectively. The primary abnormality of type 1 pseudohypoaldosteronism has been postulated to be a specific defect in the renal response to mineralocorticoid hormone, which accounts for the coexistence of salt wasting and potassium retention and acidosis. The primary abnormality in type 2 pseudohypoaldosteronism has been postulated to be an ion transport defect that limits the kaliuretic response to mineralocorticoid hormone but not the sodium and chloride reabsorptive effect of the hormone.

A. Type 1 Pseudohypoaldosteronism (Classic Pseudohypoaldosteronism of Infancy)

The term pseudohypoaldosteronism has been employed to designate clinical conditions in which the signs and symptoms are suggestive of aldosterone deficiency but in which aldosterone levels are supernormal and administration of exogenous mineralocorticoid is not ameliorative. A clinically distinctive form of pseudohypoaldosteronism occurs in infants as an apparently congenital and in some cases a familial disorder characterized by failure to thrive, dehydration, and hyponatremia due to renal salt wasting, hyperkalemia due to renal potassium retention, and renal tubular acidosis (30,57-81). Plasma renin activity and plasma and urinary aldosterone concentrations are markedly elevated, plasma deoxycorticosterone and corticosterone concentrations are normal, and neither glucocorticoid deficiency nor excess is present. Mineralocorticoid refractoriness of renal sodium wasting and potassium retention is evident even during prolonged periods of parenteral administration of large amounts of deoxycorticosterone and aldosterone and oral administration of fludrocortisone. Supplementation of the diet with large amounts of sodium chloride can reverse hyponatremia and hyperkalemia, relieve symptomatology, and permit normal or improved growth. Characteristically the severity of renal sodium wasting and potassium retention diminishes after the period of infancy, permitting discontinuation of sodium chloride supplements without recurrence of overt hyponatremia or hyperkalemia. Disordered renal handling of sodium and potassium persists, however, evidenced by recurrence of hyponatremia and hyperkalemia in response to restriction of dietary sodium chloride (99).

The pathogenesis of classic pseudohypoaldosteronism of infancy has not been elucidated. In the signal case reported by Cheek and Perry in 1958 (57), it was postulated "... that the defect may be due to a refractory state on the part of the [renal] tubules to endogenous salt-active steroids or mineralocorticoids." Generalized glomerular and tubular dysfunction is not present, and examination of biopsied renal tissue has usually revealed only the presence of mild hyperplasia of the juxtaglomerular apparatus. These patients are thus distinguishable from patients with pseudohypoaldosteronism associated with generalized renal parenchymal structural damage (e.g., salt-losing nephritis caused by methicillan nephritis, medullary cystic disease).

The pathophysiological manifestations of the disorder are consistent with a cellular defect that interferes with the action of aldosterone in those segments of the renal tubule normally responsive to aldosterone, specifically the collecting tubules and ducts. According to current concepts of the mechanism of action of aldosterone, induced alterations in transepithelial ion transport occur consequent to the binding of aldosterone to high-affinity stereospecific receptors in the cytoplasm, an event which leads to modulation of DNA-dependent messenger RNA synthesis and consequent alterations in the cellular content of specific proteins, so-called aldosterone-induced proteins, which modulate or mediate the ion transport mechanism (155,156) (Fig. 19). In the only study of a patient with pseudohypoaldosteronism in which an attempt to examine binding of aldosterone in a target tissue was performed, the amount of tritiated aldosterone binding to mucosal cells obtained from the sigmoid colon was found to be similar to that observed in control subjects (79). In another report, a mineralocorticoid-responsive defect in transepithelial transport of sodium and potassium was demonstrated in multiple target organs of aldosterone, including the salivary glands, sweat glands, and colon as well as the kidney (75). Available data on the electrolyte composition of sweat in other reported cases of pseudohypoaldosteronism suggest that the sweat glands

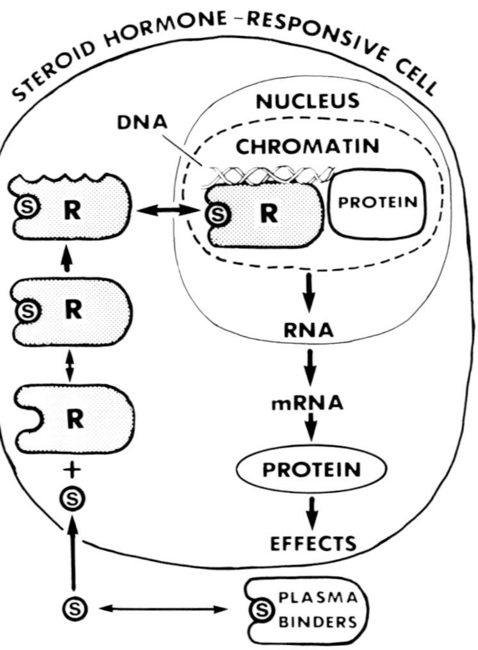

Fig. 19 Steps in steroid hormone action. After penetrating the cell membrane, steroid (S) combines with receptor (R), altering its conformation. SR then binds chromatin, and stimulates (or possibly represses) mRNA synthesis. The resulting changes in specific mRNAs result in alterations in the synthesis of specific proteins that mediate or reflect the steroid hormone response. (From Ref. 147.)

are either unresponsive to mineralocorticoid or subnormally responsive given the prevailing supernormal levels of circulating aldosterone (57,58,75). In no reported case, however, has the cellular mechanism of the defect in electrolyte transport been defined. Therefore, it remains to be determined whether a defect exists in the sequence of biochemical reactions initiated by binding of aldosterone to its receptor and culminating in the generation of aldosterone-induced proteins (Fig. 19).

It has been suggested that the renal tubule dysfunction of classic pseudohypoaldosteronism results from a deficiency of Na^+-K^+-ATPase, the ubiquitous membrane-bound enzyme that provides the fundamental cellular mechanism for maintaining the normally low concentrations of sodium and high concentrations of potassium in the cytoplasm relative to those in the extracellular fluid compartment (77). In the kidney, Na^+-K^+-ATPase is localized to the basolateral membranes of renal tubular cells in virtually every segment of the nephron, and it plays a critical role in net reabsorption of filtered sodium and net secretion of potassium by the renal tubule (157,158). Recent evidence suggests that it also plays a role in the acidification process of the distal nephron (159). Virtually no renal Na^+-K^+-ATPase activity was detectable in either proximal or distal nephron segments obtained by microdissection of biopsied renal tissue from one patient with classical pseudohypoaldosteronism (77). However, interpretation of this finding as indicative of a primary defect in renal Na^+-K^+-ATPase is questionable, since the specific activity of renal Na^+-K^+-ATPase is known to decrease under a variety of physiological circumstances that reduce net renal sodium reabsorption. In adrenalectomized animals the rate of net renal sodium reabsorption as varied by alterations in sodium chloride intake appears to be a major determinant of the specific activity of Na^+-K^+-ATPase, and mineralocorticoid-induced increases in Na^+, -K^+-ATPase activity appear to be secondary to stimulation of tubular sodium transport (160).

In classic pseudohypoaldosteronism the spontaneously occurring apparent amelioration of renal sodium wasting and potassium retention in the postinfancy period is associated with persisting supernormal levels of plasma renin and aldosterone. In one patient with classic pseudohypoaldosteronism and persisting hyperaldosteronism who was studied at age 9 years, normonatremia and normokalemia were maintained without dietary supplements of sodium chloride, but hyponatremia and hyperkalemia recurred in response to administration of the mineralocorticoid antagonist spironolactone (79). By contrast, normal subjects administered spironolactone chronically do not develop overt hyponatremia or hyperkalemia (161). Presumably, renal resistance to the action of aldosterone was incomplete in the patient with pseudohypoaldosteronism, and the supernormal levels of circulating aldosterone observed prior to spironolactone administration contributed to the maintenance of normokalemia and normonatremia.

It is not certain that the same fundamental pathogenetic disturbance underlies classic pseudohypoaldosteronism of infancy in all reported cases. The familial occurrence of the disorder has been documented in only a small fraction of the reported cases.

Systematic studies of the systemic acid-base disturbance in classic pseudohypoaldosteronism of infancy have not been carried out. In some cases severe metabolic acidosis is present as indicated by values of plasma bicarbonate concentration less than 10 meq/liter; in other cases metabolic acidosis is less severe or inapparent. The urine has been reported to be highly acidic in some cases; in other cases the pH of the urine has been reported to be abnormally high. Critical evaluation of urine acidity in relation to urine buffer content has not been carried out. It might be presumed that the renal acidification defect in patients with a specific impairment of renal aldosterone responsiveness would have physiolocial characteristics like those in patients with aldosterone deficiency states, but direct evidence to support such a presumption is lacking. If classic pseudohypoaldosteronism of infancy is a heterogeneous disorder, it is possible that more than one kind of acidification impairment underlies the occurrence of metabolic acidosis in reported cases.

B. Type 2 Pseudohypoaldosteronism (Aldosterone Resistance Without Salt-Wasting)

Renal tubular responsiveness to the action of aldosterone also appears to be impaired in a rare syndrome characterized by hyperkalemia, hyperchloremic metabolic acidosis, hypertension, hyporeninemia, and abnormally reduced aldosterone production (87-96). Glomerular filtration rate is in the normal range. Mineralocorticoid resistance is apparent by persistence of hyperkalemia and a markedly reduced kaliuretic response to large amounts of exogenously administered mineralocorticoid steroids. The antinatriuretic and antichloruretic responses to mineralocorticoid steroids may be intact. A primary defect in renal K^+ secretion has been proposed.

In one reported patient, during normal NaCl intake, fractional renal K^+ excretion was subnormal and increased only minimally during administration of large amounts of mineralocorticoid steroids (96). However, distal tubule K^+ secretion increased greatly when distal Na^+ delivery was increased with anions other than Cl^- (sulfate or bicarbonate) (Fig. 20). Thus, hyperkalemia and mineralocorticoid resistance did not appear to be due to an intrinsic defect in renal K^+ secretion. The finding of normal salivary and fecal secretion of K^+ further mitigated against a generalized defect in transepithelial transport of K^+.

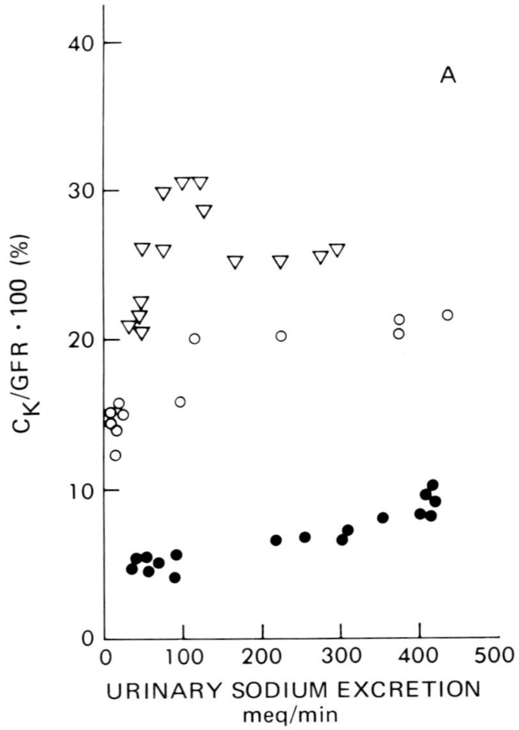

Fig. 20 Relationship between fractional renal potassium clearance (C_K/GFR 100) and (A) urinary sodium excretion during infusion of sodium chloride and (B) sodium sulfate in a patient with type 2 pseudohypoaldosteronism (filled circles) and normal subjects (unfilled symbols). Mineralocorticoid hormone (DOCA, 10 mg I.M.) was given 12 and 2 hr before the study.

The results of these studies indicate that mineralocorticoid-resistant renal hyperkalemia and acidosis in type 2 pseudohypoaldosteronism cannot be attributed to the absence of a renal potassium secretory mechanism, but instead may be dependent upon the amount of chloride available for reabsorption in the distal nephron (96). The findings suggest that the primary abnormality in this syndrome is a defect of the distal nephron that increases the reabsorptive avidity of the distal nephron for chloride, which (1) limits the sodium and mineralocorticoid-dependent voltage driving force for potassium and hydrogen secretion, resulting in hyperkalemia and acidosis, and (2) augments distal NaCl reabsorption, resulting in hyperchloremia, volume expansion, and hypertension (Fig. 21). Such a "chloride shunt" might arise as a result of an abnormal increase in the permeability of the distal nephron to chloride. Consistent with the presence of such a chloride shunt, restriction of dietary sodium chloride or administration of a chloruretic diuretic (furosemide, thiazide) ameliorates hyperkalemia and acidosis (90-92,94-96).

The occurrence of hyperchloremic metabolic acidosis can be readily explained as a consequence of abnormally enhanced absorption of chloride. In dogs in which renal chloride absorptive avidity is markedly increased by prior diuretic-induced extracellular fluid (ECF) volume depletion and sustained dietary chloride restriction, administration of chloride impairs renal acidification and induces hyperchloremic metabolic acidosis (162) (Fig. 22). In

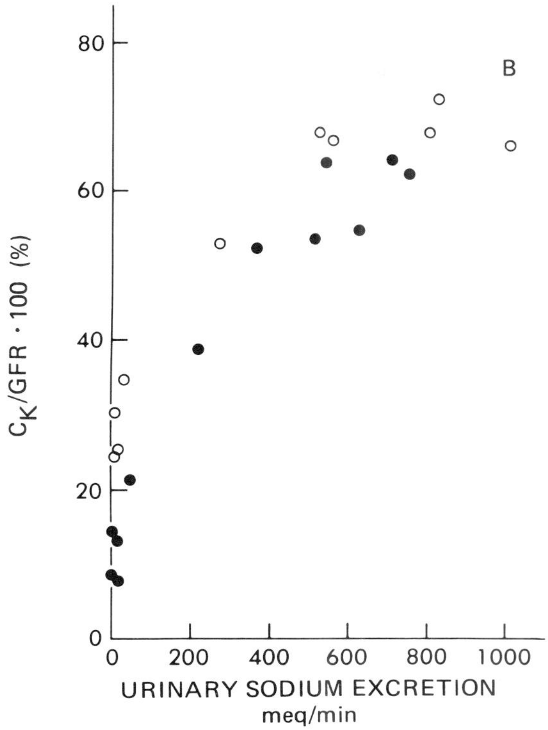

the patient the finding of a highly acidic urine (Fig. 23) might be interpreted as evidence against a reduction in transtubular potential in the distal nephron. However, in the turtle bladder, where the relationship between transepithelial potential and hydrogen ion secretion has been studied, elimination of the transepithelial potential has had little effect on the maximal hydrogen ion concentration gradient that can be generated, whereas it substantially reduces the net rate of transepithelial hydrogen ion secretion when an opposing hydrogen ion concentration gradient is not present (127). For any given H^+-secretory rate capacity, the acidity of the urine might be augmented by reduced availability of ammonia for diffusion into urine secondary to suppression of renal ammoniagenesis by hyperkalemia.

Hyperkalemia and hypervolemia may also contribute to the pathogenesis of metabolic acidosis in this disorder. Hyperkalemia is a potential renal acidosis-producing factor by virtue

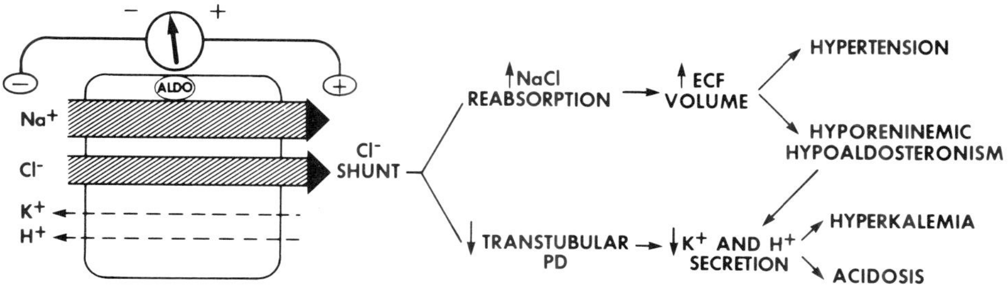

Fig. 21 Pathophysiologic consequences of abnormally increased distal nephron chloride reabsorption. (From Ref. 22.)

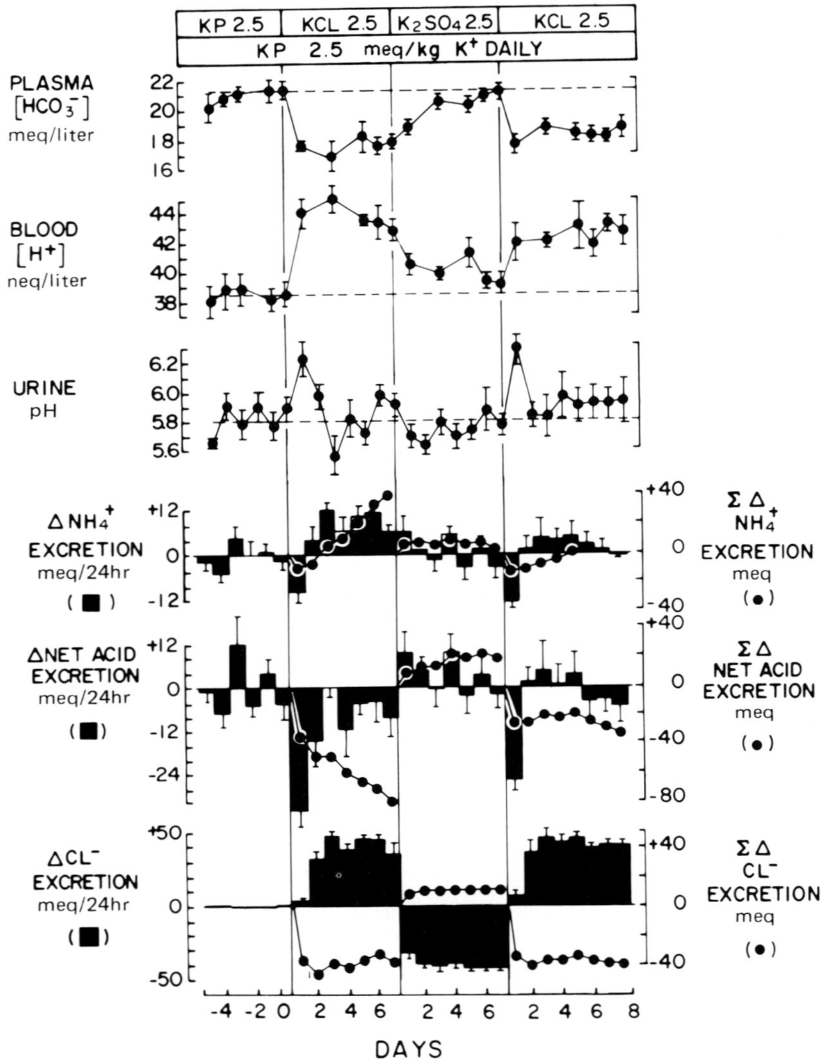

Fig. 22 Dietary chloride-induced renal tubular acidosis in dogs in which renal chloride absorptive avidity was markedly increased by prior diuretic induced ECF volume depletion and sustained dietary chloride restriction.

of its ability to reduce renal bicarbonate reabsorptive capacity (141) and to suppress renal production of ammonia (123). The availability of ammonia for diffusion into the tubular lumen is reduced, as indicated by the finding of subnormal urinary ammonium excretion during chronic acidosis despite highly acidic urine (10,19) (Fig. 23). Extracellular fluid volume expansion suppresses renal bicarbonate reabsorptive capacity (141,163,164) and may account in part for the observed reduction in renal bicarbonate reabsorption measured at normal plasma bicarbonate concentration after sustained correction of hyperkalemia observed in some patients (96).

It is possible that the occurrence of renal hyperkalemia and acidosis in this disorder is in part a consequence of hyporeninemia, which imposes a limitation on aldosterone secre-

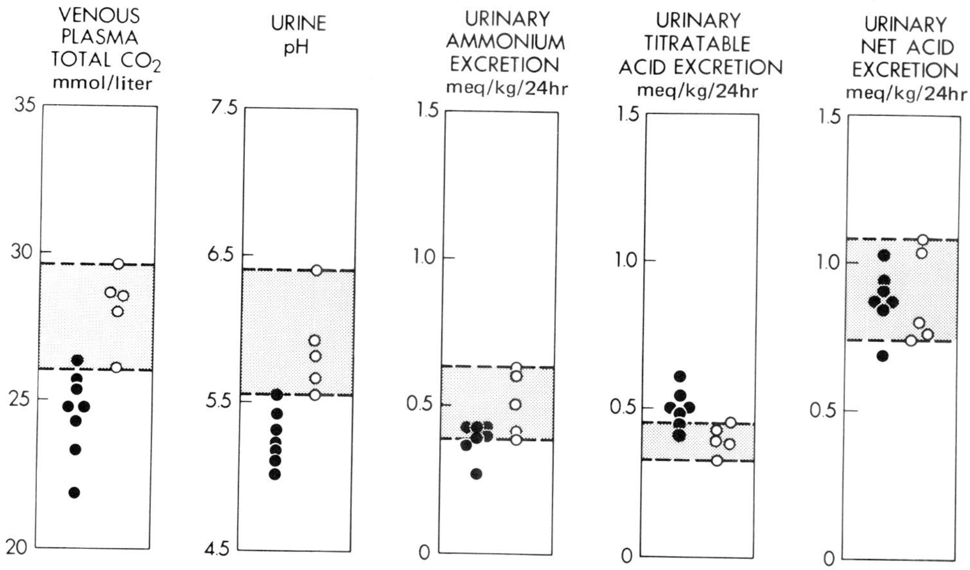

Fig. 23 Plasma and urine acid-base composition under steady-state conditions in a patient with type 2 pseudohypoaldosteronism who ingested a constant diet (filled circles). Steady-state values obtained in five similarly studied normal subjects are included for purposes of comparison (unfilled circles). Shaded areas delimit the range of values in normal subjects. The range of values in the patient reflect the degree of intraindividual variation in the steady-state inasmuch as there was no trend in the values during the 7-day period of observation represented in the figure. The finding that urinary net acid excretion in the steady-state is not supernormal indicates that the maintenance of systemic metabolic acidosis is not due to an increased systemic acid load but to a reduced set point at which the kidney is regulating plasma bicarbonate concentration. The finding that urinary ammonium excretion is not supernormal despite systemic acidosis and highly acidic urine suggests that the availability of ammonia for diffusion into urine is subnormal, presumably because renal production of ammonia is suppressed.

tion and consequently on aldosterone stimulation of renal potassium and hydrogen ion transport. Although plasma and urinary aldosterone levels may be in the upper limits of or above the normal range, much higher values than those observed would have been expected if plasma renin levels had not been suppressed, inasmuch as aldosterone secretion ordinarily increases in response to hyperkalemia (106-109). The possibility that such relative hypoaldosteronism contributed to the degree of hyperkalemia is suggested by the finding that the lowest levels of serum potassium are observed during chronic treatment with large doses of mineralocorticoid hormones.

Gordon et al. (90) suggested that hyporeninemia and hypoaldosteronism in this syndrome occurred as a consequence of extracellular fluid volume expansion due to abnormally increased reabsorption of sodium by the renal tubule proximal to the aldosterone-responsive segment of the nephron. It was postulated that sodium balance was reestablished by a "tubular escape mechanism" initiated and maintained by hypervolemia and that persistent hyperkalemia was due to aldosterone deficiency. However, aldosterone deficiency cannot account for the persistence of hyperkalemia observed during treatment with mineralocorticoid hormone or for the subnormal kaliuretic response when delivery of sodium to the distal nephron is increased further by infusion of sodium chloride. The findings are compatible with abnormally increased tubular reabsorption of sodium as suggested by Gordon et al. (90) if it is postulated that the abnormality resides in the aldosterone-responsive segment of the nephron and is the consequence of an abnormality such as enhanced renal tubular reabsorption of chloride that limits potassium-sodium exchange independent of the level of aldosterone.

It is possible that the primary abnormality in this disorder is a defect in the transport mechanism for potassium. A defect in the active (electrogenic) component of potassium secretion in the collecting tubule would be expected to enhance lumen negativity and thereby increase the electrical driving force for chloride reabsorption (165,166). The observation in rats that depletion of body potassium impairs chloride permeability in the distal nephron raises the possibility that increased renal cellular potassium content secondary to a defective potassium secretory pump on the luminal membrane would have the opposite effect, i.e., enhance chloride permeability (167). Hence, alterations in renal cellular potassium content secondary to a primary defect in potassium transport may be accompanied by alterations in cellular metabolism and membrane structure that conceivably could cause enhancement of chloride reabsorption (123,168,169). It remains to be determined whether the same primary abnormality underlies type 2 pseudohypoaldosteronism in all reported cases.

V. HYPERKALEMIA IN PATIENTS WITH TYPE 1 RTA

A. Diagnostic Considerations

Batlle and co-workers (43) have suggested that in some patients with hyperkalemic RTA, impaired renal hydrogen ion secretion results not from aldosterone deficiency or a chloride shunt but from a defect of the distal nephron like that which underlies type 1 (classic, distal) RTA. This suggestion was based on the results of studies carried out in patients in whom hyperkalemic RTA was associated with obstructive uropathy and reduced glomerular filtration rate. Despite the presence of spontaneous metabolic acidosis, in some patients the pH of the urine was greater than 5.5 and it did not decrease below 5.5 in response to acute administration of fludrocortisone and sodium sulfate. In normal subjects, acute administration of fludrocortisone and sodium sulfate decreases urine pH to values less than 5.5, presumably because of an increase in lumen-negative transtubular electrical potential difference in the distal nephron induced by fludrocortisone-stimulated reabsorption of sodium under conditions of increased delivery of sodium with an anion (sulfate) that is poorly reabsorbable by the distal nephron. In the patients studied by Batlle and co-workers (43), the impairment of renal hydrogen ion secretion (and of potassium secretion) was considered to be the consequence of a defect of the sodium reabsorption mechanism in the distal nephron. The kind and severity of the defect was believed to be such as to reduce the normally present lumen-negative transtubular electrical potential difference that ordinarily provides the major driving force for distal nephron hydrogen and potassium secretion, and it was believed that the defect was not corrected by administration of fludrocortisone and sodium sulfate. Batlle and co-workers (43) designated this group of patients as having hyperkalemic distal renal tubular acidosis, and considered their renal acidification defect to be physiologically distinct from that occurring in selective aldosterone deficiency.

However, the finding of values of urine pH greater than 5.5 in the presence of spontaneous metabolic acidosis is not diagnostic of type 1 renal tubular acidosis. Rather, the characteristic feature of type 1 RTA is the finding that an inappropriately high urine pH (usually >5.5) is present irrespective of the severity of systemic acidosis, in particular, when the severity of acidosis is exacerbated by exogenous (or endogenous) acid loading. In a patient with RTA of unidentified type, the finding of values of urine pH greater than 5.5 during spontaneous acidosis does not exclude the possibility that the pH of the urine would decrease to values considerably less than 5.5 with an increased severity of acidosis consequent to exogenous acid loading or ingestion of a diet that causes a higher rate of endogenous acid production. This proposition is supported by the data shown in Table 3, which summarizes the results of a metabolic balance study in a 53-year-old woman with chronic tubulointerstitial disease and hyperkalemic RTA in whom a constant diet of normal sodium (104 meq/24 hr) and potassium (49 meq/24 hr) content was initiated beginning on day 1 of the study. Evidently, the endogenous acid production resulting from metabolism of the imposed diet exceeded that resulting from the patient's self-selected diet ingested prior to initiation of the study, since the severity of the initial spontaneous acidosis progressively worsened in association with a progressive increase in net acid excretion following day 1 of the study. Yet, despite the presence of spontaneous acidosis, urine pH exceeded 5.5 at least for 4 successive days of observation (days 1-4). However, this criterion cannot be taken as sufficient for the diagnosis of type 1 RTA inasmuch as there was a subsequent reduction of urine pH to values approaching 5 when a more severe degree of acidosis developed in response to the endogenous acid load from the imposed diet (days 5-12).

Furthermore, nonreduction of urine pH below 5.5 following fludrocortisone and sodium sulfate administration cannot be taken as a reliable criterion for the diagnosis of type 1 RTA. The reason for this is that in patients with reduced numbers of functional nephrons the osmotic load of sodium sulfate, added to that resulting from azotemia, may sweep bicarbonate-rich luminal fluid from more proximal segments of the nephron to the more distal segments, with the result that the urine pH-lowering effect of fludrocortisone-stimulated distal hydrogen ion secretion is offset by increased bicarbonate delivery (171). Indeed, in patients with

Table 3 Plasma and Urine Acid-Base and Electrolyte Composition Following Discontinuation of an Ad Lib Diet and Initiation of a Constant Diet in a Patient with Chronic Tubulointerstitial Disease[a]

	Serum			Urine				
	Na^+	K^+	HCO_3^-	pH	NAE	Na^+	K^+	C_{creat}
Day	meq/liter				meq/24 hr			ml/min
1	144	5.4	19	6.29	25	144	44	22
2	142	5.0	17	6.08	26	110	38	22
3	144	5.3	16	5.73	27	80	35	20
4	140	5.2	16	5.60	31	94	38	19
5	140	5.4	16	5.29	32	59	34	19
6	138	4.7	15	5.28	42	90	37	18
7[b]	145	5.1	9	5.24	47	98	42	20
8	141	5.1	11	5.17	46	80	37	19
9	140	4.8	11	5.10	52	78	38	19
10	143	5.0	13	5.05	48	72	34	16
11	141	4.8	15	5.07	52	80	42	18
12	140	4.9	11	5.09	54	84	37	19

[a]Beginning on day 1, the patient ingested a constant diet consisting of 104 meq Na^+ and 49 meq K^+ per 24 hr.

[b]Arterial blood pH 7.32, PCO_2 24 torr.

chronic renal insufficiency, urine pH almost invariably increases, rather than decreases, in response to fludrocortisone and sodium sulfate administration when the preadministration value of urine pH is between 5.5 and 6.8 (n = 12) (171), precisely a range of values over which the question of the diagnosis of type 1 RTA arises. (At lower initial values of urine pH in the same patients, the urine pH characteristically decreases [usually to values well below 5.5] in response to fludrocortisone and sodium sulfate administration [171].) Therefore, nonreduction of urine pH below 5.5 following fludrocortisone and sodium sulfate administration is not a reliable indicator of a type 1 RTA defect in patients with reduced glomerular filtration rate. In such patients, small differences in plasma bicarbonate concentration in the acidotic range may be associated with relatively large differences in urine pH over the relatively broad range from 5 to 7 (172). With a lesser as opposed to a greater degree of acidosis in the same patient, the plasma bicarbonate concentration, the filtered load and luminal concentration of bicarbonate, and the urine pH will be higher, and the urine pH response to fludrocortisone and sodium sulfate may fail to reflect an unimpaired ability of the distal nephron to acidify the urine. As noted above (Table 3), such differences in degree of acidosis may be determined by corresponding differences in net endogenous acid production. The latter in turn depends on differences in the composition of the diet, in particular whether or not alkali salts have been added to the diet to partially neutralize metabolic acid and minimize the degree of metabolic acidosis (171,172).

These considerations should not be construed as an argument that in patients with chronic glomerular insufficiency the finding of values of urine pH less than 5.5 excludes the presence of a distal nephron acidification defect like that of type 1 RTA. The finding that a patient with renal acidosis can lower urine pH to values less than 5.5 during spontaneously worsening acidosis (as in the patient in Table 3) is not incompatible with the presence of a distal nephron acidification defect like that in patients with type 1 RTA, since, however low urine pH may be, it may still be abnormally high in relation to the expected values of urine pH in normal subjects studied under the same physiological conditions that promote urine acidification. By comparison with the patient in Table 3, normal subjects might have substantially lower values of urine pH than the lowest value (5.05) achieved by the patient if their degree and duration of systemic acidosis, their bicarbonate delivery rate to the distal nephron, their ammonia production rate, their non-NH_3 buffer delivery rate to the distal nephron, and their aldosterone level and responsiveness were similar to those in the patient. Unfortunately, criteria are not available for ascertaining the normality of urine pH in relation to the coordinate effect of the complex of these factors that modulate urine pH. Thus, the considerations in the previous paragraphs do not imply that a distal nephron acidification defect like that in patients with type 1 RTA can be excluded in patients such as the patient in Table 3, but assert only that a positive diagnosis of type 1 RTA is unwarranted. As noted previously, the characteristic feature of type 1 RTA is the finding that an inappropriately high urine pH (*usually* >5.5) is present irrespective of the severity of systemic acidosis, in particular, when the severity of acidosis is exacerbated by exogenous or endogenous acid loading.

Notwithstanding these considerations, the possibility remains that in at least some of the patients studied by Batlle and co-workers (43), there was an intrinsic impairment of distal nephron acidification and urine pH-lowering ability like that occurring in patients with classic, type 1 RTA. As noted by Batlle and co-workers (43), a model of hyperkalemic RTA with physiological characteristics like that of type 1 RTA can be induced experimentally by administration of amiloride, a pharmacological agent that inhibits sodium reabsorption and potassium secretion in post-macula densa segments of the distal nephron. The weight of evidence suggests that amiloride-induced renal tubular acidosis results secondary to amiloride's action to inhibit sodium reabsorption (see below). The character of amiloride-induced renal tubular acidosis and the role of sodium reabsorption in mammalian acidification is discussed in the following section.

B. Hyperkalemic RTA Induced by Amiloride Administration: Interrelation of H^+ Secretion and Na^+ Reabsorption in Mammalian Distal Nephron

The results of clearance and balance studies in dogs and man have suggested a close association between hydrogen ion secretion and sodium reabsorption in the distal nephron. Net acid excretion has been shown to increase under conditions in which distal sodium reabsorption is enhanced due to increased distal sodium delivery and/or sodium reabsorptive avidity (173). Whether, under ordinary physiological circumstances, basal rates of distal hydrogen ion secretion and net acid excretion are dependent of distal sodium reabsorption is not known, however. Reduction of basal sodium reabsorption by experimental induction of aldosterone deficiency is associated with a reduction in net acid excretion (19,25,122), but this relationship cannot be interpreted as a causal one since in vitro studies have indicated that aldosterone stimulates hydrogen ion secretion even when changes in transepithelial sodium transport are prevented (130). Stimulation of hydrogen ion secretion secondary to increased sodium reabsorption in the distal nephron may be mediated through changes in transepithelial electrical potential difference, inasmuch as the stimulation of acidification is augmented when distal delivery of sodium occurs with anions less reabsorbable than chloride, a maneuver which amplifies stimulation of potential difference (170,174). Voltage-driven acidification in the mammalian distal nephron has been recently demonstrated (132) and has been demonstrated in vertebrate urinary epithelia, which originates embryologically from the same anlage as the mammalian collecting duct (124,129).

Perhaps the best evidence that distal hydrogen ion secretion is dependent on basal sodium reabsorption under ordinary physiological conditions is the finding that net acid excretion decreases following administration of amiloride or triamterene, distally acting natriutetic agents known to inhibit directly sodium transport at the cell membrane (175). Extensive studies of the mechanism of action of amiloride in transcellular sodium transport have indicated that the agent binds to the mucosal membrane of the cell, blocks passive entry of sodium down its electrochemical gradient (176,177), and thereby diminishes the transepithelial electrical potential difference (178-180). Inhibition of acidification by amiloride has been demonstrated in toad urinary bladder (178). The results indicate that the inhibition of acidification is mediated by inhibition of the mucosa-negative transepithelial potential difference and that acidification is restimulated on application of the transepithelial potential despite the continued presence of amiloride.

Hulter and co-workers (145) investigated the effects of long-term administration of a demonstrably maximal dose of amiloride on plasma and urine acid-base and electrolyte composition in adrenalectomized dogs receiving glucocorticoid and mineralocorticoid steroids in fixed physiological replacement doses. Amiloride administration resulted in potassium retention and hyperkalemia and reduced net acid excretion and caused chronic hyperchloremic metabolic acidosis (Fig. 24). The cumulative reduction in net acid excretion and severity of systemic acidosis were not significantly different in additional groups in which potassium retention was prevented by restriction of dietary potassium during amiloride administration or in which amiloride was administered to animals with preexisting dietary potassium depletion. The response of urine pH and ammonium excretion, however, differed among groups.

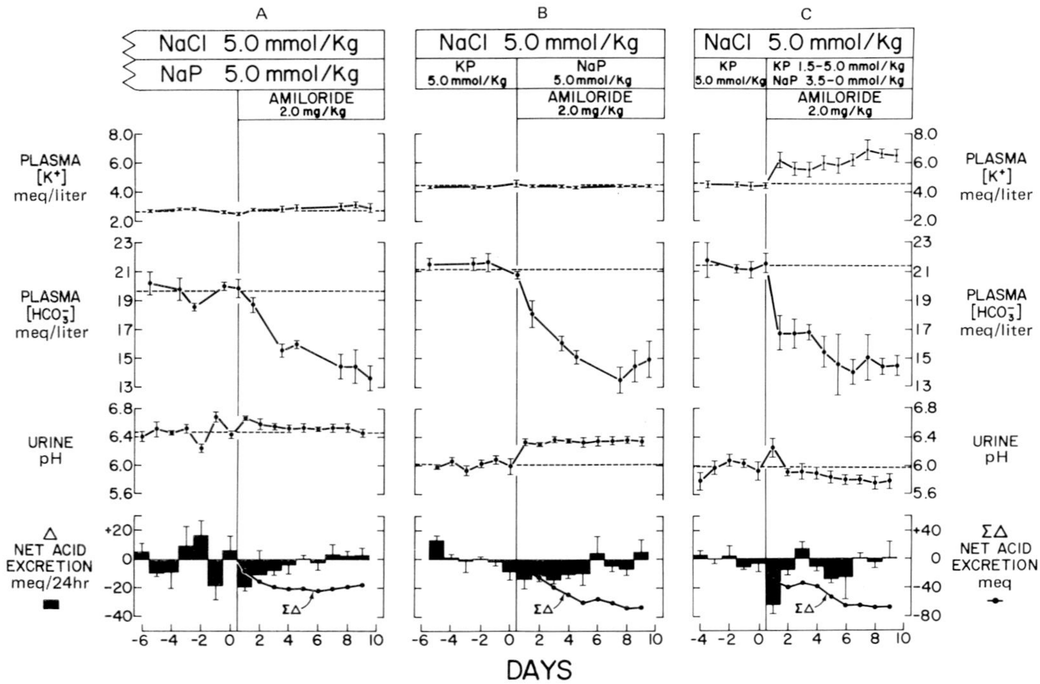

Fig. 24 Effects of long-term amiloride administration on plasma and urinary acid-base and electrolyte composition in adrenalectomized dogs maintained on fixed-steroid replacement. (B) Response in dogs maintained normokalemic both prior to and during amiloride administration (group I, n = 5); (A) response in previously potassium-depleted dogs (group II, n = 4); (C) response in dogs permitted to develop chronic hyperkalemia and potassium retention (group II, n = 4). Brackets represent standard error of the mean. (From Ref. 137.)

In the steady state of chronic acidosis, urine pH and ammonium concentration were lowest in the hyperkalemic group and highest in the hypokalemic group, and among the three groups pH and ammonium were positively correlated ($r = 0.67$, $p<0.001$). Ammonium concentration varied inversely with plasma potassium concentration. Net acid excretion rates returned to control levels during the steady-state of chronic amiloride-induced acidosis in the three groups (Fig. 24). During continued amiloride administration, sustained correction of acidosis by long-term oral administration of sodium bicarbonate did not result in negative values of net acid excretion; that is, amiloride did not cause net wasting of base at normal plasma bicarbonate concentration.

The results of these studies suggest that chronic amiloride administration results in a sustained impairment of renal hydrogen ion secretion restricted to the distal nephron and not dependent on alterations in potassium balance (145). Differences in potassium balance (positive or negative) appeared to influence only the availability of ammonia for diffusion into urine and steady-state urine pH, but not the steady-state net rate of renal hydrogen ion secretion during amiloride.

Based on the known cellular mechanism of action of amiloride, the results of these studies suggest that basal sodium reabsorption in the distal nephron provides a tonic stimulatory effect on distal nephron hydrogen ion secretion. Studies of isolated epithelia (frog skin and toad bladder) indicate that amiloride inhibits passive cellular entry of sodium from mucosal fluid. This effect of amiloride presumably explains the observed drug-induced decrease in cellular sodium content (177), increase in cellular negative charge (180), and decrease in mucosa-negative (or lumen-negative) transepithelial potential difference (178,179,181). In toad bladder, the amiloride-induced decrease in mucosa-negative voltage has been shown to account fully for the observed reduction in mucosal acidification (178), inasmuch as acidification rates normalized in response to an applied mucosa-negative voltage despite the continued presence of amiloride. In the turtle bladder, however, it has been shown that amiloride inhibits acidification even in the absence of transepithelial electrochemical gradients (182). But an electrophysiological inhibition of acidification is not excluded, inasmuch as an amiloride-induced increase in cellular negativity might inhibit acidification despite maintained absence of transepithelial potential difference (183). In isolated rabbit cortical collecting tubules, amiloride has recently been shown to inhibit bicarbonate absorption in association with a reduction in lumen-negative potential difference (184).

C. Classification of Distal RTA and Comparison of Type 1 RTA vs. Type 4 RTA

Some investigators restrict the designation distal RTA to those cases in which the pH of the urine remains inappropriately high (usually greater than 5.5) despite severe degrees of acidosis or acidosis that is exacerbated by exogenous (or endogenous) acid loading. Evidence that the acidification defect in these cases is localized to the distal nephron, and specifically to the collecting ducts, is reviewed in another chapter in this book and has previously been reviewed by other investigators. But the rationale for restriction of the designation distal RTA to these cases can be questioned since an acidosis-causing impairment of hydrogen ion secretion in the distal nephron can be present even though the urine pH-lowering ability of the distal nephron does not appear to be impaired, as in the example of the distal nephron acidification dysfunction resulting from aldosterone deficiency. It is perhaps more rational to employ a typological classification of RTA based not on nephronal localization (or inferred cellular mechanism) of acidification defect but rather on clinical and laboratory findings. Patients with type 1 RTA and patients with type 4 RTA both have distal RTA, but the clinical and laboratory findings differ.

Patients with type 1 RTA and those with type 4 RTA may share not only a common site of nephronal localization of acidification impairment but also a common cellular mechanism of the acidification impairment. In both, the ability of the kidney to generate steep blood to urine hydrogen ion concentration gradients is not lost, with the result that values of urine pH considerably lower than 5.5 can be generated. Such an extant urine pH-lowering ability of the distal nephron in some patients with type 1 RTA is revealed during the administration of pharmacological agents that inhibit renal tubular chloride reabsorption (185, 186), and in some cases, during administration of mineralocorticoid and sodium sulfate (187, 188). Furthermore, both in some patients with type 1 RTA and in patients with type 4 RTA, there appears to be a "rate defect" of distal nephron hydrogen ion secretion: The ability of the distal nephron to secrete hydrogen ion at normal rates is impaired even under conditions in which the blood to lumen hydrogen ion concentration gradient opposing hydrogen ion secretion has been eliminated or minimized by bicarbonate loading. In patients with type 1 RTA, such a rate defect of distal nephron hydrogen ion secretion has been inferred from the finding of an abnormally low urine to blood gradient of carbon dioxide tension during bicarbonate loading (189,190). In patients with type 4 RTA, evidence of a rate defect of distal nephron hydrogen ion secretion, unaccompanied by impairment of urine pH-lowering

Table 4 Determinants of the Rate of Collecting Duct Active Hydrogen Ion Secretion

1. Magnitude of transtubular H^+ concentration gradient
   a. Availability of luminal buffers (NH_3, HPO_4^{2-})
   b. Concentration of cellular H^+
2. Magnitude of transtubular electrical gradient
   a. Rate of Na^+ reabsorption
   b. Rate of Cl^- reabsorption
3. Production/transduction of metabolic energy for activity of H^+ secretory pumps
4. Integrity of H^+ secretory pumps
5. Number of H^+ secretory pumps

Table 5 Hypothetical Mechanisms of Impaired Collecting Duct Function Resulting in Renal Tubular Acidosis[a]

I. Decreased cell to lumen unidirectional active H^+ secretion
   A. Impaired function or reduced number of H^+ secretory pumps on luminal membrane
      1. Decreased strength (proton motive force) of pumps
      2. Decreased conductance of protons
         a. Decreased number of pumps
         b. Defect in active transport pathway
            (1) Defect in metabolic energy production
            (2) Defect in metabolic energy utilization
            (3) Structural defect of pump
   B. Reduction in electrochemical gradient that ordinarily promotes H^+ secretion
      1. Reduced lumen-negative transtubular electrical potential
         a. Reduced sodium reabsorption
         b. Enhanced potassium secretion
         c. Enhanced chloride reabsorption
      2. Reduced availability of cellular H^+
         a. Impaired exit of cellular bicarbonate or OH^- to peritubular fluid
         b. Carbonic anhydrase defect
      3. Increased luminal $[H^+]$ secondary to reduced concentration of luminal proton acceptors
         a. Impaired ammoniagenesis
         b. Impaired medullary ammonia delivery
         c. Hypophosphaturia
II. Impaired luminal acidification despite normal or increased cell to lumen unidirectional active H^+ secretion
   A. Permeability defect
      1. Backleak of luminal H^+ through cell membrane or between cells
      2. Increased luminal entry of HCO_3^-, CO_3^{2-}, or OH^-
   B. Abnormal stimulation of active HCO_3^- secretion or HCO_3^-/Cl^- exchange

[a]Precedent for many of the hypothetical mechanisms outlined in this table can be found in publications cited in an earlier version of the table (23).

ability, has been presented in earlier sections of this chapter. Thus, both patients with type 1 RTA and patients with type 4 RTA can be described as having distal RTA characterized by a rate defect of distal nephron hydrogen ion secretion unassociated with an obligatory loss of hydrogen ion concentration gradient-generating ability (blood to lumen).

These considerations support the view that given the present state of our knowledge it is perhaps more rational to employ a typological classification of renal tubular acidosis based on clinical and laboratory findings rather than an anatomical or mechanistic classification based on inferred nephronal localization or cellular mechanism of acidification defect. With respect to the cellular mechanism of acidification in the renal collecting duct, there are at least five separable determinants of the rate of hydrogen ion secretion that must be taken into consideration (Table 4). For each of these separate determinants of the rate of collecting duct hydrogen ion secretion there may be several alternative physiologically distinct disturbances that might lead to clinical renal tubular acidosis (Table 5). It is not possible on the basis of current knowledge to distinguish among these alternatives unequivocally from the results of in vivo studies in humans with renal tubular acidosis.

ACKNOWLEDGMENTS

These studies were supported by U.S. Public Health Service research grants AM 21605, AM 06415, AM28643, and AM 31626 from the National Institute of Arthritis, Diabetes, Digestive and Kidney Diseases, and HL 11046 and HL 06285 from the National Heart, Lung, and Blood Institute. Dr. Hulter is supported in part from grant SF 76-83, Public Health Service Central Clinical Investigation Committee. Dr. Kurtz is supported by a Fellowship from the Medical Research Council of Canada. Additional support was provided by the Academic Senate Committee on Research at the University of California, San Francisco Medical Center. The studies in humans were carried out on the General Clinical Research Centers at Moffitt and San Francisco General Hospitals, University of California, San Francisco, supported by the Division of Research Resources (RR 79, RR 83), National Institutes of Health.

We wish to express special thanks to Patricia Douglass for numerous contributions in all phases of these studies from inception to preparation of the final manuscript. We thank Vivien Ho, Joan Colman, Kenneth Kwang-Soo Son, Margaret Murphy, Bernadina Serena, Joann Schweiger, Keith Slater, Norma Brust, Barbara Chang, Joy Hirai, and Irene Agasid for technical assistance; and the nursing and dietary staff of the General Clinical Research Centers.

REFERENCES

1. Seldin, D. W.; Carter, N. W.; and Rector, F. C., Jr. Consequences of renal failure and their management. In: Diseases of the Kidney, 2nd ed., edited by Strauss, M. B., and Welt, L. G. Boston, Little, Brown, 1971, pp. 211-272.
2. Hodler, J. Etude de l'acidose au cours de pyelonephrites, de glomerulonephrites et de nephroscleroses avancees. Proceedings of the 1st International Congress of Nephrology. Geneva, Evian Publishers, 1961, pp. 611-615.
3. Elkinton, J. R. Hydrogen ion turnover in health and in renal disease. Ann. Int. Med. 57: 660-684, 1962.
4. Widmer, B.; Gerhardt, R. E.; Harrington, J. T.; and Cohen, J. J. Serum electrolyte and acid base composition. The influence of graded degrees of chronic renal failure. Arch. Intern. Med. 139:1099-1102, 1979.

5. Schambelan, M.; Sebastian, A.; and Biglieri, E. G. Prevalence, pathogenesis, and functional significance of aldosterone deficiency in hyperkalemic patients with chronic renal insufficiency. Kidney Int. 17:89-101, 1980.
6. Berl, T.; Katz, F. H.; Henrich, W. L.; DeTorrente, A.; and Schrier, R. W. Role of aldosterone in the control of sodium excretion in patients with advanced chronic renal failure. Kidney Int. 14:228-235, 1978.
7. Weidmann, P.; Maxwell, M. H.; Rowe, P.; Winer, R.; and Massry, S. G. Role of the renin-angiotensin-aldosterone system in the regulation of plasma potassium in chronic renal disease. Nephron 15:35-49, 1975.
8. Leaf, A.; and Camara, A. A. Renal tubular secretion of potassium in man. J. Clin. Invest. 28:1526-1533, 1949.
9. Hene, R. J.; Boer, P.; Koomans, H. A.; and Mees, E. J. D. Plasma aldosterone concentrations in chronic renal disease. Kidney Int. 21:98-101, 1982.
10. Sebastian, A.; Schambelan, M.; Lindenfeld, S.; and Morris, R. C., Jr. Amelioration of metabolic acidosis with fludrocortisone therapy in hyporeninemic hypoaldosteronism. N. Engl. J. Med. 297:576-583, 1977.
11. Carroll, H. J.; and Farber, S. J. Hyperkalemia and hyperchloremic acidosis in chronic pyelonephritis. Metabolism 13:808-817, 1964.
12. Phelps, K. R.; Lieberman, R. L.; Oh, M. S.; and Caroll, H. J. Pathophysiology of the syndrome of hyporeninemic hypoaldosteronism. Metabolism 29:186-199, 1980.
13. Perez, G. O.; Oster, J. R.; and Vaamonde, C. A. Renal acidosis and renal potassium handling in selective hyperaldosteronism. Am. J. Med. 57:809-815, 1974.
14. Sebastian, A.; McSherry, E.; Schambelan, M.; Connor, D.; Biglieri, E.; and Morris, R. C., Jr. Renal tubular acidosis (RTA) in patients with hypoaldosteronism caused by renin deficiency. Clin. Res. 21:706, 1973.
15. Sebastian, A.; McSherry, E.; and Morris, R. C., Jr. Metabolic acidosis with special reference to the renal acidoses. In: The Kidney, edited by Brenner, B. M., and Rector, F. C., Jr., Philadelphia, Saunders, 1976, pp. 615-660.
16. Sebastian, A.; Hulter, H. N.; and Schambelan, M. Renal hyperchloremic acidosis with hyperkalemia: Type 4 renal tubular acidosis (RTA). Proceedings of the VIIth International Congress of Nephrology. Montreal, Karger, 1978, pp. 351-360.
17. Sebastian, A.; and Morris, R. C., Jr. Renal tubular acidosis. In: Strauss and Welt's Diseases of the Kidney, 3rd ed., edited by Early, L. E., and Gottschalk, C. G. Boston, Little, Brown, 1979, pp. 1029-1054.
18. Schambelan, M.; Sebastian, A.; and Hulter, H. N. Mineralocorticoid excess and deficiency syndrome. In: Contemporary Issues in Nephrology, Acid-Base and Potassium Homeostasis, vol. 2, edited by Brenner, B. M., and Stein, J. H. New York, Churchill Livingstone, 1978, pp. 232-268.
19. Hulter, H. N.; Ilnicki, L. P.; Harbottle, J. A.; and Sebastian, A. Impaired renal H^+ secretion and NH_3 production in mineralocorticoid-deficient glucocorticoid-replete dogs. Am. J. Physiol. 232:F136-F146, 1977.
20. Arruda, J. A. L.; Batlle, D. C.; Sehy, J. T.; Roseman, M. K.; Baronowski, R. L.; and Kurtzman, N. A. Hyperkalemia and renal insufficiency: Role of selective aldosterone deficiency and tubular unresponsiveness to aldosterone. Am. J. Nephrol. 1:160-167, 1981.
21. Batlle, D. C. Hyperkalemic hyperchloremic metabolic acidosis associated with selective aldosterone deficiency and distal renal tubular acidosis. Semin. Nephrol. 1:260-274, 1981.
22. Sebastian, A.; Hulter, H. N.; Kurtz, I.; Maher, T.; and Schambelan, M. Disorders of distal nephron function. Am. J. Med. 72:289-307, 1982.
23. Morris, R. C., Jr.; and Sebastian, A. Renal tubular acidosis and Fanconi's syndrome. In: The Metabolic Basis of Inherited Disease, 5th ed., edited by Stanbury, J. B., Wyngaarden, J. B., and Fredrickson, D. S. New York, McGraw-Hill, 1982, pp. 1808-1843.

24. Perez, G. O.; Oster, J. R.; and Vaamonde, C. A. Renal acidification in patients with mineralocorticoid deficiency. Nephron 17:461-473, 1976.
25. Sebastian, A.; Sutton, J. M.; Hulter, H. N.; Schambelan, M.; and Poler, S. M. Effect of mineralocorticoid replacement therapy on renal acid-base homeostasis in adrenalectomized patients. Kidney Int. 18:762-773, 1980.
26. Oetliker, O. H.; and Zurbrugg, R. P. Renal tubular acidosis in salt-losing syndrome of congenital adrenal hyperplasia (CAH). J. Clin. Endocrinol. Metab. 31:447-450, 1970.
27. Imai, M.; Igarashi, Y.; and Sokabe, H. Plasma renin activity in congenital virilizing adrenal hyperplasia. Pediatrics 41:897-904, 1968.
28. Oetliker, O. H.; and Zurbrugg, R. P. Renal regulation of fluid, electrolyte, and acid-base homeostasis in the salt-losing syndrome of congenital adrenal hyperplasia (SL-CAH). ECF volume: A compensating factor in aldosterone deficiency. J. Clin. Endocrinol. Metab. 46:543-551, 1978.
29. DiBona, F. J.; and Kelsch, R. C. Severe uncompensated metabolic acidosis secondary to ammonium chloride loading. J. Pediatr. 91:263-265, 1979.
30. Rosler, A.; Theodor, R.; Boichis, H.; Gerty, R.; Ulick, S.; Alagem, M.; Tabachnik, E.; Cohen, B.; Rabinowitz, D. Metabolic responses to the administration of angiotensin II, K and ACTH in two salt-wasting syndromes. J. Clin. Endocrinol. Metab. 44:292-301, 1977.
31. Rosler, A.; Rabinowitz, D.; Theodor, R.; Ramirez, L. C.; and Ulick, S. The nature of the defect in a salt-wasting disorder in Jews of Iran. J. Clin. Endocrinol. Metab. 44: 279-281, 1977.
32. Ulick, S. Diagnosis and nomenclature of the disorders of the terminal portion of the aldosterone biosynthetic pathway. J. Clin. Endocrinol. Metab. 43:92-96, 1976.
33. David, R.; Golan, S.; and Drucker, W. Familial aldosterone deficiency: Enzyme defect, diagnosis, and clinical course. Pediatrics 41:403-412, 1968.
34. Rosler, A.; Gazit, E.; Theodor, R.; Biochis, H.; and Rabinowitz, D. Salt wastage, raised plasma-renin activity, and normal or high plasma-aldosterone: A form of pseudohypoaldosteronism. Lancet 1:959-962, 1973.
35. Veldhuis, J. D.; Kulin, H. E.; Santen, R. J.; Wilson, T. E.; and Melby, J. C. Inborn error in the terminal step of aldosterone biosynthesis: Corticosterone methyl oxidase type II deficiency in a North American pedigree. N. Engl. J. Med. 303:117-121, 1980.
36. Katznelson, D.; Sack, J.; Kraiem, Z.; and Lunenfeld, B. Congenital hypoaldosteronism. Thirteen year follow-up in identical twins. Hormone Res. 11:22-28, 1979.
37. Wilson, I. D.; and Goetz, F. C. Selective hypoaldosteronism after prolonged heparin administration. A case report, with postmortem findings. Am. J. Med. 36:635-640, 1964.
38. Schambelan, M.; Stockigt, J. R.; and Biglieri, E. G. Isolated hypoaldosteronism in adults, a renin deficiency syndrome. N. Engl. J. Med. 287:573-578, 1972.
39. Perez, G.; Siegel, L.; and Schreiner, G. E. Selective hypoaldosteronism with hyperkalemia. Ann. Intern. Med. 76:757-763, 1972.
40. Brown, J. J.; Chinn, R. H.; Fraser, R.; Lever, A. F.; Morton, J. J.; Robertson, J. I. S.; Three, M.; Waite, M. A.; and Park, D. M. Recurrent hyperkalaemia due to selective aldosterone deficiency. Correction by angiotensin infusion. Br. Med. J. 1:650-653, 1973.
41. Weidmann, P.; Reinhart, R.; Maxwell, M. H.; Rowe, P.; Coburn, J. W.; and Massry, S. G. Syndrome of hyporeninemic hypoaldosteronism and hyperkalemia in renal disease. J. Clin. Endocrinol. Metab. 36:965-977, 1973.
42. Oh, M. S.; Carroll, H. J.; Clemmons, J. E.; Vagnucci, A. H.; Levison, S. P.; and Whang, E. S. M. A mechanism for hyporeninemic hypoaldosteronism in chronic renal disease. Metabolism 23:1157-1165, 1974.
43. Batlle, D. C.; Arruda, J. A. L.; and Kurtzman, N. A. Hyperkalemic distal renal tubular acidosis associated with obstructive uropathy. N. Engl. J. Med. 304:373-380, 1981.

44. Perez, G. O.; and Oster, J. R. Hyporeninemic hypoaldosteronism after renal transplantation. South. Med. J. 70:363-364, 1977.
45. DeFronzo, R. A. Hyperkalemia and hyporeninemic hypoaldosteronism. Kidney Int. 17: 118-134, 1980.
46. Goldszer, R. C.; Coodley, E. L.; Rosner, M. J.; Simons, W. M.; and Schwartz, A. B. Hyperkalemia associated with indomethacin. Arch. Intern. Med. 141:802-804, 1981.
47. Tan, S. Y.; Shapiro, R.; Franco, R.; Stockard, H.; and Mulrow, P. J. Indomethacin-induced prostaglandin inhibition with hyperkalemia. Ann. Int. Med. 90:783-785, 1979.
48. Schambelan, M.; and Sebastian, A. Pathogenesis of indomethacin-induced hyperkalemia and type 4 renal tubular acidosis. Proceedings of the 5th International Conference on Prostaglandins, Florence, May, 1982, p. 772.
49. Warren, S. E.; and O'Connor, D. T. Hyperkalemia resulting from captopril administration. J.A.M.A. 244:2551-2552, 1980.
50. Morimoto, S.; Kim, K. S.; Yamamoto, I.; Uchida, K.; Takeda, R.; and Kornel, L. Selective hypoaldosteronism with hyperreninemia in a diabetic patient. J. Clin. Endocrinol. Metab. 49:742-747, 1979.
51. Marieb, N. J.; Melby, J. C.; and Lyall, S. S. Isolated hypoaldosteronism associated with idiopathic hypoparathyroidism. Arch. Intern. Med. 134:424-429, 1974.
52. Mellinger, R. C.; Petermann, F. L.; and Jurgenson, J. C. Hyponatremia with low urinary aldosterone occurring in an old woman. J. Clin. Endocrinol. Metab. 34:85-91, 1972.
53. McGiff, J. C.; Muzzarelli, R. E.; Duffy, P. A.; Gonzalez, Y.; Pierce, C. E.; and Frawley, T. F. Interrelationships of renin and aldosterone in a patient with hypoaldosteronism. Am. J. Med. 48:247-253, 1970.
54. Russell, A.; Levin, B.; Sinclair, L.; and Oberholzer, V. G. A reversible salt-wasting syndrome of the newborn and infant. Arch. Dis. Child. 38:313-325, 1963.
55. Vagnucci, A. H. Selective aldosterone deficiency. J. Clin. Endocrinol. Metab. 29:279-289, 1969.
56. Hudson, J. B.; Chobanian, A. V.; and Relman, A. S. Hypoaldosteronism. A clinical study of a patient with an isolated adrenal mineralocorticoid deficiency, resulting in hyperkalemia and Stokes-Adams attacks. N. Engl. J. Med. 257:529-536, 1957.
57. Cheek, D. B.; and Perry, J. W. A salt wasting syndrome in infancy. Arch. Dis. Child. 33:252-256, 1958.
58. Donnell, G. N.; Litman, N.; and Roldan, M. Pseudohypoadrenalocorticism. Am. J. Dis. Child. 97:813-828, 1959.
59. Lelong, M.; Alagille, D.; Philippe, A.; Gentil, C.; and Gabilan, J.-C. Diabete salin par insensibilite congenitale du tubule a l'aldosterone: "Pseudo-hypo-adrenocorticisme." Rev. Fr. Etudes Clin. et Biol. 5:558-565, 1960.
60. Raine, D. N.; and Roy, J. A salt-losing syndrome in infancy. Pseudohypoadrenocorticalism. Arch. Dis. Child. 37:548-556, 1962.
61. Royer, P.; Bonnette, J.; Mathieu, H.; Gabilan, J.-C.; Klutchko, G.; and Zittoun, R. Pseudo-hypoaldosteronisme. Ann. de Pédéatr. 54:596-605, 1963.
62. Trung, P. H., Piussan, C.; Rodary, C.; Legrand, S.; Attal, C.; and Mozziconacci, P. Etude du taux de secretion de l'aldosterone et de l'activite de la renine plasmatique d'un cas de pseudo-hypoaldosteronisme. Arch. Fr. Pediatr. 27:603-615, 1970.
63. Barakat, A. Y.; Papadopoulou, Z. L.; and August, G. P. A hyperkalemic, salt-wasting syndrome in infancy. Pediatr. Res. 6:394, 1972.
64. Proesmans, W.; Geussens, H.; Corbeel, L.; and Eeckels, R. Pseudohypoaldosteronism. Am. J. Dis. Child. 126:510-516, 1973.
65. Alvarez, M. N.; Barnes, N. D.; and Stickler, G. B. Salt wasting nephropathy of "pseudohypoaldosteronism" in twins. Pediatr. Res. 8:453, 1974.
66. Savitt, H.; Molitch, M.; Kawaoka, E.; and Leake, R. Pseudohypoaldosteronism. Clin. Res. 23:165A, 1975.

67. Roy, C. Pseudohypoaldosteronisme familial (a propos de 5 cas). Arch. Fr. Pediatr. 34: 37-54, 1977.
68. Bonnici, F. Pseudohypoaldosteronisme familial. A transmission autosomique recessive. Arch. Fr. Pediatr. 34:915-919, 1977.
69. Kaufman, E.; Hayek, A.; and Greenberg, R. Pseudohypoaldosteronism in triplets. Pediatr. Res. 11:426, 1977.
70. Lauras, B.; Ravussin, J.-J.; David, M.; Freycon, F.; and Jeune, M. Pseudo-hypoaldosteronisme chez l'enfant. A propos de quatre observations dont deux concernant des freres. Pediatrie 33:119-135, 1978.
71. Limal, J. M.; Rappaport, R.; Dechaux, M.; Riffaud, C.; and Morin, C. Familial dominant pseudohypoaldosteronism. Lancet 1:51, 1978.
72. Hanukoglu, A.; Fried, D.; and Gotlieb, A. Inheritance of pseudohypoaldosteronism. Lancet 1:1359, 1978.
73. Blacher, Y.; Kaplan, B. S.; Griffel, B.; and Levin, S. Pseudohypoaldosteronism. Clin. Nephrol. 11:281, 1979.
74. Rosenberg, S.; Franks, R. C.; and Ulick, S. Mineralocorticoid unresponsiveness with severe neonatal hyponatremia and hyperkalemia. J. Clin. Endocrinol. Metab. 50:401-404, 1980.
75. Oberfield, S. E.; Levine, L. S.; Carey, R. M.; Bejar, R.; and New, M. I. Pseudohypoaldosteronism: Multiple target organ unresponsiveness to mineralocorticoid hormones. J. Clin. Endocrinol. Metab. 48:228-234, 1979.
76. Hogg, R. J.; Frolich, J.; Marver, D.; and Marks, J. F. The basic defect in pseudohypoaldosteronism. Clin. Res. 26:828A, 1978.
77. Bierich, J. R.; and Schmidt, U. Tubular Na K-ATPase deficiency the cause of the congenital renal salt-losing syndrome. Europ. J. Pediatr. 121:81-87, 1976.
78. Anand, S. K.; Froberg, L.; Northway, J. D.; Weinberger, M.; and Wright, J. C. Pseudohypoaldosteronism due to sweat gland dysfunction. Pediatr. Res. 10:677-682, 1976.
79. Postel-Vinay, M-C.; Alberti, G. M.; Ricour, C.; Limal, J-M.; Rappaport, R.; and Royer, P. Pseudohypoaldosteronism: Persistence of hyperaldosteronism and evidence for renal tubular and intestinal responsiveness to endogenous aldosterone. J. Clin. Endocrinol. Metab. 39:1038-1044, 1974.
80. Popovtzer, M. M.; Rosler, A.; Cerasi, E.; Sherzer, P.; and Czaczkes, J. W. Na^+-K^+-ATPase deficiency: A possible mechanism of renal salt-wasting in a newborn baby with "pseudohypoaldosteronism." Clin. Res. 28:536A, 1980.
81. Petersen, S.; Giese, J.; Kappelgaard, A. M.; Lund, H. T.; Lund, J. O.; Nielsen, M. D.; and Thomsen, A. C. Pseudohypoaldosteronism. Clinical, biochemical and morphological studies in a long-term follow-up. Acta Paediatr. Scand. 67:255-261, 1978.
82. Cogan, M. G.; and Arieff, A. I. Sodium wasting, acidosis and hyperkalemia induced by methicillin interstitial nephritis: Evidence for selective distal tubular dysfunction. Am. J. Med. 64:500-507, 1978.
83. Popovtzer, M. M.; Katz, F. H.; Pinggera, W. F.; Robinette, J.; Halgrimson, C. G.; and Butkus, D. E. Hyperkalemia in salt-wasting nephropathy. Study of the mechanism. Arch. Intern. Med. 132:203-208, 1973.
84. Stanbury, S. W.; and Mahler, R. F. Salt-wasting renal disease. Metabolic observations on a patient with salt-losing nephritis. Q. J. Med. 28:425-447, 1959.
85. Horner, J. M.; Hintz, R. L.; and Luetscher, J. A. The role of renin and angiotensin in salt-losing 21-hydroxylase-deficient congenital adrenal hyperplasia. J. Clin. Endocrinol. Metab. 48:776-783, 1979.
86. Keenan, B. S.; Holcombe, J. H.; Kirkland, R. T.; Potts, V. E.; and Clayton, G. W. Sodium homeostasis and aldosterone secretion in salt-losing congenital adrenal hyperplasia. J. Clin. Endocrinol. Metab. 48:430-436, 1979.
87. Paver, W. K. A.; and Pauline, G. J. Hypertension and hyperpotassaemia without renal disease in a young male. Med. J. Aust. 2:305-306, 1964.

88. Stokes, G. S.; Gentle, J. L.; Edwards, K. D. G.; and Stewart, J. H. Syndrome of idiopathic hyperkalaemia and hypertension with decreased plasma renin activity: Effects on plasma renin and aldosterone of reducing the serum potassium level. Med. J. Aust. 2:1050-1054, 1968.
89. Arnold, J. E.; and Healy, J. K. Hyperkalemia, hypertension and systemic acidosis without renal failure associated with a tubular defect in potassium excretion. Am. J. Med. 47:461-472, 1969.
90. Gordon, R. D.; Geddes, R. A.; Pawsey, C. G. K.; and O'Halloran, M. W. Hypertension and severe hyperkalaemia associated with suppression of renin and aldosterone and completely reversed by dietary sodium restriction. Aust. Ann. Med. 4:287-294, 1970.
91. Spitzer, A.; Edelmann, C. M., Jr.; Goldberg, L. D.; and Henneman, P. H. Short stature, hyperkalemia and acidosis: A defect in renal transport of potassium. Kidney Int. 3: 251-257, 1973.
92. Weinstein, S. F.; Allan, D. M. E.; and Mendoza, S. A. Hyperkalemia, acidosis, and short stature associated with a defect in renal potassium excretion. J. Pediatr. 85:355-358, 1974.
93. Brautbar, N.; Levi, J.; Rosler, A.; Leitesdorf, E.; Djaldeti, M.; Epstein, M.; and Kleeman, C. R. Familial hyperkalemia, hypertension, and hyporeninemia with normal aldosterone levels: A tubular defect in potassium handling. Arch. Intern. Med. 138: 607-610, 1978.
94. Farfel, Z.; Iaina, A.; Rosenthal, T.; Waks, U.; Shibolet, S.; and Gafni, J. Familial hyperpotassemia and hypertension accompanied by normal plasma aldosterone levels. Possible hereditary cell membrane defect. Arch. Intern. Med. 138:1828-1832, 1978.
95. Lee, M. R.; Ball, S. G.; Thomas, T. H.; and Morgan, D. B. Hypertension and hyperkalaemia responding to bendrofluazide. Q. J. Med. 48:245-258, 1979.
96. Schambelan, M.; Sebastian, A.; and Rector, F. C., Jr. Mineralocorticoid-resistant renal hyperkalemia without salt wasting (type II pseudohypoaldosteronism): Role of increased renal chloride reabsorption. Kidney Int. 19:716-727, 1981.
97. Szylman, P.; Better, O. S.; Chaimowitz, C.; and Rosler, A. Role of hyperkalemia in the metabolic acidosis of isolated hypoaldosteronism. N. Engl. J. Med. 294:361-365, 1976.
98. Rado, J. P.; Szende, L.; and Szucs, L. Hyperkalemia unresponsive to massive doses of aldosterone in a patient with renal tubular acidosis. Endokrinologie 68:183-188, 1976.
99. Batlle, D. C.; Mozes, M. F.; Manaligod, J.; Arruda, J. A. L.; and Kurtzman, N. A. The pathogenesis of hyperchloremic metabolic acidosis associated with kidney transplantation. Am. J. Med. 70:786-796, 1981.
100. DeFronzo, R. A.; Cooke, R.; Goldberg, M.; Cox, M.; Myers, A. R.; and Agus, Z. S. Impaired renal tubular potassium secretion in systemic lupus erythematosus. Ann. Intern. Med. 86:268-271, 1977.
101. Lathem, W. Hyperchloremic acidosis in chronic pyelonephritis. N. Engl. J. Med. 258: 1031-1036, 1958.
102. Hadler, N. M.; Gill, J. R., Jr.; and Gardner, J. D. Impaired renal tubular secretion of potassium, elevated sweat sodium chloride concentration and plasma inhibition of erythrocyte sodium outflux as complications of systemic lupus erythematosus. Arthritis Rheum. 15:515-523, 1972.
103. Gyory, A. Z.; Stewart, J. H.; George, C. R. P.; Tiller, D. J.; and Edwards, K. D. G. Renal tubular acidosis, acidosis due to hyperkalemia, hypercalcemia, disordered citrate metabolism and other tubular dysfunctions following human renal transplantation. Q. J. Med. 38:231-254, 1969.
104. Rubini, M. E.; Sanford, J. P.; and Meroney, W. H. Studies of potassium secretion in glomerulonephritis. Am. J. Med. 17:790-797, 1977.
105. Luke, R. G.; Allison, M. E. M.; Davidson, J. F.; and Duguid, W. P. Hyperkalemia and renal tubular acidosis due to renal amyloidosis. Ann. Intern. Med. 70:1211-1217, 1969.

106. Cannon, P. J.; Ames, R. P.; and Laragh, J. H. Relation between potassium balance and aldosterone secretion in normal subjects and in patients with hypertensive or renal tubular disease. J. Clin. Invest. 45:865-879, 1966.
107. Dluhy, R. G.; Axelrod, L.; Underwood, R. H.; and Williams, G. H. Studies of the control of plasma aldosterone concentration in normal man. II. Effect of dietary potassium and acute potassium infusion. J. Clin. Invest. 51:1950-1957, 1972.
108. Laragh, J. H. Potassium, angiotensin and the dual control of aldosterone secretion. N. Engl. J. Med. 289:745-747, 1973.
109. Himathongkam, T.; Dluhy, R. G.; and Williams, G. H. Potassium-aldosterone-renin interrelationships. J. Clin Endocrinol. Metab. 41:153-159, 1975.
110. Schambelan, M.; and Sebastian, A. Adrenocortical hormone response to metabolic acidosis in normal man. Clin. Res. 25:301A, 1977.
111. Perez, G. O.; Oster, J. R.; Vaamonde, C. A.; and Katz, F. H. Effect of NH_4Cl on plasma aldosterone cortisol and renin activity in supine man. J. Clin. Endocrinol. Metab. 45:762-767, 1977.
112. Relman, A. S.; and Schwartz, W. B. The effect of DOCA on electrolyte balance in normal man and its relation to sodium chloride intake. Yale. J. Biol. Med. 24:540-548, 1952.
113. Liddle, G. W. Aldosterone antagonists. Arch. Intern. Med. 102:998-1004, 1958.
114. Mills, J. N.; Thomas, S.; and Williamson, K. S. The acute effect of hydrocortisone deoxycorticosterone and aldosterone upon the excretion of sodium, potassium and acid by the human kidney. J. Physiol. (Lond.) 151:312-331, 1960.
115. Mills, J. N.; Thomas, S.; and Williamson, K. S. The effects of intravenous aldosterone and hydrocortisone on the urinary electrolytes of the recumbent human subject. J. Physiol. (Lond.) 156:415-423, 1961.
116. Sonnenblick, E. H.; Cannon, P. J.; and Laragh, J. H. The nature of the action of intravenous aldosterone: Evidence for a role of the hormone in urinary dilution. J. Clin. Invest. 40:903-913, 1961.
117. Crabbe, J.; and Thorn, G. W. Effects de l'aldosterone sur la fonction renale de l'homme normal. Rev. Frc. Etudes Clin. et Biol. 9:729-735, 1964.
118. Lemann, J., Jr.; Piering, W. F.; and Lennon, E. J. Studies of the acute effects of aldosterone and cortisol on the interrelationship between renal sodium, calcium and magnesium excretion in normal man. Nephron 7:117-130, 1970.
119. Kassirer, J. P.; London, A. M.; Goldman, D. M.; and Schwartz, W. B. On the pathogenesis of metabolic alkalosis in hyperaldosteronism. Am. J. Med. 49:306-315, 1970.
120. Kurtzman, N. A.; White, M. G.; and Rogers, P. W. Pathophysiology of metabolic alkalosis. Arch. Intern. Med. 131:702-708, 1973.
121. Hulter, H. N.; Sigala, J. F.; and Sebastian, A. K^+ Deprivation potentiates the renal alkalosis-producing effect of mineralocorticoid. Am. J. Physiol. 235:F298-F309, 1978.
122. Hulter, H. N.; Licht, J. H.; Glynn, R. D.; and Sebastian, A. Renal acidosis in mineralocorticoid deficiency is not dependent on NaCl depletion or hyperkalemia. Am. J. Physiol. 236:F283-F294, 1979.
123. Tannen, R. L. Relationship of renal ammonia production and potassium homeostasis. Kidney Int. 11:453-465, 1977.
124. Steinmetz, P. R. Cellular mechanisms of urinary acidification. Physiol. Rev. 54:890-955, 1974.
125. Al-Awqati, Q. H. H^+ Transport in urinary epithelia. Am. J. Physiol. 235:F77-F88, 1978.
126. Steinmetz, P. R. Cellular defects in urinary acidification and renal tubular acidosis. In: Physiology of Membrane Disorders, edited by Andreoli, T. E., Hoffman, J. F., and Fanestil, D. D. New York, Plenum, 1978, pp. 987-1018.
127. Steinmetz, P. R. Characteristics of hydrogen ion transport in urinary bladder of water turtle. J. Clin. Invest. 46:1531-1540, 1967.

128. Steinmetz, P. R.; Omachi, R. S.; and Frazier, H. C. Independence of hydrogen ion secretion and transport of other electrolytes in turtle bladder. J. Clin. Invest. 46: 1541-1548, 1967.
129. Al-Awqati, Q.; Mueller, A.; and Steinmetz, P. R. Transport of H^+ against electrochemical gradients in turtle urinary bladder. Am. J. Physiol. 233:F502-F508, 1977.
130. Al-Awqati, Q.; Norby, L. H.; Mueller, A.; and Steinmetz, P. R. Characteristics of stimulation of H^+ transport by aldosterone in turtle urinary bladder. J. Clin. Invest. 58: 351-358, 1976.
131. Berry, C. A.; and Warnock, D. G. Acidification in the in vitro perfused tubule. Kidney Int. 22:507-518, 1982.
132. Koeppen, B. M.; and Helman, S. I. Acidification of luminal fluid by the rabbit cortical collecting tubule perfused in vitro. Am. J. Physiol. 242:F521-F531, 1982.
133. Laski, M. D.; and Kurtzman, N. A. Characterization of acidification in the cortical and medullary collecting tubule of the rabbit. J. Clin. Invest. 72:2050-2059, 1983.
134. Stokes, J. B.; Ingram, M. J.; Williams, A. D.; and Ingram, D. Heterogeneity of the rabbit collecting tubule: Localization of mineralocorticoid hormone action to the cortical portion. Kidney Int. 30:341-347, 1981.
135. Lombard, W. E.; Jacobson, H. R.; and Kokko, J. P. Collecting duct bicarbonate transport: Comparison of cortical and medullary segments. Kidney Int. 16:827, 1979.
136. Stone, D. K.; Kokko, J. P.; and Jacobson, H. R. Sodium independence of proton secretion in medullary collecting duct. Clin. Res. 30:464A, 1982.
137. Stone, D. K.; Seldin, D. W.; Kokko, J. P.; and Jacobson, H. R. Chloride dependence of medullary collecting duct acidification. Kidney Int. 23:239, 1983.
138. Stone, D. K.; Kokko, J. P.; and Jacobson, H. R. In-vitro stimulation of proton secretion by aldosterone. Kidney Int. 21:240, 1982.
139. Madsen, K. M.; and Tisher, C. C. Evidence for hydrogen ion (H^+) secretion in rat outer medullary collecting duct (OMCD). Kidney Int. 23:236, 1983.
140. Daughaday, W. H.; and Rendleman, D. Severe symptomatic hyperkalemia in an adrenalectomized woman due to enhanced mineralocorticoid requirement. Ann. Int. Med. 66:1197-1203, 1967.
141. Kurtzman, N. A.; White, M. G.; and Rogers, P. W. The effect of potassium and extracellular volume on renal bicarbonate reabsorption. Metabolism 22:481-492, 1973.
142. Levine, D. Z.; Walker, T.; and Nash, L. A. Effects of KCl infusions on proximal tubular function in normal and potassium-depleted rats. Kidney Int. 4:318-325, 1973.
143. Tannen, R. L.; Wedell, E.; and Moore, R. Renal adaptation to a high potassium intake. The role of hydrogen ion. J. Clin. Invest. 52:2089-2101, 1973.
144. Hulter, H. N.; Toto, R. D.; Ilnicki, L. P.; and Sebastian, A. Chronic hyperkalemic renal tubular acidosis induced by KCl loading. Am. J. Physiol. 244:F255-F264, 1983.
145. Hulter, H. N.; Licht, J. H.; Glynn, R. D.; and Sebastian, A. Pathophysiology of chronic renal tubular acidosis induced by administration of amiloride. J. Lab. Clin. Med. 95: 637-653, 1980.
146. Maher, T.; Schambelan, M.; Kurtz, I.; Hulter, H. N.; Jones, J. W.; and Sebastian, A. Correction of metabolic acidosis by dietary potassium restriction in hyperkalemic patients with chronic renal insufficiency. J. Lab. Clin. Med. 103:432-445, 1984.
147. Horwitz, D.; Margolius, H. S.; and Keiser, H. R. Effects of dietary potassium and race on urinary excretion of kallikrein and aldosterone in man. J. Clin. Endocrinol. Metab. 47:296-299, 1978.
148. Dusing, R.; Gill, J. R., Jr.; Bartter, F. C.; and Gullner, H.-G. The effect of potassium depletion on urinary prostaglandins in normal man. Adv. Prostaglandin Thromboxane Res. 7:1189-1192, 1980.
149. Jones, J. W.; Sebastian, A.; Hulter, H. N.; Schambelan, M.; Sutton, J. M.; and Biglieri, E. G. Systemic and renal acid-base effects of chronic dietary potassium depletion in humans. Kidney Int. 21:402-410, 1982.

150. DeFronzo, R. A. Hyperkalemia and hyporeninemic hypoaldosteronism. Kidney Int. 17:118-134, 1980.
151. Madias, N. E.; Adrogue, H. J.; Horowitz, G. L.; Cohen, J. J.; and Schwartz, W. B. A redefinition of normal acid-base equilibrium in man: Carbon dioxide tension as a key determinant of normal plasma bicarbonate concentration. Kidney Int. 16:612-618, 1979.
152. Sebastian, A.; Schambelan, M.; and Sutton, J. M. Amelioration of hyperchloremic acidosis with furosemide therapy in patients with chronic renal insufficiency and type 4 renal tubular acidosis. Am. J. Nephrol. 4:287-300, 1984.
153. Jacobson, H. R.; and Kokko, J. P. Diuretics: Sites and mechanisms of action. Ann. Rev. Pharm. Tox. 16:201-214, 1976.
154. Bosch, J. P.; Goldstein, M. H.; Levitt, M. F.; and Kahn, T. Effect of chronic furosemide administration on hydrogen and sodium excretion in the dog. Am. J. Physiol. 232:F397-F404, 1977.
155. Baxter, J. D.; and Funder, J. W. Hormone receptors. N. Engl. J. Med. 301:1149-1161, 1979.
156. Ludens, J. H.; and Fanestil, D. D. The mechanism of aldosterone function. Pharmacol. Ther. 2:371-412, 1976.
157. Katz, A. I.; and Epstein, F. H. The role of sodium-potassium activated adenosine triphosphatase in the reabsorption of sodium by the kidney. J. Clin. Invest. 46:1999-2011, 1967.
158. Silva, P.; Hayslett, J. P.; and Epstein, F. H. The role of Na-K activated adenosine triphosphatase in potassium adaptation. J. Clin. Invest. 52:2665-2671, 1973.
159. Westenfelder, C.; Birch, F. M.; and Baranowski, R. L. Effect of Na-K-ATPase inhibition on hydrogen ion and potassium secretion. Pflugers Arch. 386:161-171, 1980.
160. Westenfelder, C.; Arevalo, G. J.; Baranowski, R. L.; Kurtzman, N. A.; and Katz, A. I. Relationship between mineralocorticoids and renal Na^+-K^+-ATPase: Sodium reabsorption. Am. J. Physiol. 233:F593-F599, 1977.
161. Manuel, M. A.; Beirne, G. J.; Wagnild, J. P.; and Weiner, M. W. An effect of spironolactone on urinary acidification in normal man. Arch. Intern. Med. 134:472-474, 1974.
162. Toto, R. D.; Hulter, H. N.; Mackie, S.; and Sebastian, A. Renal tubular acidosis induced by dietary chloride. Kidney Int. 25:26-32, 1984.
163. Kurtzman, N. A. Regulation of renal bicarbonate reabsorption by extracellular volume. J. Clin. Invest. 49:586-595, 1970.
164. Slatopolsky, E.; Hoffsten, P.; Purkerson, M.; and Bricker, N. S. On the influence of extracellular fluid volume expansion and of uremia on bicarbonate reabsorption in man. J. Clin. Invest. 49:988-998, 1970.
165. Garcia-Filho, E.; Malnic, G.; and Giebisch, G. Effects of changes in electrical potential difference on tubular potassium transport. Am. J. Physiol. 238:F235-F246, 1980.
166. Boudry, J. F.; Stoner, L. C.; and Burg, M. B. Effect of acid lumen pH on potassium transport in renal cortical collecting tubules. Am. J. Physiol. 230:239-244, 1976.
167. Luke, R. G.; Wright, F. S.; Fowler, N.; Kashgarian, M.; and Giebisch, G. H. Effects of potassium depletion on renal tubular chloride transport in the rat. Kidney Int. 14:414-427, 1978.
168. Ordonez, N. G.; Toback, F. G.; Aithal, H. N.; and Spargo, B. H. Zonal changes in renal structure and phospholipid metabolism during reversal of potassium depletion nephropathy. Lab. Invest. 36:33-47, 1977.
169. Morris, D. J.; Douglis, F.; and DeConti, G. Effect of potassium loading on metabolism of aldosterone in rats. Metabolism 27:737-744, 1978.
170. Schwartz, W. B.; Jenson, R. L.; and Relman, A. S. Acidification of the urine and increased ammonium excretion without change in acid-base equilibrium: Sodium reabsorption as a stimulus to the acidifying process. J. Clin. Invest. 34:673-680, 1955.
171. Seldin, D. W.; Coleman, A. J.; Carter, N. W.; and Rector, F. C., Jr. The effect of Na_2SO_4 on urinary acidification in chronic renal disease. J. Lab. Clin. Med. 69:893-903, 1967.

172. Schwartz, W. B.; Hall, P. W.; Hays, R. M.; and Relman, A. S. On the mechanism of acidosis in chronic renal disease. J. Clin. Invest. 38:39-52, 1959.
173. De Sousa, R. C.; Harrington, J. T.; Ricanati, E. S.; Shelkrot, J. W.; and Schwartz, W. B. Renal regulation of acid-base equilibrium during chronic administration of mineral acid. J. Clin. Invest. 53:465-476, 1974.
174. Clapp, J. R.; Rector, F. C., Jr.; and Seldin, D. W. Effect of unreabsorbed anions on proximal and distal transtubular potentials in rats. Am. J. Physiol. 202:781-786, 1962.
175. Guignard, J.-P.; and Peters, G. Effects of triamterene and amiloride on urinary acidification and potassium excretion in the rat. Eur. J. Pharmacol. 10:255-267, 1970.
176. Cuthbert, A. W.; and Shum, W. K. Effects of vasopressin and aldosterone on amiloride binding in toad bladder epithelial cells. Proc. R. Soc. Lond. 189:543-575, 1975.
177. Dorge, A.; and Nagel, W. Effect of amiloride on sodium transport in frog skin. II. Sodium transport pool and unidirectional fluxes. Pflugers Arch. 321:91-101, 1970.
178. Ziegler, T. W.; Fanestil, D. D.; and Ludens, J. H. Influence of transepithelial potential difference on acidification in the toad urinary bladder. Kidney Int. 10:279-286, 1979.
179. Barratt, L. J. The effect of amiloride on the transtubular potential difference of the distal tubule of the rat kidney. Pflugers Arch. 361:251-254, 1976.
180. Sudou, K.; and Hoshi, T. Mode of action of amiloride in toad urinary bladder. J. Membr. Biol. 32:115-132, 1977.
181. O'Neil, R. G.; and Helman, S. I. Transport characteristics of renal collecting tubules: Influences of DOCA and diet. Am. J. Physiol. 233:F544-F558, 1977.
182. Lief, P. D.; and Mutz, B. Inhibition of H^+ secretion by amiloride in turtle urinary bladder: Dependence on Na^+ transport. Clin. Res. 25:440A, 1977.
183. Husted, R. F.; and Steinmetz, P. R. The effects of amiloride and ouabain on urinary acidification by turtle bladder. J. Pharmacol. Exp. Ther. 210:264-268, 1979.
184. McKinney, T. D.; and Burg, M. B. Bicarbonate absorption by rabbit cortical collecting tubules in vitro. Am. J. Physiol. 234:F141-F145, 1978.
185. Gyory, A. Z.; and Edwards, K. D. G. Effect of mersalyl, ethacrynic acid and sodium sulphate infusion on urinary acidification in hereditary renal tubular acidosis. Med. J. Aust. 2:940-945, 1971.
186. Davies, H. E. F. Renal tubular acidosis. Excretion of acid urine by patients given mersalyl. Lancet 1:565-566, 1962.
187. Buckalew, V. M., Jr.; McCurdy, D. K.; Ludwig, G. D.; Chaykin, L. B.; and Elkinton, J. R. Incomplete renal tubular acidosis. Physiologic studies in three patients with a defect in lowering urine pH. Am. J. Med. 45:32-42, 1968.
188. Tannen, R. L.; Falls, W. F., Jr.; and Brackett, N. C., Jr. Incomplete renal tubular acidosis: Some clinical and physiological features. Nephron 15:111-123, 1975.
189. Halperin, M. L.; Goldstein, M. B.; Haig, A.; Johnson, M. D.; and Stinebaugh, B. J. Studies on the pathogenesis of type 1 (distal) renal tubular acidosis as revealed by the urinary PCO_2 tensions. J. Clin. Invest. 53:669-677, 1974.
190. Stinebaugh, B. J.; Schloeder, F. X.; Tam, S. C.; Goldstein, M. B.; and Halperin, M. L. Pathogenesis of distal renal tubular acidosis. Kidney Int. 19:1-7, 1981.

11

The Pathophysiology of Distal (Type 1) Renal Tubular Acidosis

VARDAMAN M. BUCKALEW, JR., and RALPH J. CARUANA
Bowman Gray School of Medicine of Wake Forest University, Winston-Salem, North Carolina

In 1936, Butler et al. (1) described four infants in whom severe, hyperchloremic acidosis was found in association with diffuse calcification of the renal medulla. In the same paper they also reported in a footnote the case of a 10-year-old boy with growth retardation, a history of "rickets" since age 1½ years, hyperchloremic acidosis, and calcium deposits in the renal medulla. Extensive metabolic evaluation was not performed on these patients.

Subsequently, Albright et al. (2,3) published detailed metabolic studies on several adolescents with growth retardation, "rickets," hyperchloremic acidosis, and nephrocalcinosis and neperolithiasis, in which they correctly attributed the metabolic acidosis to a defect in the ability of the renal tubule to lower urine pH and first recognized the excessive renal excretion of potassium, sodium, and calcium. Albright and his colleagues (2,3) referred to this condition as tubular insufficiency without glomerular insufficiency. However, this cumbersome designation was subsequently replaced by the currently accepted term renal tubular acidosis (RTA), as suggested by Pines and Mudge (4). Further progress occurred with the recognition of the difference between distal (type 1) and proximal (type 2) (5-8), and the description of the forme frust of type 1 RTA (incomplete RTA) by Wrong and Davies (9).

Albright et al. (3) originally suggested that all the major clinical manifestations of type 1 RTA might be explained by a single abnormality in tubular function, as outlined in Fig. 1. According to their hypothesis, the metabolic acidosis caused by the inability to acidify the urine caused a shortage of base (ammonia) with which to excrete mineral acids (chloride), leading to an increased excretion of other bases (calcium, sodium, and potassium). This hypothesis was based on Arrhenius' theory of ionization in which anions were acids and cations bases. In the more modern Bronsted system acids are hydrogen ion donors and bases are hydrogen ion acceptors, and renal acidosis is caused by a failure of the kidney to regenerate base utilized in buffering the "fixed" acid generated by ingestion of phosphoproteins and sulfur containing amino acids (10). The resultant chronically positive balance of hydrogen ion is buffered by calcium phosphate in bone, resulting in hypercalciuria (11). It can be appreciated, however, that reformulation of Albright's hypothesis (3) into the Bronsted framework does not provide an explanation for the monovalent cation (Na-K) wasting.

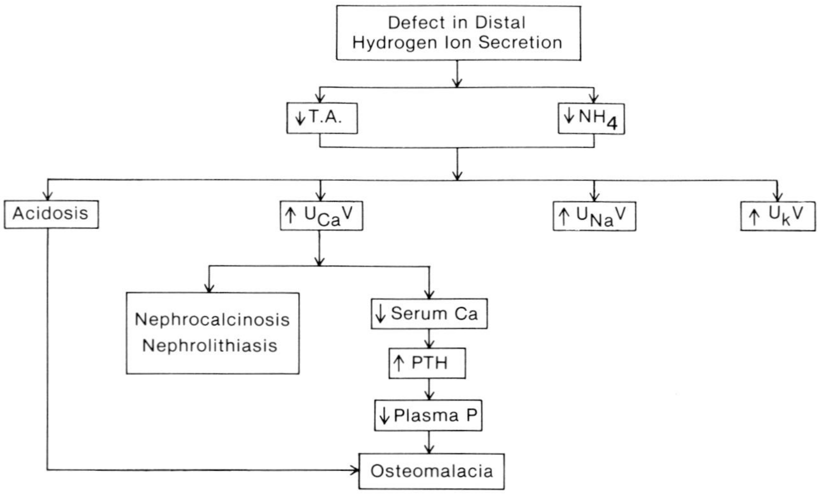

Fig. 1 Albright's original hypothesis (3) suggested that a single defect in distal hydrogen ion secretion lead to all of the observed abnormalities in distal RTA.

As knowledge of RTA has increased over the years, much has been learned which supports the original Albright hypothesis, However, it is now clear that type 1 RTA is not a single, homogeneous entity, but a complex group of disorders with similar clinical manifestations resulting from multiple pathophysiologies. In this chapter we will discuss the current understanding of the pathophysiology of the major clinical manifestations of type 1 RTA (Table 1), with an emphasis on the therapeutic implications of these new concepts.

I. HYPERCHLOREMIC ACIDOSIS

The classic manifestation of RTA, from which its name was derived, is hyperchloremic metabolic acidosis. The earliest investigations correctly surmised that metabolic acidosis resulted from a defect in lowering urine pH (2). As knowledge of the mechanisms of urine acidification has expanded it has become clear that several types of defects, discussed in detail in Ch. 9, may lead to the clinically recognizable syndrome of type 1 RTA. The consequences

Table 1 Major Clinical Manifestations of Type 1 RTA

1. Hyperchloremic acidosis
2. Hyperexcretion of cation
   a. Calcium
   b. Potassium
   c. Sodium
3. Nephrocalcinosis
4. Nephrolithiasis
5. Growth retardation
6. Osteomalacia
7. Renal insufficiency

of a limitation in ability to lower urine pH seem reasonably clear from numerous studies over the past 25 years.

Ingestion of sulfur containing amino acids and phosphoproteins by meat-eating humans results in the production of 60-100 meq/day of "fixed" acid (10). Fixed acid, as opposed to "volatile acid" (i.e., carbonic acid) must be neutralized by the blood buffers. Accordingly, maintenance of acid-base balance requires that 60-100 meq/day of bicarbonate must be regenerated by the kidney, which excretes hydrogen ions produced in renal tubular cells from carbonic acid, generating the appropriate amount of new base as bicarbonate. Excretion of hydrogen ions is accomplished by reabsorption of all filtered bicarbonate and titration of urinary buffers, principally phosphate and ammonia. Net acid excretion, the total amount of new bicarbonate generated by the kidney, is defined as the sum of urinary titratable acid and ammonium minus the amount of bicarbonate excreted. Careful studies of acid balance have demonstrated that net acid excretion on a day to day basis equals the amount of fixed acid generated primarily by the combustion of foodstuffs (12). Reabsorption of all filtered bicarbonate, titration of urinary buffers, and excretion of ammonia is dependent upon acidification of the urine, a function of the distal tubule. Therefore, when the ability to lower urine pH is limited, the amount of hydrogen ion which can be excreted as titratable acid and ammonia may be reduced, and a small leak of bicarbonate may occur.

Urinary ammonia is derived from deamination of amino acids in renal tubular cells. The free base ammonia diffuses into tubular fluid where, if tubular fluid pH is appropriately acid, it is converted to ammonium, a cation which will not diffuse back into tubular cells. Patients with type 1 RTA who do not have advanced renal insufficiency excrete ammonia in amounts which are appropriate for the urine pH, but which are quantitatively low in absolute terms because of the abnormally high urine pH (9).

In normal subjects, titration of phosphate accounts for about 25% and ammonia approximately 75% of the daily acid excretion. Therefore, it appears that the principal cause of metabolic acidosis in type 1 RTA is an inability to excrete adequate hydrogen ion as ammonia (9). Bicarbonate wasting in type 1 RTA is usually less than 5% of the filtered load, and contributes little to the genesis of acidosis (8). However, some children with type 1 RTA have been found to waste large amounts of bicarbonate when treated with bicarbonate (13). The cause of this phenomenon is not clear, but it clearly increases the alkali requirement for adequate therapy (see below).

Since the anion gap is normal in type 1 RTA, acidosis is invariably associated with hyperchloremia. Very few studies have been performed to elucidate the mechanism of hyperchloremia. In two patients with type 1 RTA, Seldin et al. (14,15) found that when alkali therapy was withdrawn while dietary sodium was rigidly restricted plasma bicarbonate fell with no rise in plasma chloride. (Although not reported, serum sodium concentration presumably fell as well, assuming no rise in anion gap.) Adding salt to the diet without alkali caused a marked rise in serum chloride and a further decrement in bicarbonate. Therefore, it appeared from this study that hyperchloremia resulted from accelerated reabsorption of sodium chloride by the kidney, diluting plasma bicarbonate and aggravating the acidosis. Alternatively, feeding sodium chloride could aggravate acidosis by expanding plasma volume, thereby decreasing tubular bicarbonate reabsorption. The effect of sodium intake on tubular bicarbonate reabsorption in type 1 RTA has not been studied.

A. Incomplete RTA

In 1959, Wrong and Davies (9) described three patients with a defect in lowering urine pH without systemic acidosis. They found that these patients had the following characteristics:

(1) ammonia excretion in response to ammonium chloride loading was high relative to urine pH, and was therefore quantitatively normal, so that net acid excretion was normal; and (2) glomerular filtration rate (GFR) tended to be higher than in patients with complete RTA. They attributed the normal ammonia excretion to the higher GFR, since generalized renal failure was invariably accompanied by impaired ammonia excretion. These observations lead to the hypothesis outlined in Fig. 2 that incomplete RTA was a preacidotic stage of complete RTA, and that incomplete patients were those with normal or near normal GFRs and ammonia excretion. Generalized renal damage secondary to recurrent pyelonephritis and/or nephrocalcinosis would then lead to a reduction in GFR and ammonia excretion, and together with the impairment in excretion of titratable acid, produce systemic acidosis.

The concept of an incomplete form of RTA is now well established, since large numbers of patients have been described with an inability to lower urine pH without systemic acidosis. In addition, families have been reported in which both the complete and incomplete forms of RTA have been observed (16,17). However, the question of how incomplete RTA relates to acidotic RTA is not entirely clear. It is striking that very few patients have been reported in which an evolution from incomplete to complete RTA has been observed. One of the original cases described by Wrong and Davies was followed for 2½ years, with no sign of acidosis developing (9). Buckalew et al. (18) reported one case in which incomplete RTA was observed to evolve into acidotic RTA, but studies of renal function were not reported after the onset of acidosis.

In the absence of longitudinal observations on patients before and after development of acidosis, one must rely on studies of renal function in complete versus incomplete RTA to ascertain how some patients with a defect in urine acidification are able to avoid acidosis. Buckalew et al. (18) reported three cases of primary incomplete RTA, all of whom had normal GFRs. Net acid excretion on the third day of ammonium chloride loading was within

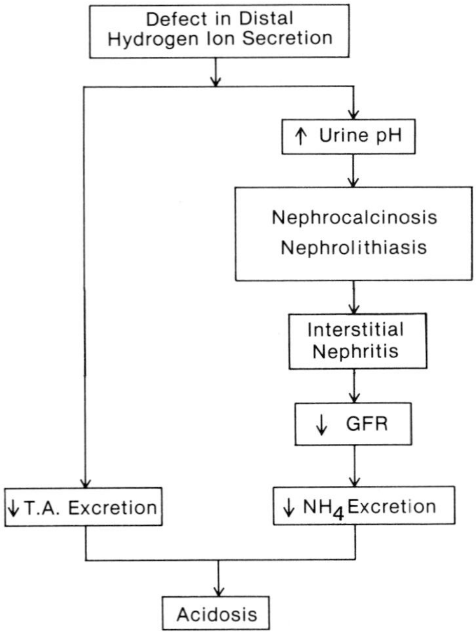

Fig. 2 Wrong and Davies (9) proposed that metabolic acidosis occurred only in those individuals with enough generalized renal disease to cause impairment in renal ammonia excretion.

the normal range in two patients, and only slightly reduced in a third. Ammonia excretion was appropriate for the urinary pH in two, and higher than expected in a third. Absolute values for ammonia excretion were within the normal range in all three patients. Two of these patients were able to lower urine pH to less than 5.5 in response to sodium sulfate infusion, with one of these two reaching a low of 4.62. In these three patients, the lack of acidosis seems readily explainable by the ability to excrete normal amounts of ammonia and net acid.

Tannen et al. (19) studied four patients with incomplete and four with complete primary RTA using the short ammonium chloride loading test. Although urine ammonia excretion was higher in the incompletes, net acid excretion in one incomplete patient with a minimum urine pH of 6.54 was in the same range as the completes. The glomerular filtration rate tended to be higher in the incompletes, possibly accounting for the difference in ammonia excretion. Three patients with incomplete RTA were able to lower urine pH below 5.5 in response to sodium sulfate infusion, whereas two patients with complete RTA could not. In addition, one incomplete patient lowered urine pH to 5.13 in response to progressive ammonium chloride loading with severe systemic acidosis (pH 7.12, plasma bicarbonate 14 meq/liter), whereas one complete patient could not go below 6.11 in response to a similar challenge. Tannen et al. (19) interpreted these results to indicate that patients with incomplete RTA had a less severe defect in lowering urine pH and were therefore better able to excrete acid.

The differences in response of urine pH to various stimuli observed in the study of Buckalew et al. (18) and Tannen et al. (19) have formed the basis for more extensive studies and classification of type 1 RTA into various pathophysiological types, as discussed in Ch. 9. According to the scheme of Batlle and Kurtzman, RTA patients with a normal response to sodium sulfate, but an abnormal response to ammonium chloride could have either an acid backleak or a voltage-dependent defect. However, a voltage-dependent defect, as defined by Batlle and Kurtzman, would be expected to cause hyperkalemia, which was not present in those patients studied by Buckalew et al. (18) and Tannen et al. (19). Whether patients such as this have an acid backleak, and whether this abnormality is confined to the incomplete form of RTA remains to be determined.

Batlle et al. (20) have recently reported three patients without acidosis who lowered urine pH normally in response to the three day ammonium chloride loading test, but who did not raise urine PCO_2 normally in response to bicarbonate loading. Ammonia, titratable acid, and net acid excretion were normal during acidosis. They suggested these patients have a rate-dependent defect in distal hydrogen ion secretion, which is only observed during bicarbonate loading when the stimulus for hydrogen ion secretion is reduced. Interestingly, one other patient with the same defect had metabolic acidosis. They proposed that the nonacidotic patients should be classified as having incomplete RTA, but had no explanation for why one of the patients was acidotic.

Other studies of renal acid excretion have been reported in patients with incomplete RTA. In seven patients with lithium-induced incomplete RTA (21), urinary ammonia excretion was normal in all patients, titratable acid excretion was normal in four of seven, and net acid excretion was normal in six of seven. Five patients with incomplete RTA after renal transplant had reduced net acid excretion during the 2-hr period 6-8 hr after an acute ammonium chloride load when compared to 15 normals studied by the same group (22). Two of these five had low ammonia excretion when compared to normal. In seven patients with hyperglobulinemia and incomplete RTA, ammonia excretion tended to be normal in association with higher GFR than the acidotic patients (23). However, net acid excretion appeared to be markedly reduced in two of the incomplete patients (cases 2 and 3) and moderately reduced in two others (cases 5 and 10). In the family reported by Buckalew et al. (16) only one subject had acidotic RTA, whereas three had incomplete RTA. The patients with incomplete RTA had only modest reductions in GFR, whereas the acidotic patient had severe renal failure with a creatinine clearance of 6 ml/min. Urine ammonia excretion was not measured, but would have been expected to be very low in that patient.

It is possible that some patients could avoid acidosis despite reduced net acid excretion if net acid production were decreased. Camien and Gonick (24) showed that net acid production calculated from net acid excretion as conventionally defined (10) was in error by the amount of organic anion excreted in the urine. They contended that organic anion excretion represents loss of base and should, like bicarbonate, be subtracted from the sum of titratable acid and ammonia in calculating net acid excretion. According to this suggestion, decreased citrate excretion, such as occurs in some patients with both complete and incomplete RTA (see below), would reduce net acid production and allow acid-base balance to be maintained in the presence of an apparent decrease in the conventionally defined net acid excretion.

To summarize, the overall results of cases published to date tend to support the original hypothesis of Wrong and Davies. This might explain why so few patients have been observed to progress from incomplete to complete RTA, since progressive renal failure is rare in type 1 RTA. However, a substantial number of cases with incomplete RTA associated with a variety of diseases have been reported with markedly reduced ammonia and/or net acid excretion, whose glomerular filtration rates are not markedly reduced (19,22,23). The mechanism by which these patients avoid metabolic acidosis is still not clear, nor is it clear why some patients who do avoid acidosis may lose that ability with the passage of time. Changes in renal function other than a decline in ability to generate and excrete ammonia might occur, such as a worsening of the defect in lowering urine pH, or the development of significant bicarbonate wasting, or there might be some changes in net acid production. Additional studies of patients before and after the transition from incomplete to complete RTA will be necessary before these questions can be answered.

II. HYPERCALCIURIA

A. Metabolic Acidosis as a Cause of Hypercalciuria

The early investigations of Albright et al. (2,3) clearly demonstrated that alkali therapy in patients with type 1 RTA not only reduced calcium excretion, but also lessened the degree of roentgenographically demonstrable nephrocalcinosis. These observations lead to the hypothesis that metabolic acidosis somehow contributed to the hypercalciuria, which in turn caused the nephrocalcinosis and nephrolithiasis.

Albright's hypothesis (3) that metabolic acidosis causes hypercalciuria has received some support from studies both in patients with RTA, and in normal subjects with experimental acidosis. Nash et al. (25) showed in two children with type 1 RTA that correction of acidosis reduced calcium excretion from a value greater than 4 mg/kg per day to less than 2 mg/kg per day. These studies have lead to the suggestion that alkali therapy should be given to children with type 1 RTA in an amount sufficient to decrease calcium excretion to less than 2 mg/kg per day. More recently McSherry and Morris (13) studied the effect of two doses of alkali on urinary calcium excretion in five children with type 1 RTA. In four of the five, calcium excretion was lower on high dose alkali sufficient to correct the acidosis than on a lower dose of alkali insufficient to correct acidosis. However, calcium excretion was less than 2 mg/kg per day in only three of the five on high-dose alkali.

Using a technique for quantitating hydrogen ion balance, Goodman et al. (11) and Lemann et al. (26,27) found that patients with chronic metabolic acidosis of severe renal failure and normal subjects made chronically acidotic by the administration of ammonium chloride were in chronically positive hydrogen ion balance. Since the plasma bicarbonate concentration was stable in these individuals, it appeared that retained hydrogen ion was being buffered somewhere outside the extracellular fluid. The magnitude of the hydrogen ion balance was such that buffering by bone seemed the only possible mechanism. This was reinforced by the observations that chronic ammonium chloride-induced acidosis resulted in a strongly negative calcium balance due to a marked increase in urinary calcium excretion without an increase in net intestinal calcium absorption. However, further studies by this group (28) demonstrated that ammonium chloride acidosis increased urine calcium excretion without an increase in glomerular filtration rate, and with no increase in filtered load of calcium, indicating decreased tubular reabsorption of calcium. This occurred even in patients with hypoparathyroidism (28). Furthermore, chronic acidosis was not accompanied by increments in serum parathyroid hormone (PTH) or 1,25-dihydroxyvitamin D (29,30) in normal subjects, suggesting that metabolic acidosis or a reduced plasma bicarbonate concentration per se might inhibit tubular calcium reabsorption.

These studies suggest that hypercalciuria in type 1 RTA may be due both to a direct effect of acidosis on tubular calcium reabsorption and to dissolution of bone by a chronic hydrogen ion balance. However, it should be noted that all patients with type 1 RTA do not have hypercalciuria (16,31,32), nor do patients with type 2 (5,33), or type 4 RTA (34), suggesting that factors other than acid-base balance may be important in determining the absolute rate of calcium excretion in any given patient with RTA.

The question as to why patients with type 2 RTA do not have hypercalciuria is of some interest with regard to the pathophysiology of hypercalciuria and bone disease in type 1 RTA. Sutton et al. (35) showed that dogs with chronic ammonium chloride acidosis exhibited increased fluid reabsorption in the proximal nephron and a dissociation of calcium from sodium reabsorption distally, resulting in an increased delivery of calcium relative to sodium to the distal tubule and final urine. When the acidosis was corrected by sodium bicarbonate infusion proximal fluid reabsorption was decreased and a selective increase in distal reabsorption of calcium relative to sodium occurred. The same results were obtained in both intact and thyroparathyroidectomized animals. It therefore appeared that delivery of bicarbonate distally modulated calcium reabsorption in that portion of the nephron. These studies have been invoked as an explanation for the difference in calcium excretion between type 2 and type 1 RTA (36). Thus, in type 2 RTA, proximal bicarbonate reabsorption is impaired such that enhanced distal delivery of bicarbonate might augment distal calcium reabsorption, preventing hypercalciuria. In contrast, in type 1 RTA proximal bicarbonate reabsorption is complete, as in normal subjects given ammonium chloride, allowing metabolic acidosis to decrease distal calcium reabsorption. However, according to current concepts, when patients with type 2 RTA are in a steady state of chronic metabolic acidosis, without alkali therapy, proximal bicarbonate reabsorption is complete and little or no bicarbonate is delivered distally which could increase distal calcium reabsorption (37,38). Thus, the effect of bicarbonate on distal calcium reabsorption might explain the effect of alkali therapy to decrease calcium excretion in type 2 RTA (5), but it would not explain the absence of hypercalciuria in acidotic patients with type 2 RTA who are not on alkali.

Another possible explanation for the lack of hypercalciuria in type 2 RTA has been suggested (36). It is possible that in contrast to type 1 RTA patients with type 2 RTA may be in acid balance at low, steady-state plasma bicarbonate concentrations, since renal acid excretion may be normal in this situation (39), so that titration of bone salts is not necessary to maintain acid-base balance. Even if this situation exists the question remains as to why chronic acidosis does not decrease renal tubular calcium reabsorption.

B. Hypercalciuria as a Cause of Type 1 RTA

Several lines of evidence have developed in recent years to indicate that metabolic acidosis is not the sole cause of hypercalciuria in type 1 RTA. In 1959, Wrong and Davies (9) described the syndrome of incomplete RTA discussed above in Sect. I.A. The original cases of incomplete RTA had nephrocalcinosis but did not have hypercalciuria. Subsequently, Buckalew et al. (18) reported three additional cases of incomplete RTA; all had recurrent nephrolithiasis, two had nephrocalcinosis, and two had hypercalciuria. The presence of hypercalciuria without metabolic acidosis in two patients with a defect in lowering urine pH suggested that hypercalciuria in at least some cases of type 1 RTA must be due to some mechanisms other than chronic acidosis. An alternate explanation for hypercalciuria in type 1 RTA was suggested by studies of a 64 member kindred from the Atlanta, Georgia, area with hereditary type 1 RTA reported in 1974 by Buckalew et al. (16). Four cases of RTA were found in the family, three with incomplete RTA, and a fourth with the classic, acidotic form of the syndrome. All four had hypercalciuria, nephrocalcinosis, and a history of recurrent nephrolithiasis. In addition, 15 members of this kindred had hypercalciuria, none of whom had RTA. Two of the hypercalciuric individuals without RTA had nephrocalcinosis, one of whom had a history of nephrolithiasis. Of the remaining 13 hypercalciuric individuals, two had a history of nephrolithiasis. Therefore, most of the affected persons in this kindred had asymptomatic hypercalciuria.

These findings were interpreted to indicate that hypercalciuria was inherited as an autosomal dominant trait in this family, and that nephrocalcinosis, nephrolithiasis, and type 1 RTA developed as a secondary consequence of prolonged hypercalciuria. This hypothesis was supported by longitudinal observations in one of the affected males. When first observed at age 10, he was found to have hypercalciuria without RTA or roentgenographically demonstrable nephrocalcinosis. However, at age 13, incomplete RTA had developed in addition to readily observable nephrocalcinosis.

In 1979, Hamed et al. (17) reported another large kindred from the Okalhoma City, Oklahoma, area in which type 1 RTA occurred in eight family members, whereas hypercalciuria was present without RTA in six other studied family members. These investigators found that the hypercalciuric subjects without RTA were statistically significantly younger than affected individuals with RTA, and concluded, as had Buckalew et al. (16), that hypercalciuria was the primary defect and that RTA was secondary to the hypercalciuria. Fig. 3 contrasts the apparent difference in pathophysiology between the Atlanta and Oklahoma City families. In the Atlanta family all patients with RTA had hypercalciuria, and RTA did not occur in the absence of nephrocalcinosis. However, three patients in the Oklahoma City family with RTA did not have nephrocalcinosis. They were younger than the five patients with RTA who did have nephrocalcinosis. This finding suggested the hypothesis that hypercalciuria caused sufficient tubular damage in the absence of nephrocalcinosis to cause type 1 RTA, and that the presence of RTA may then have promoted the development of nephrocalcinosis. Hamed et al. (17) explained the absence of hypercalciuria in some of the older patients with RTA by the presence of some type of unspecified further renal damage.

The differences between these two families are of interest. While the data in both families supports the notion that chronic hypercalciuria may cause type 1 RTA, the data do suggest that there may be unknown factors which determine the sequence of events in individuals who inherit a tendency to hypercalciuria.

The mechanism of the hypercalciuria in these individuals is a question of considerable importance, since it might have therapeutic implications. According to current concepts, hypercalciurias can be classified as absorptive, in which hyperabsorption of dietary calcium

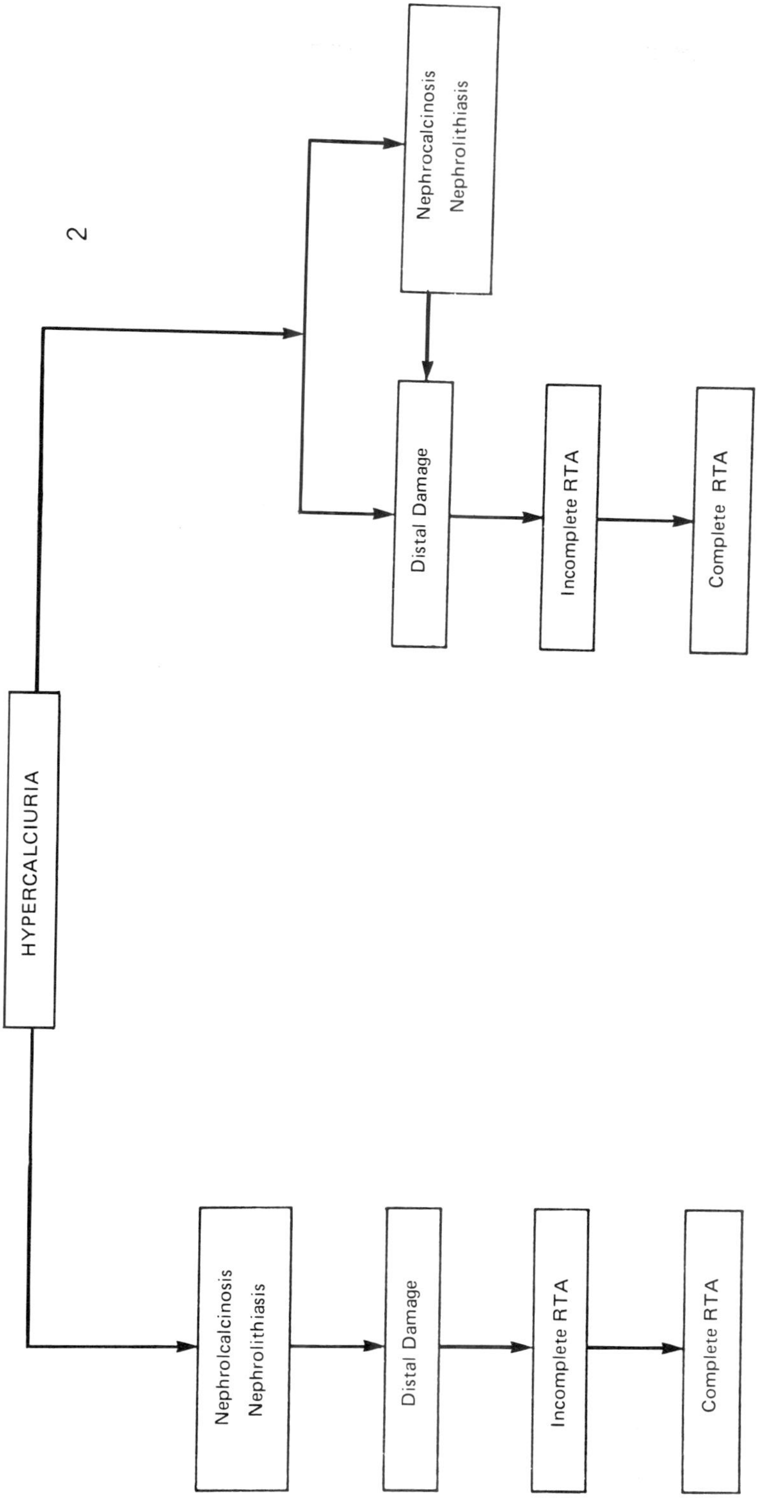

Fig. 3 Pathophysiology of RTA in two reported families with hypercalciuria. In family 1 (16) all patients with RTA had nephrocalcinosis, suggesting that distal tubular damage was caused by nephrocalcinosis. In family 2 (17) some patients with RTA did not have nephrocalcinosis, suggesting that hypercalciuria alone was sufficient to cause distal damage.

occurs, and renal, in which renal tubular calcium reabsorption is impaired (40-42). Unfortunately, only one member of the Atlanta family was studied, but the data in that individual suggested an absorptive type hypercalciuria (16). Eighteen members of the Oklahoma City family were studied by the method of Pak et al. (43), in an attempt to classify the hypercalciuria. Unfortunately, some discrepancies in the data reported by Hamed et al. (17) make their interpretation difficult (44). The authors concluded that most individuals had absorptive hypercalciuria, although inspection of the data suggests that some had tubular hypercalciuria as well (44). Over the past several years we have studied two families, similar to the one reported by Buckalew et al. (16), in which absorptive hypercalciuria has been found (45).

It is our tenative hypothesis that families such as those reported by Buckalew et al. (16) and Hamed et al. (17) represent a variant of the poorly characterized syndrome of hereditary idiopathic hypercalciuria. Hypercalciuria in childhood has been frequently reported (46-52), and Moore et al. (52) found the incidence of idiopathic hypercalciuria in children (2.9%) to be only slightly less than that usually found in adult populations. This observation suggests that idiopathic hypercalciuria may have its origins in childhood. Beilin and Clayton (49) reported a 6-year-old boy with hypercalciuria and nephrocalcinosis whose father and brother both had hypercalciuria. More recently, Coe et al. (53) studied the frequency of hypercalciuria in the families of nine adults with idiopathic hypercalciuria and recurrent calcium oxalate kidney stones. They found that 19 of 44 first-degree relatives and seven of 29 other relatives of the stone formers also had idiopathic hypercalciuria. Five of 19 first-degree relatives with hypercalciuria were below the age of 20. Their data suggested that idiopathic hypercalciuria may be inherited as an autosomal dominant trait, but the incidence of hereditary idiopathic hypercalciuria in the total population of patients with idiopathic hypercalciuria is not clear from this limited study.

If idiopathic hypercalciuria frequently begins in childhood as a hereditary disorder (52, 53) and if the families reported by Buckalew et al. (16) and Hamed et al. (17) represent variants of hereditary idiopathic hypercalciuria, one would expect more families of this type to have been detected. It could be that these families represent the extreme end of a spectrum of the syndrome of hereditary idiopathic hypercalciuria, being more severely affected because of environmental or other poorly defined factors. Alternatively, these families may be the end result of a fundamentally different type of hereditary abnormality which expresses itself initially as hypercalciuria.

III. NEPHROLITHIASIS

Recurrent formation of calcium containing stones occurs in both the complete and incomplete forms of type 1 RTA, although the exact incidence is difficult to ascertain. In one recently reported series (54), only two of 27 adults (7%) and none of 17 children had nephrolithiasis. In our institution, a referral center for stone-forming patients, 29 of 38 adults (76%) presented with stones (45). The problem of stone disease in type 1 RTA is an extremely important one, since it accounts for a considerable degree of morbidity associated with this syndrome. Recurrent nephrolithiasis with its attendant complications may be partly responsible for the generalized renal disease seen in some patients with type 1 RTA.

The incidence of type 1 RTA among the population of calcium stone formers has been recorded in several series between 0.3 and 8% (31,55-60). This is undoubtedly an overestimate of the true incidence, since most of these series have been reported from referral centers where highly selected populations are seen.

The mechanism of stone formation in RTA can be considered in the context of current concepts of the pathophysiology of nephrolithiasis. Significant advances have been made in the understanding of this process over the past 5-10 years. We will review this subject briefly here, but an extensive discussion is beyond the scope of this chapter. The reader is referred to several excellent reviews for an in depth discussion of this topic (59,61).

Calcium stone formation is fundamentally a physiochemical process in which the salts of calcium precipitate from a supersaturated solution. Supersaturation can be defined by the activity product ratio (APR), as follows. The product of the chemical activities of two ions in solutions, such as calcium and oxalate or calcium and phosphate, is the activity product (A_i). The thermodynamic solubility product (A_o) is the product of the concentration of two ions in solution at the point where the solution is in thermodynamic equilibrium with a solid phase of the two ions. The APR is the ratio of A_i to A_o. Supersaturation with respect to any salt is present when the APR exceeds one: that is, when the product of the activities of the two ions in solution exceeds the product of the activities of these two ions if they were in equilibrium with a solid phase of the salt.

A solution in which the APR exceeds one is said to be metastable as long as precipitation of salts does not occur. When the APR exceeds some critical limit, called the formation product ratio (FPR), precipitation of crystals may occur by a process called nucleation. Once nucleation has occurred, stone growth will proceed as long as the APR of the solution exceeds the FPR. Homogeneous nucleation occurs when nucleation is spontaneous; in heterogeneous nucleation crystallization occurs on the surface of some impurity or foreign substance in the solution. The FPR for homogenous nucleation is higher than for heterogenous nucleation. Thus, the presence of certain foreign surfaces in urine might promote stone formation.

Stone formation in humans is thought to be due to heterogeneous nucleation (59,61). Thus, while the APR for calcium oxalate is elevated in various types of stone formers (62), it has also been shown that the FPR for calcium oxalate is lower in stone formers than in normal subjects (62). This suggests the absence of inhibitors or the presence of promoters of heterogeneous nucleation in urine of stone formers. Substances which have been implicated as forming the nidus of stones and as such are promoters of heterogeneous nucleation include brushite ($CaHPO_4 \cdot 2H_2O$)(63-65), hydroxyapatite [$Ca_{10}(PO_4)_6(OH)_2$] (66), monosodium urate (66-70), and a yet to be identified, low-molecular-weight protein (71-73).

Other studies have also provided evidence for a deficiency of inhibitors of crystallization in urine of stone formers (74,75). When both the degree of supersaturation of urine with respect to calcium oxalate and the lack of inhibitors of crystallization are taken into account, almost complete separation between stone formers and normals can be shown (76). Substances which have been identified as potential inhibitors of stone formation in urine include pyrophosphate (77-79), citrate (80,81), magnesium (81,82), zinc (83), and some poorly defined macromolecules (84-86).

Patients with type 1 RTA have three abnormalities in renal function which might be expected to increase the likelihood of stone formation (Table 2). The elevated urine pH increases the activity products of the calcium phosphate salts such as brushite, octocalcium phosphate, and hydroxyapatite, since the concentration of the phosphate-containing anion of these salts increases with increasing pH. Increased activity products for calcium salts might also occur because of the hypercalciuria in many patients with type 1 RTA. In addition, citrate, a putative inhibitor of nucleation, is low in urine of many patients with type 1 RTA (88-90). However, there have been no quantitative studies of the relative contributions of these three stone-promoting abnormalities to the formation of stones in patients with type 1 RTA. Robertson et al. (87) found activity products for octocalcium phosphate and hydroxyatite exceeded the solubility products for those salts in urine of patients with type 1

Table 2 Abnormalities Promoting Stone Formation in Type 1 RTA

Abnormality	Mechanism of stone generation
1. Increased urine pH	Increased APR for phosphate salts of calcium (brushite, octocalcium phosphate, hydroxyapatite)
2. Hypercalciuria	Increased APR[a] for calcium salts
3. Hypocitraturia	? Decreased FPR[b] for calcium salts

[a]Activity product ratio (see text).
[b]Formation product ratio (see text).

RTA. This abnormality was apparently due entirely to the increased pH of urine; however, its contribution to the formation of stones is not clear, since there was considerable overlap between patients and normal controls. The possible role of the low urine citrate found in these patients on stone formation was not considered.

The effect of urine pH on the type of stone formed in both idiopathic stone formers and in patients with type 1 RTA has received some attention. Melick and Henneman (31) analyzed the type of stone formed in relation to urine pH in a large group of patients. Fourteen calcium stone formers had spontaneous urine pH persistently less than 5.5, and 25 had spontaneous urine pH persistently greater than 6.0. In the former group (low pH), eight (57%) had calcium oxalate stones, four (29%) had mixed calcium oxalate-calcium phosphate stone, but only two (14%) had calcium phosphate stones. In the high pH group, the percentages were reversed. Ten (40%) had calcium phosphate stones, 12 (48%) had mixed stones, while only three (12%) had calcium oxalate stones. A possible explanation for this observation was provided by Marshall et al. (91), who found that patients with mixed calcium oxalate-calcium phosphate stones had elevated urinary activity product for octocalcium phosphate and a higher urine pH than normal subjects. Patients with "pure" calcium oxalate stones, on the other hand, had normal maximum urinary octocalcium phosphate activity product, normal urine pH, and a high urinary calcium oxalate activity product. Pak et al. (66) found that urine APR for brushite increases with increasing urine pH in normal subjects and in idiopathic stone formers, becoming greater than 1 at urine pH above 6.5. However, in patients with idiopathic hypercalciuria, the APR for brushite was above 1 at any urine pH, presumably due to the increased urine concentration of calcium. Thus, increased urine saturation with respect to calcium phosphate (at least for brushite) may result either from increased urine pH or increased urine calcium concentration, both of which may be present in patients with type 1 RTA.

Based on these observations, one might expect, as suggested by Coe (59) that patients with type 1 RTA would have calcium phosphate stones. However, the few reports of stone composition in patients with type 1 RTA do not indicate this clear-cut association. In the earliest report, Melick and Henneman (31) found that all six patients with RTA had calcium phosphate stones. Similarly, Lee et al. (92) reported three patients with type 1 RTA, all of whom had calcium phosphate stones, and Coe and Parks (93) reported six patients, five of whom had calcium phosphate stones. On the other hand, Wilansky and Schneiderman (94) and Buckalew et al. (18) reported cases in which mixed calcium phosphate and calcium oxalate stones were found. Even more surprising, Bachman et al. (58) found that 34% of patients with RTA and stones had calcium oxalate as the major component, while 37% had calcium phosphate and 26% had mixed calcium phosphate-calcium oxalate stones. This incidence of calcium oxalate stones is approximately the same as in the stone-forming population at large (95). It should be noted, however, that the criteria for definition of RTA in the series of Bachman et al. (58) is questionable, since a large number of patients were included who were said to have incomplete type 2 RTA. According to current concepts of type 2 RTA, an incomplete or nonacidotic form of this condition cannot exist; and furthermore, most experience indicates that patients with type 2 RTA do not or only rarely form kidney stones (see Ch. 8). Be that as it may, we have also seen several patients with incomplete RTA and hypercalciuria who formed stones composed primarily of calcium oxalate. Thus, it would appear that factors other than high urine pH play a role in the pathophysiology of stone formation in type 1 RTA. This conclusion is strengthened by the observation that alkali therapy decreases stone formation in RTA (93). The possible explanation for this will be discussed in more detail below.

The role of citrate in the pathogenesis of stones in type 1 RTA has received little attention. As discussed above, if citrate is an inhibitor of nucleation, it is possible that low urine citrates found in many patients with type 1 RTA might contribute to stone formation. This question has more than theoretical interest, since it has been shown that citric acid excretion can be increased to normal levels by the administration of sodium bicarbonate (89,90). Thus, it is possible that the beneficial effects of bicarbonate therapy on stone disease in type 1 RTA might be due in part to the effect of bicarbonate on citrate excretion. Coe and Parks (93) reported six patients with complete type 1 RTA in whom alkali therapy sufficient to correct metabolic acidosis caused by a dramatic reduction in the incidence of nephrolithiasis, without an increase in urine citrate excretion. However, bicarbonate therapy caused marked reductions in urinary calcium excretion in these patients, which may explain the decreased stone formation. The complexities of the pathophysiology of the various abnormalities that predispose to stones preclude the generalization from this small series that alkali therapy is the best or only modality for treatment of stones in type 1 RTA, or that low urine citrate excretion is not a factor in stone pathogenesis. As we have pointed out above, not all patients with type 1 RTA and stones have hypercalciuria, and in those that do, alkali therapy does not always reduce calcium excretion. Our approach to therapy of stones in patients with type 1 RTA will be discussed in detail in Sect. XI.B.

Hypocitraturia is common but not ubiquitous in type 1 RTA, and stone formation may occur in patients with normal urine citrate as well as in those with hypocitraturia (16). In our experience, adult patients with type 1 RTA who form stones have either hypercalciuria, hypocitraturia, or both. We have seen three patients with incomplete type 1 RTA in whom hypocitraturia was present in the absence of hypercalciuria (45). Alkali therapy in these patients raised urine citrate to normal, and caused a marked reduction in stone formation. On the other hand, we have seen patients with hypercalciuria and normal urine citrate in whom alkali had no effect on calcium excretion. These patients have responded to treatment proposed for those with idiopathic hypercalciuria, such as thiazide diuretics, orthophosphate, and calcium-restricted diets (59,61) as will be discussed in more detail in Sect. XI.B.

The mechanism of hypocitraturia in type 1 RTA is of some interest. The clearance of citrate never exceeds the creatinine clearance (96), indicating that citrate is filtered and reabsorbed by the tubules. However, these clearance studies do not rule out some component of tubular secretion, and Runeberg and Lotspeich (97) have in fact provided some evidence for such a mechanism. Tubular reabsorption of citrate is markedly inhibited by metabolic alkalosis and increased by metabolic acidosis (96,98,99). An explanation for this effect was provided by Simpson (100), who showed that citrate oxidation by kidney slices and renal metochondria was an inverse function of pH (in slices) or bicarbonate (in mitochondria). Thus, metabolic alkalosis decreases renal cellular citrate oxidation, increasing intracellular citrate concentration, which presumably inhibits tubular reabsorption. The opposite of these events occurs during metabolic acidosis, suggesting a possible mechanism for hypocitraturia in type 1 RTA. Hypocitraturia may also be caused by potassium depletion (101), and decreased GFR (102,103), both of which may be present in type 1 RTA, suggesting two other possible explanations. However, the demonstration of hypocitraturia in patients with incomplete RTA without acidosis, renal failure, or hypokalemia (18,45) indicates an abnormality which has not yet been fully elucidated. Whatever the mechanism of this interesting abnormality, it is clear that urine levels of citrate can be increased to normal by adequate alkali administration (90), with potentially beneficial effects.

IV. NEPHROCALCINOSIS

Nephrocalcinosis is a common feature of type 1 RTA, particularly in its hereditary form. In some families it is present in virtually all patients with RTA, whereas in other families the incidence may be as low as 25% (16). The overall incidence of nephrocalcinosis in hereditary cases of RTA published up to 1974 was 55% (16). A more recent survey from a single center by Brenner et al. found that 56% of 27 patients with type 1 RTA had nephrocalcinosis (54). Interestingly, these investigators found that 73% of adults but only 29% of children had nephrocalcinosis. This suggests that nephrocalcinosis is related to the duration of the disease process. A similar conclusion results from our series, where none of 15 children with type 1 RTA had nephrocalcinosis, whereas 20 of 38 adults (53%) had this abnormality (45).

In one series of 41 patients with nephrocalcinosis reported in 1974 from the New York Hospital, six or 15% had RTA (104). Nephrocalcinosis in non-RTA patients usually occurs in conditions associated with chronic hypercalcemia, such as hyperparathyroidism, sarcoidosis, or carcinomatosis. Patients with medullary sponge kidney may have nephrocalcinosis without type 1 RTA (105), although some of these patients have been found to have incomplete RTA.

Nephrocalcinosis has been produced experimentally in rats by the chronic administration of the carbonic anhydrase inhibitor acetazolamide (106,107), by the chronic administration of vitamin D (108), and by magnesium depletion (109). Gyory et al. (106) found in rats that the major effect of acetazolamide causing nephrocalcinosis was the production of a chronically alkaline urine. Although hypocitraturia was produced by acetazolamide, when urine pH was reduced by the administration of calcium chloride nephrocalcinosis was prevented despite the presence of hypocitraturia. In the study by Gough et al. (108) the effect of vitamin D administration to produce nephrocalcinosis was augmented by feeding an alkaline ash diet.

Magnesium deficiency in rats is associated with hyperparathyroidism, hypercalcemia, hypocalciuria, hyperphosphaturia, and hypocitraturia (109). Hypocitraturia could be ameliorated by alkali administration, a maneuver which prevented nephrocalcinosis. Nephrocalcinosis was also prevented by reducing phosphate excretion by a low phosphate diet.

Patients with type 1 RTA and nephrocalcinosis may have many of the factors demonstrated experimentally to cause nephrocalcinosis, namely chronically alkaline urine, hypocitraturia, hypercalciuria, and hyperphosphaturia. While all of these abnormalities are not present in all patients with nephrocalcinosis, all patients will have at the very least a chronically alkaline urine. When this abnormality is combined with one or more of the other identified risk factors, it is not surprising that nephrocalcinosis is so commonly observed.

Several authors have reported that alkali treatment of type 1 RTA may be associated with reduction in the apparent degree of nephrocalicnosis as observed by radiological assessment (2,93,94). It has also been reported that adequate alkali therapy of infants with type 1 RTA predictably prevents the development of nephrocalicnosis (34). This effect occurs despite the fact that urine becomes more alkaline during chronic therapy. The beneficial effect of alkali on nephrocalcinosis must be due to decreased calcium excretion and/or increased citrate excretion.

V. OSTEOMALACIA

Bone disease was a prominent feature of the first reported cases of RTA (1-3), but is now rarely observed (54). Albright originally characterized this bone condition as a form of renal rickets, but different from the common type of renal rickets associated with chronic renal failure. Clinically, the bone disease in type 1 RTA is typical of osteomalacia, and is characterized by failure of calcification of newly formed osteoid. This leads to the clinical picture of classic rickets in children. In adults, the typical radiographic picture of osteomalacia is seen with generalized decreased calcification and pseudofractures. Bone pain may be prominent and the serum alkaline phosphatase is elevated.

A major difference between osteomalacia in type 1 RTA and in chronic renal failure is that in the latter healing occurs only with large-dose vitamin D therapy. In type 1 RTA, however, bicarbonate therapy alone has been reported to cause healing of osteomalacia (110,111). This observation has lead to the suggestion that the osteomalacia of type 1 RTA is secondary to metabolic acidosis. Various abnormalities produced by metabolic acidosis may contribute to osteomalacia, such as decreased gut calcium absorption (2,11,112), and increased renal excretion of calcium (26-28,36). Acidosis may also decrease the synthesis of 1,25-dihydroxyvitamin D_3 (113,114), increase phosphate excretion (115,116), and stimulate PTH secretion (116), although these effects are not always demonstrable (117).

The role of acidosis in the pathophysiology of type 1 RTA osteomalacia is further supported by the fact that no cases of incomplete RTA have been reported with osteomalacia. However, it is also true that chronic metabolic acidosis in other acidotic conditions such as type 2 RTA may not be associated with bone disease. In addition, it has been observed that osteomalacia in type 1 RTA heals more quickly when alkali is given with high-dose vitamin D than when alkali is given alone (111), but that only bicarbonate is needed to prevent recurrence. This observation has lead Dent and Stamp to suggest that calcium deposits in the renal tubules lead to decreased synthesis of 1,25-dihydroxyvitamin D_3, contributing to the osteomalacia (111). According to this hypothesis, alkali therapy promotes bone healing by diminishing nephrocalcinosis and improving the defect in vitamin D synthesis. Although the suggestion that abnormal vitamin D synthesis may play a role in type 1 RTA osteomalacia is reasonable, it seems unlikely that the presence or absence of nephrocalcinosis is the critical feature, since nephrocalcinosis is common in type 1 RTA but osteomalacia is rare. In our extensive experience with adult type 1 RTA, we have seen only two cases of osteomalacia, one of which was associated with end-stage renal disease (16) and was probably not due to the RTA per se. When observed, osteomalacia seems most likely to be found in patients who have had the acidotic form of type 1 RTA since infancy or early childhood, have been inadequately treated for metabolic acidosis, and who have concomitant growth retardation.

VI. GROWTH RETARDATION

Growth retardation is a regular feature of most children with chronic acidosis of whatever etiology (118), and type 1 RTA is no exception to this generalization. The question of whether factors other than acidosis might contribute to short stature in type 1 RTA seems to have been settled in the negative by the very important study of McSherry and Morris (13). These investigators treated 10 children with both hereditary and acquired type 1 RTA with sustained alkali therapy, and in all cases growth accelerated and either became normal or nearly normal.

The difference between the study of McSherry and Morris (13) and a previously published study of Nash et al. (25) which showed persistence of growth retardation despite alkali was the amount of alkali used. Whereas Nash et al. (25) used a standard dose of bicarbonate, McSherry and Morris (13) gave bicarbonate in whatever amount was necessary to completely correct acidosis. In so doing, they uncovered the previously unrecognized fact that bicarbonate wasting is a regular occurrence in children with type 1 RTA treated with bicarbonate. They found that complete correction of acidosis required varying amounts of bicarbonate at different ages, ranging from 4.8 to as high as 14.1 meq/kg per day. In all but one patient, at least 6 meq/kg per day was required during some period to correct acidosis. In general, the alkali requirement was lower during the initial treatment phase, with requirements increasing as growth accelerated. This phenomenon may be due primarily to bicarbonate wasting, as argued by McSherry and Morris (13), but also to accelerated acid production associated with rapid growth.

The cause of bicarbonate wasting in bicarbonate-treated patients is not clear from these studies. It did not appear to be due to suppression of tubular bicarbonate reabsorption by volume expansion, since measured values of blood and plasma volume were not increased, and plasma and urine and aldosterone levels were not suppressed (13). Although absolute plasma volume was not increased, it is possible that the increase in plasma volume associated with bicarbonate therapy suppressed, for some unknown reason, tubular bicarbonate reabsorption. One other interesting question which has not yet been explored is whether tubular reabsorption of bicarbonate is decreased in the proximal tubule, the distal tubule, or both.

The mechanism by which chronic acidosis retards growth is still a matter of some uncertainty. As discussed above (see Sect. V), acidosis decreases gut calcium absorption, and may interfere with the metabolism of vitamin D. It has been shown by McSherry that metabolic acidosis suppresses the normal release of growth hormone (34). This latter observation may provide the best explanation for growth failure in acidotic patients, since it would explain why children with acidosis may have growth retardation without osteomalacia. Both calcium deficiency and decreased levels of 1,25-dihydroxyvitamin D_3 would be expected to produce osteomalacia.

VII. MONOVALENT CATION WASTING

Frequent features of type 1 RTA in children such as lethargy, muscle weakness, and polyuria are the consequences of sodium and potassium wasting, the mechanism of which is not entirely clear.

A. Hyperkaliuria

Albright's original hypothesis (3) that monovalent cations were excreted in excess as bases to cover the excretion of mineral acids is no longer tenable, as discussed above. Gill et al.

(119), modifying Albright's original proposal, suggested that potassium wasting in type 1 RTA might be secondary to the defect in hydrogen ion secretion. This hypothesis was based on the view that Na-H exchange in the tubule is linked to Na-K exchange, such that a decrease in Na-H exchange leads to an increase in Na-K exchange (120). Thus, potassium wasting and hypokalemia were said to be corrected by treatment with alkali or sodium phosphate (4,119). These data were interpreted to mean that bicarbonate-rich or phosphate-rich tubular fluid allowed the tubule to secrete more hydrogen in exchange for sodium, and to secrete less potassium in exchange for sodium. However, later studies showed that both sodium and potassium wasting were ameliorated but not completely eliminated by sustained correction of metabolic acidosis (121).

Excessive potassium wasting could be due in part to the hyperreninemia and hyperaldosteronism observed in many patients with type 1 RTA (119,121). Some studies suggest that hyperaldosteronism in type 1 RTA is due to chronic volume depletion, since alkali therapy was shown to significantly reduce aldosterone secretion (119,121). However, Sebastian et al. (121) pointed out that although aldosterone secretion was suppressed by alkali therapy, it remained inappropriately high for the serum potassium concentration. These investigators suggested that inappropriate secretion of renin and aldosterone might be sustained in alkali-treated patients by the persistence of a sodium wasting defect, despite correction of acidosis (see below), with continued chronic volume depletion.

One patient with incomplete RTA has been reported in whom indomethacin administration was associated with return of plasma renin activity to normal (122), with amelioration but not elimination of potassium wasting. This observation suggests that hyperreninemia in at least some cases of type 1 RTA may be due to increased synthesis of renal prostaglandins. Why prostaglandin synthesis might be increased in type 1 RTA is not clear, but it could be secondary to potassium wasting, as may occur in Bartter's syndrome (44,123). If this were the case, potassium wasting could not be attributed entirely to hyperprostaglandinism or to its attendant hyperreninemia. Rather, a more specific defect in renal potassium handling, perhaps at the tubular level, would be necessary, as has been suggested in Bartter's syndrome (123).

Whatever the mechanism of hyperkaliuria, potassium depletion appears to be the most likely explanation for severe muscle weakness when it occurs in type 1 RTA. Potassium depletion may also contribute to the concentrating defect and polyuria, although medullary nephrocalcinosis may also be an important factor.

B. Hypernatriuria

Overt sodium wasting is not a common feature of type 1 RTA. However, inability to conserve sodium on a restricted sodium intake has been demonstrated in some patients with type 1 RTA (124), an abnormality which persisted despite correction of metabolic acidosis. Thus, as noted above with respect to potassium, the defect in sodium reabsorption cannot be attributed directly to the defect in hydrogen ion secretion or to the effects of metabolic acidosis (124). It is, however, possible that the defect in sodium reabsorption could be a manifestation of the same abnormality causing the defect in hydrogen ion secretion, since both abnormalities probably reside in the same segment of the nephron (124,125). Alternatively, the defect may be secondary to tubular damage resulting from nephrocalcinosis or the interstitial nephritis observed in some patients (124). In addition, a possible role for increased bicarbonate concentration in the distal tubule in alkali treated patients has not been fully evaluated.

It should be noted that a primary defect in sodium reabsorption in the distal tubule may lead to a reduction in distal tubule potential difference, and hence to an impaired hydrogen ion secretion. However, such an abnormality also leads to impaired potassium secretion and hyperkalemia, or type 4 RTA (see Ch. 9).

VIII. CHRONIC RENAL FAILURE

Although mild impairment in GFR is common in type 1 RTA, severe renal failure requiring replacement therapy is unusual in the primary form. We have seen a number of cases of end-stage renal disease due to problems such as analgesic nephropathy and other forms of chronic interstitial nephritis who had acquired type 1 RTA. However, we have only seen one case of primary, hereditary type 1 RTA who required dialysis (16).

The cause of chronic renal failure is not entirely clear, but it is likely due in most cases to interstitial nephritis resulting from the combination of medullary nephrocalcinosis and recurrent urinary tract infections (126-128). The latter are usually the consequence of recurrent nephrolithiasis. Thus, chronic renal failure in primary type 1 RTA may be similar to that which occurs in the general population of renal stone formers.

It has also been suggested that interstitial nephritis in type 1 RTA may be due to an autoimmune mechanism (129). In that case, both the defect in lowering urine pH and the interstitial nephritis could be due to a single immunological process. The occurrence of type 1 RTA in diseases with immunological abnormalities such as Sjorgren's syndrome (130,131) and idiopathic hypergammaglobulinemia (23,132) supports the immunological hypothesis, whereas the lack of evidence of immunoglobulins in the renal insterstitium (128) is against the hypothesis.

IX. SUMMARY OF PATHOPHYSIOLOGY OF RTA

An approach to pathophysiology of the various clinical abnormalities in RTA as presently viewed is summarized in Fig. 4. In contrast to Albright's original proposal outlined in Fig. 1, we suggest that five primary abnormalities may contribute to a complex pathophysiology. The defect in lowering urine pH is clearly the only abnormality present in all patients, and certainly leads to metabolic acidosis, which in turn may cause growth retardation and hypercalciuria and contribute to osteomalacia. Acidosis may also contribute to the formation of stones and nephrocalcinosis by reducing citrate excretion and increasing calcium excretion. However, hypercalciuria may occur in some patients as a primary abnormality, leading to nephrolithiasis, nephrocalcinosis, distal tubular damage, and a defect in lowering urine pH. Low urine citrate may be present in some cases as a primary abnormality, contributing to the development of nephrocalcinosis and nephrolithiasis. Renal failure due to interstitial nephritis may be secondary to recurrent nephrolithiasis, infection, and nephrocalcinosis. However, interstitial nephritis may be present in some cases as a separate primary disorder of uncertain etiology. Renal failure, when present, leads to a reduction in ammonia excretion, which contributes to the development of metabolic acidosis. Renal failure, if severe, may also lead to decreased synthesis of 1,25-dihydroxyvitamin D_3, contributing to the osteomalacia. Sodium and potassium wasting, the other major manifestations of type 1 RTA, are probably due to a multiplicity of factors, possibly including a primary defect in tubular potassium reabsorption, acidosis, secondary hyperaldosteronism of uncertain cause, and increased production of renal prostaglandins.

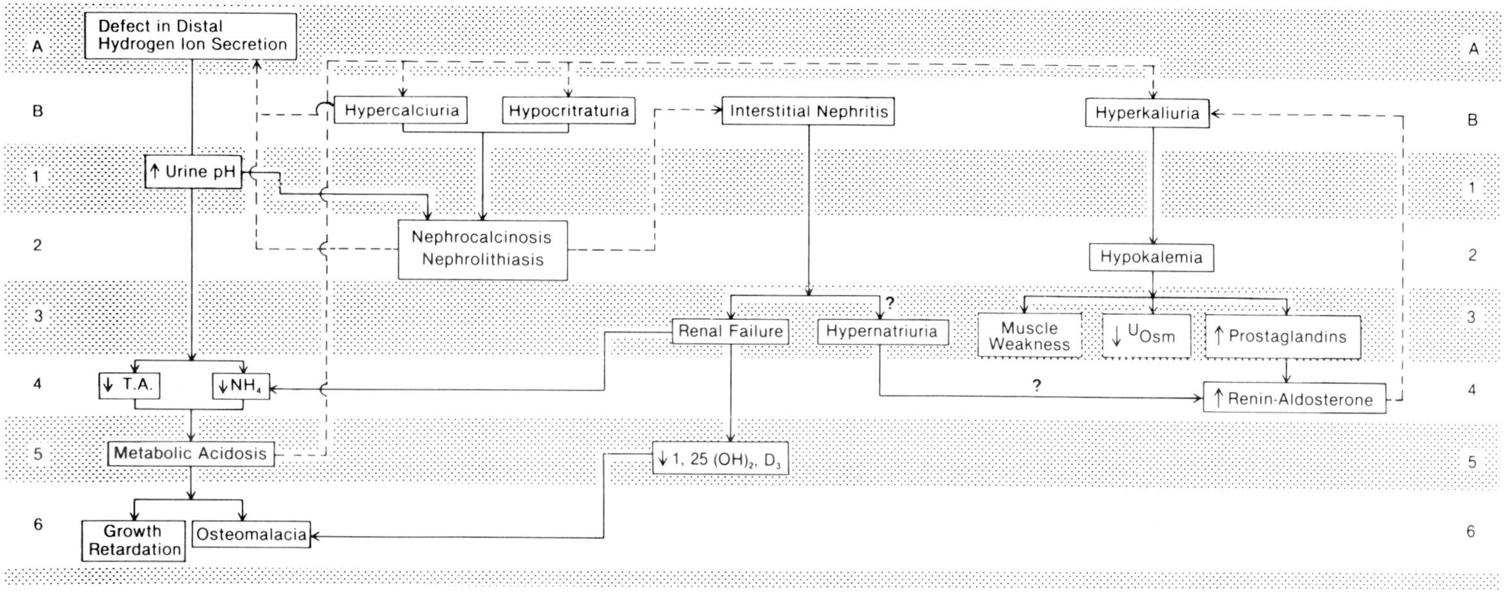

Fig. 4 A new multitiered pathophysiological model is proposed based on current evidence. Lettered tiers (A and B) are primary abnormalities in renal function, defined as those which appear to develop spontaneously, without recognizable cause. Tier A is the only primary abnormality which is invariably present in all cases. Tier B contains those primary abnormalities which are not invariably present. Numbered tiers (1-6) are secondary abnormalities, variably present, which result directly or indirectly from the primary defects. Those abnormalities on the same tier occur independently of each other. Abnormalities on lower tiers may be caused by those on higher tiers as indicated by solid lines. Secondary abnormalities may amplify or cause defects which are also primary as indicated by dotted lines.

X. DIAGNOSIS OF TYPE 1 RTA

A. Presenting Signs and Symptoms

Type 1 RTA presents in infants and young children as failure to thrive, often accompanied by vomiting, diarrhea, polyuria, and muscle weakness. In older children, growth retardation may be the presenting problem.

The primary syndrome in adolescents and adults has a more varied presentation. In our population, the most common complaint is passage of kidney stones (45). Nephrocalcinosis may be discovered incidentally on radiological examination of the abdomen. Some patients are discovered on workups for mild, chronic renal insufficiency, or for asymptomatic proteinuria. Occasionally, patients may present with severe hypokalemia resulting in profound muscle weakness. Metabolic acidosis is usually mild and is only discovered as an incidental finding. Osteomalacia, the prominent feature of the early cases (2,3), is only rarely seen.

In patients with acquired type 1 RTA the same presenting symptoms as in the primary form may be seen. However, in many cases the diagnosis of RTA is made in the course of investigation of the primary disease. A list of diseases causing acquired type 1 RTA can be found in a recent review (133).

B. Diagnostic Criteria

The diagnosis of RTA is established by demonstrating a defect in the ability to acidify the urine. Controversy exists as to what criteria to use for demonstrating the defect. Elkinton et al. (134) and Wrong and Davies (9) described standardized tests of ammonium chloride loading. Both groups agreed that subjects whose urine pH did not fall below 5.35 in response to 3 days of ammonium chloride (100 mg/kg per day) or to 100 mg/kg given acutely were abnormal and had type 1 RTA. However, other authors have argued that standard tests of ammonium chloride may be misleading, and that the response in urine pH must be related to the plasma bicarbonate concentration (6). These authors believe that patients with type 1RTA have a fixed defect in lowering urine pH in response to metabolic acidosis, so that urine pH will never fall below 5.4, no matter how severe the acidosis.

The problem arises in patients with mild, spontaneous metabolic acidosis whose urine pH is greater than 5.4. Some contend that this finding is adequate for the diagnosis of type 1 RTA. However, others argue that these findings may be observed in patients with type 2 RTA, and that patients presenting with mild metabolic acidosis and a urine pH of 5.4 or greater should be acid loaded, and only those who remain above 5.4 in response to severe acidosis can be considered to have type 1 RTA (see Ch. 8).

It is clear that patients exist who do not lower urine pH below 5.4 in the presence of mild acidosis, either spontaneous or secondary to the standard ammonium chloride load, but who can lower urine pH to less than 5.4 in the presence of more severe, ammonium chloride-induced acidosis (19). However, it is not yet clear whether these patients have type 1 RTA, as we believe, or type 2 RTA, as Edelmann believes (Ch. 8). If it is type 2, they should excrete greater than 15% of the filtered load of bicarbonate at normal plasma bicarbonate concentrations (8). On the other hand, if they have type 1 RTA, they should fail to raise urine PCO_2 normally in response to bicarbonate loading (Ch. 9). No group of patients exhibiting the abnormality in question has been studied in such a way as to make this distinction. Until this is done, the controversy will remain.

Our approach to the diagnosis of type 1 RTA is as follows. If the patient has hyperchloremia and a low serum total CO_2, an arterial blood gas must be obtained to distinguish between metabolic acidosis and respiratory alkalosis. Assuming the former is present, all alkali therapy should be withheld for 24-48 hr, and a urine collected under oil for pH determination by pH meter. If the urine pH is greater than 5.4, we believe the criteria for type 1 RTA are satsified and that no further studies need be done. However, if one wants to be absolutely certain the patient does not have type 2 RTA, the plasma bicarbonate can be normalized by alkali therapy, at which time patients with type 1 RTA will excrete less than 15% of the filtered load. This approach is safer than inducing more severe metabolic acidosis and provides an unequivocal result.

If a patient with normal acid-base balance is suspected of having incomplete RTA, the standard ammonium chloride test of Elkinton et al. (134) or Wrong and Davies (9) can be utilized. The long test of Elkinton et al. is somewhat more palatable to the patient, since the daily ammonium chloride load is taken in four divided doses. This test also stimulates maximal ammonium excretion and gives more reliable information on that aspect of renal function. The patient collects a 24-hr urine under oil on the third day of acid loading, at which time the urine pH by pH meter should be less than 5.4.

We frequently use the acute test of Wrong and Davies (9) for three reasons. First, the shorter time involved is important to minimize length of stay in hospitalized patients. Second, the short test does not depend on a 24-hr urine collection by the patient under non-controlled conditions. Although some patients are unable to tolerate the acute load because of nausea and vomiting, we find this problem to be minimal when the ammonium chloride is given in gelatin capsules after a light breakfast.

Another advantage of the short test is that the normal response to acute ammonium chloride loading involves not only the absolute urine pH, but the time course and pattern of the fall in urine pH. As Wrong and Davies (9) originally demonstrated, confirmed by many investigators, urine pH falls progressively to less than 5.4 within 2 hr after the acid ingestion, and remains at that value for at least 4-6 hr. Table 3 illustrates the type of mild abnormality we have observed in a number of cases of incomplete RTA. The patient is a 17-year-old male who had passed three kidney stones and whose father has classic type 1 RTA with recurrent nephrolithiasis and nephrocalcinosis. The patient was normal by the absolute pH criteria, in that urine pH in the fourth hour after the acid load was 5.39. However, the pattern of response was distinctly abnormal in that pH fell erratically, not progressively, and the lowest urine pH was not reached until 4 hr after the load, and could not be maintained. We are not certain that mild abnormalities such as the one illustrated in Table 3 will be picked up by the 3-day test. It is possible that 3 days of ammonium chloride loading might have caused his urine pH to fall to 5.4 or thereabouts. Thus, the short test may be more sensitive in detecting mild abnormalities in acidification.

Table 3 Abnormal Response to Acute Ammonium Chloride Load

Time (min)	Specimen	pH
0	U0	7.05
0-45	100 mg/kg NH_4Cl by mouth	
60	U1	6.04
120	U2	5.80
180	U3	5.94
240	U4	5.39
300	U5	5.85

XI. TREATMENT OF TYPE 1 RTA

A. Metabolic Acidosis, Growth Retardation, and Osteomalacia

Treatment of metabolic acidosis is best accomplished by the use of sodium bicarbonate. Since the amounts sufficient to correct acidosis in children are unpredictable, close monitoring of the acid-base status of patients is necessary. An initial dose of 3 meq/kg per day in infants and children would seem reasonable, with additional increments as necessary. This can be given conveniently as a solution containing 1 meq/ml. Most adults will not require more than 1 meq/kg per day to correct acidosis. Some patients develop abdominal bloating on sodium bicarbonate, in which case sodium citrate may be more palatable. Sodium citrate has no other advantage over sodium bicarbonate, since urine citrate excretion increases following alkali therapy in whatever form.

Complete correction of acidosis can be expected to correct growth retardation in children and osteomalacia in children and adults. However, complete healing of osteomalacia may require many months if alkali is used alone. Accordingly, it seems advisable to treat patients with severe osteomalacia with both bicarbonate and vitamin D, being careful to monitor the serum calcium concentrations. Dihydrotachysterol (DHT) can be recommended as reliable and the most economical preparation to use. Since patients with type 1 RTA may demonstrate vitamin D resistance, as do patients with chronic renal failure, large doses (0.2-0.6 mg/day) may be necessary.

B. Nephrolithiasis, Hypercalciuria, and Hypocitraturia

In our opinion, the approach to treatment of nephrolithiasis in type 1 RTA depends upon whether the patients have hypocitraturia and/or hypercalciuria, and upon the mechanism of hypercalciuria, if present. Accordingly, we advocate investigation of these parameters in stone-forming type 1 RTA patients. Since recurrent nephrolithiasis may occur in both complete and incomplete RTA, essentially all patients with severe stone disease should be investigated for type 1 RTA.

In our experience in adults, most but not all patients with type 1 RTA who form stones have either hypocitraturia or hypercalciuria, or both. This may not be the case in children. If the patient is acidotic, bicarbonate therapy sufficient to correct acidosis will probably be sufficient to cure recurrent nephrolithiasis. However, if urine citrate is low, bicarbonate therapy should be instituted, regardless of whether the patient is acidotic or not, in a dose adequate to raise urine citric acid to normal. A dose of 1 meq/kg per day is usually sufficient; however, as much as 3-6 meq/kg per day may be required in some patients (90), and repeated monitoring of urine citrate excretion is necessary. We now have three patients with incomplete type 1 RTA, hypocitraturia, and severe, recurrent nephrolithiasis who have formed no stones since institution of bicarbonate therapy (45).

Patients with type 1 RTA should be evaluated for the presence of hypercalciuria by one of the several published approaches. The calcium loading test developed by Pak et al. (43) is useful for identifying hypercalciuria and distinguishing between absorptive and renal types. The problem with this test is that it requires the patient to be on a low calcium diet (300 mg/day) for several days prior to the test. In our experience, this is difficult for many patients to accomplish at home. Patients who undergo the test on less than adequate calcium restriction appear to have tubular hypercalciuria by the normal values developed by Pak et al. (43). Accordingly, we have found it necessary to perform this test on patients who have been on a hospital-prepared metabolic diet for several days in order to obtain reliable results.

Perhaps the easiest test to perform on adult outpatients is the one described by Broadus and Thier (40). Their approach allows the patient to eat a diet low in dairy products, supplemented by 600 mg of calcium as calcium gluconate so that total calcium intake is approximately 1000 mg. Adults excreting more than 4.0 mg/kg per day of calcium on a 1000-mg calcium diet have hypercalciuria.

A rational approach to treatment of hypercalciuria in type 1 RTA can be based on the varied causes of hypercalciuria outlined in Fig. 3. If the patient has acidotic RTA with hypercalciuria, adequate alkali treatment can be expected to reduce both calcium excretion and stone formation (93). In those patients with incomplete RTA with hypercalciuria and in those acidotic patients who continue to have hypercalciuria despite adequate alkali, other approaches may be necessary. If some patients with type 1 RTA have a form of idiopathic hypercalciuria, as discussed above, the same treatment modalties developed for that condition may be efficacious. These are essentially dietary calcium restriction, thiazide diuretics, and orthophosphate (59,61). As noted in Sect. II.B, we have studied two families with type 1 RTA in which hypercalciuria seemed to be due to hyperabsorption of dietary calcium (16). We previously reported one patient from one of these families in which a thiazide diuretic was shown to reduce renal calcium excretion (122). In another unreported case from one of these families, stone formation has been eliminated by the use of thiazide diuretics (45).

We recommend that incomplete RTA patients with absorptive hypercalciuria without hypocitraturia be tried first on a 300-mg calcium diet with a high fluid intake. If stone formation continues, either a thiazide diuretic or orthophosphate can then be added. We have found this approach to virtually eliminate stone formation in several patients of this type (45).

Mild hyperparathyroidism has been reported in type 1 RTA, the cause of which is uncertain (92,135). Coe and Firpo (135) suggested that it was secondary to either metabolic acidosis or hypercalciuria, both of which are corrected by alkali therapy. Lee et al. (92) reported one case, however, in which alkali therapy reduced calcium excretion and parathyroid hormone (PTH) levels, but not to normal, and did not reduce stone formation. This patient was subjected to subtotal parathyroidectomy, which resulted in marked improvement in nephrolithiasis. We have treated one patient with absorptive hypercalciuria, nephrocalcinosis and incomplete RTA who continued to form large numbers of stones despite a combination of calcium restriction, sodium bicarbonate, and thiazide diuretics or orthophosphate (45). Following subtotal parathyroidectomy, calcium excretion fell with reduction in incidence of nephrolithiasis.

We have reported one patient in which calcium excretion fell in conjunction with indomethacin administration (122). It is not clear how many patients would demonstrate this phenomenon or whether this approach has any real therapeutic value.

C. Chronic Renal Failure

As noted above, severe renal failure is uncommon in type 1 RTA. However, in light of the proposed pathophysiology, severe renal failure is probably preventable in those few cases in which it occurs secondary to stone disease. It seems likely that adequate therapy of acidosis and/or treatment of nephrocalcinosis and recurrent nephrolithiasis and its attendant urinary tract infections will prevent severe renal damage of this type.

XII. GENETIC CONSIDERATIONS

All indications are that hereditary type 1 RTA is usually an autosomal dominant trait (136), although recessive type inheritance has been reported occasionally (137,138). Therefore, a careful family history should be taken in patients with an apparent primary type 1 RTA. The possible history of nephrolithiasis and/or recurrent urinary tract infection in relatives should be explored. Even if the family history is negative, there is the possibility that some relatives might have asymptomatic involvement. Identification of these cases would be important, both therapeutically and from the standpoint of genetic counseling. Therefore, we believe that investigation of family members should be offered to those who are interested.

Investigation of family members can be done in several ways. Measurement of serum electrolytes will certainly detect overt cases, but will not uncover those affected individuals with incomplete RTA. If the index patient has hypocitraturia, measurement of 24-hr urine citrate excretion has been shown to be an effective method of detecting other cases (90). If the index patient has hypercalciuria, we recommend that all willing family members be investigated for idiopathic hypercalciuria, especially those with a history of renal stones. It seems likely that early detection and effective therapy of idiopathic hypercalciuria in asymptomatic cases may prevent the development of nephrocalcinosis and recurrent nephrolithiasis. Similarly, identification and therapy of undetected cases of acidotic RTA in children will certainly prevent the development of growth retardation and nephrocalcinosis.

REFERENCES

1. Butler, A. M.; Wilson, J. L.; and Farber, S. Dehydration and acidosis with calcification at renal tubules. J. Pediatr. 8:489-499, 1936.
2. Albright, F.; Consolazio, W. V.; Coombs, F. S.; Sulkowitch, H. W.; and Talbot, J. H. Metabolic studies and therapy in a case of nephrocalcinosis and dwarfism. Bull. Johns Hopkins Hosp. 66:7-33, 1940.
3. Albright, F.; and Reifenstein, E. C., Jr. In: The Parathyroid Glands and Metabolic Bone Disease. Baltimore, Williams & Wilkins, 1948.
4. Pines, K. L.; and Mudge, G. H. Renal tubular acidosis with osteomalacia. Report of three cases. Am. J. Med. 11:302-311, 1951.
5. Soriano, J. R.; Boichis, H.; Stark, H.; and Edelmann, C. M., Jr. Proximal renal tubular acidosis: A defect in bicarbonate reabsorption with normal urinary acidification. Pediatr. Res. 1:81-98, 1967.
6. Soriano, J. R.; Boichis, H.; and Edelmann, C. M., Jr. Bicarbonate reabsorption and hydrogen ion excretion in children with renal tubular acidosis. J. Pediatr. 71:802-813, 1967.
7. Morris, R. C., Jr. An experimental renal acidification defect in patients with hereditary fructose intolerance. II. Its distinction from classic renal tubular acidosis; its resemblance to the renal acidification defect associated with the Fanconi syndrome of children with cystinosis. J. Clin. Invest. 47:1648-1663, 1968.
8. Morris, R. C., Jr. Renal tubular acidosis. Mechanisms, classification and implications. N. Engl. J. Med. 281:1405-1413, 1969.
9. Wrong, O.; and Davies, H. E. F. The excretion of acid in renal disease. Q. J. Med. 28: 259-313, 1959.
10. Elkinton, J. R. Hydrogen ion turnover in health and in renal disease. Ann. Int. Med. 57: 660-684, 1962.
11. Goodman, A. D.; Lemann, J., Jr.; Lennon, E. J.; and Relman, A. S. Production, excretion and net balance of fixed acid in patients with renal acidosis. J. Clin. Invest. 44:495-506, 1965.
12. Relman, A. S.; Lennon, E. J.; and Lemann, J., Jr. Endogenous production of fixed acid and the measurements of the net balance of acid in normal subjects. J. Clin. Invest. 40: 1621-1630, 1961.

13. McSherry, E.; and Morris, R. C., Jr. Attainment and maintenance of normal stature with alkali therapy in infants and children with classic renal tubular acidosis. J. Clin. Invest. 61:509-527, 1978.
14. Seldin, D. W.; Rector, F. C.; Portwood, R.; and Carter, N. Pathogenesis of hyperchloremic acidosis in renal tubular acidosis. In: Proceedings of the Ist International Congress of Nephrology, Geneva, 1961, p. 725.
15. Seldin, D. W.; and Wilson, J. D. Renal tubular acidosis. In: The Metabolic Basis of Inherited Disease, 2nd ed., edited by Stanbury, J. B., Wyngaarden, J. B., and Fredrickson, D. S. New York, McGraw-Hill, 1966, p. 1230.
16. Buckalew, V. M., Jr.; Purvis, M. L.; Shulman, M. G.; Herndon, C. N.; and Rudman, D. Hereditary renal tubular acidosis. Report of a 64 member kindred with variable clinical expression including idiopathic hypercalciuria. Medicine 53:229-254, 1974.
17. Hamed, I. A.; Czerwinski, A. W.; Coats, B.; Kaufman, C.; and Altmiller, D. H. Familial absorptive hypercalciuria and renal tubular acidosis. Am. J. Med. 67:385-391, 1979.
18. Buckalew, V. M., Jr.; McCurdy, D. K.; Ludwig, G. D.; Chaykin, L. B.; and Elkinton, J. R. Incomplete renal tubular acidosis. Physiologic studies in three patients with a defect in lowering urine pH. Am. J. Med. 45:32-42, 1968.
19. Tannen, R. L.; Falls, W. F.; and Brackett, N. C., Jr. Incomplete renal tubular acidosis: Some clinical and physiological features. Nephron 15:111-123, 1975.
20. Batlle, D.; Grupp, M.; Gaviria, M.; and Kurtzman, N. A. Distal renal tubular acidosis with intact capacity to lower urine pH. Am. J. Med. 72:751-758, 1982.
21. Perez, G. O.; Oster, J. R.; and Vaamonde, C. A. Incomplete syndrome of renal tubular acidosis induced by lithium carbonate. J. Lab. Clin. Med. 86:386-394, 1975.
22. Better, O. S.; Chaimowitz, C.; Naveh, Y.; Stein, A.; Nahir, A. M.; Barzilai, A.; and Erlik, D. Syndrome of incomplete renal tubular acidosis after cadaver kidney transplantation. Ann. Int. Med. 71:39-46, 1969.
23. Morris, R. C., Jr.; and Fudenberg, H. H. Impaired renal acidification in patients with hypergammaglobulinemia. Medicine 46:57-69, 1967.
24. Camien, M. N.; and Gonick, H. C. Relationship of renal "net acid" excretion to titratable ash-acidity (ash-TA) in diet and feces. Proc. Soc. Exp. Biol. Med. 126:45-51, 1967.
25. Nash, M. A.; Torrado, A. D.; Greifer, I.; Spitzer, A.; and Edelmann, C. M., Jr. Renal tubular acidosis in infants and children. J. Pediatr. 80:738-748, 1972.
26. Lemann, J., Jr.; Lennon, E. J.; Goodman, A. D.; Litzow, J. R.; and Relman, A. S. The net balance of acid in subjects given large loads of acid or alkali. J. Clin. Invest. 44:507-517, 1965.
27. Lemann, J., Jr.; Litzow, J. R.; and Lennon, E. J. The effects of chronic acid loads in normal man: Further evidenced for the participation of bone mineral in the defense against chronic metabolic acidosis. J. Clin. Invest. 45:1608-1614, 1966.
28. Lemann, J., Jr.; Litzow, J. R.; and Lennon, E. J. Studies of the mechanism by which chronic metabolic acidosis augments urinary calcium excretion in man. J. Clin. Invest. 46:1318-1326, 1967.
29. Weber, H. P.; Gray, R. W.; Dominguez, J. H.; and Lehmann, J., Jr. The lack of effect of chronic metabolic acidosis on 25-OH-vitamin D metabolism and serum parathyroid hormone in humans. J. Clin. Endocrinol. Metab. 43:1047-1055, 1976.
30. Adams, N. D.; Gray, R. W., Jr.; and Lemann, J., Jr. The calciuria of increased fixed acid production in humans: Evidence against a role for parathyroid hormone and 1,25-$(OH)_2$-vitamin D. Calcif. Tissue Int. 28:233-238, 1979.
31. Melick, R. A.; and Henneman, P. H. Clinical and laboratory studies of 207 consecutive patients in a kidney stone clinic. N. Engl. J. Med. 259:307-314, 1958.
32. Seedat, Y. K. Renal tubular acidosis. S. Afr. Med. J. 41:1007-1012, 1967.
33. Brenes, L. G.; Brenes, J. N.; and Hernandez, M. M. Familial proximal renal tubular acidosis. A distinct clinical entity. Am. J. Med. 63:244-252, 1977.
34. McSherry, E. Renal tubular acidosis in childhood. Kidney Int. 20:799-809, 1981.

35. Sutton, R. A. L.; Wong, N. L. M.; and Dirks, J. H. Effects of metabolic acidosis and alkalosis on sodium and calcium transport in the dog kidney. Kidney Int. 15:520-533, 1979.
36. Lemann, J., Jr.; Adams, N. D.; and Gray, R. W. Urinary calcium excretion in human beings. N. Engl. J. Med. 301:535-541, 1979.
37. Sebastian, A.; and Morris, R. C., Jr. Renal tubular acidosis. Clin. Nephrol. 7:216-230, 1977.
38. Nairns, R. G.; and Goldberg, M. Renal tubular acidosis: Pathophysiology, diagnosis and treatment. Disease-a-Month 23 (6):March, 1977.
39. Lemann, J., Jr.; Wilz, D. R.; and Brenes, L. G. Acid, calcium and phosphorus balances in proximal renal tubular acidosis. Kidney Int. 10:561, 1976.
40. Broadus, A. E.; and Thier, S. O. Metabolic basis of renal stone disease. N. Engl. J. Med. 300:839-845, 1979.
41. Pak, C. Y. C. Physiological basis for absorptive and renal hypercalciurias. Am. J. Physiol. 237:F415-F423, 1979.
42. Pak, C. Y. C.; Ohata, M.; Lawrence, E. C.; and Snyder, W. The hypercalciurias. Causes, parathyroid function and diagnostic criteria. J. Clin. Invest. 54:387-400, 1974.
43. Pak, C. Y. C.; Kaplan, R.; Bone, H.; Townsend, J.; and Waters, O. A simple test for the diagnosis of absorptive, resorptive and renal hypercalciurias. N. Engl. J. Med. 292:497-500, 1975.
44. Buckalew, V. M., Jr.; Lorentz, W. B.; and Frazer, D. S. Renal tubular disorders. In: Current Nephrology, vol. 4, edited by Gonick, H. C. Boston, Houghton-Mifflin, 1980, pp. 39-75.
45. Caruana, R. J.; and Buckalew, V. M., Jr. Unpublished observations.
46. Zetterstrom, R. Idiopathic hypercalcemia and hypercalciuria. Bibl. Paediat. 66:478-489, 1958.
47. Royer, P.; Mathieu, H.; Gerbeaux, S.; Frederich, A.; Rodriquez-Soriano, J.; Dartois, A. M.; and Cuisinier, P. L'hypercalciurie idiopathique avec manisme et atteinte renal chez l'enfant. Semin. Hop. Paris 38:767-783, 1962.
48. Fanconi, V. A. Idiopathishe hypercalciurie im kindersalter. Helvet Paediatr. Acta 4: 306-414, 1963.
49. Beilin, L. J.; and Clayton, B. E. Idiopathic hypercalciuria in a child. Arch. Dis. Child. 39:409-414, 1964.
50. DeLuca, R.; Guzetta, F. L'ipercalciuria idiopatica infantile. Pediatr. (Napoli) 73:613-619, 1965.
51. Royer, P.; and Balsan, S. Effet d'un regime pauvre in chlorure de sodium dans le "syndrome d'hypercalciurie idiopathique avec nanisme et troubles renaux" de l'enfant. Schweiz. Med. Wochenschr. 96:412-415, 1966.
52. Moore, E. S.; Coe, F. L.; McMann, B. J.; and Favus, M. J. Idiopathic hypercalciuria in children: Prevalence and metabolic characteristics. J. Pediatr. 92:906-910, 1978.
53. Coe, F. L.; Parks, J. H.; and Moore, E. S. Familial idiopathic hypercalciuria. N. Engl. J. Med. 300:337-340, 1979.
54. Brenner, R. J.; Spring, D. B.; Sebastian, A.; McSherry, E. M.; Genant, H. K.; Palubinskas, A. J.; and Morris, R. C., Jr. Incidence of radiographically evident bone disease, nephrocalcinosis and nephrolithiasis in various types of renal tubular acidosis. N. Engl. J. Med. 307:217-221, 1982.
55. Coe, F. L.; and Kavalach, A. G. Hypercalciuria and hyperuricosuria in patients with calcium nephrolithiasis. N. Engl. J. Med. 291:1344-1350, 1974.
56. Cintron-Nadal, E.; Lespier, L. E.; Roman-Miranda, A.; and Martinez-Maldonado, M. Renal acidifying ability in subjects with recurrent stone formation. J. Urol. 118:704-706, 1977.
57. Drach, G. W.; Perin, R.; and Jacobs, S. Outpatient evaluation of patients with calcium urolithiasis. J. Urol. 121:564-567, 1979.

58. Backman, U.; Danielsen, B. G.; Johansson, G.; Ljunghall, S.; and Wikstrom, B. Incidence and clinical importance of renal tubular defects in recurrent renal stone formers. Nephron 25:96-101, 1980.
59. Coe, F. L. Nephrolithiasis. Pathogenesis and Treatment. Chicago, Year Book, 1978.
60. Rapado, A.; Mancha, A.; Castrillo, J. M.; Traba, M. L.; Santos, M.; and Cifuentes Delatte, L. Etiological classification of renal lithiasis: A study based on 1936 patients. In: Urolithiasis Research, edited by Fleisch, H., Robertson, W. G., Smith, L. H., and Vahlensieck, W. New York, Plenum, 1976, pp. 495-498.
61. Pak, C. Y. C. Calcium Urolithiasis. Pathogenesis, Diagnosis and Management. New York, Plenum, 1978.
62. Pak, C. Y. C.; and Holt, K. Nucleation and growth of brushite and calcium oxalate in urine of stone formers. Metabolism 25:665-673, 1976.
63. Prien, L. Studies in urolithiasis. III. Physicochemical principles in stone formation and prevention. J. Urol. 73:627-652, 1955.
64. Pak, C. Y. C.; Eanes, E. D.; and Ruskin, B. Spontaneous precipitation of brushite: Evidence that brushite is the nidus of renal stones originating as calcium phosphate. Proc. Natl. Acad. Sci. U.S.A. 68:1456-1460, 1971.
65. Pak, C. Y. C. Quantitative assessment of various forms of therapy for nephrolithiasis. In: Urinary Calculi: Proceedings of the International Symposium on Renal Stone Research, Madrid, edited by Cifuentes Delatte, L., Rapado, A., and Hodkinson, A. Basel and New York, Karger, 1972, pp. 177-187.
66. Pak, C. Y. C.; Hayashi, Y.; and Arnold, L. H. Heterogeneous nucleation between urate, calcium phosphate and calcium oxalate. Proc. Soc. Exp. Biol. Med. 153:83-87, 1976.
67. Coe, F. L.; Lawton, R. L.; Goldstein, R. B.; and Tembe, V. Sodium urate accelerates precipitation of calcium oxalate in vitro. Proc. Soc. Exp. Biol. Med. 149:926-929, 1975.
68. Pak, C. Y. C.; and Arnold, L. H. Heterogeneous nucleation of calcium oxalate by seeds of monosodium urate. Proc. Soc. Exp. Biol. Med. 149:930-932, 1975.
69. Pak, C. Y. C.; Waters, O.; Arnold, L.; Holt, K.; Cox, C.; and Barilla, D. Mechanism for calcium urolithiasis among patients with hyperuricosuria: Supersaturation of urine with respect to monosodium urate. J. Clin. Invest. 59:426-431, 1977.
70. Coe, F. L.; and Kavalich, A. G. Hypercalciuria and hyperuricosuria in patients with calcium nephrolithiasis. N. Engl. J. Med. 291:1344-1350, 1974.
71. Boyce, W. H.; and King, J. S., Jr. Present concepts concerning the origin of matrix and stones. Ann. N.Y. Acad. Sci. 104:563-578, 1963.
72. Boyce, W. H. Organic matrix of human urinary concretions. Am. J. Med. 45:673-683, 1968.
73. Resnick, M. I.; and Boyce, W. H. Low molecular weight urinary proteins and renal lithiasis. Invest. Urol. 16:270-273, 1979.
74. Robertson, W. G.; and Peacock, M. Calcium oxalate crystalluria and inhibitors of crystallization in recurrent renal stone formers. Clin. Sci. 43:499-506, 1972.
75. Dent, C. E.; and Sutor, D. J. Presence or absence of inhibitor of calcium oxalate crystal growth in urine of normals and of stone formers. Lancet 2:775-778, 1971.
76. Robertson, W. G.; Peacock, M.; Marshall, R. W.; Marshall, D. H.; and Nordin, B. E. C. Saturation-inhibition index as a measure of the risk of calcium oxalate stone formation in the urinary tract. N. Engl. J. Med. 294:249-252, 1976.
77. Fleisch, H.; and Bisaz, S. Isolation from urine of pyrophosphate, a calcification inhibitor. Am. J. Physiol. 203:671-675, 1962.
78. Robertson, W. G.; Peacock, M.; and Nordin, B. E. C. Inhibitor of growth and aggregation of calcium oxalate crystals in vitro. Clin. Chim. Acta 43:31-37, 1973.
79. Hansen, N. M.; Felix, R.; Bisaz, S.; and Fleisch, H. Aggregation of hydroxyapatite crystals. Biochim. Biophys. Acta 451:549-559, 1976.
80. Meyer, J. L.; and Smith, L. H. Growth of calcium oxalate crystals. II. Inhibition by natural urinary crystal growth inhibitors. Invest. Urol. 13:36-39, 1975.

81. Bisaz, S.; Felix, R.; Neuman, W. F.; and Fleisch, H. Quantitative determination of inhibitors of calcium phosphate precipitation in whole urine. Miner. Electrolyte Metab. 1:74-83, 1978.
82. Smith, L. H.; Meyer, J. L.; and McCall, J. T. Chemical nature of crystal inhibitors isolated from human urine. In: Urinary Calculi: Proceedings of the International Symposium on Renal Stone Research, Madrid, edited by Cifuentes Delatte, L., Rapado, A., and Hodkinson, A. Basel and New York, Karger, 1972, pp. 318-327.
83. Byrd, E. D.; and Thomas, W. C., Jr. Effects of various metals on mineralization in vitro. Proc. Soc. Exp. Biol. Med. 112:640-643, 1963.
84. Howard, J. E.; Thomas, W. C.; Barker, L. M.; Smith, L. H.; and Wadkins, C. L. The recognition and isolation from urine and serum of a peptide inhibitor to calcification. Johns Hopkins Med. J. 120:119-136, 1967.
85. Smith, L. H.; and McCall, J. T. Isolation of nucleation inhibitor from urine. In: Urolithiasis—Physical Aspects, edited by Finlayson, B., Hench, L. L., and Smith, L. H. Washington, D. C., National Academy of Sciences, 1972, pp. 157-160.
86. Robertson, W. G.; Knowles, F.; and Peacock, M. Urinary acid mucopolysaccharide inhibitors of calcium oxalate crystallization. In: Urolithiasis Research, edited by Fleisch, H., Robertson, W. G., Smith, L. H., and Vahlensieck, W. London, Plenum, 1976, pp. 331-340.
87. Robertson, W. G.; Peacock, M.; and Nordin, B. E. C. Activity products in stone-forming and non-stone-forming urine. Clin. Sci. 34:579-594, 1968.
88. Nordin, B. E. C.; and Smith, D. A. Citric acid excretion in renal stone disease and in renal tubular acidosis. Br. J. Urol. 35:438-444, 1963.
89. Morrissey, J. F.; Ochoa, M.; Lotspeich, W. D.; and Waterhouse, C. Citrate excretion in renal tubular acidosis. Ann. Int. Med. 58:159-166, 1963.
90. Norman, M. E.; Feldman, N. I.; Cohn, R. M.; and McCurdy, D. K. Urinary citrate excretion in the diagnosis of distal renal tubular acidosis. J. Pediat. 92:394-400, 1978.
91. Marshall, R. W.; Cochran, M.; Robertson, W. G.; Hodkinson, A.; and Nordin, B. E. C. The relation between the concentration of calcium salts in the urine and renal stone composition in patients with calcium-containing renal stones. Clin. Sci. 43:433-441, 1972.
92. Lee, D. N. B.; Drinkard, J. P.; Gonick, H. C.; Coulson, W. F.; and Cracchiolo, A. Pathogenesis of renal calculi in distal renal tubular acidosis. Clin. Orthop. 121:234-242, 1976.
93. Coe, F. L.; and Parks, J. H. Stone disease in hereditary distal renal tubular acidosis. Ann. Int. Med. 93:60-61, 1980.
94. Wilansky, D. L.; and Schneiderman, C. Renal tubular acidosis with recurrent nephrolithiasis and nephrocalcinosis. N. Engl. J. Med. 257:399-403, 1957.
95. Prien, E. L.; and Prien, E. L., Jr. Composition and structure of urinary stone. Am. J. Med. 45:654-672, 1968.
96. Grollman, A. P.; Harrison, H. C.; and Harrison, H. E. The renal excretion of citrate. J. Clin. Invest. 40:1290-1296, 1961.
97. Runeberg, L.; and Lotspeich, W. D. Krebs cycle acid excretion with isotopic split renal function techniques. Am. J. Physiol. 211:467-475, 1966.
98. Crawford, M. A.; Milne, M. D.; and Scribner, B. H. The effect of changes in acid-base balance on urinary citrate in the rat. J. Physiol. (Lond.) 149:413-423, 1959.
99. Simpson, D. P. Influence of plasma bicarbonate concentration and pH on citrate excretion. Am. J. Physiol. 206:875-882, 1964.
100. Simpson, D. P. Regulation of renal citrate metabolism by bicarbonate ion and pH: Observations in tissue slices and mitochondria. J. Clin. Invest. 46:225-238, 1967.
101. Fourman, P.; and Robinson, J. R. Diminished urinary excretion of citrate during deficiencies of potassium in man. Lancet 2:656-657, 1953.
102. Hodgkinson, A. Citric acid excretion in normal adults and in patients with renal calculus. Clin. Sci. 23:203-212, 1962.

103. Gyory, A. Z.; Edwards, K. D. G.; Alcock, N. W.; and Armstrong, C. Abnormal citrate metabolism in patients with renal tubular defects, including renal tubular acidosis. Bull. Post-Grad. Comm. Med. Univ. Sydney 23:241-262, 1967.
104. Farrell, R. M.; Horwith, M.; and Muecks, E. C. Renal tubular acidosis and nephrocalcinosis: Diagnosis and clinical management. J. Urol. 111:429-433, 1974.
105. Morris, R. C.; Yamauchi, H.; Oalubinskas, A. J.; and Howenstine, J. Medullary sponge kidney. Am. J. Med. 38:883-892, 1965.
106. Gyory, A. Z.; Edwards, K. D. G.; Robinson, J.; and Palmer, A. A. The relative importance of urinary pH and urinary content of citrate, magnesium and calcium in the production of nephrocalcinosis by diet and acetazolamide in the rat. Clin. Sci. 39: 605-623, 1970.
107. Harrison, H. E.; and Harrison, H. C. Inhibition of urine citrate excretion and production of renal calcinosis in the rat by acetazolamide (Diamox) administration. J. Clin. Invest. 34:1662-1670, 1955.
108. Gough, J.; Duguid, J. B.; and Davies, D. R. The renal lesions in hypervitaminosis D; observations on the urinary calcium and phosphorus excretion. Br. J. Exp. Pathol. 14:137-145, 1933.
109. Lifshitz, F.; Harrison, H. C.; Bull, E. C.; and Harrison, H. E. Citrate metabolism and the mechanism of renal calcification induced by magnesium depletion. Metabolism 16:345-357, 1967.
110. Richards, P.; Chamberlain, M. J.; and Wrong, O. M. Treatment of osteomalacia of renal tubular acidosis by sodium bicarbonate alone. Lancet 2:994-997, 1972.
111. Dent, C. E.; and Stamp, T. C. B. Vitamin D, rickets and osteomalacia. In: Metabolic Bone Disease, vol. I, edited by Avioli, L. V., and Krane, S. M. New York, Academic Press, 1977, pp. 237-305.
112. Greenberg, A. J.; McNamara, H.; and McCrory, W. W. Metabolic balance studies in primary renal tubular acidosis: Effect of acidosis on external calcium and phosphorus balances. J. Pediatr. 69:610-618, 1966.
113. Lee, S. W.; Russell, J. E.; and Avioli, L. V. $25OHD_3$ to $1,25\text{-}(OH)_2D_3$: Conversion impaired by systemic acidosis. Science 195:994-996, 1977.
114. Sauveur, B.; Garabedian, M.; Fellot, C.; Mongin, P.; and Balsan, S. The effect of induced metabolic acidosis on vitamin D_3 metabolism in rachitic chicks. Calcif. Tissue Res. 23:121-124, 1977.
115. Pitts, R. F.; Lotspeich, W. D.; Schiess, W. A.; and Ayer, A. L. The renal regulation of acid-base balance in man. 1. The nature of the mechanism of acidifying the urine. J. Clin. Invest. 27:48-61, 1948.
116. Coe, F. L.; Firpo, J. J., Jr.; Hollandsworth, D. L.; Segil, L.; Canterbury, J. M.; and Reiss, E. Effect of acute and chronic metabolic acidosis on serum immunoreactive parathyroid hormone in man. Kidney Int. 8:262-273, 1975.
117. Weber, H. P.; Gray, R. W.; Dominguez, J. H.; and Lemann, J. The lack of effect of chronic metabolic acidosis on 25-OH-vitamin D metabolism and serum parathyroid hormone in humans. J. Clin. Endocrinol. Metab. 43:1047-1055, 1976.
118. McSherry, E. Acidosis and growth in nonuremic renal disease. Kidney Int. 14:349-354, 1978.
119. Gill, J. R., Jr.; Bell, N. H.; and Bartter, F. D. Impaired conservation of sodium and potassium in renal tubular acidosis and its corrections by buffer anions. Clin. Sci. 33: 577-592, 1967.
120. Berliner, R. W. Renal mechanisms for potassium excretion. Harvey Lect. 55:141-171, 1960.
121. Sebastian, A.; McSherry, E.; and Morris, R. C., Jr. Renal potassium wasting in renal tubular acidosis (RTA). Its occurrence in types 1 and 2 RTA despite sustained correction of systemic acidosis. J. Clin. Invest. 50:667-678, 1971.

122. Caruana, R. J.; and Buckalew, V. M., Jr. Improvement of hypercalciuria, potassium wasting and hyperreninemia in incomplete distal renal tubular acidosis by indomethacin. Nephron 24:232-235, 1979.
123. Ferris, T. F. Prostaglandins, potassium and Bartter's syndrome. J. Lab. Clin. Med. 92: 663-668, 1978.
124. Sebastian, A.; McSherry, E.; and Morris, R. C., Jr. Impaired renal conservation of sodium and chloride during sustained correction of systemic acidosis in patients with type 1, classic renal tubular acidosis. J. Clin. Invest. 58:454-469, 1976.
125. Rodriguez-Soriano, J. R.; Vallo, A.; Castillo, G.; and Oliveros, R. Renal handling of water and sodium in children with proximal and distal renal tubular acidosis. Nephron 25:193-198, 1980.
126. Milne, M. D. Renal tubular dysfunction. In: Diseases of the Kidney, 2nd ed., edited by Straus, M. B., and Welt, L. G. Boston, Little, Brown, 1971, pp. 1071-1138.
127. Chan, J. C. M. Acid-base, calcium, potassium and aldosterone metabolism in renal tubular acidosis. Nephron 23:152-158, 1979.
128. Feest, T. G.; Lockwood, C. M.; Morley, A. R.; and Uff, J. S. Renal histology and immunopathology in distal renal tubular acidosis. Clin. Nephrol. 10:187-190, 1978.
129. Pasternack, A.; and Linder, E. Renal tubular acidosis: An immunopathological study on four cases. Clin. Exp. Immunol. 7:115-123, 1970.
130. Tu, W. H.; Shearn, M. A.; Lee, J. C.; and Hopper, J. Interstitial nephritis in Sjogren's syndrome. Ann. Intern. Med. 69:1163-1170, 1968.
131. Shioji, R.; Furuyama, T.; Onodera, S.; Saito, H.; Ito, H.; and Sasaki, Y. Sjogren's syndrome and renal tubular acidosis. Am. J. Med. 48:456-463, 1970.
132. Wilson, I.; Williams, R. C.; and Tobian, L. Renal tubular acidosis—Three cases with immunoglobulin abnormalities in the patients and their kindred. Am. J. Med. 43:356-370, 1967.
133. Caruana, R. J.; Buckalew, V. M., Jr.; and Lorentz, W. B. Renal tubular disorders. In: Current Nephrology, vol. 6, edited by Gonick, H. C. New York, Wiley, 1983.
134. Elkinton, J. R.; Huth, E. J.; Webster, G. D.; and McCance, R. A. The renal excretion of hydrogen ion in renal tubular acidosis. I. Quantitative assessment of the response to ammonium chloride as an acid load. Am. J. Med. 29:554-575, 1960.
135. Coe, F. L.; and Firpo, J. J. Evidence for mild reversible hyperparathyroidism in distal renal tubular acidosis. Arch. Intern. Med. 135:1485-1489, 1975.
136. Seldin, D. W.; and Wilson, J. D. Renal tubular acidosis. In: The Metabolic Basis of Inherited Disease, 3rd ed., edited by Stanbury, J. B., Wyngaarden, J. B., and Fredrickson, D. S. New York, McGraw-Hill, 1973, p. 1548.
137. Kuhlencordt, F.; Lenz, W.; Seemann, N.; and Zukswerdt, L. Renal tubular acidosis and bilateral nephrocalcinosis in uniovular twins. Germ. Med. Month. 12:565-570, 1967.
138. Simon, H.; Orive, B.; Zamora, I.; and Mendizabal, S. The acidification defect in the syndrome of renal tubular acidosis with nerve deafness. Acta Pediatr. Scand. 68:291-295, 1979.

12

Nephrogenic Diabetes Insipidus

GREGORY L. BRADEN,* IRWIN SINGER, and MALCOLM COX
University of Pennsylvania School of Medicine, Philadelphia Veterans Administration Medical Center, and Hospital of the University of Pennsylvania, Philadelphia, Pennsylvania

Nephrogenic diabetes insipidus has been recognized with increasing frequency during the last 10 years. Although familial renal concentrating defects that are unresponsive to the administration of exogenous vasopressin (antidiuretic hormone; ADH) have been recognized for many years, and although similar defects had been demonstrated in patients with hypokalemia or hypercalcemia, it is only recently that several commonly used drugs have also been shown to produce nephrogenic diabetes insipidus. In fact, drugs account for most cases of nephrogenic diabetes insipidus now encountered clinically.

This chapter will focus on the mechanisms by which renal water handling is impaired in the various kinds of nephrogenic diabetes insipidus. Some agents which cause nephrogenic diabetes insipidus have clearly defined mechanisms of action. Other kinds of nephrogenic diabetes insipidus are not nearly as well characterized, primarily because there is insufficient evidence to incriminate a particular defect in renal water handling with certainty.

A clear understanding of normal renal water handling is a prerequisite for a discussion of the multiple pathophysiological mechanisms involved in the different kinds of nephrogenic diabetes insipidus. In this chapter the mechanisms by which renal unresponsiveness to ADH could occur will be delineated, and a description of how nephrogenic diabetes insipidus is distinguished clinically from other polyuric disorders will be presented. This will be followed by an in-depth discussion of the pathophysiology of the different etiologies of nephrogenic diabetes insipidus. Finally the therapy of nephrogenic diabetes insipidus will be discussed.

I. RENAL WATER EXCRETION

In order to appreciate how interference with water and/or solute reabsorption may diminish renal concentrating ability it is necessary to consider the normal mechanisms which control renal water excretion, particularly those processes that are ADH dependent. The homeostatic system that regulates renal water excretion consists of two components: (1) a central com-

**Current affiliation*: Tufts University School of Medicine, Boston, and Baystate Medical Center, Springfield, Massachusetts

ponent which involves the release of ADH from the posterior pituitary (and/or hypothalamus), and (2) a peripheral component which involves the kidney and the response of the kidney to ADH.

Antidiuretic hormone is synthesized in the supraoptic and paraventricular nuclei in the hypothalamus and stored in the posterior pituitary. Under most circumstances, ADH is released into the circulation in response to a rise in body fluid tonicity; however, effective arterial blood volume also has an important role in the physiological regulation of ADH release (1-4). Effective arterial blood volume depletion enhances the release of ADH in response to a given change in plasma osmolality and effective arterial blood volume expansion has the opposite effect.

An increase in plasma osmolality to the highest level that normally occurs (~295 mOsm/kg H_2O) produces maximal circulating levels of ADH. Under such circumstances, provided that the renal component of the homeostatic system is intact, urine osmolality reaches maximal values (800-1200 mOsm/kg H_2O) and urine volume becomes minimal. In contrast, as plasma osmolality decreases, ADH release is progressively inhibited until, at about 280 mOsm/kg H_2O, circulating ADH levels become undetectable. Under these conditions, urine osmolality reaches minimal values (50-100 mOsm/kg H_2O) and urine volume increases dramatically. Thus, variable circulating levels of ADH are translated into variable degrees of renal water excretion. As a result, body fluid tonicity is maintained within extremely precise limits.

The processes responsible for variable renal water excretion can be conveniently divided into two parts: (1) the generation (and maintenance) of an osmotic gradient, and (2) the utilization of this gradient (Table 1). The osmotic gradient in the renal medullary and papillary interstitium provides the driving force for water reabsorption from the collecting duct, but water reabsorption occurs rapidly only after the collecting duct has been rendered water permeable by ADH.

A. Generation and Maintenance of an Osmotic Gradient

Generation of the osmotic gradient is dependent on normal functioning of the countercurrent multiplier system, the central features of which are: (1) the "hairpin" arrangement of the loop of Henle, and (2) the transport of sodium chloride out of the relatively water-impermeable ascending limb of Henle's loop into the renal interstitium (5,6). As electrolyte is reabsorbed along the course of the ascending limb the tubular fluid that remains becomes

Table 1 Factors That Influence Urinary Concentration

A. Generation and maintenance of an osmotic gradient
   1. Delivery of NaCl to the ascending limb of Henle's loop
      a. Glomerular filtration rate
      b. Proximal tubular reabsorption
   2. Reabsorption of NaCl in the ascending limb of Henle's loop
   3. Urea trapping in the medullary interstitium
      a. Dietary protein intake
      b. Urea reabsorption in the medullary collecting duct
   4. Renal medullary blood flow

B. Utilization of the osmotic gradient
   1. Circulating ADH levels
   2. ADH-responsiveness of the collecting duct
   3. Collecting duct flow rate

progressively more dilute, reaching an osmolality of about 150 mOsm/kg H_2O as it enters the early distal convoluted tubule. The transfer of a small amount of electrolyte without water from the initial portion of the ascending limb to the interstitium creates a small osmotic gradient between the tubular lumen and the interstitium. As the tubular fluid passes to the next portion of the ascending limb an additional small amount of electrolyte is transferred against a similar small gradient. Repetitive transfer of small amounts of electrolyte against small osmotic gradients occurs at each successive level of the ascending limb. The countercurrent arrangement of the loop of Henle "multiplies" the effect of the small "horizontal" osmotic gradient so that a large "vertical" osmotic gradient is generated from the renal cortex to the tip of the papilla.

Several factors influence the production and maintenance of the corticopapillary osmotic gradient (Table 1). First, sufficient glomerular filtrate must be produced so that adequate amounts of sodium chloride can be delivered to the ascending limb. Second, proximal tubular reabsorption must not be so great that delivery to the ascending limb is compromised. Third, NaCl reabsorption in the ascending limb must be of sufficient magnitude to allow for the establishment of the corticopapillary osmotic gradient. Fourth, since urea also contributes to medullary hypertonicity (accounting for up to 50% of the osmotic gradient), the trapping of sufficient amounts of urea in the renal medulla must be ensured. Urea accumulation requires the ingestion of adequate amounts of protein (so that normal amounts of urea are produced in the liver) and the transport of urea out of the medullary collecting duct into the renal interstitium.

The integrity of the vasa rectae and the rate of the medullary blood flow are crucial factors in the maintenance of the corticopapillary osmotic gradient. These blood vessels course through the renal medulla in a similar fashion to the loops of Henle and equilibrate osmotically with the medullary interstitium, a process termed countercurrent exchange. The net result is that blood exiting from the vasa rectae into the renal venous system has an osmolality only slightly greater than plasma and, since large amounts of medullary interstitial solute are not removed, the medullary osmotic gradient is maintained. In addition, less than 10% of total renal blood flow is normally directed to the medulla; this low regional blood flow also serves to maintain the corticopapillary osmotic gradient.

B. Utilization of the Osmotic Gradient

The corticopapillary osmotic gradient provides the driving force for the reabsorption of water in the ADH-responsive portions of the distal nephron (cortical collecting tubule and collecting duct). When ADH levels are undetectable (e.g., when body fluid tonicity is subnormal) these portions of the nephron are relatively water impermeable and hypotonic fluid leaving the ascending limb of Henle's loop is excreted virtually unchanged as dilute urine. In contrast, in the presence of high levels of ADH (e.g., when body fluid tonicity is above normal) collecting ducts become much more permeable to water and the tubular fluid is progressively concentrated as it passes down the collecting system and equilibrates with the hypertonic medullary interstitum. Since the degree of water permeability of the ADH-responsive portions of the nephron is dependent on the amount of ADH present, widely variable amounts of water (at varying urine osmolalities) can be excreted.

In addition to the circulating level of ADH and the ability of the distal nephron to respond to ADH, tubular fluid flow rate is also an important determinant of urine osmolality; the flow rate through the collecting duct must allow sufficient time for osmotic equilibration between tubular fluid and renal interstitium.

Water extracted from the cortical collecting tubule is rapidly removed by the abundant cortical blood supply. Water extracted from the medullary and papillary collecting ducts (where the final phase of urinary concentration is completed) is removed by the vasa rectae. The latter process is another aspect of the "maintenance" function of the medullary microcirculation: Water removal ensures that the hypertonicity of the medullary interstitium is not progressively dissipated.

C. The Cellular Action of Antidiuretic Hormone

Recent work has greatly enhanced our understanding or the mechanism of action of ADH and has clarified some of the biochemical steps involved, in particular the role of cyclic adenosine-3',5'-monophosphate (cAMP) (Fig. 1). In ADH-responsive epithelia, ADH enhances cAMP synthesis and exogenous cAMP mimics the hydro-osmotic effect of ADH (7,8). Consequently, cAMP is felt to be an essential biochemical intermediate (or "second messenger") in ADH-stimulated water flow. It is convenient to divide the ADH-second messenger system into two major components: (1) a proximal component that includes those processes that determine the intracellular concentration of cAMP, and (2) a distal component that includes those processes by which cAMP exerts the physiological effect of the hormone.

The first step in the proximal component of ADH action involves binding of the hormone to specific receptors located at the outer surface of the basolateral cell membrane. The receptor appears to be an individual protein (or group of proteins) that is (are) distinct

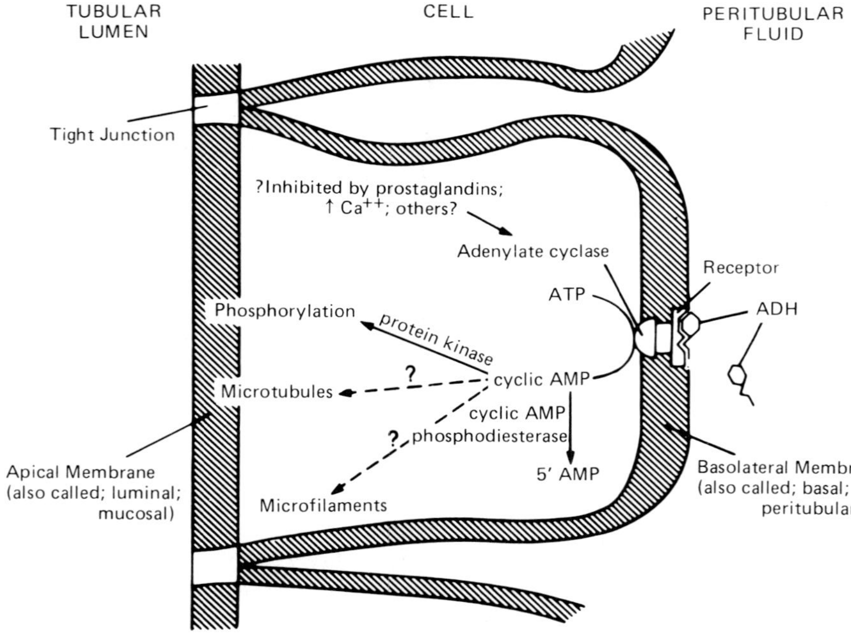

Fig. 1 Cellular action of antidiuretic hormone (ADH). See text for details. ATP, adenosine triphosphate; 5' AMP, 5'-adenosine monophosphate; cyclic AMP, cyclic adenosine-3',5'-monophosphate. (From Ref. 8. Reprinted from Kidney International 10:46-63, 1976, with permission.)

from the adenylate cyclase enzyme complex per se (9). Receptor occupancy has recently been correlated with cellular cAMP production in porcine kidney cells in culture (10,11): The threshold concentrations of ADH necessary for hormone binding and for increasing cellular cAMP content were similar, the time course of the increase in intracellular cAMP levels was compatible with the time needed for binding to the receptor, and there was good agreement between the concentration of hormone that produced 50% receptor occupancy and a half-maximal increase in cAMP levels (10 and 2-6 nmol/liter, respectively). These values are remarkably close to the concentration of ADH that produces half-maximal urine osmolality in humans, about 2.5 nmol/liter (1).

Hormone-receptor binding is followed by activation of adenylate cyclase, which catalyzes the formation of cAMP from its precursor, adenosine triphosphate (ATP). This enzyme complex is located at the inner surface of the cell membrane and is composed of at least two subunits: a magnesium-dependent catalytic subunit which, when activated, is responsible for the synthesis of cAMP and a guanine nucleotide-binding regulatory subunit which modulates the activity of the catalytic subunit (9). The exact role of guanine nucleotides in the regulation of adenylate cyclase activity has not been defined, but the presence of some guanine (or related purine) nucleotide is an absolute requirement for the stimulation of adenylate cyclase activity by hormones (9).

The intracellular concentration of cAMP at any given time is a function not only of its rate of synthesis but also of its rate of catabolism. The most important determinant of the latter is the activity of the cyclic nucleotide phosphodiesterases, a group of enzymes found in virtually all cells that degrade cyclic nucleotides to their 5'-monophosphate counterparts (12). Several different forms of phosphodiesterase have been identified on the basis of differences in kinetic behavior, substrate specificity, subcellular localization, and susceptibility to activation by calcium (12,13). The two major forms of phosphodiesterase—the soluble "high-K_m" enzyme that is calcium sensitive and the membrane-associated "low-K_m" enzyme that is not activated by calcium—have both been identified in renal epithelia (12,14), but the relative importance of these enzymes in the modulation of cAMP metabolism in such epithelia remains to be clarified.

Much less is known about the distal component of ADH action, i.e., the mechanism(s) by which ADH-induced increases in intracellular cAMP levels are translated into increased epithelial water permeability (15). Since a variety of physiological and morphological studies have indicated that the apical cell membrane is the critical barrier to water flow, it is widely assumed that alterations in apical membrane function represent the ultimate expression of the hormone's effects. In this regard, ADH and cAMP have been shown to stimulate the aggregation of intramembranous particles in the apical cell membrane of ADH-responsive epithelia (16) and these changes have been correlated with the hydro-osmotic effects of the hormone (17,18). Thus, it appears that the ultrastructural expression of the ultimate effect of ADH (a change in the permeability of the apical cell membrane) is a rearrangement of intramembranous particles.

The processes that translate elevated intracellular cAMP levels into alterations in apical cell membrane structure and function remain controversial. By analogy with other systems (19), a popular working hypothesis is that the hydro-osmotic effects of cAMP are mediated by reversible phosphorylation of specific cellular proteins (20), a process that is under the control of two groups of enzymes—cAMP-dependent protein kinases and phosphoprotein phosphatases. The former are magnesium-dependent enzymes that exist as tetramers composed of two dissimilar subunits: Binding of cAMP to the regulatory subunits of the inactive holoenzyme results in the dissociation of the tetramer into a regulatory subunit dimer and two active catalytic subunit monomers which catalyze the side-chain phosphorylation of proteins using ATP as the phosphate group donor (21). Both cytosolic and membrane-associated cAMP-dependent protein kinases have been described in renal epithelia (14,22). Phosphoprotein phosphatases, which catalyze the dephosphorylation of proteins, also appear to be widespread in renal epithelia (14).

In the phosphoprotein hypothesis of ADH action it is assumed that cAMP regulates water permeability by activating a cAMP-dependent protein kinase that controls the phosphorylation of critical cellular effector proteins (8). This reaction could be reversed by phosphoprotein phosphatase-catalyzed dephosphorylation of the effector proteins. Thus, reversible phosphorylation is regarded as providing a cyclical mechanism (an on-off switch) for the precise modulation of ADH-induced water flow. In this regard, ADH has been shown to activate cAMP-dependent protein kinase in the toad urinary bladder and mammalian collecting tubule in a dose-dependent fashion and such activation has been correlated with the hydro-osmotic effect of the hormone (15).

The putative effector phosphoproteins have proven extremely difficult to identify. Reports of specific cAMP-dependent phosphorylation of apical (as opposed to basolateral) cell membrane proteins in bovine renal medulla (23) have not been confirmed. The dephosphorylation of a 50,000-dalton protein in toad urinary bladders has been linked to the cellular actions of ADH and cAMP (24,25), but it is unclear whether this event is involved in the hydro-osmotic or the natriferic effects of these agents. In addition, this protein is apparently ubiquitous in all vertebrate tissues (26) and may be nothing more than the regulatory subunit of a cAMP-dependent protein kinase (27). It seems unlikely, therefore, that it is also an apical membrane protein whose degree of phosphorylation influences epithelial water permeability.

Microtubules and microfilaments have been implicated in the hydro-osmotic response to ADH and cAMP (28,29). Microtubules are cylindrical organelles composed of longitudinally aligned protofilaments, whose major constituent is the protein, tubulin. Tubulin is a substrate for cAMP-dependent protein kinases and so is a microtubule-associated protein that may be involved in microtubule assembly (30,31). However, it is not known whether phosphorylation regulates microtubule structure and function. Microfilaments are fine, fibrillar organelles composed primarily of an actinlike protein. Both organelles comprise important parts of the cytoskeleton and are involved in the maintenance of cell shape and in the movement of cell components (32).

Colchicine, podophyllotoxin, and vinblastine, all of which inhibit microtubule aggregation, inhibit ADH- and cAMP-induced water flow in the amphibian urinary bladder (28). Cytochalasin B, a microfilament inhibitor, has similar effects (29,33,34). Despite these interesting observations, the precise role of microtubules and microfilaments in the hydro-osmotic response to ADH has yet to be delineated. In amphibian epithelia, there is indirect evidence that microtubules are necessary for the initiation of intramembranous particle aggregation and that microfilaments are required for the maintenance of these aggregates in the apical membrane (29). It has been suggested that microtubules provide the effector mechanism for assembly of the intramembranous aggregates and that microfilaments provide the "anchor" to keep the aggregates in place within the apical cell membrane. It is well to remember, however, that the evidence that the cytoskeleton has a specific role in the hydro-osmotic response to ADH is derived almost entirely from inhibitor studies and that it is very likely that agents such as colchicine and cytochalasin B have a variety of cellular effects unrelated to their interactions with cytoskeletal elements.

Although the central role of cAMP in the hydro-osmotic response to ADH has been well defined, there is increasing evidence that other intracellular second messengers (e.g., Ca^{2+}, prostaglandins) may modulate the actions of the hormone. The cellular effects of cyclic nucleotides and Ca^{2+} are closely intertwined throughout biology (35). Calmodulin serves as an intracellular Ca^{2+} receptor and appears to mediate many of the cellular effects of this ion, including those on cyclic nucleotide metabolism (13,36,37).

Calcium has multiple potential sites of action within the ADH-responsive epithelial cell. One is the adenylate cyclase complex per se; however, the relationship between Ca^{2+} and ADH-responsive adenylate cyclase activity is a complex one. Enzyme activity is decreased both in the absence of Ca^{2+} and in the presence of 10^{-5} to 10^{-3} Ca^{2+} (38). Thus, a low ($\sim 10^{-6}$ nmol/liter), but critical, Ca^{2+} concentration is necessary for optimal adenylate cyclase activation—deviations from this value in either direction impair enzyme activity. The activation of ADH-responsive adenylate cyclase by micromolar concentrations of Ca^{2+} in porcine kidney cells in culture has recently been shown to be dependent on the presence of calmodulin (39). Another site at which Ca^{2+} may modulate the hydro-osmotic effect of ADH is the phosphodiesterase reaction. The soluble high-K_m enzyme is activated by Ca^{2+}, a process that is critically calmodulin dependent (12,13,36). Finally, microtubule metabolism is known to be affected by calmodulin (13,36), so that the cytoskeleton may also be a site at which Ca^{2+} modulates epithelial water permeability. Despite these provocative interrelationships the precise role of Ca^{2+} in the hydro-osmotic response to ADH has yet to be defined.

Prostaglandins may also have important roles in the modulation of water permeability in renal epithelia (40). Low concentrations of prostaglandin E (PGE) inhibit ADH-induced water flow in renal epithelia but have no effect on the hydro-osmotic response to exogenous cAMP. In addition, the accumulation of cyclic AMP in renal epithelial cells exposed to ADH is decreased by PGE. Furthermore, inhibitors of prostaglandin synthesis enhance cAMP accumulation and the hydro-osmotic effect of submaximal concentrations of ADH. There seems little doubt, therefore, that alterations in renal epithelial prostaglandin metabolism can profoundly influence ADH's effect on water flow. However, it is less clear whether changes in prostaglandin metabolism have a physiological role in the hydro-osmotic response to ADH.

The original suggestion that prostaglandins, formed within ADH-sensitive renal epithelial cells, serve to dampen the hydro-osmotic effect of the hormone (41) remains to be proven. Some investigators (42,43) have provided evidence that ADH stimulates PGE synthesis in toad urinary bladders, but this has not been confirmed by others (44,45). In addition, although there is no question that mammalian kidneys can synthesize a variety of prostaglandins (and related compounds), there is at present no evidence that ADH affects prostaglandin synthesis in those portions of the nephron that respond to the hormone with an increase in water permeability. Collecting duct cells have recently been shown to have the capacity to synthesize prostaglandins (46,47), but the effects of ADH on this process remain to be examined. The urinary excretion of PGE is increased by ADH in some species but not in others (40). In any event, the urinary excretion of locally active compunds, such as prostaglandins, is unlikely to provide useful information either on their site of synthesis or on their site of action.

II. PATHOPHYSIOLOGICAL MECHANISMS

In considering defects in water homeostasis, it is important to recall that there are two limbs to the servomechanism regulating body fluid tonicity (Fig. 2). The normal response to a body water deficit (hypertonicity) is an increase in water intake and a decrease in renal water excretion. The normal response to an increase in total body water (hypotonicity) is a decrease

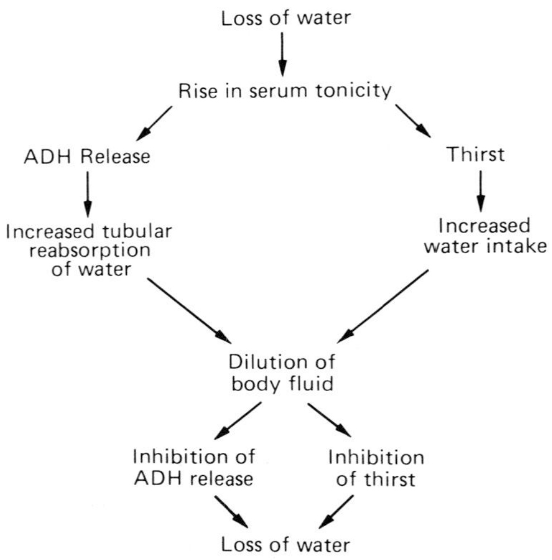

Fig. 2 Regulation of body fluid tonicity. See text for details. (From Leaf, A.; and Cotran, R. S. Renal Pathophysiology. New York, Oxford University Press, 1976.)

in water intake and an increase in renal water excretion. Polyuria* can arise from defects in either limb of this servomechanism: Primary polyuria results from inadequate renal water conservation (diabetes insipidus) and secondary polyuria results from excessive water intake (primary polydipsia). Failure of water conservation can be due to inadequate circulating amounts of ADH (central diabetes insipidus) or to an inadequate end-organ response to ADH (nephrogenic diabetes insipidus). Consequently, the concentrating defect in patients with central diabetes insipidus is improved by the administration of exogenous ADH, whereas patients with complete nephrogenic diabetes insipidus are unresponsive to the administration of the hormone.

Nephrogenic diabetes insipidus can result from abnormalities in the production and maintenance of the renal medullary osmotic gradient (i.e., from loss of the driving force for water reabsorption from the collecting duct) or from abnormalities in the utilization of the osmotic gradient (i.e., from an inability of collecting duct epithelial cells to respond to ADH with an appropriate increase in water permeability) (Table 2). An appreciation of the potential mechanisms that could give rise to nephrogenic diabetes insipidus (and of the techniques used to define these mechanisms) will be important in understanding the detailed discussions of the pathophysiology of the various causes of nephrogenic diabetes insipidus.

A. Defects in Gradient Formation and Maintenance

The existence of the medullary osmotic gradient is dependent on the delivery of appropriate amounts of NaCl to the ascending limb of Henle's loop (Table 2). Decreased delivery could be due to a decrease in glomerular filtration rate (GFR) or to an increase in proximal tubular NaCl reabsorption; the resulting decrement in salt delivery to the ascending limb, and there-

*Polyuria means increased urine volume, which may be due primarily to increased water excretion (as in this case) or to increased solute excretion, or both. A polyuric state due to increased water excretion alone is called a water diuresis.

Table 2 Pathophysiological Mechanisms of Nephrogenic Diabetes Insipidus

A. Abnormalities in the generation and/or maintenance of the osmotic gradient
  1. Decreased glomerular filtration rate
  2. Increased proximal tubular reabsorption
  3. Decreased reabsorption of NaCl by the ascending limb of Henle's loop
  4. Decrease urea trapping in the medullary interstitium
  5. Abnormal medullary blood flow

B. Abnormalities in the utilization of the osmotic gradient
  1. Decreased cAMP accumulation in response to ADH (proximal component of ADH action)
    a. Defective ADH-receptor binding
    b. Decreased adenylate cyclase activity
    c. Decreased ATP availability
    d. Increased cAMP phosphodiesterase activity
  2. Decreased hydro-osmotic response to cAMP (distal component of ADH action) e.g., alterations in:
    a. Phosphoprotein turnover
    b. Microtubule and/or microfilament function
    c. Cellular calcium homeostasis
    d. Cellular prostaglandin metabolism

fore in the ability to generate an osmotic gradient, would lead to decreased renal concentrating ability and polyuria. The GFR is usually estimated from the clearances of creatinine or inulin and proximal tubular reabsorption is frequently measured in experimental animals by micropuncture techniques.

Decreased NaCl reabsorption by the ascending limb of Henle's loop would also lead to a decrement in the osmotic gradient and, thereby, be associated with decreased renal concentrating ability. Decreased loop solute reabsorption could also contribute to polyuria by overwhelming the rather limited reabsorptive capacity of more distal portions of the nephron. The adequacy of loop solute transport is generally evaluated in an indirect fashion by measuring: (1) solute-free water clearance (C_{H_2O}) and minimum urine osmolality (minimum U_{osm} or U_{min}) during a steady-state water diuresis; (2) some index of total urinary electrolyte excretion, e.g., urinary Na^+ plus K^+ excretion (U_{Na+K}) under hydropenic conditions; and (3) negative solute-free water clearance ($T^c_{H_2O}$) during the infusion of hypertonic saline and ADH.

Agents that decrease C_{H_2O} (and have no effect on GFR) are presumed to act by inhibiting NaCl reabsorption in the ascending limb of Henle's loop. Such agents would, of course, also increase U_{min} and U_{Na+K}. Since $T^c_{H_2O}$ is a measure of overall renal concentrating ability (and as such is affected by defects either in gradient generation or in gradient utilization), it would be expected to be decreased in such circumstances. Conversely, if $T^c_{H_2O}$ is decreased, but C_{H_2O}, U_{min}, and U_{Na+K} are all normal, electrolyte (and urea) delivery and transport are assumed to be adequate to allow for generation of the osmotic gradient; therefore, the abnormality in $T^c_{H_2O}$ is presumed to be due to a defect in the response of the collecting duct to ADH.

Although these tests are of considerable value because they can be performed in vivo, they cannot exclude subtle defects in ascending limb function. More direct measurement of ascending limb NaCl reabsorption can be obtained either by examing the composition of early distal convoluted tubular fluid after micropuncture or by measuring the electrolyte and urea content of medullary tissue; the latter may best reflect the overall integrity of the mechanism that determines the medullary osmotic gradient. However, the interpretation of measurements of medullary solute concentrations must take into account the finding that the absolute amount of water reabsorbed from the medullary collecting duct during water diuresis is actually greater than the amount of water reabsorbed during antidiuresis (49). Consequently, in the presence of diabetes insipidus (which is characterized by an ongoing water diuresis) the medullary NaCl concentration (measured as meq per unit of tissue water) might be decreased despite normal NaCl reabsorption in the ascending limb of Henle's loop. More accurate medullary solute determinations can be obtained by first drying the tissue and then expressing the concentration as meq per unit of dry tissue weight (50). Since none of the studies of medullary solute concentration in experimental models of nephrogenic diabetes insipidus have employed the latter method, their results must be interpreted with caution.

B. Tubular Resistance to ADH

If the renal medullary osmotic gradient is normal (and circulating levels of ADH are appropriate) an ADH-resistant concentrating defect must be due to an inability of the collecting duct epithelium to respond appropriately to the hormone. Some classifications of diabetes insipidus exclude abnormalities in formation and maintenance of the osmotic gradient from the diagnosis of "true" nephrogenic diabetes insipidus. In these schemes the term nephrogenic diabetes insipidus is reserved for those situations in which only the ability of the collecting duct to respond to ADH is impaired. However, there are diseases in which such distinctions are very difficult to make or in which more than one defect is present. For example, diseases in which the renal medullary and papillary interstitium are heavily involved (e.g., amyloidosis, Sjogren's syndrome, sickle cell anemia, radiation nephritis, polycystic kidney disease, medullary cystic disease, chronic interstitial nephritis, obstructive nephropathy) are often associated with ADH-resistant concentrating defects (51). Since these diseases are generally associated with a decreased medullary osmotic gradient (and often also with a decreased GFR), the intrinsic ability of the collecting duct epithelium to respond to ADH cannot be easily assessed. Such diseases are not discussed in this chapter. Rather, we will focus on those disorders in which a defect in the cellular response to ADH is the major or the sole factor in the genesis of the concentrating defect.

Abnormalities in the cellular response to ADH could be due to defects in the proximal or the distal component of the ADH-cAMP system (Table 2). Defects in the proximal component (those processes that determine the intracellular concentration of cAMP, the mediator of ADH action) would include: (1) interference with the binding of ADH to its plasma membrane receptor, with inadequate stimulation of adenylate cyclase, (2) inhibition of adenylate cyclase activity per se, (3) decreased production or availability of ATP, the substrate for cAMP formation by adenylate cyclase; and (4) enhancement of cAMP-phosphodiesterase activity, which would increase the degradation of cAMP to AMP. Defects in the distal component (those processes by which cAMP produces a hydro-osmotic response) are not as well characterized, but could include abnormalities in: (1) phosphoprotein metabolism (e.g., inhibition of cAMP-dependent protein kinases); (2) intramembranous particle aggregation; (3) microtubule and/or microfilament function; and (4) cellular calcium homeostasis.

The initial approach to exploring the pathophysiology of ADH-resistance is to determine whether the primary abnormality is in the proximal or the distal component of the ADH-cAMP system. The urinary excretion of cAMP after the administration of ADH has been utilized to obtain such information; theoretically, subnormal ADH-induced urinary cAMP excretion would indicate a defect in at least the proximal component of the system. Unfortunately, even under normal circumstances, it is often difficult to demonstrate a consistent increase in urinary cAMP excretion in response to ADH (52). The administration of cAMP, or of cAMP analogues, has been utilized to define the existence of defects in the distal component of the system. Unfortunately, the intravenous or intramuscular administration of cAMP (or its analogs) is followed by rapid inactivation of these compounds by many extrarenal tissues, making such studies extremely difficult to interpret. Thus, although in vivo studies provide some insight into the mechanisms underlying nephrogenic diabetes insipidus, the events leading to ADH resistance cannot be well delineated in intact organisms.

Important advances in the understanding of the cellular mechanisms involved in ADH resistance were coincident with the development of in vitro techniques for the study of water transport. Such model systems include: (1) anuran epithelia (toad urinary bladder and frog skin) which have become classic models of the mammalian distal nephron; (2) renal cortical and medullary slices; and (3) isolated perfused mammalian collecting tubules. In anuran epithelia or isolated perfused collecting tubules, the effects of ADH and/or cAMP on water transport can be examined directly under rigorously controlled conditions. If an agent inhibits the hydro-osmotic response to ADH but not to cAMP, then it is presumed to act by inhibiting one or more steps in the proximal component of the ADH-cAMP system. In contrast, an agent that inhibits both ADH- and cAMP-mediated water transport is presumed to act either exclusively on the distal component of the system or on both components of the system.

Further delineation of abnormalities in the two components of the ADH-cAMP system can be provided by biochemical studies of anuran epithelia and of renal cortical and medullary slices incubated under conditions which produce ADH-resistance in clinical settings. In these studies, direct measurements of enzyme activities (e.g., adenylate cyclase, cAMP phosphodiesterase, cAMP-dependent protein kinases, protein phosphatases, calmodulin) and of tissue concentrations of cAMP, ATP, and other substances can be used to determine whether or not a proximal or distal biochemical abnormality may play a role in hormone resistance. In addition, anatomical studies of these same tissues can be useful in determining whether disruptions of microtubules, of microfilaments or of intramembranous particle aggregates are factors in producing hormone resistance.

III. DIFFERENTIAL DIAGNOSIS

Although a diagnosis of nephrogenic diabetes insipidus may be suspected in a patient presenting with polyuria and polydipsia, other causes of polyuria such as primary polydipsia and central diabetes insipidus must always be excluded. The most easily available test to define the cause of polyuria is the so-called standard dehydration test (53). Older tests, such as the Hickey-Hare hypertonic saline infusion test and the nicotine stimulation test have largely been replaced by the standard dehydration test (54).

A. The Standard Dehydration Test

The standard dehydration test is performed in two parts (Table 3). The first part evaluates the patient's ability both to release ADH when stimulated to do so by an increase in plasma osmolality (P_{osm}) and/or a decrease in extracellular fluid (ECF) volume, and to respond to the released *endogenous* ADH with an appropriate increase in urine osmolality (U_{osm}). Baseline values for body weight, P_{osm} and U_{osm} are obtained, and then no fluid intake is permitted for the next 12-18 hr. The test is usually started after the evening meal, so that most of the period of fluid deprivation occurs while the patient is asleep. The patient is weighed

Table 3 Differential Response to Fluid Deprivation and Exogenous ADH in the Diagnosis of Polyuric States

	U_{max}	U_{max}-ADH	P_{osm}
Normal volunteers (10)	1068 ± 69	979 ± 79	290 ± 2
Central diabetes insipidus			
Complete (19)	168 ± 14	445 ± 52	306 ± 3
Partial (13)	438 ± 34	549 ± 28	294 ± 1
Nephrogenic diabetes insipidus			
Complete (5)	186 ± 31	213 ± 24	305 ± 4
Partial (5)	501 ± 40	530 ± 27	297 ± 4
Primary polydipsia (5)	738 ± 53	780 ± 73	289 ± 2

Values are means ± SEM; number of subjects in parentheses. U_{max}, U_{osm} after dehydration alone; U_{max}-ADH, U_{osm} after dehydration and exogenous ADH; P_{osm} was obtained after dehydration and prior to administration of ADH. Patients were studied without reconstitution of medullary solutes. The distinction between complete and partial diabetes insipidus is necessarily arbitrary and is based on the relationship between U_{max} and P_{osm}: the complete disorder is characterized by $U_{max} < P_{osm}$ and the partial disorder is characterized by $U_{max} > P_{osm}$. The patients with complete nephrogenic diabetes insipidus had either the congenital form of the disease (n = 2) or severe lithium-induced diabetes insipidus (n = 3). All the patients with partial nephrogenic diabetes insipidus had lithium-induced concentrating defects. [Two patients with lithium-induced diabetes insipidus in Ref. 55 (nos. 1 and 6) were excluded from analysis because of the possibility that they had combined central and nephrogenic diabetes insipidus.]
Source: Data from Refs. 53, 55.

upon arising in the morning and the first urine specimen is discarded. U_{osm} is then measured at approximately hourly intervals until both parts of the test are completed. Patients suspected of having severe diabetes insipidus (urine volume > 4-5 liters/day or $U_{osm} < 250$ mOsm/kg H_2O) should be closely observed during the dehydration test. Such individuals may rapidly become volume depleted and it is wise to follow them with hourly weights and frequent observations of supine and erect blood pressure. Children present special problems and also need to be observed more closely; a pediatric modification of the standard dehydration test has been described (56).

The proper interpretation of this part of the test requires that two conditions be satisfied: (1) a rise in P_{osm} and/or a 5% decrement in body weight must be documented, either of which would indicate that an appropriate stimulus for the release of ADH has been provided; and (2) the U_{osm} must reach a plateau (less than 5% change on two successive determinations), which assures that partial defects in ADH release (partial central diabetes insipidus) will be identified. In the latter disorder, ADH may be released very slowly and may never reach a level that is appropriate to the stimulus. As shown in Table 3, in normal humans after 12-18 hr of fluid deprivation urinary osmolality (maximum U_{osm} or U_{max}) is $\geqslant 850$ mOsm/kg. Although failure to achieve a $U_{max} > 850$ mOsm/kg at this point indicates that diabetes insipidus (or primary polydipsia; see below) is present, it does not distinguish central from nephrogenic diabetes insipidus. Therefore, if $U_{max} < 850$ mOsm/kg, the second part of the dehydration test should be completed.

The second part consists of the administration of *exogenous* ADH (5 I.U. of aqueous vasopressin subcutaneously) and the determination of U_{osm} for 2 additional hr (maximal U_{osm} after ADH or U_{max}-ADH). The second part of the test is not required if the normal U_{max} ($\geqslant 850$ mOsm/kg) has already been achieved, no further increase in U_{osm} would be expected under such circumstances (Table 3). Failure to respond to exogenous ADH suggests that nephrogenic diabetes insipidus (or both central and nephrogenic diabetes insipidus) is (are) present.

By definition, all patients with diabetes insipidus are unable to maximally concentrate their urine during the first part of the dehydration test ($U_{max} < 850$ mOsm/kg) (Table 3). In patients with *complete central* diabetes insipidus U_{max} is less than P_{osm}, but after the administration of vasopressin U_{osm} increases to a value greater than P_{osm} (i.e., U_{max}-ADH $> P_{osm} > U_{max}$). Patients with *partial central* diabetes insipidus have a U_{max} greater than P_{osm} and the administration of vasopressin results in a further increase in U_{osm} (i.e., U_{max}-ADH $> U_{max} > P_{osm}$). (High urinary flow rates in diabetes insipidus can cause "washout" of the medullary osmotic gradient. Thus, the administration of exogenous ADH to patients with untreated *central* diabetes insipidus may not elevate U_{osm} to the normal range. Reconstitution of the gradient by correction of the polyuria with therapeutic doses of vasopressin for several days and by solute replacement will usually allow such patients to raise their U_{osm} to ≥ 850 mOsm/kg.)

In patients with *complete nephrogenic* diabetes insipidus, U_{max} is less than P_{osm} and there is little or no improvement after the administration of vasopressin (i.e., U_{max}ADH = $U_{max} < P_{osm}$). Patients with *partial nephrogenic* diabetes insipidus have a U_{max} greater than P_{osm}, and U_{osm} does not increase after the administration of vasopressin (i.e., U_{max}-ADH = $U_{max} > P_{osm}$). Thus, the hallmark of patients with *nephrogenic* diabetes insipidus is unresponsiveness to the administration of vasopressin (i.e., U_{max}-ADH = U_{max}) at a time when the renal concentrating mechanism has already been maximally stimulated by a prolonged period of water deprivation.

One of the greatest sources of difficulty in using the dehydration test is in the discrimination of partial nephrogenic diabetes insipidus from primary polydipsia. (Urine-concentrating ability in patients with primary polydipsia is impaired by a washout of the medullary osmotic gradient, similar to that described above, that results from the secondary polyuria.) In both disorders U_{max} will be greater than P_{osm} (but <850 mOsm/kg), and in patients with primary polydipsia there may be no increase in U_{osm} following the administration of vasopressin (i.e., U_{max}-ADH = U_{max}). The latter circumstance is of course the hallmark of nephrogenic diabetes insipidus. In such situations, the specific cause of the polyuria can only be determined after the medullary solute gradient has been reconstituted. This is best achieved by correcting the polyuria with a long-acting ADH preparation while providing adequate solute intake, as described above; after reconstitution of the gradient, patients with primary polydipsia will have a normal U_{max} (or will become hyponatremic if allowed free access to water during the period of vasopressin administration). In contrast, the dehydration test in patients with partial nephrogenic diabetes insipidus will remain abnormal. Examination of the baseline P_{osm} may also be helpful in differentiating primary polydipsia from diabetes insipidus: Patients with primary polydipsia tend to have a P_{osm} in the low-normal range, whereas patients with diabetes insipidus tend to have P_{osm} in the high-normal or high range.

B. Radioimmunoassay of ADH

With the development of reliable methods for the radioimmunoassay of ADH, plasma ADH levels (obtained during the performance of the standard dehydration test) have been utilized in an attempt to improve the diagnostic accuracy of the test. When the relationships between plasma ADH concentration, plasma osmolality, and urine osmalality are examined (Fig. 3) patients with varying degrees of central diabetes insipidus, patients with complete nephrogenic diabetes insipidus, and normal subjects can generally be identified accurately (57). Such

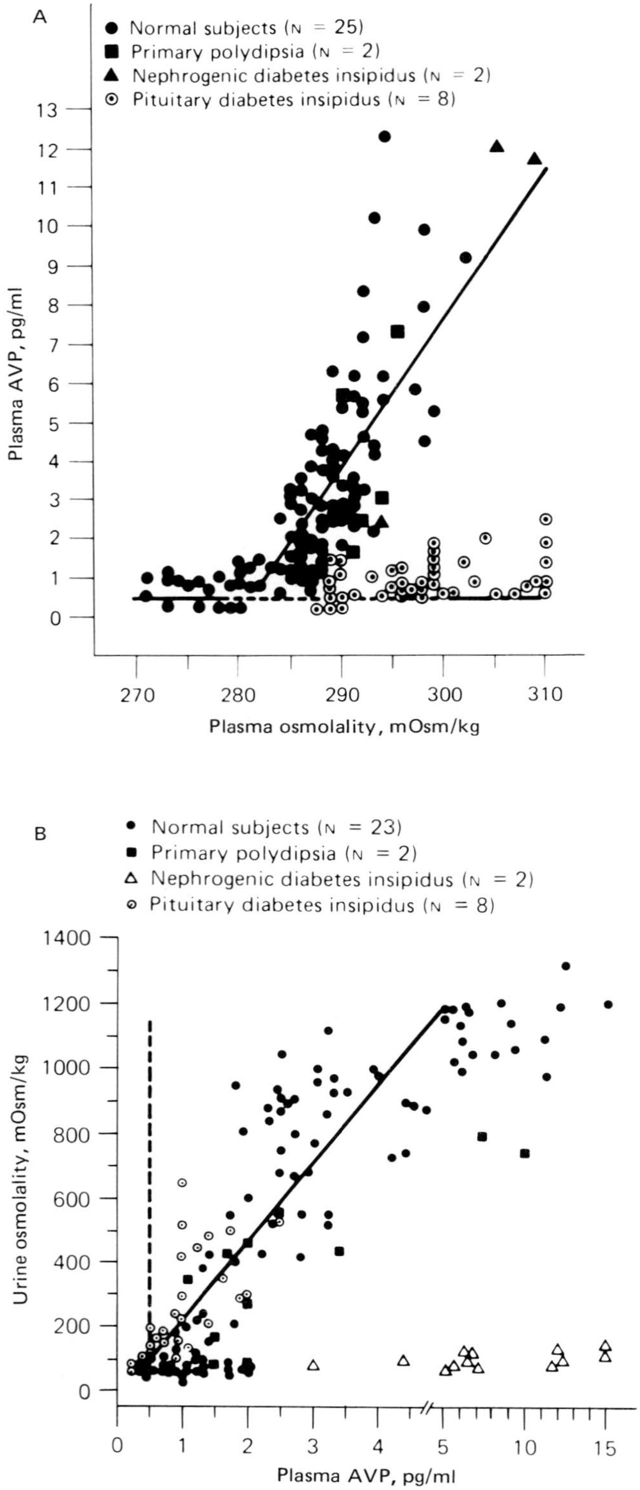
A
Normal subjects (N = 25)
Primary polydipsia (N = 2)
Nephrogenic diabetes insipidus (N = 2)
Pituitary diabetes insipidus (N = 8)
Plasma AVP, pg/ml
Plasma osmolality, mOsm/kg
B
Normal subjects (N = 23)
Primary polydipsia (N = 2)
Nephrogenic diabetes insipidus (N = 2)
Pituitary diabetes insipidus (N = 8)
Urine osmolality, mOsm/kg
Plasma AVP, pg/ml

analyses are most useful in the detection of partial central diabetes insipidus. However, as one would predict, it remains difficult to separate patients with primary polydipsia from normal subjects, and to discriminate between primary polydipsia and partial nephrogenic diabetes insipidus.

The plasma ADH response to hypertonic (5%) saline infusion has also been used as an adjunct to the standard dehydration test (58). As expected, patients with nephrogenic diabetes insipidus have a plasma ADH response to hypertonic saline infusion that is similar to that of normal subjects, patients with complete central diabetes insipidus do not have any response (Fig. 4), and patients with partial central diabetes have a subnormal increase in ADH levels (Fig. 4). This type of evaluation is most useful in separating patients with partial central diabetes insipidus from those with primary polydipsia, since the latter have a normal plasma ADH response to hypertonic saline infusion (Fig. 4). However, as one would predict, it is not helpful in differentiating patients with partial nephrogenic diabetes insipidus from patients with primary polydipsia (or from normal subjects): In all three instances the plasma ADH response is normal.

In summary, while the development of reliable and sensitive assays for ADH has improved our ability to discriminate between the underlying causes of polyuria, the standard dehydration test continues to be widely employed in the evaluation of clinically significant polyuria. In the vast majority of patients, the results of a carefully performed dehydration test will enable the physician to establish a diagnosis of central or nephrogenic diabetes insipidus, and to separate these disorders from primary polydipsia. In those instances where the diagnosis is in doubt, a therapeutic trial of ADH (and solute replacement) will generally delineate the problem. Measurement of ADH levels is only needed in uncommon circumstances.

IV. CLINICAL MANIFESTATIONS

Polyuria, nocturia, and polydipsia are the clinical hallmarks of diabetes insipidus of any etiology. In addition, patients with diabetes insipidus may develop symptoms related to increased body fluid tonicity (hypernatremia), the result of excessive renal water losses. However, hypernatremia is uncommon unless the thirst mechanism is simultaneously compromised. With free access to water and normal thirst sensation, patients with diabetes insipidus can easily compensate for the excessive water losses. Thus, patients with nephrogenic diabetes insipidus who present with hypernatremia almost always have an inappropriately low water intake (hypodipsia). Primary hypodipsia is an extremely uncommon disorder; much more often, the hypernatremia is a consequence of inadequate water intake in bedridden, senile, or comatose individuals, in young children, in patients permitted nothing by mouth, or in patients who cannot retain ingested water.

Fig. 3 Relationship between plasma ADH concentration (plasma AVP, arginine vasopressin) and plasma osmolality (A) and between urine osmolality and plasma AVP (B) in normal subjects and in patients with polyuria of different etiologies. Plasma (for osmolality and AVP determination by radioimmunoassay) was obtained from recumbent subjects in three states of water balance: (1) ad lib fluid intake, (2) 90 min after an acute water load, and (3) after variable periods of fluid restriction. Urine was collected simultaneously with the plasma sample. The numbers of individuals in each group are shown in the parentheses. The horizontal (A) and vertical (B) broken lines represent the sensitivity limit of the assay. The solid lines were derived from regression analysis of all samples from normal subjects in whom plasma osmolality was > 280 mOsm/kg H_2O (A) and in whom plasma AVP was $\leqslant 5$ pg/ml (B) (n = 87). (From Ref. 57.)

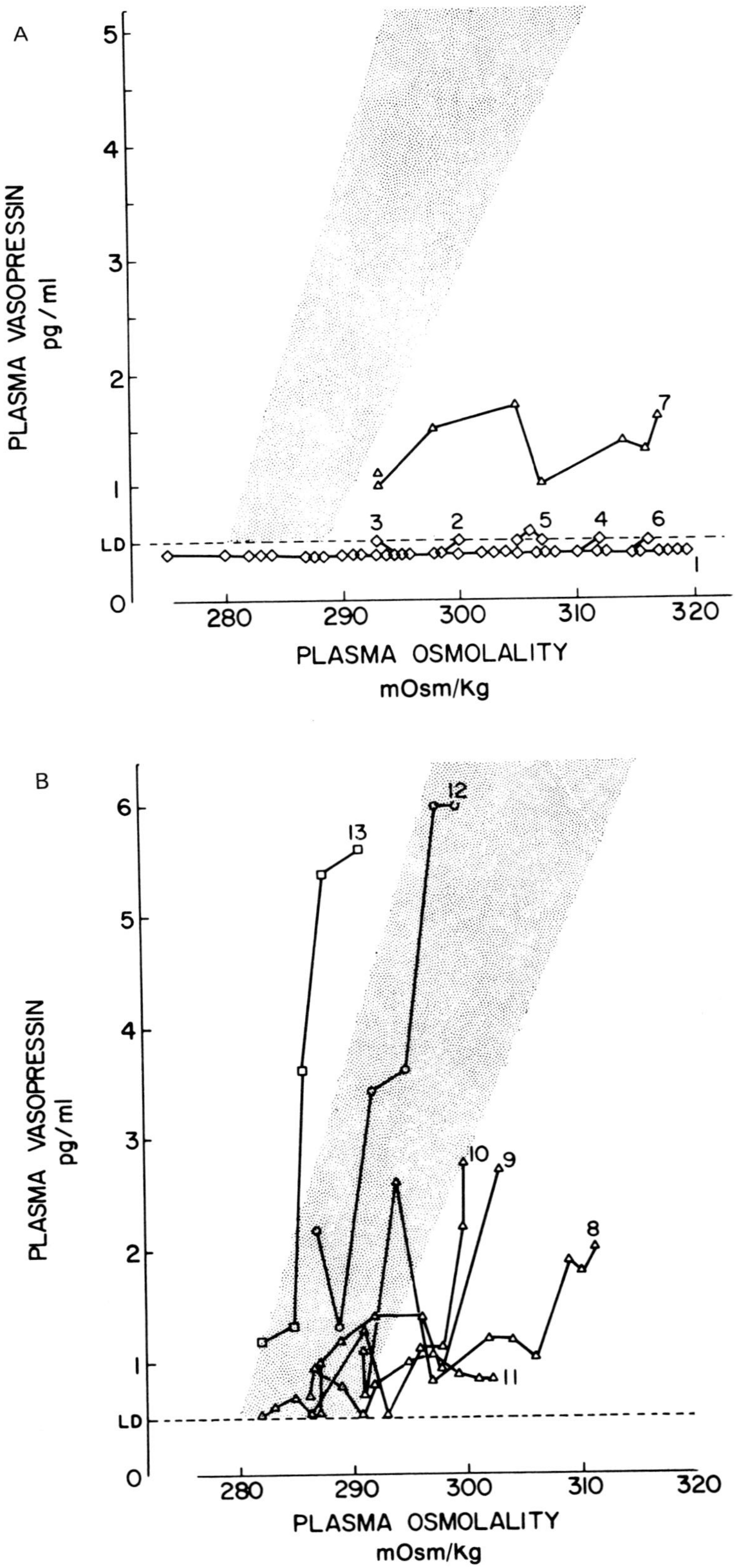
A
PLASMA VASOPRESSIN
pg/ml
5
4
3
2
1
LD
0
3
2
5
4
6
7
1
280
290
300
310
320
PLASMA OSMOLALITY
mOsm/Kg
B
PLASMA VASOPRESSIN
pg/ml
6
5
4
3
2
1
LD
0
13
12
10
9
8
11
280
290
300
310
320
PLASMA OSMOLALITY
mOsm/Kg

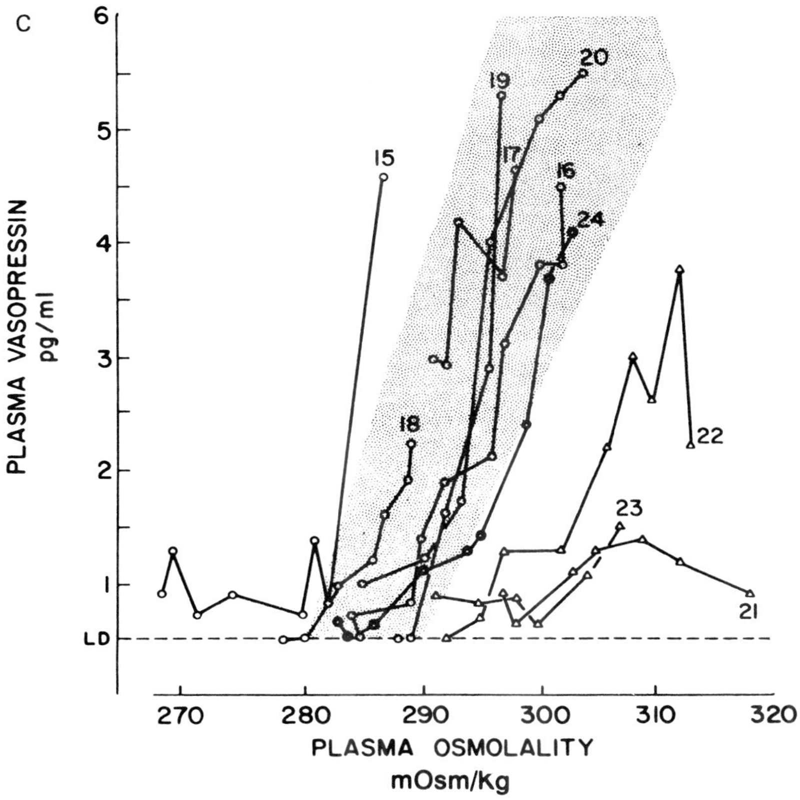

Fig. 4 Use of plasma ADH (vasopressin) response to hypertonic saline infusion in the differential diagnosis of polyuric states. Twenty-three patients underwent a standard dehydration test which was used to classify their polyuria into one of three categories: complete central diabetes insipidus (seven patients), partial central diabetes insipidus (six patients), or primary polydipsia (10 patients). The relationship of plasma vasopressin concentration to plasma osmolality during the infusion of 5% saline is shown for the patients with (A) complete central diabetes insipidus, (B) partial central diabetes insipidus, and (C) primary polydipsia. In each case, the shaded area represents the range of values observed in a large group of healthy adults in various states of hydration and the dotted line (designated LD) represents the lower limit of detectability of the assay. One of the seven patients classified as complete central diabetes was shown to have partial central diabetes insipidus (no. 7, A). Two of the six patients classified as partial central diabetes insipidus were shown to have essentially normal ADH responses (nos. 12,13, B). Three of the 10 patients classified as primary polydipsia were shown to have defects in ADH release (nos. 21-23, C). (From Ref. 58. Reprinted by permission of the New England Journal of Medicine 305:1539-1546, 1981.)

The symptoms associated with hypertonicity are the result of cellular dehydration (most especially of the central nervous system) and are rather nonspecific (59). In children, cerebral dehydration is manifested by irritability, vomiting, fever, a high-pitched cry, depression of the sensorium (varying from lethargy to coma), muscle rigidity, and muscle twitching. Seizures are rare and are most often seen during therapy, particularly if rehydration proceeds too rapidly. Vomiting, fever, and constipation are common symptoms in children with congenital nephrogenic diabetes insipidus (60). In adults, the symptoms are less well delineated, but some depression of the sensorium is usually present; muscular rigidity and twitching are rare in adults, as are seizures.

The signs of hypertonicity include decreases in skin turgor, in ocular firmness, in mucous membrane hydration and in axillary sweat, as well as a depressed sensorium. Since only one-twelfth of a pure water loss is derived from the intravascular fluid compartment, signs of intravascular volume contraction (tachycardia, orthostatic hypotension, shock) are rare in patients with diabetes insipidus. However, if present, such findings are almost always indicative of a very large deficit in total body water. One common sign of intravascular volume contraction that is almost never present in patients with diabetes insipidus is oliguria; the inability of the nephron to concentrate the urine obligates excessive renal water losses (polyuria) even in the presence of severe intravescular volume contraction. However, a decrease in the degree of polyuria may occur if severe intravascular volume contraction is present.

V. CLASSIFICATION

The many causes of nephrogenic diabetes insipidus can be grouped into two categories: familial and acquired (Table 4). Familial nephrogenic diabetes insipidus is most commonly inherited as a sex-linked disorder which is completely expressed in males but only partially expressed in females. Acquired nephrogenic diabetes most commonly is drug induced or is associated with hypercalcemia or potassium depletion. In addition, several drugs have been shown to inhibit ADH-mediated water transport in animals and/or in in vitro model systems (such as the toad urinary bladder), but they have not been reported to produce nephrogenic diabetes insipidus in humans. Since several of these drugs have had important roles in the

Table 4 Classification of Nephrogenic Diabetes Insipidus

A. Familial
B. Acquired
    1. Drugs
        (a) Lithium
        (b) Demeclocycline
        (c) Methoxyflurane
        (d) Amphotericin B
        (e) Gentamicin[a]
        (f) Cisplatin[a]
        (g) Propoxyphene[b]
        (h) Isophosphamide[b]
        (i) Clonidine[a]
        (j) Guanabenz[a]
        (k) Colchicine[a]
        (l) Vinca alkaloids[a]
        (m) Vasopressin analogues[a]
    2. Electrolyte Disorders
        (a) Potassium depletion
        (b) Hypercalcemia
    3. Tumors[b]

[a]Not established in humans (data from animal and/or in vitro studies).
[b]Not well established.

definition of the cellular mechanism of action of ADH, a discussion of their effects is included in this chapter.

VI. FAMILIAL NEPHROGENIC DIABETES INSIPIDUS

A. Clinical Manifestations

Familial nephrogenic diabetes insipidus usually presents in males shortly after birth. Symptoms include polyuria, polydipsia, vomiting, constipation, high skin resistance, and recurrent erratic febrile episodes (61-74). The latter appear to correlate with the state of hydration and body temperature can generally be normalized by rehydration (61,65,69,72). Since the detection of polyuria and polydipsia in an infant is often difficult, the diagnosis is frequently not made until early childhood. Nocturia and enuresis are frequent complaints later in childhood.

Unfortunately, growth impairment and mental retardation are common. Growth impairment is thought to result from malnutrition because so much feeding time early in life is devoted to maintaining hydration that adequate caloric intake cannot always be maintained (61-64,66,67,71,72,75-78). Mental retardation is a common but not invariable finding in children who survive infancy (62,63,65,67-69,71,75,78-80); abnormalities range from mild memory deficits to imbecility. The mental retardation is not genetically determined, but probably results from repeated episodes of severe dehydration, from cerebral edema due to overzealous attempts at rehydration, from cerebral hypoxia, and from malnutrition (67,71, 79-87).

Although most cases of complete, familial, nephrogenic diabetes insipidus are males, a few females have also been reported with full expression of the disease (72,88-90). More commonly, however, affected females have partial nephrogenic diabetes insipidus, and consequently are less symptomatic (62,73,88,91,92). In a 1963 report, a male who was presumed to have complete ADH-resistant polyuria was found to be partially responsive to pharmacological doses of ADH (74). His mother had partial nephrogenic diabetes insipidus, and by history, his maternal grandfather and great-uncle had complete nephrogenic diabetes insipidus. Thus, complete or partial nephrogenic diabetes insipidus can occur in both males and females, but the complete disorder is much more common in males and the incomplete disorder usually occurs in females.

B. Heredity

Although numerous attempts have been made to classify all families with familial nephrogenic diabetes insipidus into a single pattern of inheritance, it is clear that no single pattern can explain the findings in every family. The majority of family trees indicate that this disorder is transmitted in a sex-linked fashion, either an X-linked recessive trait or as an X-linked dominant trait with variable penetrance in females.

In many families the disease skips generations, affects only males, and is transmitted from asymptomatic mothers to their sons (61-63,93-96); no cases of male to male or female to female transmission are observed in such families. Taken together, these features strongly suggest an X-linked recessive mode of inheritance. After an extensive genealogical review of these families it was proposed that these North Americans with hereditary nephrogenic diabetes insipidus are all descendants of a single Scottish family who migrated from the Ulster Province of Ireland to Nova Scotia on the ship *Hopewell* in 1761 (the Hopewell Hypothesis) (96).

In other families, although only males demonstrate complete nephrogenic diabetes insipidus, some females have polyuria, nocturia, and polydipsia as well (68,73,91,97). In these families, both symptomatic and asymptomatic females have been found to have mild ADH-resistant concentrating defects (partial nephrogenic diabetes insipidus). Male to male transmission excludes an X-linked recessive mode of inheritance. An X-linked dominant mode of inheritance with variable penetrance in females appears to best explain the genetic pattern in this second group of families.

In one family the presence of complete nephrogenic diabetes in a few females and the possibility of male to male transmission in a minority of affected males led to the conclusion that the mode of inheritance may be autosomal dominant, with variable penetrance in females (72,88-90,98). However, since complete expression of the disease in females is still compatible with an X-linked dominant pattern of inheritance, and since all five cases of alleged male to male transmission were based solely on historical data, this conclusion may not be justified. In addition, the family in question did not fit the classic autosomal dominant mode of inheritance because of an improper distribution of affected males and females.

C. Pathophysiology

Postmortem anatomical studies have found no structural abnormalities either in Henle's loop or in the collecting ducts of patients with familial nephrogenic diabetes insipidus (61,68-70, 88). In some patients, the number of convolutions in the proximal tubules appear to be decreased (69,99), but such an abnormality can not explain ADH resistance.

Abnormalities in glomerular filtration rate and renal blood flow have been reported in patients with this disorder (61,63,66,69,72,73,100), but after rehydration these parameters characteristically return to normal (61,65,69,73). The few patients who did manifest persistent decrements in filtration rate and blood flow (despite volume expansion) also had hyperuricemia, gout, and hypertension (101,102). Although chronically elevated ADH levels in such patients could potentially cause renal vasoconstriction, it is much more likely that the renal hemodynamic abnormalities are the result of gouty and/or hypertensive nephropathy (93).

Renal sodium conservation is normal in patients with familial nephrogenic diabetes insipidus and no abnormalities in potassium, calcium, or phosphate homeostasis have been reported (61). Tests of proximal tubular function (e.g., Tm glucose, Tm phosphate, urinary amino acid excretion, and phenolsulfophthalein excretion) are normal (61,63,69,72,73, 100,101), as are tests of distal tubular function (e.g., acidifying ability, ammonia excretion) (61,69,92,100). Hyperuricemia, due to decreased renal urate clearance (101,103), has been reported in some patients, but this finding can easily be explained by the presence of chronic, mild volume contraction.

Numerous reports of bladder dilatation, hydroureter, and hydronephrosis have appeared in association with familial nephrogenic diabetes insipidus (61,63,88,104,105). However, studies of the urethra, bladder, and ureterovesicular valves have not found any anatomical abnormalities which could lead to obstruction of urinary flow (104,106,107). Thus, it is likely that the "obstruction" reflects an increased hydrostatic pressure in the urinary outflow tract that is the consequence of increased urine production in the face of a fixed bladder storage capacity. In summary, despite extensive evaluation of renal morphology and function, the only abnormality that is consistently found in patients with familial nephrogenic diabetes insipidus is an inability to elaborate a maximally concentrated urine.

In order to definitively establish that the polyuria in patients with familial nephrogenic diabetes insipidus is exclusively due to renal resistance to ADH, the coexistence of central diabetes insipidus had first to be rigorously excluded. Early studies of this disorder, in which a bioassay was utilized, revealed the presence of ADH-like activity in serum and urine obtained from patients with familial nephrogenic diabetes insipidus (63,65,69,72,74,88,108). More recently, when a sensitive radioimmunoassay for ADH has been employed in such studies, all the patients were found to have a normal threshold for ADH release and a plasma antidiuretic activity that was immunologically identical to normal human ADH (57). Thus, no defects in ADH synthesis or release have been found in any of the patients with familial nephrogenic diabetes insipidus studied to date. In addition, anti-ADH antibodies are absent from the plasma of these patients (57,62,109). Consequently, familial nephrogenic diabetes insipidus appears to be exclusively due to renal resistance to the action of ADH.

Since humans with familial nephrogenic diabetes are able to dilute their urine appropriately (i.e., U_{min} and C_{H_2O} are normal during a steady-state water diuresis) (101), sodium chloride reabsorption in the ascending limb of Henle's loop must be grossly normal. Of course, such studies do not exclude more subtle defects in gradient generation. For example, as may be the case in certain strains of mice (102,110), anatomical and/or functional abnormalities in the countercurrent system may contribute to the concentration defect in humans with this disorder. However, since diluting capacity was not tested and since direct measurements of the medullary solute concentration were not made, firm conclusions cannot be drawn from this study. Indeed, more recent studies of one particular strain of mice (the so-called DI +/+ severe strain), which provides a most useful model of the human disorder, have indicated that the major abnormality causing the defect in urinary concentration in these animals is tubular resistance to ADH (111,112).

The intravenous infusion of ADH during a steady-state water diuresis increases U_{osm} and urinary cAMP excretion in normal subjects and in patients with central diabetes insipidus, but it has no effect on these parameters in patients with familial nephrogenic diabetes insipidus (113-115). In addition, tolbutamide (which enhances the hydro-osmotic effect of submaximal concentrations of ADH, and which increases urinary cAMP excretion in normal humans) did not increase urinary cAMP excretion in a patient with familial nephrogenic diabetes insipidus (113). These studies strongly suggest that there is a defect in the proximal component of the ADH-cAMP system in patients with nephrogenic diabetes insipidus (i.e., in the generation and/or maintenance of appropriate intracellular cAMP levels). In addition, since intravenous infusions of cAMP do not increase U_{osm} in these patients (113,116,117), it has been suggested that additional defects may exist in the distal component of the ADH-cAMP system (i.e., in the cellular action of cAMP). However, because cAMP is rapidly metabolized by extrarenal tissues and is slowly taken up by cells, a lack of response to exogenous cAMP need not imply the presence of a distal effect.

Biochemical studies in mice with hereditary nephrogenic diabetes insipidus (the DI +/+ severe strain) have helped to delineate the specific defects responsible for the ADH resistance in this animal model. Initial studies with mouse medullary homogenates demonstrated decreased ADH-stimulated adenylate cyclase activity (111). This was not due to a defect in receptor binding because the affinity of the receptor for physiological concentrations of ADH was perfectly normal (111). In addition, cAMP phosphodiesterase and cAMP dependent protein kinase activities were no different than those of normal mice. More recently, similar studies were carried out in microdissected tubules, and ADH-stimulated cAMP accumulation was found to be markedly decreased in medullary collecting tubules (112). This was due to a large increase in cAMP phosphodiesterase activity (Fig. 5), and to a small decrease in ADH-stimulated adenylate cyclase activity (Fig. 6) (112). However, ADH-stimulated adenylate cyclase activity was found to be markedly diminished in the medullary thick

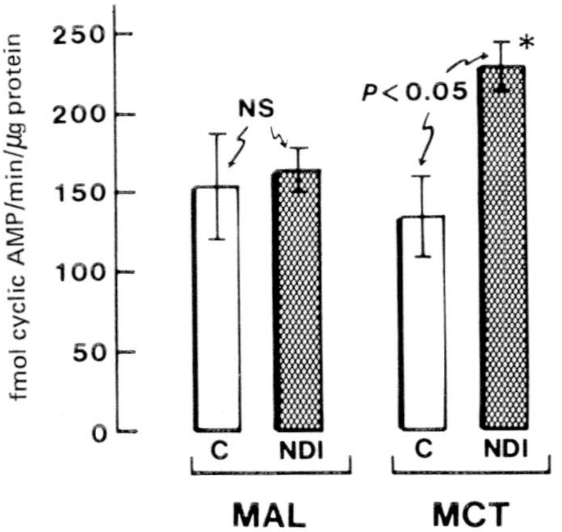

Fig. 5 Activity of cAMP phosphodiesterase in medullary thick ascending limb (MAL) (left panel) and medullary collecting tubule (MCT) (right panel) of normal mice (C) and mice with nephrogenic diabetes insipidus (NDI). Each column represents the mean ± SEM from five animals; the value for each animal being the mean of at least four to six samples. *, indicates value significantly higher ($p < 0.05$) than in C mice, as well as higher than the value in MAL of NDI mice. NS, not significant. Values for control MCT and control MAL were not significantly different from each other. (From Ref. 112.)

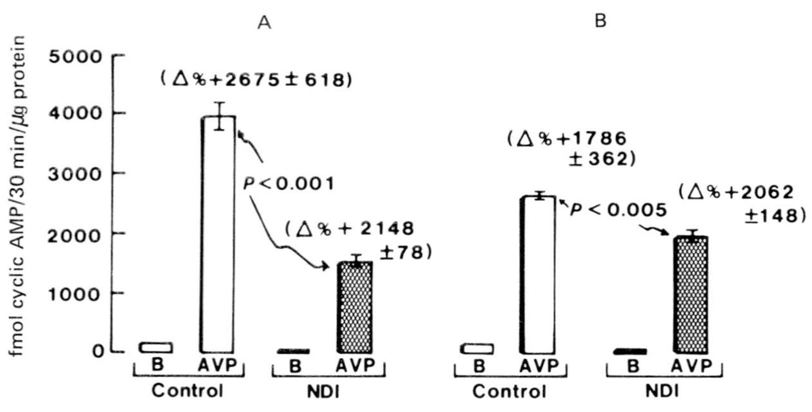

Fig. 6 Stimulation of adenylate cyclase activity by ADH (AVP) in (A) medullary thick ascending limb (MAL) and (B) medullary collecting tubule (MCT) of normal (control) mice and mice with nephrogenic diabetes insipidus (NDI). B, basal activity; AVP, activity in the presence of 1 μmol/liter AVP. Each bar represents the mean ± SEM from four animals; the value for each animal is the mean of four to six samples. AVP-stimulated adenylate cyclase in MAL of control mice is significantly higher ($p < 0.005$) than in MCT of control mice. In contrast, AVP-stimulated adenylate cyclase activity in MAL of NDI mice is significantly less ($p < 0.05$) than in MCT of NDI mice. AVP-stimulated adenylate cyclase activites in both MAL and MCT of control mice are significantly higher ($p < 0.001$ and $p < 0.005$, respectively) than in the corresponding segments of NDI mice. (From Ref. 112.)

ascending limb of Henle's loop (Fig. 6), and the decreased adenylate cyclase activity noted in the previous study (111) was ascribed to decreased activity of this enzyme in the thick ascending limb rather than in the collecting ducts. Thus, the major biochemical defect in the collecting duct of mice with hereditary nephrogenic diabetes insipidus is decreased intracellular cAMP accumulation, a problem which appears to be primarily due to increased cAMP degradation (as the result of the presence of an abnormally active cAMP phosphodiesterase) rather than being primarily due to decreased cAMP synthesis.

Recent studies have demonstrated that ADH stimulates sodium transport in the thick ascending limb of Henle's loop in a number of different experimental animals (118-121). Such a process could have an important role in the renal concentrating mechanism (by enhancing solute accumulation in the medullary interstitium). The decrease in ADH-stimulated adenylate cyclase activity in the thick ascending limb of mice with hereditary nephrogenic diabetes insipidus (112) may, therefore, represent the biochemical basis of a second abnormality in the concentrating mechanism of these animals (i.e., a defect in gradient formation). However, since an ADH-sensitive adenylate cyclase has not been detected in the human thick ascending limb (122), the relevance of these findings to hereditary nephrogenic diabetes insipidus in humans is unclear.

VII. LITHIUM

Polydipsia and polyuria are frequently reported side effects in psychiatric patients treated with lithium, but their exact prevalence is unknown. Forrest et al. (55) noted polydipsia in 40% and polyuria in 12% of lithium-treated patients, and Baylis and Heath (123) reported figures of 20% and 10%, respectively. Despite the relatively high prevalence of polyuria, however, urine volume does not often exceed 3 liters/day and is only rarely of sufficient magnitude to require cessation of lithium therapy.

Although lithium may directly stimulate thirst in animals (124-126), there is no evidence that lithium-induced primary polydipsia has an important role in the genesis of the polyuria in humans (55,123,127). However, the presence of psychogenic polydipsia may coincidentally influence water homeostasis in some psychiatric patients receiving maintenance lithium therapy.

Lithium-induced polyuria is generally characterized by normal solute-free water generation (C_{H_2O}) and by impaired solute-free water reabsorption ($T^c_{H_2O}$) (128-130). These findings strongly suggest that lithium has a major effect on the ADH-dependent aspects of water homeostasis (i.e., that is causes diabetes insipidus). Lithium may also produce polyuria by affecting processes that are ADH independent. For example, by decreasing fluid reabsorption in the proximal tubule (128,131,132), lithium could increase solute-free water generation and, thereby, increase the delivery of water to the collecting duct. Such a mechanism may explain the observations that Brattleboro rats become more polyuric after treatment with lithium (133,134) and that the administration of lithium to these animals during a steady-state water diuresis increases solute-free water clearance (135). Whether these findings are relevant to lithium-induced polyuria in humans is unknown.

Most humans and animals with lithium-induced polyuria are unresponsive to the administration of exogenous ADH (55,129,133,136,141). Urinary and plasma ADH levels are generally elevated or normal during chronic lithium administration (123,127,134,138,142,143) (Fig. 7) and increase after dehydration (143). Lithium has also been shown to impair ADH-stimulated osmotic water flow in amphibian epithelia such as the toad urinary bladder and frog skin (129,137,144). Consequently, nephrogenic diabetes insipidus is the major cause of lithium-induced polyuria.

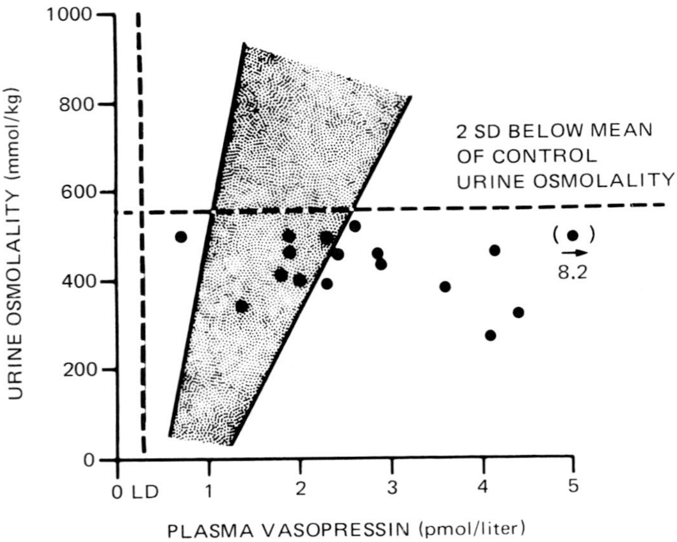

Fig. 7 Relationship of urine osmolality to plasma ADH (vasopressin) concentration in 17 patients with lithium-induced polyuria. The shaded area represents the 95% confidence limits of data from normal subjects. The vertical broken line (LD) represents the limit of detection of the radioimmunoassay employed. All of the patients had a significant impairment of renal concentrating ability which, with a single exception, was associated with normal or elevated plasma ADH levels. (From Ref. 123.)

Although most humans with lithium-induced polyuria are completely unresponsive to the administration of exogenous ADH, a few do respond by concentrating their urine, albeit submaximally (55,129,138). Similar observations have been made in animals (55,128,133, 139). While such results could be explained by the presence of *partial* nephrogenic diabetes insipidus, in some cases the ADH was administered after a period of prolonged water deprivation had led to weight loss and/or hypertonicity, i.e., at a time when endogenous ADH levels (and, consequently, renal concentrating ability) should already have been maximal. In addition, although ADH levels are generally normal or increased during chronic lithium administration, at least one patient with lithium-induced polyuria has been described whose plasma ADH concentration was abnormally low (123). Thus, lithium can cause central diabetes insipidus, but this appears to be extremely uncommon.

The glomerular filtration rate is normal during lithium-induced polyuria (128,129,145-148) and lithium does not grossly alter the normal corticopapillary osmotic gradient (55, 137,139,147,149). In addition, solute-free water generation is normal during lithium-induced polyuria (128-130), indicating that sodium reabsorption in the ascending limb of Henle's loop is grossly unimpaired by lithium. Consequently, it seems unlikely that lithium has a clinically significant effect on the generation or maintenance of the renal medullary osmotic gradient.

Lithium is concentrated in the renal medulla (55,139,147,149,150) and ADH stimulates the uptake of lithium into amphibian renal epithelia (151,152). The uptake of lithium is a prerequisite for its cellular effects. Amiloride blocks the uptake of lithium into amphibian renal epithelial cells (152-154) and reverses the inhibitory effect of lithium on ADH-induced water flow (144). In addition, pretreatment of animals with amiloride partially restores the lithium-related reduction in $T^c_{H_2O}$ to normal (130,155), an effect that appears to be specifically related to partial restoration of the sensitivity of the collecting duct to ADH (156). Amiloride has also recently been shown to ameliorate polyuria in patients receiving lithium maintenance therapy (157).

The mechanisms by which lithium impairs the hydro-osmotic response to ADH are not entirely clear, but there is evidence that defects exist both proximal and distal to the ADH-induced generation of cAMP. The normal antidiuretic response to the infusion of cAMP (or dibutyryl cAMP) is inhibited in lithium-treated rats (55,128,136), suggesting at least a distal site of action. However, in one of these studies, the antidiuretic response to dibutyryl cAMP was only partially inhibited, whereas under the same circumstances the antidiuretic response to ADH was completely eliminated (55) (Fig. 8); these results suggest that lithium acts at loci both proximal and distal to cAMP generation.

Physiological studies in in vitro systems have not been able to resolve this issue. In the toad urinary bladder, Singer et al. (129,144) found that lithium inhibited the hydro-osmotic response to ADH but not that to dibutyryl cAMP, suggesting a single site of action of lithium proximal to cAMP generation. In contrast, in the same tissue, Harris and Jenner (137) reported that both ADH- and cAMP-stimulated water flow were inhibited, suggesting that lithium also acts distal to cAMP generation. The reasons for these conflicting results are unclear, but they may be related to the inhibitory effect certain cAMP analogs (such as dibutyryl cAMP) have on cAMP phosphodiesterase. Alternatively, they may be related to the absence of potassium in the incubation medium used by Harris and Jenner (137); potassium is known to modulate water transport in the toad urinary bladder (158-160). The situation is further complicated by the failure of Bentley and Wasserman (161) to detect an effect of lithium on

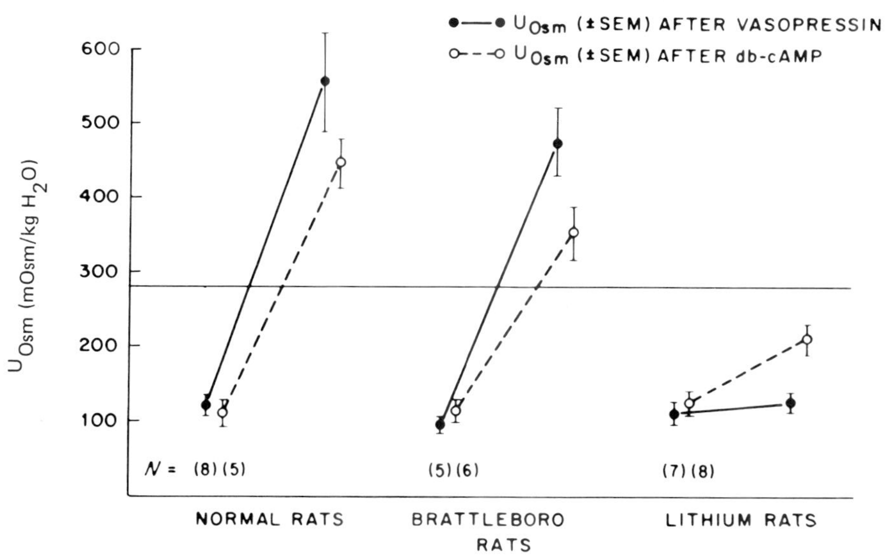

Fig. 8 Maximal effect of a single intravenous injection of ADH (vasopressin) (5-10 mU/kg) and dibutyryl cAMP (db cAMP) (15-20 mg/kg) on urine osmolality (U_{osm}) during water diuresis in normal, Brattleboro, and lithium polyuric rats. Lithium-induced polyuria is unresponsive to ADH and only partially responsive to db cAMP, suggesting defects both proximal and distal to cAMP generation. (From Ref. 55.)

ADH-stimulated osmotic water flow in toad urinary bladders, and by the observations of Carney et al. (162) in the isolated perfused papilla of the rat. The latter investigators found that diffusional water permeability increased normally following the administration of ADH to rats with lithium-induced polyuria.

Biochemical studies have also suggested that lithium has multiple sites of action, including at least adenylate cyclase, phosphodiesterase, and protein kinase. Many of the diverse biological effects of the lithium ion have been ascribed to interference with hormone-stimulated adenylate cyclase activities (163). In the case of the renal medulla, the evidence in this regard is substantial. In a medium of high osmolality (such as exists in the renal medulla in vivo) lithium inhibits ADH-stimulated adenylate cyclase activity in membrane-rich homogenates prepared from normal human or rabbit renal medulla (133,164-167). Relatively high concentrations of lithium (5-25 mmol) were required in these studies, but such concentrations are achievable in the renal medullary interstitium in vivo (55,139,147,149,150). Although Beck and Davis (168) were unable to detect an effect of 10 mmol/liter lithium on ADH-stimulated adenylate cyclase in normal rat renal medullary homogenates, this may have been due to the use of an incubation medium of considerably lower osmolality than that employed by other investigators (133,164-167). Indeed, in more recent studies using microdissected rat medullary collecting tubules (169) 15-50 mmol/liter lithium was shown to inhibit ADH-stimulated adenylate cyclase activity provided that a hyperosmolar incubation medium was employed.

The effects of chronic treatment with lithium in vivo on ADH-stimulated adenylate cyclase activity have also been examined. Using whole kidney homogenates, Geisler et al. (165) observed that rats with lithium-induced polyuria had decreased ADH-stimulated adenylate cyclase activity and Wraae et al. (166) showed that this was reversible following discontinuation of the lithium and resolution of the polyuria. More recently, similar findings were obtained in microdissected medullary collecting tubules obtained from rats with lithium-induced polyuria (169).

Whether lithium affects cAMP-phosphodiesterase activity is controversial. Lithium had no effect on phosphodiesterase activity in human renal medullary tissue or in microdissected rat medullary collecting tubules (167,169). In contrast, relatively low concentrations of lithium (10 mmol/liter) were found to stimulate putative high-K_m phosphodiesterase activity in rat renal medullary slices (168), leading to the suggestion that lithium inhibits ADH-stimulated cAMP accumulation by augmenting the catabolism of cAMP rather than by inhibiting its synthesis. Further studies will be needed to resolve this issue.

Since the tissue level of cAMP is also related to the availability of its precursor (ATP), lithium could act by stimulating one or more of the ATPase group of enzymes (170,171). However, Wraae et al. (166) found that the lithium-related decrease in cAMP accumulation in rat renal medullary tissue could still be observed when an ATP-regenerating system was added to the incubation medium. In addition, the K_m for ATP in this reaction is such that the intracellular ATP concentration probably never becomes rate limiting. Thus, it is unlikely that depletion of ATP has an important role in the inhibition of ADH-induced water flow by lithium.

Since prostaglandins modulate the hydro-osmotic effect of ADH, a potential mechanism for lithium-induced tubular resistance to the hormone could be the stimulation of renal PGE synthesis. Although the acute administration of lithium to dogs increased urinary PGE excretion (and caused polyuria), and although these effects were abolished by indomethacin (172), the polyuria was probably not due to antagonism of the hydro-osmotic effect of ADH because solute-free water reabsorption increased normally (as a function of osmolar clearance). The antidiuretic effect of indomethacin could be best ascribed to hemodynamic factors, rather than to decreased prostaglandin synthesis per se. Two recent reports in humans have described partial attenuation of lithium-induced polyuria with indomethacin, but detailed hemodynamic analyses were not performed (173,174). Furthermore, the fact that indomethacin directly inhibits cAMP phosphodiesterase in amphibian epithelia (175) makes the findings in humans even more difficult to interpret.

Lithium has a variety of other effects in renal epithelia, but their relevance to the concentrating defect in humans is uncertain. Lithium has been shown to inhibit cAMP-dependent protein kinase activity in human renal medulla (167), but the effect is small. In addition, in concentrations that may well occur in the medulla in vivo, lithium inhibits microtubule assembly in rabbit renal medullary homogenates (176). Forrest et al. (177) have recently demonstrated the presence of aggregates of intermediate microfilaments in the principal cells of the cortical collecting ducts of lithium-treated rats with polyuria; such aggregates were absent in normal rats and in rats with comparable degrees of polyuria induced by drinking glucose and water. Finally, since lithium has been shown to affect several Ca^{2+}-dependent processes (163), it may influence the hydro-osmotic effect of ADH by interacting with some aspect of cellular Ca^{2+} metabolism.

In summary, lithium affects both thirst and water conservation. Lithium-induced polyuria is due to a major disturbance in water conservation (primary polyuria); lithium-induced polydipsia, at least in humans, appears to be a consequence of the defect in water conservation (secondary polydipsia). The polyuria is largely, if not entirely, due to a disturbance in the ADH-dependent aspects of the water conservation system (diabetes insipidus). Nephrogenic diabetes insipidus is the predominant defect induced by lithium, but central diabetes insipidus may also have a role in the occasional patient. At the cellular level, lithium has a major effect on the proximal component of the ADH-cAMP second messenger system, most probably by inhibiting hormone-stimulated adenylate cyclase activity. However, there is also evidence for other sites of action, including cAMP-dependent protein kinase, microtubules, and cellular Ca^{2+} and prostaglandin metabolism. Further work will be necessary to definitively include or exclude these possibilities.

Lithium-induced nephrogenic diabetes insipidus has generally been considered to be readily reversible following the discontinuation of lithium therapy. Recently, however, several reports have suggested that it may persist for many months (and perhaps indefinitely) (178-182). The persistence of a renal concentrating defect after lithium withdrawal suggests that, at least in some patients, the chronic administration of the drug might lead to long-term renal damage. Indeed, it has been suggested that lithium maintenance therapy may be associated with the development of chronic interstitial nephritis and renal insufficiency (183). At this point in time, however, there is no definitive evidence in this regard. This controversy has been recently reviewed in detail (184,185) and will not be further elaborated here.

VIII. DEMECLOCYCLINE

In 1965 the first in a series of reports appeared linking the use of the tetracycline antibiotic demeclocycline to the development of a dose-related reversible form of nephrogenic diabetes insipidus (186-189). If a sufficient dose of demeclocycline is employed (usually 900-1200 mg/day), the urinary concentrating ability of virtually all subjects will be affected; occasionally, however, clinically significant effects are manifest with even lower doses (189). The ADH unresponsiveness generally develops gradually and polyuria may not become clinically apparent for a week or more, even when high doses of the drug are employed (189,190).

Similarly, several weeks may pass after the drug is discontinued before renal concentrating ability returns to normal (189,190). Since demeclocycline is eliminated by the kidneys (191), patients with renal insufficiency might be expected to be more susceptible to the development of nephrogenic diabetes insipidus unless appropriate adjustments in drug dosage are made. However, no information is presently available in this regard. With the exception of tetracycline itself, which has a very much smaller effect than demeclocycline (188), the effects of other tetracyclines on water homeostasis in humans have not been evaluated. There are no reports of polyuria following the use of these agents in the clinical literature, however.

Antagonism of the hydro-osmotic effect of ADH provided the rationale for the successful use of demeclocycline in the treatment of the hyponatremia associated with the chronic syndrome of inappropriate ADH secretion (SIADH) (190,192). The administration of demeclocycline (600-1200 mg/day) is associated with the production of hypotonic urine and restores the serum Na^+ concentration to normal within 1-2 weeks. Such therapy permits unrestricted water intake in most patients and side effects in patients with otherwise normal renal function appear to be minimal. The concentrating defect is reversible within several weeks of discontinuing the drug (Fig. 9).

Patients with demeclocycline-induced polyuria have a reduction in solute-free water clearance ($T^c_{H_2O}$) and are essentially unresponsive to the administration of exogenous ADH (188, 189). In otherwise normal individuals, this defect in renal function appears to be quite selec-

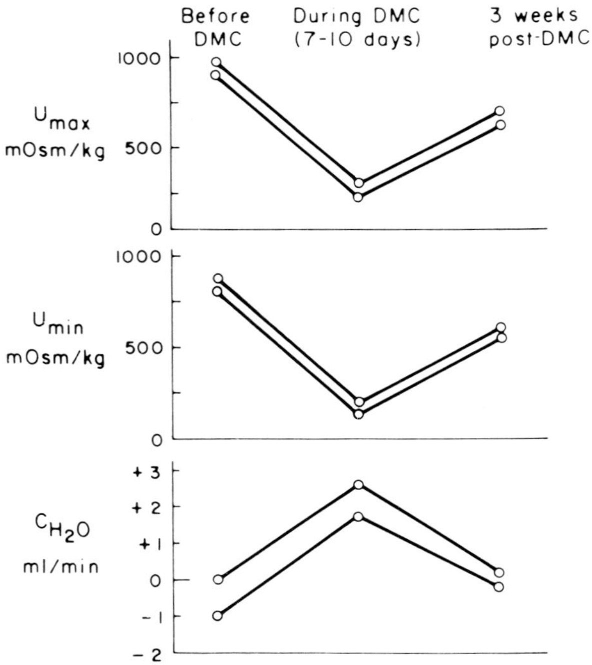

Fig. 9 Maximum urinary concentrating (U_{max}) and diluting (U_{min}) ability and electrolyte-free water clearance (C_{H_2O}) before, during, and 3 weeks after demeclocycline (DMC) therapy in two patients with the chronic syndrome of inappropriate ADH secretion. Note that the concentrating defect is reversible after the drug is discontinued. (From Ref. 190. Reprinted by permission of The New England Journal of Medicine 298:173-177, 1978.)

tive: glomerular filtration rate is normal and there are no gross alterations in sodium or potassium balance (188,189). In addition, solute-free water clearance (C_{H_2O}) and minimum urine osmolality (U_{min}) are normal (189). In patients with SIADH who are treated with demeclocycline, sodium balance also remains grossly normal (190). In such patients, a small but definite increase in the serum creatinine concentration and a modest increase in the blood urea nitrogen concentration are sometimes observed (190,192). This is rarely of clinical significance, however, and may be due to extracellular fluid volume depletion (secondary to drug-induced water loss) and/or to the antianabolic effect of the tetracyclines (193). Thus, at least in normal humans and in patients with uncomplicated SIADH, there is no evidence that demeclocycline directly affects the generation or maintenance of the medullary osmotic gradient.

In contrast, in patients with preexisting renal insufficiency, hepatic cirrhosis, or congestive heart failure, demeclocycline-induced polyuria is associated not only with ADH unresponsiveness, but often also with marked renal sodium wasting and decrements in glomerular filtration rate (194-201). The pathogenesis of demeclocycline-induced natriuresis and renal insufficiency is unclear (193), but until such time as this problem is resolved, the use of demeclocycline (either as an antibiotic or as a diuretic) in these clinical situations should be avoided.

It should be clear from the human studies described above that the major factor leading to demeclocycline-induced polyuria is tubular resistance to the hydro-osmotic effect of ADH. Demeclocycline has also been shown to produce polyuria and ADH-unresponsiveness in normal and in ADH-treated Brattleboro rats (202), but these models have not been exploited in any detail. At present, most of the information concerning the cellular site(s) of action of demeclocycline has been derived from in vitro studies, largely utilizing the toad urinary bladder.

Demeclocycline inhibits both ADH- and cAMP-induced water flow in toad urinary bladders (189,203), but since inhibition of the effect of ADH can be out of proportion to inhibition of the effect of cAMP (203), the drug may act proximal as well as distal to cAMP generation. Biochemical studies have also suggested a dual site of action. Demeclocycline inhibits ADH-stimulated adenylate cyclase and cAMP-dependent protein kinase activities in human renal medullary homogenates (204). In the same study, tetracycline and chlortetracycline were shown to have similar effects. Since neither of these two drugs has been associated with clinically significant nephrogenic diabetes insipidus, another explanation may be needed to relate these biochemical findings to the physiological observations.

Recent studies in the toad urinary bladder may have provided some insight into the apparently selective behavior of demeclocycline. Only those tetracycline congeners that bound strongly to proteins in a crude 10,000-g supernatant fraction derived from toad urinary bladder epithelial cells were effective ADH antagonists (193). The degree of tetracycline-protein binding varied directly with the inhibitory effect of the particular tetracycline on ADH-induced water flow. Of the clinically available tetracyclines tested, demeclocycline was most strongly bound and was the most potent ADH antagonist. In contrast, there was no correlation between protein binding and the inhibitory effect of the tetracycline on cAMP-induced water flow. These results suggest that demeclocycline-induced inhibition of osmotic water flow in renal epithelia may involve the binding of the drug to a cellular protein (or proteins) that has (have) a major role in the proximal component of the ADH-cAMP second messenger system. Further studies will be necessary to establish the specificity of tetracycline-protein binding and to identify the protein(s) involved.

Prostaglandin metabolism has also been considered as a potential locus of demeclocycline's cellular effect(s). Demeclocycline had no effect on PGE synthesis in toad urinary bladders at a time when ADH-induced water flow was inhibited (205). In addition, indomethacin failed to alter the magnitude of demeclocycline-induced polyuria in rats despite reducing urine PGE excretion. Consequently, the concentrating defect induced by demeclocycline appears to be independent of alterations in prostaglandin synthesis.

Since tetracyclines chelate a variety of divalent cations, including Ca^{2+} and Mg^{2+} (207-209), the role of chelation in their effects on ADH-induced water flow warrants more careful investigation. Chelation may alter the divalent cation microenvironment in a critical subcellular compartment in renal epithelia. Alternatively, divalent cations may be involved in the binding of tetracyclines to proteins or to other macromolecules (210-211). In the latter regard, preliminary studies have shown that Ca^{2+} markedly influences the binding of tetracyclines to toad urinary bladder epithelial cell proteins (193).

Whether antibiotic activity is a prerequisite for ADH antagonism has also been examined in the toad urinary bladder model system. 4-Dedimethylaminotetracycline has a small but definite effect on ADH-induced water flow and 5a,6-anhydro-demeclocycline is several-fold more potent than equimolar concentrations of its parent compound, demeclocycline (193). Since neither of these congeners has significant tetracycline antibiotic activity (212), the latter is not required for their effects on epithelial water transport.

In summary, demeclocycline produces a dose-dependent, reversible form of nephrogenic diabetes insipidus. Although this has been shown to be due to interference with the cellular action of ADH, the precise locus of demeclocycline's action is unknown. Demeclocycline appears to influence both proximal and distal components of the ADH-cAMP second messenger system and binding of the drug to specific renal epithelial cell proteins may be important. Inhibition of the hydro-osmotic effect of ADH in the human kidney accounts for the therapeutic efficacy of demeclocycline in patients with hyponatremia associated with the chronic syndrome of inappropriate ADH secretion.

IX. METHOXYFLURANE

Shortly after the introduction of methoxyflurane as an anesthetic in the early 1960s, reports began to appear linking its use with the development of a postoperative toxic nephropathy (213-224). Although some of the patients were oliguric, the majority developed polyuric renal failure and were unresponsive (or markedly hyporesponsive) to the administration of exogenous ADH (214-224). The polyuria generally begins in the immediate postoperative period and its severity and duration are highly variable. The incidence of methoxyflurane-induced polyuric renal failure is unknown but the anesthetic is now little used.

The two major metabolites of methoxyflurane are oxalic acid and inorganic fluoride, both of which have been implicated in methoxyflurane nephrotoxicity. However, each has been associated with a different syndrome (225,226). In those patients with oliguric renal failure, urinary excretion of oxalate is markedly increased. Biopsies obtained from such patients reveal extensive oxalate deposition in the renal medulla, along with changes consistent with acute tubular necrosis (215,220,221,227-229). Poisoning with oxalic acid or with ethylene glycol (3-10% of ethylene glycol is metabolized to oxalic acid) is also associated with acute oliguric renal failure and with similar histological findings (230).

Although acute renal failure of any cause may be associated with oxalate deposition in the kidneys, that seen in methoxyflurane-induced *oliguric* renal failure is much more marked. In fact, the amount of oxalate apparent on renal biopsy has been correlated with the severity of the renal failure (220,231). The majority of patients with this syndrome either die or require chronic dialysis. The few patients who improve sufficiently to no longer need dialysis, and those whose renal failure is not severe enough to require dialysis, are often left with some degree of renal insufficiency; biopsies in such patients generally reveal chronic intestitial nephritis (220,223,224,227,229).

In contrast, in patients with methoxyflurance-induced *polyuric* renal failure, the ADH-unresponsiveness appears to be related, at least in part, to the marked increase in the serum concentration and/or the urinary excretion of inorganic fluoride (232,233). Following methoxyflurane anesthesia, the serum inorganic fluoride concentration peaks on the first or second postoperative day and the concentration achieved is directly related to the amount of methoxyflurane administered (234,235). Concentrations of more than 90 μmol/liter are associated with polyuria, while concentrations of less than 50 μmol/liter are generally not associated with renal dysfunction (233,234,236,237). In both experimental animals and humans, the intravenous infusion of sodium fluoride induces a prompt water diuresis which, at least in the rat, has been shown to be ADH resistant (235,238-240).

A variety of studies have been performed in order to determine the mechanisms by which methoxyflurane and/or its metabolite, inorganic fluoride, produce ADH-resistant polyuria. In humans, methoxyflurane-induced polyuria can occur in association with widely different glomerular filtration rates. Some patients have been reported to have significant polyuria in the absence of renal insufficiency (222,234), while others have polyuria with only modest decrements in glomerular filtration rate (213,215,218,221). Still others have polyuria and severe acute renal failure and several patients have either died with end-stage renal failure or have required maintenance dialysis (213,215,217,219-221,223,224,228). Consequently, alterations in glomerular filtration rate do not appear to have a significant role in the genesis of methoxyflurane-induced polyuria.

Renal medullary electrolyte concentrations have been reported to be decreased in animals infused with sodium fluoride (238,239), suggesting that generation or maintenance of the osmotic gradient is abnormal. However, fluoride does not appear to grossly impair sodium chloride reabsorption in the ascending limb of Henle's loop. For example, patients with methoxyflurane-induced polyuria generally do not manifest a natriuresis (222) and inorganic fluoride infusions in animals are not associated with sodium-wasting or with an increase in osmolar clearance (238,239). In addition, despite the polyuria and a reduction in solute-free water reabsorption, solute-free water clearance in such animals is normal (Fig. 10) (239, 241).

Since gradient formation appears to be normal, it has been suggested that inorganic fluoride may disrupt the corticopapillary gradient by affecting renal medullary blood flow. Indeed, fluoride, which may accumulate in the renal medulla (238,242), has been shown to be a peripheral vasodilator (243). However, direct measurements of cortical and medullary blood flow in fluoride-treated animals have not yet been made. Thus, it remains speculative as to whether alterations in renal blood flow contribute to the concentrating direct in methoxyflurane-induced polyuria.

The presence of a persistently hypotonic urine (after the administration of ADH) in humans with methoxyflurane-induced polyuria (215,218) and the finding of decreased free-water reabsorption in animals infused with inorganic fluoride (239,241) are indicative of a defect in water reabsorption in the ADH-responsive segments of the distal nephron. Several studies have provided evidence of ADH-resistance produced either by fluoride or by methoxyflurane itself.

As discussed above, rats treated with fluoride develop an ADH-resistant concentrating defect and polyuria (241). Both basal and ADH-stimulated urinary cAMP excretion are decreased in such animals (241), findings consistent with effects of fluoride on adenylate cyclase activity

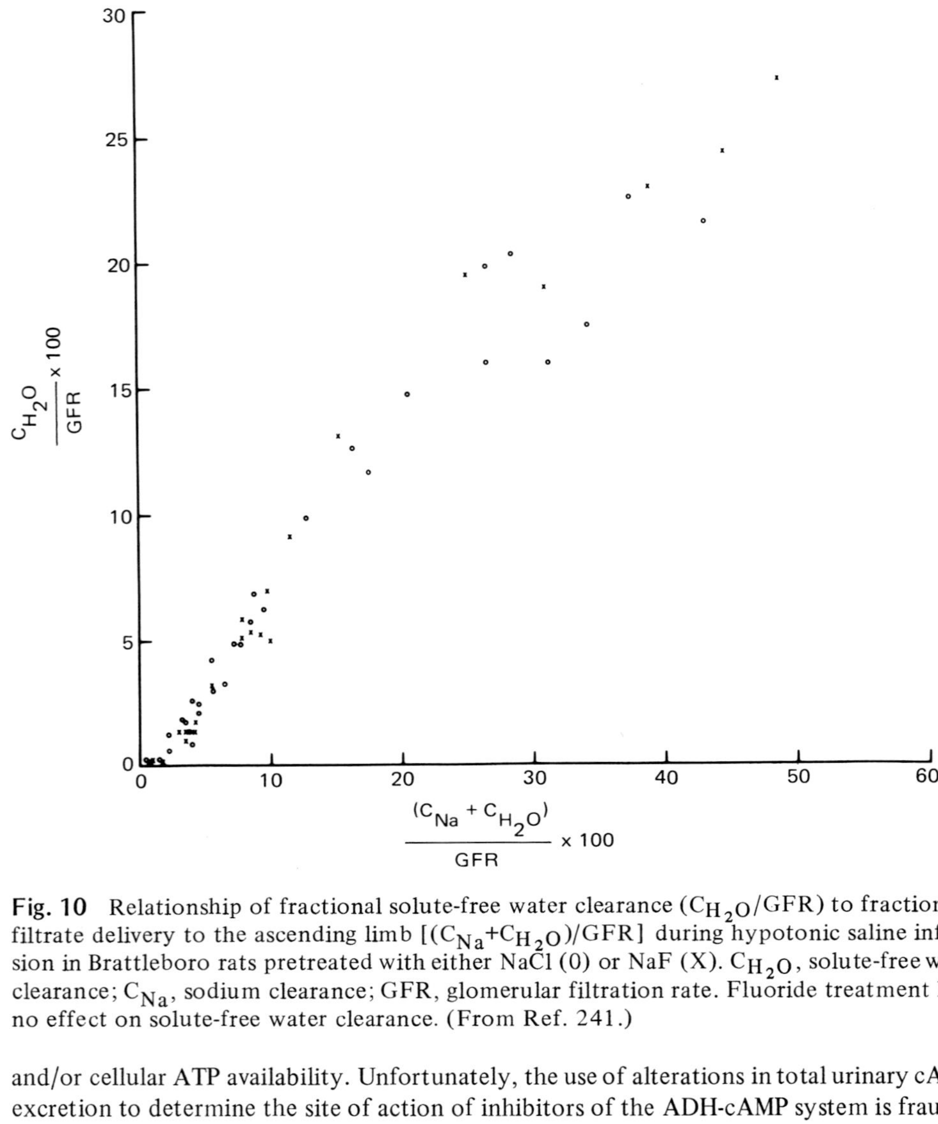

Fig. 10 Relationship of fractional solute-free water clearance (C_{H_2O}/GFR) to fractional filtrate delivery to the ascending limb [(C_{Na}+C_{H_2O})/GFR] during hypotonic saline infusion in Brattleboro rats pretreated with either NaCl (0) or NaF (X). C_{H_2O}, solute-free water clearance; C_{Na}, sodium clearance; GFR, glomerular filtration rate. Fluoride treatment has no effect on solute-free water clearance. (From Ref. 241.)

and/or cellular ATP availability. Unfortunately, the use of alterations in total urinary cAMP excretion to determine the site of action of inhibitors of the ADH-cAMP system is fraught with problems (see Sect. II.B). Moreover, inorganic fluoride is well known to increase cAMP levels in a wide variety of tissues by directly activating adenylate cyclase (9,244), an action which further complicates interpretation of these data.

The effects of methoxyflurane and inorganic fluoride have been examined in the toad urinary bladder model system. Methoxyflurane gas reversibly inhibits ADH-stimulated water flow, but it has no effect on cAMP-stimulated water flow (245). In addition, methoxyflurane has been shown to blunt the ADH-dependent increase in intracellular cAMP levels, probably by directly inhibiting ADH-dependent adenylate cyclase (246). Indeed, in these studies, ADH-stimulated adenylate cyclase activities were decreased over a wide range of ADH concentrations.

Inorganic fluoride also inhibits ADH-stimulated water flow in toad urinary bladders (245, 247,248). This occurs despite the fact that ADH-induced elevations of intracellular cAMP levels are increased (not decreased) by fluoride (247,248). Fluoride appears to exert this effect not only by way of activating adenylate cyclase (see above) but also by blocking calmodulin-dependent phosphodiesterase activity (248). These findings, taken together with the observation that cAMP-induced water flow is inhibited by fluoride (248), indicate that fluoride probably has an important site of action distal to the generation of cAMP.

Anaerobic glycolysis is an important energy source in the renal medulla and provides the bulk of the ATP generated in this tissue (249). One of the rate-limiting enzymes in the glycolytic pathway is enolase. The finding that fluoride inhibits this enzyme (250) suggests a possible mechanism for ADH resistance, at least in the medullary portions of the collecting duct. However, in the toad urinary bladder, both fluoride and 2-deoxyglucose inhibit glycolysis, but only fluoride inhibits ADH-induced water flow (248).

In summary, although there is no doubt that the use of methoxyflurane can be associated with clinically significant nephrogenic diabetes insipidus, the underlying mechanisms have not been completely defined. A decrease in the osmotic gradient for water reabsorption (perhaps due to fluoride-related alterations in renal medullary blood flow) and defects in the cellular response to ADH have both been suggested. The latter have been ascribed to inhibition of ADH-stimulated adenylate cyclase activity by methoxyflurane, and to inhibition of the cellular action of cAMP by inorganic fluoride. Obviously, more work is needed before these diverse observations can be integrated into a coherent schema of the cellular effects of these two compounds. Only then will their relationship to the polyuria associated with methoxyflurane anesthesia become clear.

X. AMPHOTERICIN B

Amphotericin B is currently the most effective agent available for the treatment of serious fungal infections. Unfortunately, it is a rather toxic drug, frequently producing headaches, nausea, vomiting, diarrhea, chills, fever, and superficial phlebitis. The major limitation in its use, however, is nephrotoxicity. Renal dysfunction occurs to some extent in virtually all patients and includes early evidence of tubular disorders (distal renal tubular acidosis, potassium wasting, concentrating defects) and, with continued therapy, depression of the glomerular filtration rate.

Several early reports of clinical experience with the drug described reduced renal concentrating ability (251-254). This defect frequently became evident before the onset of azotemia and appeared to be a common manifestation of amphotericin B therapy. However, clinically significant polyuria was distinctly unusual. Indeed, in one large series (254), only two of 81 patients treated with amphotericin B were noted to be polyuric. In a more recent study (255), polyuria and nocturia developed in two patients treated with the drug, but in both cases urine volumes were less than 5 liters/day. Unfortunately, most of the animal studies of amphotericin B nephrotoxicity have been limited to the acute effects of the drug. However, Gouge and Andreoli (256) administered the drug to rats for a period of 25 days and confirmed the clinical observation that tubular dysfunction, including hyposthenuria, often precedes the development of azotemia.

Butler et al. (254) were the first to report that the concentrating defect induced by amphotericin B was unresponsive to pharmacological doses of ADH. Since that time three other studies have demonstrated that amphotericin B can produce nephrogenic diabetes insipidus (255,257,258) (Fig. 11). Although the factors responsible for the ADH resistance have not been completely elucidated, it seems likely that amphotericin B has multiple effects on the renal concentrating mechansim.

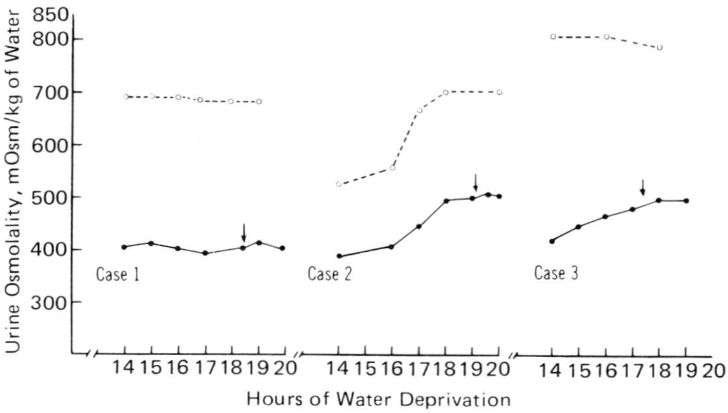

Fig. 11 Evaluation of renal concentrating ability in three patients during (●——●), and 3-4 months after completion (○- - -○) of amphotericin B therapy. The arrows indicate the administration of exogenous ADH; see (Ref. 255) for details. In all three cases, during amphotericin B therapy there was a subnormal response to dehydration and an insignificant response to the administration of exogenous ADH. Marked improvement in renal concentrating ability occurred after amphotericin B was stopped. (From Ref. 255. Arch. Int. Med. 139:86-88. Copyright 1979, American Medical Association.)

A decrement in glomerular filtration rate is a common manifestation of amphotericin B therapy (251-254,257-259). Mild azotemia occurs frequently, but it is usually reversible when the drug is discontinued. However, about 40% of patients receiving greater than 4 g of amphotericin and about 90% of patients receiving more than 5 g of the drug develop some degree of irreversible renal insufficiency (254,260,261). Amphotericin B has been shown to produce marked renal vasoconstriction in acute studies in experimental animals (262-264), and consequently at least part of the decrement in filtration rate may be explicable purely on hemodynamic grounds. Whether additional mechanisms (e.g., tubular necrosis) are also involved is unknown. Whatever the case, however, since renal concentrating defects can be manifest prior to the onset of azotemia or in the presence of only mild renal insufficiency (251,255), it is unlikely that they can be fully explained by a reduction in the glomerular filtration rate.

Studies of the medullary osmotic gradient in patients with amphotericin-induced concentrating defects have yielded conflicting results. Butler et al. (254) reported that two of their patients could not excrete an oral water load normally and suggested that NaCl reabsorption in the ascending limb of Henle's loop was impaired. However, these patients had significant degrees of renal insufficiency and, consequently, a reduction in glomerular filtration rate may have contributed to the defective water excretion. Indeed, Barbour et al. (255) found U_{min}, C_{H_2O}, and Na^+ delivery to the diluting sites to be normal in a patient whose filtration rate was only minimally reduced.

Acute studies in the dog revealed a decrement in C_{H_2O} that could not be completely accounted for by the amphotericin B-related fall in glomerular filtration rate or the associated decrease in Na^+ delivery to the diluting sites (263). Unfortunately, however, despite the development of a chronic model of amphotericin B nephrotoxicity in the rat (256), animal studies have not yet been performed to evaluate the adequacy of osmotic gradient generation and/or maintenance. Further studies will be needed in order to define whether abnormalities in the medullary osmotic gradient have a role in the ADH-unresponsive hyposthenuria associated with amphotericin B therapy.

The effects of amphotericin B on the cellular response to ADH have also been incompletely examined. In the only study in humans reported to date (255), a single patient with amphotericin-induced hyposthenuria and ADH-unresponsiveness was shown to have a reduction in solute-free water reabsorption ($T^c_{H_2O}$) in the absence of abnormalities in solute-free water clearance (C_{H_2O}) and glomerular filtration rate. Such findings are of course compatible with a defect in the response of the distal nephron to ADH. However, they do not exclude subtle defects in osmotic gradient generation and/or maintenance as possible etiological factors in the ADH unresponsiveness.

The effects of amphotericin B on solute and water transport have been examined in the toad urinary bladder but, unfortunately, only limited insight into the clinical problem of amphotericin B-related polyuria has been provided. Although the effects of the drug are quite variable, there is general agreement that this polyene antibiotic, which disrupts cell membranes by interacting with sterol groups (265), increases the permeability of the toad bladder to a variety of small solutes (e.g., sodium, potassium, chloride, urea) and to water (266-269). However, it is less certain whether amphotericin affects osmotic (net) water flow; although, in some hands, the drug has little or no effect on osmotic water flow (266,269), it clearly has the ability to markedly increase osmotic water flow under certain conditions (268).

The effect of amphotericin B on the hydro-osmotic response to ADH is also not entirely clear. When tested within 60 min of exposure to the drug (and in its continued presence), the response to ADH was essentially normal (269); this finding was accompanied by a marked blunting of the effect of the hormone on short-circuit current (presumably reflecting net sodium transport). In contrast, when tested several hours following a 30-min exposure to the drug, the hydro-osmotic responses to both ADH and cAMP were markedly diminished (268).

Since amphotericin B may irreversibly damage membranes (270,271), the question can justifiably be raised as to whether these effects of amphotericin B on ADH responsiveness are specific or whether they simply represent irreversible tissue damage. This concern has been strengthened by a recent study of the effects of amphotericin B on the morphology of the toad urinary bladder. Numerous abnormalities in cellular membranes were noted after as short as an 8-min exposure to the drug, abnormalities which progressed to frank necrosis over a period of several hours (272). Whether such findings are pertinent to the polyuric syndrome associated with the use of amphotericin B is unknown. Although biopsies from patients treated with amphotericin have revealed some distal tubular damage, primarily manifested by nephrocalcinosis, it is difficult to implicate the nephrocalcinosis as a cause of the concentrating defect, since it may persist after normalization of renal function (251-254,273,274).

In summary, it must be admitted that the etiology of the concentrating defect associated with amphotericin B therapy is unknown. A decrement in glomerular filtration rate, in and of itself, does not seem to be sufficient to explain the defect. Further studies will be needed before we are able to ascribe the ADH unresponsiveness to abnormalities in the osmotic gradient or to alterations in the cellular response to the hormone.

XI. MISCELLANEOUS DRUGS

A. Sulfonylureas

Glyburide, tolazamide, and acetohexamide produce polyuria in humans, an effect initially postulated to be due to inhibition of the hydro-osmotic effect of ADH (275-281). In contrast, two other sulfonylureas, chlorpropamide and tolbutamide, are antidiuretic (282-287). Indeed, chlorpropamide has been used successfully in the treatment of partial central diabetes insipidus (288-290). In addition, dilutional hyponatremia, simulating the syndrome of inappropriate ADH, has been reported in patients with diabetes mellitus treated with chlorpropamide (283-287). The rather surprising finding that drugs of the same class apparently have markedly different effects on renal water excretion has prompted many studies of their interactions with this system.

Glyburide is the best studied "diuretic" sulfonylurea. The initial studies on the mechanism of glyburide-induced diuresis were performed on patients with central diabetes insipidus. In contrast to chlorpropamide, glyburide produced an increase in urine volume and solute-free water clearance and a decrease in urine osmolality; there was no change in osmolar clearance (276). Glyburide had similar effects during the administration of submaximal doses of ADH; increasing the dose of ADH decreased the magnitude of the glyburide effect (280). In general, these findings were reproduced in normal subjects and similar findings have been obtained with tolazamide and acetohexamide (277-279,281). These data were interpreted to mean that the diuretic sulfonylureas have a peripheral (renal) action to decrease ADH effectiveness when the hormone is present at submaximal concentrations.

However, such a mechanism of action cannot explain glyburide-induced polyuria in water-loaded normal subjects or in patients with complete central diabetes insipidus, circumstances where circulating ADH levels would be minimal or absent. The fact that glyburide produces a diuresis in the Brattleboro rat (291), which lacks endogenous ADH, also implies that ADH-independent mechanisms must be operative. Furthermore, glyburide and acetohexamide have been shown to increase (not decrease) the hydro-osmotic effect of submaximal doses of ADH in the toad urinary bladder (292,293). In this respect, the diuretic sulfonylureas have essentially the same in vitro action as chlorpropamide (293-299), the paradigm "antidiuretic" sulfonylurea. This enhancement of the hydro-osmotic effect of submaximal doses of ADH has recently been shown to be secondary to the ability of sulfonylureas to inhibit ADH-induced prostaglandin synthesis (300); prostaglandins inhibit the effect of ADH on water flow by decreasing ADH-stimulated adenylate cyclase activity (40). Neither glyburide nor chlorpropamide has any effect on basal water flow or on water flow induced by maximal doses of ADH. Paradoxically, however, both drugs inhibit cAMP-induced osmotic water flow (292).

These in vitro studies have lent credence to the suggestion that antidiuretic sulfonylureas such as chlorpropamide derive their efficacy in the treatment of partial central diabetes insipidus (288-290) from the enhancement of the renal effects of ADH (289,301-303). A similar mechanism may explain chlorpropamide-induced dilutional hyponatremia in normal subjects (283-287). It has also been suggested that chlorpropamide may increase endogenous ADH release (289,301-303), but in the only study in which plasma ADH levels were actually measured chlorpropamide decreased (rather than increased) the already low circulating levels of the hormone in patients with central diabetes insipidus (304).

It seems likely that the diuretic sulfonylureas have qualitatively (but not necessarily quantitatively) similar effects in the collecting duct to chlorpropamide, namely, that they enhance the hydro-osmotic effect of submaximal concentrations of ADH. The manner in which the diuretic sulfonylureas increase water excretion, despite enhancing the ADH sensitivity of the collecting duct, is unclear but decreased ADH release and increased solute-free water generation need to be considered. Decreased release of ADH has not been rigorously excluded, but it seems unlikely, since normal subjects treated with these agents while undergoing a sustained water diuresis (which itself should have completely suppressed ADH release) still had detectable urinary ADH levels (277).

Sulfonylurea-induced alterations in glomerular filtration rate leading to increased fluid delivery to the distal nephron have not been documented (276-280). Indeed, solute excretion in hydrated normal subjects or in patients with central diabetes insipidus is not increased by either glyburide or tolazamide (276-278). However, the latter observation does not exclude the possibility that the administration of these agents is associated with redistribution of solute reabsorption within the nephron. For example, inhibition of proximal tubular reabsorption and increased delivery of fluid to the high-capacity ascending limb of Henle's loop (where the extra solute could be reabsorbed) would lead to enhanced solute-free water generation. In the presence of low circulating ADH levels this sequence of events would result in a water diuresis, a decrease in urine osmolality, and little or no change in electrolyte excretion. In this regard, it is of interest that both glyburide and chlorpropamide have been shown to increase the magnitude of a water diuresis in rats under certain circumstances (305).

Such a mechanism is of course speculative and does not account for the ADH-enhancing action displayed by all sulfonylureas in the toad urinary bladder or the markedly different effects of the diuretic and the antidiuretic sulfonylureas in humans. However, it is possible that sensitization of the human collecting duct to the hydro-osmotic effect of ADH is relatively slight in the case of the diuretic sulfonylureas, whereas it is much more marked in the case of the antidiuretic sulfonylureas. Congeners in the former category (glyburide, tolazamide, acetohexamide) would increase solute-free water generation and their weak ADH-enhancing action would, at best, only attenuate the resultant polyuria. Congeners in the latter category (chlorpropamide, tolbutamide) would increase solute-free water generation to a similar extent, but their more potent ADH-enhancing action would lead to increased water reabsorption in the collecting duct and, ultimately, would lead to antidiuresis and water retention.

Clearly, more work will be needed before the diverse effects of the sulfonylureas on water homeostasis are understood. At this time it seems safe to conclude, however, that the diuretic sulfonylureas do not produce polyuria by producing nephrogenic diabetes insipidus.

B. Gentamicin

Many patients with gentamicin-induced acute renal failure are nonoliguric; indeed, urine volume may increase prior to the appearance of renal insufficiency (306-309). Studies to determine the etiology of polyuria in such patients have not yet been carried out. However, in experimental animals, gentamicin can produce a vasopressin-resistant concentrating defect before changes in filtration rate, renal blood flow, free-water clearance, or sodium excretion are evident (310-315). Consequently, a defect in the cellular response to ADH may have a role in the genesis of the polyuria. This suggestion is supported by the observation that nephrogenous cAMP excretion does not increase following the administration of exogenous vasopressin to rats with early gentamicin nephrotoxicity (312). The hydro-osmotic response to ADH in the toad urinary bladder is inhibited by gentamicin (316-318), an effect that was overcome by the prostaglandin inhibitor, ibuprofen, and by exogenous cAMP. Although such findings are provocative and, if confirmed, may shed light on the cellular mechanisms by which gentamicin affects osmotic water flow in the distal nephron, a recent report (319) has ascribed these results with toad urinary bladders to drug-induced alterations in medium pH rather than to specific tissue effects of the aminoglycoside.

C. Cisplatin

Cis-dichlorodiammine (II) platinum (cisplatin) is the first of a group of platinum coordination complexes with antineoplastic activity to achieve widespread use in the therapy of solid tumors. Although cisplatin has a variety of adverse effects, nephrotoxicity has emerged as the major factor limiting its use (320-323). Adverse renal effects range from generalized renal insufficiency of varying degree and duration to isolated renal tubular defects, most notably urinary magnesium wasting with resulting hypomagnesemia, hypokalemia, and hypocalcemia (324-326). Indeed, magnesuria appears to be a common expression of cisplatin nephrotoxicity and may occur more commonly than azotemia. Unlike cisplatin-induced azotemia, the magnesuria is not dose dependent. Magnesuria may occur in the presence of a normal glomerular filtration rate.

It has been claimed (327), but to our knowledge not substantiated (306,320-323), that the most common form of cisplatin-induced nephrotoxicity is a polyuric state associated with mild renal insufficiency. It is possible, however, that a defect in renal concentration is "masked" by the common practice of volume expansion prior to cisplatin administration. Such expansion, with resultant polyuria, is employed to reduce the incidence of cisplatin-induced azotemia (322). In contrast, in experimental animals, the administration of cisplatin has, indeed, been associated with decreased renal concentrating ability and polyuria (327-331).

Recent studies in the rat have indicated that cisplatin-induced polyuria is multifactorial in etiology. Urine output increases, and urine osmolality decreases, within 1-3 days of the intraperitoneal administration of a single dose (~ 5 mg/kg) of the drug; these changes may persist for several weeks with or without concomitant mild azotemia (327,331). The very early polyuria, occurring within 1 day of drug administration, may be due to transient partial central diabetes insipidus (327,329), but after a week the polyuria is vasopressin unresponsive and circulating ADH levels are elevated (327,331). Although water restriction reduces the polyuria, urine volume remains greater in water-restricted, cisplatin-treated animals than in controls receiving comparable water intake. In addition, water restriction does not lead to an improvement in renal concentrating ability. Thus, while polydipsia may contribute to the polyuria, the defect in renal concentration can not be ascribed to polydipsia alone (327).

The mechanisms underlying the development of ADH unresponsiveness in this rodent model system are not entirely clear but abnormalities in gradient generation appear to have a major role. Medullary electrolyte and urea concentrations are decreased in rats with cisplatin-induced polyuria in the face of apparently normal medullary blood flow (327,331). Micropuncture studies have revealed an abnormality in urea recycling (between the collecting duct and loop of Henle), which is manifest by a reversal of the normal addition of urea to the tubular fluid along Henle's loop (331). The etiology of this defect in gradient generation remains to be determined.

D. Propoxyphene

Only a single case report (332) of polyuria secondary to the ingestion of large amounts of propoxyphene has been reported, despite the publication of several series of patients with propoxyphene intoxication (333,334). This patient developed clinically significant hypernatremia and polyuria (up to 5 liters/day), which was partially resistant to the administration of exogenous vasopressin. Although a solute diuresis was excluded in this study, the possible role of other factors such as hypokalemia (which was present) and hypercalcemia (which was not determined) were not rigorously excluded. Concentrations of propoxyphene intended to approximate the levels obtainable in the mammalian kidney were found to decrease the response to ADH in the toad urinary bladder (335), but the clinical significance of these in vitro findings is unknown. Further studies are needed to determine whether propoxyphene-induced polyuria is a real phenomenon and, if so, whether nephrogenic diabetes insipidus is the underlying cause of the polyuria.

E. Isophosphamide

Isophosphamide is a derivative of cyclophosphamide which has been tested for therapeutic efficacy against a variety of tumors. An initial report noted azotemia, hematuria, and urinary frequency in some patients treated with this agent (336). A more detailed study of the effects of isophosphamide on renal function in a patient with metastatic breast cancer demonstrated several proximal and distal tubular abnormalities: polyuria, nocturia, and an ADH-resistant concentrating defect developed shortly after the intravenous administration of the drug (337). A decrement in glomerular filtration rate and marked natriuresis were also noted. The solute diuresis may of course have contributed to the polyuria. The reduction in glomerular filtration rate as well as inhibition of sodium reabsorption in the ascending limb of Henle's loop (if this was the source of the excess urinary sodium) may have led to abnormalities in gradient generation and/or maintenance. Definitive conclusions must, however, await further studies. Interestingly, cyclophosphamide (the parent compound) has been reported to produce water intoxication, either by stimulating the release of ADH or by enhancing the peripheral action of the hormone (338).

F. Clonidine and Guanabenz

Two centrally acting antihypertensives, the α_2-agonists clonidine and guanabenz, have been reported to produce a diuresis in experimental animals under certain conditions (339,340). The polyuria is multifactoral in etiology, with both increased filtration rate and decreased tubular fluid reabsorption having roles. Both drugs can decrease ADH release (339-342) but, at least in the case of guanabenz, this is probably not of sufficient degree to interfere with urine concentration. Both drugs inhibit the hydro-osmotic effect of ADH in toad urinary bladders (343), but the relevance of this observation to the experimentally induced diuresis is uncertain. Neither clonidine nor guanabenz have been reported to produce clinically significant polyuria in humans.

G. Colchicine and Vinca Alkaloids

Colchicine and the vinca alkaloids, vincristine and vinblastine, inhibit the hydro-osmotic effect of ADH in experimental animals (344) and in toad urinary bladders (28,29,345-348). In rats, the chronic administration of colchicine or vinblastine produces vasopressin-resistant polyuria that cannot be explained by alterations in glomerular filtration rate or tubular sodium reabsorption (344). Neither drug affects adenylate cyclase, cAMP phosphodiesterase, or cAMP-dependent protein kinase activities (344). The hydro-osmotic response to exogenous cAMP is inhibited by these agents, both in the rat (344) and in the toad urinary bladder in vitro (345,346).

Taken together, these observations localize the inhibition of the cellular effect of ADH to a step distal to the generation of cAMP. Since these agents are potent inhibitors of microtubule assembly, it has generally been assumed that they inhibit the action of the second messenger by disrupting microtubule function. Colchicine has been shown to bind to tubulin (the major protein constituent of microtubules) prepared from toad urinary bladder epithelial cells (347). In addition, electron microscopical studies have demonstrated decreased numbers of microtubules in colchicine- or vinblastine-treated bladders (348).

Despite the obvious potential for the development of ADH unresponsiveness in humans treated with these agents, no cases of nephrogenic diabetes insipidus have been reported. In fact, the use of vinca alkaloids as antineoplastic agents has occasionally been associated with the syndrome of inappropriate ADH (349). The latter appears to be due to increased ADH release rather than to increased renal sensitivity to the hormone, and it may be secondary to disruption of hypothalamic microtubules (350,351).

H. Vasopressin Analogs

Numerous analogs of vasopressin have been synthesized but relatively few have proven to inhibit the antidiuretic activity of the naturally occurring hormone (8-arginine vasopressin, in humans). Recently, however, four effective antidiuretic antagonists have been developed, the most potent of which is (1-[β-mercapto-β,β-cyclopentamethylenepropionic acid], 2-O-ethyltyrosine, 4-valine)arginine vasopressin or d$(CH_2)_5$Tyr(Et)VAVP (352,353). While some of these compounds retain agonist activity, this is generally weak and only transiently expressed. They antagonize both exogenous and endogenous vasopressin and the inhibition

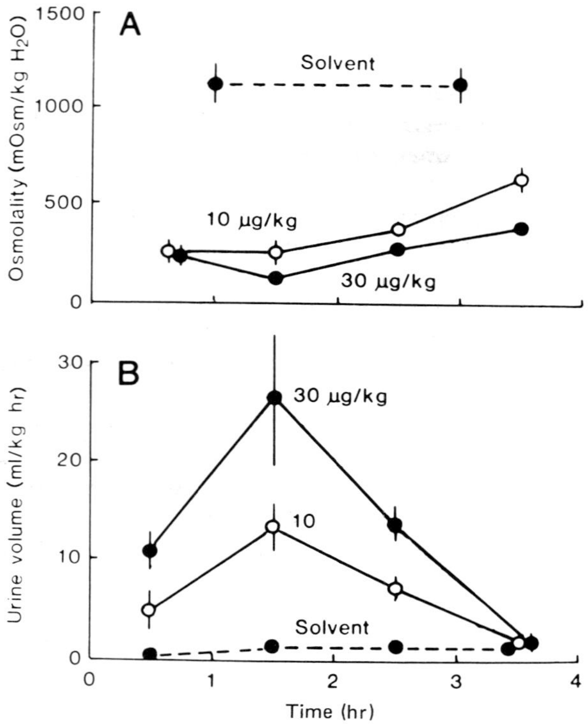

Fig. 12 Responses of normal rats to intraperitoneal injections of solvent (●– –●) and 10 (○—○) and 30 (●—●) µg/kg of the vasopressin antagonist, d$(CH_2)_5$Tyr(Et)VAVP. Rats were provided free access to water, and following injection, urine osmolality (upper panel) and urine volume (lower panel) were measured hourly for 4 hr. Each point represents the mean ± SEM from six animals. d$(CH_2)_5$Tyr(Et)VAVP reversibly inhibits renal concentrating ability. (From Ref. 352. Copyright 1981, American Association for the Advancement of Science.)

is competitive in nature. In normal rats, the intraperitoneal administration of d$(CH_2)_5$Tyr-(Et)VAVP, produces hyposthenuria and polyuria (Fig. 12) that is indistinguishable from that seen in Brattleboro rats (352).

These analogs have not been tested in humans. However, d$(CH_2)_5$ Tyr(Et)VAVP displaces tritiated lysine-vasopressin from human renal medullary receptors and blocks the activation of vasopressin-stimulated renal medullary adenylate cyclase (354). If free of significant side effects, such specific antiduiretic hormone antagonists will prove invaluable in the evaluation and treatment of hypotonic states such as the syndrome of inappropriate ADH.

XII. POTASSIUM DEPLETION

The most common abnormality in renal function associated with severe potassium depletion is an inability to maximally concentrate the urine, a defect which is refractory to the administration of exogenous vasopressin (355,356). Most patients with potassium depletion are able to increase their urine osmolality above that of plasma; consequently, polyuria and polydipsia are relatively mild. Experimental potassium depletion in animals is also associated with an ADH-resistant concentrating defect (357-370).

Renal biopsies in patients with potassium depletion and defects in concentrating ability have revealed vacuolization of proximal tubular epithelial cells (371-373). Such lesions are thought to be characteristic of potassium depletion nephropathy. More commonly, however, mild nonspecific degenerative changes are found in the proximal tubule (356). The glomeruli and more distal portions of the nephron are usually normal, although tubular basement membrane thickening and mitochondrial swelling have been reported (356). In contrast to the human disease, the early lesion in animals is characterized by hydropic swelling and marked epithelial hyperplasia of the collecting duct; this is often of sufficient magnitude to obliterate the lumen and lead to dilatation of more proximal portions of the nephron (357, 372,374-376). PAS-Positive droplets (that resemble lysosomes on electron microscopy) have also been described in the medullary and papillary collecting duct (377). The vacuoles characteristic of the human lesion are not consistently found in experimental animals. Thus, the primary site of anatomical tubular injury in human potassium depletion nephropathy appears to be the proximal tubule, whereas in experimental animals the distal nephron may be more involved.

The relevance of these anatomical lesions to the concentrating defect associated with potassium depletion (either in humans or in experimental animals) is not clear. The lack of consistent structural changes in the human distal nephron suggests that functional defects may exist in the absence of overt morphological changes. In addition, potassium repletion reverses the renal concentrating defect in rats well before the proliferative lesion in the collecting duct resolves, again suggesting the presence of a functional defect that is poorly correlated with the morphological changes (378).

The role of primary polydipsia in the polyuria of human potassium depletion has not been completely delineated (379,380). Mahler and Stanbury reported a woman with potassium deficiency and chronic interstitial nephritis who had intense thirst that was almost immediately relieved when potassium therapy was begun (379). However, it is unclear (either in this case or in other reports of experimentally induced potassium depletion in humans) whether the thirst and polydipsia antedated the polyuria. Consequently, primary polydipsia has not been proven to result from potassium depletion in humans.

Polyuria and polydipsia occur early in the course of potassium depletion in experimental animals, but in initial studies it was unclear whether the polydipsia preceded the polyuria (358,381,382). This uncertainty was resolved by the studies of Blythe et al. (360) and of

Berl et al. (359) in potassium-depleted rats. These investigators showed that by the end of the first week of potassium depletion the polyuria was solely due to increased fluid intake; however, after 2 weeks of potassium depletion, a vasopressin-resistant concentrating defect was also present. The latter is not due to washout of the medullary osmotic gradient, since water-restricted nonpolyuric hypokalemic rats develop a similar concentrating defect to rats on an ad libitum water intake (359,360). Thus, at least in rats, polydipsia appears to be an important cause of polyuria and nephrogenic diabetes insipidus occurs only after more prolonged potassium deprivation. The relevance of these studies to the polyuria associated with chronic potassium depletion in humans is presently uncertain.

The role of central diabetes insipidus in the polyuria associated with potassium depletion has been incompletely evaluated. Plasma ADH levels have not been measured in potassium-depleted humans or animals, but in one carefully studied patient (whose urine remained hypotonic despite dehydration and hypertonic saline infusion) the administration of exogenous ADH produced a marked (albeit submaximal) increase in urine osmolality (383). These findings are compatible with central diabetes insipidus, which may have coexisted with some degree of nephrogenic diabetes insipidus in this patient. With this one possible exception, however, there is no evidence that central diabetes insipidus is an important or common concomitant of potassium depletion.

The postulated mechanisms underlying the ADH-unresponsive concentrating defect associated with potassium depletion include defects in generation, maintenance, and utilization of the osmotic gradient. With regard to gradient generation and maintenance, the direct measurement of medullary and papillary solute content in potassium-depleted animals has revealed decreased sodium (and in one study, decreased urea) concentrations (384-386). However, the mechanisms limiting gradient generation (and/or maintenance) have not been well defined.

Some patients with severe potassium depletion have a decreased glomerular filtration rate (371,387,388), and it has been suggested that this may limit gradient generation. Unfortunately, glomerular filtration rate has not been measured in the majority of studies of experimental potassium depletion in humans (389-391). Thus, it is uncertain whether potassium depletion is associated with a decrement in glomerular filtration rate in humans and, if so, whether this has a role in the concentrating defect.

Animal studies do not support such a role, however. Although experimental potassium depletion in rats is associated with a fall in glomerular filtration rate, these animals do not gain weight as rapidly as controls (361,392), a fact that was not always taken into account. With a single exception (362), when glomerular filtration rate has been corrected for body weight, no difference between control and potassium-depleted rats has been found (363-365). In a single study of potassium depletion in dogs, the glomerular filtration rate decreased in six of nine animals; however, this probably did not contribute to the concentrating defect, since solute-free water generation (C_{H_2O}) was normal in these animals (367).

Since experimental potassium depletion in humans is associated with sodium retention (389-391), decreased delivery of fluid to the ascending limb of Henle's loop could limit gradient generation. Early micropuncture and microinjection studies in potassium-depleted rats suggested that this may be the case (362,368). However, subsequent studies of the same type have failed to support this hypothesis (365,369,370). In fact, in one micropuncture study (365), fluid reabsorption in the proximal tubule was decreased (rather than being increased). In addition, in vitro experiments (utilizing either the split droplet technique or isolated proximal tubule perfusion) have failed to reveal an increase in proximal tubular fluid reabsorption when the peritubular potassium concentration is reduced to physiologically obtainable levels (393,394). Thus, most of the available data do not support the concept that potassium depletion leads to decreased delivery of fluid to the ascending limb by increasing proximal tubular fluid reabsorption.

Humans with mild degrees of potassium depletion have no abnormalities in C_{H_2O} or U_{min}, yet they may still have a mild concentrating defect (395). In contrast, in subjects with more severe potassium depletion (total body losses of > 350 meq), C_{H_2O}, $T^c_{H_2O}$, and U_{max} are still all decreased, and U_{min} is increased (395), indicating abnormalities in both diluting and concentrating ability. The latter findings are consistent with decreased NaCl reabsorption in the thick ascending limb of Henle's loop. Unfortunately, glomerular filtration rate was not measured in this study and a decrease in filtration rate could also explain these results. Consequently, definitive conclusions concerning the function of the thick ascending limb in potassium-depleted humans cannot be drawn at the present time.

Animal studies have, likewise, been inconclusive in this regard. Early clearance studies in potassium-depleted rats yielded conflicting results; moreover, the glomerular filtration rate was not measured (382,396-398). In subsequent clearance studies in rats, C_{H_2O} decreased out of proportion to any change in glomerular filtration rate (361,364). In contrast, in potassium-depleted dogs, C_{H_2O} did not change, or even increased (367,399). Micropuncture studies have also produced conflicting results. Initial studies found a normal early distal tubular fluid to plasma osmolality ratio in potassium-depleted rats (362,398). This led to the conclusion that NaCl reabsorption in the thick ascending limb was unimpaired. However, such an analysis does not evaluate the transport capacity of the ascending limb; in this regard C_{H_2O} is much more informative (see above). In other micropuncture studies, fractional chloride reabsorption was found to be decreased in the thick ascending limb of potassium-depleted rats (365).

It has also been suggested that defects in the maintenance of the osmotic gradient have a role in the ADH unresponsiveness of potassium depletion. Two groups of investigators have found decreased papillary plasma flow rates in potassium-depleted rats (400,401). In this regard, it is of interest that prostaglandin E_2 (a vasodilator) and thromboxane B_2 (a vasoconstrictor) were shown to be decreased and increased, respectively, in extracts of renal papillae from potassium-depleted rats (402).

Thus, it is difficult to incriminate defective gradient formation and/or maintenance in the renal concentrating defect of potassium depletion with any degree of certainty. The evidence in humans is clearly inconclusive and data from animal studies have been conflicting. In rats, both decreased reabsorption of NaCl in the ascending limb and decreased papillary blood flow may impair medullary solute accumulation, and may have roles in the concentrating defect. In dogs, decreased accumulation of medullary solute may also have a role but the responsible factors are unknown.

Several studies have evaluated potential mechanisms for defective gradient utilization in potassium depletion. The excretion of urinary cAMP after the administration of exogenous ADH was normal in six modestly hypokalemic patients (403), but renal concentrating ability was not formally evaluated. Both basal and ADH-induced urinary cAMP excretion were decreased in potassium-depleted rats (404,405) and potassium repletion returned concentrating ability and ADH-stimulated cAMP excretion to normal (404). Thus, at least in rats, the in vivo evidence suggests the presence of a defect in the proximal portion of the ADH-second messenger system.

In vitro studies with renal medullary preparations from potassium-depleted rats have led to similar conclusions. In one study, the normal increase in medullary cAMP content that follows an in vivo infusion of pharmacological doses of ADH was blunted (403). In another,

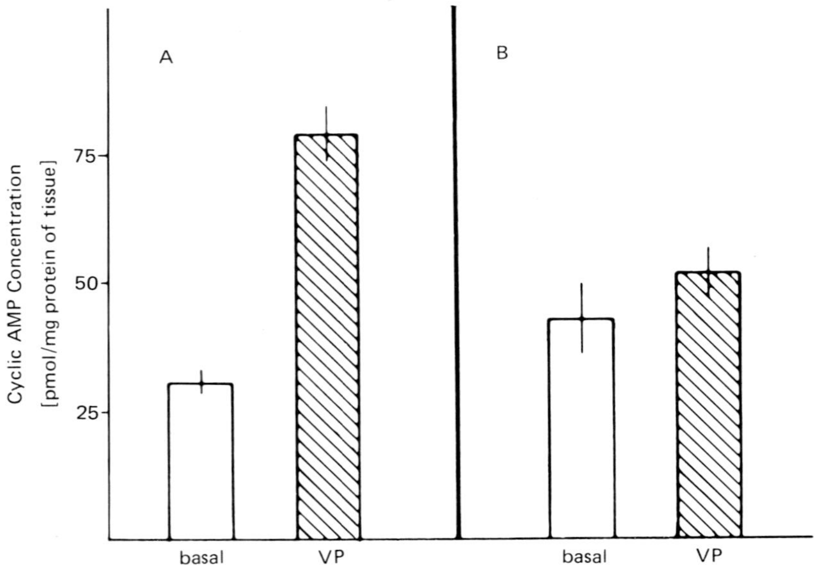

Fig. 13 Effect of prior potassium depletion on basal and ADH (VP)-stimulated cAMP accumulation in rat renal medullary slices incubated in vitro. Each bar represents the mean ± SEM of 12 kidneys from six rats. Data from (A) control and (B) potassium-depleted animals are illustrated. Potassium depletion did not affect basal cAMP accumulation. However, ADH-stimulated cAMP accumulation was significantly less in the slices obtained from potassium-depleted rats than in those obtained from control rats ($p < 0.01$). These results are compatible with a defect in the proximal component of the ADH-cAMP second messenger system in potassium-depleted rats (From Ref. 404.)

the cAMP concentration did not increase normally after addition of ADH to the incubation medium in vitro (404) (Fig. 13). In a third study, basal cAMP levels were decreased and there was no increase in renal medullary cAMP content following dehydration (with presumably, elevated endogenous ADH levels) (406). In addition, since phosphodiesterase activity was decreased, increased catabolism of cAMP could not be implicated as a cause for the low cAMP concentration. Therefore, at least in rats, it seems clear that potassium depletion induces vasopressin-resistant diabetes insipidus, at least in part, by inhibiting the generation of cAMP.

The effects of potassium on ADH-induced water flow have also been examined in the toad urinary bladder model system. Early studies demonstrated that ADH-mediated water flow was blunted when potassium was decreased in (or eliminated from) the bathing medium (158,159), and that inhibition of ADH-mediated water flow could be correlated with a decrease in the cellular potassium concentration (160); cAMP-mediated water flow was likewise inhibited (160). These data are consistent with the suggestion that renal tubular resistance to ADH has a role in the polyuria associated with potassium depletion. In addition, they indicate that there may be a defect in the ADH-second messenger system at a step distal to the generation of cAMP.

Potassium has recently been shown to modulate the synthesis of prostaglandins by renal interstitial cells in vitro: a decrease in medium potassium concentration being associated with increased prostaglandin synthesis (407,408). Since prostaglandin E inhibits the hydro-osmotic effect of ADH by inhibiting adenylase cyclase activity (40), the ADH-resistance associated with potassium depletion may result from increased renal prostaglandin synthesis. In one study, prostaglandin E excretion increased in potassium-depleted dogs (409). However, subsequent studies showed that indomethacin returned prostaglandin excretion to normal without correcting the concentrating defect (410). In addition, urinary prostaglandin E excretion and renal medullary prostaglandin E content were not increased in potassium-depleted rats (405,411,412). Moreover, in a recent study of experimental potassium depletion in humans, the urinary excretion of prostaglandins was not increased and indomethacin did not reverse the concentrating defect (413). Thus, alterations in prostaglandin production do not appear to be responsible for the nephrogenic diabetes insipidus associated with potassium depletion.

In summary, the overall effects of potassium depletion on water homeostasis and the pathophysiology of the nephrogenic diabetes insipidus associated with this disorder are incompletely understood. With regard to the concentrating defect, there is evidence for abnormalities in the production (and/or maintenance) of the medullary osmotic gradient, and for tubular resistance to the hydro-osmotic effect of ADH. However, definitive conclusions cannot be drawn at this time. Further studies in both humans and animals will be required to pinpoint the mechanisms responsible for the nephrogenic diabetes insipidus associated with potassium depletion.

XIII. HYPERCALCEMIA

Since Allan first noted polyuria and polydipsia in a patient with hyperparathyroidism in 1931, this association has been repeatedly confirmed (414-418). However, it was not until 1957 that ADH resistance was documented in polyuric patients with hyperparathyroidism and hypercalcemia (416). Polyuria and polydipsia have also been reported in other disorders associated with hypercalcemia and hypercalciuria, including idiopathic hypercalcemia, vitamin D intoxication, and the hypercalcemia that occurs during prolonged immobilization (417-420).

Chronic hypercalcemia can result in renal interstitial calcification and fibrosis (416,421-423). Consequently, ADH-resistant polyuria may be secondary to anatomical disruption of the renal concentrating mechanism. However, while anatomical damage may have a role in certain situations, renal concentrating ability has been noted to improve within several days of correction of chronic hypercalcemia in some patients (416,418) and acute hypercalcemia can also impair concentrating ability (see below). Consequently, the polyuria undoubtedly has functional components as well.

Whether primary polydipsia contributes to the polyuria is unknown. A patient with hyperparathyroidism has been described who had intense thirst (even in the absence of overt polyuria) which was promptly relieved by removal of the parathyroid adenoma (380). However, since the serum calcium remained elevated after surgery, parathyroid hormone, rather than hypercalcemia, may have been the dipsogenic factor involved. Studies of chronically hypercalcemic animals have not reported an increased ingestion of water prior to the development of the renal concentrating defect, but this possibility has not been specifically evaluated (399,424,425).

Plasma ADH levels have not been measured in hypercalcemic humans. However, the half-life of exogenous ADH is increased (not decreased) in hypercalcemic rabbits (426). In addition, studies with rat pituitary glands in vitro have shown that increased medium calcium concentrations enhance (rather than inhibit) ADH release (427-431). It seems unlikely, therefore, that central diabetes insipidus has a role in the polyuria associated with hypercalcemia in humans. Nonetheless, definitive conclusions must await further studies.

The mechanisms responsible for the ADH-unresponsive concentrating defect associated with hypercalcemia have not been completely defined. Bank and Aynedjian (432), using micropuncture techniques, were unable to demonstrate an osmotic gradient between the collecting duct and renal medulla in chronically hypercalcemic animals and postulated a defect in gradient generation and/or maintenance. Unfortunately, the direct measurement of medullary and papillary solute content in (vitamin D-intoxicated) hypercalcemic rats has produced conflicting results: decreased sodium and urea concentrations in one study (425), normal sodium concentrations in a second study (384), and an increased solute concentration in a third study (433). The protocols and methodologies employed in these studies were so different that meaningful comparison is impossible. Consequently, no definitive conclusions concerning the integrity of the corticopapillary osmotic gradient can be drawn from these data.

Hypercalcemia has variable effects on the glomerular filtration rate. In humans, acute hypercalcemia has been associated with no change or with an increase in filtration rate (434-437), whereas chronically hypercalcemic individuals may have normal or decreased filtration rates (416,418). Prolonged hypercalcemia may irreversibly depress the filtration rate because of the development of chronic interstitial nephritis. However, in patients with hyperparathyroidism, hypercalcemia, and renal insufficiency, renal concentrating ability can improve after removal of the parathyroid adenoma in the absence of an increase in glomerular filtration rate (416,418).

In animals, the glomerular filtration rate may remain normal or fall in the presence of acute hypercalcemia (438-443). More prolonged hypercalcemia is associated with normal or decreased filtration rates (399,424,432,439). However, in almost all these studies, even when the filtration rate was decreased, this abnormality was insufficient, in and of itself, to explain the renal concentrating defects. In only a single instance (432), was the decrement in filtration rate thought to have a major role in the genesis of the concentrating defect. In summary, alterations in glomerular filtration rate probably do not have an important role in the concentrating defect either in humans or in animals. This conclusion is perhaps best substantiated by the reversibility of the concentrating defect (after correction of the hypercalcemia) in the face of persistent renal insufficiency (399,416,418).

From the time that acute hypercalcemia was first shown to produce a natriuresis in dogs (444), it has been suggested that hypercalcemia may impair sodium chloride reabsorption in the ascending limb of Henle's loop and, thereby, limit gradient generation. This could be so even though balance studies in chronically hypercalcemic humans have shown that dietary sodium restriction leads to an appropriate decrease in urinary sodium excretion (418); such studies cannot exclude subtle defects in ascending limb function. Clearance studies in humans have shown that both acute and chronic hypercalcemia are associated with a reduction in $T^c_{H_2O}$ (418,436), but since C_{H_2O} was not measured in these studies, defects in ascending limb function could not be separated from defects in gradient utilization.

Acute hypercalcemia in animals is generally associated with a reduction in $T^c_{H_2O}$ (438-441), but C_{H_2O} has been examined in only one study (441). In the latter, C_{H_2O} was markedly impaired, indicating that ascending limb function was abnormal (Fig. 14). In contrast, C_{H_2O} was found to be normal in animals with more prolonged hypercalcemia (399); however, since $T^c_{H_2O}$ was not invariably depressed, the etiology of the concentrating defect observed in this study is unclear. Micropuncture studies of tubular sodium reabsorption during acute hypercalcemia have not demonstrated abnormalities in NaCl reabsorption in the ascending limb (445,446), and similar findings have been obtained in animals with more prolonged hypercalcemia as well (432). Thus, a definitive case for abnormalities in gradient generation in hypercalcemic animals has yet to be made.

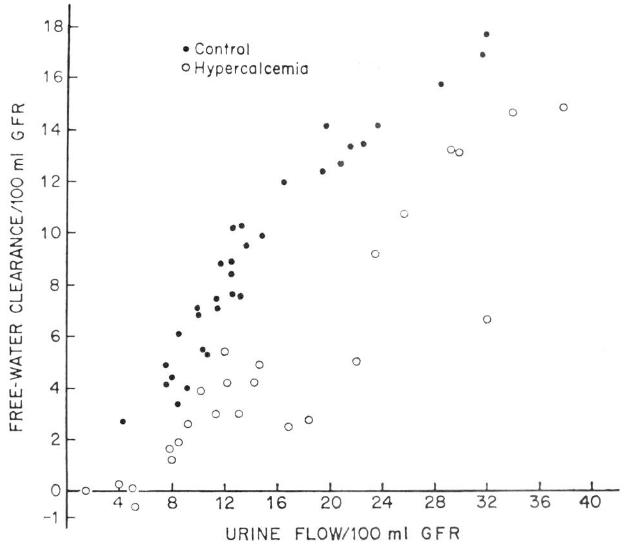

Fig. 14 Effect of acute hypercalcemia in dogs on fractional solute-free water clearance expressed as a function of fractional urine flow rate. The data from five experiments are illustrated, with hypercalcemic periods (○) and compared to control (nonhypercalcemic) periods (●) in the same animals. Note that there was a marked impairment of solute-free water clearance at all levels of urine flow rate. (From Ref. 441.)

There has been only a single study of the effects of hypercalcemia on gradient maintenance. Both acute and chronic hypercalcemia were shown to markedly increase medullary blood flow (447), an event which would be expected to lead to dissolution of the corticopapillary gradient. This could explain the reduction in $T^c_{H_2O}$ and the ADH unresponsiveness generally associated with hypercalcemia. However, the possibility of such a mechanism must remain speculative until further data are available.

There is considerable physiological evidence that hypercalcemia impairs the cellular action of ADH. Some polyuric, hypercalcemic patients continue to produce urine that is hypotonic to plasma despite the administration of ADH (416,436,448), indicating that tubular resistance to the hormone must have a role in the genesis of the polyuria. Studies in acutely hypercalcemic rats have shown decreased urinary cAMP excretion in response to submaximal doses of ADH (449). In amphibian epithelia, increases in the serosal calcium concentration ($>$5 mmol/liter) impair ADH-induced osmotic water flow, but have no effect on the increase in water permeability induced by exogenous cAMP (450-452). These observations suggest that increased calcium concentrations impair ADH-induced water flow in renal epithelia, perhaps by inhibiting one or more steps in the proximal component of ADH action. In contrast, in recent microperfusion studies of the cortical collecting tubule of the rabbit (453), increases in the serosal calcium concentration were found to increase (rather than to decrease) ADH-induced water flow. The reasons for these apparently contradictory results are unknown, but it is possible that species differences exist. In addition, it should be noted that water transport in the medullary collecting duct was not examined in this study.

As discussed in Sect. I.C, the interactions between calcium and renal epithelial water transport are complex and may be biphasic. Calcium has multiple potential sites of action within the ADH-responsive cell including (among others) the adenylate cyclase complex, cAMP phosphodiesterase, and microtubule metabolism. It is important to appreciate that it is intracellular (not extracellular) calcium that is the critical determinant of the influences of this ion on cellular transport processes. It is equally important to realize that a particular process may be both calcium dependent and inhibited by excessive amounts of the ion. Unfortunately, there is little information on the effects of alterations in medium calcium concentration on the concentration of calcium in the various subcellular compartments. Nor have the effects of ADH (or cAMP) on the subcellular concentrations of calcium been examined. For example, ADH has been shown to increase the efflux of calcium from toad urinary bladder epithelial cells into the mucosal medium (454), but the effects of the hormone on cytosolic or mitochondrial calcium levels are unknown.

A variety of recent studies in amphibian epithelia utilizing agents that alter cellular calcium uptake and/or mitochondrial calcium release (calcium ionophores, verapamil, quinidine) have confirmed the existence of a complex system in which presumed changes in intracellular calcium levels produce unpredictable responses in ADH- and cAMP-induced water flow (455-458). This should not be surprising when one considers the myriad potential cellular effects of these agents; certainly, their specificity for only affecting calcium activity has not been established.

The mechanisms by which calcium could inhibit ADH-induced water flow have been examined in a number of biochemical studies. Antidiuretic hormone-stimulated cAMP accumulation is reduced in renal medullary slices prepared from acutely hypercalcemic rats (449) and in toad bladder epithelial cells incubated in the presence of high concentrations of calcium (459). Medium calcium concentrations from 0.1 to 2.0 mmol/liter inhibit basal, ADH-stimulated, and NaF-activated adenylate cyclase activity in rat and/or hamster renal medullary homogenates (449,460). In similar experiments with rat renal medullary homogenates, increasing the medium calcium concentration had no effect on cAMP phosphodiesterase activity (449). These observations are consistent with the hypothesis that hypercalcemia impairs the cellular response to ADH by inhibiting the generation of cAMP, presumably by directly inhibiting the adenylate cyclase complex.

Since prostaglandin E may inhibit adenylate cyclase activity in renal epithelia (40), it has been suggested that a calcium-related increase in prostaglandin synthesis could account for the decrease in adenylate cyclase activity. Vitamin D-intoxicated, hypercalcemic, polyuric rats have increased urinary prostaglandin E excretion (461). Indomethacin normalizes the excretion of prostaglandin E in these animals, while at the same time reducing the polyuria and partially restoring ADH responsiveness. In addition, the intrarenal arterial infusion of $CaCl_2$ increases the renal prostaglandin E secretion rate in dogs, an event which was shown to be both verapamil- and indomethacin-sensitive (462). Finally, prostaglandin E synthesis and release from rat renal medullary slices is dependent on the medium calcium concentration and is enhanced by calcium ionophores (463,464). Thus, prostaglandins may, indeed, have a role in the nephrogenic diabetes insipidus associated with hypercalcemia. Further studies of calcium-prostaglandin interactions in ADH-responsive renal epithelia are clearly warranted.

In summary, it is clear that hypercalcemia can lead to a primary defect in renal concentrating ability. Although structural damage to the renal interstitium (and concomitant renal insufficiency) may contribute to the defect in certain cases, the polyuria appears to be largely functional in origin. There is evidence that hypercalcemia impairs the generation and maintenance of the corticopapillary osmotic gradient, but the underlying mechanisms are unclear. There is also substantial evidence that hypercalcemia impairs the cellular action of ADH, possibly at the level of the adenylate cyclase complex. Consequently, it is likely that the nephrogenic diabetes insipidus associated with hypercalcemia is multifactorial in etiology.

XIV. TUMORS

Vasopressin-resistant hyposthenuria and polyuria have recently been reported in a patient with metastatic ileal leiomyosarcoma (465). Urine output averaged 12 liters/day; despite marked dehydration and weight loss during water deprivation (P_{osm} increased from 291 to 318 mOsm/kg H_2O, and body weight decreased 2.5 kg, in 6 hr), U_{osm} never rose above 100 mOsm/kg H_2O. Plasma vasopressin levels were normal relative to P_{osm} and, following the infusion of hypertonic saline (P_{osm} increased from 291 to 325 mOsm/kg H_2O), reached a concentration fivefold that needed to produce maximal antidiuresis in normal individuals. Known causes of nephrogenic diabetes insipidus were excluded and antibodies to vasopressin were not demonstrable. The patient received a course of chemotherapy, but there was no regression of the tumor or amelioration of the polyuria; he died with persistent nephrogenic diabetes insipidus. The underlying cause of the vasopressin unresponsiveness is unknown. Indeed, while provocative, its relationship to the neoplastic process remains speculative.

XV. THERAPY

Initial therapy of nephrogenic diabetes insipidus should include rehydration (if clinically significant water losses are present), correction of potentially etiological electrolyte abnormalities (hypercalcemia, potassium depletion), and withdrawal of offending drugs (if possible). Unless access to water is limited or there are concurrent defects in thirst, most adults with nephrogenic diabetes insipidus are able to maintain normal water balance. Consequently, hypernatremia is usually mild and rehydration is generally not required. Of course, the ongoing need for increased water ingestion must be recognized and appropriately provided for. If rehydration is necessary the oral route is preferable. Otherwise, intravenous hypotonic fluids (e.g., 5% dextrose in water) can be employed.

Since renal sodium conservation is normal in most patients with nephrogenic diabetes insipidus, symptoms and signs of extracellular fluid volume depletion are characteristically absent. However, severe body water deficits (usually in excess of 9 liters) are associated with losses of plasma water of sufficient magnitude to threaten intravascular volume. In severe instances, where shock supervenes, volume considerations should take precedence over tonicity considerations and therapy with volume expanders (colloids, isotonic saline) should be initiated without delay. Once intravascular volume has been stabilized, the hypernatremia and water deficit can be corrected with hypotonic fluids.

Correction of hypercalcemia and potassium depletion or withdrawal of an offending drug is frequently the only therapy necessary to reverse the concentrating defect. However, in some patients vasopressin hyporesponsiveness may persist for months after chronic electrolyte disorders are corrected or offending drugs are withdrawn. Such individuals should be followed closely and their requirement for increased water intake should be recognized and provided for. In some instances, it may not be possible to withdraw the drug. For example, the considerable morbidity and mortality of manic-depressive psychosis, and the recognized effectiveness of lithium in the treatement of this disorder, often make it difficult to discontinue lithium maintenance therapy simply because of the development of nephrogenic diabetes insipidus.

In such circumstances, or in the case of hereditary nephrogenic diabetes insipidus (where no other therapy is available), the polyuria can sometimes be attenuated by decreasing obligatory urinary solute excretion. This is achieved by restricting dietary protein and sodium intake (which decreases urea and sodium excretion) while simultaneously administering a thiazide diuretic. Diuretic-induced sodium losses (combined with continued dietary sodium restriction) lead to mild extracellular fluid volume depletion. As a consequence, proximal tubular reabsorption is enhanced, fluid delivery to the distal nephron is decreased, electrolyte-free water generation is decreased, and the polyuria is attenuated (466-468). Such management may, however, result in orthostatic hypotension.

REFERENCES

1. Robertson, G. L.; Shelton, R. L.; and Athar, S. The osmoregulation of vasopressin. Kidney Int. 10:25, 1976.
2. Robertson, G. L. The regulation of vasopressin function in health and disease. Recent Prog. Horm. Res. 33:333, 1977.
3. Robertson, G. L.; Aycinean, P.; and Zerbe, R. L. Neurogenic disorders of osmoregulation. Am. J. Med. 72:339, 1982.
4. Schrier, R. W.; Berl, T.; and Anderson, R. J. Osmotic and non-osmotic control of vasopressin release. Am. J. Physiol. 236:F321, 1979.
5. Jamison, R. L. Urine concentration and dilution. In: The Kidney, edited by Brenner, B. M., and Rector, F. C., Jr. Philadelphia, Saunders, 1981, p. 495.
6. Jamison, R. L.; and Oliver, R. E. Disorders of urinary concentration and dilution. Am. J. Med. 72:308, 1982.
7. Handler, J. S.; and Orloff, J. The mechanism of action of antidiuretic hormone. In: Handbook of Physiology, Sect. 8, Renal Physiology, edited by Orloff, J., and Berliner, R. W. Washington, D. C., American Physiological Society, 1973, p. 791.
8. Dousa, T. P.; and Valtin, H. Cellular actions of vasopressin in the mammalian kidney. Kidney Int. 10:46, 1976.
9. Ross, E. M.; and Gilman, A. G. Biochemical properties of hormone-sensitive adenylate cyclase. Ann. Rev. Biochem. 49:533, 1980.
10. Roy, C.; and Ausiello, D. A. Characterization of (8-lysine) vasopressin binding sites on a pig kidney cell line (LLC-PK_1). J. Biol. Chem. 256:3415, 1981.
11. Roy, C.; Hall, D.; Karish, M.; and Ausiello, D. A. Relationship of (8-lysine) vasopressin receptor transition to receptor functional properties in a pig kidney cell line (LLC-PK_1). J. Biol. Chem. 256:3423, 1981.
12. Wells, J. N.; and Hardman, J. G. Cyclic nucleotide phosphodiesterases. Adv. Cyclic Nucleotide Res. 8:119, 1977.
13. Klee, C. B.; Crouch, T. H.; and Richman, P. G. Calmodulin. Ann. Rev. Biochem. 49: 489, 1980.
14. Dousa, T. P. Cyclic nucleotides in renal pathophysiology. Contemp. Issues Nephrol. 4: 251, 1979.
15. Handler, J. S.; and Orloff, J. Antidiuretic hormone. Ann. Rev. Physiol. 43:611, 1981.
16. Kachadorian, W. A.; Wade, J. B.; and DiScala, V. A. Vasopressin-induced structural changes in toad bladder luminal membrane. Science 190:67, 1975.
17. Kachadorian, W. A.; Wade, J. B.; Uiterwyk, C. C.; and DiScala, V. A. Membrane structural and functional responses to vasopressin in toad bladder. J. Membr. Biol. 30:381, 1977.
18. Kachadorian, W. A.; Levine, S. D.; Wade, J. B.; DiScala, V. A.; and Hays, R. M. Relationship of aggregated intramembranous particles to water permeability in vasopressin-treated toad urinary bladder. J. Clin. Invest. 59:576, 1977.
19. Cohen, P. (ed.). Recently discovered systems of enzyme regulation by reversible phosphorylation. In: Molecular Aspects of Cellular Regulation, vol. 1. Amsterdam, Elsevier North-Holland, 1980.
20. Strewler, G. J.; and Orloff, J. Role of cyclic nucleotides in the transport of water and electrolytes. Adv. Cyclic Nucleotide Res. 8:311, 1977.
21. Glass, D. B.; and Krebs, E. G. Protein phosphorylation catalyzed by cyclic AMP-dependent and cyclic GMP-dependent protein kinases. Ann. Rev. Pharmacol. Toxicol. 20:363, 1980.

22. Ausiello, D. A.; Hall, D. H.; and Dayer, J.-M. Modulation of cyclic AMP-dependent protein kinase by vasopressin and calcitonin in cultured porcine renal LLC-PK_1 cells. Biochem. J. 186:773, 1980.
23. Schwartz, I. L.; Shlatz, L.; Kinne-Saffron, E.; and Kinne, R. Target cell polarity and membrane phosphorylation in relation to the mechanism of action of antidiuretic hormone. Proc. Natl. Acad. Sci. U.S.A. 71:2595, 1974.
24. Walton, K. D.; DeLorenzo, R. J.; Curran, P. F.; and Greengard, P. Regulation of protein phosphorylation and sodium transport in toad bladder. J. Gen. Physiol. 65:153, 1975.
25. Ferguson, D. R.; and Twite, B. R. Effects of vasopressin on toad bladder membrane proteins: Relationship to transport of sodium and water. J. Endocrinol. 61:501, 1974.
26. Malkinson, A. M.; Krueger, B. K.; Rudolph, S. A.; Casnellia, J. E.; Haley, B. E.; and Greengard, P. Widespread occurrence of a specific protein in vertebrate tissues and regulation by cyclic AMP of its endogenous phosphorylation and dephosphorylation. Metabolism 24:331, 1975.
27. Schwartz, I. L.; Huang, C. J.; Reisman, L.; Scalettar, E.; Wyssbrod, H. R.; Cort, J. H.; Roth, L. B.; Li, H. C.; and Ripoche, P. A. Cyclic AMP mediated dephosphorylation in renal collecting duct epithelial cell plasma membrane: a substrate level phenomenon. In: Hormonal Control of Epithelial Transport, edited by Bourget, J., Chevalier, J., Parisi, M., and Ripoche, P. Paris, INSERM, 1979, p. 71.
28. Taylor, A. Role of microtubules and microfilaments in the action of vasopressin. In: Disturbances in Body Fluid Osmolality, edited by Andreoli, T. E., Grantham, J. J., and Rector, F. C. Washington, D. C., American Physiological Society, 1977, p. 97.
29. Kachadorian, W. A.; Ellis, S. J.; and Muller, J. Possible roles for microtubules and microfilaments in ADH action on toad urinary bladder. Am. J. Physiol. 236:F14, 1979.
30. Stephens, R. E.; and Edds, K. T. Microtubulules: Structure, chemistry and function. Physiol. Rev. 56:709, 1976.
31. Sloboda, R. D.; Rudolph, S. A.; Rosenbaum, J. L.; and Greengard, P. Cyclic AMP-dependent endogenous phosphorylation of a microtubule-associated protein. Proc. Natl. Acad. Sci. U.S.A. 72:177, 1975.
32. Dedman, J. R.; Brinkley, B. R.; and Means, A. R. Regulation of microfilaments and microtubules by calcium and cyclic AMP. Adv. Cyclic Nucleotide Res. 11:131, 1979.
33. DeSousa, R. C.; Grosso, A.; and Rufener, C. Blockade of the hydrosmotic effect of vasopressin by cytochalasin B. Experientia 30:175, 1974.
34. Davis, W. L.; Goodman, D. B. P.; Schuster, R. J.; Rasmussen, H.; and Martin, J. W. Effects of cytochalasin B on the response of toad urinary bladder to vasopressin. J. Cell Biol. 63:986, 1974.
35. Rasmussen, H.; and Goodman, D. B. P. Relationships between calcium and cyclic nucleotides in cell activation. Physiol. Rev. 57:422, 1977.
36. Means, A. R.; and Dedman, J. R. Calmodulin—An intracellular calcium receptor. Nature 285:73, 1980.
37. Cheung, W. Y. Calmodulin: An overview. Fed. Proc. 41:2253, 1982.
38. Jard, S.; and Bockaert, J. Stimulus-response coupling in neurohypophysial peptide target cells. Physiol. Rev. 55:489, 1975.
39. Ausiello, D. A.; and Hall, D. Regulation of vasopressin-sensitive adenylate cyclase by calmodulin. J. Biol. Chem. 256:9796, 1981.
40. Handler, J. S. Vasopressin-prostaglandin interactions in the regulation of epithelial cell permeability to water. Kidney Int. 19:831, 1981.
41. Grantham, J.; and Orloff, J. Effect of prostaglandin E_1 on the permeability response of the isolated collecting tubule to vasopressin, adenosine 3',5'-monophosphate, and theophylline. J. Clin. Invest. 47:1154, 1968.
42. Zusman, R. M.; Keiser, H. R.; and Handler, J. S. Vasopressin-stimulated prostaglandin E biosynthesis in the toad urinary bladder. Effect on water flow. J. Clin. Invest. 60: 1339, 1977.

43. Burch, R. M.; Knapp, D. R.; and Halushka, P. V. Vasopressin stimulated thromboxane synthesis in the toad urinary bladder: Effects of imidazole. J. Pharmacol. Exp. Ther. 210:344, 1979.
44. Bisordi, J. E.; Schlondorff, D.; and Hays, R. M. Interaction of vasopressin and prostaglandins in the toad urinary bladder. J. Clin. Invest. 66:1200, 1980.
45. Forrest, J. N., Jr.; Schneider, C. J.; and Goodman, D. B. P. Role of prostaglandin E_2 in mediating the effects of pH on the hydroosmotic response to vasopressin in the toad urinary bladder. J. Clin. Invest. 69:499, 1982.
46. Jackson, B. A.; Edwards, R. M.; and Dousa, T. P. Vasopressin-prostaglandin interactions in isolated tubules from rat outer medulla. J. Lab. Clin. Med. 96:119, 1980.
47. Smith, W. L.; and Bell, T. Immunohistochemical localization of the prostaglandin-forming cyclooxygenase in renal cortex. Am. J. Physiol. 235:F451, 1978.
48. Singer, I. Differential diagnosis of polyuria and diabetes insipidus. Med. Clin. North Am. 65:303, 1981.
49. Jamison, R. L.; Buerkert, J.; and Lacy, F. A micropuncture study of collecting tubule function in rats with hereditary diabetes insipidus. J. Clin. Invest. 50:2444, 1971.
50. Gardner, K. D., Jr.; and Vierling, J. M. Solids, water and solutes in papillary region of the rat kidney. Am. J. Physiol. 217:58, 1969.
51. Berl, T.; Anderson, R. J.; McDonald, K.; and Schrier, R. W. Clinical disorders of water metabolism. Kidney Int. 10:117, 1976.
52. Bia, M. J.; Dewitt, S.; and Forrest, J. N., Jr. Dissociation between plasma, urine, and renal papillary cAMP content following vasopressin and DDAVP. Am. J. Physio. 237: F218, 1979.
53. Miller, M.; Dalakos, T.; Moses, A. M.; Fellerman, H.; and Streeten, D. H. P. Recognition of partial defects in antidiuretic hormone secretion. Ann. Intern. Med. 73:721, 1970.
54. Hays, R. M.; and Levine, S. D. Pathophysiology of water metabolism. In: The Kidney, edited by Brenner, B. M., and Rector, F. C., Jr. Philadelphia, Saunders, 1981, p. 777.
55. Forrest, J. N., Jr.; Cohen, A. D.; Torretti, J.; Himmelhoch, J. M.; and Epstein, F. H. On the mechanism of lithium-induced diabetes insipidus in man and the rat. J. Clin. Invest. 53:1115, 1974.
56. Frasier, S. D.; Kutnick, L. A.; Schmidt, R. T.; and Smith, F. G., Jr. A water deprivation test for the diagnosis of diabetes insipidus in children. Am. J. Dis. Child. 114:157, 1967.
57. Robertson, G. L.; Mahr, E. A.; Athar, S.; and Sinha, T. Development and clinical application of a new method for the radioimmunoassay of arginine vasopressin in human plasma. J. Clin. Invest. 52:2340, 1973.
58. Zerbe, R. L.; and Robertson, G. L. A comparison of plasma vasopressin measurements with a standard indirect test in the differential diagnosis of polyuria. N. Engl. J. Med. 305:1539, 1981.
59. Arieff, A. I.; and Guisado, R. Effects on the central nervous system of hypernatremic and hyponatremic states. Kidney Int. 10:104, 1976.
60. Schrager, G. O.; Josephson, B. H.; Fine, B. F.; and Berger, G. Nephrogenic diabetes insipidus presenting as fever of unknown origin in the neonatal period. Clin. Pediatr. 15: 1070, 1976.
61. Waring, A. J.; Laslo, K.; and Tappan, V. A congenital defect of water metabolism. Am. J. Dis. Child. 69:323, 1945.
62. Forssman, H. On hereditary diabetes insipidus: With special reference to a sex-linked form. Acta Med. Scand. 121:(Suppl. 159)1, 1945.
63. Williams, R. H.; and Henry, C. Nephrogenic diabetes insipidus: Transmitted by females and appearing during infancy in males. Ann. Intern. Med. 27:84, 1947.
64. Kao, M. Y.; and Steiner, M. M. Diabetes insipidus in infancy resistant to pitressin. Pediatrics 12:400, 1953.
65. Luder, J.; and Burnett, D. A congenital renal tubular defect. Arch. Dis. Child. 29:44, 1954.

66. Girard, H. L. Pitressin resistant diabetes insipidus nephrogenic function defect. Report of a case. Med. Bull. U.S. Army 10:185, 1953.
67. Ellborg, A.; and Forssman, H. Nephrogenic diabetes insipidus in children. Acta Paediatr. 44:209, 1955.
68. Kirman, B. H.; Black, J. A.; Wilkinson, R. H.; and Evans, P. R. Familial pitressin-resistant diabetes insipidus with mental defect. Arch. Dis. Child. 31:59, 1955.
69. MacDonald, W. B. Congenital pitressin-resistant diabetes insipidus of renal origin. Pediatrics 15:298, 1955.
70. Wattiez, P. R.; Loeb, H.; Bellens, R.; and Van Geffel, R. Diabete insipide pitressino-resistant. Helv. Paediatr. Acta 12:643, 1957.
71. Gautier, E.; and Simpkiss, M. The management of nephrogenic diabetes insipidus in early life. Acta Paediatr. 46:354, 1957.
72. Daneis, J.; Birmingham, J. R.; and Leslie, S. H. Congenital diabetes insipidus resistant to treatment with pitressin. Am. J. Dis. Child. 75:316, 1949.
73. Schoen, E. J. Renal diabetes insipidus. Pediatrics 26:808, 1960.
74. Holliday, M. A.; Burstin, C.; and Harrah, J. Evidence that the antidiuretic substance in the plasma of children with nephrogenic diabetes insipidus is antidiuretic hormone. Pediatrics 32:384, 1963.
75. DeLange, L. Ulser erblichen diabetes insipidus. Jahrb. Kinderheilkd. 145:1, 1935.
76. West, C. D.; and Smith, W. C. An attempt to elucidate the course of growth retardation in renal disease. Am. J. Dis. Child. 91:460, 1956.
77. Uttley, W. S.; Paxton, J.; and Thistlethwaite, D. Urinary concentrating ability and growth failure in urinary tract disorders. Arch. Dis. Child. 47:436, 1972.
78. Hillman, D. A.; Neyzi, O.; Porter, P.; Cushman, A.; and Talbot, N. B. Renal (vasopressin-resistant) diabetes insipidus: Definition of the effects of a homeostatic limitation in capacity to conserve water on the physical, intellectual, and emotional development of a child. Pediatrics 21:430, 1958.
79. Forssman, H. Is hereditary diabetes insipidus of the nephrogenic type associated with mental deficiency? Acta Psychiatr. Neurol. Scand. 30:577, 1955.
80. Reuss, A. L.; and Rosenthal, I. M. Intelligence in nephrogenic diabetes insipidus. Am. J. Dis. Child. 105:358, 1963.
81. Finberg, L.; Luttrell, C.; and Redd, H. Pathogenesis of lesions in the central nervous system in hypernatremic states. II. Experimental studies of gross anatomic changes and alterations of chemical concentrations of tissues. Pediatrics 23:46, 1959.
82. Luttrell, C. N.; and Finberg, L. Hemorrhagic encephalopathy induced by hypernatremia. I. Clinical, laboratory and pathological observations. Arch. Neurol. Psychiatr. 81:424, 1959.
83. Sotos, J.; Dodge, P. R.; Mearoy, P.; and Talbot, N. B. Studies in experimental hypertonicity. I. Pathogenesis of the clinical syndrome, biochemical abnormalities and cause of death. Pediatrics 26:925, 1960.
84. Dodge, P. R.; Sotos, J.; Gainstorp, I.; DeVivo, D.; Levy, M.; and Rabe, T. Neurophysiologic disturbances in hypertonic dehydration. Trans. Am. Neurol. Assoc. 87:33, 1962.
85. Macaulay, D.; and Watson, M. Hypernatremia in infants as a cause of brain damage. Arch. Dis. Child. 42:485, 1967.
86. Holliday, M. A.; Kalayci, M. N.; and Harrah, J. Factors that limit brain volume changes in response to acute and sustained hyper- and hyponatremia. J. Clin. Invest. 47:1916, 1968.
87. Hogan, G. R.; Dodge, P. R.; Gill, S. R.; Master, S.; and Sotos, J. Pathogenesis of seizures occurring during restoration of plasma tonicity to normal in animals previously chronically hypernatremic. Pediatrics 43:54, 1969.
88. Cannon, J. F. Diabetes insipidus: Clinical and experimental studies with consideration of genetic relationships. Arch Intern. Med. 96:215, 1955.

89. Orloff, J.; and Walser, M. Water and solute excretion in pitressin-resistant diabetes insipidus. Clin. Res. Proc. 4:136, 1956.
90. Crawford, J. D.; and Kennedy, G. C. Chlorthiazide in diabetes insipidus. Nature 183: 891, 1959.
91. Carter, C.; and Simpkiss, M. The "carrier state" in nephrogenic diabetes insipidus. Lancet 2:1069, 1956.
92. Childs, B.; and Sedbury, J. B. A survey of genetics as it applies to problems in medicine. Pediatrics 20:177, 1957.
93. Messerli, F. H.; Frohlich, E. D.; Dreslinski, G. R.; Suarez, D. H.; and Aristimuno, G. G. Serum uric acid in essential hypertension: An indicator of renal vascular involvement. Ann. Intern. Med. 93:817, 1980.
94. Perry, T. L.; Robinson, G. C.; Teasdale, J. M.; and Hansen, S. Concurrence of cystathionuria, nephrogenic diabetes insipidus and severe anemia. N. Engl. J. Med. 276: 721, 1967.
95. Walker, N. F.; and Ranee, C. P. Inheritance of nephrogenic diabetes insipidus. Am. J. Hum. Genet. 6:354, 1954.
96. Bode, H. H.; and Crawford, J. D. Nephrogenic diabetes insipidus in North America—the Hopewell hypothesis. N. Engl. J. Med. 280:750, 1969.
97. Flax, L. J.; and Gersh, P. Congenital renal tubular dysfunction (nephrogenic diabetes insipidus). Am. J. Dis. Child. 89:602, 1955.
98. Robinson, M. G.; and Kaplan, S. A. Inheritance of vasopressin-resistant (nephrogenic) diabetes insipidus. Am. J. Dis. Child. 99:164, 1960.
99. Darmady, E.; Prince, J.; and Stranack, F. The proximal convoluted tubule in the renal handling of water. Lancet 2:1254, 1964.
100. West, J. R.; and Kramer, J. G. Nephrogenic diabetes insipidus. Pediatrics 15:424, 1955.
101. Cutler, R. E.; Kleeman, C. R.; Maxwell, M. H.; and Dowling, J. T. Physiologic studies in nephrogenic diabetes insipidus. J. Clin. Endocrinol. Metab. 22:827, 1962.
102. Naik, W. V.; and Valtin, H. Hereditary vasopressin-resistant urinary concentrating defects in mice. Am. J. Physiol. 217:1183, 1969.
103. Gorden, P.; Robertson, G. L.; and Seegmiller, J. E. Hyperuricemia, a concomitant of congenital vasopressin-resistant diabetes insipidus in the adult: Studies of uric acid metabolism and plasma vasopressin. N. Engl. J. Med. 284:1057, 1971.
104. Silverstein, E.; and Tobian, L. Pitressin-resistant diabetes insipidus with massive hydronephrosis. Am. J. Med. 30:819, 1961.
105. Ten Bensel, R. W.; and Peters, E. R. Progressive hydronephrosis, hydroureter, and dilatation of the bladder in siblings with congenital neprhogenic diabetes insipidus. J. Pediatr. 77:439, 1970.
106. Carter, R. D.; and Goodman, A. D. Nephrogenic diabetes insipidus accompanied by massive dilatation of the kidneys, ureters and bladder. J. Urol. 89:366, 1963.
107. Miller, S. S.; and Winston, M. C. Nephrogenic diabetes insipidus. Radiology 87:893, 1966.
108. Dicker, S. E.; and Eggleton, M. G. Nephrogenic diabetes insipidus. Clin. Sci. 24:81, 1963.
109. Robertson, G. L.; and Scheidler, J. A. A newly recognized variant of familial nephrogenic diabetes insipidus distinguished by partial resistance to vasopressin. Clin. Res. 29:555A, 1981.
110. Kettyle, W. M.; and Valtin, H. Chemical and dimensional characterization of the renal countercurrent system in mice. Kidney Int. 1:135, 1972.
111. Dousa, T. P.; and Valtin, H. Cellular action of antidiuretic hormone in mice with inherited vasopressin-resistant urinary concentrating defects. J. Clin. Invest. 54:753, 1974.
112. Jackson, B. A.; Edwards, C. M.; Valtin, H.; and Dousa, T. P. Cellular action of vasopressin in medullary tubules of mice with hereditary nephrogenic diabetes insipidus. J. Clin. Invest. 66:110, 1980.

113. Fichman, M. P.; and Brooker, G. Deficient renal cyclic adesnosine 3'-5' monophosphate production in nephrogenic diabetes insipidus. J. Clin. Endocrinol. Metab. 35: 35, 1972.
114. Bell, N. H.; Clark, C. M.; Avery, S.; Sinha, T.; Trygstad, C.; and Allen, D. O. Demonstration of defects in the formation of and response to cyclic adenosine monophosphate in vasopressin resistant diabetes insipidus. Clin. Res. 8:223A, 1974.
115. Jones, N. R.; Barraclough, M. A.; Barnes, M. A.; and Cotton, D. C. Nephrogenic diabetes insipidus: Effects of 3'-5'-cyclic adenosine monophosphate. Arch. Dis. Child. 47:794, 1972.
116. Levine, R. A. Antidiuretic response to exogenous adenosine 3'-5'-monophosphate in man. Clin. Sci. 34:253, 1968.
117. McConnell, R. F., Jr.; Lorentz, W. B., Jr.; Berger, M.; Smith, E. H.; Carvajal, H. F.; and Travis, L. B. The mechanism of urinary concentration in nephrogenic diabetes insipidus. Pediatr. Res. 11:33, 1977.
118. Hall, D. A.; and Varney, D. M. Effect of vasopressin on electrical potential difference and chloride transport in mouse medullary thick ascending limb of Henle's loop. J. Clin. Invest. 66:792, 1980.
119. Sasaki, S.; and Imai, M. Effects of vasopressin on water and NaCl transport across the in vitro perfused medullary thick ascending limb of Henle's loop of mouse, rat, and rabbit kidneys. Pflugers Arch. 383:215, 1980.
120. Herbert, S. C.; Culpepper, R. M.; and Andreoli, T. E. NaCl transport in mouse medullary thick ascending limbs. I. Functional nephron heterogeneity and ADH-stimulated NaCl cotransport. Am. J. Physiol. 241:F412, 1981.
121. Herbert, S. C.; Culpepper, R. M.; and Andreoli, T. E. NaCl transport in mouse medullary thick ascending limbs. II. ADH enhancement of transcellular cotransport; origin of transepithelial voltage. Am. J. Physiol. 241:F432, 1981.
122. Chabardes, D.; Gagnan-Brunette, M.; Imbert-Teboul, M.; Gontcharevskaia, O.; Montegut, M.; Clique, A.; and Morel, F. Adenylate cyclase responsiveness to hormones in various portions of the human nephron. J. Clin. Invest. 65:439, 1980.
123. Baylis, P. H.; and Heath, D. A. Water disturbances in patients treated with oral lithium carbonate. Ann. Intern. Med. 88:607, 1978.
124. Smith, D. F.; and Balogura, S. Sodium appetite in rats given lithium. Life Sci. 11:1021, 1972.
125. Mishkind, M. H.; Greenspan, R. E.; Borg, W. H.; and Ferris, T. F. Studies on lithium-induced polyuria. Clin. Res. 25:596A, 1977.
126. Galla, J. N.; Forrest, J. N.; Hecht, B.; Kashgarian, M.; and Hayslett, J. P. Effect of lithium on water and electrolyte metabolism. Yale J. Biol. Med. 48:305, 1975.
127. Miller, P. D.; Dubovsky, S. L.; McDonald, K. M.; Katz, F. H.; Robertson, G. L.; and Schrier, R. W. Central, renal, and adrenal effects of lithium in man. Am. J. Med. 66: 797, 1979.
128. Martinez-Maldonado, M.; Stavroulaki-Tsapara, A.; Tasparas, N.; Suki, W. N.; and Eknoyan, G. Renal effects of lithium in rats: Alterations in water and electrolyte metabolism and the response to vasopressin and cyclic adenosine monophosphate during prolonged administration. J. Lab. Clin. Med. 86:445, 1975.
129. Singer, I.; Rotenberg, D.; and Puschett, J. B. Lithium-induced nephrogenic diabetes insipidus: In vivo and in vitro studies. J. Clin. Invest. 51:1081, 1972.
130. Webb, R. K.; Woodhall, P. B.; Tisher, C. C.; and Robinson, R. R. Acute effects of lithium on the renal concentrating mechanism in a primate. Am. J. Physiol. 228:909, 1975.
131. Hecht, B.; Kashgarian, M.; Forrest, J. N., Jr.; and Hayslett, J. P. Micropuncture study on the effects of lithium on proximal and distal tubule function in the rat kidney. Pflugers Arch. 377:69, 1978.
132. Carney, S. L.; Wong, N. L. M.; and Dirks, J. H. Effect of lithium treatment on rat renal tubule function. Nephron 25:293, 1980.

133. Hochman, S.; and Gutman, Y. Lithium: ADH antagonism and ADH-independent action in rats with diabetes insipidus. Eur. J. Pharmacol. 28:100, 1974.
134. Balment, R. J.; Jones, P. C.; and Henderson, I. W. Time course of lithium-induced alterations in renal and endocrine function in normal and Brattleboro rats with hypothalamic diabetes insipidus. Br. J. Pharmacol. 59:627, 1977.
135. Rahn, D. W.; and Forrest, J. N., Jr. Lithium-enhancement of water excretion in the absence of vasopressin. Clin. Res. 23:602A, 1975.
136. Jenner, F. A.; and MacNeil, S. The effects of lithium ions on the antidiuretic action of vasopressin in the rat. Br. J. Pharmacol. 55:527, 1975.
137. Harris, C. A.; and Jenner, F. A. Some aspects of the inhibition of the action of antidiuretic hormone by lithium ions in the rat kidney and bladder of the toad, *Bufo marinus*. Br. J. Pharmacol. 44:223, 1972.
138. MacNeil, S.; Jennings, G.; Eastwood, P. R.; Paschalis, C.; and Jenner, F. A. Lithium and the antidiuretic hormone. Br. J. Clin. Pharmacol. 3:305, 1976.
139. Christensen, S. Acute and chronic effects of vasopressin in rats with lithium polyuria. Acta Pharmacol. Toxicol. 38:241, 1976.
140. Christensen, S. Effect of antidiuretic drugs in rats with lithium-induced polyuria. Acta Pharmacol. Toxicol. 38:81, 1976.
141. Christensen, S.; and Geisler, A. Antidiuretic and urinary cyclic AMP response of vasopressin in normal rats and in rats with lithium polyuria. Acta Pharmacol. Toxicol. 40: 447, 1977.
142. Padfield, P. L.; Park, S. J.; Morton, J. J.; and Braidwood, A. E. Plasma levels of antidiuretic hormone in patients receiving prolonged lithium therapy. Br. J. Phychiatry 130:144, 1977.
143. Padfield, P. L.; Morton, J. J.; Lindop, G. B. M.; and Timbury, G. C. Lithium-induced nephrogenic diabetes insipidus; changes in plasma vasopressin and angiotensin II. Clin. Nephrol. 3:220, 1975.
144. Singer, I.; and Franko, E. A. Lithium-induced ADH resistance in toad urinary bladders. Kidney Int. 3:151, 1973.
145. Baer, L.; Platman, S. R.; Kassir, S.; and Fieve, R. R. Mechanisms of renal lithium handling and their relationship to mineralocorticoids: A dissociation between sodium and lithium ions. J. Psychiatr. Res. 8:91, 1971.
146. Thomsen, K. The effect of sodium chloride on kidney function in rats with lithium intoxication. Acta Pharmacol. Toxicol. 33:92, 1973.
147. Thomsen, K. Lithium-induced polyuria in rats. Int. Pharmacopsychiatry 5:233, 1970.
148. Thomsen, K. Renal elimination of lithium in rats with lithium intoxication. J. Pharmacol. Exp. Ther. 199:483, 1976.
149. Solomon, S. Action of alkali metals on papillary-cortical sodium gradient of dog kidney. Proc. Soc. Exp. Biol. Med. 125:1183, 1967.
150. Dousa, T. P.; and Barnes, L. D. Lithium-induced diuretic effect of antidiuretic hormone in rats. Am. J. Physiol. 231:1754, 1976.
151. Natochin, Y. V.; and Leontev, V. G. Pituitrin stimulation of active transport of lithium by wall of frog urinary bladder. Fiziol. Zh. S.S.S.R. 50:618, 1964.
152. Leblanc, G. The mechanism of lithium accumulation in the isolated frog skin epithelium. Pflugers Arch. 337:1, 1972.
153. Reinach, P. S.; Candia, D. A.; and Siegal, G. J. Lithium transport across isolated frog skin epithelium. J. Membr. Biol. 25:75, 1975.
154. Herrera, F. C. Inhibition of lithium transport across toad bladder by amiloride. Am. J. Physiol. 222:499, 1972.
155. Martinez-Maldonado, M.; and Opava-Stitzer, S. Distal nephron function of the rat during lithium chloride infusion. Kidney Int. 12:17, 1977.
156. March, T. W.; and Forrest, J. N., Jr. Amiloride reverses chronic lithium-induced polyuria by a mechanism dependent on antidiuretic hormone. Clin. Res. 28:455A, 1980.

157. Kosten, T. R.; and Forrest, J. N., Jr. Treatment of severe lithium-induced nephrogenic diabetes insipidus with amiloride. Clin. Res. 30:540A, 1982.
158. Bentley, P. J. The effects of ionic changes on water transfer across the isolated urinary bladder of the toad, Bufo marinus. J. Endocrinol. 18:327, 1959.
159. Hays, R. M.; and Leaf, A. The problem of clinical vasopressin resistance: In vitro studies. Ann. Intern. Med. 54:700, 1961.
160. Finn, A. L.; Handler, J. S.; and Orloff, J. Relation between toad bladder potassium content and permeability response to vasopressin. Am. J. Physiol. 210:1279, 1966.
161. Bentley, P. J.; and Wasserman, A. The effects of lithium on the permeability of an epithelial membrane, the toad urinary bladder. Biochim. Biophysiol. Acta 266:285, 1972.
162. Carney, S.; Rayson, B.; and Morgan, T. The effect of lithium on the permeability response induced in the collecting duct by antidiuretic hormone. Pflugers Arch. 366: 19, 1976.
163. Cox, M.; and Singer, I. Lithium. In: Disorders of Mineral Metabolism, vol. 1, Trade Minerals, edicated by Bronner, F., and Coburn, J. W. New York, Academic Press, 1981, p. 370.
164. Dousa, T. P.; and Hechter, O. The effect of NaCl and LiCl on vasopressin-sensitive adenyl cyclase. Life SCi. 9:765, 1970.
165. Geisler, A.; Wraae, O.; and Olesen, O. V. Adenyl cyclase activity in kidneys of rats with lithium-induced polyuria. Acta Pharmacol. Toxicol. 31:203, 1972.
166. Wraae, O.; Geisler, A.; and Olesen, O. V. The relation between vasopressin stimulation of renal adenyl cyclase and lithium-induced polyuria in rats. Acta Pharmacol. Toxicol. 31:314, 1972.
167. Dousa, T. P. Interaction of lithium with vasopressin-sensitive cyclic AMP system of human renal medula. Endocrinology 95:1359, 1974.
168. Beck, N.; and Davis, B. B. Effects of lithium on vasopressin-dependent cyclic AMP in rat renal medulla. Endocrinology 97:202, 1975.
169. Jackson, B. A.; Edwards, R. M.; and Dousa, T. P. Lithium-induced polyuria: Effect of lithium on adenylate cyclase and adenosine 3',5'-monophosphate phosphodiesterase in medullary ascending limb of Henle's loop and in medullary collecting tubules. Endocrinology 107:1693, 1980.
170. Willis, J. S.; and Fang, L. S. T. Li^+ stimulation of ouabain-sensitive respiration and (Na^+-K^+)-ATPase of kidney cortex of ground squirrels. Biochim. Biophys. Acta 219: 486, 1970.
171. Gutman, Y.; Hochman, S.; and Wald, H. The differential effect of Li^+ on microsomal ATPase in cortex, medulla, and papilla of rat kidney. Biochim. Biophys. Acta 298: 284, 1973.
172. Nally, J. V.; Rutecki, G. W.; and Ferris, T. F. The acute effect of lithium on renal renin and prostaglandin E synthesis in the dog. Circ. Res. 46:739, 1980.
173. Walker, R. M.; Brown, R. S.; and Stoff, J. S. Role of renal prostaglandins during antidiuresis and water diuresis in man. Kidney Int. 21:365, 1981.
174. Rapoport, J.; Chaimovitz, C.; Alroy, G. G.; and Better, O. S. Lithium-induced nephrogenic diabetes insipidus: Studies of tubular function and pathogenesis. Isr. J. Med. Sci. 15:765, 1979.
175. Flores, A. G. A.; and Sharp, G. W. G. Endogenous prostaglandins and osmotic water flow in the toad bladder. Am. J. Physiol. 233:1392, 1972.
176. Dousa, T. P.; Hui, Y. S. F.; and Barnes, L. D. Microtubule assembly in renal medullary slices: Effects of vasopressin, vinblastine, and lithium. J. Lab. Clin. Med. 92:252, 1978.
177. Forrest, J. N., Jr.; Marcy, T. W.; Biemesderfer, D.; and Kashgarian, M. Cytoskeletal defect in cortical collecting duct cells in lithium-induced polyuria. Abstract of the 13th Annual Meeting of the American Society of Nephrology, Washington, D. C., 1980, p. 93A.

178. Simon, N. M.; Garber, E.; and Arieff, A. J. Persistent nephrogenic diabetes insipidus after lithium treatment. Ann. Intern. Med. 86:446, 1977.
179. Epstein, F. H. Disturbances in renal concentrating ability. In: Disturbances in Body Fluid Osmolality, edited by Andreoli, T. E., Grantham, J. J., and Rector, F. C. Washington, D. C., American Physiological Society, 1977, p. 255.
180. Rabin, E. Z.; Garston, R. G.; Weir, R. V.; and Posen, G. A. Persistent nephrogenic diabetes insipidus associated with long-term lithium carbonate treatment. Can. Med. Assoc. J. 121:194, 1979.
181. Price, T. R. P.; and Beisswenger, P. J. Lithium and diabetes insipidus (letter to the editor). Ann. Intern. Med. 88:576, 1978.
182. Bucht, G.; and Wahlin, A. Renal concentrating capacity in long-term lithium treatment and after withdrawal of lithium. Acta Med. Scand. 207:309, 1980.
183. Hestbech, J.; Hansen, H. E.; Amdisen, A.; and Olsen, S. Chronic renal lesions following long-term treatment with lithium. Kidney Int. 12:205, 1977.
184. Singer, I. Lithium and the kidney. Kidney Int. 19:374, 1981.
185. Ramsey, T. A.; and Cox, M. Lithium and the kidney: A review. Am. J. Physiol. 139: 443, 1982.
186. Castell, D. O.; and Sparks, H. A. Nephrogenic diabetes insipidus due to demethylchlortetracycline hydrochloride. J.A.M.A. 193:237, 1965.
187. Roth, H.; Becker, K. L.; Shalhoub, R. J.; and Katz, S. Nephrotoxicity of demethylchlortetracycline hydrochloride. Arch. Intern. Med. 120:433, 1967.
188. Wilson, D. M.; Perry, H. O.; Sams, W. M., Jr.; and Dousa, T. P. Selective inhibition of human distal tubular function by demeclocycline. Curr. Ther. Res. 15:734, 1973.
189. Singer, I.; and Rotenberg, D. Demeclocycline-induced nephrogenic diabetes insipidus: In-vivo and in-vitro studies. Ann. Intern. Med. 79:679, 1973.
190. Forrest, J. N., Jr.; Cox, M.; Hong, C.; Morrison, G.; Bia, M.; and Singer, I. Superiority of demeclocycline over lithium in the treatment of chronic syndrome of inappropriate secretion of antidiuretic hormone. N. Engl. J. Med. 298:173, 1978.
191. Appel, G. B.; and Neu, H. C. The nephrotoxicity of antimicrobial agents. Part II. N. Engl. J. Med. 296:722, 1977.
192. DeTroyer, A. Demeclocycline treatment for syndrome of inappropriate antidiuretic hormone secretion. J.A.M.A. 237:2723, 1977.
193. Cox, M. Tetracycline nephrotoxicity. In: Nephrotoxic Mechanisms of Drugs and Environmental Toxins, edited by Porter, G., New York, Plenum, 1982, p. 165.
194. Oster, J. R.; Epstein, M.; and Ulano, H. B. Deterioration of renal function with demeclocycline administration. Curr. Ther. Res. 20:794, 1976.
195. DeTroyer, A.; Pilloy, W.; Broeckaert, I.; and Demanet, J.-C. Demeclocycline treatment of water retention in cirrhosis. Ann. Intern. Med. 85:336, 1976.
196. Carrilho, F.; Bosch, J.; Arroyo, V.; Antoni, M.; Viver, J.; and Rodes, J. Renal failure associated with demeclocycline in cirrhosis. Ann. Intern. Med. 87:195, 1977.
197. Cox, M.; Guzzo, J.; Morrison, G.; and Singer, I. Demeclocycline and therapy of hyponatremia. Ann. Intern. Med. 86:113B, 1977.
198. Zegers de Beyl, D.; Naeije, R.; and DeTroyer, A. Demeclocycline treatment of water retention in congestive heart failure. Br. Med.J. 1:760, 1978.
199. Miller, P. D.; Linas, S. L.; and Schrier, R. W. Plasma demeclocycline levels and nephrotoxicity—Correlation in hyponatremic cirrhotic patients. J.A.M.A. 243:2513, 1980.
200. Geheb, M.; and Cox, M. Renal effects of demeclocycline. J.A.M.A. 243:2519, 1980.
201. Braden, G.; Geheb, M.; and Cox, M. Renal toxicity of demeclocycline in patients with edematous disorders. Clin. Res. 28:655A, 1980.
202. Chan, S. Water diuretic activity of demeclocycline in rats. Fed. Proc. 38:749A, 1979.
203. Feldman, H.; and Singer, I. Comparative effects of tetracyclines on water flow across toad urinary bladders. J. Pharmacol. Exp. Ther. 190:358, 1974.

204. Dousa, T. P.; and Wilson, D. M. Effects of demethylchlortetracycline on cellular action of antidiuretic hormone in vitro. Kidney Int. 5:279, 1974.
205. Zusman, R. M.; Keiser, H. R.; and Handler, J. S. Effect of adrenal steroids on vasopressin-stimulated PGE synthesis and water flow. Am. J. Physiol. 234:F532, 1978.
206. Serros, E. R.; Lowe, A. G.; and Kirschenbaum, M. A. Effect of prostaglandin inhibition on demeclocycline administration in conscious rats. Prostaglandins Med. 5:175, 1980.
207. Albert, A.; and Rees, C. W. Avidity of the tetracyclines for the cations of metals. Nature 177:433, 1956.
208. Dolusio, J. T.; and Martin, A. N. Metal complexation of the tetracycline hydrochlorides. J. Med. Chem. 6:16, 1963.
209. Martin, S. R. Equilibrium and kinetic studies on the interactions of tetracyclines with calcium and magnesium. Biophys. Chem. 10:319, 1979.
210. Kohn, K. W. Mediation of divalent metal ions in the binding of tetracycline to macromolecules. Nature 191:1156, 1961.
211. Doluisio, J. T.; and Martin, A. N. The binding to tetracycline analogs to conalbumin in the absence and presence of cupric ions. J. Med. Chem. 6:20, 1963.
212. Blackwood, R. K.; and English, A. R. Structure-activity relationships in the tetracycline series. In: Advances in Applied Microbiology, vol. 13, edited by Perlman, D., and Umbreit, W. New York, Academic Press, 1977, p. 237.
213. Paddock, R. B.; Parker, J. W.; and Guadagni, N. P. The effects of methoxyflurane on renal function. Anesthesiology 25:707, 1964.
214. Pezzi, P. J.; Frobese, A. S.; and Greenberg, S. R. Methoxyflurane and renal toxicity. Lancet 1:823, 1966.
215. Crandell, W. B.; Pappas, S. G.; and MacDonald, A. Nephrotoxocity associated with methoxyflurane anesthesia. Anesthesiology 27:591, 1966.
216. Austin, W. H.; and Villandry, P. J. Methoxyflurane and renal function. Anesthesiology 28:637, 1967.
217. Elkington, S. G.; Goffinet, J. A.; and Conn, H. E. Renal and hepatic injury associated with methoxyflurane anesthesia. Ann. Intern. Med. 69:1229, 1968.
218. Lebowitz, M. H. Nephrogenic diabetes insipidus following methoxyflurane anesthesia. Anesth. Analg. 48:233, 1969.
219. Panner, B. J.; Freeman, R. B.; Roth-Moyo, L. A.; and Markowitch, W., Jr. Toxicity following methoxyflurane anesthesia. I. Clinical and pathological observations in two cases. J.A.M.A. 214:86, 1970.
220. Kuzucu, E. Y. Methoxyflurane, tetracycline, and renal failure. J.A.M.A. 211:1162, 1970.
221. Frascino, J. A.; Varramee, P.; and Rosen, P. P. Renal oxalosis and azotemia after methoxyflurane anesthesia. N. Engl. J. Med. 283:676, 1970.
222. Mazze, R. I.; Shue, G. L.; and Jackson, S. H. Renal dysfunction associated with methoxyflurane anesthesia. J.A.M.A. 216:278, 1971.
223. Wong, E. G. C.; Rowe, P. H.; Blumenkrantz, M. J.; and Coburn, J. W. Nephrotoxicity associated with use of methoxyflurane. Nephron 13:174, 1974.
224. Churchill, D.; Knaack, J.; Chirito, E.; Barre, P.; Cole, C.; Muercke, R.; and Gault, M. H. Persisting renal insufficiency after methoxyflurane anesthesia. Am. J. Med. 56:575, 1974.
225. Holaday, D. A.; Rudofsky, S.; and Treubaft, P. S. The metabolic degradation of methoxyflurane in man. Anesthesiology 33:579, 1970.
226. Mazze, R. I.; and Hitt, B. A. Methoxyflurane metabolism. Anesthesiology 44:369, 1976.
227. Halpern, B. A.; Kempson, R. L.; and Coplon, N. S. Interstitial fibrosis and chronic renal failure following methoxyflurane anesthesia. J.A.M.A. 233:1239, 1973.

228. Hollenberg, N. K.; MacDonald, F. D.; Cotran, R.; Galvanck, E. G.; Warhol, M.; Vandam, L. D.; and Merrill, J. P. Irreversible acute oliguric renal failure. A complication of methoxyflurane anesthesia. N. Engl. J. Med. 286:877, 1972.
229. Bullock, J. D.; and Albert, D. M. Generalized oxalosis with retinal involvement following methoxyflurane anesthesia. Anesthesiology 41:296, 1974.
230. Jeghers, H.; and Murphy, R. Practical aspects of oxalate metabolism. Am. J. Med. 45:715, 1968.
231. Aufderheide, A. C. Renal tubular calcium oxalate crystal deposition. Arch. Pathol. 92:162, 1971.
232. Toves, D. R.; Fry, B. W.; Freeman, R. B.; and Gillies, A. J. Toxicity following methoxyflurane anesthesia. II. Fluoride concentrations in nephrotoxicity. J.A.M.A. 214: 91, 1970.
233. Mazze, R. I.; Trudell, J. R.; and Cousins, M. J. Methoxyflurane metabolism and renal dysfunction: Clinical correlation in man. Anesthesiology 35:247, 1971.
234. Cousins, M. J.; and Mazze, R. I. Methoxyflurane nephrotoxicity. A study of dose response in man. J.A.M.A. 225:1611, 1973.
235. Mazze, R. I.; Cousins, M. J.; and Kosek, J. C. Dose-related methoxyflurane nephrotoxicity in rats. Anesthesiology 36:571, 1972.
236. Hetrick, W. D.; Wolfson, B.; Garcia, D. A.; and Siker, E. S. Renal response to light methoxyflurane anesthesia. Anesthesiology 38:30, 1973.
237. Tobey, R. E.; and Clubb, R. J. Renal function after methoxyflurane and halothane anesthesia. J.A.M.A. 223:649, 1973.
238. Whitford, G. M.; and Taves, D. R. Fluoride-induced diuresis: Renal-tissue solute concentrations, functional, ehmodynamic, and histologic correlates in the rat. Anesthesiology 39:416, 1973.
239. Frascino, J. A. Effect of inorganic fluoride on the renal concentrating mechanism; possible nephrotoxicity in man. J. Lab. Clin. Med. 79:192, 1972.
240. Goldenberg, L. Tratemiento de la enfermedad de Basedow y del hipertirodismo por fluor. Rev. Soc. Med. Int. Soc. Fisiol. 6:217, 1931.
241. Wallin, J. D.; and Kaplan, R. A. Effect of sodium fluoride on concentrating and diluting ability in the rat. Am. J. Physiol. 232:F335, 1977.
242. Smith, F. A. Metabolism of inorganic fluoride. In: Handbook of Experimental Pharmacology, vol. 20, part 2, edited by Smith, F. A., New York, Springer-Verlag, 1966, p. 53.
243. Caruso, F. S.; Maynard, E. A.; and DiStefano, V. Pharmacology of fluorides. In: Handbook of Experimental Pharmacology, vol. 20, part 2, edited by Smith, F. A., New York, Springer-Verlag, 1966, p. 144.
244. Sutherland, E. W.; Rall, T. W.; and Menon, T. Adenyl cyclase. I. Distribution, preparation and properties. J. Biol. Chem. 237:1220, 1962.
245. Levine, S. D.; Levine, R. D.; Worthington, R. E.; and Hays, R. M. Selective inhibition of osmotic water flow by general anesthetics in toad urinary bladder. J. Clin. Invest. 58:980, 1976.
246. Levine, S. D.; Weber, H.; and Schlondorff, D. Inhibition of adenylate cyclase by general anesthetics in toad urinary bladder. Am. J. Physiol. 237:F372, 1979.
247. Chakabe, S.; Handler, J. S.; and Orloff, J. Release of cyclic AMP by toad urinary bladder. Am. J. Physiol. 228:954, 1975.
248. Yorio, T.; Sinclair, R.; and Henry, S. Fluoride inhibition of the hydro-osmotic response of the toad urinary bladder to antidiuretic hormone. J. Pharmacol. Exp. Ther. 219: 459, 1981.
249. Bernanke, D.; and Epstein, F. H. Metabolism of the renal medulla. Am. J. Physiol. 208:541, 1965.
250. Warburg, O.; and Christian, W. I. Solierungund kristallisation des garungsferments enolase. Biochem. Z. 310:384, 1942.

251. Beard, H. W.; Richert, J. H.; and Taylor, R. R. The treatment of deep mycotic infections with amphotericin B. Am. Rev. Respir, Dis. 81:43, 1960.
252. Bell, N. H.; Andriole, V. T.; Sabesin, S. M.; and Utz, J. P. On nephrotoxicity of amphotericin B in man. Am. J. Med. 33:64, 1962.
253. Holeman, C. W., Jr.; and Einstein, H. Toxic effects of amphotericin B in man. Calif. Med. 99:90, 1963.
254. Butler, W. T.; Bennett, J. E.; Alling, D. W.; Wertlake, P. T.; Utz, J. P.; and Hill, G. J. Nephrotoxicity of amphotericin B: Early and late effects in 81 patients. Ann. Intern. Med. 61:175, 1964.
255. Barbour, G. L.; Straub, K. D.; O'Neal, B. L.; and Leatherman, J. W. Vasopressin-resistant nephrogenic diabetes insipidus: A result of amphotericin B therapy. Arch. Intern. Med. 139:86, 1979.
256. Gouge, T. H.; and Andrioli, V. T. An experimental model of amphotericin B nephrotoxicity with renal tubular acidosis. J. Lab. Clin. Med. 78:713, 1971.
257. McCurdy, D. K.; Federic, M.; and Elkinton, J. R. Renal tubular acidosis due to amphotericin B. N. Engl. J. Med. 278:124, 1968.
258. Douglas, J. B.; and Healy, J. K. Nephrotoxic effects of amphotericin B, including renal tubular acidosis. Am. J. Med. 46:154, 1969.
259. Rhoades, E. R.; Ginn, H. E.; Muchmore, H. G.; Smith, W. O.; and Hammarsten, J. F. The effect of amphotericin B upon renal function in man. In: Antimicrobial Agents Manual, edited by Gray, P., Tabenkin, B., and Bradley, S. G. New York, Plenum, 1961, p. 539.
260. Winn, W. A. Coccidiomycosis and amphotericin B. Med. Clin. North Am. 47:1131, 1963.
261. Takacs, F. J.; Tomkiewicz, Z. M.; and Merril, J. P. Amphotericin B nephrotoxicity with irreversible renal failure. Ann. Intern. Med. 59:716, 1963.
262. Butler, W. T.; Hill, G. J.; Szwed, C. F.; and Knight, V. Amphotericin B renal toxicity in dog. J. Pharmacol. Exp. Ther. 143:47, 1964.
263. Jose, P. A.; Eisner, G. M.; Hollerman, C. E.; and Calcagno, P. L. Acute renal effects of amphotericin B. Proc. Soc. Exp. Biol. Med. 137:224, 1971.
264. Gerrens, J. F.; and Branch, R. A. The influence of sodium status and furosemide on canine acute amphotericin B nephrotoxicity. J. Pharmacol. Exp. Ther. 214:306, 1980.
265. Andreoli, T. On the anatomy of amphotericin B-cholesterol pores in lipid bilayer membranes. Kidney Int. 4:337, 1973.
266. Lichtenstein, N. S.; and Leaf, A. Effect of amphotericin B on the permeability of the toad bladder. J. Clin. Invest. 44:1328, 1965.
267. Lichtenstein, N. S.; and Leaf, A. Evidence for a double series permeability barrier at the mucosal surface of the toad bladder. Ann. N.Y. Acad. Sci. 137:556, 1966.
268. Mendoza, S. A.; Handler, J. S.; and Orloff, J. Effect of amphotericin B on permeability and short-circuit current in toad bladder. Am. J. Physiol. 213:1263, 1967.
269. Singer, I.; Civan, M. M.; Baddour, R. F.; and Leaf, A. Interactions of amphotericin B, vasopressin, and calcium in toad urinary bladder. Am. J. Physiol. 217:938, 1969.
270. Lampen, J. O.; Arnow, P. M.; and Safferman, R. S. Mechanism of protection by sterols against polyene antibiotics. J. Bacteriol. 80:200, 1960.
271. van Zutphen, H.; van Deenen, L. L. M.; and Kinsky, S. C. The action of polyene antibiotics on bilayer lipid membranes. Biochem. Biophys. Res. Commun. 22:393, 1966.
272. Saladino, A. J.; Bentley, P. J.; and Trump, B. F. Ion movements in cell injury. Effect of amphotericin B on the ultrastructure and function of the epithelial cells of the toad bladder. Am. J. Pathol. 54:421, 1969.
273. Reynolds, E. S.; Tomkiewicz, Z. M.; and Dammin, G. J. Renal lesion related to amphotericin B treatment for coccidiomycosis. Med. Clin. North Am. 47:1149, 1963.
274. Wertlake, P. T.; Butler, W. T.; Hill, G. J.; and Utz, J. P. Nephrotoxic tubular damage and calcium deposition following amphotericin B therapy. Am. J. Pathol. 43:449, 1963.

275. Rado, J. P.; and Borbely, L. Enhancement of polyuria by glybenclamide in diabetes insipidus. Lancet 2:216, 1971.
276. Rado, J. P.; and Borbely, L. Glybenclamide enhancement of polyuria in patients with pituitary diabetes insipidus. Endokrinologie 59:397, 1972.
277. Moses, A. M.; Howazwitz, J.; and Miller, M. Diuretic action of three sulfonylurea drugs. Ann. Intern. Med. 78:541, 1973.
278. Tuma, S.; Syzlman, P.; and Better, O. S. Augmented urinary dilution following administration of tolinase in man. Nephron 13:145, 1974.
279. Rado, J. P.; Borbely, L.; Szende, L.; Fischer, J.; and Tako, J. Investigation of the diuretic effect of glybenclamide in healthy subjects and in patients with pituitary and nephrogenic diabetes insipidus. Horm. Metab. Res. 6:289, 1974.
280. Rado, J. P.; Szende, L.; and Marosi, J. Influence of glyburide on the antidiuretic response induced by 1-deamino-8-D-arginine vasopressin (DDAVP) in patients with pituitary diabetes insipidus. Metabolism 23:1057, 1974.
281. Rado, J. P.; and Borbely, L. Inhibition of the antidiuretic effect of 1-deamino-8-D-arginine vasopressin (DDAVP) by glybenclamide in water-loaded healthy subjects. Endokrinologie 66:88, 1975.
282. Zuethi, A.; and Studer, H. Antidiuretic action of chlorpropamide and tolbutamide. Minn. Med. 52:33, 1969.
283. Weissman, P. N.; Shenkman, L.; and Gregerman, R. I. Chlorpropamide hyponatremia. Drug-induced inappropriate antidiuretic-hormone activity. N. Engl. J. Med. 284:65, 1971.
284. Hagen, G. A.; and Frawley, T. F. Hyponatremia due to suflonylurea compounds. J. Clin. Endocrinol. 31:570, 1970.
285. Garcia, M.; Miller, M.; and Moses, A. M. Chlorpropamide-induced water retention in patients with diabetes mellitus. Ann. Intern. Med. 75:549, 1971.
286. Lichtenberg, L.; and Abraira, C. Tolbutamide-associated hyponatremia. J.A.M.A. 240: 2433, 1978.
287. Moore, T. D.; and Bechtel, T. P. Hyponatremia secondary to tolbutamide and chlorthiazide. Am. J. Hosp. Pharm. 36:1107, 1979.
288. Arduino, F.; Ferraz, F. P. J.; and Rodrigues, J. Antidiuretic action of chlorpropamide in idiopathic diabetes insipidus. J. Clin. Endocrinol. Metab. 26:1325, 1966.
289. Miller, M.; and Moses, A. M. Mechanism of chlorpropamide action in diabetes insipidus. J. Clin. Endocrinol. 30:488, 1970.
290. Bode, H. H.; Harley, B. M.; and Crawford, J. D. Restoration of normal drinking behavior by chlorpropamide in patients with hypodipsia and diabetes insipidus. Am. J. Med. 51:304, 1971.
291. Moses, A. M.; Van Gemert, M.; and Miller, M. Evidence that glyburide-induced diuresis is not mediated by inhibition of ADH. Horm. Res. 5:359, 1974.
292. Fernandez, P.; and Singer, I. Enhancement of ADH-induced water flow in isolated toad urinary bladders by two new sulfonylureas. Clin. Res. 23:219A, 1975.
293. Urakabe, S.; Shirai, D.; Ando, A.; Takamitsu, Y.; Orita, Y.; and Abe, H. Effect of sulfonylureas on the permeability to water and electrical properties of the urinary bladder of the toad. Jpn. Circ. J. 34:595, 1970.
294. Ingelfinger, J. R.; and Hays, R. M. Evidence that chlorpropamide and vasopressin share a common site of action. J. Clin. Endocrinol. 29:738, 1969.
295. Mendoza, S. Effect of chlorpropamide on the permeability of the urinary bladder of the toad and the response to vasopressin, adenosine-3',5'-monophosphate and theophylline. Endocrinology 84:411, 1969.
296. Danisi, G.; Genta, E. N.; Timoner, J.; and Marcondes, M. Effect of chlorpropamide on urinary excretion of water and solute in patients with diabetes insipidus and on water flow across isolated toad bladder. J. Clin. Endocrinol. Metab. 30:528, 1970.

297. Wales, J. K. The effect of chlorpropamide and related compounds on water transport across the toad bladder. J. Endocrinol. 49:551, 1971.
298. Lozada, E. S.; Gouaux, J.; Franki, N.; Appel, G. B.; and Hays, R. M. Studies of the mode of action of the sulfonylureas and phenylacetamides in enhancing the effect of vasopressin. J. Clin. Endocrinol. Metab. 34:704, 1972.
299. Mendoza, S. A.; and Brown, C. A., Jr. Effect of chlorpropamide on osmotic water flow across toad bladder and the response to vasopressin, theophylline and cyclic AMP. J Clin. Endocrinol. Metab. 38:883, 1974.
300. Zusman, R. M.; Keiser, H. R.; and Handler, J. S. Inhibition of vasopressin-stimulated prostaglandin E biosynthesis by chlorpropamide in the toad urinary bladder. J. Clin. Invest. 60:1348, 1977.
301. Miller, M.; and Moses, A. M. Potentiation of vasopressin action by chlorpropamide in vivo, Endocrinology 86:1024, 1970.
302. Zweig, S. M.; Ettinger, B.; and Earley, L. E. Mechanism of antidiuretic action of chlorpropoamide in the mammalian kidney. Am. J. Physiol. 221:911, 1971.
303. Moses, A. M.; Numann, P.; and Miller, M. Mechanism of chlorpropamide-induced antidiuresis in man: Evidence for release of ADH and enhancement of peripheral action. Metabolism 22:59, 1973.
304. Meinders, A. E.; Van Leeuwen, A. M.; Borst, J. G.; and Cejka, V. Paradoxical diuresis after vasopressin administration to patients with neurohypophysial diabetes insipidus treated with chlorpropamide, carbamazepine or clofibrate. Clin. Sci. Molec. Med. 49: 283, 1975.
305. Foy, J. M.; and Lucas, P. D. Modification of diuresis in the rat by chlorpropamide, glibenclamide, and tolbutamide. Experientia 31:570, 1975.
306. Porter, G. A.; and Bennett, W. M. Toxic nephropathies. In: The Kidney, edited by Brenner, B. M., and Rector, F. C. Philadelphia, Saunders, 1981, p. 2045.
307. Bennett, W. M.; Luft, F. C.; and Porter, G. A. Pathogenesis of renal failure due to aminoglycosides and radiographic contrast media. Am. J. Med. 69:767, 1980.
308. Cronin, R. E. Aminoglycoside nephrotoxicity: Pathogenesis and prevention. Clin. Nephrol. 11:251, 1979.
309. Bennett, W. M. Aminoglycoside nephrotoxicity. Experimental and clinical considerations. Miner. Electrolyte Metab. 6:277, 1981.
310. Kosek, J. C.; Mazze, R. I.; and Cousins, M. J. Nephrotoxicity of gentamicin. Lab. Invest. 30:48, 1974.
311. Luft, F. C.; Patel, V.; Yum, M. N.; Patel, B.; and Kleit, S. A. Experimental aminoglycoside nephrotoxicity. J. Lab. Clin. Med. 86:213, 1975.
312. Plamp, C.; Reger, K.; Bennett, W.; McClung, M.; and Porter, G. Vasopressin-resistant polyuria in gentamicin nephrotoxicity. Clin. Res. 26:141A, 1978.
313. Appel, G. B.; Siegel, N. J.; Appel, A. S.; and Hayslett, J. P. Gentamicin induced non-oliguric acute renal failure. Proceedings of the 11th Annual Meeting of the American Society of Nephrology. New Orleans, 1978, p. 87A.
314. Houghton, D. C.; Hartnett, M. N.; Campbell-Boswell, M.; Porter, G. A.; and Bennett, W. M. A light and electron microscopic analysis of gentamicin nephrotoxicity in rats. Am. J. Pathol. 82:589, 1976.
315. Cronin, R. E.; Bulger, R. E.; Southern, P.; and Henrich, W. L. Natural history of aminoglycoside nephrotoxicity in the dog. J. Lab. Clin. Med. 95:463, 1980.
316. Parker, R. A.; Porter, G. A.; and Bennett, W. M. Gentamicin induced resistance to ADH stimulated water flow in the toad urinary bladder: Partial correction by prostaglandin inhibition. Clin. Res. 27:499A, 1979.
317. Souliere, C. R.; Goodman, D. B. P.; Appel, G. B.; and Forrest, J. N., Jr. Gentamicin selectively inhibits antidiuretic hormone induced water flow in the toad urinary bladder. Proceedings of the 11th Annual Meeting of the American Society of Nephrology., New Orleans, 1978, p. 99A.

318. Humes, H. D.; and Weinberg, J. M. Importance of membrane bound calcium to the hydro-osmotic water flow response to antidiuretic hormone in toad urinary bladder. Clin. Res. 28:449A, 1980.
319. Ross, M.; Parker, R. A.; Elliott, W. C.; Porter, G. A.; and Bennett, W. M. Gentamicin-induced resistance to ADH-stimulated water flow in the toad urinary bladder explained by drug-induced pH changes. Clin. Res. 28:64A, 1980.
320. Madias, N. E.; and Harrington, J. T. Platinum nephrotoxicity. Am. J. Med. 65:307, 1978.
321. Blachley, J. D.; and Hill, J. B. Renal and electrolyte disturbances associated with cisplatin. Ann. Intern. Med. 95:628, 1981.
322. Walker, E. M., Jr.; and Gale, G. R. Methods of reduction of cisplatin nephrotoxicity. Ann. Clin. Lab. Sci. 11:397, 1981.
323. Porter, G. A.; and Bennett, W. M. Nephrotoxic acute renal failure due to common drugs. Am. J. Physiol. 241:F1, 1981.
324. Schilsky, R. L.; and Anderson, T. Hypomagnesemia and renal magnesium wasting in patients receiving cisplatin. Ann. Intern. Med. 90:929, 1979.
325. Hill, J. B.; Blachley, J. D.; and Trotter, M. Hypomagnesemia, hypocalcemia, and hypokalemia with cis-platinum treatment. Clin. Res. 26:780A, 1978.
326. Anderson, T.; Javadpour, N.; Schilsky, R.; Barlock, A.; and Young, R. C. Chemotherapy for testicular cancer: Current status of the National Cancer Institute combined modality trial. Cancer Treat. Rep. 63:1687, 1979.
327. Gordon, J. A.; Peterson, L. N.; and Anderson, R. J. Water metabolism after cisplatin in the rat. Am. J. Physiol. 243:F36, 1982.
328. Schaeppi, U.; Heyman, I. A.; Fleischman, R. W.; Rosenkrantz, H.; Ilievski, V.; Phelan, R.; Cooney, D. A.; and Davis, R. D. cis-Dichlorodiammine-platinum(II)(NSC-119875): Preclinical toxicologic evaluation of intravenous infection in dogs, monkeys and mice. Toxicol. Appl. Pharmacol. 25:230, 1973.
329. Clifton, G.; Pearce, C.; O'Neill, W. M., Jr.; and Wallin, J. D. cis-Diamminedichloroplatinum decreases both neurohypophysial and plasma concentrations of vasopressin in the rat. Clin. Res. 29:458A, 1981.
330. Chopra, S.; Kaufman, J. S.; Chase, D.; and Flamenbaum, W. Initiation phase of cis-diamminedichloroplatinum-induced acute renal failure in rats. Abstract of the 13th Annual Meeting of the American Society of Nephrology, Washington, D. C., 1980, p. 89A.
331. Safirstein, R.; Miller, P.; Dikman, S.; Lyman, N.; and Shapiro, C. Cisplatin nephrotoxicity in rats: Defect in papillary hypertonicity. Am. J. Physiol. 241:F175, 1981.
332. McCarthy, W. H.; and Keenan, R. L. Propoxyphene hydrochloride poisoning. J.A.M.A. 187:460, 1964.
333. Gustafson, A.; and Gustafson, B. Acute poisoning with dextropropoxyphene. Acta Med. Scand. 200:241, 1976.
334. Hudson, P.; Barringer, M.; and McBay, A. J. Fatal poisoning with propoxyphene: Report from 100 consecutive series. South. Med. J. 70:938, 1977.
335. Bower, B. F.; Wegienka, L. C.; and Forsham, P. H. In vitro studies of the mechanism of polyuria induced by dextropropoxyphene (Darvon). Proc. Soc. Exp. Biol. Med. 120:155, 1965.
336. Van Dyk, J. J.; Folkson, H. C.; and Van der Merwe, A. M. Unexpected toxicity in patients treated with isophosphamide. Cancer Res. 32:921, 1972.
337. DeFronzo, R. A.; Abeloff, M.; Braine, H.; Humphrey, R. L.; and Davis, P. J. Renal dysfunction after treatment with isophosphamide. Cancer Chem. Rep. 58:375, 1974.
338. DeFronzo, R. A.; Braine, H.; Colvin, O. M.; and Davis, P. J. Water intoxication in man after cyclophosphamide therapy. Ann. Intern. Med. 78:861, 1973.
339. Strandloy, J. W.; Morris, M.; and Buckalew, V. M., Jr. Renal effects of the antihypertensive, guanabenz, in the dog. J. Pharmacol. Exp. Ther. 221:347, 1982.

340. Roman, R. J.; Cowley, A. W., Jr.; and Lechene, C. Water diuretic and natriuretic effect of clonidine in the rat. J. Pharmacol. Exp. Ther. 211:385, 1979.
341. Chrysant, S. G.; and Lavender, A. P. Direct renal hemodynamic effects of clondine. Arch. Int. pharmacodyn. Ther. 218:207, 1975.
342. Humphrey, M. H.; and Reid, I. A. Acute effect of clonidine on renal water excretion. Clin. Res. 22:532, 1974.
343. Strandloy, J. W.; Steg, B. D.; and Buckalew, V. M., Jr. Antagonism of the hydro-osmotic effect of vasopressin by the antihypertensive, guanabenz. Life Sci. 27:2513, 1980.
344. Dousa, T. P.; and Barnes, L. D. Effects of colchicine and vinblastine on the cellular action of vasopressin in mammalian kidney. A possible role for microtubules. J. Clin. Invest. 54:252, 1974.
345. Yuasa, H.; Urakabe, S.; Kimura, G.; Shirai, D.; Takamitsu, R.; Orita, Y.; and Abe, H. Effect of colchicine on the osmotic water flow across the toad urinary bladder. Biochim. Biophys. Acta 413:277, 1975.
346. Taylor, A.; Mamelak, M.; Golbetz, H.; and Maffly, R. Evidence for involvement of microtubules in the action of vasopressin in toad urinary bladder. J. Membr. Biol. 40: 213, 1978.
347. Wilson, L.; and Taylor, A. Evidence for involvement of microtubules in the action of vasopressin in toad urinary bladder. II. Colchicine binding properties of toad bladder epithelial cell tubulin. J. Membr. Biol. 40:237, 1978.
348. Reaven, E.; Maffly, R.; and Taylor, A. Evidence for involvement of microtubules in toad urinary bladder. III. Morphological studies on the content and distribution of microtubule in bladder epithelial cells. J. Membr. Biol. 40:251, 1978.
349. Cutting, H. O. Inappropriate secretion of antidiuretic hormone secondary to vincrestine therapy. Am. J. Med. 51:269, 1971.
350. Robertson, G. L.; Bhoopalam, N.; and Zelkowitz, L. J. Vincristine neurotoxicity and abnormal secretion of antidiuretic hormone. Arch. Intern. Med. 132:717, 1973.
351. Rosenthal, S.; and Kaufman, S. Vincristine neurotoxicity. Ann. Intern. Med. 80:733, 1974.
352. Sawyer, W. H.; Pang, P. K. T.; Seto, J.; McEnroe, M.; Lammek, B.; and Manning, M. Vasopressin analogs that antagonize antidiuretic responses by rats to the antidiuretic hormone. Science 212:49, 1981.
353. Sawyer, W. H.; Grzonka, Z.; and Manning, M. Neurohypophysial peptides. Design of tissue-specific agonists and antagonists. Mol. Cell. Endocrinol. 22:117, 1981.
354. Jard, S. Personal communication, quoted in: Manning, M.; and Sawyer, W. H. Antagonists of vasopressor and antidiuretic responses to arginine vasopressin. Ann. Intern. Med. 96:520, 1982.
355. Relman, A. S.; and Schwartz, W. B. The kidney in potassium depletion. Am. J. Med. 24:764, 1958.
356. Schwartz, W. B.; and Relman, A. S. Effects of electrolyte disorders on renal structure and function. N. Engl. J. Med. 276:383, 1965.
357. Oliver, J.; MacDowell, M.; Welt, L. G.; Holiday, M. A.; Hollander, W.; Winters, R. W.; Williams, T. F.; and Segar, W. E. The renal lesions of electrolyte imbalance. I. The structural alterations in potassium-depleted rats. J. Exper. Med. 106:563, 1957.
358. Hollander, W.; Winters, R. W.; Williams, T. F.; Bradley, J.; Oliver, J.; and Welt, L. G. Defect in the renal tubular reabsorption of water associated with potassium depletion in rats. Am. J. Physiol. 189:557, 1957.
359. Berl, T.; Linas, S. L.; Aisenberry, G. A.; and Anderson, R. J. On the mechanism of polyuria in potassium depletion. J. Clin. Invest. 60:620, 1977.
360. Blythe, W. B.; Newton, M.; Lazcano, F.; and Welt, L. G. Effect of water restriction on urinary concentrating ability of K-depleted rats. Am. J. Physiol. 199:912, 1960.

361. Holliday, M. A.; and Egan, T. J. Changes in GFR and C_{H_2O} before and after repair of K deficiency in rats. Am. J. Physiol. 202:773, 1962.
362. Bank, N.; and Aynedjian, H. S. A micropuncture study of the renal concentrating defect of potassium depletion. Am. J. Physiol. 206:1347, 1964.
363. Buckalew, V. M., Jr.; Ramirez, M. A.; and Goldberg, M. Free water reabsorption during solute diuresis in normal and potassium-depleted rats. Am. J. Physiol. 212:381, 1967.
364. Eknoyan, G.; Martinez-Maldonado, M.; Suki, W. N.; and Richie, Y. Renal diluting capacity in the hypokalemic rat. Am. J. Physiol. 219:933, 1970.
365. Luke, R. G.; Wright, F. S.; Fowler, N.; Kashgarian, M.; and Giebisch, G. H. Effects of potassium depletion on renal tubular chloride transport in the rat. Kidney Int. 14: 414, 1978.
366. Whinnery, M. A.; and Kunau, R. T. Effect of potassium deficiency on papillary plasma flow in the rat. Ann. J. Physiol. 6:F226, 1979.
367. Kunau, R. T. Function of ascending loop of Henle in the potassium deficient dog. Am. J. Physiol. 219:1071, 1970.
368. Jones, N. F.; Mylle, M.; and Gottschalk, C. W. Renal tubular microinjection studies in normal and potassium-depleted rats. Clin. Sci. 29:261, 1965.
369. Malnic, G.; Klose, R. M.; and Giebisch, G. Micropuncture study of renal potassium excretion in rat. Am. J. Physiol. 206:674, 1964.
370. Levine, D. Z.; Walker, T.; Nash, L. A.; and Raman, S. Effects of KCl infusions on proximal tubular function in normal and potassium-depleted rats. Kidney Int. 4:318, 1973.
371. Relman, A. S.; and Schwartz, W. B. The nephropathy of potassium depletion. N. Engl. J. Med. 255:195, 1956.
372. Muhrcke, R. C.; and Rosen, S. R. Hypokalemic nephropathy in rat and man: A light and electron microscopic study. Lab. Invest. 13:1359, 1964.
373. Darmady, E. M.; and Stranack, F. Microdissection of nephron in disease. Br. Med. Bull. 13:21, 1957.
374. Spongs, B.; Strous, F.; and Fitch, F. Zonal renal papillary droplet change with potassium. Arch. Pathol. 70:599, 1960.
375. Evan, A.; Huser, J.; Bengele, H. H.; and Alexander, E. A. The effect of alterations in dietary potassium on collecting system morphology in the rat. Lab. Invest. 42:668, 1980.
376. Stetson, D. L.; Wade, J. B.; and Giebisch, G. Morphologic alterations in the rat medullary collecting duct following potassium depletion. Kidney Int. 17:45, 1980.
377. Morrison, A. B.; and Panner, B. J. Lysosome induction in experimental potassium deficiency. Am. J. Pathol. 45:295, 1964.
378. Hollander, W.; Winters, R. W.; Bradley, J.; Williams, T. F.; Loring, W. E.; Oliver, J.; and Welt, L. G. The effect of potassium repletion on the renal concentrating defect, the renal structural changes, and the cardiac and skeletal muscle lesions produced by potassium depletion in rats. Clin. Res. 6:287, 1958.
379. Mahler, R. F.; and Stanbury, W. S. Potassium-losing renal disease; renal and metabolic observations on a patient sustaining renal wastage of potassium. Q. J. Med. 25:21, 1956.
380. Fourman, P.; and Leeson, P. M. Thirst and polyuria with a note on the effects of potassium deficiency and calcium excess. Lancet 1:268, 1959.
381. Smith, S. G.; and Kasater, T. E. A diabetes insipidus-like condition produced in dogs by a potassium deficient diet. Proc. Soc. Exper. Biol. Med. 74:427, 1950.
382. Brokaw, A. Renal hypertrophy and polydipsia in potassium-deficient rats. Am. J. Physiol. 172:333, 1953.
383. Kleeman, C. R.; and Maxwell, M. H. Contributory role of extrarenal factors in the polyuria of potassium depletion. N. Engl. J. Med. 260:268, 1959.

384. Eigler, J. O. C.; Salassa, R. M.; Bohn, R. C.; and Owen, C. A. Renal distribution of sodium in potassium depleted vitamin D-intoxicated rats. Am. J. Physiol. 202:1115, 1962.
385. Manitius, A.; Levitin, H.; Beck, D.; and Epstein, F. H. On the mechanism of impairment of renal concentrating ability in potassium depletion. J. Clin. Invest. 39:684, 1960.
386. Wilson, D. M.; and Kissane, J. M. The distribution of electrolytes in the kidneys of potassium deficient and normal rats in varying states of hydration. Lab. Invest. 11: 45, 1962.
387. Schwartz, W. B.; and Relman, A. S. Metabolic and renal studies in chronic potassium depletion resulting from overuse of laxatives. J. Clin. Invest. 32:258, 1953.
388. Pereira, V. G.; Wajchenberg, B. L.; Quintao, E. R.; and Machado, M. M. Electrolyte and renal changes in severe potassium depletion. Metabolism 14:800, 1965.
389. Black, D. A. K.; and Milne, M. D. Experimental potassium depletion in man. Clin. Sci. 11:397, 1952.
390. Blahd, W. H.; and Bassett, S. H. Potassium deficiency in man. Metabolism 2:218, 1953.
391. Fourman, P.; and Hervey, G. R. An experimental study of oedema in potassium deficiency. Clin. Sci. 14:75, 1955.
392. Muntwyler, E.; and Griffin, G. E. Creatinine clearance in normal and potassium deficient rats. Am. J. Physiol. 173:145, 1953.
393. Maude, D. L. Effects of K and ouabain on fluid transport and cell Na in proximal tubule in vitro. Am. J. Physiol. 216:1199, 1969.
394. Cardinal, J.; and Duchesneau, D. Effect of potassium on proximal tubular function. Am. J. Physiol. 234:F381, 1978.
395. Rubini, M. Water excretion in potassium-deficient man. J. Clin. Invest. 40:2215, 1961.
396. Levitin, H.; Manitius, A.; and Epstein, F. H. Urinary dilution in potassium deficiency. Yale J. Biol. Med. 32:390, 1960.
397. Holliday, M. A.; Segar, W. E.; Bright, M. D.; and Egan, T. The effect of potassium deficiency on the kidney. Pediatrics 26:950, 1960.
398. Gottschalk, C. W.; Mylle, M.; Jones, N. F.; Winters, R. W.; and Welt, L. G. Osmolality of renal tubular fluids in potassium-depleted rodents. Clin. Sci. 29:249, 1965.
399. Bennett, C. M. Urine concentration and dilution in hypokalemic and hypercalcemic dogs. J. Clin. Invest. 49:1447, 1970.
400. Whinnery, M. A.; and Kunau, R. T. Effect of potassium deficiency on papillary plasma flow. Am. J. Physiol. 6:F226, 1979.
401. Petersen, L. N. On the mechanism of the concentrating defect in potassium depletion: The role of papillary plasma flow. Proceedings of the 13th Annual Meeting of the American Society of Nephrology, Washington, D. C., 1980, p. 145A.
402. Beck, N.; and Shaw, J. O. Thromboxane and prostaglandin E in K depleted rat kidney. Proceedings of the 12th Annual Meeting of the American Society of Nephrology, Boston, 1979, p. 78A.
403. Pawlson, L. G.; Taylor, A.; Mintz, D. H.; Field, J. B.; and Davis, B. B. Effect of vasopressin on renal cyclic AMP generation in potassium deficiency and patients with sickle hemoglobin. Metabolism 19:694, 1970.
404. Beck, N.; and Webster, S. K. Impaired urinary concentrating ability and cyclic AMP in K-depleted rat kidney. Am. J. Physiol. 231:1204, 1976.
405. Gullner, H. G.; and Bartter, F. L. The role of urinary prostaglandin E and cyclic-AMP in the polyuria of hypokalemia in rats. Prostaglandins Med. 4:13, 1980.
406. Kim, J. K.; Schrier, R. W.; and Berl, T. Effect of hypokalemia on renal medullary cyclic AMP generation, metabolism and action. Clin. Res. 27:420A, 1979.
407. Zusman, R. M.; and Keiser, H. R. Prostaglandin biosynthesis by rabbit renomedullary interstitial cells in tissue culture. Stimulation by angiotensin II, bradykinin, and arginine vasopressin. J. Clin. Invest. 60:251, 1977.

408. Dusing, R. A.; Attallah, A. A.; Prezyna, A. P.; and Lee, J. B. Renal biosynthesis of prostaglandin E_2 and $F_{2\alpha}$: Dependence on extracellular potassium. J. Lab. Clin. Med. 92:669, 1978.
409. Galvez, O. G.; Roberts, B. W.; Bay, W. H.; and Ferris, T. F. Studies of the mechanism of polyuria with hypokalemia. Kidney Int. 10:583A, 1976.
410. Rutecki, G.; Greenspan, R.; Cox, J. W.; Robertson, G.; and Ferris, T. F. Studies of the diabetes insipidus with K-deficiency. Clin. Res. 27:499A, 1979.
411. Hood, V. L.; and Dunn, M. J. Urinary excretion of PGE_2 and $PGF_{2\alpha}$ in potassium-deficient rats. Prostaglandins 15:273, 1978.
412. Berl, T.; Aisenbrey, G. A.; and Linas, S. L. Renal concentrating defect in the hypokalemic rat is prostaglandin independent. Am. J. Physiol. 238:F37, 1980.
413. Stoff, J. S.; Rosa, R. M.; and Epstein, F. H. The concentrating defect of acute potassium depletion in man is independent of renal prostaglandins. Kidney Int. 16:874, 1979.
414. Allan, F. N. Hyperparathyroidism: Report of a case. Proc. Staff Meet. Mayo Clin. 6: 684, 1931.
415. Gutman, A. B.; Swenson, P. C.; and Parsons, W. B. The differential diagnosis of hyperparathyroidism. J.A.M.A. 103:87, 1934.
416. Cohen, S. I.; Fitzgerald, M. G.; Fourman, P.; Griffiths, W. J.; and deWardener, H. E. Polyuria in hyperparathyroidism. Q. J. Med. 26:423, 1957.
417. Dorhout Mees, E. J. Disturbed water-reabsorption by the renal tubules in two patients with hypercalcemia. Acta Med. Scand. 157:199, 1957.
418. Gill, J. R.; and Bartter, F. C. On the impairment of renal concentrating ability in prolonged hypercalcemia and hypercalciuria in man. J. Clin. Invest. 40:716, 1961.
419. Lightwood, R. Idiopathic hypercalcemia in infants with failure to thrive. Arch. Dis. Child. 27:302, 1952.
420. Dietrick, J. E.; Whedon, G. D.; and Shorr, E. Effect of immobilation upon various metabolic and physiological functions of normal man. Am. J. Med. 4:3, 1948.
421. Anderson, W. A. D. The renal lesion in hyperparathyroidism. Endocrinology 24:372, 1939.
422. Mulligan, R. M. Metastatic calcification associated with hypervitaminosis D haliphagia. Am. J. Pathol. 22:1293, 1946.
423. Becker, D. L.; Boggenstoss, A. H.; and Weir, J. F. Parenchymal calcification of the kidneys in patients with duodenal ulcer. Am. J. Clin. Pathol. 22:843, 1952.
424. Epstein, F. H.; Rivera, M. J.; and Carone, F. A. The effect of hypercalcemia induced by calciferol upon renal concentrating ability. J. Clin. Invest. 37:1702, 1958.
425. Manitius, A.; Levitin, H.; Beck, D.; and Epstein, F. H. On the mechanism of impairment of renal concentrating ability in hypercalcemia. J. Clin. Invest. 39:693, 1960.
426. Hasan, S. H. The clearance of vasopressin and deaminovasopressin from the circulation of normal and hypercalcemic rabbits. J. Endocrinol. 47:135, 1970.
427. Douglas, W. W.; and Poisner, A. M. Stimulus-secretion coupling in a neurosecretory organ: The role of calcium in the release of vasopressin from the neurohypophysis. J. Physiol. (Lond.) 172:1, 1964.
428. Douglas, W. W.; and Poisner, A. M. Calcium movement in the neurohypophysis of the rat and its relation to the release of vasopressin. J. Physiol. (Lond.) 172:19, 1964.
429. Mikiten, T. M.; and Douglas, W. W. Effect of calcium and other ions on vasopressin release from rat neurohypophysis stimulated electrically in vitro. Nature 207:302, 1965.
430. Russell, J. T.; and Thorn, N. A. Calcium and stimulus-secretion coupling in the neurohypophysis. I. 45-Calcium transport and vasopressin release in slices from ox neurohypophysis stimulated electrically or by a high potassium concentration. Acta Endocrinol. 76:449, 1974.

431. Nakazato, Y.; and Douglas, W. W. Vasopressin release from the isolated neurohypophysis induced by a calcium ionophore, X-537A. Nature 249:479, 1974.
432. Bank, N.; and Aynedjian, H. S. On the mechanism of hypothesnuria in hypercalcemia. J. Clin. Invest. 44:681, 1965.
433. Gardner, K. D.; and Vierling, J. M. Solids, water, and solutes in papillary region of the kidney. Am. J. Physiol. 217:58, 1969.
434. Levitt, M. F.; Halperin, M. H.; Polineros, D. P.; Sweet, A. Y.; and Gribetz, D. The effect of abrupt changes in plasma calcium concentrations on renal function and electrolyte excretion in man and monkey. J. Clin. Invest. 37:294, 1958.
435. Freedman, P.; Moulton, R.; and Spencer, A. G. The effect of intravenous calcium gluconate on the renal excretion of water and electrolytes. Clin. Sci. 17:247, 1958.
436. Grossman, J.; Mines, M. F.; Goldman, A. G.; and Wolfman, M. Effects of calcium on urine concentrating ability. J. Clin. Invest. 37:899, 1958.
437. Lindeman, R. D.; Lee, T. D.; Yiengst, M. J.; and Shock, N. W. Influence of age, renal disease, hypertension, diuretics, and calcium on the antidiuretic responses to suboptimal infusions of vasopressin. J. Lab. Clin. Med. 68:206, 1966.
438. Epstein, F. H.; Beck, D.; Carone, F. A.; Levitin, H.; and Manitius, A. Changes in renal concentrating ability produced by parathyroid extract. J. Clin. Invest. 38:1214, 1959.
439. Guignard, J. P.; Jones, N. F.; and Barraclough, M. A. Effect of brief hypercalcemia on free water reabsorption during solute diuresis. Evidence for impairment of sodium transport in Henle's loop. Clin. Sci. 39:337, 1970.
440. Beck, D.; Levitin, H.; and Epstein, F. H. Effect of intravenous infusions of calcium on renal concentrating ability. Am. J. Physiol. 197:1118, 1959.
441. Suki, W. N.; Eknoyan, G.; Rector, F. C.; and Seldin, D. W. The renal diluting and concentrating mechanism in hypercalcemia. Nephron 6:50, 1969.
442. DiBona, G. F. Effect of hypercalcemia on renal tubular sodium handling in the rat. Am. J. Physiol. 220:49, 1971.
443. Massry, S. G.; Coburn, J. W.; Chapman, L. W.; and Kleeman, C. R. Role of serum calcium, parathyroid hormone, and sodium chloride infusion on renal calcium and sodium clearances. Am. J. Physiol. 214:1403, 1968.
444. Wolf, A. V.; and Ball, S. M. Effect of intravenous calcium salts on renal excretion in the dog. Am. J. Physiol. 158:205, 1949.
445. Edwards, B. R.; Sutton, R. A. L.; and Dirks, J. H. Effect of calcium infusion on renal tubular reabsorption in the dog. Am. J. Physiol. 227:13, 1974.
446. LeGrimellec, C.; Roinel, N.; and Morel, F. Simultaneous Mg, Ca, P, K, Na, and Cl analysis in rat tubular fluid. III: During acute Ca plasma loading. Pflugers Arch. 346:171, 1974.
447. Brunette, M. G.; Vary, J.; and Carriere, S. Hypothenuria in hypercalcemia: A possible role of intrarenal blood flow (IRBF) redistribution. Pflugers Arch. 350:9, 1974.
448. Fourman, P.; Smith, J. W. G.; and McConkey, B. Defects of water reabsorption and of hydrogen ion excretion by the renal tubules in hyperparathyroidism. Lancet 1: 619, 1960.
449. Beck, N.; Singh, H.; Reed, S. W.; Murdaugh, H. V.; and Davis, B. B. Pathogenic role of cyclic-ADP in the impairment of urinary concentrating ability in acute hypercalcemia. J. Clin. Invest. 54:1049, 1974.
450. Bentley, P. J. The effects of ionic changes on water transfer across the isolated urinary bladder of the toad, Bufo marinus. J. Endocrinol. 18:327, 1959.
451. Petersen, M. J.; and Edelman, I. S. Calcium inhibition of the action of vasopressin on the urinary bladder of the toad. J. Clin. Invest. 43:583, 1964.
452. Argy, W. P.; Handler, J. S.; and Orloff, J. Ca^{++} and Mg^{++} effects on toad bladder response to cyclic AMP, theophylline, and ADH analogues. Am. J. Physiol. 213:803, 1967.

453. Goldfarb, S. Effects of calcium on ADH action in the cortical collecting tubule perfused in vitro. Am. J. Physiol. 243:F481, 1982.
454. Cuthbert, A. W.; and Wong, P. Y. D. Calcium release in relation to permeability changes in toad bladder epithelium following antidiuretic hormone. J. Physiol. 241: 407, 1974.
455. Arruda, J. A. L.; and Sabatini, S. Effect of quinidine on Na^+, H^+ and water transport by the turtle and toad bladders. J. Membr. Biol. 55:141, 1980.
456. Humes, H. D.; Simmons, C. F., Jr.; and Brenner, B. M. Effect of verapamil on the hydroosmotic response to antidiuretic hormone in toad urinary bladder. Am. J. Physiol. 239:F250, 1980.
457. Hardy, M. A. Intracellular calcium as a modulator of transepithelial permeability to water in frog urinary bladder. J. Cell. Biol. 76:787, 1978.
458. Taylor, A. E.; Eich, E.; Pearl, M.; and Brem, A. Role of cytosolic Ca^{++} and Na-Ca exchange in the action of vasopressin. INSERM 85:167, 1979.
459. Omachi, R. S.; Robbie, D. E.; Handler, J. S.; and Orloff, J. Effects of ADH and other agents on cyclic AMP accumulation in toad bladder epithelium. Am. J. Physiol. 226: 1152, 1974.
460. Marumo, F.; and Edelman, I. S. Effects of Ca and prostaglandin E on vasopressin activation of renal adenyl cyclase. J. Clin. Invest. 50:1613, 1971.
461. Serros, E. R.; and Kirschenbaum, M. A. Prostaglandin-dependent polyuria in hypercalcemia. Am. J. Physiol. 241:F224, 1981.
462. Okahara, T.; Abe, Y.; Imanishi, M.; Yukimura, T.; and Yamamoto, K. Effect of calcium on prostaglandin E_2 release in dogs. Am. J. Physiol. 241:F77, 1981.
463. Zenser, T. V.; and Davis, B. B. Effects of calcium on prostaglandin E_2 synthesis by rat inner medullary slices. Am. J. Physiol. 235:F213, 1978.
464. Zenser, T. V.; Herman, C. A.; and Davis, B. B. Effects of calcium and A23187 on renal inner medullary prostaglandin E_2 synthesis. Am. J. Physiol. 238:E371, 1980.
465. Feibusch, J.; Barbosa-Saldivas, J. L.; Bernstein, R. S.; and Robertson, G. L. Tumor-associated nephrogenic diabetes insipidus. Ann. Intern. Med. 92:797, 1980.
466. Crawford, J. D.; and Kennedy, G. C. Chlorothiazide in diabetes insipidus. Nature 183:891, 1959.
467. Earley, L. E.; and Orloff, J. The mechanism of antidiuresis associated with the administration of hydrochlorothiazide to patients with vasopressin-resistant diabetes insipidus. J. Clin. Invest. 41:1988, 1962.
468. Shirley, D. G.; Walter, S. J.; and Laycock, J. F. The role of sodium depletion in hydrochlorothiazide-induced antidiuresis in Brattleboro rats with diabetes insipidus. Clin. Sci. Molec. Med. 54:209, 1978.

13

Bartter's Syndrome

JOHN R. GILL, JR.
National Heart, Lung and Blood Institute, National Institutes of Health, Bethesda, Maryland

Bartter's syndrome was first described in two patients with growth retardation, hypertrophy, and hyperplasia of the juxtaglomerular apparatus of the kidney, increased amounts of circulating angiotensin II, normal blood pressure with decreased pressor responsiveness to angiotensin II, aldosteronism, hypokalemic alkalosis, and impaired urinary concentrating ability that was resistant to vasopressin (Pitressin) (1). Other abnormalities usually or occasionally present in these patients have been hyperreninemia, decreased pressor responsiveness to norepinephrine (2), hypomagnesemia (3), supranormal plasma bradykinin, supranormal urinary kallikrein, subnormal urinary kinins (4), hyperuricemia (5), supranormal urinary prostaglandins (PGs) (6-9), and decreased distal fractional chloride reabsorption (10). Bartter's syndrome occurs in patients of both sexes, but it may have a greater predilection for females; in one series of 25 patients only nine were males (11). Although Bartter's syndrome has been observed in patients of various racial backgrounds from different geographical areas, it continues to be a relatively rare disorder of unknown prevalence.

The presence of Bartter's syndrome at birth or during early life and its occurrence in two or more siblings (3,12) are features that suggest that the syndrome may be inherited. It should be noted, however, that in all of the reported families with Bartter's syndrome only one generation has been affected. In a family in which six of 13 siblings have Bartter's syndrome, five of the affected siblings have had children and none of them have signs or symptoms of the syndrome (12). Bartter's syndrome usually presents as a sporadic rather than as a familial disorder, however. In the sporadic cases the syndrome may develop in childhood or during adult life as late as the fifth decade (13). Whether the sporadic cases represent the same disorder as the familial cases is not presently known and probably cannot be answered until more detailed knowledge about the etiology of the syndrome becomes available.

The clinical features of Bartter's syndrome may also occur as a complication of certain renal disorders such as cystinosis (14,15) and glomerulonephritis (16). The syndrome presumably developed because damage to the kidney caused by the primary disease led to potassium wasting. Whether the excessive urinary potassium excretion was associated with a defect in distal fractional chloride reabsorption, as is the case in Bartter's syndrome (10), is unknown.

I. RENAL HISTOLOGY

Juxtaglomerular hypertrophy and hyperplasia was the most striking histological abnormality noted in renal tissue obtained from the two index cases (1). This renal abnormality was such a consistent finding in patients with Bartter's syndrome that it was considered a hallmark of the disorder. Indeed, when patients with the clinical features of Bartter's syndrome did not have this histological feature they were considered to have another disorder. It is now clear that juxtaglomerular hyperplasia is not unique to Bartter's syndrome; it has been observed in familial chloride diarrhea (17), chronic laxative abuse (18), and chronic covert vomiting (19). Thus, the juxtaglomerular hyperplasia appears to represent a renal response to biochemical and physiological changes which these gastrointestinal disorders and Bartter's syndrome have in common. The stimulatory effects of hypokalemia on renin secretion (20,21) suggest that potassium depletion may be a factor in the juxtaglomerular hyperplasia. The considerable variation in juxtaglomerular histology from normal (22) to striking hyperplasia and hypertrophy (1) in patients with potassium-losing nephropathy and hypokalemia suggests that a factor or factors other than potassium depletion may also be involved. One such factor may be decreased chloride transport at the macula densa resulting from either decreased delivery of chloride to the macula densa, as occurs during chronic hypochloremic alkalosis associated with gastrointestinal loss of chloride, or impaired chloride transport by macula densa cells, as may be the case in Bartter's syndrome (10). Experimental evidence suggests that chloride may be involved in the regulation of renin release by the macula densa (23). If this is, indeed, the case, then decreased chloride transport by the macula densa may contribute to the hyperreninemia in Bartter's syndrome and, long term, stimulate juxtaglomerular hyperplasia.

Other histopathological changes such as periglomerular fibrosis, glomerulosclerosis, and thickened and hypercellular arterial and arteriolar walls with perivascular sclerosis may be observed in patients with Bartter's syndrome. As these changes, like juxtaglomerular hyperplasia, may also be observed in extrarenal disorders (17-19), they presumably represent a renal response to the biochemical and physiological changes that the disorders show.

II. RENAL TUBULAR FUNCTION

A variety of abnormalities in renal tubular function have been observed in Bartter's syndrome. The most prominent and a hallmark of the disorder is increased secretion of potassium by the distal tubule; this causes excessive urinary potassium excretion and potassium depletion. Although initially the increased tubular secretion of potassium was attributed to overproduction of aldosterone (1), the failure of treatment with aminoglutethimide, an inhibitor of aldosterone biogenesis (24), or of bilateral adrenalectomy (25,26) to correct potassium wasting suggested that potassium hypersecretion was a primary tubular abnormality and that aldosterone was an aggravating factor. This hypothesis received additional support when studies of prolonged treatment with prostaglandin synthetase inhibitors showed correction of hyperreninemia and aldosteronism but not hypokalemia (27).

The cause of the increase in potassium secretion has been postulated to reside in another tubular abnormality, defective reabsorption of sodium chloride (10). Although patients with Bartter's syndrome have for the most part responded to a low sodium intake with normal sodium conservation (1,28), they have shown an exaggerated natriuresis in response to intravenous saline (12,28). This finding of an abnormality in the tubular handling of sodium chloride during sodium loading prompted a number of investigators to examine the status of tubular transport of sodium chloride in Bartter's syndrome in more detail. Renal clearance studies performed during infusion of hypotonic saline solution (13,29-32) or dextrose and water (10,32) showed a decrease in proximal tubular reabsorption (13,32), in distal tubular reabsorption (10,29,31), or in both (10,30,32). The decrease in proximal reabsorption was variable and usually present in patients with impaired glomerular filtration (10,13). In such patients, a relatively greater expansion of extracellular fluid volume may have contributed to the decrease in proximal reabsorption of sodium chloride via effects on renal hemodynamics and peritubular Starling forces (33). The decrease in distal sodium chloride reabsorption was a more consistent finding, being present in virtually all of the patients studied (10). Impaired solute-free water formation accompanied the impairment in distal tubular sodium chloride reabsorption (10); this suggested that the ascending limb of the loop of Henle was the site of abnormal sodium chloride transport.

Considerable data point to the thick ascending limb of the loop of Henle as the segment of the nephron responsible for dilution of tubular fluid (34). The epithelium of this portion of the nephron is impermeable to water and appears to reabsorb chloride actively, with sodium and potassium following passively (35). These concepts of the behavior of the diluting segment have been successfully adapted to determine maximal diluting capacity in vivo and, thereby, to assess chloride reabsorption by the thick ascending limb (36). Thus, during maximal water diuresis distal fractional chloride reabsorption can be estimated by the formula $C_{H_2O}/C_{H_2O} + C_{Cl}$, where C_{H_2O} is the clearance of solute-free water and C_{Cl} is the clearance of chloride (36). Values for distal fractional chloride reabsorption in patients with Bartter's syndrome were significantly lower than those in normal subjects, in patients with hypokalemia secondary to gastrointestinal loss (10), and in patients with another form of potassium-losing nephropathy (22). The ability of patients with Bartter's syndrome to conserve sodium normally in response to a restricted sodium intake could be explained if the defect in chloride reabsorption were limited to the thick ascending limb and a compensatory increase in absorption of sodium chloride occurred in unaffected, more distal tubule segments.

The cause of defective chloride reabsorption by the loop of Henle is unknown. Prostaglandin E has been shown to inhibit chloride transport by the thick ascending limb in vitro (37), and because it is overproduced by the kidney in Bartter's syndrome (7-9) PGE has been considered as a possible mediator of the impairment in distal fractional chloride reabsorption. This does not appear to be the case, however, as treatment of patients with Bartter's syndrome with a prostaglandin synthetase inhibitor does not affect distal fractional chloride reabsorption (10). In fact, distal fractional chloride reabsorption may be normal despite an overproduction of PGE by the kidneys, as is the case in a sibship with familial tubulopathy (22).

A defect in chloride transport in the thick ascending limb may increase potassium excretion by two mechanisms: First, passive reabsorption of potassium by the thick ascending limb depends on the transtubular potential difference generated by chloride reabsorption and will decrease when chloride reabsorption is decreased (35). Second, medullary hypertonicity depends on reabsorption of sodium chloride by the ascending limb of Henle's loop and will decrease when chloride reabsorption is decreased. A consequence of the decrease in osmotic gradient across the decending limb of Henle's loop is the delivery of a larger volume of more dilute tubule fluid to the ascending limb, thereby further limiting chloride reabsorption and increasing flow of tubular fluid through the distal convoluted tubule where potassium secretion is highly flow dependent (38). Although, in theory, an impairment in the function of the thick ascending limb may stimulate potassium loss as outlined above, an abnormality in tubular handling of sodium chloride is not essential for an increase in tubular potassium secretion to occur: three siblings with a familial tubulopathy secret potassium excessively despite apparently normal renal tubular handling of sodium chloride (22). Thus, alternatively, Bartter's syndrome could represent a primary defect in potassium secretion with the defect in chloride reabsorption stimulating further loss. Additional study is required to characterize the nature of the potassium loss more precisely.

Hypermagnesiuria and hypomagnesemia are usually but not always present in Bartter's syndrome. The increased excretion of magnesium has been attributed to defective magnesium reabsorption by the thick ascending limb because it is this segment of the tubule that regulates the rate of magnesium excretion in urine. The mechanism of magnesium transport by cells of the thick ascending limb has not been elucidated but there is some evidence that, like sodium and potassium, it may depend on chloride transport (39).

Magnesium depletion of renal or gastrointestinal origin can lead to potassium depletion and alkalosis (40). Although this interrelationship is not well understood, there is some evidence that aldosterone may play a role (41). Thus, in those patients with Bartter's syndrome who exhibit hypomagnesemia, the magnesium depletion may be an additional factor in the potassium loss. In one patient, correction of hypomagnesemia by infusing magnesium sulfate for several days was associated with partial correction of the hypokalemia (42). Administration of magnesium did not appear to affect the defect in chloride reabsorption, however (42).

Occasionally, hypercalciuria may be associated with the clinical features of Bartter's syndrome (14,43-46). As the tubular reabsorption of calcium is quite similar to that of magnesium, it is possible that the underlying abnormality that impairs magnesium reabsorption may sometimes impair calcium reabsorption. Serum magnesium was normal in these patients (14,44,45), however, and suggests the more likely alternative possibility that renal calcium loss was the primary event. In this case, the defect in the transport of calcium that leads to nephrocalcinosis may also lead to hyperreninemia (47), aldosteronism, and hypokalemia. Values for distal fractional chloride reabsorption were normal in five siblings with hypercalciuria (46), suggesting that this variable is probably normal in calcium-losing nephropathy.

The frequent occurrence of hyperuricemia and acute gouty arthritis in Bartter's syndrome (5) suggests that the tubular handling of uric acid may be impaired. As hypokalemic alkalosis and hyperreninemia associated with a variety of disorders, some of them extrarenal, have been reported to increase the concentration of serum uric acid, biochemical and physiological changes rather than an intrinsic tubular abnormality in urate transport appear to be a more probable cause of this abnormality in Bartter's syndrome (19,48-50). The observations that alkalosis (5) and angiotensin II (51) can each decrease the clearance of uric acid support this assumption.

Chondrocalcinosis may also be a cause of arthritis in Bartter's syndrome (52). The affected patients were hypomagnesemic and this was considered a factor in the deposition of pyrophosphate crystals in their joints. Improvement in symptoms and decrease in intra-articular calcium deposits have been observed following magnesium treatment (53).

The abnormalities in tubular transport cited above may mediate other derangements in renal function. The impairment in chloride reabsorption may explain in part the decreased ability of patients with Bartter's syndrome to concentrate their urine, as reabsorption of sodium chloride by the ascending limb of the loop of Henle is required to generate and maintain a hypertonic medullary interstitium and provide the osmotic gradient necessary to abstract water from tubular fluid (54). Potassium depletion, a well-established cause of impaired renal concentrating ability, may also be a factor leading to the loss of concentrating ability in Bartter's syndrome. Although it is not known how hypokalemia affects the renal concentrating process, there is some evidence that it may impair cyclic adenosine monophosphate (cAMP) generation (55) (see Ch. 12). Although PGs, which are overproduced in many hypokalemic disorders, including Bartter's syndrome (56), may antagonize the stimulation of adenylate cyclase by vasopressin (57), hypokalemia may also directly impair the formation of cAMP by adenylate cyclase (55). In any event, the failure of treatment with a prostaglandin synthetase inhibitor to affect maximal urinary osmolality in patients with Bartter's syndrome suggests that prostaglandins probably do not play an important role in the pathogenesis of the concentrating defect in this disorder (54).

Potassium depletion is a major determinant of the hyperreninemia of Bartter's syndrome. An association of hypokalemia and hyperreninemia has been observed in other hypokalemic disorders of renal and extrarenal origin (14,18,19,22,43-46,48-50,53,56) and in animal studies in which potassium loss has been experimentally produced (58,59). Although studies in the potassium-depleted rat indicate that the hyperreninemia may be suppressed by dilatation of the renal afferent arteriole by papaverine (60) or by expansion of intravascular volume by hyperoncotic albumin (61), the precise mechanism whereby potassium depletion stimulates renin release is still to be elucidated. Whatever the initiating stimulus may be, studies to date indicate that PGs play an important modulating role in the hyperreninemia that results; treatment with a prostaglandin synthetase inhibitor corrects the hyperreninemia despite persistence of hypokalemia (58). The renal excretion of both PGE_2 and 6-keto-$PGF_{1\alpha}$, a metabolite of prostacyclin, are increased in Bartter's syndrome (62) and in experimental potassium depletion (59). Whereas infusion of either PGE_2 or prostacyclin into a renal artery increases release of renin, prostacyclin appears to be the PG responsible for modulating renin release in vivo (63).

For the most part, the disorders of potassium depletion characterized by an increase in urinary PGs such as potassium-losing nephropathies (7-9,22), psychogenic vomiting (18,49, 56), diuretic abuse (50,56), and experimental potassium depletion (58,59) usually show an increase in plasma renin activity. The hyperreninemia could be an important stimulus for renal PG synthesis in these conditions as angiotensin II and bradykinin, which may be increased also in Bartter's syndrome (4), can stimulate PGE_2 synthesis by renal tissue (64,65). The observation that treatment of dogs with desoxycorticosterone can increase urinary PGE despite suppression of plasma renin activity (66) suggests that factors other than angiotensin II stimulate renal synthesis of PGE_2 in potassium depletion. One such factor may be the direct effects of subnormal potassium concentration on PG synthesis. In vitro studies have shown a release of PGs from renal tissue into incubation media at low potassium concentrations (67).

A growing body of evidence also suggests that chloride reabsorption by the macula densa may be a determinant of renin release. Stimulation of renin release by selective chloride depletion has been observed to occur independently of a change in arterial pressure, glomerular filtration rate, plasma volume, or plasma potassium concentration (23). Conversely, when renin release has been stimulated by sodium deprivation, administration of either sodium chloride or choline chloride are more effective than other sodium salts in suppressing renin release. When chloride reabsorption in the thick ascending limb, which includes the macula densa, is blocked by a diuretic such as furosemide, renin release is stimulated before sodium loss occurs and when contraction of extracellular fluid is prevented (23). This mechanism of renin release, like that of baroreceptor-mediated renin release (47), may depend upon prostaglandins. Thus, in Bartter's syndrome, if the thick ascending limb is the locus of impaired chloride reabsorption, as is thought to be the case, then the macula densa may also be sufficiently involved to stimulate renin release.

III. CARDIOVASCULAR FUNCTION

Experimental potassium deletion in the dog is associated with a decrease in peripheral resistance and an increase in cardiac output and plasma volume without a change in blood pressure (58). These changes appear to represent effects of hypokalemia on vascular function as plasma renin activity (58,59) and sympathoadrenal activity (68) are increased in this and other experimental models of potassium depletion. That an increase in activity of these vasopressor systems was important in the maintenance of a normal blood pressure was indicated by the significant decline in pressure that occurred when an angiotensin II antagonist was given to potassium-depleted dogs (58). Furthermore, these dogs also showed a decrease in vascular responsiveness to infusions of angiotensin II (58). Thus, the increases in plasma renin activity and in plasma catecholamines appear to be primarily compensatory changes that occur to stabilize blood pressure in response to vascular vasodilation. The possibility that hypokalemia may also stimulate the renin-angiotensin or sympathetic systems directly cannot be excluded, however.

The vascular resistance to vasopressors appears to be mediated by PGs which increase pari passu with potassium depletion (58,59); treatment with a PG synthetase inhibitor corrects both the overproduction of PGs and the vascular resistance but not the hypokalemia (58). The observation that the formation of PGs by vascular strips increases when potassium concentration of the bathing media is decreased (69) provides further support for the notion that hypokalemia stimulates synthesis of PGs by vascular tissue and that these vasodilator PGs are responsible for the decrease in peripheral resistance and, in part, the diminished vascular responsiveness to vasopressors. The high circulating angiotensin II may itself contribute to the vascular resistance to angiotensin II through down regulation of its receptors (70). Whether or not circulating angiotensin II constitutes an additional stimulus for vascular synthesis of PGs in potassium depletion is uncertain. Although peptides such as antiotensin II and bradykinin stimulate the synthesis of PGs by vascular tissue in vitro (64), the increase in PG synthesis induced by hypokalemia together with a reduction in angiotensin II receptors may limit any further effect of angiotensin II on PG synthesis. A summary of the pathophysiological changes that can be induced by experimental potassium depletion are presented in Table 1.

The findings in patients with Bartter's syndrome tend to mirror those of experimental potassium depletion. Although data are inadequate to draw definitive conclusions about peripheral resistance in Bartter's syndrome, the observations that plasma volume is normal (71), that pressor resistance to angiotensin II and norepinephrine is increased (2), that plasma renin activity and pressor resistance to angiotensin II may decrease in response to expansion of intravascular volume (13,24,28,31), and that a large decrease in blood pressure may occur in response to an angiotensin II antagonist (72-74) are consistent with an underlying

Table 1 Pathophysiological Changes Induced by Experimental Potassium Depletion

Increased urinary prostaglandins (PGE_2, 6-keto-$PGF_{1}\alpha$)
Decreased peripheral resistance
Increased pressor resistance to angiotensin II
Increased plasma renin activity
Increased sympathetic nervous system activity
Impaired urinary concentrating ability

state of vasodilatation. The increase in adrenergic activity that usually accompanies the hyperreninemia (75) and the large falls in blood pressure that follow the administration of an angiotensin II antagonist (72-74) support the notion that increases in activity of these two vasopressor systems are counteracting vasodilatory stimuli to maintain blood pressure. The stimuli for vascular dilatation are, presumably, the increase in plasma bradykinin (4) and an increase in vasodilator PGs in blood vessels. The foregoing pathogenetic schema and the hypothesis that increased formation of PGs by vascular tissue is the proximate cause of these changes are also supported by the observation that inhibition of prostaglandin synthesis corrects the pressor resistance, supranormal plasma bradykinin, hyperreninemia, and increased adrenergic activity (4,8,71,75).

The specific PG (or PGs) synthesized by vascular tissue in response to potassium depletion is uncertain. Supranormal urinary PGE and 6-keto-$PGF_{1\alpha}$, a metabolite of prostacyclin, observed in hypokalemic states have been attributed to increased synthesis of PGE and prostacyclin by the kidney (7-9,59,62). As the synthesis of prostacyclin by vascular strips in vitro may be stimulated by a low potassium concentration (69), it has been postulated that potassium deficiency may stimulate the synthesis of PGs by vascular tissue in vivo. This hypothesis has not been supported by the estimates of systemic production of PGE (8) or of prostacyclin (76) in Bartter's syndrome; they have both been normal. Another vasodilator PG such as PGD_2, which is also increased in Bartter's syndrome (77), may mediate the vasodilatation induced by potassium depletion. Alternatively, it may be that current methods for estimating systemic production can not detect an increase in synthesis of PGE or prostacyclin in vascular tissue.

Although inhibition of prostaglandin synthesis restores pressor responsiveness to angiotensin II to normal, PGs and bradykinin may not be the only determinants of pressor resistance to angiotensin II in Bartter's syndrome. Treatment with captopril, an angiotensin-converting enzyme inhibitor, lowered plasma angiotensin II to normal and partially corrected the pressor resistance to angiotensin II (78,79). The reduction in pressor resistance following captopril was not as great as that following indomethacin, however (78). These results

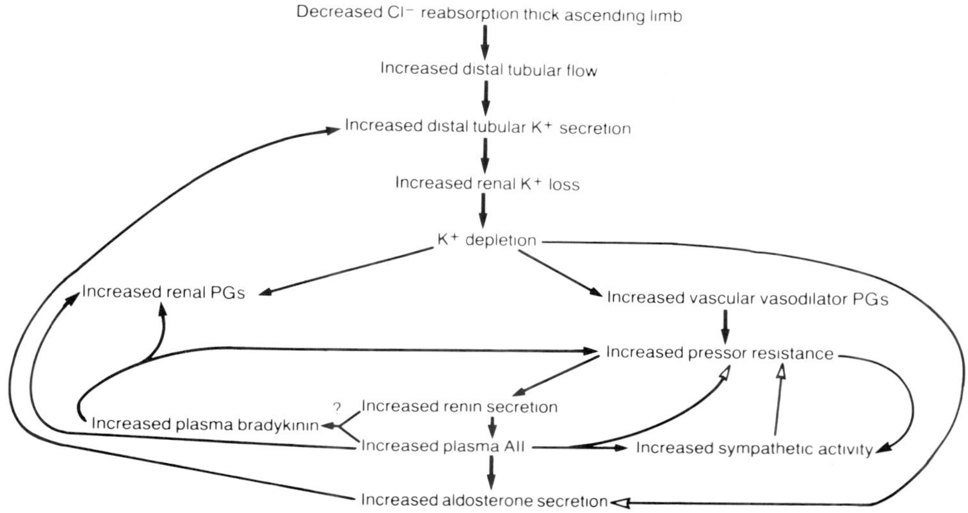

Fig. 1. Proposed schema for the pathogenesis of Bartter's syndrome. The solid arrows indicate a stimulatory action and the open arrows an inhibitory action.

Table 2 Effects of Indomethacin on the Abnormalities of Bartter's Syndrome

Persistent Abnormalities
Impaired distal fractional chloride reabsorption
Renal potassium wasting
Renal magnesium wasting
Impaired urinary concentrating ability
Corrected Abnormalities
Overproduction of renal prostaglandins
Increased pressor resistance to angiotensin II and norepinephrine
Increased plasma renin activity
Increased sympathetic nervous system activity
Increased plasma bradykinin
Increased plasma aldosterone
Increased urinary kallikrein

suggest that the high concentrations of angiotensin II in Bartter's syndrome may reduce angiotensin II receptors and represent an additional determinant of the pressor resistance to angiotensin II (70).

Although the increase in plasma bradykinin is linked to the increase in PG synthesis, the precise cause of the increase in bradykinin is unknown. A direct relationship between plasma bradykinin and plasma renin activity has been observed in normal subjects and has been thought to represent modulatory regulation of the pressor activity of angiotensin II by bradykinin (80). What relationship, if any, the increase in plasma bradykinin has to the reduction in urinary kinins that also occur in Bartter's syndrome is also unknown (4). Urinary kallikrein is high, and this is most likely caused by the high aldosterone. The increase in urinary kallikrein probably is not responsible for the change in urinary kinins as an increase in kallikrein is usually associated with an increase in kinins (4).

The abnormalities in renal tubular and cardiovascular function discussed above may be interrelated as depicted in the pathogenetic schema in Fig. 1. Treatment with indomethacin does not affect the impairment in distal fractional chloride reabsorption (10) and produces only a transient decrease in renal potassium loss, presumably as a result of renal hemodynamic changes (8), but it does correct many other features of the syndrome (Table 2). The sequence of events in Fig. 1 assumes that the prostaglandin-independent renal abnormalities are the basis for prostaglandin overproduction and those prostaglandin-dependent abnormalities.

IV. RED BLOOD CELL FUNCTION

The membranes of the red blood cell contain mechanisms for transport of ions which are similar to those in epithelial tissues such as the kidney. The possibility that the abnormal transport of ions in the renal tubule in Bartter's syndrome might be a manifestation of a generalized membrane defect has led investigators to study red blood cells from patients with the syndrome. An increase in sodium concentration in red blood cells was the most consistent finding in these studies (81-85). The reported transport abnormalities associated with high intracellular sodium have been more variable, however, and these differences may be attributable, for the most part, to differences in methodology. Some investigators used ouabain to define active sodium efflux (83), some used ethacrynic acid (82), and some used ouabain and either ethacrynic acid (81,84) or furosemide (85). In some studies the red blood cells were loaded with sodium before study (85), in others they were not (84). Although one study reported a decrease in sodium efflux (82), most of the studies reported an increase (81,83-85). The two most recent studies observed an increase in the rate constant for passive sodium efflux and hypothesized an increase in passive sodium permeability in red cells in Bartter's syndrome (84,85). It has not been possible to confirm this latter finding, however. In studies of red blood cells from nine patients with Bartter's syndrome, sodium concentration, ouabain-sensitive and furosemide-sensitive sodium effluxes were all increased, but the rate constant for ouabain- and furosemide-resistant sodium efflux (so-called passive permeability) was normal (86). Correction of hypokalemia in these patients by treatment with supplemental potassium restored sodium concentration, ouabain-sensitive and furosemide-sensitive sodium effluxes to normal without a change in the rate constant for passive sodium efflux (86). Such results suggest that the abnormalities in sodium concentration and efflux in red blood cells in Bartter's syndrome result from a low potassium milieu inhibiting function of the sodium-potassium ATPase and not from an intrinsic abnormality of membrane transport processes.

Although the studies in red blood cells do not support the presence of a transport defect such as that in the kidney, a study of parotid saliva is compatible with the presence of such a defect in the parotid gland. Sodium concentrations in parotid saliva were low in patients with primary aldosteronism and extrarenal potassium loss but high in those with Bartter's syndrome (87). These results await confirmation and explanation.

V. PLATELET FUNCTION

Studies of platelet function in Bartter's syndrome have shown defective platelet aggregation in patients with a normal bleeding time (88). This abnormality was corrected by transferring the platelets to plasma from normal subjects. It was further observed that defective aggregation by normal platelets could be induced by transferring them to plasma from patients with Bartter's syndrome. These observations suggested that a "plasma factor" was responsible for abnormal aggregation. Since treatment with a prostaglandin synthetase inhibitor improved defective platelet aggregation, it was further suggested that this plasma factor was probably a prostaglandin or metabolite (88). A supranormal content of cyclic AMP found in the platelet-rich plasma from Bartter's syndrome was thought to mediate the effect of the plasma factor on aggregation (88).

In other studies, patients with Bartter's syndrome who also exhibited a defect in platelet aggregation had subnormal basal cyclic AMP production by their platelets (89). Furthermore, adenylate cyclase stimulation with PGE_1 increased cyclic AMP less than the normal stimulated control value (89). Although the cause of the impairment in cyclic AMP formation is not known, it is possible that potassium depletion, which has been shown to impair cyclic AMP formation by the kidney (55), was responsible. Whether potassium depletion also mediated the defect in platelet aggregation is unknown. Why these two studies of platelet function in Bartter's syndrome yielded different results is not clear and must await further study.

VI. GROWTH AND DEVELOPMENT

Delayed growth and development was a prominent feature of the index cases of Bartter's syndrome (1) and proportional dwarfism has been a cardinal feature of the syndrome when it has occurred in early childhood (90). Also, many patients who developed the syndrome during the first year of life showed some degree of mental retardation. The onset of puberty may also be delayed, usually until the adolescent growth spurt begins in the late teens, with normal sexual function and normal height attained by the twentieth year. Although measurements of plasma growth hormone in these patients have not shown a consistent abnormality, plasma insulin has frequently been high in association with normal as well as abnormal carbohydrate tolerance (90). Although the abnormalities of growth and development are probably a reflection of potassium depletion, potassium administration has usually had little effect on them (90). In recent studies, the addition of a prostaglandin synthetase inhibitor to the treatment regimen has appeared to stimulate catch-up growth in children with Bartter's syndrome, probably because it has also enhanced potassium retention (91).

VII. DIFFERENTIAL DIAGNOSIS

Many features of Bartter's syndrome such as hyperreninemia, aldosteronism, increased adrenergic activity, increased pressor resistance to angiotensin II and norepinephrine, and increased urinary PGE are the result of potassium depletion (56) and are not unique to Bartter's syndrome. Consequently, the various disorders shown in Table 3 can produce potassium loss and may exhibit any or all of the above features which we associate with Bartter's syndrome. Hyperplasia of the juxtaglomerular apparatus is present in some of these disorders (14-19, 43-45,50,53) but not in others (22,92,93). The occurrence of juxtaglomerular hyperplasia in a variety of hypokalemic disorders indicates that it is not unique to Bartter's syndrome and further suggests that its presence is not a sufficient criterion for diagnosis of the syndrome. On the other hand, juxtaglomerular hyperplasia has always been considered a requirement for the diagnosis of Bartter's syndrome and in the absence of this finding a diagnosis of the syndrome probably should not be made. Decreased distal fractional chloride reabsorption appears to be a consistent feature of Bartter's syndrome that, with few exceptions, does not occur in patients with hypokalemia of other etiologies. Until the molecular basis for the disordered tubular function has been elucidated, measurement of distal fractional chloride reabsorption appears to be the best available tool to distinguish Bartter's syndrome from other potassium-losing nephropathies. An important exception is the potassium-losing nephropathy induced by diuretics. The covert abuse of diuretics, especially furosemide,

Table 3 Differential Diagnosis of Bartter's Syndrome

1. Potassium-losing nephropathy
   a. Bartter's syndrome
   b. Covert diuretic abuse
   c. Familial tubulopathy
2. Magnesium-losing nephropathy
3. Calcium-losing nephropathy
4. Chronic renal disease
   a. Nephritis
   b. Cystinosis
5. Gastrointestinal disorders
   a. Covert vomiting
   b. Covert laxative abuse
   c. Familial chloride diarrhea

ethacrynic acid, and bumetamide that inhibit chloride reabsorption in the thick ascending limb of Henle's loop (35), can mimic the defect in tubular chloride transport and simulate Bartter's syndrome (50,94). Thus, adults who appear to have Bartter's syndrome and show subnormal distal fractional chloride reabsorption should have their urine tested for diuretics to confirm a suspicion of covert diuretic abuse or to establish a diagnosis of Bartter's syndrome.

Renal potassium wasting has recently been observed in three of four siblings (22). Renal tissue from the affected children showed normal glomeruli and juxtaglomerular apparatus, but proximal tubule cells with hypertrophy of the basement membrane and dense-staining cytoplasm. Evaluation of renal sodium chloride handling by clearance techniques showed normal proximal and distal reabsorption. This familial tubulopathy also exhibited a genetic linkage with the histocompatibility system and a low serum uric acid, additional features that distinguish this disorder from Bartter's syndrome. The prevalence of this tubulopathy is unknown but examination of renal tissue and measurement of distal fractional chloride reabsorption in children with potassium-losing nephropathy should uncover additional patients with this disorder.

Magnesium depletion can lead to renal potassium loss (40,53,95-98). Whether the increase in potassium excretion is the consequence of hyperreninemia and aldosteronism or some other effect of hypomagnesemia on tubular function is unclear. The juxtaglomerular apparatus is usually normal (96-98), although it may be prominent (53). When magnesium-losing nephropathy is associated with prominence of the juxtaglomerular apparatus, it can be difficult to distinguish from Bartter's syndrome. The response of serum and urinary potassium to treatment with magnesium may be a useful distinguishing feature, but Bartter's syndrome can also show potassium retention when treated with magnesium (42). In some patients the hypermagnesuria was accompanied by hypocalciuria (53,96) which improved with magnesium administration (53). When estimated, distal fractional chloride reabsorption has been normal, but more patients need to be studied to establish this finding as a reliable differential feature.

Calcium-losing nephropathy may also be associated with hyperreninemia and aldosteronism and juxtaglomerular hyperplasia (14,43-45,98,99), although the latter finding may not be present in all cases (99). Why the defect in tubular transport of calcium is associated with hyperreninemia is unknown but the inverse relationship between calcium and renin secretion (47) suggests that regulation of calcium content of renin-secreting cells may be abnormal. Blood pressure may be normal or high (44). These patients can usually be recognized by their hypercalciuria and frequently have nephrocalcinosis and a history of stone (14,43-45,97). Estimates of distal fractional chloride reabsorption in six siblings were normal (46).

Some patients with chronic renal diseases such as cystinosis (14,15) or glomerulonephritis (16) may develop secondary renal potassium wasting, hyperreninemia with aldosteronism, and juxtglomerular hyperplasia. Presumably, the renal potassium loss is the result of tubular damage caused by the primary disorder. The underlying diseases responsible for the potassium loss can usually be recognized without difficulty.

Gastrointestinal loss of potassium by covert vomiting (19,49) or covert laxative abuse (18) can produce severe hypokalemic alkalosis, hyperreninemia with aldosteronism, and juxtaglomerular hyperplasia. Despite hypokalemia, renal excretion of potassium may be inappropriately high because of the high filtered load of bicarbonate delivered to the distal nephron. These patients can usually be recognized by their low urinary chloride excretion relative to that of sodium or by their low urinary sodium and chloride excretion during a constant normal intake of these ions (approximately 100 meq/day of sodium and of chloride). Rarely, the gastrointestinal loss of potassium and chloride can be caused by familial chloride diarrhea, an inherited disorder of gastrointestinal ion transport (48). This disease can usually be readily diagnosed by history, character of the stools, and measurement of chloride in the urine.

VIII. MANAGEMENT

Therapy of Bartter's syndrome is directed toward correction of hypokalemia and, when present, hypomagnesemia and improvement of the associated symptoms of tiredness, easy fatigability, muscle weakness, and muscle cramps. The amount of potassium usually required to bring serum potassium into the normal range is 30-40 meq every 3-4 hr. Although this regimen can be managed for short periods of time in hospital, it is unrealistic for prolonged treatment because of gastrointestinal irritation, and the logistical demands of such frequent dosing. These problems can be resolved by giving less potassium supplementation, 90-160 meq/day given in three or four divided doses, and by adding therapeutic agents that decrease the renal excretion of potassium. It is also difficult to raise serum magnesium into the normal range by oral supplementation. The administration of magnesium, 30-60 meq/day in three or four divided doses, is usually adequate to relieve the symptoms of tetany and muscle cramps despite persistence of a subnormal plasma magnesium.

Many of the abnormalities in Bartter's syndrome that are mediated by prostaglandins such as hyperreninemia and aldosteronism can be corrected by treatment with a prostaglandin synthetase inhibitor (6-9). When first administered, prostaglandin inhibitors produce considerable potassium retention, apparently as a result of renal hemodynamic changes (7, 8), and some improvement does persist, although this initial decrease in renal potassium excretion is not sustained (27). Prolonged administration of full therapeutic dosages of these inhibitors is not feasible because of abdominal discomfort or peptic ulceration, fluid retention, or other distressing side effects. Most patients can tolerate a smaller dose and with the addition of supplemental potassium it is possible to improve the potassium deficiency with few side effects. This is especially so in children where the combination of aspirin or other prostaglandin synthetase inhibitors and supplemental potassium has proven to be very effective therapy (9,91,99).

In some patients supplemental potassium and treatment with a prostaglandin synthetase inhibitor may not provide adequate correction of the hypokalemia. When this is the case a potassium-sparing diuretic such as triamterene or amiloride may be added to the regimen (100).

The approach to management outlined above can foster catch-up growth and development in children (91) and allow most patients with Bartter's syndrome to lead a relatively normal life. With appropriate adjustments in therapy, patients with Bartter's syndrome may be managed through pregnancy (101) or a major operation without experiencing any untoward effects of hypokalemia.

REFERENCES

1. Bartter, F.C.; Pronove, P.; Gill, J. R., Jr.; and MacCardle, R.C. Hyperplasia of the juxtaglomerular complex with hyperaldosteronism and hypokalemic alkalosis. Am. J. Med. 33:811-828, 1962.
2. Gill, J. R., Jr.; and Bartter, F. C. Hyperplasia of the juxtaglomerular complex with hyperaldosteronism and hypokalemic alkalosis. In: Water and Electrolyte Metabolism II, edited by DeGraeff, J., and Leijnse, B. Amsterdam, Elsevier, 1964, pp. 119-124.

3. Sutherland, L. E.; Hartroft, P.; Balis, U.; Bailey, J. D.; and Lynch, M. J. Bartter's syndrome. Acta Paediatr. Scand. (Suppl) 201:1-24, 1970.
4. Vinci, J. M.; Gill, J. R., Jr.; Bowden, R. E.; Pisano, J. J.; Izzo, J. L., Jr.; Radfar, N.; Taylor, A. A.; Zusman, R. M.; Bartter, F. C.; and Keiser, H. R. The kallikrein-kinin system in Bartter's syndrome and its response to prostaglandin synthetase inhibition. J. Clin. Invest. 61:1671-1682, 1978.
5. Meyer, W. J., III; Gill, J. R., Jr.; and Bartter, F. C. Gout as a complication of Bartter's syndrome. Ann. Intern. Med. 83:56-59, 1975.
6. Verberckmoes, R.; VanDamme, B.; Clement, J.; Avery, A.; and Michielsen, P. Bartter's syndrome with hyperplasia of renomedullary cells: Successful treatment with indomethacin. Kidney Int. 9:302-397, 1976.
7. Fichman, M. P.; Telfer, N.; Zia, P.; Speckart, P.; Golub, M.; and Rude, R. Role of prostaglandins in the pathogenesis of Bartter's syndrome. Am. J. Med. 60:785-797, 1976.
8. Gill, J. R., Jr.; Frolich, J. C.; Bowden, R.; Taylor, A. A.; Keiser, H. R.; Seyberth, H. W.; Oates, J. A.; Bartter, F. C. Bartter's syndrome: A disorder characterized by high urinary prostaglandins and a dependence of hyperreinemia on prostaglandin synthesis. Am. J. Med. 61:43-51, 1976.
9. Norby, L.; Flamenbaum, N.; Lentz, R.; and Ramwell, P. Prostaglandins and aspirin therapy in Bartter's syndrome. Lancet 2:604-606, 1976.
10. Gill, J. R., Jr.; and Bartter, F. C. Evidence for a prostaglandin-independent defect in chloride reabsorption in the loop of Henle as a proximal cause of Bartter's syndrome. Am. J. Med. 65:766-772, 1978.
11. Gill, J. R., Jr. Bartter's syndrome. Ann. Rev. Med. 31:405-419, 1981.
12. Delaney, V. B.; Oliver, J. F.; Simms, M.; Costello, J.; and Bourke, E. Bartter's syndrome: Physiological and pharmacological studies. Q. J. Med. 198:213-232, 1981.
13. Tomko, D. J.; Yeh, B. P. Y.; and Falls, W. F., Jr. Bartter's syndrome. Study of a 52 year old man with evidence for a defect in proximal tubular sodium reabsorption and comments on therapy. Am. J. Med. 61:111-117, 1976.
14. Godard, C.; Vallotton, M. B.; Broyer, M.; and Royer, P. A study of the inhibition of the renin-angiotensin system in renal potassium wasting syndromes, including Bartter's syndrome. Helv. Paediat. Acta 27:495-511, 1972.
15. Berio, A. Considerazioni Sullanefropatio della cistinosi con s. di Bartter secondari. Minerva Pediatr. 30:1825-1831, 1978.
16. LaGareca, G.; Bazzato, G.; Bisioli, S.; Coli, V.; Fabris, A.; Gaianigo, P.; Mantero, F.; Olivetti, G.; Pisani, E.; and Bonanno, A. Bartter's syndrome associated with sponge disease. Kidney Int. 73:192, 1978.
17. Pasternack, A.; Perheentupa, J.; Launiala, K.; and Hallman, N. Kidney biopsy findings in familial chloride diarrhoea. Acta Endocrinol. 55:1-9, 1967.
18. Fleischer, N.; Brown, H.; Graham, D. Y.; and Delena, S. Chronic laxative-induced hyperaldosteronism and hypokalemia simulating Bartter's syndrome. Ann. Intern. Med. 70: 791-798, 1969.
19. Ramos, E.; Hall-Craggs, M.; and Demers, L. M. A case of surreptitious, habitual vomiting simulating Bartter's syndrome. J.A.M.A. 43:1070-1072, 1980.
20. Sealey, J. E.; Clark, I.; Bull, M. R.; and Laragh, J. H. Potassium balance and the control of renin secretion. J. Clin. Invest. 49:2119-2127, 1970.
21. Brunner, H. R.; Baer, L.; Sealey, J. E.; Ledingham, J. G. G.; and Laragh, J. H. The influence of potassium administration and of potassium deprivation on plasma renin in normal and hypertensive subjects. J. Clin. Invest. 49:2128-2138, 1970.
22. Gullner, H.-G.; Bartter, F. C.; Gill, J. R., Jr.; Dickman, P. S.; Wilson, C. B.; and Tiwari, J. L. A sibship with hypokalemic alkalosis and renal proximal tubulopathy. Arch. Int. Med. 143:1534-1540, 1983.

23. Kotchen, T. A.; Luke, R. G.; Ott, C. E.; Galla, J. H.; and Whitescarver, S. Effect of chloride on renin and blood pressure responses to sodium chloride. Inn. Intern. Med. 98:817-822, 1983.
24. Goodman, A. D.; Vagnucci, A. H.; and Hartroft, P. M. Pathogenesis of Bartter's syndrome. N. Engl. J. Med. 281:1435-1439, 1969.
25. Trygstad, C. W.; Mangos, J. A.; Bloodworth, J. M. B.; and Lobeck, C. C. A sibship with Bartter's syndrome: Failure of total adrenalectomy to correct the potassium wasting. Pediatrics 44:234-242, 1969.
26. Takayasu, H.; Aso, Y.; and Lakanchi, K. A case of Bartter's syndrome with surgical treatment followed for four years. J. Clin. Endocrinol. Metab. 32:842-845, 1971.
27. Bowden, R. E.; Gill, J. R., Jr.; Radfar, N.; Taylor, A. A.; and Keiser, H. R. Prostaglandin synthetase inhibitors in Bartter's syndrome. J.A.M.A. 239:117-121, 1978.
28. White, M. G. Bartter's syndrome. A manifestation of renal tubular defects. Arch. Intern. Med. 129:41-47, 1972.
29. Chaimovitz, C.; Levi, J.; Better, O. S.; Oslander, L.; and Benderli, A. Studies on the site of renal salt loss in a patient with Bartter's syndrome. Pediatr. Res. 7:89-94, 1973.
30. Chan, J. C. M.; Malekzedeh, M. H.; and Anand, S. L. Defect in renal tubular sodium reabsorption in a patient with Bartter's syndrome. Clin. Proc. Child. Hosp. Natl. Med. Cent. 31:67-71, 1975.
31. Fujita, T.; Sakuguchi, H.; Shibagaki, M.; Fukui, T.; Nomura, M.; and Sekiguchi, S. The pathogenesis of Bartter's syndrome. Am. J. Med. 63:467-474, 1977.
32. Bartter, F. C.; Delea, C. S.; Kawasaki, T.; and Gill, J. R., Jr. The adrenal cortex and the kidney. Kidney Int. 6:272-280, 1974.
33. Knox, F. G.; Mertz, J. I.; Burnett, J. C., Jr.; and Harmati, A. Role of hydrostatic and oncotic pressures in renal sodium reabsorption. Circ. Res. 52:491-500, 1983.
34. Eknoyan, G.; Suki, W. N.; Rector, F. C., Jr.; and Seldin, D. W. Functional characteristics of the diluting segment of the dog nephron and the effect of extracellular volume expansion on its reabsorptive capacity. J. Clin. Invest. 46:1178-1188, 1967.
35. Burg, M. B.; and Bourdeau, J. E. Function of the thick ascending limb of Henle's loop. In: Newer Aspects of Renal Function, edited by Cogel, H. G., and Ullrich, K. J. Amsterdam, Excerpta Medica, 1978, pp. 91-102.
36. Danovitch, G. M.; and Bricker, N. S. Influence of volume expansion on NaCl reabsorption in the diluting segments of the nephron. A study using clearance methods. Kidney Int. 10:229-238, 1976.
37. Stokes, J. B. Effect of prostaglandin E_2 on chloride transport across the rabbit thick ascending limb of Henle. J. Clin. Invest. 64:495-502, 1979.
38. Wright, F. C.; and Giebisch, G. Renal potassium transport: Contributions of individual nephron segments and populations. Am. J. Physiol. 235:F515-F527, 1978.
39. Shareghi, S. R.; and Agus, Z. S. Magnesium transport in the cortical thick ascending limb of Henle's loop of the rabbit. J. Clin. Invest. 69:759-769, 1982.
40. Shils, M. E. Experimental human magnesium depletion. Medicine 48:61-85, 1969.
41. Dibona, G. F. Mechanism of negative potassium balance in the magnesium deficient rat. Proc. Soc. Exp. Biol. Med. 168:382-388, 1981.
42. Baehler, R. W.; Work, J.; Kotchen, T. A.; McMorrow, G.; and Guthrie, G. Studies on the pathogenesis of Bartter's syndrome. Am. J. Med. 69:933-938, 1980.
43. Fanconi, A.; Schachenmann, G.; Nussli, R.; and Prader, A. Chronic hypokalemia with growth retardation, normotensive hyperrenin-hyperaldosteronism ("Bartter's syndrome"), and hypercalciuria. Helv. Paediatr. Acta 26:144-163, 1971.
44. Meyer, W. J., III; Middler, S. A.; Delea, C. S.; and Bartter, F. C. Hypercalciuria and increased plasma renin activity. In: Control of Renin Secretion, edited by Assaykeen, A. New York, Plenum, 1972, pp. 245-262.
45. McCredie, D. A.; Rotenbert, E.; and Williams, A. C. Hypercalciuria in potassium-losing nephropathy: A variant of Bartter's syndrome. Aust. Paediatr. J. 10:286-295, 1974.

46. Kurtz, I.; Maher, T.; Jones, J. W.; Sutton, J. M.; Schambelan, M.; Hulter, H. N.; Rector, F. C., Jr.; Moris, R. C., Jr.; and Sebastian, A. Familial chloride-resistant renal alkalosis and hypokalemia with fasting hypercalciuria and medullary nephrocalcinosis: A unique variant of Bartter's syndrome without impaired renal diluting ability. Clin. Res. 29: 555A, 1981.
47. Keeton, T. K.; and Campbell, W. B. The pharmacologic alteration of renin release. Pharmacol. Rev. 32:81-227, 1980.
48. Pearson, A. J. G.; Sladen, G. E.; Edmonds, C. J.; Tavill, A. S.; Wills, M. R.; and McIntyre, N. The pathophysiology of congenital chloridorrhoea. Q. J. Med. 167:453-456, 1973.
49. Veldhuis, J. C.; Bardin, C. W.; and Demers, L. M. Metabolic mimicry of Bartter's syndrome by covert vomiting. Am. J. Med. 66:361-363, 1979.
50. Jamison, R. L.; Ross, J. C.; Kempson, R. L.; Sufit, C. R.; and Parker, T. E. Surreptitious diuretic ingestion and pseudo-Bartter's syndrome. Am. J. Med. 73:142-147, 1982.
51. Ferris, T. F.; and Gorden, P. Effect of angiotensin and norepinephrine upon urate clearance in man. Am. J. Med. 44:359-365, 1968.
52. Bauer, F. C.; Glasson, P.; Vallotton, M. B.; and Courvoisier, B. Syndrome de Bartter, Chondrocalcinose et Hypomagnesemie. Schweiz. Med. Wochenschr. 109:1251-1256, 1979.
53. Runeberg, L.; Collan, Y.; Jokinen, E. J.; Lahdevirta, J.; and Aro, A. Hypomagnesemia due to renal disease of unknown etiology. Am. J. Med. 59:873-881, 1975.
54. Chan, J. C. M.; Gill, J. R., Jr.; and Bartter, F. C. Lack of evidence for a role for prostaglandins in the mediation of impaired urinary concentrating ability in Bartter's syndrome. Nephron 35:116-119, 1983.
55. Beck, N.; and Webster, S. K. Impaired urinary concentrating ability and cyclic AMP in K^+-depleted rat kidney. Am. J. Physiol. 231:1204-1208, 1976.
56. Gill, J. R., Jr. Prostaglandins in Bartter's syndrome and in potassium-deficient disorders that mimic it. Miner. Electrolyte Metab. 6:76-81, 1981.
57. Lum, G. M.; Aisenbrey, G. A.; Dunn, M. J.; Berl, T.; Schrier, R. W.; and McDonald, K. M. In vivo effect of indomethacin to potentiate the renal medullary cyclic AMP response to vasopressin. J. Clin. Invest. 59:8-13, 1977.
58. Galvez, O. G.; Bay, W. H.; Roberts, B. W.; Ferris, T. F. The hemodynamic effects of potassium deficiency in the dog. Circ. Res. 40(Suppl. I):I11-I16, 1977.
59. Gullner, H.-G.; Graf, A. K.; Gill, J. R., Jr.; and Mitchell, M. D. Hypokalemia stimulates prostacyclin synthesis in the rat. Clin. Sci. 65:43-46, 1983.
60. Linas, S. L. Mechanism of hyperreninemia in the potassium-depleted rat. J. Clin. Invest. 68:347-355, 1981.
61. Kotchen, T. A.; Guthrie, G. P., Jr.; Galla, J. H.; Luke, R. G.; Welch, W. J. Effects of NaCl on renin and aldosterone responses to potassium depletion. Am. J. Physiol. 244: E164-E169, 1983.
62. Gullner, H.-G.; Bartter, F. C.; Cerletti, C.; Smith, J. B.; and Gill, J. R., Jr. Prostacyclin overproduction in Bartter's syndrome. Lancet 2:767-770, 1979.
63. Gerber, J. C.; Branch, R. A.; Nies, A. S.; Gerkens, J. F.; Shand, D. G.; Hollifield, J. W.; and Oates, J. A. Prostaglandins and renin release: II. Assessment of renin secretion following infusion of PGI_2, E_2, and D_2 into the renal artery of anesthetized dogs. Prostaglandins 15:81-88, 1978.
64. Zusman, R. M.; and Keiser, H. R. Prostaglandin biosynthesis by rabbit renomedullary interstitial cells in tissue culture: Stimulation by angiotensin II, bradykinin and arginine vasopressin. J. Clin. Invest. 60:215-223, 1977.
65. Nadler, J.; Zipser, R. D.; Coleman, R.; and Horton, R. Stimulation of renal prostaglandins by pressor hormones in man: Comparison of prostaglandin E_2 and prostacyclin (6 keto prostaglandin $F_{1\alpha}$). J. Clin. Endocrinol. Metab. 56:1260-1265, 1983.

66. Dusing, R.; Gill, J. R., Jr.; Gullner, H.-G.; and Bartter, F. C. The role of prostaglandins in diabetes insipidus produced by desoxycorticosterone in the dog. Endocrinology 110: 644-649, 1982.
67. Dusing, R.; Attallah, A. A.; Prezyna, A. P.; and Lee, J. B. Renal biosynthesis of prostaglandin E_2 and F_2: Dependence on extracellular potassium. J. Lab. Clin. Med. 92: 669-677, 1978.
68. Gullner, H.-G.; Lake, C. R.; Gill, J. R., Jr.; and Lakatua, D. J. Hypokalemia stimulates plasma epinephrine and norepinephrine in the rat. Arch. Int. Pharmacodyn. 260:78-82, 1982.
69. Dusing, R.; Scherhag, R.; Tippelmann, R.; Budde, U.; Glanzer, K.; Kramer, H. J. Arachidonic acid metabolism in isolated rat aorta: Dependence of prostacyclin biosynthesis on extracellular potassium concentration. J. Biol. Chem. 257:1993-2001, 1982.
70. Gunther, S.; Gimbrone, M. A., Jr.; Alexander, R. W. Regulation by angiotensin II of its receptors in resistance blood vessels. Nature 287:230, 1980.
71. Radfar, N.; Gill, J. R., Jr.; Bartter, F. C.; Bravo, E.; Taylor, A. A.; Bowden, R. E. Hypokalemia, in Bartter's syndrome and other disorders, produces resistance to vasopressors via prostaglandin overproduction. Proc. Soc. Exp. Biol. Med. 158:502-507, 1978.
72. Kono, T.; Oseko, F.; Shimbo, S.; Nanno, M.; Ikeda, F.; Endo, J. Blood pressure fall by angiotensin II antagonist in patients with Bartter's syndrome. J. Clin. Endocrinol. 43: 692-695, 1976.
73. Sasaki, H.; Okumura, M.; Asano, T.; Arakawa, K.; Kawasaki, T. Responses to angiotensin II antagonist before and after treatment with indomethacin in Bartter's syndrome. Br. Med. J. 2:975-1038, 1977.
74. Rudin, A.; Aurell, M.; Hansson, L.; and Westberg, G. Effect of Sar^1-ala^8-angiotensin II on blood pressure and renin in Bartter's syndrome, before and after treatment with prostaglandin synthetase inhibitors. Scand. J. Clin. Lab. Invest. 39:543-550, 1979.
75. Gullner, H.-G.; Gill, J. R., Jr.; Bartter, F. C.; Lake, C. R.; Lakatua, D. J. Correction of increased sympathoadrenal activity in Bartter's syndrome by inhibition of prostaglandin synthesis. J. Clin. Endocrinol. Metab. 50:857, 1980.
76. Watson, M. L.; Branch, R. A.; Gill, J. R., Jr.; Oates, J. A.; and Brash, A. R. Systemic prostaglandin I_2 synthesis is normal in patients with Bartter's syndrome. Lancet 2: 368-370, 1983.
77. Gullner, H.-G.; Smith, J. B.; and Bartter, F. C. The principal metabolites of arachidonic acid are overproduced in Bartter's syndrome. Adv. Prostaglandin Thromboxane Res. 7:1185-1187, 1980.
78. Fujita, T.; Ando, K.; Sato, Y.; Yamashita, K.; Normura, M.; and Fukui, T. Independent roles of prostaglandins and the renin and angiotensin system in abnormal vascular reactivity in Bartter's syndrome. Am. J. Med. 73:71-76, 1982.
79. Aurell, M.; and Rudin, A. Effect of captopril on blood pressure, renal function, the electrolyte balance and the renin-angiotensin system in Bartter's syndrome. Nephron 33:274-278, 1983.
80. Wong, P. Y.; Talamo, R. C.; Williams, G. H.; and Coleman, R. W. Response of kallikrein-kinin-angiotensin systems to saline infusion and upright posture. J. Clin. Invest. 55: 691-698, 1975.
81. Gall, G.; Vaitukaitis, J.; Haddow, J. E.; and Klein, R. Erythrocyte Na flux in a patient with Bartter's syndrome. J. Clin. Endocrinol. Metab. 32:562-567, 1971.
82. Gardner, J. D.; Simopoulos, A. P.; Lapey, A.; and Shibolet, S. Altered membrane sodium transport in Bartter's syndrome. J. Clin. Invest. 51:1065-1071, 1972.
83. Oliver, J. F.; Delaney, V. B.; and Bourke, E. Increased erythrocyte sodium permeability in patients with Bartter's syndrome. Miner. Electrolyte Metab. 1:225-230, 1978.
84. Cole, C. H.; and O'Regan, S. Effect of treatment with prostaglandin synthetase inhibitors on the erythrocyte sodium transport abnormality of Bartter's syndrome. Pediatr. Res. 15:926-929, 1981.

85. Mongeau, J.-G.; Garay, M.; deMendonca, M.; Broyer, M.; and Meyer, P. Erythrocyte Na^+ and K^+ transport systems in children with Bartter's syndrome: Increase in passive sodium permeability. Kidney Int. 23:530-535, 1983.
86. Korff, J. M.; Siebens, A. W.; and Gill, J. R., Jr. Correction of hypokalemia corrects the abnormalities in erythrocyte sodium transport in Bartter's syndrome. J. Clin. Invest. 74:1724-1729, 1984.
87. Heidland, A.; Kreusser, W.; Hennemann, H.; Kanuf, H.; and Wigand, M. E. Excretion of the mono- and divalent ions in relation to flow in Bartter's and pseudo-Bartter's syndrome in parotid saliva. Comparative studies to the syndrome of Conn. Klin. Wochenschr. 50:959-966, 1972.
88. Stoff, J. S.; Stemerman, M.; Steer, M.; Salzman, E.; Brown, R. S. A defect in platelet aggregation in Bartter's syndrome. Am. J. Med. 68:171-180, 1980.
89. Gullner, H.-G.; Kafka, M. S.; Gill, J. R., Jr. Insensitivity of platelet adenylate cyclase to prostaglandin E_1 in patients suffering from diseases involving hypokalemia. Ann. Intern. Med. 101:342-343, 1984.
90. Simopoulos, A. P. Growth characteristics in patients with Bartter's syndrome. Nephron 23:131-136, 1979.
91. Littlewood, J. M.; Lee, M. R.; Meadow, S. R. Treatment of Bartter's syndrome in early childhood with prostaglandin synthetase inhibitors. Arch. Dis. Child. 53:43-48, 1978.
92. Kornerup, H. J.; Pedersen, E. B.; and Petersen, V. P. Bartter's syndrome without hyperplasia of the juxtaglomerular apparatus, treated with indomethacin. Acta Med. Scand. 204:235-239, 1978.
93. Bergstein, J. M.; and Weinberger, M. H. Hypokalemia, normal blood pressure and hyperreninemia with hypoaldosteronism. J. Pediatr. 99:561-564, 1981.
94. Nielsen, I.; Hesse, B.; and Christensen, P. On the pathogenetic role of prostaglandins in Bartter's syndrome. Acta Med. Scand. 625:135-140, 1979.
95. Gitelman, H. J.; Graham, J. B.; and Welt, L. G. A new familial disorder characterized by hypokalemia and hypomagnesemia. Trans. Assoc. Am. Phys. 79:221-223, 1966.
96. Evans, R. A.; Carter, J. N.; George, C. R. P.; Walls, R. S.; Newland, R. C.; McDonnell, G. D.; and Lawrence, J. R. The congenital magnesium-losing kidney. Q. J. Med. 197: 39-52, 1981.
97. Paunier, L.; and Sizonenko, P. C. Asymptomatic chronic hypomagnesemia and hypokalemia in a child: Cell membrane disease. J. Pediatr. 88:51-55, 1976.
98. McCredie, D. A.; Blair-West, J. R.; Scoggins, B. A.; Shipman, R. Potassium-losing nephropathy of childhood. Med. J. Aust. 1:129-135, 1971.
99. Dillon, M. J.; Shah, V.; and Mitchell, M. D. Bartter's syndrome: 10 cases in childhood. Q. J. Med. 48:429-446, 1979.
100. Griffing, G. T.; and Melby, J. C. The therapeutic use of a new potassium-sparing diuretic, amiloride and a converting enzyme inhibitor, MK-421 in preventing hypokalemia associated with primary and secondary hyperaldosteronism. Clin. Exper. Hypertens. A5:779-801, 1983.
101. Stokes, G. S.; Andrews, B. S.; Hagon, E.; Thornell, I. R.; Palmer, A. A.; and Posen, S. Bartter's syndrome presenting during pregnancy. Med. J. Aust. 2:360-365, 1974.

14
The Fanconi Syndrome: Clinical Disorders

EILEEN D. BREWER
University of Utah School of Medicine, Salt Lake City, Utah

The Fanconi syndrome is a renal tubular disorder characterized by multiple transport dysfunctions, classically including impaired reabsorption of amino acids, glucose, bicarbonate, and phosphate, but also uric acid, low-molecular-weight (tubular) proteins, citrate and other organic acids, calcium, magnesium, sodium, potassium, and water. When present chronically, metabolic bone disease occurs, either as rickets in children or osteomalacia in adults. The syndrome appears to be the final expression of many types of functional and morphological injury to the renal tubule, especially its proximal segment. The multiple clinical diseases and disorders associated with this syndrome are listed in Tables 1 and 2. When not associated with an identifiable disorder, the Fanconi syndrome is usually designated as primary or idiopathic. Many of the disorders may affect both children and adults, and in some instances the syndrome is reversible. When the Fanconi syndrome occurs in childhood, however, it is usually hereditary and related to inborn errors of metabolism which continue lifelong.

I. HISTORICAL PERSPECTIVES

Fanconi first described a child with rickets, stunted growth, nondiabetic glucosuria, and albuminuria in 1931 (1). Reports of two other dwarfed children with glucosuria, albuminuria, and rickets as well as hypophosphatemia, acidosis, and organic aciduria were published by De Toni in 1933 (2) and Debre et al. in 1934 (3). In 1936, Fanconi suggested that this complex of symptoms occurred together often enough that it ought to be designated by a special name, which he called nephrotic glycosuric dwarfism with hypophosphatemic rickets (4-5). McCune et al. (6) shortened the name to the Fanconi syndrome in 1943. McCune and coworkers (6) also confirmed Fanconi's speculation that the organic aciduria was primarily comprised of amino acids. In 1947, Dent (7) demonstrated the generalized nature of the aminoaciduria in an adult patient with the Fanconi syndrome.

In 1924, Lignac described three children with dwarfism, rickets, polyuria, albuminuria, and glucosuria, who were found at autopsy to have cystine accumulation in numerous tissues (8). In 1937, Beumer and Wepler pointed out the similarity between Lignac's cystine

Table 1 Familial and Hereditary Disorders Associated with the Fanconi Syndrome

Primary or idiopathic (No identifiable associated disorder)
1. Familial
2. Sporadic

Hereditary
1. Cystinosis (Lignac-Fanconi disease)
2. Lowe's syndrome
3. Heretiary fructose intolerance
4. Tyrosinemia, type 1 (tyrosinosis)
5. Galactosemia
6. Glycogen storage disease
7. Wilson's disease
8. Others
   a. Hereditary mitochrondial myopathy with lactic acidemia
   b. Metachromatic leukodystrophy
   c. Subacute necrotizing encephalomyelopathy (Leigh's syndrome)
   d. Hereditary nephritis (Alport's syndrome)
   e. Medullary cystic disease

storage disease cases and Fanconi's clinical cases (9). In 1959, Freudenberg reviewed 17 cases of cystine storage disease, all of whom had the Fanconi syndrome (10). Since then, cystinosis (Lignac-Fanconi disease) has been identified as the disease most commonly associated with the Fanconi syndrome in childhood.

Adult-onset Fanconi syndrome may have been reported as early as 1934 by Milkman, who described a 42-year-old woman with spontaneous fractures, the radiological features of osteomalacia, hypophosphatemia, and renal glycosuria (11). In 1947, Stowers and Dent reported the first studies of adult-onset renal tubular dysfunction designated as the Fanconi syndrome (12). Since then many cases of adult-onset Fanconi syndrome associated with a variety of acquired (Table 2) or accasionally genetically inherited disorders (Table 1) have been described.

II. DEFINITION

A. Complex Renal Tubular Transport Dysfunction

Fanconi's original description of the renal tubular transport dysfunction included only polyuria, renal glucosuria, phosphaturia and hypophosphatemia, generalized aminoaciduria (organic aciduria), albuminuria, and acidosis (1,4-5). The acidosis was later characterized as renal tubular acidosis caused in most patients by defective proximal tubular reabsorption and increased urinary excretion of bicarbonate (type 2 renal tubular acidosis) (13-15). Decreased tubular reabsorption and increased urinary excretion of many other substances, besides those originally described by Fanconi, are now known to be characteristic of the Fanconi syndrome. These substances include uric acid (15-16), calcium (16-19), magnesium (19), citrate (17,18,20), proteins of low molecular weight (10,000-50,000 daltons) (21-25), and sodium and potassium (16,20,26-28).

Table 2 Acquired Disorders Associated with the Fanconi Syndrome

1. Disorders of protein metabolism/excretion
   a. Multiple myeloma
   b. Benign monoclonal gammopathy
   c. Light chain nephropathy
   d. Amyloidosis
   e. Sjogren's syndrome
   f. Nephrotic syndrome
2. Immunological disorders
   a. Interstitial nephritis with anti-TBM antibody
   b. Renal transplantation
   c. Malignancy
3. Drug-related
   a. Outdated, degraded tetracycline
   b. Methyl-3-chromone
   c. 6-Mercaptopurine
   d. Gentamicin and aminoglycoside antibiotics
   e. Valproic acid
   f. Streptozotocin
   g. Isophthalanilide
4. Heavy metal exposure
   a. Cadmium
   b. Lead
   c. Mercury
   d. Uranium
   e. *Cis*-platinum
5. Other toxin exposure
   a. Paraquat poisoning
   b. Lysol burn
   c. Toluene inhalation (glue sniffing)
6. Other renal disorders
   a. Balkan nephropathy
   b. Paroxysmal nocturnal hemoglobinuria
   c. Renal vein thrombosis in newborn infant
7. Vitamin D disorders with secondary hyperparathyroidism
   a. Vitamin D deficiency
   b. Vitamin D-dependent rickets

The tubular reabsorption of many of these same substances, except amino acids, is reduced in patients with chronic renal failure (Fig. 1) (19,29). Decreased reabsorption in uremic patients is a pathophysiological adaptation of the renal tubules to reduction in the glomerular filtration rate. This adaptation may be related to the presence of a volume-responsive circulating inhibitor of renal transport (natriuretic hormone) (30), which has a proximal tubular site of action (31). No such circulating generalized inhibitor of renal tubular transport has been identified for patients with the Fanconi syndrome.

Progressive renal failure often occurs in patients with the Fanconi syndrome. When an affected patient presents for diagnosis at a time when chronic renal failure is already present, the diagnosis of the underlying Fanconi syndrome may be difficult (19). The magnitude of the urinary excretion of characteristic substances will differentiate many, but not all patients with the Fanconi syndrome from those with chronic renal failure of other etiologies

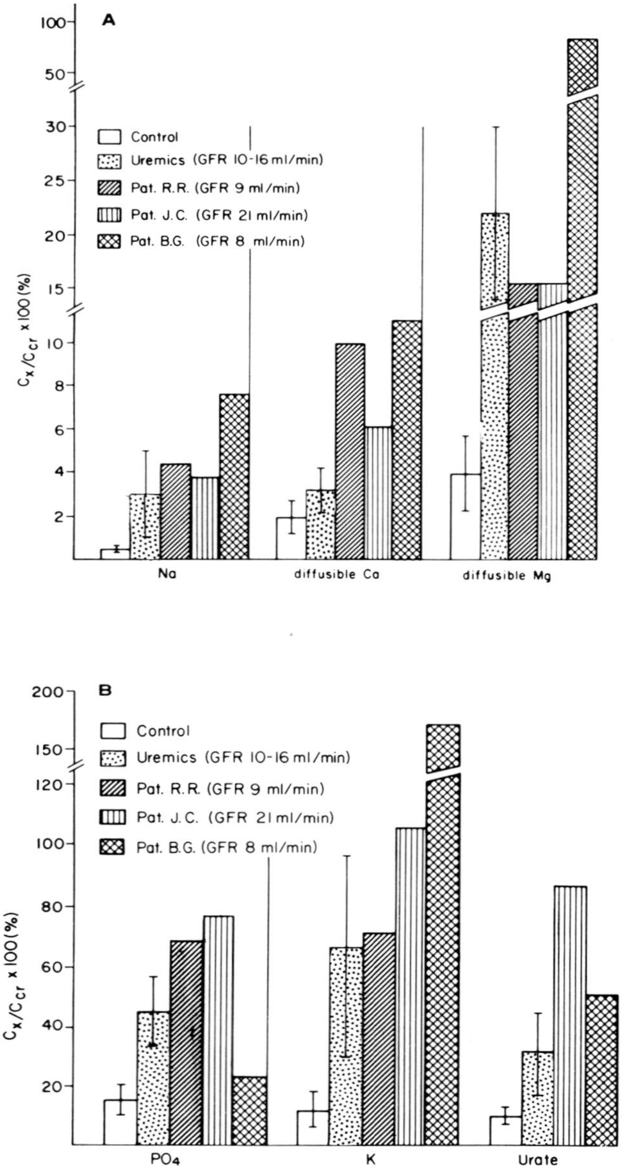

Fig. 1 Comparison of the fractional excretion of electrolytes (A,B) and urate (B) in adult patients with the Fanconi syndrome, uremic patients with a similar degree of reduction in glomerular filtration rate (GFR), and normal controls. Patient R.R., 19-year-old male with idiopathic Fanconi syndrome, onset in early childhood; patient J.C., 34-year-old female with a variant of light chain disease; patient B.G., 38-year-old female chronic abuser of mercury-containing laxatives. (From Ref. 19.)

(Fig. 1). The presence of generalized aminoaciduria, however, will correctly identify patients with the Fanconi syndrome, since increased excretion of amino acids does not occur with chronic renal failure from other causes (19).

The exact site along the nephron at which transport dysfunction occurs and results in the expression of the Fanconi syndrome continues to be a subject of speculation and debate. Early investigators suggested that the most likely site was the proximal tubule, where quantitatively most of the filtered phosphate, bicarbonate, glucose, and amino acids are reabsorbed (12,15-16). To support this speculation, they and others noted that major morphological changes, such as the swan-neck deformity and vacuolar degeneration of tubular cells, occurred in the proximal tubule, while few morphological abnormalities were present in the distal tubule (5-6,12,32). More recently, other investigators studying the experimental Fanconi syndrome in animal models have questioned this point of view (33-35). Their studies suggest that distal nephron dysfunction may also contribute importantly to the expression of the complex tubular transport dysfunction (33-35), even when that segment appears morphologically normal (Fig. 2) (36). Both points of view may be valid. Since the Fanconi syndrome is associated with a variety of inherited, acquired and experimentally induced disorders, it is quite possible that in some instances only the proximal tubule is dysfunctional, whereas in others, especially those caused by tubular toxins, both the proximal and distal nephron may be adversely affected. The specific pathogenesis of complex tubular dysfunction as it occurs in each of the clinical (Tables 1 and 2) and experimental (Table 3) disorders will be discussed later in this chapter and in Ch. 15.

B. Bone Disease

Metabolic bone disease, either rickets in children (1-5) or osteomalacia in adults (11-12,37), almost always occurs with chronic untreated Fanconi syndrome and should be considered a characteristic finding of the clinical Fanconi syndrome. Affected patients are hypophosphatemic but usually have normal serum calcium concentrations (6,13,18) and often normal circulating parathyroid hormone levels (38). The radiographic appearance of the bond disease does not differ from that of rickets or osteomalacia of other etiologies (13). The bone disease is resistant to therapy with low doses of vitamin D_2, which would be curative of vitamin D deficiency. A secondary, reversible Fanconi syndrome occurs in patients with vitamin D deficiency and vitamin D-dependent rickets (Table 2), but is always associated with secondary hyperparathyroidism (13) (see below).

C. Generalized Epithelial Transport Dysfunction

Defective transport of amino acids in both kidney and intestine has been observed in the absence of the Fanconi syndrome in hereditary aminoacidurias, such as cystinuria and Hartnup disease (39). A more generalized epithelial transport defect, which affects cells of the intestine and perhaps bone as well as kidney, has been proposed for the Fanconi syndrome (19,40). The observation of impaired intestinal absorption as well as renal tubular reabsorption of amino acids in some patients with the Fanconi syndrome associated with Lowe's syndrome lends support to this proposal (41). In hereditary fructose intolerance, the enzyme deficiency for aldolase B, which occurs in small intestine as well as kidney (13), could give rise to transport dysfunction in the intestine, although this has not been systematically studied. In a study of the Fanconi syndrome experimentally induced by maleic acid in rats, jejunal absorption of sodium and potassium was decreased; transport of amino acids and glucose, however, appeared to be intact (42). In balance studies of patients with the Fanconi

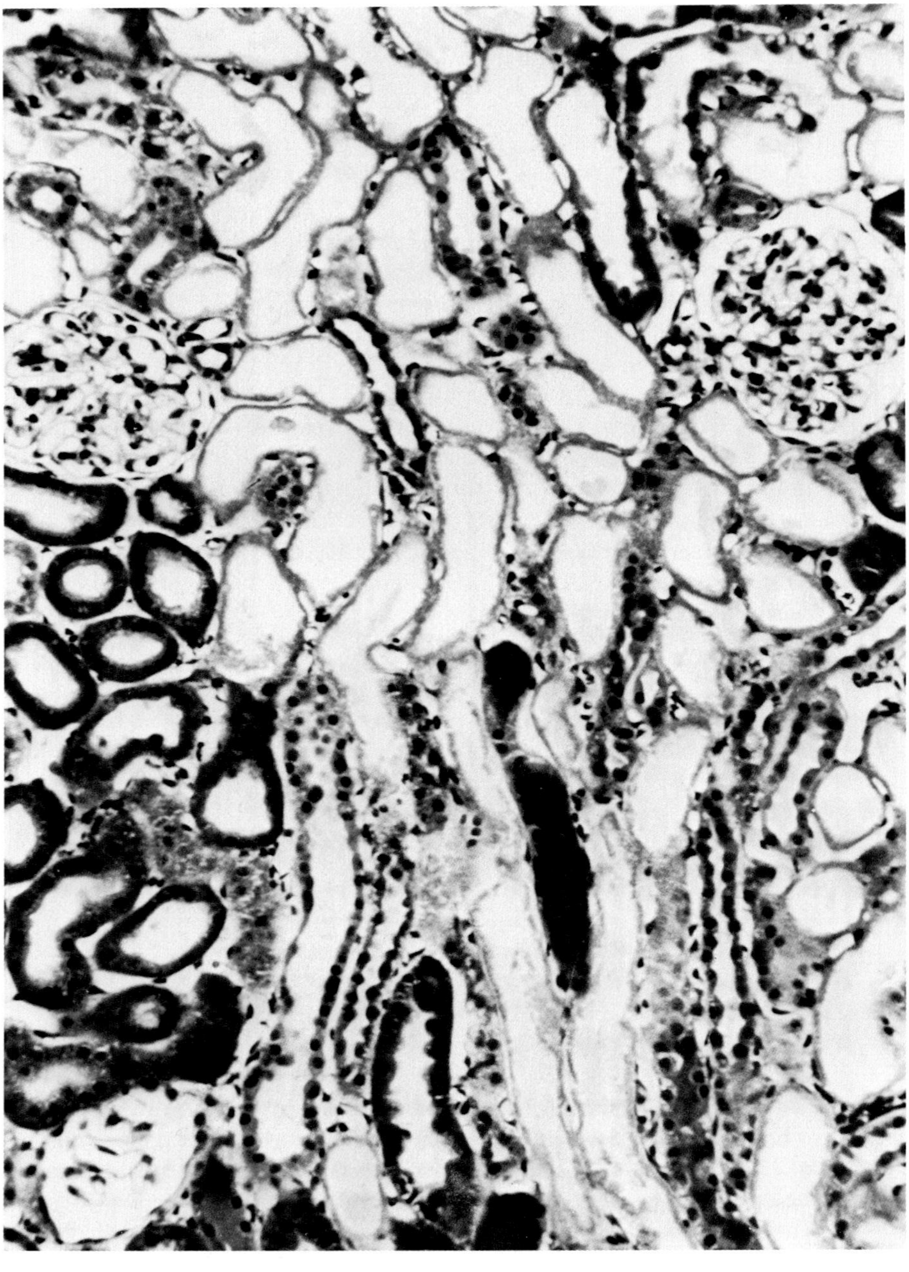

(A)

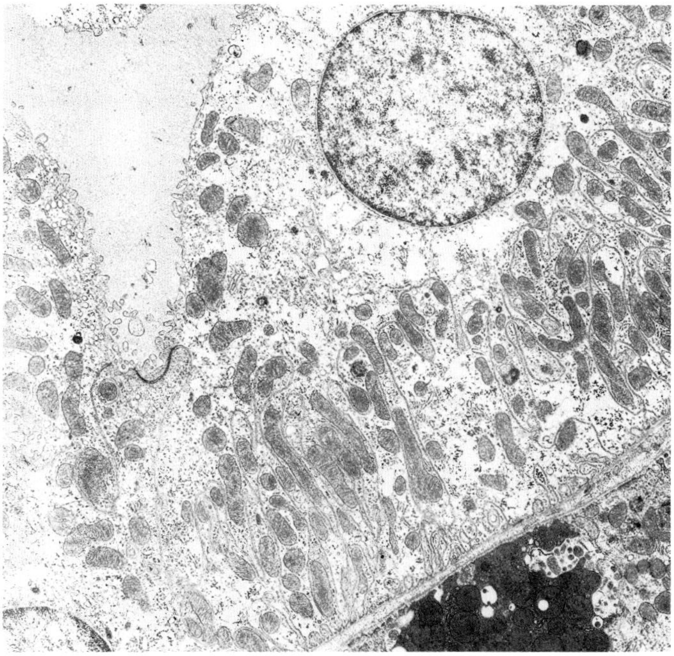

(B)

Fig. 2 Kidney tissue from rats that had the Fanconi syndrome induced 24 hr previously by intravenous administration of maleic acid, 200-400 mg per kg for one hr. (A) Light microscopy of a cortical medullary ray. Proximal pars recta segments are almost completely necrotic. Early proximal convoluted tubules, distal tubules, and glomeruli appear normal. (Periodic acid-Schiff stain, X 100.) (B) Electron micrograph of a distal convoluted tubular cell showing normal appearance of short microvilli, apically located nucleus and elongated mitochondria next to normal basal enfoldings. (X 5,600.) (From Ref. 36.)

syndrome from a variety of causes, increased fecal excretion of calcium and phosphorus has been observed, suggesting the possibility that the intestinal transport of these substances may also be affected (19,40,43). In experimental cadmium-induced Fanconi syndrome, reduced intestinal transport of calcium and phosphorous has actually been demonstrated (44).

Cellular transport of calcium and phosphorus in bone may also be affected in some patients with the Fanconi syndrome. In patients with itai-itai disease, for example, bone disease is more severe than expected for the mild degree of renal tubular dysfunction (45), perhaps because of a cadmium-induced membrane transport defect in the bone itself.

Table 3 Experimental Models of the Fanconi Syndrome

1. Maleic acid
2. Chronic cadmium
3. Degraded tetracycline
4. Spontaneous occurrence in adult Basenji dogs
5. Hereditary fructose intolerance, acute intravenous fructose administration

III. GENERAL CLINICAL SIGNS AND SYMPTOMS

The general clinical manifestations of the Fanconi syndrome depend on the age of the patient and the type and chronicity of the underlying disease. Infants and children usually present as failures to thrive, with stunted growth and often delayed psychomotor development (41,46-50). Some cases have been discovered incidentally during well child care, when a routine urinalysis revealed a dipstick positive for glucose when the blood glucose concentration was normal. Episodic vomiting, anorexia, polydipsia and polyuria, chronic constipation and unexplained fevers are nonspecific symptoms of the chronic Fanconi syndrome in childhood (4,41). Constipation probably results from chronic volume depletion caused by polyuria and the chronic acidosis of untreated Fanconi syndrome. The unexplained fevers, which occur especially frequently in infants and young children with cystinosis, are thought to reflect episodic dehydration (4,5,46).

Rachitic bone disease is a common presenting complaint of children with the Fanconi syndrome. If the child has been crawling or walking, bowing deformities of the legs will be noticed first. Non-weight-bearing children may have straight legs even when x-ray examina-

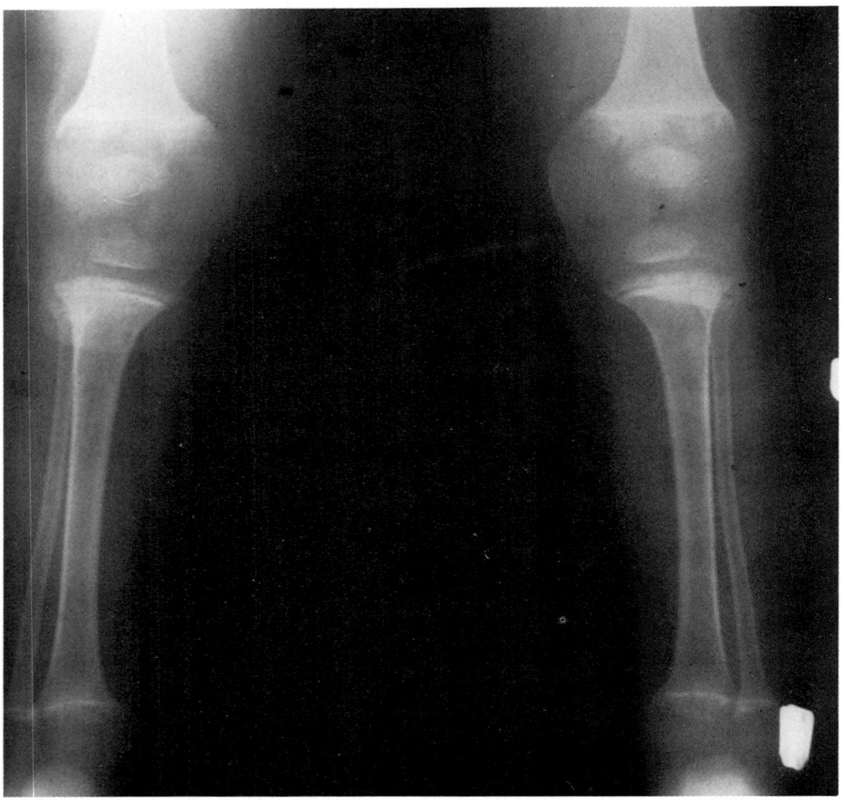

A

tion reveals severe rachitic bone changes (Fig. 3A). Other clinical findings characteristic of rickets, but often not appreciated because of the rarity with which clinical rickets is now seen, include a rachitic rosary, frontal bossing, metaphyseal widening at the knees, ankles, or wrists (Figs. 3B and C) and hypotonia. Infants less than 6 months old rarely have the clinical findings of rickets (46).

The age at which a child with the Fanconi syndrome becomes symptomatic often aids in correctly diagnosing the associated underlying disorder. Children with nephropathic cystinosis, for example, generally do not become symptomatic before the age of 6 months or after the age of 2-3 years (46). Infants with galactosemia (47) or hereditary fructose intolerance (48) can be acutely symptomatic within the first few days of life if exposed to foods or formula containing lactose or fructose, respectively. Continued exposure to the offending sugar, even in small amounts, can result in chronic symptoms or failure to thrive in later infancy and childhood (47,49). Children with Wilson's disease may present with polyuria and/or rickets, but not until late in the first decade of life (50). Idiopathic familial or nonfamilial Fanconi syndrome can become symptomatic with vomiting and failure to thrive in early

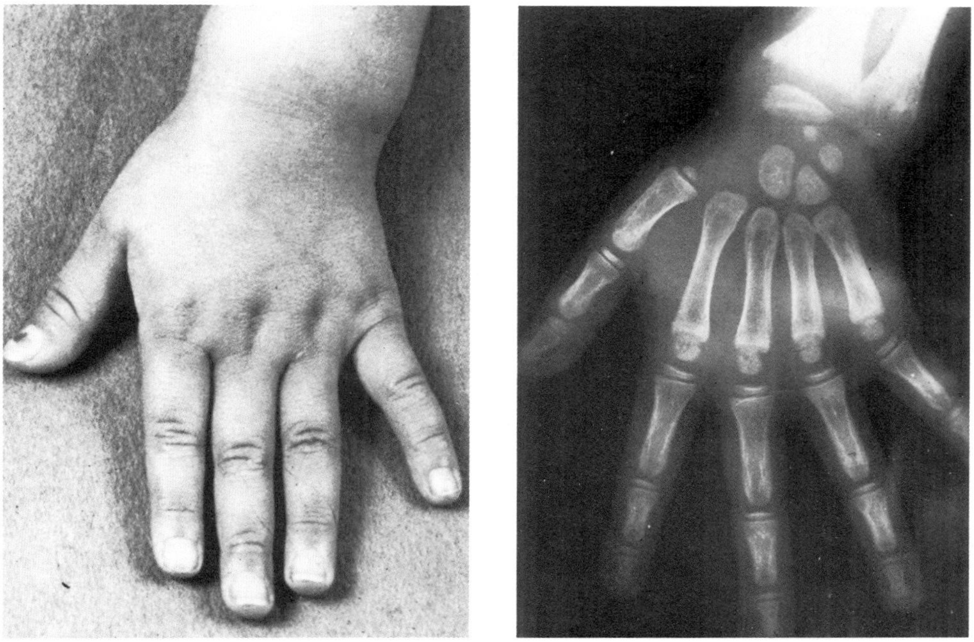

B C

Fig. 3 Rickets in children with the Fanconi syndrome. (A) Radiograph of the lower extremities of a 1-year-old boy with cystinosis, who was not yet walking and clinically had no bowing deformity of his legs, but he had evidence of severe radiographic rickets, including epiphyseal widening, metaphyseal fraying, and marked demineralization. (B) Clinically apparent metaphyseal widening of the wrist of a 6-year-old girl with vitamin D-dependent rickets. (C) Radiographic findings of rickets in the same hand as that shown in B.

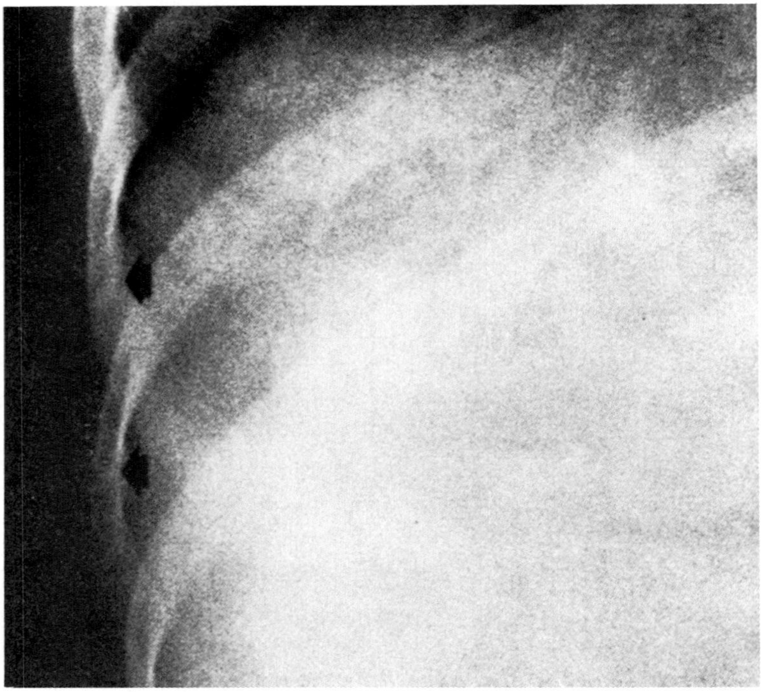

A

Fig. 4 Pseudofractures (Looser's lines) in (A) ribs and (B) femoral shaft of adults with the Fanconi syndrome.

infancy or may not become apparent until later in childhood when growth retardation and bone disease are prominent (41). Symptoms from acquired or renal toxin-associated Fanconi syndrome may occur at any age.

Patients with adult-onset Fanconi syndrome commonly present in the fourth or fifth decade of life with severe bone pain and muscle weakness that has been present for a number of years (37). The pain occurs most often in the lower back, hips, and thighs, but it also occurs in the shoulders and ribs. Pain and progressive bony deformities may interfere with walking. Fractures often occur spontaneously or after minor trauma. The earliest radiographic changes of bone are pseudofractures (Looser's lines) and osteopenia (Fig. 4). Muscle weakness and episodic paralysis are manifestations of the severe hypokalemia that can occur with the Fanconi syndrome (16,37). Proximal myopathy in some patients has also been related to phosphate depletion and hypophosphatemia (17,51).

When neither bone pain nor muscle weakness is present, the only clinical symptoms in the adult with the Fanconi syndrome may be general malaise, weight loss, polyuria, or symptoms of an associated underlying disease such as the neurological abnormalities of Wilson's disease.

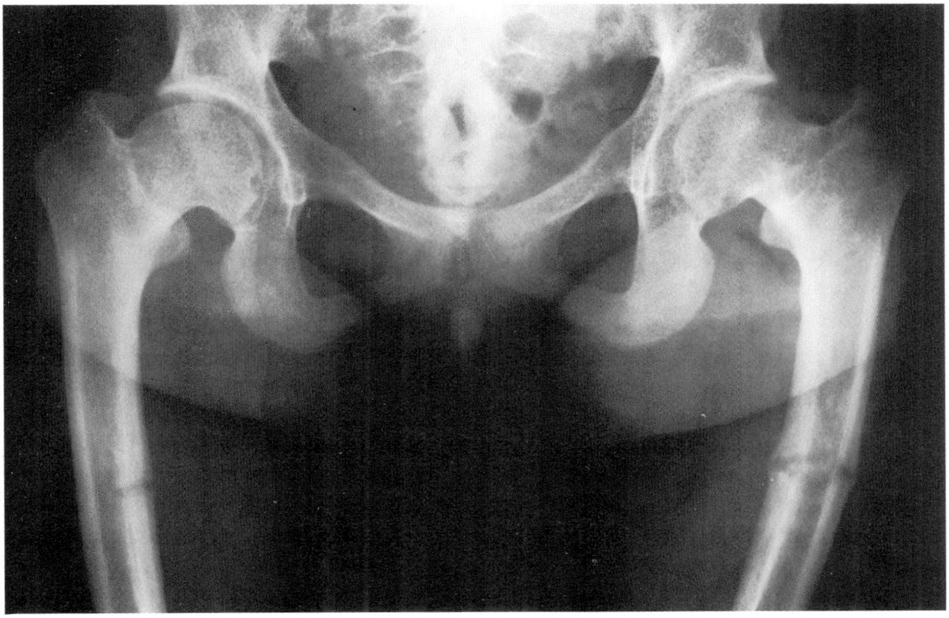

B

IV. CLINICAL DISORDERS ASSOCIATED WITH THE FANCONI SYNDROME

A. Primary or Idiopathic

The diagnosis of primary or idiopathic Fanconi syndrome is one of exclusion and no doubt includes cases with a variety of as yet unidentified etiologies. The literature pertaining to primary Fanconi syndrome is well reviewed by Brodehl (41). The diagnosis was first applied to adults without cystinosis, some of whom had had symptoms dating from childhood (52). The diagnosis of primary Fanconi syndrome in childhood was made first by von Illig and Prader (53). Most cases of primary Fanconi syndrome are sporadic (41). Those that are familial are most often genetically transmitted in an autosomal dominant fashion (52,54-58). Autosomal recessive inheritance has been suggested for some families (53,58), but in at least one instance was proved wrong after 30-year follow-up revealed the appearance of the disorder in three generations (58). Although the complete Fanconi syndrome with clinical symptoms was not expressed in affected members of this family until the third or fourth decade of life, the earliest manifestations may have been aminoaciduria in the second decade and lactic aciduria and tubular proteinuria in the first decade.

Patients with the familial and sporadic forms of primary Fanconi syndrome are at risk for the development of chronic renal failure within 10-30 years of diagnosis (19,57,59,60). Some progress to end-stage renal function and require dialysis or transplantation (57,59,60). One affected adult, who received a cadaver renal graft, had no recurrence of the Fanconi syndrome in the 6 years after transplantation (57). However, the Fanconi syndrome recurred almost immediately in a transplanted kidney implanted in another patient from his mother (60).

Aside from the usual features of the Fanconi syndrome common to all patients, some patients with primary Fanconi syndrome have abnormalities of carbohydrate metabolism, including ketosis and ketonuria (6,61,62), glucose intolerance typical of diabetes mellitus (6,56,57,61,62), blunted insulin-releasing response to intravenous glucose or glucagon (61, 62), and galactose intolerance (61,62). The relationship of these abnormalities to the Fanconi syndrome is unknown, but similar abnormalities occur in patients with an unusual form of glycogen storage disease and the Fanconi syndrome (see below).

B. Hereditary Disorders (Table 1)

Cystinosis (Lignac-Fanconi Disease)

Cystinosis is a group of genetically transmitted diseases characterized by the accumulation of cystine within cells of many tissues, including the kidney, liver, gut, spleen, lymph nodes, bone marrow, peripheral leukocytes, skin fibroblasts, choroid plexus, conjunctiva, cornea, and thyroid (46). It is not related to the disease cystinuria, which is a genetically transmitted defect for transport of the dibasic amino acids in the renal tubule and intestine, resulting in massive urinary cystine excretion and cystine nephrolithiasis (see Ch. 4). Three clinical types of cystinosis are recognized: infantile nephropathic, adolescent or juvenile, and adult. The inheritance of all forms is autosomal recessive (46).

Infantile nephropathic cystinosis is the most common form. The clinical course of this form begins between the ages of 6 months and 2 years and is dominated by the abnormalities of renal tubular function. Initially the electrolyte abnormalities resulting from the Fanconi syndrome may be quite severe and difficult to normalize with oral supplementation of alkali, potassium, and phosphorus. Glomerular filtration, which is initially normal, declines during the first decade. End-stage renal failure is reached before the age of 10 and as early as the age of 2 (46). As glomerular filtration decreases, the electrolyte abnormalities become easier to treat. Successful renal transplantation from either a living related donor, including a heterozygote parent, or a cadaver donor is possible (60,63-67). Cystine accumulates in the interstitium of the transplanted kidney and occasionally in the mesangium of the glomeruli, but not in the tubular cells (63,65,67), and the Fanconi syndrome does not recur (60,63-67).

Caucasian children with cystinosis usually have fair skin and hair (Fig. 5), but black, Mexican, and Arabian children have not been found to be noticeably different in pigmentation from their parents (68). Photophobia is a common complaint of older children and is thought to be related to cystine crystal deposition in the conjunctiva and cornea (46). A characteristic peripheral retinopathy with patchy temporal depigmentation has been described (69). The retinopathy appears to be present at birth and has allowed correct diagnosis of cystinosis at 5 weeks of age, before any clinical signs of cystinosis were apparent (70). The retinopathy has not been associated with decreased visual acuity to date, but the long-term outcome is still unknown. Some patients with cystinosis have hepatomegaly and mild elevations of serum glutamic oxalacetic transaminase (SGOT) concentration (71). Occasionally at autopsy livers have shown fatty infiltration or periportal fibrosis with chronic lymphocyte infiltration (71). Whether liver disease will be a part of the later clinical manifestations of cystinosis remains to be seen. The oldest patients with infantile nephropathic cystinosis are now only in their 20s.

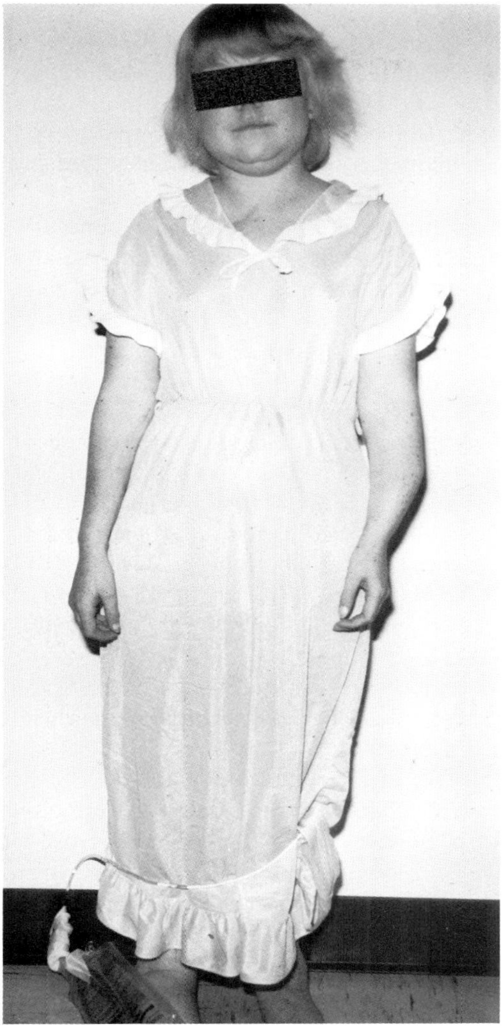

Fig. 5 22-year-old with cystinosis since infancy. End-stage renal disease occurred at age 8 years, after which she was maintained for many years with renal transplants and at this time with chronic ambulatory peritoneal dialysis (dialysate fluid bag and tubing next to foot). She has the typical blond hair and fair skin of cystinosis. No pubertal development has yet occurred.

Growth retardation is severe in infantile nephropathic cystinosis despite correction of acidosis, healing of rickets, and correction of hypothyroidism (46,72). Hypothyroidism occurs in some patients from destruction of the thyroid follicles by cystine crystals (73,74). The occurrence is not predictable; the author has cared for both a clinically hypothyroid 3 year old and a euthyroid 22 year old with normal circulating thyroid-stimulating hormone concentration. Other endocrine functions relating to growth, including adrenal and growth hormone responses and somatomedinlike activity, have been found to be normal (74). Growth retardation is accompanied by quite delayed bone age (74). Catch-up growth after successful renal transplantation and low dose steroid therapy has been observed (63,64), but it is not universal (74). In general, patients remain severely stunted, and most have emotional and social problems in adolescence and adulthood because of their dwarfed size (75,76).

Pubertal development may also be quite delayed (75). The author has cared for a 22-year-old female patient who had no pubertal development (Fig. 5). After further testing, she appeared to have primary ovarian failure.

A number of patients with infantile nephropathic cystinosis have reached adulthood with the aid of chronic dialysis and renal transplantation. Recently, cerebral atrophy and a destructive brain parenchymal process have been noted in older children and a young adult with cystinosis (77,78). Until more is known about the extent of brain involvement with age, the long-term outcome for the older nephropathic cystinotic remains guarded.

Adolescent cystinosis appears to differ from infantile nephropathic cystinosis only in the later age of onset of symptoms (late childhood or adolescence) and the progression to end-stage renal failure after the age of 10 (79-84). The renal tubular histology is similar to that of infantile nephropathic cystinosis, but glomerular lesions are more prominent and associated clinically with near-nephrotic range proteinuria (81,82,84). The characteristic retinopathy of infantile nephropathic cystinosis is usually not present (81), but all have corneal crystal deposition (79-84). Growth retardation may not occur, presumably due to the onset of clinical symptoms after good growth is achieved (79). Even infants with nephropathic cystinosis grow normally in the first 6 months of life before the onset of symptoms (46).

The adult form of cystinosis is benign and characterized by moderately increased accumulation of intracellular cystine (30-50 times normal compared to 100 times normal for nephropathic cystinosis) and the absence of the Fanconi syndrome (46,85). The kidney appears to be free of cystine crystals (85). Corneal crystals are easily observable by slit-lamp examination; their observation on routine eye examination usually is the only reason these patients come to medical attention (46,85). The bone marrow, peripheral leukocytes, and skin fibroblasts are the other known sites of cystine accumulation in these patients (46). This form of cystinosis has only been observed in adults and is not accompanied by renal dysfunction or failure (46,85).

The pathology of the kidneys in cystinosis has been well reviewed (46,86). Nonspecific changes have been seen in proximal as well as distal tubules by light and electron microscopy (86). The swan-neck deformity, described as atrophy and shortening of the earliest segment of the proximal tubule (32), is not specific for cystinosis. This lesion occurs in other disorders associated with the Fanconi syndrome and in chronic interstitial nephritis (41,86). Glomerular changes, including multinucleate giant cell transformation, are also nonspecific (86). Cystine crystals have been identified in glomerular epithelial cells, cells lining atrophic tubules, and interstitial cells. The scant accumulation of cystine crystals in tubular cells does not appear to alter morphology to explain the functional aberrations of the Fanconi syndrome (86). Morphologically, the intracellular location of cystine is lysosomal and has added to the speculation that cystinosis may be a lysosomal storage disease (87).

The cause of cystinosis remains elusive. An inborn error of metabolism is suspected because of the autosomal recessive inheritance pattern. Recent evidence suggests that the basic defect is abnormal lysosomal transport of cystine, resulting in intralysosomal accumulation of cystine (88-90). How this basic defect results in the Fanconi syndrome and progressive renal failure is unknown.

Measurement of the accumulated cystine in peripheral leukocytes and skin fibroblasts in culture has been used and is currently the definitive way to diagnose cystinosis (46). The magnitude of cystine accumulation can also distinguish the infantile nephropathic type (100 times normal values) from the benign adult form (50 times normal values) (91). Cells from heterozygotes for nephropathic cystinosis usually have cystine concentrations five to six times those of normals (92,93). These values, however, are not completely reliable for identifying heterozygotes, as they occasionally overlap control values, especially when measured in skin fibroblasts (46,92,93). Heterozygote leukocytes preloaded with ^{35}S-cystine dimethyl ester can be reliably distinguished from normals, but the laboratory procedure is not easy to carry out and shipped leukocyte samples cannot be used for this test (94). Currently, this technique is not readily available in most centers for aid in identifying heterozygotes.

Prenatal diagnosis of nephropathic cystinosis is also possible (46,95,96). The cystine content of amniotic fluid cells grown in culture can distinguish homozygotes from normals, especially if a pulse-labeling technique is used to enhance the counting accuracy for the small numbers of cells (46,96). The ability to accurately diagnose a pregnancy at risk is important for genetic counseling for families affected by nephropathic cystinosis. In most laboratories, even when pulse labeling is employed, the cystine values are usually not sufficiently different for heterozygotes and normals to differentiate the two (46,96).

The treatment of cystinosis, besides the symptomatic treatment of the Fanconi syndrome, has been directed toward depleting the cells of cystine. Penicillamine, anabolic hormones, dithiothreitol, and ascorbic acid have failed to alter the course of cystinosis (41). Cysteamine has been shown to deplete cystinotic white cells and skin fibroblasts of cystine to the levels of normal cells, but the clinical use of cysteamine for up to 30 months in five patients with nephropathic cystinosis resulted in no improvement in renal tubular function or somatic growth (97). Creatinine clearance, however, did improve in two patients. A multicenter collaborative study of the clinical use of cysteamine is still in progress. Preliminary results from that study indicate that growth may be enhanced and renal function may deteriorate less rapidly in treated patients (98). Cysteamine is not very palatable; phosphocysteamine or pantethine may prove to be better tolerated by the patients and as effective in depleting cystinotic cells of cystine as is cysteamine (98). Curative therapy for cystinosis, though, has still not been found.

Lowe's Syndrome

Individuals with the oculocerebrorenal syndrome described by Lowe et al. (100) in 1952 are characteristically males who present in infancy with dense congenital cataracts and glaucoma without neurological or renal dysfunction. The full-blown syndrome, including growth failure, developmental delay, generalized muscular hypotonia, areflexia and the Fanconi syndrome, usually becomes apparent during the first year of life (Fig. 6) (101). Mental retardation is usually severe. Seizures are uncommon. Visual acuity even after cataract removal is poor, and most patients have only limited light perception. The testes are often undescended. In rare instances, tenosynovitis and arthritis have been described as late manifestations appearing after the first decade of life (102,103).

The disorder is familial and probably genetically transmitted as an X-linked recessive trait (101,104), although the evidence for this mode of transmission is not completely convincing. The preponderance of males, a one-to-one frequency of affected to unaffected brothers and the appearance of the syndrome in sons of apparently unaffected sisters support X-linked recessive transmission (101,104). Of the more than 100 cases of Lowe's syndrome described in the literature, however, at least six have been girls (105,106). The Lyon

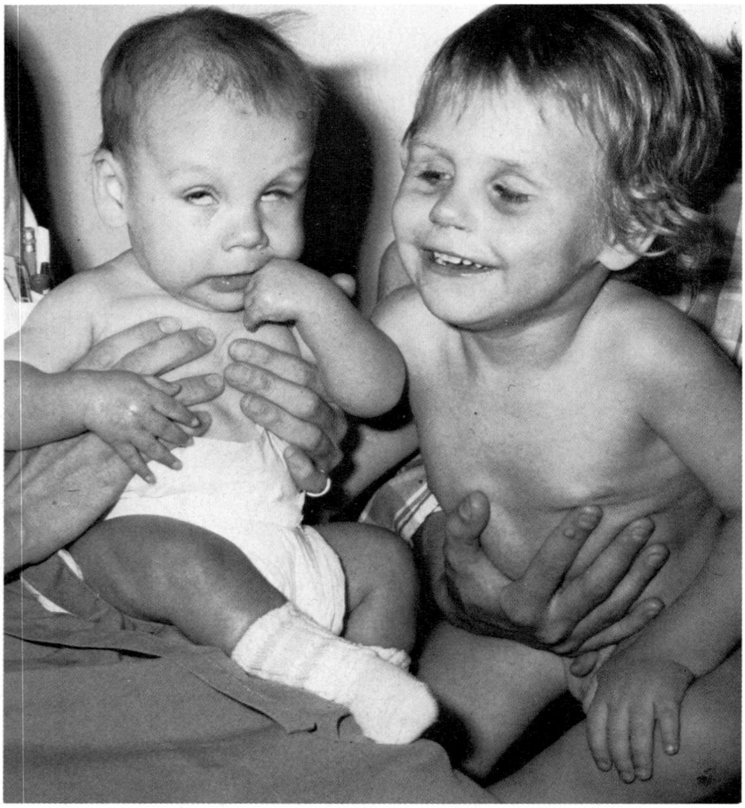

Fig. 6 Half-brothers (different fathers) with Lowe's syndrome. Both had dense cataracts and glaucoma noted in the first month of life. The 2½-year-old brother (right) has growth failure, developmental delay, hypotonia, areflexia, and the complete Fanconi syndrome. The 6-month-old brother (left) has only mild hypotonia, aminoaciduria, and hyperphosphaturia with hypophosphatemia.

hypothesis, i.e., random inactivation of one X-chromosome in each cell in females, has been invoked to explain the expression of an X-linked recessive trait in these females (41,106). By the Lyon hypothesis, if the majority of the heterozygote female's normal X-chromosomes are inactivated, the complete clinical expression of the disorder can occur, whereas if the majority of the affected X-chromosomes are inactivated, the heterozygote female will appear perfectly normal. Gradations between these two extremes should give rise to mild clinical expressions of the disorder in some females. When looked for, however, mild cases have been uncommon. Some mothers, sisters, and maternal grandmothers have been found to have punctate lenticular opacities of the eyes (104,107-109), but so have some fathers and one uncle (101,104,110). Thus, lens opacities are either not specific for the heterozygote state or the syndrome is not really X-linked recessive. No evidence for renal tubular dysfunction, as assessed by generalized aminoaciduria, has been found in presumed heterozygote females, although two mothers and one father had the appearance of generalized aminoaciduria after ornithine loading (111-113). While X-linked recessive transmission remains one explanation of the genetics of Lowe's syndrome, the final answer is not in.

Renal dysfunction in Lowe's syndrome begins as tubular dysfunction and may progress to renal failure in late childhood or adolescence (41,101). A mildly affected 20-year-old male with two-thirds normal glomerular function and 18- and 28-year-old males with normal glomerular filtration function have been reported (102,111,114). Whether all children with Lowe's syndrome will eventually develop end-stage renal disease is unknown.

The Fanconi syndrome may range from mild and incomplete to severe. Generalized aminoaciduria and tubular proteinuria appear first, usually in the first few months of life (101,115). Albuminuria, probably initially from decreased tubular reabsorption, also occurs early, but it may reach nephrotic proportions in later childhood (41,114). Glucosuria is an intermittent and inconstant finding (101). Hyperchloremic metabolic acidosis, organic aciduria, hyperphosphaturia and hypophosphatemia, and rickets may all appear within the first year of life (101).

The hyperchloremic metabolic acidosis appears to be caused by decreased proximal tubular reabsorption of bicarbonate (101,104,116,117), typical of the type 2 renal tubular acidosis characteristically associated with the Fanconi syndrome. Distal tubular acidification appears intact to the extent that an acid urine pH can be achieved (101,104,105,111, 112,116,117), and when urine pH is below 5.4 during ammonium chloride-induced acidosis, ammonia and titratable acid excretion increase to values similar to those of normal controls (116,117). Even when urine pH is greater than 6, a two- to fivefold increase in ammonia and titratable acid excretion can be seen during phosphate loading (101), suggesting appropriate function of the distal nephron.

Renal biopsies of patients with Lowe's syndrome are normal early in the course of the disease and progressively show tubular and glomerular damage (101,118). The changes are nonspecific and may be the result, not the cause of the renal metabolic dysfunction. The tubules first become dilated and filled with proteinaceous casts, then atrophic and surrounded by interstitial fibrosis. The tubular basement membrane may show focal thickening. When viewed with electron microscopy, early injury appears in proximal, but not distal tubular cells; the brush border becomes shortened and cristae of the mitochondria appear swollen or disrupted (105,119). The glomeruli first show focal, nodular thickening of the basement membranes and fusion of the podocytes, then increased mesangial cellularity, focal fibrosis, and hyalinization (101,118,119). In at least two patients the pathological renal lesion was found to be progressive despite symptomatic treatment of the Fanconi syndrome (118).

The biochemical-metabolic defect underlying the multisystem dysfunction of Lowe's syndrome is unknown. A generalized cellular transport defect may be present. Besides renal transport dysfunction, the intestinal transport of dibasic amino acids has been shown to be impaired (41,120). Bone disease, identified as radiographic osteopenia, may persist after treatment for and radiographic healing of rickets (101). At autopsy, the histological lesions of osteoporosis have been diagnosed (102), suggesting primary bone disease in addition to the treatable osteomalacia-rickets usually associated with the chronic Fanconi syndrome.

The recent reports of increased urinary excretion of mucopolysaccharides, especially undersulfated chondroitin sulfate A, and hydroxyproline suggest that Lowe's syndrome is a disorder of connective tissue metabolism (114,121,122). However, increased excretion of these substances may also occur due to the presence of metabolic bone disease per se (114, 121) or to decreased renal tubular reabsorption of these substances by a dysfunctional proximal renal tubule. Abnormal connective tissue metabolism in Lowe's syndrome has been suggested by in vitro studies of skin fibroblasts of affected patients (123). During incubation in special culture medium, these skin fibroblasts accumulate increased amounts of proline compared to controls. The significance of this in vitro phenomenon for the pathogenesis or expression of Lowe's syndrome is not yet known.

Therapy for Lowe's syndrome is entirely symptomatic. The ophthalmologist is usually the first physician to become involved. Later in infancy oral supplements with alkali, phosphate, and vitamin D metabolites may be required to treat the Fanconi syndrome. Later in childhood the metabolic abnormalities may diminish (101), probably because glomerular filtration decreases. Patients with Lowe's syndrome die from chronic renal insufficiency or intercurrent infections (41,103). Chronic dialysis and transplantation have not been attempted or recommended because of the severe mental retardation present in these patients.

Hereditary Fructose Intolerance

Hereditary fructose intolerance (HFI) is an inborn error of fructose metabolism caused by deficiency of adolase B activity in the liver, renal cortex, and small intestine (48,124). The enzyme deficiency appears to be rate limiting for glycolysis or gluconeogenesis only when an affected individual is loaded with fructose, either by oral ingestion or intravenous infusion (124). When fructose is avoided, affected patients appear normal and healthy.

The incidence of HFI is at least as common as 1 in 20,000 (125). Definite data on this point are not available, however, because affected individuals can survive infancy and live undiagnosed in the general population by avoidance of fructose-containing foods. The enzyme deficiency is inherited as an autosomal recessive trait (48). Infrequently the disorder has occurred in a parent and child, suggesting autosomal dominant transmission (48,124,126). This phenomenon can also be explained as the chance mating of a homozygote parent with a heterozygote parent (pseudodominant transmission) (124,126). In the past heterozygotes have been difficult to identify, even when enzyme activity was measured in liver biopsy tissue (127). Recently, however, Cox et al. (126) convincingly and accurately diagnosed the heterozygote state by comparing enzyme activity in intestinal mocosal biopsies of individuals at risk with those of eight normal controls. A father and all three of his children had markedly deficient intestinal aldolase B activity as well as clinical evidence of HFI. The clinically normal mother and three of the father's four siblings who were tested had enzyme activity intermediate between controls and the affected family members, a finding diagnostic of the heterozygote state. This study marked the first identification of heterozygotes for HFI and confirmed the suspected pseudodominant transmission of this autosomal recessive trait. The study also suggested that measurement of enzyme activity in intestinal tissue instead of liver biopsy tissue may be the best way to identify HFI heterozygotes.

The clinical symptoms of HFI are those of liver, gut, and kidney dysfunction, reflecting the fact that these are the tissues which normally contain aldolase B activity. The clinical expression of HFI varies with the degree of exposure to fructose. Within 30 min acute ingestion of a large amount of fructose will lead to nausea, vomiting, abdominal pain, excessive sweating, pallor, tremor, and possibly seizures or disrupted consciousness varying from lethargy to frank coma (48). Ingestion of small amounts of fructose may cause little or no symptomatology (49). Newborns who are fed fructose or sucrose-containing infant formulas as their only source of nutrition may have severe acute liver failure and hemorrhagic diathesis within a few days to weeks of exposure (128, 129). Death can ensue if fructose is not withdrawn early enough.

The most common symptoms of chronic ingestion of fructose in the first year of life are poor feeding, vomiting, and failure to thrive (130). Hepatomegaly, jaundice, abdominal distension, subarachnoid or gastrointestinal hemorrhage from the bleeding diathesis associated with liver failure, diarrhea, episodic dehydration, seizures, edema, oliguria, splenomegaly, and fever occur, but less frequently. Rickets, although uncommon, has been described in at least three infants (130). If an infant is breast-fed (breast milk contains lactose and not fructose), he will thrive until the introduction of fructose-containing cereal, fruits, or vegetables or weaning to a milk formula containing fructose, sucrose, or added honey. Commercially available corn syrup (primarily dextrins), used to sweeten infant formula may not be fructose-free because sucrose is often added by the manufacturer. Affected infants may show aversion to sweet foods as early as 4 months of age (129). Mothers of these infants often find it easier to breast-feed longer and not force-feed fructose-containing foods to their unwilling children.

Most patients with HFI are diagnosed in the first year of life (129-130). Those who learn to successfully avoid fructose, however, may not come to medical attention until later in childhood. Hepatomegaly and growth failure are then the most common clinical presentations (49,129-130). Growth failure was the only finding leading to the diagnosis in one 5-year-old boy who had voluntarily restricted his fructose intake to 130-160 mg/kg per day; he had no hepatomegaly or other obvious symptoms (49). A careful medical history did reveal that he had always refused sweets, fruits, and fruit juices and had had episodic mild abdominal pain with periods of decreased physical activity for several days at a time. Physicians who suspect the diagnosis of HFI can often elicit this type of history from affected patients or their parents, but only if very specific questions are asked. Additionally, the absence of dental caries, probably because children with HFI avoid ingestion of caries-producing fructose (124), may be helpful in pointing the physician to the diagnosis.

Some affected individuals reach adulthood without ever being diagnosed. These undiagnosed patients are at great risk if they receive routine intravenous infusions of fructose, sorbitol, or invert sugar as part of treatment for unrelated medical problems. Administration of these solutions has not only caused severe acute symptoms, but also death in some patients with HFI (131,132).

The renal manifestation of HFI is a reversible Fanconi syndrome with maintenance of normal glomerular filtration rate (13,133,134). The occurrence of the Fanconi syndrome is temporally related to actual exposure to fructose. Within minutes of the intravenous administration of fructose or slightly longer for the oral ingestion, urine pH will rise (even during ammonium chloride-induced acidosis) and urinary excretion of bicarbonate, amino acids, phosphate, urate, lactate, glucose, tubular proteins, sodium, potassium, calcum, and magnesium will markedly increase (48,49,132-137). When fructose administration ceases even temporarily, renal tubular function will return to normal within minutes to hours (132,133,135). Renal tubular dysfunction will recur again only when the patient is next exposed to fructose. Rickets occurs only rarely in infants with HFI (130), probably because of the intermittent nature of the renal tubular dysfunction interspersed with periods of normal function.

Ten to 20% of an administered dose of fructose will be excreted in the urine (124) and may be identified as a nonglucose-reducing substance. A similar percentage of administered fructose is excreted in the urine by patients with essential fructosuria (fructokinase deficiency), but the Fanconi syndrome does not occur in these patients (124).

Renal tubular abnormalities other than the reversible Fanconi syndrome have been described in two patients. A 52-year-old male patient of Steiner et al. (135) had HFI, but also persistent hypercalciuria and renal calculi with normal distal tubular acidification. Mass et al. (138) described a 41-year-old woman with HFI, who had nephrocalcinosis and distal (type 1) renal tubular acidosis. Her identical twin sister, however, had only proximal (type 2) renal tubular acidosis like that usually associated with the Fanconi syndrome and HFI (137). The unusual tubular abnormalities found in these patients most likely represent the coincidental occurrence of other renal abnormalities, and not characteristic renal manisfestations of HFI.

Since the acute intravenous administration of fructose induces a dose-dependent, reversible Fanconi syndrome in patients with HFI, it can be used as an experimental model of the Fanconi syndrome and is the only model accessible to study directly in human subjects. Using this model, Morris and his colleagues have extensively investigated the pathogenesis of the Fanconi syndrome in patients with HFI (13,49,133-134,137,139-142). They have suggested that the following sequence of events leads from the primary biochemical abnormality to the clinical expression of this disorder: In patients with HFI the renal cortex is deficient in aldolase B activity toward fructose-1-phosphate (140). When presented with a fructose load, the renal cortex rapidly converts fructose to fructose-1-phosphate under the enzymatic stimulus of fructokinase. Because of the deficiency of aldolase B, the rapid sequence of reactions to convert fructose into glucose, as shown in Fig. 7, cannot continue. Fructose-1-phosphate rapidly accumulates, depleting the cell of available inorganic phosphate, which limits the cell's ability to regenerate ATP and triggers the degradation of preformed adenine nucleotides through activation of AMP deaminase (Fig. 7) (49,139). The abnormality in adenine nucleotide metabolism may in turn impair the transepithelial transport of multiple

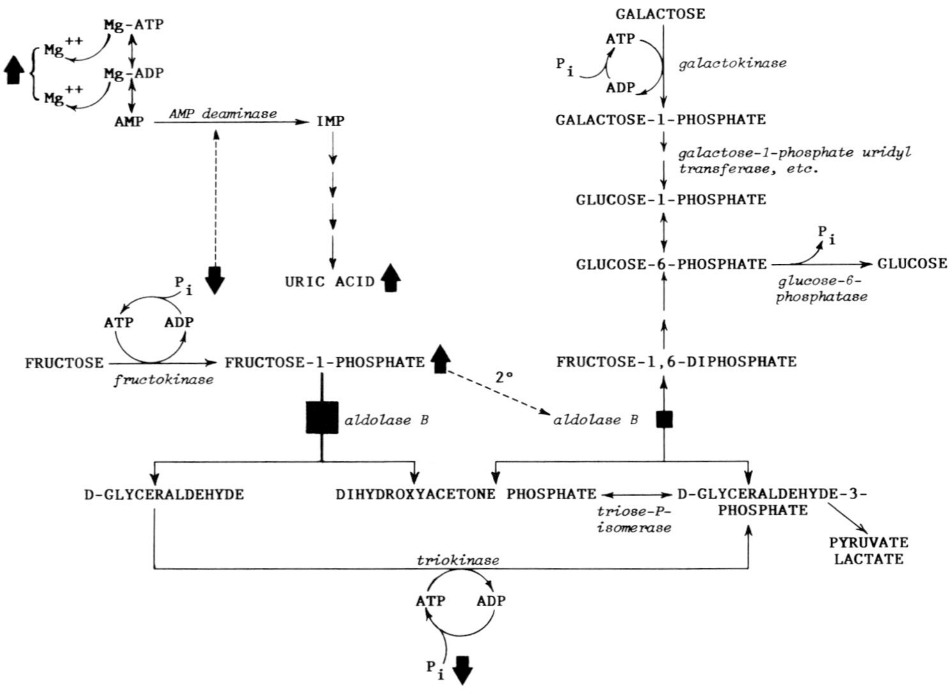

Fig. 7 Biochemical abnormalities induced by fructose in patients with hereditary fructose intolerance. A primary deficiency (■) of aldolase B activity leads to accumulation of fructose-1-phosphate, depleting the cytoplasm of inorganic phosphate (P_i), which limits regeneration of ATP and activates AMP deaminase, increasing degradation of preformed adenine nucleotides (Mg-ATP, Mg-ADP, AMP) to inosine monophosphate (IMP) and uric acid. Magnesium (Mg^{++}) is released from degraded Mg-ATP and Mg-ADP and may escape to the circulation to cause hypermagnesemia. A secondary impairment (2°) in aldolase activity toward condensing dihydroxyacetone phosphate and D-glyceraldehyde-3-phosphate to fructose-1,6-diphosphate may cause further cytoplasmic depletion of P_i. (Modified from Ref. 49.)

substances, leading to the expression of the Fanconi syndrome. When sufficient time lapses for fructose-1-phosphate to be nonenzymatically metabolized, inorganic phosphorus is released, the abnormality reverses, and transport returns to normal.

In fructose-loaded rats these events occur only in the proximal tubule, that portion of the nephron where activities of fructokinase and aldolase B exclusively reside (143). If in patients with HFI these events also occur exclusively in the proximal tubule, then only proximal tubular transport dysfunction would be expected to occur, and distal nephron function would remain intact, as has been documented for most patients in previous studies (134, 136). Recent studies suggest that the bicarbonaturia is the result of proximal dysfunction only (139,141). In patients with HFI studied during water diuresis, the bicarbonaturia induced by fructose could be completely accounted for by the quantity of bicarbonate which escaped reabsorption in the proximal tubule.

The earliest measured consequences of the biochemical events in patients with HFI are hypophosphatemia, hyperuricemia, and hyperinosinuria (139). These events occur within 10 min of intravenous fructose administration and just precede the occurrence of bicarbonaturia and type 2 renal tubular acidosis. Prior phosphate loading significantly attenuates the severity of the hyperuricemia, hyperinosinuria, and bicarbonaturia caused by fructose (13,139,142). These observations provide further evidence that cellular inorganic phosphorus depletion is the critical event in the expression of the Fanconi syndrome in patients with HFI.

The type 2 renal tubular acidosis which occurs as part of the Fanconi syndrome in patients with HFI only partially accounts for the observed metabolic acidosis. Richardson et al. (136) have shown that lactate accumulation accounts for most of it. The mechanism of lactic acidosis is not entirely understood, but inhibition of gluconeogenesis by fructose-1-phosphate and depletion of cellular ATP in liver and intestine as well as kidney are probably major contributors (124).

Hypouricemia with increased urinary urate excretion occurs in children with cystinosis and in patients with idiopathic Fanconi syndrome. In HFI, however, serum uric acid predictably increases within minutes of fructose exposure (132-136,144). An explanation for this apparent discrepancy in the expression of the Fanconi syndrome is that in HFI the biochemical disturbance in adenine nucleotide metabolism triggered by fructose also leads to markedly increased production of uric acid (Fig. 7). The production of uric acid probably exceeds the increased uric acid excretion resulting from the fructose-induced proximal tubular dysfunction (136,139), so the serum uric acid concentration is increased.

Hypermagnesemia in the presence of a proximal tubular defect for reabsorption of magnesium probably has a similar origin (49,124). Magnesium is complexed with ATP in the cell (Fig. 7). When cellular ATP is depleted, magnesium may be released from the cell to the circulation to account for the observed increase in serum magnesium concentration.

Generalized hyperaminoacidemia often results from hepatic failure of any cause and may lead to hyperaminoaciduria. Although hyperaminoacidemia may occur in patients with HFI and liver disease (41,124,145), generalized hyperaminoaciduria occurs even when serum amino acid concentrations are normal (133,134,146), clearly implicating dysfunction of the proximal tubule. In some patients chronically ingesting fructose, the plasma concentrations of tyrosine and methionine are elevated out of proportion to other amino acids, making the diagnosis of HFI difficult to distinguish from that of tyrosinemia, type 1 (see below) (41, 129,130,145,146). These patients may also have excessive urinary excretion of *p*-hydroxyphenylacetic and *p*-hydroxyphenyllactic acids (41,145,146). Unlike for patients with tyrosinemia, type 1, however, these abnormalities resolve when fructose exposure ceases.

Hypoglycemia is observed within 30-60 min after exposure to fructose and occurs more promptly and profoundly in affected children than in adults (48,124,135). The hypoglycemia probably results from several abnormalities, including markedly decreased glucose production caused by fructose-1-phosphate inhibition of gluconeogenesis, depletion of cellular ATP, and a block in glycogenolysis at the level of phosphorylase (124). Hypoglycemia can be prevented by intravenous infusion of glucose begun shortly after fructose administration has been initiated (49).

When HFI is suspected, the diagnosis should be confirmed by an intravenous fructose tolerance test performed several days to weeks after all fructose-containing substances are eliminated from the diet and from medications (124). Clinical improvement after elimination of exposure to fructose is very supportive of the diagnosis. The results of a typical fructose tolerance test, using a test dose of 500 mg/kg body weight administered intravenously over 5 min, is shown in Table 4. Gitzelmann et al. (124,125) recommend a lower test dose, 200 mg/kg body weight, for children because the chemical changes appear to be more pronounced in children than in adults. Mock et al. (49) have administered glucose, 100 mg/kg per hr intravenously, to prevent hypoglycemia during the fructose tolerance test. The diagnosis was made on the basis of fructose-induced hyperuricemia, hypophosphatemia, hypermagnesemia, and the occurrence of the Fanconi syndrome. The patient did not have to be subjected to the potential ill effects of severe hypoglycemia while undergoing a diagnostic test.

If the diagnosis is in doubt, aldolase B activity should be measured in tissue from a biopsy of the liver (49,124) or small bowel (126). Activity toward fructose-1-phosphate is less than 15% of normal in patients with HFI (124,125). Values almost this low have also been measured in liver tissue of patients with tyrosinemia, type 1 (147). Rickets is a prominent clinical feature of tyrosinemia, type 1, however, and may help distinguish it from HFI; only a few patients with HFI have had rickets (130).

Treatment of any of the manifestations of HFI begins by withdrawal of fructose, sucrose, sorbitol, and invert sugar from the diet and from medications or intravenous infusion solu-

Table 4 Results of a Diagnostic Intravenous Fructose Tolerance Test

	Before	60 min after
Serum		
Glucose (mg/dl)	78.0	38.0
Uric acid (mg/dl)	4.8	11.6
Phosphate (mg/dl)	5.5	3.8
	Before	**35 min after**
Urine		
pH	6.7	7.6
α-amino nitrogen (mg/dl)	4.35	11.86
Citrate (μmol/liter)	584.0	2493.0
Lysozyme (μg/ml)	1.9	10.5
Glucose (Labstix)	Neg	1+

A 20% solution of fructose, 500 mg/kg, was administered over 5 minutes to a 6 1/2 month old male with hereditary fructose intolerance, who presented with growth failure, vomiting after feeds, and hepatomegaly.

tions. Acidosis and the Fanconi syndrome will self-correct within a few days and often within 24-48 hr of discontinuing fructose (124,132). Recovery of hepatic function depends upon the degree of hepatic failure prior to withdrawal of fructose. If the diagnosis is made too late, the patient may succumb to irreversible hepatic failure, even several days after fructose exposure has been eliminated (124,130). Hepatomegaly in infants may persist for months to years after fructose restrction (129,130). Liver biopsies in these patients show persistent fatty vacuolization of the periportal hepatocytes. Mental retardation does not develop (129). Growth will usually return to normal after institution of a fructose-restricted diet (49,129). Mild growth retardation may persist if dietary restriction of fructose is not maintained well below 130 mg/kg per day (49).

Tyrosinemia, Type 1 (Tyrosinosis, Hereditary Tyrosinemia)

Of the various clinical disorders of tyrosine metabolism, in which plasma and urinary levels of tyrosine are increased, only tyrosinemia, type 1, is associated with the Fanconi syndrome (148). This disorder appears in the literature under many different names, including tyrosinosis, hereditary tyrosinemia, tyrosyluria and hypermethioninemia, hypermethioninemia, tyrosinose congenitale, and inborn hepatorenal dysfunction (41,148). The disorder is clearly distinct from transient tyrosinemia of the neonate and from tyrosinemia, type 2, which is an oculocutaneous syndrome without hepatic or renal dysfunction (148). Tyrosinemia, type 2, is associated with genetic deficiency of hepatic tyrosine aminotransferase (148).

Tyrosinemia, type 1, is genetically transmitted as an autosomal recessive trait with a high prevalance in the French-Canadian population of Quebec, especially in the Chicoutini Lac-St. Jean region where almost all of the residents are descendents of the original settlers (149). Many patients have also been identified in the Scandinavian countries (148,150). The disease manifests itself clinically in two forms, acute and chronic, both of which may occur within the same family (150).

The acute form of tyrosinemia, type 1, occurs in infants, usually within the first 6 months of life, and if untreated is characterized by a rapid decline to death from liver failure (148). The earliest clinical symptoms are vomiting and diarrhea with failure to thrive. The infants may emit a peculiar cabbagelike odor (147-150). A bleeding tendency with easy bruisability occurs within weeks to months after the onset of symptoms. Abdominal distension, hepatomegaly, ascites, and enlarged kidneys are usually present on physical examination. Jaundice occurs, but it is not prominent (147,151). The Fanconi syndrome may or may not be noted initially (41,147,151,152). When the Fanconi syndrome is present early on, clinical signs of rickets are often pronounced, even in infants as young as 3-4 months of age (150).

Patients with the chronic form of the disease usually present between the ages of 1 and 3 years with failure to thrive and the Fanconi syndrome, hepatomegaly with early nodular cirrhosis, and/or severe rickets resistant to therapy with low doses of vitamin D_2 (150,153). Hypoglycemia resistant to glucagon may occur (151). Mild mental retardation occurs in some but not all patients (150).

Affected patients usually die within the first decade of life, most often from liver cirrhosis or hepatoma (41). The hepatomas are either hepatocellular carcinomas or malignant hepatomas (153). They occur in one-third of the patients with tyrosinemia, type 1, and are the cause of death in over half of those who have these tumors.

During the chronic course some patients have experienced symptoms resembling those of acute intermittent porphyria, i.e., abdominal crisis, fever, and polyneuropathy, with increased urinary excretion of δ-aminolevulinic acid, but not porphobilinogen (155,156). In general, patients with tyrosinemia have increased urinary excretion of δ-aminolevulinic acid and catecholamines (155-157). An explanation for the increased urinary excretion of δ-aminolevulinic acid has been suggested based on the finding of succinylacetone and succinylacetoacetate in the urine of patients with tyrosinemia, type 1 (157). These abnormal metabolites inhibit the in vitro activity of prophobilinogen synthetase toward δ-aminolevulinic acid. Serum from these patients also inhibits the enzyme in vitro. If this inhibition also occurs in vivo, accumulation of δ-aminolevulinic acid could result and lead to its increased urinary excretion. How or if δ-aminolevulinic acid participates in causing the symptoms of acute intermittent porphyria in some patients is unknown.

The Fanconi syndrome of tyrosinemia, type 1, usually occurs within a few months of the onset of symptoms and is reversible after reduction of tyrosine and phenylalanine in the diet (41,150,152,154,158). Glomerular filtration rate is always normal or increased (41,151). Hematuria occurs in about a third of the patients (149). The first evidence of tubular dysfunction may be just generalized aminoaciduria, usually with a pronounced increase in tyrosine, methionine, ornithine, arginine, phenylalanine, lysine, proline, and threonine excretion, and normal or decreased cystine excretion (41,147,152,153). The plasma cystine concentration is often decreased (148). Increased plasma concentrations of tyrosine and methionine may be partly responsible for their prominent urinary excretion (41,149,152, 153). Glucosuria evident on urinalysis occurs intermittently (41). Fructose and galactose have also been identified in the urine of some patients with tyrosinemia, type 1 (147,150, 155); the significance of their presence is unknown. Mild proteinuria, probably of tubular origin, has been reported (41). Urinary concentrating ability may be normal or decreased (41,158).

Hyperchloremic metabolic acidosis and hypokalemia with hyperkaluria have been reported, but without simultaneous urine pH values (153,154,156,158). To date, no careful studies of proximal or distal tubular acidification have been done. Sass-Kortsak et al. (151) reported that an acidification defect was present in one patient, but they gave no details.

Hypophosphatemia, phosphaturia, and severe rickets with normocalcemia are prominent features of acute or chronic tyrosinemia, type 1 (41,150-156,158). Hypophosphatemia may appear months before rickets is clinically manifest (151,152). As with the Fanconi syndrome of other etiologies, high dosages of vitamin D_2 (50,000-200,000 IU daily) have led to improvement, but not complete healing of the rickets (150,158). Institution of a low tyrosine-phenylalanine diet alone or with a low dose of supplemental vitamin D_2 (3000 IU/day) has resulted in healing of rickets without a recurrence (150,152).

The kidneys are often enlarged on physical examination or on radiographs or at autopsy (150,151,153,155). Histologically, the tubules show moderate to marked dilatation, mainly in the proximal convoluted and straight segments, with some granular degeneration and occasional calcium deposits (41,147,150,153-154). Glomeruli appear normal. Interstitial edema may be very prominent and is perhaps the cause of the renal enlargement.

Markedly increased urinary excretion of *p*-hydroxyphenylpyruvate (*p*-HPPA), *p*-hydroxyphenyllactate (*p*-HPLA), and *p*-hydroxyphenylacetate (*p*-HPAA) originally led investigators to postulate that a deficiency of *p*-HPPA oxidase (hydrolase) (Fig. 8) was the underlying abnormality in tyrosinemia, type 1 (147,150). When measured in liver and kidney from affected patients, *p*-HPPA oxidase activity was greatly reduced (159), but so were activities of other liver enzymes, including tyrosine aminotransferase, aldolase B, cystathionine synthase, and cystathionase (147,159). The occurrence of reduced activity of all these enzymes would be more compatible with nonspecific generalized liver dysfunction than with a specific deficiency of *p*-HPPA oxidase. A genetically determined deficiency of *p*-HPPA oxidase would also not explain why in one patient, whose hepatic *p*-HPPA oxidase activity was only moder-

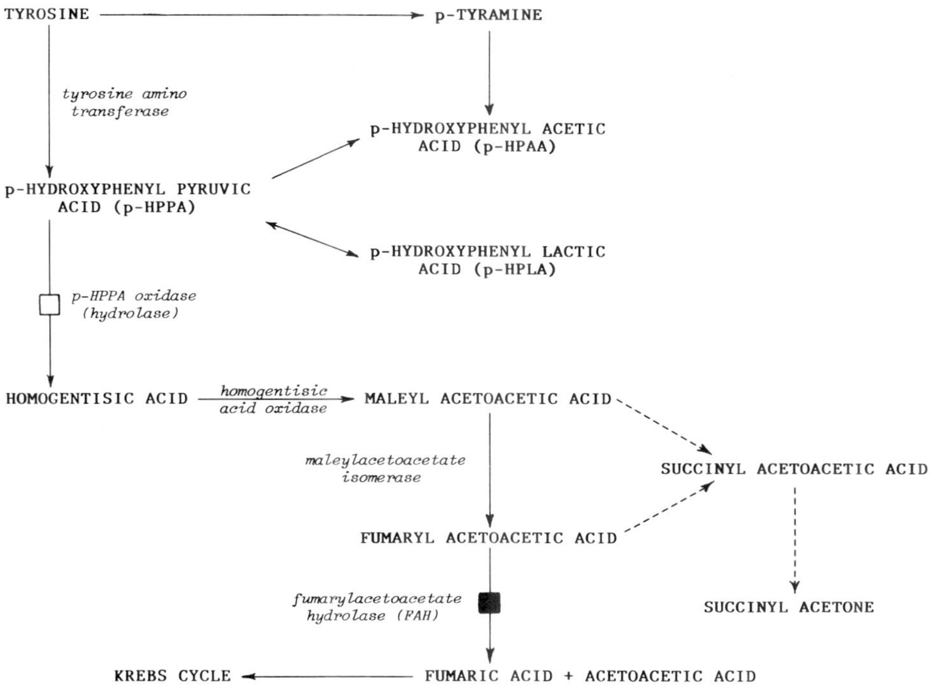

Fig. 8 Biochemical abnormalities in the degradation of tyrosine in patients with tyrosinemia, type 1. Primary (■) deficiency of fumarylacetoacetate hydrolase (FAH) activity leads to the accumulation of fumaryl acetoacetic acid and maleyl acetoacetic acid, which are converted to the abnormal metabolies, succinyl acetoacetic acid and succinyl acetone, found in the blood and urine of affected patients. A secondary (□) deficiency of *p*-HPPA oxidate activity may also occur.

ately decreased, the clinical manifestations of the disease were not different from those of other patients with severely deficient hepatic *p*-HPPA oxidase (158).

The question of the primary enzyme deficiency in tyrosinemia, type 1, remained unresolved until 1977, when Linblad et al. (157) first reported that urinary excretion of large amounts of succinylacetone and succinylacetoacetate occurred in patients with tyrosinemia, type 1. These investigators were the first to postulate that a deficiency of fumarylacetoacetate fumaryl hydrolase (FAH) might be the long sought after primary enzyme deficiency. Deficient activity of FAH could lead to accumulation of fumarylacetoacetic acid and maleylacetoacetic acid, which would be converted to the abnormal metabolites succinylacetoacetic acid and succinylacetone found in the urine (Fig. 8).

Subsequent to these studies, FAH activity has been measured in a variety of normal tissues and found to be most abundant in those organs which are most dysfunctional in patients with tyrosinemia, type 1, namely in the liver and in the kidney (160). In the liver, FAH activity is 50-fold greater than in the lung, heart, spleen, pancreas, and muscle; and in kidney, fivefold greater. Fumarylacetoacetate fumaryl hydrolase activity in lymphocytes, skin fibroblasts, and amniotic fluid cells is intermediate between kidney and other tissues. When FAH activity has been measured in tissues from patients with tyrosinemia, type 1, it is almost undectable in liver (160-163) and kidney (160) and reduced to less than 10% of control values in skin fibroblasts and lymphocytes (160). Seventeen parents of affected patients have also been tested (160). Fumarylacetoacetate fumaryl hydrolase activity in their lymphocytes and skin fibroblasts was 50% of control values, a finding compatible with a heterozygote state. Only 5% of the control determinations overlapped the heterozygote range of values for lymphocyte FAH activity.

The evidence above strongly favors a deficiency of FAH activity as the primary biochemical abnormality in tyrosinemia, type 1. Reduced activities of other enzymes, such as *p*-HPPA oxidase and tyrosine aminotransferase, are probably secondary abnormalities resulting from the disruption of tyrosine metabolism (Fig. 8) and the consequent organ failure. Lindblad et al. (157) have suggested that a genetically variable secondary deficiency of *p*-HPPA oxidase could account for the acute and chronic expressions of this disease. If *p*-HPPA oxidase were more deficient, less tyrosine would be metabolized to fumarylacetoacetate and a less acute clinical picture might result. More investigation in this area is needed before any conclusions can be drawn.

The linking events between FAH deficiency and organ dysfunction are as yet unknown. Hostetter et al. (164) have argued that accumulation of tyrosine and methionine is probably not the mechanism for liver dysfunction, since the blood levels of these amino acids may be normal when α-fetoprotein, a marker for liver disease, is already elevated. These investigators have also pointed out that even when patients adhere to a low tyrosine diet progressive hepatic failure occurs and urinary excretion of succinylacetone is not eliminated (165). On the other hand, tyrosine does cause or at least exaccerbate the renal tubular dysfunction. The Fanconi syndrome resolves during low tyrosine and phenylalanine intake (150, 152,154,158) and reappears when tyrosine and phenylalanine are reintroduced into the diet (158). Perhaps the difference in the liver and kidney responses to tyrosine restriction reflects the fact that FAH activity in kidney is 10-fold less than it is in the liver (160).

The diagnosis of tyrosinemia, type 1, should be suspected in any infant or child with hepatic dysfunction and the Fanconi syndrome, especially if plasma and urinary concentrations of tyrosine and methionine are elevated and urinary excretion of the hydroxyphenolic acids is increased (41,148). The recent biochemical discoveries suggest that assaying the urine for succinylacetone (166) or measuring FAH activity in lymphocytes, skin fibroblasts, or liver biopsy tissue (160) is the best means of establishing the diagnosis. Assaying for succinylacetone in a dried blood spot may be useful for neonatal mass screening, especially in high-risk geographical areas (166).

Prenatal diagnosis is now possible. The assay for succinylacetone in amniotic fluid (the δ-aminolevulinate dehydratase-inhibition test) appears to have a high degree of accuracy for mass screening (166-168). To be certain of the diagnosis in pregnancies known to be at risk, however, FAH activity should also be measured in cultured amniotic fluid cells (168).

A low tyrosine-low phenylalanine diet successfully treats the Fanconi syndrome and rickets, but does not prevent progressive hepatic failure in this disorder (41,150,152,154,158). In addition, a tyrosine-phenylalanine deficiency syndrome can occur if dietary intake is too low (169). Improvement in therapy will depend upon further characterizing the biochemical abnormalities of tyrosenemia, type 1. Perhaps efforts to prevent the accumulation of fumarylacetoacetate, maleylacetoacetate, or succinylacetoacetate and succinylacetone will be the effective therapy of the future (157).

Galactosemia

Galactosemia is the result of any of several autosomal recessively inherited enzyme deficiencies in the metabolic pathway for galactose (Fig. 9) (47). Only galactose-1-phosphate uridyl transferase deficiency is associated with the Fanconi syndrome (41,47). Renal tubular dysfunction does not occur with galactokinase or epimerase deficiencies.

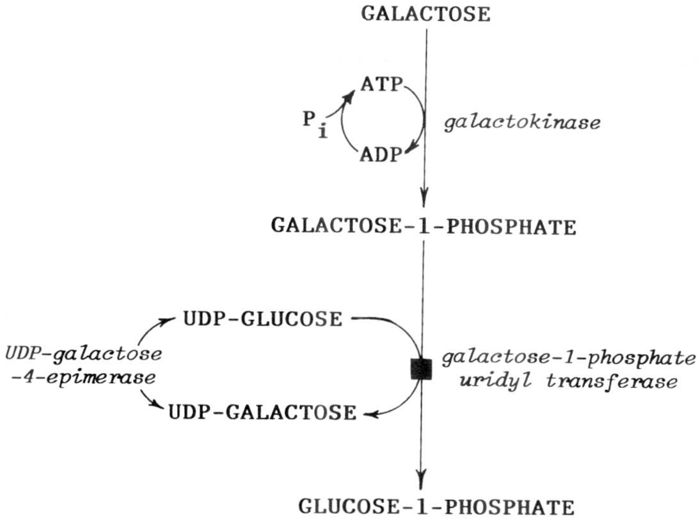

Fig. 9 Biochemical abnormality in galactose metabolism for patients with galactosemia associated with the Fanconi syndrome. Deficiency (■) of galactose-1-phosphate uridyl transferase activity, but not galactokinase or epimerase activity, occurs in patients with galactosemia and renal tubular dysfunction.

In transferase deficiency, the clinical presentation can be either an acute toxicity syndrome with vomiting, diarrhea, severe jaundice, hepatomegaly, bleeding diathesis, and *Escherichia coli* sepsis, or a chronic set of symptoms associated with growth failure (170-171). Patients with the acute form usually present during the newborn period within a few days of intake of breast milk or lactose-containing infant formula. Punctate cataracts in the fetal lens nucleus may be identifable at birth (47). Patients with the more chronic course present during the first year of life with failure to thrive, occasional vomiting, hepatomegaly, delayed development, and cataracts (47,170). The cataracts result from the accumulation in the lens of excessive galactitol, probably in the same fashion as occurs in galactokinase deficiency (47).

In patients with transferase deficiency, the reversible complex renal tubular dysfunction occurs after several days of galactose intake and ceases several days after intake has stopped (41,172). The dysfunction is best characterized as an incomplete Fanconi syndrome. Tubular proteinuria and generalized aminoacidura with normal plasma amino acid concentrations are always present (21,41,170,172-174). Glucosuria is always absent, but galactosuria and hypergalactosemia are present (170,172). Galactose-induced hyperphosphaturia may occur in association with a slight decrease in serum phosphate concentration; severe hypophosphatemia and rickets, however, have not been observed (41,171). Normal adults receiving an intravenous galactose load may have increased excretion of phosphate and amino acids (175), so the significance of these findings in galactosemia is uncertain.

The hyperchloremic metabolic acidosis and hypokalemia observed in some patients with transferase deficiency (170,172) may be secondary to chronic diarrhea (47) or renal tubular acidosis (172) or both. An attempt was made by Komrower et al. (172) to carefully study renal acidification in two patients. Both patients had a fall in urine pH to less than 5.5 in response to ammonium chloride loading during galactose ingestion. After one patient was treated with a galactose-free diet for many months, a 10-day period of galactose feeding failed to induce severe acidosis, but it did induce a slight decrease in serum CO_2-combining power, an increase in serum chloride concentration, and a concomitant large increase in bicarbonaturia with a decrease in urinary excretion of ammonia and titratable acidity. These findings are suggestive of proximal (type 2) renal tubular acidosis. Other careful studies still need to be done before the question of the etiology of the metabolic acidosis in transferase deficiency galactosemia can be settled.

Galactose-1-phosphate uridyl transferase catalyzes the conversion of galactose-1-phosphate to glucose-1-phosphate (Figs. 7 and 9). When transferase activity is deficient, galactose-1-phosphate and galactitol accumulate in the deficient tissues, including the kidney (176,177). The exact role of these metabolites, especially galactose-1-phosphate, in the pathogenesis of the Fanconi syndrome is unknown. Tedesco and Miller (178) demonstrated a galactose-induced alteration in sulfate uptake as well as a large accumulation of galactose-1-phosphate by transferase-deficient skin fibroblasts. They suggested that an abnormality in sulfate metabolism might play a role in the expression of organ dysfunction.

Another possibility for the role of galactose-1-phosphate in the pathogenesis of renal tubular dysfunction might be one analogous to that of fructose-1-phosphate in the pathogenesis of hereditary fructose intolerance. If accumulation of galactose-1-phosphate also depletes the cellular supply of inorganic phosphorus, triggering the loss of adenine nucleotides via the activation of AMP deaminase (Fig. 7), then transepithelial transport function could be disrupted. In support of this hypothesis are the observations that when an affected patient receives an acute galactose load, serum uric acid concentration increases, serum phosphate concentration decreases, and erythrocyte intracellular inorganic phosphorus concentration decreases as galactose-1-phosphate concentration increases (144,172,174). These changes slowly reverse when galactose administration is stopped (144). The sequence of events is not as dramatic as with fructose administration to patients with aldolase B deficiency, but then galactose is normally phosphorylated more slowly than is fructose (179).

The diagnosis of transferase deficiency should be suspected in any infant with failure to thrive, hepatomegaly, and non-glucose-reducing substance in the urine (47). Blood galactose levels will be high if an affected infant is chronically ingesting galactose. The definitive diagnosis is made by measuring galactose-1-phosphate uridyl transferase activity in red blood cells (180).

The elements of the Fanconi syndrome completely reverse when galactose is eliminated from the diet (47,170,172). Renal failure does not occur. Maintenance of a life-long galactose-free diet will promote normal growth (47,181,182) and prevent further liver damage and cataracts (47). Cataracts present before therapy will often regress. Long-term therapy becomes more difficult as children grow older and find it harder to strictly adher to the dietary restrictions (182). Mild to moderate mental retardation, speech and language deficits, tremor, and ataxia may become apparent with time, even when dietary galactose restriction is begun in the newborn period (183-185). Maternal lactose restriction during pregnancy has not prevented the occurrence of these neurological deficits (185). Another long-term sequela of transferase deficiency galactosemia in girls has been primary ovarian failure, even in those who received dietary therapy from birth (186,187). A postnatal effect of abnormal galactose metabolism has been postulated, based on the finding at autopsy of a histologically normal ovary in a five-day-old neonate who died of sepsis (186).

Glycogen Storage Disease

The classic Fanconi syndrome is associated with only one type of glycogen storage disease (GSD), for which the enzyme deficiency, if any, has not yet been identified (189-198).

Glycogen stores are increased in liver and kidney, as in von Gierke's disease (GSD, type I), but the kidneys are not enlarged, and in all but one case (193), hepatic glucose-6-phosphatase activity has been normal (190,191,194-196). A single patient with GSD, type III (debrancher enzyme deficiency), has been observed to have mild tubular proteinuria, renal glucosuria, and proximal (type 2) renal tubular acidosis, without aminoaciduria or phosphaturia (199). Glycogen storage disease, type III, clinically also closely resembles von Gierke's disease, but like GSD with the classic Fanconi syndrome, the kidneys are not enlarged.

Glycogen storage disease with the classic Fanconi syndrome appears to be genetically transmitted in an autosomal recessive fashion (41). Clinically, these patients may be idenfified in infancy, as early as the first 2 months of life, with manifestations of the Fanconi syndrome, followed by the onset of clinical rickets (196). Hepatomegaly, episodic fever, increased thirst, and failure to thrive occur later (191,194-196). Fasting hypoglycemia has been observed (41,191), but the oral glucose tolerance test usually produces a diabetic-type response with insulinopenia (191,192,196,198). Hyperlipidemia, acetonuria, and mild lactic acidemia may also occur (191,192,194,196-198). The hyperglycemic response to glucagon is variable (191,192,196,198). Garty et al. (196) found that the response was normal before the onset of hepatomegaly. Fructose tolerance tests are normal (196,198).

Galactose intolerance occurs in all patients and has been an identifying characteristic of GSD with the classic Fanconi syndrome (191,193,194,196-198). Activities of galactose-1-phosphate uridyl transferase, galactokinase, and epimerase in erythrocytes and liver are normal (196,198). Nonetheless, an oral galactose load produces prolonged galactosemia and galactosuria (196,198), further decrease in the already low serum phosphate concentration (197), and worsening of the Fanconi syndrome, manifested by an increase in glucosuria, phosphaturia, and uricosuria (197). Brivet et al. (198) demonstrated a marked reduction in galactose oxidation in liver tissue, but not in erythrocytes. They suggested that a localized abnormality of galactose transport, confined to the liver (and perhaps the kidney), might explain the galactose intolerance in patients with GSD and the classic Fanconi syndrome.

The carbohydrate (glucose and galactose) intolerance of these patients is similar to that described by Chesney et al. (61,62) in three patients with idiopathic Fanconi syndrome without GSD. It is possible that the Fanconi syndrome could result from bichemical events common to both of these disorders.

The striking feature of the Fanconi syndrome in patients with GSD is their massive glucosuria, even during hypoglycemia (41,192,195). Glucose excretion may approach 75% of the filtered load of glucose, a much higher level than occurs in the Fanconi syndrome of other etiologies. On this basis, Broedehl et al. (41,195) have suggested that an appropriate name for this disorder might be renal glucose-losing syndrome.

Generalized aminoacidura and phosphaturia may also be massive (41,191,195,197). Plasma amino acid concentrations are not increased when aminoaciduria occurs (191,196). Phosphaturia precedes the onset of hypophosphatemia (196). Hypophosphatemia, presumably from chronic urinary phosphate loss, and rickets are usually prominent, however, by the time the patient presents for medical care (190-195,197,198). Urinary excretion of uric acid may also be massive (191,197), and serum uric acid concentration is decreased (196). Hypouricemia is another feature distinquishing these patients from those with von Gierke's disease, who always have hyperuricemia. Metabolic acidosis may not be present when a patient presents with other features of the Fanconi syndrome (196), but it usually occurs with time and is moderate to severe (41,196). Careful studies of renal acidification have not been reported to assess whether the acidosis results from proximal tubular dysfunction alone.

Glomerular function remains normal (41). Histologically, the glomeruli also appear normal. Morphological changes occur in the tubules. Giant mitochondria with abnormal crystal patterns, like those seen in some patients with idiopathic Fanconi syndrome, have been observed in proximal tubules examined by electron microscopy (41,200). Both proximal and distal tubules have been found to have increased intracellular glycogen, although not as massively as in von Gierke's disease (41,190,191), which perhaps accounts for the lack of renal enlargement as compared to that usually found in patients with von Gierke's disease. The significance of the increased renal glycogen stores is unknown.

Treatment of patients with GSD and the classic Fanconi syndrome consists primarily of controlling the symptoms of the Fanconi syndrome and preventing episodic hypoglycemia. The rickets is not responsive to low doses of vitamin D or 25-hydroxycholecalciferol, but has healed with high doses and phosphate supplements (195,196,198). Therapy with either dihydrotachysterol or 1,25-dihydroxycholecalciferol is probably a more specific form of vitamin D metabolite therapy, but the use of these metabolites in this disorder has not yet been reported.

The tubular defects of these patients may improve with age (41). Growth retardation may persist (196,200). Mental retardation does not occur (41). The oldest patient, described originally at age 4 years by Fanconi and Bickel (189), has survived to his 30s and has done well (41).

Wilson's Disease (Hepatolenticular Degeneration)

Wilson's disease is a genetically transmitted, autosomal recessive disorder of copper metabolism that primarily affects the function of the liver and brain (50,201-203). Markedly increased amounts of copper are found in these tissues as well as in the kidneys and some other organs. Serum ceruloplasmin concentration is usually quite low, but ceruloplasmin deficiency is not the underlying genetic abnormality. The accumulation of copper in affected tissues appears to be related directly to the disturbances in function. The variability of tissue accumulation may account for the variability of symptomatology.

The classic clinical triad is hepatic cirrhosis, Kayser-Fleischer rings (greenish-brown deposits of copper in Descemet's membrane of the cornea), and neurological symptoms ranging from behavioral and psychiatric disorders to flapping tremors and dystonia. Hepatic symptoms are the major mode of presentation in childhood, usually between the ages of 6 and 14 years (202). Fulminant hepatitis may occur suddenly, but chronic hepatitis is more common. Kayser-Fleischer rings and neurological symptoms may be absent at this time. Neurological and psychiatric symptoms are the most common clinical presentation of the disease in general, usually with onset between the ages of 12 and 32 years (202). Kayser-Fleischer rings are always present when neurological disease becomes apparent.

Renal manifestations, including both glomerular and tubular dysfunction, are clinically less important, but are often present when liver disease predominates. In some patients, hematuria or renal calculi have been the clinical presentation, preceding appearance of the classic features of the disease (50,203,204). Glomerular filtration rate is usually mildly reduced (205,206); severe renal failure has not appeared before the patients succumb to other manifestations of their disease.

Renal tubular dysfunction is more prominent than glomerular insufficiency. The clearance of *p*-aminohippurate is reduced out of proportion to the decrease in inulin clearance (205,206). Typical abnormalities of the Fanconi syndrome usually occur, including generalized aminoaciduria with normal plasma amino acid concentrations and increased urinary excretion of phosphate, urate, bicarbonate, glucose, sodium, potassium, calcium, peptides, and tubular proteins (203-207). Distal tubular dysfunction also occurs (203-206).

Phosphaturia is often associated with hypophosphatemia and rickets or osteomalacic bone disease (203,208,209). Rickets is occasionally the presenting symptom (209). Serum calcium is almost always normal (203). Besides the classic radiographic changes of rickets, osteomalacia, or pseudofractures commonly associated with the Fanconi syndrome, other bone and joint abnormalities have been observed (50,203,209). These include osteochondritis dissecans and subchondral changes of the knees and spine, marginal bone fragmentation around joints, multilocular bone cysts, and evidence of osteoarthritis. These changes could be due to the recurrent minor trauma associated with the neurological dysfunction of Wilson's disease (203), but they could also represent direct toxicity of copper within the skeletal system.

Glucosuria is often absent when tested by a urine dipstick, but tubular reabsorption of glucose is reduced when compared to normals (203,205). Blood glucose concentration is normal.

Patients with Wilson's disease are usually hypouricemic (203-206,210). Values for the 24-hr urinary excretion of uric acid often fall within the normal range, but because of the low serum concentration of uric acid, renal clearance may actually be increased. A question has been raised regarding whether the increased urate excretion may reflect distal as well as proximal tubular dysfunction (210).

Distal renal acidification is abnormal in some patients with Wilson's disease, especially those with renal calculi (204-206). The distal tubular functions of concentration and dilution may also be impaired (203,206).

The etiology of hypercalciuria in Wilson's disease may be multifactorial, reflecting decreased proximal tubular reabsorption of calcium, defective distal renal acidification, hypoparathyroidism, or any combination of the three. Decreased proximal tubular reabsorption of calcium and hypercalciuria associated with the Fanconi syndrome of other disorders is usually accompanied by an increase in urinary excretion of citrate (139). On the other hand, the hypercalciuria of patients with distal (type 1) renal tubular acidosis is usually associated with decreased urinary excretion of citrate (139). Urinary citrate excretion has not been measured in patients with Wilson's disease, but might be particularly useful to help clarify the pathogenesis of the nephrocalcinosis and renal calculi which occur in some of these patients. Nephrolithiasis and nephrocalcinosis are commonly associated with distal renal tubular acidosis, but they are very uncommon in patients with the Fanconi syndrome of various etiologies (17,139).

Hypoparathyroidism, perhaps secondary to the toxic effects of copper accumulation in the parathyroid gland, has been described in an 11-year-old girl with Wilson's disease and the Fanconi syndrome (211). This patient had hypocalcemic tetany as well as hypercalciuria. Glucosuria, generalized aminoaciduria, tubular proteinuria, and phosphaturia with hypophosphatemia but not radiographic bone disease were also present. Serum immunoreactive parathyroid hormone concentration was undetectable, even during an episode of hypocalcemia.

Serum non-ceruloplasmin-bound copper is increased and urinary copper excretion is usually elevated in untreated patients with Wilson's disease (50,201,203). Values for urinary excretion range from 100-1000 μg/24 hr (201). Treatment with D-penicillamine mobilizes tissue copper and increases urinary copper excretion to even greater magnitudes (1500-3000 μg in 24 hr).

The renal pathology in patients with renal tubular dysfunction is confined predominantly to the proximal tubules (212,213). The tubular epithelium may be focally flattened with loss of the brush border and degenerative changes in the mitochondria (212), similar to changes observed after administrations of other tubular toxins like maleic acid (36). Histochemically, copper has been localized to the cytoplasm and nuclei of proximal tubular cells; some intranuclear deposition may appear in glomerular cells and rarely in distal tubular cells (212,213). Glomeruli and the distal tubules were normal in a patient who had the Fanconi syndrome, but normal distal tubular function and a mildly reduced inulin clearance (212). Renal tissue from patients with distal acidification dysfunction has not been studied, but might be expected to show marked accumulation of copper in distal tubular epithelial cells.

The pathogenesis of Wilson's disease is still unknown, despite the fact that the clinical entity has been known since 1912 and many cases have been described. The two abnormalities of copper metabolism which are currently thought to be the most important in this disease are the decreased biliary excretion of copper and the prolonged retention of copper in the liver (201). These features are very similar to the normal hepatic metabolism of copper in the fetus and newborn infant, who appear to need a positive hepatic copper balance (214). Neonates also usually have a decreased concentration of serum ceruloplasmin. Failure to switch soon after birth from the fetal-neonatal pattern of copper metabolism to the normal child-adult pattern might be the explanation for the abnormal copper metabolism in patients with Wilson's disease (214). The genetic abnormality might be a defect in the controller gene or genes which induce normal copper metabolism. Accumulation of copper in other organs could result from overflow of hepatic copper into the general circulation (201). Further studies are needed before the mystery of the pathogenesis of Wilson's disease is solved.

The diagnosis can usually be made in the patient with neurological disease by the identification of Kayser-Fleischer rings (either on observation or slit-lamp examination) and the measurement of a decreased concentration of serum ceruloplasmin (<20 mg/dl). The diagnosis is more difficult in the child with liver disease (201,215). Measurement of the hepatic concentration of copper in an adequate tissue specimen from a needle biopsy may be necessary to distinguish Wilson's disease from chronic active hepatitis (215). A tissue concentration greater than 400 μg/g dry weight is usually diagnostic, although there may be overlap with values for patients with primary biliary cirrhosis (215,216). Serum ceruloplasmin concentration and 24-hr urinary excretion of copper may not be helpful in distinguishing these two diseases (201,215,216). In this circumstance demonstration of negligible incorporation of radioactive copper into the patient's serum ceruloplasmin after oral administration of a tracer dose is the most definitive test for Wilson's disease (215).

The mainstay of treatment for Wilson's disease has been oral administration of the chelating agent D-penicillamine (50,201,217). Early diagnosis and treatment yield the best outcome, but early diagnosis is often not possible unless the physician has a high index of suspicion for this disease (202). Renal tubular and glomerular dysfunctions are completely reversible with therapy (213,217). When the development of side effects of D-penicillamine therapy prevents its continuation, as it does in about 10% of patients, triethylene tetramine dihydrochloride may be used as an effective alternative chelator (218).

Other Inborn Errors of Metabolism

Several other hereditary diseases have been associated with the complete or partial Fanconi syndrome. Classic Fanconi syndrome has been described in one infant with a lethal form of hereditary mitochondrial myopathy, in which skeletal muscle mitochondria were very large and had abnormal cristae (219). Muscle mitochondrial cytochromes aa_3 and b were found to be absent. Renal tissue was not available for testing, but a similar abnormality in renal mitochondria might be the underlying biochemical abnormality leading to the observed proximal tubular transport dysfunction.

A partial Fanconi syndrome has been described in a patient with the late infantile form of metachromatic leukodystrophy (lysosomal arylsulfatase A deficiency) (220). Proximal (type 2) renal tubular acidosis and increased clearance of ornithine, threonine, glycine, alanine, and leucine were noted, but tubular reabsorption of glucose, phosphate, and uric acid was normal. In this severe neurological disorder, galactosyl and lactosyl sulfatides accumulate mainly in cerebral white matter and peripheral nerves, but also in other tissues, including the kidney. Although the sulfatide accumulation has been observed morphologically in cells of the distal nephron (loop of Henle to the collecting duct) (220,221), only proximal tubular dysfunction has been reported.

Proximal (type 2) renal tubular acidosis with and without generalized aminoaciduria and phosphaturia has been described in a few patients several months into their course of subacute necrotizing encephalomyelopathy (Leigh's syndrome) (222-224). Rickets has not been observed prior to death in the first few years of life. A deficiency of pyruvate carboxylase activity has been demonstrated in kidney tissue obtained at autopsy (223). Deficiency of this enzyme could interfere with ATP generation in the proximal tubule and contribute to the pathogenesis of the observed tubular transport dysfunction.

An occasional patient with hereditary nephritis (225) or medullary cystic disease (226) has also had the Fanconi syndrome. In each case renal biopsies showed significant tubular basement membrane structural abnormalities (thickening, splitting) and tubular atrophy. Whether these tubular changes were more severe than in other patients with the same disorder is not certain. Histological abnormalities of the tubules occur often in these patients, but the Fanconi syndrome has only occurred in a few. A separate, acquired injury in the rare patient with the Fanconi syndrome cannot be ruled out.

C. Acquired Disorders

Immunological and toxic injury to the renal tubule from a variety of sources may result in the clinical Fanconi syndrome (Table 2). Most of these disorders affect adults more often than children, but some can occur at any age. Many are reversible when the underlying abnormality is treated successfully or when exposure to the toxin ceases. The Fanconi syndrome is often partial and frequently associated with abnormalities of distal tubular function, especially defective distal renal acidification.

Disorders of Protein Metabolism-Excretion

Disorders of protein metabolism and excretion have in common the urinary excretion of abnormal quantities of protein either from excessive extrarenal production and an increased filtered load of proteins (multiple myeloma and other dysproteinemias) or increased glomerular permeability to circulating proteins (nephrotic syndrome). Direct toxicity to the proximal tubule by the filtered proteins is a speculative, but attractive hypothesis to explain the pathogenesis of these forms of the Fanconi syndrome, although, clearly, other factors are also important in patients with the nephrotic syndrome.

Multiple Myeloma and Other Dysproteinemias

The Fanconi syndrome is an occasional, but important clinical manifestation of dysproteinemias, often preceding the diagnosis of the underlying disease by many years (227-229). Multiple myeloma is the most common of the dysproteinemias and also the most common identifiable cause of the Fanconi syndrome in adulthood (37). Patients with myeloma and the Fanconi syndrome usually develop signs and symptoms after the fourth decade of life (227-232). Renal glycosuria or mild proteinuria are often the first observable signs (227, 228). The full-blown Fanconi syndrome with generalized aminoaciduria, uricosuria and hypouricemia, tubular proteinuria, phosphaturia, hypophosphatemia, and debilitaing osteomalacic bone disease may develop slowly over years. Renal tubular acidosis is usually mild or absent (227,231,232). Renal failure may be a late manifestation, probably related to multiple myeloma per se and not to the Fanconi syndrome (227,233).

In the patients with multiple myeloma and the Fanconi syndrome, Bence Jones (light chain) proteinuria is always present, although it may be missed if a urine protein electrophoresis is not done (227). When the Bence Jones protein has been typed, it has always been of the kappa variety (227-230).

At the time of diagnosis of the Fanconi syndrome, the bone marrow plasma cells may be normal in morphology, except for the presence of crystalline cytoplasmic inclusion bodies seen with the electron microscope (227). Similar inclusion bodies have been observed in proximal renal tubular cells (Fig. 10) (227,229,232). Degenerative changes of the renal tubular cells, especially in the proximal convoluted segment, have been seen by light microscopy (227,231,232). Whether the degenerative proximal tubular changes are more striking in patients with myeloma and the Fanconi syndrome than in those with myeloma alone (233) has not been determined by a systematic study.

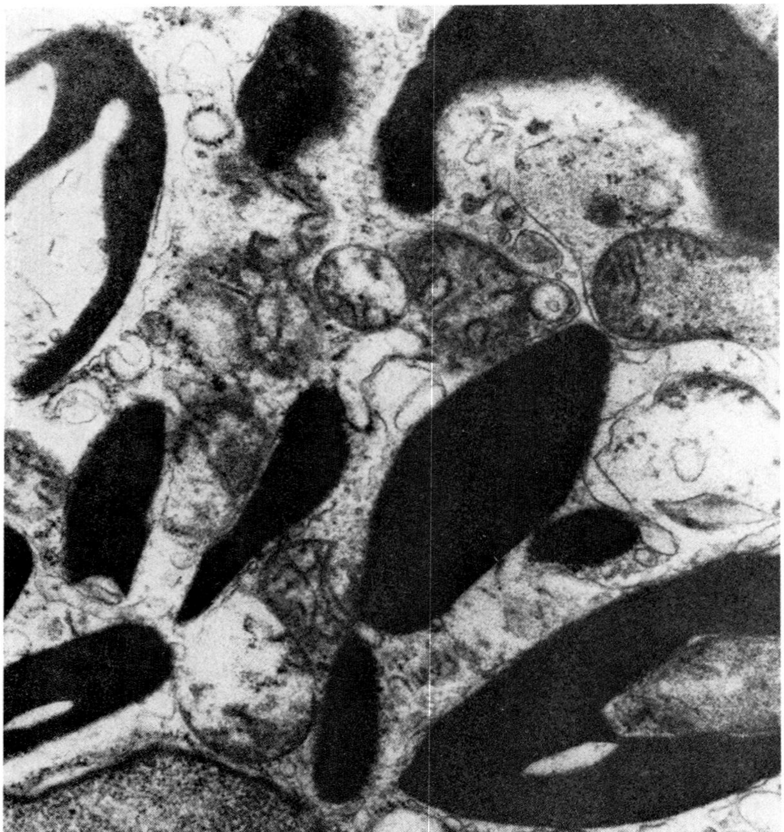

Fig. 10 Electron micrograph of a proximal renal tubular cell of a 34-year-old woman with light chain nephropathy. The dense crystalline deposits in the cytoplasm are characteristic of those observed in plasma cells and proximal renal tubular cells of patients with multiple myeloma and other dysproteinemias. (X 34,000.) (From Ref. 19.)

Partial or complete Fanconi syndrome also occurs infrequently in patients with benign monoclonal gammopathy (234,235), light chain nephropathy (19,236-239), amyloidosis (227,239,240), and, very rarely, Sjogren's syndrome (234,241-243). All of these patients have had Bence Jones proteinuria (19,227,234-240,242), just like patients with multiple myeloma and the Fanconi syndrome (227-230). However, unlike the patients with multiple myeloma, who all had kappa light chainuria, two of these patients had predominately lambda light chainuria (234,242). Crystalline cytoplasmic inclusion bodies, like those found in patients with multiple myeloma, have also been observed in proximal renal tubular cells of patients with these other kinds of dysproteinemia (Fig. 10) (19, 236,240).

An attractive hypothesis to explain the occurrence of the Fanconi syndrome in patients with dysproteinemia is that filtered light chains exert a direct toxic effect on the proximal tubules, where light chains are reabsorbed in large quantity (19,227,237). The finding of crystalline inclusion bodies, probably representing light chain accumulation, within proximal tubular cells in patients with these disorders is supportive of this hypothesis. Clyne et al. (244) have shown that kappa light chain administered to rats accumulates in crystalline inclusion bodies in the proximal tubule. Direct renal toxicity of light chains has also been demonstrated in vitro: Gluconeogenesis and uptake of *p*-aminohippurate by rabbit kidney cortex slices are inhibited by light chains (245), and both kappa and lambda light chains inhibit Na-K-ATPase in plasma membranes of rat renal cortical tubules (246). If these events occur in vivo, multiple proximal tubular transport abnormalities, like those characteristic of the Fanconi syndrome, might be expected to occur. If the toxic damage to the tubule were not severe and if the toxin, in this case light chains, were removed, the lesion might also be reversible. In one 41-year-old woman with kappa light chainuria, who was treated with a single course of melphalan, renal glucosuria did disappear parallel to the resolution of the light chainuria (238).

Why only a few patients with dysproteinemias and Bence Jones proteinuria have the Fanconi syndrome is unknown. The long duration of relatively benign Bence Jones proteinuria, asymptomatic except for the Fanconi syndrome in most affected patients, may be a partial explanation (227,237). Other factors, such as the magnitude of the excretion of light chains and the solubility characteristics of the light chain itself, must also play a role. The significance of the predominance of kappa over lambda light chainuria in these patients is not yet known.

Nephrotic Syndrome

Occasional patients with the nephrotic syndrome may develop the Fanconi syndrome (247-253). These patients are usually children with onset of their nephrotic syndrome between the ages of 1 and 10 years. Proteinuria, when analyzed, has been nonselective (251), and the nephrotic syndrome has usually been steroid resistant, if not initially, then later in the course (249-254). In two families siblings have been affected (250), but most cases have been sporadic.

The Fanconi syndrome usually develops progressively within months to a few years after clinical presentation of the nephrotic syndrome. Renal glycosuria or renal tubular acidosis appears first, often followed in time by generalized aminoaciduria, then hyperphosphaturia and hypophosphatemia, hyperkaluria and hypokalemia, and occasionally tubular proteinuria and hyperuricosuria and hypouricemia (247,251,252). Rickets occurs in some, but not all patients (247,250,251,253,254). Some patients have evidence of distal tubular dysfunction expressed as distal (type 1) renal tubular acidosis and nephrocalcinosis (250-252). Maximum urinary concentrating capacity may be decreased (251,252). After the onset of tubular dysfunction, most patients develop progressive renal insufficiency, which usually leads to end stage renal disease within a few years (250-252).

In some patients renal biopsies obtained early in the clinical course may suggest minimal change disease, with or without mesangial hyperplasia and with normal or focally dilated tubules (250-252). Follow-up biopsies in these patients and initial biopsies in other affected children, however, usually show the histological features of focal glomerulosclerosis (250-252). Tubular atrophy and interstitial fibrosis are prominent. Immunofluorescence is usually negative.

Another group of young nephrotic children with a similar clinical course have a different pathological lesion by renal biopsy. These patients have membranous glomerulopathy with severe interstitial nephritis and positive immunoflourescence for IgG and C_3 deposited in a linear pattern along the tubular basement membrane (253,254). The Fanconi syndrome in these patients is more likely related to their interstitial nephritis and antitubular basement membrane antibody deposition than to their nephrotic syndrome. They are discussed in more detail in the section below (Immunological Disorders) along with other cases of antitubular basement membrane antibody disease.

The renal biopsy of one 6-year-old girl who had the simultaneous onset of the nephrotic syndrome and the Fanconi syndrome showed severe acute tubulointerstitial nephritis and mesangial and endothelial proliferative glomerulonephritis (255). Immunofluorescent staining was positive for IgG and complement along the glomerular basement membrane and within the proximal tubular cells. Renal tubular epithelial antigen was demonstrated in the glomeruli and the proximal tubules, and the antigen and its specific antibody were isolated from the patient's serum. This patient, unlike other patients with the primary nephrotic syndrome and Fanconi syndrome, may have had a primary tubular injury which caused the Fanconi syndrome and released renal tubular epithelial antigen to the circulation to cause immune complex-mediated glomerulonephritis and secondary nephrotic syndrome.

The pathogenesis of the Fanconi syndrome in patients with focal glomerulosclerosis and the nephrotic syndrome is uncertain. Excessive filtered protein might be directly toxic to the proximal tubule, but this seems unlikely, since heavy proteinuria occurs often in association with other glomerular lesions, but the Fanconi syndrome does not. The incidence of proximal tubular dysfunction in children with focal glomerulosclerosis has been reported to be as high as 12.5% (eight of 64 cases) (256). Whether the underlying abnormality of focal glomerulosclerosis affects the tubule as well as the glomerulus awaits further investigation.

Immunological Disorders

Tubulointerstitial nephritis may be immunologically mediated by autoantibodies (antitubular basement membrane antibody disease), by accumulation of immune complexes along the tubular basement membrane and within the interstitium (immune complex-mediated disease), and by delayed hypersensitivity reactions to autologous or exogenous substances (cell-mediated tubulointerstitial disease) (257,258). Patients with antitubular basement membrane disease, renal transplants, and some lymphomatous malignancies fall into this category. These patients occasionally develop the Fanconi syndrome.

Interstitial Nephritis with Antitubular Basement Membrane Antibody

The hallmark of interstitial nephritis with anti-TBM antibody is the immunofluorescent identification of linear deposits of IgG and C_3 along the basement membrane of the cortical tubules, primarily the proximal tubules (254,258), and in the serum (253,254,259,260). Although many patients with anti-TBM disease also have antiglomerular basement membrane disease, some have anti-TBM disease alone (257-260). One such patient, a 4-year-old boy, had clinically evident tubular dysfunction (259). He presented with renal glucosuria which progressed over 2 years to the complete Fanconi syndrome, including generalized aminoaciduria, phosphaturia, bicarbonaturia, acidosis, proteinuria, and chronic renal failure.

Seven children, most of whom presented with steroid-resistant nephrotic syndrome between the ages of 10 months and 10 years and later developed the partial or complete Fanconi syndrome, including rickets, had membranous glomerulopathy and interstitial nephritis with anti-TBM antibody (253,254). The anti-TBM antibody was deposited in a granular pattern in some, but usually linearly. Most also had circulating anti-TBM antibody (254). Progressive renal failure occurred in the five patients for whom follow-up was available.

In rats with anti-TBM interstitial nephritis produced by injection of homologous kidney suspension, glucosuria and proteinuria have also been observed (261).

Renal Transplantation

A reversible Fanconi syndrome may develop in either a cadaveric or living related donor renal allograft (262-265), usually coincident with an acute rejection episode and resolving after successful treatment of the rejection episode (264,265). The Fanconi syndrome most likely results from an immunological event which injures the tubules. Ischemic injury, hyperparathyroidism, and toxic injury from azathioprine immunosuppression appear to be unlikely contributors to the pathogenesis (264,265). Anti-TBM antibodies have been detected in a linear pattern in allografts undergoing rejection and in the serum of some transplant recipients (266,267). To date, however, no renal biopsy tissue has been available from transplant recipients with the Fanconi syndrome to assay for anti-TBM antibody. Whether anti-TBM antibody, the mononuclear cellular infiltrate of acute rejection, or both participate in the pathogenesis of the Fanconi syndrome of transplant recipients is not yet known. In one instance, a 14-year-old boy whose original disease was the idiopathic Fanconi syndrome, the Fanconi syndrome recurred and persisted after a living related donor renal transplant (60). This patient also had several acute rejection episodes, though they were thought not to be related to the persistent recurrent Fanconi syndrome.

Malignancy

The Fanconi syndrome has been described in two patients with lymphoid malignancies, one with Burkitt's lymphoma (268) and one with chronic lymphocytic leukemia, kappa light chainuria, and peritubular amyloidosis (239). Both patients had peritubular infiltrates of lymphoid cells in kidneys examined at autopsy. In the first case, the infiltrates were massive and compressed tubular and glomerular structures. In the second case, the leukemic infiltrates were focally scattered in the interstitium of the cortex and medulla, but amyloid was prominent within the tubular basement membranes. Mechanical destruction of the tubules by the massive infiltrates, toxic damage to the tubule by light chains, or tubular basement membrane injury from amyloid may have played important roles in the pathogenesis of the Fanconi syndrome in these patients. Cell-mediated immunological injury to the tubules by the lymphoid infiltrates may also have been important.

Other malignancies, including malignant hepatoma (12) and adenocarcinoma of the pancreas (269), have occurred in patients presenting with the Fanconi syndrome, but the simultaneous occurrence may have been unrelated. Two patients with carcinoma of the lung developed partial Fanconi syndrome during the latter stages of their disease; the cause of their Fanconi syndrome could not be determined (270).

Drug-Related

Drugs may induce tubular injury and dysfunction, including the Fanconi syndrome. The dysfunction is usually reversible on withdrawal of the offending agent. Examples of drugs which are known to induce the Fanconi syndrome are outdated tetracycline (271-280), methyl-3-chromone (281), 6-mercaptopurine (282), gentamicin and the aminoglycoside antibiotics (283-286), the anticonvulsant valproic acid (287), and the chemotherapeutic agents streptozotocin (288) and isophthalanilide (289).

Outdated, Degraded Tetracycline

Ingestion of outdated, degraded preparations of this drug has caused severe, but reversible Fanconi syndrome in children (272,273,275) and adults (271,273-277). Anhydro-4-epitetracycline, a breakdown product of tetracycline exposed to air, heat, moisture, and low pH, is the toxic substance (273,278). When this compound is given to dogs or rats, dose-dependent proximal tubular morphological injury becomes apparent after the Fanconi syndrome has begun (278-280). Structural abnormalities of proximal tubular mitochondria occur first (280). Tetracycline is known to accumulate within mitochondria of renal cells, and anhydro-4-epitetracycline is known to cause decreased oxidative enzyme activity concurrent with the onset of the tubular dysfunction in rats (280). Toxic injury to proximal tubular mitochondria, resulting in an inability to generate sufficient ATP to drive active transport processes, may be important in the pathogenesis of the Fanconi syndrome in patients who ingest degraded tetracyclines.

Methyl-3-Chromone

The accidental ingestion of a large dose of methyl-3-chromone (Diachrome) by a 3-year-old boy resulted in the occurrence of a reversible Fanconi syndrome (281). This spasmolytic drug, which was used by the father for treatment of coronary disease, is structurally similar to tetracycline.

6-Mercaptopurine

An adult who received 6-mercaptopurine therapy for the nephrotic syndrome associated with membranoproliferative glomerulonephritis also developed the Fanconi syndrome after prolonged therapy and the appearance of other toxic side effects, namely anemia and leukopenia (282). Other adult nephrotics not treated with 6-mercaptopurine have shown increased urinary excretion of amino acids (290,291), glucose (291), and proximal (type 2) renal tubular acidosis (291), but not hyperphosphaturia and hyperuricosuria with hypouricemia, as in this patient. Whether the Fanconi syndrome resulted from tubular injury by 6-mercaptopurine or was associated with the nephrotic syndrome per se, as in the childhood nephrotics described above, is unknown.

Gentamicin and Aminoglycoside Antibiotics

The aminoglycoside antibiotics are known to accumulate in proximal tubular cells (286, 292) and to cause dose-dependent morphological injury to that nephron segment (293-295). In animals, only netilmicin has been found to have less nephrotoxicity than the other aminoglycosides (296). Aminoglycoside toxicity is usually manifested clinically as reduced glomerular filtration rate (286), but tubular dysfunction, including tubular proteinuria (297,298), hypomagnesemia with hypokalemia and urinary hyperexcretion of magnesium and potassium (299-302), and the Fanconi syndrome (283-285) have been described. Most clinical cases have been associated with gentamicin therapy. The author has recently cared for a 23-year-old male patient with renal magnesium and potassium wasting associated with prolonged tobramycin administration. More cases of tubular toxicity from other aminoglycosides, except possibly netilmicin, may be expected with widespread use of these drugs. One case of the Fanconi syndrome occurred in a patient treated with gentamicin and cephalothin, also a potential proximal tubular toxin (283). The combination of these two drugs may have increased the likelihood of tubular dysfunction.

Valproic Acid

Valproic acid, which is used to control seizure disorders, has caused reversible Fanconi syndrome and growth arrest concurrently with some of its other known side effects in a 12-year-old boy (287). Catch-up growth and normalization of tubular function occurred after cessation of the drug. The author has observed generalized aminoaciduria without the Fanconi syndrome in another child receiving valproic acid therapy for a seizure disorder.

Heavy Metals

Chronic exposure to several of the heavy metals, including cadmium, lead, mercury, uranium, and platinum, leads to selective binding by the metal to the proximal tubule and proximal tubular dysfunction varying from generalized aminoaciduria or tubular proteinuria to the full-blown Fanconi syndrome (303,304). Cadmium is the most frequent cause of the Fanconi syndrome.

Cadmium

Cadmium has a long biological half-life (over 10 years). Prolonged exposure, even at low levels, may lead to excessive accumulation in body tissues, especially in the kidney (303). Chronic nephrotoxicity occurs in a cadmium-polluted environment (305) or from occupational exposure in the steel-plating, pigment, plastic, alloy, accumulator battery, or nuclear and electronic engineering industries (306-309). The classic example of environmentally induced cadmium renal disease is itai-itai byo, or "ouch-ouch" disease (305,310,311). This disease had its peak incidence after World War II in the Jinzu River Basin in Japan. The soil and rice fields in this area were shown to be heavily contaminated with cadmium brought with irrigation water from a polluted river. Primarily middle-aged, postmenopausal, multiparous women were affected. The patients came to medical attention because of severe pain from crippling osteomalacic bone disease. Tubular proteinuria, glucosuria, aminoaciduria, decreased tubular reabsorption of phosphorus, low phenolsulfonphthalein excretion, and decreased concentrating ability were then identified. A few had renal failure. Histological examination of kidney tissue usually showed normal glomeruli, tubular atrophy and dilatation, eosinophilic casts, and interstitial fibrosis. Autopsies of five itai-itai patients revealed liver tissue with five to 10 times the cadmium content of age-matched controls. Although kidney tissue cadmium concentration was lower than for controls, this finding probably reflected the expected decrease in cadmium concentration in damaged kidneys and kidneys from adults of advanced age (312,313).

An epidemiological study of the endemic area for itai-itai disease revealed that in adults over 70 years of age, 45% of women and 40% of men had proteinuria and glucosuria (311). Another study was carried out in adults over 35 years of age in the Hosogoe area of Kosaka, Japan, where a copper refinery has been operating since the 1870s and the soil as well as rice and vegetables grown there are heavily contaminated with cadmium (314). Twenty-two percent of those tested had proteinuria and glucosuria, and more than a third of these were age 35-60 years. All had lived in the contaminated region for 28 years or more. These two studies suggest that renal tubular dysfunction probably results from protracted exposure to environmental cadmium over many years.

Renal tubular dysfunction resulting from occupational poisoning with cadmium also occurs after years of exposure. Clinically detectable proteinuria is not seen until at least 9 and usually 25 years of exposure (306). The proteinuria is primarily of tubular origin and persists for years after cessation of exposure (306,309). Mild glomerular proteinuria may also appear after many years (usually about 20) of exposure (315,316). Increased excretion of β_2-microglobulin, a tubular protein, appears early and may be a useful screening test for subtle renal tubular damage (305,315). Other tubular abnormalities are usually found only in workers with tubular proteinuria; these include glucosuria, uricosuria, hyperchloremic acidosis, and impaired concentrating ability (306-308,316). Glomerular filtration rate is either normal or only mildly reduced (306,308,315). Hypercalciuria, renal calculi, and osteomalacia have also been observed (306-308,316,317). Nasorespiratory disease may be a prominent feature in the industrially exposed patient (307,308).

The severity of osteomalacic bone disease appears to be out of proportion to that of the renal tubular dysfunction, especially in patients with itai-itai disease (44-45,318). Whether cadmium per se or in combination with other factors, such as nutritional deficiencies, is responsible for the severe bone disease is unclear. Dietary deficiencies of calcium and protein intake in experimental animals do appear to contribute to the severe bone disease of cadmium poisoning (319). Hypercalciuria from decreased reabsorption by cadmium-damaged renal tubules may also reduce the calcium available for bone mineralization (306,315,320, 321). Whether mild dietary vitamin D deficiency is important in the development of the bone disease is unclear (320,322). Chronic cadmium poisoning in experimental animals does not appear to inhibit renal vitamin D metabolism to cause the vitamin D-deficient state (323). Cadmium itself, however, may have a direct toxic effect on bone (323,324). This possibility is considered in detail in the next chapter in the discussion of the experimental model of chronic cadmium poisoning.

Treatment of chronic cadmium nephrotoxic disease is symptomatic. The use of chelating agents has been limited. British antilewisite (BAL) appears to be more toxic, as a BAL-cadmium complex, than cadmium itself (325), so it should not be used. Patients should be removed from their toxic environment, if possible, to prevent further renal damage.

Lead

Unlike cadmium, lead causes Fanconi syndrome only in children with acute intoxication (326,327) and in experimental animals (328). The Fanconi syndrome is reversible with treatment of the lead intoxication. Chronic lead poisoning in adults usually presents as renal failure, although aminoaciduria has been found in some lead workers (329). In contrast to the hypouricemia and increased urinary urate clearance of the Fanconi syndrome, hyperuricemia and decreased urate clearance may occur in the adult lead nephropathy associated with either remote childhood lead exposure (330) or ingestion of moonshine whiskey (331). In both cases, a high incidence of saturnine gout has been noted. Evidence of distal renal tubular dysfunction, characterized by salt wasting, acidosis, and hyperkalemia, has been reported with lead nephropathy from moonshine whiskey ingestion (332,333).

Lead, like cadmium, binds selectively to the proximal tubule (334). Histologically, in lead poisoning but not poisoning with other heavy metals, a nuclear inclusion body appears in proximal tubular cells (335,336). The nuclear inclusion body contains lead and lead-binding protein and disappears with therapy.

Treatment for either acute lead intoxication or chronic lead nephropathy ordinarily consists of Ca-EDTA (ethylenediaminetetraacetic acid) chelation and removal from the lead-contaminated environment or cessation of ingestion of lead-contaminated products (337).

Mercury

Exposure to mercury either as inorganic salts or organic mercurials, like those found in mercurial diuretics, can be toxic to the kidney. Inorganic mercuric salt administered to rats accumulates in the proximal tubule and causes dose-dependent necrosis, especially in the pars recta (338,339). Organic mercurials appear to be less toxic than inorganic mercury, but still can cause tubular necrosis and renal failure (339). Acute ingestion of mercury-containing compounds by man causes severe gastrointestinal disturbances and acute renal failure

(341). Chronic ingestion usually results in the nephrotic syndrome (303,342-344) and rarely tubular dysfunction (19,345). Generalized aminoaciduria has been identified in workmen chronically exposed to mercury vapor (346). Reversible Fanconi syndrome has been found in a 38-year-old woman after years of ingestion of a mercury containing laxative (Calomel) (19) and in a 1½-year-old infant girl treated with a topical mercury-based teething solution for 12 months (345).

Uranium

In experimental animals uranyl nitrate reacts with proximal tubular cell membranes, disrupts amino acid transport, and causes necrosis, especially of the pars recta (347-349). Industrial exposure to gaseous uranium compounds has been associated with a high incidence of aminoaciduria and glucosuria, even months after exposure ceased (346). Uranium appears to be a far more potent agent in producing aminoaciduria from industrial exposure than either lead or mercury (346).

Platinum

In the past decade platinum, in the form of *cis*-diamminedichloroplatinum (cisplatin or *cis*-DDP), has found a place in anticancer therapy for solid tumors (350). The drug has become an integral part of the therapy for disseminated testicular and ovarian carcinoma and is also being used in chemotherapy regimens for other types of cancer, including bladder carcinoma, recurrent squamous cell carcinoma of the head and neck, non-oat cell carcinoma of the lung, osteogenic sarcoma, and some carcinomas of the cervix, prostate, and esophagus.

Dose-dependent nephrotoxicity in the form of decreased glomerular filtration rate, has been the limiting factor in the use of the drug (350,351). Renal failure results from tubular, and not glomerular injury. The percentage of patients developing renal failure, even after a single dose of *cis*-DDP, was high until prehydration and maintenance of a good diuresis during administration of the drug was routinely instituted. Concomitant use of other nephrotoxic drugs, like the aminoglycosides, also increases the incidence of renal failure. When renal failure occurs after chronic treatment courses, it is usually irreversible (352). Azotemia and decreasing glomerular filtration rate parallel histological changes of injury and necrosis in both proximal and distal renal tubules (352-354). Careful studies in rats demonstrated the worst injury to be in the proximal and distal tubular segments at the corticomedullary junction, the region of the kidney that also contained the highest concentration of platinum (354). The injury was maximal 7 days after a single dose of *cis*-DDP and progressed to irreversible necrosis with chronic treatment (11 weeks).

Tubular function in patients receiving *cis*-DDP treatment has been evaluated rarely, so the incidence of tubular dysfunction like that which occurs with other heavy metal intoxications is not yet known. Stark and Howell (355) prospectively studied 10 cancer patients at 5, 12, and 22 days after treatment courses that consisted of *cis*-DDP, 20 mg/m^2, for 5 consecutive days. They found no decrease in tubular reabsorption of phosphorus nor any appearance of glucosuria, renal tubular acidosis, or light chain proteinuria, even after as many as three treatment courses at 3-week intervals. Other investigators have confirmed the absence of hyperphosphaturia and hyperchloremic acidosis (304). However, evidence of proximal tubular dysfunction has been noted in more recent prospective studies. Jones et al. (356) detected proximal tubular proteinuria, including β_2-microglobulinuria and *N*-acetyl-β-glucosaminidasuria, in 12 cancer patients as long as 6 weeks after treatment with *cis*-DDP, 120 mg/m^2, as a single dose given with a mannitol-induced diuresis. Bitran et al. (304) demonstrated generalized aminoaciduria in nine of 14 cancer patients at 48-72 hr after *cis*-DDP, 30 or 50 mg/m^2, administered in a single dose with appropriate diuresis.

Aminoaciduria and tubular proteinuria may be the most sensitive markers for subtle renal tubular injury from *cis*-DDP administration.

The most important renal transport system to be affected by *cis*-DDP is probably that for absorption of magnesium. Hypermagnesuria in the presence of hypomagnesemia has been documented in a number of patients treated with *cis*-DDP (304,357). The inappropriate renal magnesium loss is not related to forced diuresis or mannitol or diuretic therapy, since in some patients hypermagnesuria has been documented 3 weeks after discontinuation of diuresis and diuretic agents (357). Hypomagnesemia resulting from the renal magnesium losses may be severe (serum magnesium < 1 meq/liter) and is often accompanied by marked hypokalemia and/or hypocalcemia (304,357).

The mechanism of platinum-induced renal tubular dysfunction is unknown. Focal proximal cellular necrosis probably cannot account for the isolated aminoaciduria, tubular proteinuria, or hypermagnesuria. Guarino et al. (358) have demonstrated inhibition of Na-K-ATPase activity in rat renal cortical slices incubated in vitro with *cis*-DDP. They suggest that platinum is a direct cellular toxin inhibiting tubular transport mechanisms through inhibition of Na-K-ATPase.

Since there is no treatment for *cis*-DDP nephrotoxicity, prevention is the goal. Careful attention to hydration and diuresis prior to, during, and at least 24 hrs after administration of the drug greatly reduces the incidence of renal failure (350,351). In the experience of the author, hydration should also be monitored during the period of vomiting that invariably occurs and may persist for days after high doses of *cis*-DDP. Avoidance of rapid infusion rates for *cis*-DDP administration and of the concommitant use of other nephrotoxic drugs is also warranted. Administration of mannitol during or just after a *cis*-DDP dose, besides inducing a diuresis may retard the rate of excretion of *cis*-DDP and, therefore, reduce the concentration of the toxin presented at any one time to the renal tubule (351). Furosemide and other diuretics appear to have no special advantage. Dissolving *cis*-DDP in sodium chloride solution, instead of a nonchloride solution like dextrose and water, in which aquation of *cis*-DDP can occur, may also have a protective effect (359). Finally, careful monitoring for reduction of renal function and for electrolyte imbalances related to *cis*-DDP are mandatory. Reduction of renal function is a relative contraindication for continued use of *cis*-DDP. Although firm recommendations have not yet been decided, reduction of the dose or discontinuation of therapy are probably warranted if the renal failure is not caused by obstruction from the tumor itself (351,355). When renal magnesium wasting occurs, correction of the hypomagnesemia with intravenous or oral magnesium supplements should also correct the associated hypokalemia and hypocalcemia, unless they are related to nutritional or other unrelated causes.

Other Toxin Exposure

Paraquat, a widely used herbicide, when ingested either accidentally or suicidally causes severe lung injury, but can also result in acute oliguric renal failure and proximal tubular dysfunction (360). Renal glucosuria, aminoaciduria, tubular proteinuria, increased sodium excretion, hyperphosphaturia with hypophosphatemia, and hyperuricosuria with hypouricemia have been documented in two patients during the recovery phase of their acute renal failure. Histological examination of the kidneys of a third patient, who died on the first day after ingestion, showed tubular epithelial cell lesions compatible with toxic injury. A severe Lysol burn to the thigh resulted in reversible aminoaciduria, glucosuria, and acute renal failure in a 58-year-old laboratory assistant (361). Toluene inhalation (glue sniffing) has also led to the reversible Fanconi syndrome without renal failure (362,363). Renal tubular acidosis, either distal (type 1) or proximal (type 2) or a combination of the two, is a more common finding than Fanconi syndrome in these substance abusers (362-365).

Other Renal Disorders

Partial or complete Fanconi syndrome occasionally occurs in a variety of other renal diseases. The exact cause of the tubular dysfunction in these disorders is not known, but tubular injury from toxins or ischemia is highly likely.

Environmental toxins have been suggested, but not yet identified, as etiological agents for the tubulointerstitial nephritis of Balkan nephropathy (366,367). These patients all come from a narrow geographic region, in adjacent areas of Bulgaria, Romania, and Yugoslavia. Their disease begins with tubular proteinuria; then hyperuricosuria, glucosuria, and aminoaciduria occur (366). Renal acidification and phosphate reabsorption are spared.

Iron appears to be a tubular toxin in some patients with hemolytic episodes associated with paroxysmal nocturnal hemoglobinuria (368). Like other heavy metals, iron is deposited preferentially in the proximal tubular cells and may result in multiple tubular functional defects, including tubular proteinuria, proximal (type 2) renal tubular acidosis, aminoaciduria, and phosphaturia. Proximal tubular function is usually normal in patients with renal hemosiderosis from other disorders, such as thalassemia minor, hereditary spherocytosis, or autoimmune hemolytic anemia (325).

Partial or complete Fanconi syndrome has been described in infants after spontaneous recovery from renal vascular accidents, clinically diagnosed as renal vein thrombosis in the newborn period (369). These infants presented between the ages of 6 months and 1 year with rickets, acidosis, and growth retardation. Further testing identified glucosuria, aminoaciduria, tubular proteinuria, phosphaturia and hypophosphatemia, and renal tubular acidosis. The tubular functional defects were chronic and required therapy in most.

Vitamin D Disorders Associated with Secondary Hyperparathyroidism

Reversible proximal tubular dysfunction, including hyperphosphaturia, generalized aminoaciduria, and proximal (type 2) renal tubular acidosis, has been observed in children and adults with dietary vitamin D deficiency (370-374), intestinal malabsorption syndromes with vitamin D deficiency and hypocalcemia (139,374,375), and the autosomal recessively transmitted disorders known as vitamin D-dependent rickets (376-380). Hypocalcemia and secondary hyperparathyroidism as well as a deficiency of or end-organ resistance to 1,25-dihydroxyvitamin D occur in all of these disorders. Whether excessive parathyroid hormone or relative deficiency of 1,25-dihydroxyvitamin D or both are necessary conditions for the expression of the Fanconi syndrome in these disorders is controversial (139,381). Complete reversal of the Fanconi syndrome has occurred with either correction of hypocalcemia and suppression of hyperparathyroidism (371,377) or administration of the appropriate metabolite of vitamin D (370,372,374-377). Parathyroid hormone is not necessary for the expression of the Fanconi syndrome in other disorders; in a child with Wilson's disease the Fanconi syndrome occurred in the absence of any detectable circulating parathyroid hormone (211).

V. PATHOPHYSIOLOGY

The specific biochemical and toxic abnormalities which are known or suspected to contribute to the pathogenesis of the Fanconi syndrome in each of the clinical disorders have been discussed in detail in the preceding section. How these abnormalities might contribute to a basic pathophysiological defect common to all the clinical and experimental expressions of the Fanconi syndrome is discussed in detail in Ch. 15. The most likely possibilities for this basic defect include impairment of the renal tubular cell's ATP-Na-K-ATPase transport system or an alteration in its cell membrane permeability, or both. Studies of experimental models of the Fanconi syndrome (Table 3) have been very important in the attempt to define a basic cellular defect.

The remainder of this section will be devoted to additional comments about the pathophysiology of the proximal (type 2) renal tubular acidosis, potassium and sodium wasting, and bone disease which occur as part of the Fanconi syndrome.

A. Proximal (Type 2) Renal Tubular Acidosis

When the proximal tubular acidification process is impaired, the urine pH is inappropriately high during mild to moderate degrees of hyperchloremic metabolic acidosis, but it is appropriately reduced (< 5.5) during severe acidosis (Fig. 11) (15,139). Bicarbonaturia occurs as urine pH increases. The magnitude of bicarbonaturia varies directly with the plasma bicarbonate concentration (15,139). At normal plasma bicarbonate levels bicarbonaturia equals or exceeds 15% of the filtered load of bicarbonate. This magnitude of excretion can occur only if bicarbonate reabsorption by the proximal tubule is impaired. If distal nephron acidi-

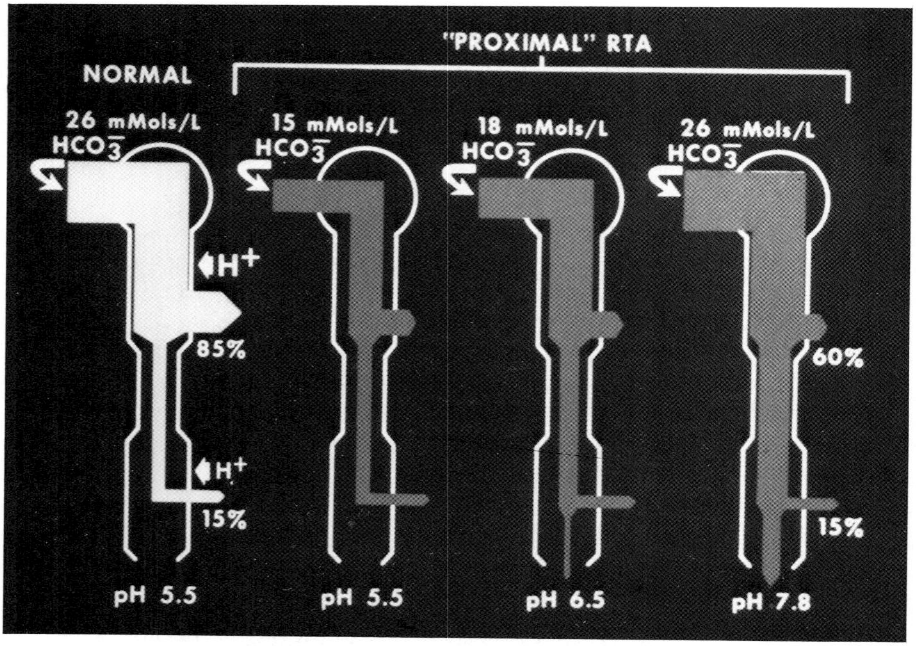

Fig. 11 Schematic representation of the renal acidification defect in proximal (type 2) renal tubular acidosis compared to normal renal acidification (nephron at far left). In affected patients during severe acidosis (e.g., plasma HCO_3 15 mmol/liter), urinary pH will be appropriately reduced (pH 5.5 or less), if the amount of HCO_3 escaping reabsorption proximally does not exceed the reabsorptive capacity of the distal nephron. If acidosis is mild or moderate (e.g., plasma HCO_3 18 mmol/liter), supernormal amounts of HCO_3 will be delivered out of the defective proximal tubule into the distal tubule, exceeding its reabsorptive capacity and resulting in bicarbonaturia and an inappropriately high urinary pH (e.g., 6.5). If the plasma HCO_3 concentration is increased to normal (26 mmol/liter), the amount of HCO_3 escaping reabsorption in the defective proximal tubule will greatly exceed the reabsorptive capacity of the distal tubule and massive bicarbonaturia (e.g., 25% of the filtered load as shown in the nephron on the far right) will occur. (From Ref. 137.)

fication is intact and only proximal acidification is impaired, then during severe degrees of acidosis urine pH will fall, bicarbonaturia will be absent, and the excretion of ammonium and titratable acidity will not be reduced. In general, this type of pure proximal tubular acidification defect almost always occurs in association with the Fanconi syndrome (14,15, 117,139). Some patients, however, especially those with toxin-induced forms of the Fanconi syndrome, may have both proximal and distal acidification defects (19,39,204-206, 250-252,362-365).

In proximal (type 2) renal tubular acidosis the magnitude of bicarbonaturia is also an important determinant of alkali therapy (139). Oftentimes, especially in children with normal glomerular filtration rates, alkali supplements of more than 10 and occasionally greater than 20 meq/kg body weight per day are required to chronically correct the metabolic acidosis. If a patient cannot tolerate such large doses, contraction of the extracellular fluid volume with hydrochlorothiazide therapy (382-384) or salt and water restriction (116,385, 386) has proved useful for sustaining correction of the acidosis. One boy with idiopathic Fanconi syndrome had such severe salt wasting, potassium depletion, and volume contraction when untreated that he actually spontaneously developed metabolic alkalosis (26). Expansion of his extracellular volume resulted in the appearance of mild proximal (type 2) renal acidosis typical of the Fanconi syndrome.

B. Potassium and Sodium Wasting

Potassium wasting occurs invariably in patients with the Fanconi syndrome and proximal (type 2) renal tubular acidosis with bicarbonaturia, especially when plasma bicarbonate is maintained in the normal range by chronic alkali therapy (Fig. 12) (26,28,386,387). Impaired proximal tubular reabsorption of potassium alone is not sufficient to account for the degree of potassium wasting. Actual net renal secretion of potassium often occurs as indicated by the observation that the fractional excretion of potassium is greater than 1 (Fig. 12) (28). The excessive secretion of potassium occurs in the intact distal nephron (388); it is the result of excessive delivery of sodium and bicarbonate out of the dysfunctional proximal tubule into the distal nephron in the presence of a continuous stimulus for distal sodium reabsorption (26,28,139). The pathogenesis of potassium wasting in proximal (type 2) renal tubular acidosis and its comparison to that associated with distal (type 1) renal tubular acidosis is discussed in greater detail in Ch. 8.

Sodium reabsorption by the proximal tubule is greatly reduced in both clinical (26-28, 386) and experimental (35,389) forms of the Fanconi syndrome. The loss of sodium often is large enough to result in volume contraction and secondary hyperaldosteronism (26,28, 139). In this circumstance, as noted above, a normal distal nephron will be stimulated to maximally reabsorb sodium and secrete potassium (26,28,388). Expansion of the extracellular volume by treatment with sodium and alkali supplements will further reduce proximal reabsorption and enhance urinary loss of sodium, potassium, and water (116,386). During alkali therapy, increased distal delivery of bicarbonate, a less permeant anion than the chloride which normally accompanies sodium exiting the proximal tubule, will also increase distal potassium secretion (28,386,388).

Renal potassium wasting is usually severe enough to cause potassium depletion. Potassium depletion per se may impair renal concentration and stimulate thirst and polydipsia to partially account for the striking polyuria of some patients (139,386). Even in the presence of dehydration, the urine usually remains dilute in patients with the Fanconi syndrome (26,27,139,386).

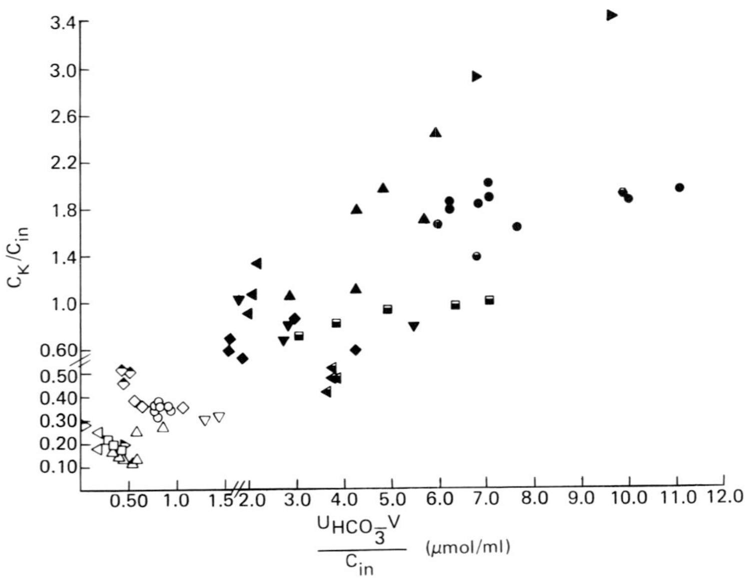

Fig. 12 Relationship between fractional potassium excretion (C_K/C_{in}) and urinary bicarbonate excretion ($U_{HCO_3}V/C_{in}$) in patients with the Fanconi syndrome and proximal (type 2) renal tubular acidosis (closed and three-quarter-closed symbols) and in patients with distal (type 1) renal tubular acidosis (open and three-quarter-open symbols). The plasma bicarbonate concentration was maintained at normal levels (22-26 mmol/liter) for more than two months (closed and open symbols) or was rapidly increased to normal levels by intravenous administration of sodium bicarbonate (three-quarter-closed and three-quarter-open symbols). Each geometric symbol represents measurements made in a single patient. (From Ref. 28.)

C. Bone Disease

Multiple factors may contribute to the pathogenesis of the metabolic bone disease (rickets-osteomalacia) which occurs with chronic forms of the Fanconi syndrome. These include impaired renal tubular synthesis of 1,25-dihydroxyvitamin D, hyperphosphaturia and hypophosphatemia, hypercalciuria, chronic metabolic acidosis, and perhaps even metabolic abnormalities of the bone itself caused by the underlying disorder. Although many patients with the Fanconi syndrome may develop chronic renal failure, their bone disease often occurs when the glomerular filtration rate is normal or only slightly reduced, distinguishing it pathogenetically from the hyperphosphatemic renal osteodystrophy of chronic renal failure.

In the normal kidney 1,25-dihydroxyvitamin D is synthesized by 1-hydroxylation of 25-hydroxyvitamin D, a reaction which occurs primarily, if not exclusively in mitochondria of the proximal tubule (390-393). The proximal tubule is also the major site of functional and morphological injury caused by the clinical and experimental disorders of the Fanconi syndrome (16,32,35,36,41,139). A reduction in the proximal tubular synthesis of 1,25-dihydroxyvitamin D might be expected to occur as part of complex proximal tubular dysfunction characteristic of the Fanconi syndrome. This possibility seems especially likely for those disorders in which proximal tubular mitochondria are known to be affected morphologically or functionally, such as in Lowe's syndrome (105,119) or the maleic acid-induced experimental model (36,394). Evidence for and against this hypothesis has been obtained from studies of experimental models and from clinical cases.

When the renal conversion of 25-hydroxyvitamin D to 1,25-dihydroxyvitamin D was studied experimentally in vitamin D-deficient rats and chicks with maleic acid-induced Fanconi syndrome a significant reduction in conversion was observed in the absence of a significant decrease in glomerular filtration rate (394). On the other hand, in rats and dogs with the chronic cadmium-induced Fanconi syndrome, synthesis of 1,25-dihydroxyvitamin D appeared to be intact (323,395), even though cadmium added in vitro to chick kidney mitochondria had been found to completely inhibit the 1-hydroxylation reaction (323,396). A difference in the degree of severity of injury to the proximal tubule could account, at least partially, for the discrepancy in findings in different experimental models. Maleic acid in the dosage used for the vitamin D studies appears to cause more severe functional and morphological changes (35,36) than does chronic cadmium administration (321,324). In the chronic cadmium model protein binding of cadmium within the renal tubular cell might have protected the mitochondria from the toxic effects of cadmium (321). If large concentrations of free cadmium had accumulated, the results might have been different.

Studies of clinical cases of the Fanconi syndrome have provided conflicting results. In cystinotic children, some of whom had previously received alkali supplements to correct their acidosis, phosphate supplements to correct their hypophosphatemia and large doses of vitamin D_2 to treat their rickets, complete healing of rickets did not occur until treatment with 1-α-hydroxyvitamin D_3 or 1,25-dihydroxyvitamin D_3 was instituted (397,398). These observations suggested that sufficient 1,25-dihydroxyvitamin D might not be synthesized even in the presence of adequate substrate for 1-hydroxylation. Serum concentrations of 1,25-dihydroxyvitamin D, to the extent that they are reflective of renal synthesis, should be decreased in patients with the Fanconi syndrome, if renal synthesis of this metabolite is impaired. When serum concentrations of 1,25-dihydroxyvitamin D were first measured in one patient with cystinosis, two with Lowe's syndrome and three with idiopathic Fanconi syndrome, the levels were reduced when compared to age-matched controls (399-401). These patients were receiving either vitamin D_2, dihydrotachysterol, or no therapy at the time of the determinations. At least three had glomerular filtration rates greater than 50% of normal. Two patients were noted to be mildly acidotic (serum CO_2 combining power 18.0 and 18.5 meq/liter), but one was not (23 meq/liter) (400).

Since these initial studies, other patients with the Fanconi syndrome have been evaluated and found to have serum levels of 1,25-dihydroxyvitamin D within the normal range for age. The reports include studies of two patients with idiopathic Fanconi syndrome and one with the Fanconi syndrome associated with severe combined immune deficiency (402). None was receiving vitamin D therapy. Two had radiographic evidence of rickets at the time of study. One was also hypophosphatemic. Moss et al. (362) studied an adult with reversible Fanconi syndrome from toluene inhalation. This patient actually had elevated values for serum 1,25-dihydroxyvitamin D concentration when she was hypophosphatemic during the recovery phase of her tubular dysfunction.

The author's clinical experience with 11 nonacidotic children with the Fanconi syndrome (six with cystinosis, three with Lowe's syndrome, and one with idiopathic Fanconi syndrome) has been that serum levels of 1,25-dihydroxyvitamin D were within the normal range for age, except for one cystinotic boy whose glomerular filtration rate was less than 25% of normal. The patients were all receiving alkali supplements to correct their acidosis. Ten were receiving no vitamin D metabolite therapy at the time of study. Eight were hypophosphatemic.

In patients with the Fanconi syndrome and hypophosphatemia, the presence of normal or low, but not supranormal concentrations of serum 1,25-dihydroxyvitamin D is consistent with the formulation that a dysfunctional proximal tubule may have impaired ability to synthesize adequate amounts of 1,25-dihydroxyvitamin in response to the usual stimuli for increased production. Hypophosphatemia is usually a potent stimulator of renal 1,25-dihydroxyvitamin D synthesis (403-405) and might be expected to be associated with the appearance of supranormal levels of circulating 1,25-dihydroxyvitamin D. In a child with vitamin D deficiency, rickets, and hypophosphatemia, Chesney et al. (406) observed that the serum 1,25-dihydroxyvitamin D concentration was normal before the patient was treated, but increased to supranormal during 3 months of therapy with vitamin D_2. Supranormal values for serum 1,25-dihydroxyvitamin D concentration were noted 3 days after cessation of toluene inhalation in the chronic substance abuser with reversible Fanconi syndrome discussed above (362). This patient might have had impaired renal synthesis of 1,25-dihydroxyvitamin D during continued toluene exposure that was reversible, just like the rest of the Fanconi syndrome, when the toxic exposure ceased. The supranormal values for serum 1,25-dihydroxyvitamin D concentration would have been appropriate for a recovery phase. Unfortunately, no comparison values were obtained during a period of toluene inhalation to know whether synthesis had been impaired.

The reduction in renal synthesis of 1,25-dihydroxyvitamin D in patients with the Fanconi syndrome could vary with the degree of metabolic injury sustained by the proximal tubule from the underlying etiology, even among patients with the same disorder. This spectrum of severity could explain some of the variation in measured concentrations of serum 1,25-dihydroxyvitamin D among patients with the Fanconi syndrome.

Hypophosphatemia resulting from decreased renal tubular reabsorption and urinary loss of phosphate may contribute directly to the pathogenesis of the metabolic bone disease. In some adults and children with Fanconi syndrome and chronic hypophosphatemia, healing of the bone disease has occurred with phosphate supplementation, even without vitamin D therapy (17,46,56,407). But, bone disease has also healed in some patients after administration of large doses of vitamin D alone (18,408), without measured improvement in hypophosphatemia (409). The presence of chronic hypophosphatemia has not been predictive of the occurrence of bone disease (139,237). Hypophosphatemia per se and the consequent deficiency of substrate for bone mineralization is probably an important pathogenetic determinant of bone disease in many patients, but certainly not a major determinant in all.

Urinary loss of calcium might reduce the availability of this substrate for bone mineralization and contribute to the pathogenesis of metabolic bone disease. Hypercalciuria occurs frequently in patients with the Fanconi syndrome (16-19,41,139,211), but hypocalcemia, except in vitamin D disorders, is rare (13,18,139). Extracellular fluid volume expansion during therapy for the electrolyte disturbances of the Fanconi syndrome enhances hypercalciuria in some patients, but without inducing hypocalcemia (18,385,386). Contraction of extracellular volume by sodium restriction (385), fluid restriction (386), or hydrochlorothiazide therapy (382,383) reduces hypercalciuria and may increase the available supply of calcium for bone mineralization. Hydrochlorothiazide therapy has improved bone mineralization in adults being chronically treated for hypertension (410).

Chronic metabolic acidosis, like that which results from the renal acidification defect of the Fanconi syndrome, promotes bone demineralization (139,411). The release of bone calcium salts to buffer the increased body hydrogen ion concentration in the chronically acidotic subject may be the major contributor to the pathogenesis of the demineralization (411). Impaired renal synthesis of 1,25-dihydroxyvitamin D does not appear to occur in chronically acidotic humans (412,413), although studies of vitamin D-deficient animals previously suggested this possibility (414,415). Renal tubular acidosis from a variety of causes besides the Fanconi syndrome may be associated with metabolic bone disease (412,416). Healing of the bone disease with alkali therapy alone has occurred in some of these patients (412,417). The effect of alkali supplements without simultaneous administration of vitamin D has not been systematically evaluated in patients with the Fanconi syndrome. The author has cared for two children with nephropathic cystinosis and the Fanconi syndrome, who received alkali therapy alone for several months. During that time rickets markedly improved in one and healed radiographically in the other. These observations suggest a direct pathogenetic role for chronic metabolic acidosis in the bone disease associated with the Fanconi syndrome.

Lee et al. (19) proposed that an abnormality in transport intrinsic to bone itself might contribute to the bone disease of some patients with the Fanconi syndrome, especially if the abnormality decreased the flux of phosphate (and calcium) into the bone. Studies in experimental animals suggest that cadmium might have this kind of toxic effect on bone as well as kidney (323,324,395). No other evidence is currently available to support or refute this hypothesis.

VI. GENERAL CLINICAL MANAGEMENT

Treatment of the underlying disease or toxin exposure has been discussed for each of the clinical disorders in Sect. III. When no specific therapy exists, symptomatic treatment of the electrolyte disturbances and bone disease of the Fanconi syndrome is the only alternative. Correction of the hyperchloremic metabolic acidosis usually requires dosages of alkali in excess of 3 meq/kg body weight per day (139). The total dose should be divided and given at frequent intervals throughout the day. When very large doses ($>$ 15-20 meq/kg per day) either cannot be tolerated or do not completely correct the acidosis, extracellular volume contraction should be considered. This may be accomplished by sodium chloride restriction (385,386) or occasionally by fluid restriction in the severely polydipsic patient (386). Hydrochlorthiazide therapy contracts extracellular volume and helps correct acidosis, but also potentiates the severity of hypokalemia and hyponatremia, which limits its usefulness (382-384).

Potassium supplementation is always a necessary part of therapy for patients with the Fanconi syndrome who have chronic acidosis which must be treated with alkali therapy (139,386,387). Administration of the potassium salts of bicarbonate, citrate, or acetate fulfills the dual purpose of treating acidosis and preventing hypokalemia. In severe cases, contraction of extracellular fluid volume may be helpful to sustain normokalemia (385,386).

The use of vitamin D metabolites instead of vitamin D_2 for treatment of the metabolic bone disease associated with the Fanconi syndrome is now widespread, at least for children. The rationale for using 1,25-dihydroxyvitamin D_3, 1-α-hydroxyvitamin D_3 or dihydrotachysterol is that their biological activity does not depend on their renal metabolism (418-420), which may be impaired in the Fanconi syndrome (see above). These metabolites also have a shorter biological half-life than vitamin D_2, minimizing the risk of toxic effects from prolonged hypercalcemia which can occur during therapy with large doses of vitamin D_2 (139).

Oral phosphate supplements are useful in some patients to initiate and help sustain healing of rickets-osteomalacia (17,46,56,139,407) and to improve or cure muscle weakness (17,51). The simultaneous administration of phosphate and alkali supplements has led to tetany (46), however, so phosphate supplements should be used with caution.

Generalized aminoaciduria, tubular proteinuria, glucosuria, and hyperuricosuria have not been associated with any clinical signs or symptoms to warrant specific therapy. Renal magnesium wasting, however, may be sufficient to cause hypomagnesemia, and if it does, should be treated with supplemental doses of magnesium salts (19,304,357).

Polyuria occurs in most patients and may be extreme in some (386). Unless the patient's therapy necessitates some degree of volume contraction, prevention of dehydration from obligatory polyuria is best handled by allowing the patient free access to fluids.

When chronic renal failure occurs and progresses in patients with the Fanconi syndrome, treatment of the electrolyte disturbances and polyuria may become easier. The magnitude of renal wasting of electrolytes and water diminishes as glomerular filtration rate falls. Chronic dialysis and renal transplantation are viable alternatives for the management of end-stage renal disease in patients whose underlying disease can be cured or controlled.

REFERENCES

1. Fanconi, G. Die nicht diabetischen Glykosurien und Hyperglykamien des altern Kindes. Jahrb. Kinderh. 133:257, 1931.
2. De Toni, G. Remarks on the relations between renal rickets (renal dwarfism) and renal diabetes. Acta Paediatr. 16:479-484, 1933.
3. Debre, R.; Marie, J.; Cleret, F.; and Messimy, R. Rachitisme tardif coexistant avec une nephrite chronique et une glycosurie. Arch. Med. Enf. 37:597, 1934.
4. Fanconi, G. Der nephrotisch-glykosurische Zwergwuchs mit hypophosphatamischer Rachitis. Dtsch. Med. Wochenschr. 62:1169-1171, 1936.
5. Fanconi, G. Der fruhinfantile nephrotisch-glykosurische Zwergwuchs mit hypophosphatamischer Rachitis. Jahrb. Kinderh. 147:299-338, 1936.
6. McCune, D. J.; Mason, H. H.; and Clarke, H. T. Intractable hypophosphatemic rickets with renal glycosuria and acidosis (the Fanconi syndrome). Am. J. Dis. Child. 65:81-146, 1943.
7. Dent, C. E. The amino-aciduria in Fanconi syndrome: A study making extensive use of techniques based on paper partition chromatography. Biochem. J. 41:240-253, 1947.
8. Lignac, G. O. E. Storung des Cystinstoffwechsels bei Kindern. Dtsch. Arch. Klin. Med. 145:139, 1924.
9. Beumer, H.; and Wepler, W. Uber die Cystinkrankheit der ersten Lebenzeit. Klin. Wochenschr. 16:8, 1937.
10. Freudenberg, E. Cystinosis: Cystine disease (Lignac's disease) in children. Adv. Pediatr. 4:265-292, 1949.
11. Milkman, L. A. Multiple spontaneous idiopathic symmetrical fractures. Am. J. Roentgenol. 32:622-634, 1934.
12. Stowers, J. M.; and Dent, C. E. Studies on the mechanism of the Fanconi syndrome. Q. J. Med. 16:275-290, 1947.
13. Morris, R.C.; McInnes, R.R.; Epstein, C.J.; Sebastian, A.; and Scriver, C.R. Genetic and metabolic injury of the kidney. In: The Kidney, edited by Brenner, B. M., and Rector, F. C. Philadelphia, Saunders, 1976, pp. 1213-1225.
14. Rodriguez-Soriano, J.; Boichis, H.; and Edelmann, C. M. Bicarbonate reabsorption and hydrogen ion excretion in children with renal tubular acidosis. J. Pediatr. 71:802-812, 1967.
15. Morris, R. C. An experimental renal acidification defect in patients with hereditary fructose intolerance. II. Its distinction from classic renal tubular acidosis; its resemblance to the renal acidification defect associated with the Fanconi syndrome of children with cystinosis. J. Clin. Invest. 47:1648-1663, 1968.
16. Sirota, J. H.; and Hamerman, D. Renal function studies in an adult subject with Fanconi syndrome. Am. J. Med. 16:138-152, 1954.

17. Wilson, D. R.; and Yendt, E. R. Treatment of the adult Fanconi syndrome with oral phosphate supplements and alkali. Am. J. Med. 35:487-511, 1963.
18. Rodriguez-Soriano, J.; Houston, I. B.; Boichis, H.; and Edelmann, C. M. Calcium and phosphorus metabolism in Fanconi syndrome. J. Clin. Endocrinol. 28:1555-1563, 1968.
19. Lee, D. B.; Drinkard, U. P.; Rosen, V. J.; and Gonick, H. C. The adult Fanconi syndrome. Medicine 51:107-138, 1972.
20. Milne, M. D.; Stanbury, S. W.; and Thomson, A. E. Observations on the Fanconi syndrome in renal hyperchloraemic acidosis in the adult. Q. J. Med. 21:61-82, 1952.
21. Butler, E. A.; and Flynn, F. V. The proteinuria of renal tubular disorders. Lancet 2: 978-980, 1958.
22. Harrison, J. F.; and Blainey, J. D. Low molecular weight proteinuria in chronic renal disease. Clin. Sci. 33:381-390, 1967.
23. Dillard, M. G.; Pesce, A. F.; Pollak, V. E.; and Boreisha, I. Proteinuria and renal protein clearance in patients with renal tubular disorders. J. Lab. Clin. Med. 78:203-215, 1971.
24. Barratt, T. M.; and Crawford, R. Lysozyme excretion as a measure of renal tubular dysfunction in children. Clin. Sci. 39:457-564, 1970.
25. Waldmann, T. A.; Strober, W.; and Mogielnicki, R. P. The renal handling of low molecular weight proteins. II. Disorders of serum protein catabolism in patients with tubular proteinuria, the nephrotic syndrome or uremia. J. Clin. Invest. 51:2162-2174, 1972.
26. Houston, I. B.; Boichis, H.; and Edelmann, C. M. Fanconi syndrome with renal sodium wasting and metabolic alkalosis. Am. J. Med. 44:638-646, 1968.
27. Rodriguez-Soriano, J.; Vallo, A.; Castillo, G.; Olivero, R. Renal handling of water and sodium in children with proximal and distal renal tubular acidosis. Nephron 25:193-198, 1980.
28. Sebastian, A.; McSherry, E.; Morris, R. C. On the mechanism of renal potassium wasting in renal tubular acidosis associated with the Fanconi syndrome (type 2 RTA). J. Clin. Invest. 50:231-243, 1971.
29. Bricker, N. S. On the meaning of the intact nephron hypothesis. Am. J. Med. 46:1-11, 1969.
30. Bricker, N. S.; Schmidt, R.W.; Favre, H.; Fine, L.; and Bourgoignie, J. J. On the biology of sodium excretion. The search for a natriuretic hormone. Yale J. Biol. Med. 48:293-303, 1975.
31. Weber, H.; Bourgoignie, J. J.; and Bricker, N. S. Effects of the natriuretic serum fraction on proximal tubular reabsorption. Am. J. Physiol. 226:419-425, 1974.
32. Clay, R. D.; Darmady, E. M.; and Hawkins, M. The nature of the renal lesion in Fanconi syndrome. J. Pathol. Bacteriol. 65:551-558, 1953.
33. Bergeron, M.; Dubord, L.; and Hausser, C. Membrane permeability as a cause of transport defects in experimental Fanconi syndrome. J. Clin. Invest. 57:1181-1189, 1976.
34. Wen, S. F. Micropuncture studies of glucose transport in the dog: Mechanism of renal glycosuria. Am. J. Physiol. 231:468-475, 1976.
35. Brewer, E. D.; Senekjian, H. O.; Ince, A.; and Weinman, E. J. Maleic acid-induced reabsorptive dysfunction in the proximal and distal tubule. Am. J. Physiol. 245:F339-F344, 1983.
36. Verani, R. R.; Brewer, E. D.; Ince, A.; Gibson, G.; and Bulger, R. E. Proximal tubular necrosis associated with maleic acid administration to the rat. Lab. Invest. 46:79-88, 1982.
37. Wallis, L. A.; and Engle, R. L. The adult Fanconi syndrome. II. Review of eighteen cases. Am. J. Med. 22:13-23, 1957.
38. Fanconi, A.; Fisher, J. A.; and Prader, A. Serum parathyroid hormone concentration in hypophosphatemic vitamin D-resistant rickets. Helv. Paediatr. Acta 29:187, 1974.

39. Scriver, C. R.; and Rosenberg, L. E. Amino Acid Metabolism and Its Disorders. Philadelphia, Saunders, 1973, pp. 159, 190-191.
40. Davies, H. E. F.; Evans, B.; Rees, H. M. N.; and Fourman, P. The defective absorption of phosphorus and calcium and the effect of vitamin D in the Fanconi syndrome. Guys Hosp. Rep. 107:486, 1958.
41. Brodehl, J. The Fanconi syndrome. In: Pediatric Kidney Disease, edited by Edelmann, C. M. Boston, Little, Brown, 1978, pp. 955-987.
42. Wapnir, R.A.; Exeni, R.A.; McVicar, M.; deRosas, F.J.; and Lifshitz, F. Inhibition of sodium intestinal transport and mucosal (Na^+-K^+)-ATPase in experimental Fanconi syndrome. Proc. Soc. Exp. Biol. Med. 150:517-520, 1975.
43. Bickel, H.; and Hickmans, E.M. Cystine storage disease with aminoaciduria and dwarfism (Lignac-Fanconi disease): Some biochemical aspects of Lignac-Fanconi disease. Acta Paediatr. 42(Suppl. 90): 137-170, 1952.
44. Raghaven, S. R. V.; Walling, M.; Mills, B.; Mirra, J.; Hartenbower, D.; Coburn, J.; and Gonick, H. Dissociation of osteodystrophy from renal tubular dysfunction in cadmium induced experimental Fanconi syndrome. Clin. Res. 25:139A, 1977.
45. Tsuchiya, K. Causation of ouch-ouch disease. Keio J. Med. 18:181-211, 1969.
46. Schneider, J. A.; Schulman, J. D.; and Seegmiller, J. E. Cystinosis. In: The Metabolic Basis of Inherited Disease, 4th ed., edited by Stanbury, J.B., Wyngaarden, J. B., and Fredrickson, D.S. New York, McGraw-Hill, 1978, pp. 1660-1682.
47. Segal, S. Disorders of galactose metabolism. In: The Metabolic Basis of Inherited Disease, 5th ed., edited by Stanbury, J. B., Wyngaarden, J. B., Fredrickson, D. S., Goldstein, J. L., and Brown, M. S. New York, McGraw-Hill, 1983, pp. 167-191.
48. Froesch, E. R. Essential fructosuria, hereditary fructose intolerance and fructose-1,6-diphosphatase deficiency. In: The Metabolic Basis of Inherited Disease, 4th ed., edited by Stanbury, J. B., Wyngaarden, J. B., and Fredrickson, D. S. New York, McGraw-Hill, 1978, pp. 121-136.
49. Mock, D. M.; Perman, J. A.; Thaler, M. M.; and Morris, R. C. Chronic fructose intoxication after infancy in children with hereditary fructose intolerance. A cause of growth retardation. N. Engl. J. Med. 309:764-770, 1983.
50. Sass-Kortsak, A.; and Bearn, A. G. Hereditary disorders of copper metabolism. In: The Metabolic Basis of Inherited Disease, 4th ed., edited by Stanbury, J. B., Wyngaarden, J. B.; and Fredrickson, D. S. New York, McGraw-Hill, 1978, pp. 1098-1126.
51. Mallette, L. E.; and Patten, B. M. Neurogenic muscle atrophy and osteomalacia in adult Fanconi syndrome. Ann. Neurol. 1:131-137, 1977.
52. Hunt, D. D.; Stearns, G.; McKinley, J. B.; Fronig, E.; Hick, P.; and Bonfiglio, M. Long-term study of family with Fanconi syndrome without cystinosis (DeToni-Debre-Fanconi syndrome). Am. J. Med. 40:492-510, 1966.
53. von Illig, R.; Prader, A. Primare Tubulopathien. II. Ein Fall von idopathischen Gluko-Amino-Phosphat-Diabetes (DeToni-Debre-Fanconi syndrome). Helvet. Paediatr. Acta 16:622-646, 1961.
54. Sheldon, W.; Luder, J.; and Webb, B. A familial tubular absorption defect of glucose and amino acids. Arch. Dis. Child. 36:90-95, 1961.
55. Ben-Ishay, D.; Dreyfuss, F.; and Ullmann, T. D. Fanconi syndrome with hypouricemia in an adult. Family study. Am. J. Med. 31:793-800, 1961.
56. Smith, R.; Lindenbaum, R. H.; and Walton, R. J. Hypophosphataemic osteomalacia and Fanconi syndrome of adult onset and dominant inheritance. Q. J. Med. 179:387-400, 1976.
57. Friedman, A.L.; Trygstad, C.W.; and Chesney, R. W. Autosomal dominant Fanconi syndrome with early renal failure. Am. J. Med. Genet. 2:225-232, 1978.
58. Brenton, D. P.; Isenberg, D. A.; Cusworth, D. C.; Garrod, P.; Krywawych, S.; and Stamp, T. C. B. The adult presenting idiopathic Fanconi syndrome. J. Inherited Metab. Dis. 4:211-215, 1981.

59. Patrick, A.; Cameron, J. S.; and Ogg, C. S. A family with a dominant form of idiopathic Fanconi syndrome leading to renal failure in adult life. Clin. Nephrol. 16:289-292, 1981.
60. Briggs, W. A.; Kominami, N.; Wilson, R. E.; and Merrill, J. P. Kidney transplantation in Fanconi syndrome. N. Engl. J. Med. 286:25, 1972.
61. Chesney, R. W.; Kaplan, B. S.; Colle, E.; Scriver, C. R.; McInnes, R. R.; Dupont, C. H.; and Drummond, K. N. Abnormalities of carbohydrate metabolism in idiopathic Fanconi syndrome. Pediatr. Res. 14:209-215, 1980.
62. Chesney, R. W.; Kaplan, B. S.; Teitel, D.; Colle, E.; McInnes, R. R.; Goldman, H.; and Scriver, C. R. Metabolic abnormalities in the idiopathic Fanconi syndrome: Studies of carbohydrate metabolism in two patients. Pediatrics 67:113-118, 1981.
63. Mahoney, C. P.; Striker, G. E.; Hickman, R. O.; Manning, G. B.; and Marchionio, T. L. Renal transplantation for childhood cystinosis. N. Engl. J. Med. 283:397-402, 1970.
64. Malekzadeh, M. H.; Nustein, H. B.; Schneider, J. A.; Pennisi, A.; Ettenger, R.; Uittenbogaart, G.; Kogut, M.; and Fine, R. Cadaver renal transplantation in children with cystinosis. Am. J. Med. 63:525-533, 1977.
65. West, J. C.; Goodman, S. I.; Schroter, G. P.; Bloustein, P. A.; Hambridge, K. M.; and Weil, R. Pediatric kidney transplantation for cystinosis. J. Pediatr. Surg. 12:651-655, 1977.
66. Barnes, B. E.; Bergan, J. J.; Braun, W. E.; Fraumeni, J. F.; Kountz, S. L.; Mickey, M. R.; Rubin, A. L.; Simmons, R. L.; Stevens, L. E.; and Wilson, R. E. Renal transplantation in congenital and metabolic diseases. J.A.M.A. 232:148-153, 1975.
67. Langlois, R. P.; O'Regan, S.; Pelletier, M.; and Robitaille, P. Kidney transplantatiion in uremic children with cystinosis. Nephron 28:273-275, 1981.
68. Jonas, A. J.; Schulman, J. D.; Matalon, R.; Velazquez, A.; Brewer, E. D.; Chen, H.; Boyer, M. G.; Brandwein, E.; Arbus, G. S.; Morris, C. R.; and Schneider, J. A. Cystinosis in non-caucasian children. J. Hopkins Med. J. 151:118-121, 1982.
69. Wong, V. G.; Lietman, P. S.; and Seegmiller, J. E. Alterations of pigment epithelium in cystinosis. Arch. Ophthalmol. 77:361-369, 1967.
70. Schneider, J. A.; Wong, V.; and Seegmiller, J. E. The early diagnosis of cystinosis. J. Pediatr. 74:114-116, 1969.
71. Gahl, W. A.; Schulman, J. D.; Thoene, J. G.; and Schneider, J. A. Hepatotoxicity of cysteamine? J. Pediatr. 103:1008-1009, 1983.
72. Rezvani, I.; DiGeorge, A. M.; and Cote, M. L. Primary hypothyroidism in cystinosis. J. Pediatr. 91:340-341, 1977.
73. Chan, A. M.; Lynch, M. J. G.; Bailey, J. D.; Exrin, C.; and Fraser, D. Hypothyroidism in cystinosis: A clinical, endocrinologic and histologic study involving sixteen patients with cystinosis. Am. J. Med. 48:678-692, 1970.
74. Lucky, A. W.; Howley, P. M.; Megyesi, K.; Spielberg, S. P.; and Schulman, J. D. Endocrine studies in cystinosis: Compensated primary hypothyroidism. J. Pediatr. 91:204-210, 1977.
75. Trompeter, R. S.; Bosque, M.; Wass, V.; Haycock, G. B.; and Chantler, C. Prognosis for children with cystinosis following renal transplantation. Evaluation of endocrine function, pubertal status and growth. Abstract. Eur. J. Pediatr. 140:191, 1983.
76. Wolff, G.; Ehrich, J. H. H.; Offner, G.; and Brodehl, J. Psychosocial and intellectual development in 12 patients with infantile nephropathic cystinosis. Acta Paediatr. Scand. 71:1007-1011, 1982.
77. Ehrich, J. H. H.; Stoeppler, L.; Offner, G.; Brodehl, J. Evidence for cerebral involvement in nephropathic cystinosis. Neuropadiatrie 10:128-137, 1979.
78. Levine, S.; and Paparo, G. Brain lesions in a case of cystinosis. Acta Neuropathol. 57:217-220, 1982.
79. Goldman, H.; Scriver, C. R.; Aaron, K.; Delvin, E.; and Canlas, Z. Adolescent cystinosis: Comparisons with infantile and adult forms. Pediatrics 47:979-988, 1971.

80. Zimmerman, T. J.; Hood, C. I.; and Gasset, A. R. Adolescent cystinosis. Arch. Ophthalmol. 92:265-268, 1974.
81. Hauglustaine, D.; Corbeel, L.; van Damme, B.; Serrus, M.; and Michielsen, P. Glomerulonephritis in late-onset cystinosis. Report of two cases and review of the literature. Clin. Nephrol. 6:529-536, 1976.
82. Weber, H. P.; Harms, E.; and Knopfle, G. Adoleszenten-Zystinose Literaturubersicht mit eigener Beobachtung. Klin. Padiatr. 191:8-19, 1979.
83. Dale, R. T.; Rao, G. N.; Aquabella, J. V.; and Metz, H. S. Adolescent cystinosis: A clinical and specular microscopic study of an unusual sibship. Br. J. Ophthal. 65:828-832, 1981.
84. Manz, F.; Harms, E.; Lutz, P.; Waldherr, R.; and Scharer, K. Adolescent cystinosis: Renal function and morphology. Eur. J. Pediatr. 138:354-357, 1982.
85. Leitman, P. S.; Frazier, P. D.; Wong, V. G.; Shotton, D.; and Seegmiller, J. E. Adult cystinosis—a benign disorder. Am. J. Med. 40:511-517, 1966.
86. Spear, G. S. Pathology of the kidney in cystinosis. In: Pathology Annual, edited by Sommers, S. C. New York, Appleton-Century-Crofts, 1974, pp. 225-237.
87. Schulman, J. D. Lysosomes and the ultrastructural pathology of cystinosis. In: Cystinosis, edited by Schulman, J. D. DHEW publication No. 72-249, Washington, D. C. 1973, pp. 95-109.
88. Chesney, R. W. Etiology and pathogenesis of the Fanconi syndrome. Miner. Electrolyte Metab. 4:303-316, 1980.
89. Jonas, A. J.; Greene, A. A.; Smith, M. L.; and Schneider, J. A. Cystine accumulation and loss in normal, heterozygous and cystinotic fibroblasts. Proc. Natl. Acad. Sci. U. S. A. 79:4442-4445, 1982.
90. Gahl, W. A.; Bashan, N.; Tietze, F.; Bernardini, I.; and Schulman, J. D. Cystine transport is defective in isolated leukocyte lysosomes from pateitns with cystinosis. Science 217:1263-1265, 1982.
91. Schneider, J. A.; Wong, V.; Bradley, K.; and Seegmiller, J. E. Biochemical comparisons of the adult and childhood forms of cystinosis. N. Engl. J. Med. 279:1253-1257, 1968.
92. Schneider, J. A.; Bradley, K.; and Seegmiller, J. E. Increased cystine in leukocytes from individuals homozygous and heterozygous for cystinosis. Science 157:1321-1322, 1967.
93. Schneider, J. A.; Rosenbloom, F. M.; Bradley, K. H.; and Seegmiller, J. E. Increased free-cystine content of fibroblasts cultured from patients with cystinosis. Biochem. Biophys. Res. Commun. 29:527-531, 1967.
94. Steinherz, R.; Tietze, F.; Triche, T.; Modesti, A.; Gahl, W. A.; and Schulman, J. D. Heterozygote detection in cystinosis, using leukocytes exposed to cystine dimethyl ester. N. Engl. J. Med. 306:1468-1470, 1982.
95. Schneider, J. A.; Verroust, F. M.; Kroll, W. A.; Garvin, A. J.; Horger, E. O.; Wong, V. G.; Spear, G. S.; Jacobson, C.; Pellett, O. L.; and Becker, F. L. Prenatal diagnosis of cystinosis. N. Engl. J. Med. 290:878-882, 1974.
96. States, B.; Blazer, B.; Hamb, D.; and Segal, S. Prenatal diagnosis of cystinosis. J. Pediatr. 87:558-562, 1975.
97. Yudkoff, M.; Foreman, J. W.; and Segal, S. Effects of cysteamine therapy in nephropathic cystinosis. N. Eng. J. Med. 304:141-145, 1981.
98. Thoene, J.; Gahl, W.; Rizzo, W.; Schulman, J. D.; Reed, G.; Denman, D.; Schlesselman, J.; Jonas, A.; and Schneider, J. A. Cysteamine therapy of nephropathic cystinosis: Evidence for effectiveness. Abstract. Pediatr. Res. 17:220A, 1983.
99. Butler, JDeb.; and Zatz, M. Pantethine depletes cystinotic fibroblasts of cystine. J. Pediatr. 102:796-798, 1983.

100. Lowe, C. U.; Terrey, M.; and McLachlan, E. A. Organic-aciduria, decreased renal ammonia production, hydrophthalmus, and mental retardation. Am. J. Dis. Child. 83: 164-184, 1952.
101. Abassi, V.; Lowe, C. U.; and Calcagno, P. L. Oculo-cerebro-renal syndrome. A review. Am. J. Dis. Child. 115:145-168, 1968.
102. Rosenblatt, D.; and Holmes, L. B. Development of arthritis in Lowe's syndrome. J. Pediatr. 84:924-925, 1974.
103. Elliman, D.; and Woodley, A. Tenosynovitis in Lowe'ssyndrome. J. Pediatr. 103:1011, 1983.
104. Richards, W.; Donnell, G. N.; Wilson, W. A.; Stowens, D.; Perry, T. The oculo-cerebro-renal syndrome of Lowe. Am. J. Dis. Child. 109:185-203, 1965.
105. Sagel, I.; Ores, R. O.; and Yuceoglu, A. M. Renal function and morphology in a girl with oculo-cerebro-renal syndrome. J. Pediatr. 77:124-127, 1970.
106. Betend, B.; Scherrer, M.; Evrard, A.; Votan-Bonnamour, B.; and Hermier, M. Syndrome oculo-cerebro-renal de Lowe chez une fille. Arch. Fr. Pediatr. 35:269-279, 1978.
107. Terslev, E. Two cases of aminociduria, ocular changes and retarded mental and somatic development (Lowe's syndrome). Acta Pediatr. 49:635-644, 1960.
108. Illig, R.; Dumermuth, G.; and Prader, A. Das oculo-cerebro-renale syndrome (Lowe): Klinische, metabolische and elektroencephelographische Befundebei 3 Fallen. Heiv. Pediatr. Acta 18:173-202, 1963.
109. Fisher, N. F.; Hallet, J.; and Carpenter, G. Oculocerebrorenalsyndrome of Lowe. Arch. Ophthalmol. 77:642-645, 1967.
110. Holmes, L. B.; McGowan, B. L.; and Efron, M. L. Lowe's syndrome: A search for the carrier state. Pediatrics 44:358-364, 1969.
111. Schwartz, R.; Hall, P. W.; and Gabuzda, G. J. Metabolism of ornithine and other amino acids in the cerebro-oculo-renal syndrome. Am. J. Med. 36:778-786, 1964.
112. Chutorian, A.; and Rowland, L. P. Lowe's syndrome. Neurology 16:115-122, 1966.
113. Matsuda, I.; Sugai, M.; and Kajii, T. Ornithine loading test in Lowe's syndrome. J. Pediatr. 77:127-129, 1970.
114. Hayasi, S.; Nagata, T.; Kimura, A.; Tsurumi, K. Urinary excretion of acid glycosaminoglycans and hydroxyproline in a patient with oculo-cerebro-renal syndrome. Tohoku J. Exp. Med. 126:215-223, 1978.
115. Hambreus, L.; Pallisgaard, G.; and Kildeberg, P. The Lowe syndrome: Observations on the amino acid metabolism in a two-year-old affected boy. Acta Paediatr. Scand. 59: 631-636, 1970.
116. Oetliker, O.; and Rossi, E. The influence of extracellular fluid volume on the renal bicarbonate threshold. A study of two children with Lowe's syndrome. Pediatr. Res. 3:140-148, 1969.
117. Matsuda, I.; Takeda, T.; Sugai, M.; and Matsuura, N. Oculocerebrorenal syndrome in a child with a normal urinary acidification and a defect in bicarbonate reabsorption. Am. J. Dis. Child. 117:205-212, 1969.
118. Witzleben, C. L.; Schoen, E. J.; Tu, W. H.; and McDonald, L. W. Progressive morphologic renal changes in the oculo-cerebro-renal syndrome of Lowe. Am. J. Med. 44: 319-324, 1968.
119. Ores, R. O. Renal changes in oculo-cerebro-renal syndrome of Lowe. Electron microscopic study. Arch. Pathol. 89:221-225, 1970.
120. Bartsocas, C. S.; Levy, H. L.; Crawford, J. D.; and Their, S. O. A defect in intestinal transport in Lowe's syndrome. Am. J. Dis. Child. 117:93-95, 1969.
121. Hayashi, S.; Nagata, T.; Kimura, A.; and Tsurumi, K. Urinary acid glycosaminoglycans in a patient with oculo-cerebro-renal syndrome. Tohuko J. Exp. Med. 126:225-234, 1978.

122. Akasaki, M.; Fukui, S.; Sakano, T.; Tanaka, T.; Usui, T.; and Yamashina, I. Urinary excretion of a large amount of bound sialic acid and of undersulfated chondroitin sulfate A by patients with the Lowe syndrome. Clin. Chim. Acta 89:119-125, 1978.
123. States, B.; Palmieri, M. J.; and Segal, S. Uptake of proline in cultured cells from patients with Lowe's syndrome. Biochem. Biophys. Res. Commun. 109:428-433, 1982.
124. Gitzelmann, R.; Steinmann, D.; and Van Den Berghe, G. Essential fructosuria, hereditary fructose intolerance and fructose-1, 6-diphosphatase deficiency. In: The Metabolic Basis of Inherited Disease, 5th ed., edited by Stanbury, J. B., Wyngaarden, J. B., Fredrickson, D. S., Goldstein, J. L., and Brown, M. S. New York, McGraw-Hill, 1983, pp. 118-140.
125. Steinmann, B.; and Gitzelmann, R. The diagnosis of hereditary fructose intolerance. Helv. Paediatr. Acta 36:297-316, 1981.
126. Cox, T. M.; Camilleri, M.; O'Donnell, M. W.; and Chadwick, V. S. Pseudodominant transmission of fructose intolerance in an adult and three offspring. N. Engl. J. Med. 307:537-540, 1982.
127. Raivio, K.; Perheentupa, J.; and Nikkila, E. A. Aldolase activities in the liver in parents of patients with hereditary fructose intolerance. Clin. Chim. Acta 17:275-279, 1967.
128. Mercier, J. C.; Bourrillon, A.; Beaufils, F.; and Odievre, M. Intolerance hereditaire au fructose a revelation precoce. Arch. Fr. Pediatr. 33:945-953, 1976.
129. Odievre, M.; Gentil, C.; Gautier, M.; and Alagille, D. Hereditary fructose intolerance in childhood. Am. J. Dis. Child. 132:605-608, 1978.
130. Baerlocher, K.; Gitzelmann, R.; Steinmann, D.; and Gitzelmann-Cumarasamy, N. Hereditary fructose intolerance in early childhood: A major diagnostic challenge. Helv. Paediatr. Acta 33:465-487, 1978.
131. Schulte, M.-J.; and Lenz, W. Fatal sorbitol infusion in patient with fructose-sorbitol intolerance. Lancet 2:188, 1977.
132. Lameire, N.; Mussche, M.; Baele, G.; Kint, J.; and Ringoir, S. Hereditary fructose intolerance: A difficult diagnosis in the adult. Am. J. Med. 65:416-423, 1978.
133. Morris, R. C. An experimental renal acidification defect in patients with hereditary fructose intolerance. I. Its resemblance to renal tubular acidosis. J. Clin. Invest. 47: 1389-1398, 1967.
134. Morris, R. C. An experimental renal acidification defect in patients with hereditary fructose intolerance. II. Its distinction from classical renal tubular acidosis; its resemblance to the renal acidification defect associated with the Fanconi syndrome of children with cystinosis. J. Clin. Invest. 47:1648-1663, 1968.
135. Steiner, G.; Wilson, D.; and Vranic, M. Studies of glucose turnover and renal function in an unusual case of hereditary fructose intolerance. Am. J. Med. 62:150-158, 1977.
136. Richardson, R. M. A.; Little, J. A.; Patten, R. L.; Goldstein, M. B.; and Halperin, M. L. Pathogenesis of acidosis in hereditary fructose intolerance. Metabolism 28:1133-1138, 1979.
137. Morris, R. C.; McSherry, E.; and Sebastian, A. Modulation of experimental renal dysfunction of hereditary fructose intolerance by circulating parathyroid hormone. Proc. Natl. Acad. Sci. U.S.A. 68:132-135, 1971.
138. Mass, R. E.; Smith, W. R.; and Walsh, J. R. The association of hereditary fructose intolerance and renal tubular acidosis. Am. J. Med. Sci. 251:516-523, 1966.
139. Morris, R. C.; and Sebastian, A. Renal tubular acidosis and Fanconi syndrome. In: The Metabolic Basis of Inherited Disease, 5th ed., edited by Stanbury, J. B., Wyngaarden, J. B., Fredrickson, D. S., Goldstein, J. L., and Brown, M. S. New York, McGraw-Hill, 1983, pp. 1808-1843.
140. Morris, R. C.; Ueki, I.; Loh, D.; Eanes, R. Z.; and McLin, P. Absence of renal fructose-1-phosphate aldolase activity in hereditary fructose intolerance. Nature 214:920-921, 1967.

141. Brewer, E. D.; Kranhold, J. F.; Sebastian, A.; McSherry, E.; and Morris, R. C. The experimental renal dysfunction of hereditary fructose intolerance (HFI): Evidence that function of the thick ascending limb is intact and HCO_3 reabsorptive capacity of the proximal tubule is reduced. Kidney Int. 12:462, 1977.
142. Morris, R. C.; Brewer, E. D.; and Brater, C. Evidence of a severe phosphate depletion dependent disturbance of cellular metabolism in patients with hereditary fructose intolerance (HFI). Clin. Res. 28:556A, 1980.
143. Burch, H. B.; Choi, S.; Dence, C. N.; Alvey, T. R.; Cole, B. R.; and Lowry, O. H. Metabolic effects of large fructose loads in different parts of the rat nephron. J. Biol. Chem. 255:8239-8244, 1980.
144. Kogut, M. D.; Roe, T. F.; Ng, W.; and Donnell, G. N. Fructose-induced hyperuricemia: Observations in normal children and in patients with hereditary fructose intolerance and galactosemia. Pediatr. Res. 9:774-778, 1975.
145. Lindemann, R.; Gjessing, L. R.; Merton, B.; Loken, A. C.; and Halvorsen, S. Amino acid metabolism in hereditary fructosemia. Acta Paediatr. Scand. 59:141-147, 1970.
146. Grant, D. B.; Alexander, F. W.; and Seakins, J. W. T. Abnormal tyrosine metabolism in hereditary fructose intolerance. Acta Paediatr. Scand. 59:432-434, 1970.
147. Carson, N. A. J.; Biggart, J. D.; Bittles, A. H.; Donovan, D. Hereditary tyrosinaemia. Clinical, enzymatic, and pathological study of an infant with the acute form of the disease. Arch. Dis. Child. 51:106-113, 1976.
148. Goldsmith, L. A. Tyrosinemia and related disorders. In: The Metabolic Basis of Inherited Disease, 5th ed., edited by Stanbury, J. B., Wyngaarden, J. B., Fredrickson, D. S., Goldstein, J. L., and Brown, M. S. New York, McGraw-Hill, 1983, pp. 287-299.
149. Larochelle, J.; Mortezai, A.; Belanger, M.; Tremblay, M.; Claveau, J. C.; and Aubin, G. Experience with 37 infants with tyrosinemia. Can. Med. Assoc. J. 97:1051-1054, 1967.
150. Halvorsen, S.; Pande, H.; Loken, A. C.; and Gjessing, L. R. Tyrosinosis. A study of 6 cases. Arch. Dis. Child. 41:238-249, 1966.
151. Sass-Kortsak, A.; Ficici, S.; Paunier, L.; Kooh, S. W.; Fraser, D.; and Jackson, S. H. Secondary metabolic derangements in patients with tyrosyluria. Can. Med. Assoc. J. 97:1079-1083, 1967.
152. Scriver, C. R.; Silverberg, M.; and Clow, C. L. Hereditary tyrosinemia and tyrosyluria: Clinical report of four patients. Canad. Med. Assoc. J. 97:1047-1050, 1967.
153. Baber, M. D. Case of congenital cirrhosis of the liver with renal tubular defects akin to those in the Fanconi syndrome. Arch. Dis. Child. 31:335-339, 1956.
154. Weinberg, A. G.; Mize, C. E.; and Worthen, H. G. The occurrence of hepatoma in the chronic form of hereditary tyrosinemia. J. Pediatr. 88:434-438, 1976.
155. Kang, E. S.; and Gerard, P. S. Hereditary tyrosinemia and abnormal pyrrole metabolism. J. Pediatr. 77:397-406, 1970.
156. Strife, C. F.; Zuroweste, E. L.; Emmett, E. A.; Finelli, V. N.; Petering, H. G.; and Berry, H. K. Tyrosinemia with acute intermittent porphyria: Aminolevulinic acid dehydratase deficiency related to elevated urinary aminolevulinic acid levels. J. Pediatr. 90:400-404, 1977.
157. Lindblad, B.; Lindstedt, S.; and Steen, G. On the enzymic defects in hereditary tyrosinemia. Proc. Natl. Acad. Sci. 74:4641-4645, 1977.
158. Jagenburg, R.; Lindblad, B.; de Mare, J. M.; and Rodjer, S. Hereditary tyrosinemia: Metabolic studies in a patient with partial p-hydroxyphenylpyruvate hydroxylase activity. J. Pediatr. 80:994-1004, 1972.
159. Taniguchi, K.; and Gjessing, L. R. Studies on tyrosinosis: 2. Activity of the transaminase, parahydroxy-phenylpyruvate oxidase, and homogentisic acid oxidase. Br. Med. J. 1:968-969, 1965.
160. Kvittingen, E. A.; Halvorsen, S.; and Jellum, E. Deficient fumarylacetoacetate fumarylhydrolase activity in lymphocytes and fibroblasts from patients with hereditary tyrosinemia. Pediatr. Res. 14:541-544, 1983.

161. Fallstrom, S. P.; Lindblad, B.; Lindstedt, S.; and Steen, G. Hereditary tyrosinemia-fumarylacetoacetase deficiency. Pediatr. Res. 13:78, 1979.
162. Berger, R.; Smit, G. P. A.; Stoker-de Vries, S. A.; Duran, M.; Ketting, D.; and Wadman, S. K. Deficiency of fumarylacetoacetase in a patient with hereditary tyrosinemia. Clin. Chim. Acta 114:37-44, 1981.
163. Kvittingen, E. A.; Jellum, E.; and Stokke, O. Assay of fumarylacetoacetate fumarylhydrolase in human liver—Deficient activity in a case of hereditary tyrosinemia. Clin. Chim. Acta 115:311-319, 1981.
164. Hostetter, M. K.; Levy, H. L.; Winter, H. S.; Knight, G. J.; and Haddow, J. E. Evidence for liver disease preceding amino acid abnormalities in hereditary tyrosinemia. N. Engl. J. Med. 308:1265-1267, 1983.
165. Gagne, R. Liver disease in hereditary tyrosinemia. (Letter reply by Levy, H. L. and Hostetter, M. K.). N. Engl. J. Med. 309:1063, 1983.
166. Grenier, A.; Lescault, A.; Laberge, C.; Gagne, R.; and Mamer, O. Detection of succinylacetone and the use of its measurement in mass screening for hereditary tyrosinemia. Clin. Chim. Acta 123:93-99, 1982.
167. Gagne, R.; Lescault, A.; Grenier, A.; Laberge, C.; Melancon, S. B.; and Dallaire, L. Prenatal diagnosis of hereditary tyrosinaemia: Measurement of succinylacetone in amniotic fluid. Prenatal. Diagn. 2:185-188, 1982.
168. Steinmann, B.; Gitzelmann, R.; Kvittingen, E. A.; and Stokke, O. Prenatal diagnosis of hereditary tyrosinemia. (Letter reply by Gagne, R.). N. Engl. J. Med. 310:855, 1984.
169. Cohn, R. M.; Yudkoff, M.; Yost, B.; and Segal, S. Phenylalanine—tyrosine deficiency syndrome as a complication of the management of hereditary tyrosinemia. Am. J. Clin. Nutr. 30:209-214, 1977.
170. Holzel, A.; Komrower, G. M.; and Schwarz, V. Galactosemia. Am. J. Med. 22:703-711, 1957.
171. Levy, H. L.; Sepe, S. J.; Shih, V. E.; Vawter, G. F.; and Klein, J. O. Sepsis due to Escherichia coli in neonates with galactosemia. N. Engl. J. Med. 297:823-825, 1977.
172. Komrower, G. M.; Schwarz, V.; Holzel, A.; and Golberg, L. A clinical and biochemical study of galactosaemia. Arch. Dis. Child. 31:254-264, 1956.
173. Holzel, A.; Komrower, G. M.; and Wilson, V. K. Amino-aciduria in galactosaemia. Br. Med. J. 1:194-195, 1952.
174. Cusworth, D. C.; Dent, C. E.; and Flynn, F. V. The amino-aciduria in galactosaemia. Arch. Dis. Child. 30:150-154, 1955.
175. Fox, M.; Thier, S.; Rosenberg, L.; and Segal, S. Impaired renal tubular function induced by sugar infusion in man. J. Clin. Endocrinol. 24:1318-1327, 1964.
176. Schwarz, V. The value of galactose phosphate determinations in the treatment of galactosaemia. Arch. Dis. Child. 35:428-432, 1960.
177. Quan-Ma, R.; Wells, H. J.; Wells, W. W.; Sherman, F. E.; and Egan, T. J. Galactitol in the tissues of a galactosemic child. Am. J. Dis. Child. 112:477-478, 1966.
178. Tedesco, T. A.; and Miller, K. L. Galactosemia: Alterations in sulfate metabolism secondary to galactose-1-phosphate uridyltransferase deficiency. Science 205:1395-1397, 1979.
179. Raivio, K. O.; Kekomaki, M. P.; and Maenpaa, P. H. Depletion of liver adenine nucleotides induced by D-fructose. Biochem. Pharmacol. 18:2615-2624, 1969.
180. Beutler, E.; and Baluda, M. C. Improved method for measuring galactose-1-phosphate uridyl transferase activity of erythrocytes. Clin. Chim. Acta 13:369-379, 1966.
181. Donnell, G. N.; Collado, M.; and Koch, R. Growth and development of children with galactosemia. J. Pediatr. 58:836-844, 1961.
182. Komrower, G. M.; and Lee, D. H. Long-term follow-up of galactosaemia. Arch. Dis. Child. 45:367-373, 1970.

183. Fishler, K.; Koch, R.; Donnell, G. N.; and Wenz, E. Developmental aspects of galactosemia from infancy to childhood. Clin. Pediatr. 19:38-44, 1980.
184. Waisbren, S. E.; Norman, T. R.; Schnell, R. R.; and Levy, H. L. Speech and language deficits in early-treated children with galactosemia. J. Pediatr. 102:75-77, 1983.
185. Lo, W.; Packman, S.; Nash, S.; Schmidt, K.; Ireland, S.; Diamond, I.; Ng, W.; and Donnell, G. Curious neurologic sequelae in galactosemia. Pediatrics 73:309-312, 1984.
186. Kaufman, F. R.; Kogut, M. D.; Donnell, G. N.; Goebelsmann, U.; March, C.; and Koch, R. Hypergonadotropic hypogonadism in female patients with galactosemia. N. Engl. J. Med. 304:994-998, 1981.
187. Chen, Y. T.; Mattison, D. R.; and Schulman, J. D. Hypogonadism and galactosemia. N. Engl. J. Med. 305:464-465, 1981.
188. Levy, H. L.; Driscoll, S. G.; Porensky, R. S.; and Wender, D. F. Ovarian failure in galactosemia. N. Engl. J. Med. 310:50, 1984.
189. Fanconi, G.; and Bickel, H. Die chronische Aminoacidurie (Aminosaure diabetes oder nephrotisch-glukosurischer Zwergwuchs) bei der Glykogenose und der Cystinkrankheit. Helv. Paediatr. Acta 4:359-396, 1949.
190. Rotthauwe, H. W.; Fichsel, H.; Heldt, H. W.; Kirsten, E.; Reim, M.; Schmidt, E.; Schmidt, F. W.; and Wesemann, W. Glykogenose der Leber mit Aminoacidurie and Glucosurie. Klin. Wochenschr. 41:818-825, 1963.
191. Odievre, M. Glycogenose hepato-renale avec tubulopathie complexe. Rev. Int. Hepatol. 16:1-70, 1966.
192. Fellers, F. X.; Piedrahita, V.; and Galan, E. M. Pseudo-phlorizin diabetes. Pediatr. Res. 1:304, 1967.
193. Lampert, F.; and Mayer, H. Glykogenose der Leber mit Galaktose-verwertungsstorung und schwerem Fanconi-Syndrom. Zeitschr. Kinderh. 98:133-145, 1967.
194. Bauer, B. Debre-de-Toni-Fanconi-Syndrom mit Clykogenose der Leber. Klin. Wochenschr. 46:317-328, 1968.
195. Brodehl, J.; Gellissen, K.; and Hagge, W. The Fanconi syndrome in hepatorenal glycogen storage disease. In: Progress in Nephrology, edited by Peters, G., and Roch-Ramel, F. New York, Springer-Verlag, 1969, pp. 241-243.
196. Garty, R.; Cooper, M.; and Tabachnik, E. The Fanconi syndrome associated with hepatic glycogenosis and abnormal metabolism of galactose. J. Pediatr. 85:821-823, 1974.
197. Houser, M.; and Angle, C. Fanconi type glycogen storage disease, a galactose sensitive tubulopathy. Clin. Res. 25:138A, 1977.
198. Brivet, M.; Moatti, N.; Corriat, A.; Lemonnier, A.; and Odievre, M. Defective galactose oxidation in a patient with glycogen storage disease and Fanconi syndrome. Pediatr. Res. 17:157-161, 1983.
199. Cohen, J.; and Friedman, M. Renal tubular acidosis associated with type III glycogenosis. Acta Paediatr. Scand. 68:779-782, 1979.
200. Brodehl, J. Tubular Fanconi syndromes with bone involvement. In: Inborn Errors of Calcium and Bone Metabolism, edited by Bickel, H., and Stern, J. Baltimore, University Park Press, 1976, pp. 191-213.
201. Danks, D. M. Hereditary disorders of copper metabolism in Wilson's disease and Menke's disease. In: The Metabolic Basis of Inherited Disease, 5th ed., edited by Stanbury, J. B., Wyngaarden, J. B., Fredrickson, D. S., Goldstein, J. L., and Brown, M. S. New York, McGraw-Hill, 1983, pp. 1251-1268.
202. Cartwright, G. E. Diagnosis of treatable Wilson's disease. N. Engl. J. Med. 298:1347-1350, 1978.
203. Strickland, G. T.; and Leu, M. L. Wilson's disease, clinical and laboratory manifestations in 40 patients. Medicine 54:113-137, 1975.

204. Wiebers, D. O.; Wilson, D. M.; McLeod, R. A.; and Goldstein, N. P. Renal stones in Wilson's disease. Am. J. Med. 67:249-254, 1979.
205. Bearn, A. G.; Yu, T. F.; and Gutman, A. B. Renal function in Wilson's disease. J. Clin. Invest. 36:1107-1114, 1957.
206. Leu, M. L.; Strickland, G. T.; and Gutman, R. A. Renal function in Wilson's disease: Response to penicillamine therapy. Am. J. Med. Sci. 260:381-398, 1970.
207. Asatoor, A. M.; Milne, M. D.; and Walshe, J. M. Urinary excretion of peptides and of hydroxyproline in Wilson's disease. Clin. Sci. Molec. Med. 51:369-378, 1976.
208. Aksoy, M.; Camli, N.; Dincol, K.; Erdem, S.; and Akgun, T. Osseous changes in Wilson's disease. Radiology 102:505-509, 1972.
209. Cavallino, R.; and Grossman, H. Wilson's disease presenting with rickets. Radiology 90:493-494, 1968.
210. Wilson, D. M.; and Goldstein, N. P. Renal urate excretion in patients with Wilson's disease. Kidney Int. 4:331-336, 1973.
211. Carpenter, T. O.; Carnes, D. L.; and Anast, C. S. Hypoparathyroidism in Wilson's disease. N. Engl. J. Med. 309:873-877, 1983.
212. Reynolds, E. S.; Tannen, R. L.; and Tyler, H. R. The renal lesion in Wilson's disease. Am. J. Med. 40:518-537, 1966.
213. Elsas, L. J.; Hayslett, J. P.; Spargo, B. H.; Durant, J. L.; and Rosenberg, L. E. Wilson's disease with reversible renal tubular dysfunction. Ann. Intern. Med. 75:427-433, 1971.
214. Epstein, O.; and Sherlock, S. Is Wilson's disease caused by a controller gene mutation resulting in perpetuation of the fetal mode of copper metabolism into childhood? Lancet 1:303-305, 1981.
215. Perman, J. A.; Werlin, S. L.; Grand, R. J.; and Watkins, J. B. Laboratory measures of copper metabolism in the differentiation of chronic active hepatitis and Wilson disease in children. J. Pediatr. 94:564-568, 1979.
216. Sternlieb, I.; and Scheinberg, I. H. The role of radiocopper in the diagnosis of Wilson's disease. Gastroenterology 77:138-142, 1979.
217. Walshe, J. M. Effect of penicillamine on failure of renal acidification in Wilson's disease. Lancet 1:775-779, 1968.
218. Walshe, J. M. Treatment of Wilson's disease with trientine (triethylene tetramine) dihydrochloride. Lancet 1:643-647, 1982.
219. Van Biervliet, J. P. G. M.; Bruinvis, L.; Ketting, D.; DeBree, P. K.; Van Der Heiden, C.; and Wadman, S. K. Hereditary mitochondrial myopathy with lactic acidemia, a DeToni-Fanconi-Debre syndrome, and a defective respiratory chain in voluntary striated muscles. Pediatr. Res. 11:1088-1093, 1977.
220. Rodriguez-Soriano, J.; Rivera, J. M.; Vallo, A.; Prats-Vinas, J. M.; and Castillo, G. Proximal renal tubular acidosis in metachromatic leukodystrophy. Helv. Paediatr. Acta 33:45-52, 1978.
221. Joosten, E.; Hoes, M.; Gabreels-Festen, A.; Hommes, O.; Stekhoven, H. S.; and Slooff, J. L. Electron microscopic investigation of inclusion material in a case of adult metachromatic leukodystrophy; observations on kidney biopsy, peripheral nerve and cerebral white matter. Acta Neuropathol. 33:165-171, 1975.
222. Worsley, H. E.; Brookfield, R. W.; Elwood, J. S.; Noble, R.; and Taylor, W. H. Lactic acidosis with necrotizing encephalopathy in two sibs. Arch. Dis. Child. 40:492-501, 1965.
223. Gruskin, A. B.; Patel, M. S.; Linshaw, M.; Ettenger, R.; Huff, D.; and Grover, W. Renal function studies and kidney pyruvate carboxylase in subacute necrotizing encephalomyelopathy (Leigh's syndrome). Pediatr. Res. 7:832-841, 1973.
224. Hirschman, G. H.; and Chan, J. C. M. Complex acid-base disorders in subacute necrotizing encephalomyelopathy (Leigh's syndrome). Pediatrics 61:278-281, 1978.

225. Passwell, J. H.; David, R.; Boichis, H.; and Herzfeld, S. Hereditary nephritis with associated defects in proximal renal tubular function. J. Pediatr. 98:85-87, 1981.
226. Fyhrquist, F. Y.; Klockars, M.; Gordin, A.; Tornroth, T.; and Kock, B. Hyperreninemia, lysozymuria, and erythrocytosis in Fanconi syndrome with medullary cystic kidney. Acta Med. Scand. 207:359-365, 1980.
227. Maldonado, J. E.; Velosa, J. A.; Kyle, R. A.; Wagoner, R. D.; Holley, K. E.; and Salassa, R. M. Fanconi syndrome in adults. A manifestation of a latent form of myeloma. Am. J. Med. 58:354-364, 1975.
228. Gailani, S.; Byeong-Kuk, S.; and Henderson, E. S. Kappa light chain-myeloma associated with adult Fanconi syndrome: Response of the nephropathy to treatment of myeloma. Med. Pediatr. Oncol. 4:141-147, 1978.
229. Walb, D.; Wohlenberg, H.; Rumpelt, H. J.; Schmidt, H.; and Thomas, L. Fanconi-Syndrom des Erwachsenen bei Fruhmyelom mit monoklonaler Gammopathie IgG, Typ kappa. Dtsch. Med. Wochenschr. 39:1355-1359, 1980.
230. Siame, J. L.; Sebert, J. L.; Delcambre, B.; and D'Eshougues, J. R. Le syndrome de Fanconi de l'adulte son association au myelome multiple a propos d'un cas. Lille Med. 23:428-430, 1978.
231. Short, I. A.; and Smith, J. P. Myelomatosis associated with glycosuria and aminoaciduria. Scott. Med. J. 4:89-93, 1959.
232. Costanza, D. J.; and Smoller, M. Multiple myeloma with the Fanconi syndrome. Am. J. Med. 34:125-133, 1963.
233. Cohen, A. H.; and Border, W. A. Myeloma kidney. An immunomorphogenetic study of renal biopsies. Lab. Invest. 42:248-256, 1980.
234. Rawlings, W.; Griffin, J.; Duffy, T.; and Humphrey, R. Fanconi syndrome with lambda light chains in urine. N. Engl. J. Med. 292:1351, 1975.
235. Dahlstrom, U.; Martensson, J.; and Lindstrom, F. D. Occurrence of adult Fanconi syndrome in benign monoclonal gammopathy. Acta Med. Scand. 208:425-429, 1980.
236. Harrison, J. F.; and Blainey, J. D. Adult Fanconi syndrome with monoclonal abnormality of immunoglobulin light chain. J. Clin. Pathol. 20:42-48, 1967.
237. Smithline, N.; Kassirer, J. P.; and Cohen, J. J. Light-chain nephropathy. Renal tubular dysfunction associated with light-chain proteinuria. N. Engl. J. Med. 294:71-74, 1976.
238. Von Scheele, C. Light chain myeloma with features of the adult Fanconi syndrome: Six years remission following one course of melphalan. Acta Med. Scand. 199:533-537, 1976.
239. Rochman, J.; Lichtig, C.; Osterweill, D.; Tatarsky, I.; and Eidelman, S. Adult Fanconi's syndrome with renal tubular acidosis in association with renal amyloidosis. Arch. Intern. Med. 140:1361-1363, 1980.
240. Finkel, P. N.; Kronenberg, K.; Pesce, A. J.; Pollak, V. E.; and Pirani, C. L. Adult Fanconi syndrome, amyloidosis and marked kappa light chain proteinuria. Nephron 10: 1-24, 1973.
241. Shearn, M. A.; and Tu, W. H. Nephrogenic diabetes insipidus and other defects of renal tubular function in Sjogren's syndrome. Am. J. Med. 39:312-318, 1965.
242. Walker, B. R.; Alexander, F.; and Tannenbaum, P. J. Fanconi syndrome with renal tubular acidosis and light chain proteinuria. Nephron 8:103-107, 1971.
243. Kamm, D. E.; and Fischer, M. S. Proximal renal tubular acidosis and the Fanconi syndrome in a patient with hypergammaglobulinemia. Nephron 9:208-219, 1972.
244. Clyne, D. H.; Brendstrup, L.; First, M. R.; Pesce, A. J.; Finkel, P. N.; Pollak, V. E.; and Pirani, C. L. Renal effects of intraperitoneal kappa chain injection. Lab. Invest. 31:131-142, 1974.
245. Preuss, H. G.; Hammack, W. J.; and Murdaugh, H. V. The effect of Bence Jones protein on the invitro function of rabbit renal cortex. Nephron 5:210-216, 1967.

246. McGeoch, J.; Smith, J. F.; Ledingham, J.; and Ross, B. Inhibition of active-transport sodium-potassium-A.T.P.ase by myeloma protein. Lancet 2:17-18, 1978.
247. Tegelaers, W. H.; and Tiddens, H. W. Nephrotic-glucosuric, amino aciduric dwarfism and electrolyte metabolism. Helv. Paediatr. Acta 10:269, 1955.
248. Hooft, C.; and Vermassen, A. DeToni-Debre-Fanconi syndrome in nephrotic children: A review. Ann. Pediatr. (Basel) 194:193, 1960.
249. Stanbury, S. W.; and Macaulay, D. Defects of renal tubular function in the nephrotic syndrome. Q. J. Med. 26:7-31, 1957.
250. Burke, E. C.; Holley, K. E.; and Stickler, G. B. Familial nephrotic syndrome with nephrocalcinosis and tubular dysfunction. J. Pediatr. 82:202-206, 1973.
251. Bouissou, F.; Barthe, P.; and Pierragi, M. T. Severe idiopathic nephrotic syndrome with tubular dysfunction (report of nine pediatric cases). Clin. Nephrol. 14:135-141, 1980.
252. McVicar, M.; Exeni, R.; and Susin, M. Nephrotic syndrome and multiple tubular defects in children: An early sign of focal segmental glomerulosclerosis. J. Pediatr. 97: 918-922, 1980.
253. Wood, E. G.; Brouhard, B. H.; Travis, L. B.; Cavallo, T.; and Lynch, R. E. Membranous glomerulonephropathy with tubular dysfunction and linear tubular basement membrane IgG deposition. J. Pediatr. 101:414-417, 1982.
254. Levy, M.; Gagnadoux, M. F.; Beziau, A.; and Habib, R. Membranous glomerulonephritis associated with anti-tubular and anti-alveolar basement membrane antibodies. Clin. Nephrol. 10:158-165, 1978.
255. Shwayder, M.; Ozawa, T.; Boedecker, E.; Guggenheim, S.; and McIntosh, R. M. Nephrotic syndrome associated with Fanconi syndrome. Ann. Intern. Med. 84:433-437, 1976.
256. Royer, P.; Habib, R.; Mathieu, H.; Broyer, M.; and Walsh, A. Pediatric nephrology. In: Major Problems in Clinical Pediatrics, edited by Schaffer, A. J. Philadelphia, Saunders, 1974, pp. 262-265.
257. Andres, G. A.; and McCluskey, R. T. Tubular and interstitial renal disease due to immunologic mechanisms. Kidney Int. 7:271-289, 1975.
258. McCluskey, R. T.; and Colvin, R. B. Immunological aspects of renal tubular and interstitial diseases. Ann. Rev. Med. 29:191-203, 1978.
259. Bergstein, J.; and Litman, N. Interstitial nephritis with anti-tubular-basement-membrane antibody. N. Engl. J. Med. 292:875-878, 1975.
260. Cattran, D. C. Circulating anti-tubular basement membrane antibody in a variety of human renal diseases. Nephron 26:13-19, 1980.
261. Sugisaki, T.; Klassen, J.; Milgrom, F.; Andres, G. A.; and McCluskey, R. T. Immunopathologic study of an autoimmune tubular and interstitial renal disease in brown Norway rats. Lab. Invest. 28:658-671, 1973.
262. Massry, S. G.; Preuss, H. G.; Maher, J. F.; and Schreiner, G. E. Renal tubular acidosis after cadaver kidney homotransplantation. Am. J. Med. 42:284-292, 1967.
263. Mookerjee, B.; Gault, M. H.; and Dossetor, J. B. Hyperchloremic acidosis in early diagnosis of renal allograft rejection. Ann. Intern. Med. 71:47-58, 1969.
264. Vertuno, L. L.; Preuss, H. G.; Argy, W. P.; and Schreiner, G. E. Fanconi syndrome following homotransplantation. Arch. Intern. Med. 133:302-305, 1974.
265. Friedman, A.; and Chesney, R. Fanconi's syndrome in renal transplantation. Am. J. Nephrol. 1:45-47, 1981.
266. Wilson, C. B.; Lehman, D. H.; McCoy, R.; Gunnells, J. C.; and Stickel, D. L. Antitubular basement membrane antibodies after renal transplantation. Transplantation 18:447-452, 1974.
267. Paul, L. C.; VanEs, L. A.; Stuffers-Herman, M.; de La Riviere, G. B.; and Kalft, M. W. Antibodies directed against tubular basement membranes in human renal allograft recipients. Clin. Immunol. Immunopathol. 14:231-237, 1979.

268. Goldsweig, H. G.; Brisson de Champlain, M. L.; and Davidman, M. Proximal tubular dysfunction associated with Burkitt's lymphoma. Cancer 41:568-577, 1978.
269. Myerson, R. M.; and Pastor, B. H. The Fanconi syndrome and its clinical variants. Am. J. Med. Sci. 228:378-387, 1954.
270. Weinstein, B.; Irreverre, F.; and Watkin, D. M. Lung carcinoma, hypouricemia and aminoaciduria. Am. J. Med. 39:520-526, 1965.
271. Gross, J. M. Fanconi syndrime (adult type) developing secondary to the ingestion of outdated tetracycline. Ann. Intern. Med. 58:523-528, 1963.
272. Ehrlich, L. I.; and Stein, H. S. Abnormal urinary findings following administration of achromycin V. J. Pediatr. 31:339, 1963.
273. Frimpter, G. W.; Timpanelli, A. E.; Eisenmenger, W. J.; Stein, H. S.; and Ehrlich, L. I. Reversible "Fanconi syndrome" caused by degraded tetracycline. J.A.M.A. 184:111-113, 1963.
274. Wegienka, L. C.; and Weller, J. M. Renal tubular acidosis caused by degraded tetracycline. Arch. Intern. Med. 114:232-235, 1964.
275. Cleveland, W. W.; Adams, W. C.; Mann, J. B.; and Nyhan, W. L. Acquired Fanconi syndrome following degraded tetracycline. J. Pediatr. 66:333-342, 1965.
276. Fulop, M.; and Drapkin, A. Potassium-depletion syndrome secondary to nephropathy apparently caused by "outdated tetracycline." N. Engl. J. Med. 272:986-989, 1965.
277. Mavromatis, F. Tetracycline nephropathy. J.A.M.A. 193:191-194, 1965.
278. Benitz, K. F.; and Diermeier, H. F. Renal toxicity of tetracycline degradation products. Proc. Soc. Exp. Biol. Med. 115:930-935, 1964.
279. Lowe, M. B.; Obst, D.; and Tapp, E. Renal damage caused by anhydro 4-epitetracycline. Arch. Pathol. 81:362-364, 1966.
280. Lindquist, R. R.; and Fellers, F. X. Degraded tetracycline nephropathy. Lab. Invest. 15:864-876, 1966.
281. Otten, J.; and Vis, H. L. Acute reversible renal tubular dysfunction following intoxication with methyl-3-chromone. J. Pediatr. 73:422-425, 1968.
282. Butler, H. E.; Morgan, J. M.; and Smythe, C. M. Mercaptopurine and acquired tubular dysfunction in adult nephrosis. Arch. Intern. Med. 116:853-856, 1965.
283. Schwartz, H. H.; and Schein, P. Fanconi syndrome associated with cephalothin and gentamicin therapy. Cancer 41:769-772, 1978.
284. Russo, J. C.; and Adelman, R. D. Gentamicin-induced Fanconi syndrome. J. Pediatr. 96:151-153, 1980.
285. Casteels-Van Daele, M.; Corbeel, L.; Van de Casseye, W.; Standaert, L. Gentamicin-induced Fanconi syndrome. J. Pediatr. 97:507, 1980.
286. Cronin, R. E. Aminoglycoside nephrotoxicity: Pathogenesis and prevention. Clin. Nephrol. 11:251-256, 1979.
287. Lenoir, G. R.; Perignon, J. L.; Gubler, M. C.; and Broyer, M. Valproic acid: A possible cause of proximal tubular renal syndrome. J. Pediatr. 98:503-504, 1981.
288. Schein, P.; Kahn, R.; Gorden, P.; Wells, S.; and DeVita, V. T. Streptozotocin for malignant insulinomas and carcinoid tumor. Arch. Intern. Med. 132:555-561, 1973.
289. Marsh, J. C.; Block, J. B.; Bentzel, C. J.; and Powell, R. D. Renal tubular reabsorption defects associated with isophthalanilide (NSC-53212). Cancer Chemother. Rep. 36:35-39, 1964.
290. Shreeve, W. W.; Hutchin, M. E.; Harper, H. A.; Miller, C. D.; Doolan, P. D. Excretion of amino acids in nephrosis. Proc. Soc. Exp. Biol. Med. 88:510-514, 1955.
291. Doolan, P. D.; Morris, M. D.; and Harper, H. A. Aminoaciduria in an elderly man with the nephrotic syndrome and in a young man with a variant of the Fanconi syndrome. Ann. Intern. Med. 56:448-456, 1962.
292. Kuhar, M. J.; Mak, L. L.; and Lietman, P. S. Autoradiographic localization of [^{3}H] gentamicin in the proximal renal tubules of mice. Antimicrob. Agents Chemother. 15:131-133, 1979.

293. Houghton, D. C.; Plamp, C. E.; DeFehr, J. M.; Bennett, W. M.; Porter, G.; and Gilbert, D. Gentamicin and tobramycin nephrotoxicity. Am. J. Pathol. 93:137-147, 1978.
294. Kosek, J. C.; Mazze, R. I.; and Cousins, M. J. Nephrotoxicity of gentamicin. Lab. Invest. 30:48-57, 1974.
295. Dobyan, D. C.; Cronin, R. E.; and Bulger, R. E. Effect of potassium depletion on tubular morphology in gentamicin-induced acute renal failure in dogs. Lab. Invest. 47:586-594, 1982.
296. Cronin, R. E.; Bulger, R. E.; Southern, P.; and Henrich, W. L. Natural history of aminoglycoside nephrotoxicity in the dog. J. Lab. Clin. Med. 95:463-474, 1980.
297. Schentag, J. J.; Sutfin, T. A.; Plaut, M. E.; and Jusko, W. J. Early detection of aminoglycoside nephrotoxicity with urinary beta-2-microglobulin. J. Med. 9:201-210, 1978.
298. Sethi, K.; and Diamond, L. H. Aminoglycoside nephrotoxicity and its predictability. Nephron 27:265-270, 1981.
299. Bar, R. S.; Wilson, H. E.; and Mazzaferri, E. L. Hypomagnesemic hypocalcemia secondary to renal magnesium wasting. A possible consequence of high-dose gentamicin therapy. Ann. Intern. Med. 82:646-649, 1975.
300. Keating, M. J.; Sethi, M. R.; Bodey, G. P.; and Samaan, N. A. Hypocalcemia with hypoparathyroidism and renal tubular dysfunction associated with aminoglycoside therapy. Cancer 39:1410-1414, 1977.
301. Kelnar, C. J. H.; Taor, W. S.; Reynolds, D. J.; Smith, D. R.; Slavin, B. M.; Brook, C. G. D. Hypomagnesaemic hypocalcaemia with hypokalaemia caused by treatment with high dose gentamicin. Arch. Dis. Child. 53:817-820, 1978.
302. Patel, R.; and Savage, A. Symptomatic hypomagnesemia associated with gentamicin therapy. Nephron 23:50-52, 1979.
303. Gonick, H. C. Trace metals and the kidney. Miner. Electrolyte Metab. 1:107-120, 1978.
304. Bitran, J. D.; Desser, R. K.; Billings, A. A.; Kozloff, M. F.; and Shapiro, C. M. Acute nephrotoxicity following cis-dichlorodiammineplatinum. Cancer 49:1784-1788, 1982.
305. Friberg, L.; Piscater, M.; Nordberg, G. F.; and Kjellstrom, T. Cadmium in the Environment, 2nd ed. Cleveland, CRC Press, 1974.
306. Adams, R. G.; Harrison, J. F.; and Scott, P. The development of cadmium-induced proteinuria, impaired renal function, and osteomalacia in alkaline battery workers. Q. J. Med. 38:425-443, 1969.
307. Kazantzis, G.; Flynn, F. V.; Spowage, J. S.; and Trott, D. G. Renal tubular malfunction and pulmonary emphysema in cadmium pigment workers. Q. J. Med. 32:165-192, 1963.
308. Friberg, L. Health hazards in the manufacture of alkaline accumulators with special reference to chronic cadmium poisoning. Acta Med. Scand. 138(Suppl. 240): 9-124, 1950.
309. Piscator, M. Proteinuria in chronic cadmium poisoning. III. Electrophoretic and immunoelectrophoretic studies on urinary proteins from cadmium workers, with special reference to the excretion of low molecular weight proteins. Arch. Environ. Health 12:335-344, 1966.
310. Nomiyama, K.; and Sugata, Y. Urinary low-molecular-weight proteins in itai-itai disease. Environ. Res. 6:373-381, 1973.
311. Effects of cadmium on human health. A review of studies mainly performed in Japan. Japan Public Health Association, 1976, pp. 1-23.
312. Perry, H. M.; Tipton, I. H.; Schroeder, H. A.; Steiner, R. L.; and Cook, H. J. Variation in the concentration of cadmium in human kidney as a function of age and geographic origin. J. Chron. Dis. 14:259-271, 1961.
313. Indraprasit, S.; Alexander, G. V.; and Gonick, H. C. Tissue composition of major and trace elements in uremia and hypertension. Autopsy studies in man. J. Chron. Dis. 27:135-161, 1972.

314. Saito, H.; Shioji, R.; Hurukawa, Y.; Nagai, K.; Arikawa, T.; Saito, T.; Sasaki, Y.; Furuyama, T.; and Yoshinaga, K. Cadmium-induced proximal tubular dysfunction in a cadmium-polluted area. Contrib. Nephrol. 6:1-12, 1977.
315. Bernard, A.; Buchet, J. P.; Roels, H.; Masson, P.; and Lauwerys, R. Renal excretion of proteins and enzymes in workers exposed to cadmium. Eur. J. Clin. Invest. 9:11-22, 1979.
316. Gompertz, D.; Fletcher, J. G.; Perkins, J.; Smith, N. J.; Chettle, D. R.; Mason, H.; Scott, M. C.; Topping, M. D.; and Blindt, M. Renal dysfunction in cadmium smelters: Relation to in-vivo liver and kidney cadmium concentrations. Lancet 1:1185-1187, 1983.
317. Scott, R.; Fitzgerald-Finch, O. P.; Cunningham, C.; Ottoway, J. M.; and Fell, G. S. The importance of chronic cadmium poisoning in renal stone formation—A five year study. In: Urolithiasis—Clinical and Basic Research, edited by Smith, L. H., Robertson, U. G., and Finlayson, B. New York, Plenum, 1981, pp. 353-357.
318. Takase, T. On the pathogenesis of so-called "itai-itai" disease patients in Toyama prefecture. Jpn. J. Clin. Med. 25:200-219, 1967.
319. Itokawa, Y.; Abe, J.; and Tamaka, S. Bone changes in experimental chronic cadmium poisoning. Arch. Environ. Health 26:241-244, 1973.
320. Nogawa, K.; Kobayashi, E.; and Konishi, F. Comparison of bone lesions in chronic cadmium intoxication and vitamin D deficiency. Environ. Res. 24:233-249, 1981.
321. Kawamura, J.; Yoshida, O.; Nishino, K.; and Itokawa, Y. Disturbances in kidney functions and calcium and phosphate metabolism in cadmium-poisoned rats. Nephron 20:101-110, 1978.
322. Kitamura, S. Etiology of itai-itai disease. In: Edited Proceedings, 1st International Cadmium Conference, San Francisco. London, Metal Bulletin Ltd., 1978, pp. 211-213.
323. Kimura, M.; Otaki, N.; Yoshiki, S.; Suzuki, M.; Horiuchi, N.; and Suda, T. The isolation of metallothionein and its prospective role in cadmium poisoning. Arch. Biochem. Biophys. 165:340-348, 1974.
324. Yoshiki, S.; Yanagisaiva, T.; Kimura, M.; Otaki, N.; Suzuki, M.; and Suda, T. Bone and kidney lesions in experimental cadmium intoxication. Arch. Environ. Health 30: 559-562, 1975.
325. Gonick, H. C. Nephropathies of heavy metal intoxication. In: Textbook of Nephrology, edited by Massry, S. G., and Glassock, R. J. Baltimore, Williams & Wilkins, 1983, pp. 6.184-6.194.
326. Chisolm, J. J.; Harrison, H. C.; Eberlein, W. R.; and Harrison, H. E. Amino-aciduria, hypophosphatemia and rickets in lead poisoning. Am. J. Dis. Child. 89:159-168, 1955.
327. Chisolm, J. J. Aminoaciduria as a manifestation of renal tubular injury in lead intoxication and a comparison with patterns of aminoaciduria seen in other diseases. J. Pediatr. 60:1-17, 1962.
328. Goyer, R. A. The renal tubule in lead poisoning. Lab. Invest. 19:71-77, 1968.
329. Goyer, R. A.; Tsuchiya, K.; Leonard, D. L.; and Kahyo, H. Aminoaciduria in Japanese workers in the lead and cadmium industries. Am. J. Clin. Pathol. 57:635-642, 1972.
330. Emerson, B. T. Chronic lead nephropathy. Kidney Int. 4:1-5, 1973.
331. Morgan, J. M.; Hartley, M. W.; and Miller, R. E. Nephropathy in chronic lead poisoning. Arch. Intern. Med. 118:17-29, 1966.
332. Morgan, J. M. Hyperkalemia and acidosis in lead nephropathy. South. Med. J. 69: 881-883, 1967.
333. Sandstead, H. H.; Michelalsis, A. M.; and Temple, T. E. Lead intoxication. Its effects on the renin-aldoterone response to sodium deprivation. Arch. Environ. Health 20: 356-363, 1970.

334. Miani, N.; and Viterbo, B. Studio isoautoradiografico sulla localizazione del plombo (RaD) in vari organi di cane. Z. Zellforsch. Mikrosk. Anat. 49:188-208, 1958.
335. Galle, P.; and Morel-Maroger, L. Les Lesiones renales du saturnisme humain et experimental. Nephron 2:273-286, 1965.
336. Goyer, R. A.; May, P.; Cates, M. M.; and Krigman, M. R. Lead and protein content of isolated intranuclear inclusion bodies from kidneys of lead-poisoned rats. Lab. Invest. 22:245-251, 1970.
337. Chisolm, J. J. Increased lead absorption and lead poisoning. In: Nelson Textbook of Pediatrics, 11th ed., edited by Behrman, R. E., and Vaughn, V. C. Philadelphia, Saunders, 1983, pp. 1801-1804.
338. McDowell, E. M.; Nagle, R. B.; Zalme, R. C.; McNeil, J. S.; Flamenbaum, W.; and Trump, B. F. Studies on the pathyphysiology of acute renal failure. I. Correlation of ultrastructure and function in the proximal tubule of the rat following administration of mercuric chloride. Virchows Arch. (Cell Pathol.) 22:173-196, 1976.
339. Clarkson, T. W. The pharmacology of mercury compounds. Ann. Rev. Pharmacol. 12:375-406, 1972.
340. Freeman, R. B.; Maher, J. F.; Schreiner, G. E.; and Mostofi, F. K. Renal tubular necrosis due to nephrotoxicity of organic mercurial diuretics. Ann. Intern. Med. 57:34-43, 1962.
341. Gerstner, H. B.; and Huff, J. E. Clinical toxicology of mercury. J. Toxicol. Environ. Health 2:491-526, 1977.
342. Wilson, V. K.; Thomson, M. C.; and Holzel, A. Mercury nephrosis in young children. Br. Med. J. 1:358-360, 1952.
343. Porter, G. A.; and Bennett, W. M. Toxic Nephropathies. In: The Kidney, 2nd ed., edited by Brenner, B. M., and Rector, F. C. Philadelphia, Saunders, 1981, pp. 2078-2079.
344. Williams, N. E.; and Bridge, H. G. T. Nephrotic syndrome after the application of mercury ointment. Lancet 2:602, 1958.
345. Rutzler, L. Passagres tubulares Syndrom durch Vergiftung mit einer organischen Quecksilberverbindung (Glyceromerfen) bei einem 1½ jahrigen Madchen. Schweiz. Med. Wochenschr. 103:678-681, 1973.
346. Clarkson, T. W.; and Kench, J. E. Urinary excretion of amino acids by men absorbing heavy metals. Biochem. J. 62:361-372, 1956.
347. Foulkes, E. C. Effects of heavy metals on renal aspartate transport and the nature of solute movement in kidney cortex slides. Biochim. Biophys. Acta 241:815-822, 1971.
348. Rothstein, A.; and Berke, H. J. Aminoaciduria in uranium poisoning; the use of amino-acid nitrogen to creatinine ratio in "spot" samples of urine. J. Pharmacol. Exp. Ther. 96:179-187, 1949.
349. Biber, T.; Mylle, M.; Baines, A. D.; Gottschalk, C. W.; Oliver, J. R.; and MacDowell, M. C. A study of micropuncture and microdissection of acute renal damage in rats. Am. J. Med. 44:664-705, 1968.
350. Cisplatin (Editorial). Lancet 1:374-375, 1982.
351. Blanchley, J. D.; and Hill, J. B. Renal and electrolyte disturbances associated with cisplatin. Ann. Intern. Med. 95:628-632, 1981.
352. Dentio, M.; Luft, R. C.; Yum, N. M.; Williams, D. S.; and Einhorn, L. H. Long term effect of cis-diamminedichloride platinum (CDDP) on renal function and structure in man. Cancer 41:1274-1281, 1978.
353. Gonzalez-Vitale, J. C.; Hayes, D. M.; Cvitkovic, E.; and Steinberg, S. The renal pathology in clinical trials of cis-platinum (II) diamminedichloride. Cancer 39:1362-1371, 1977.
354. Choie, D. D.; Longnecker, D. S.; and del Campo, A. A. Acute and chronic cisplatin nephropathy in rats. Lab. Invest. 44:397-402, 1981.

355. Stark, J. J.; and Howell, S. B. Nephrotoxicity of cis-platinum (II) dichlorodiammine. Clin. Pharmacol. Ther. 23:461-466, 1978.
356. Jones, B. R.; Bhalla, R. B.; Mladek, J.; Kaleya, R. N.; Gralla, R. J.; Alcock, N. W.; Schwartz, M. K.; Young, C. W.; and Reidenberg, M. M. Comparison of methods of evaluating nephrotoxicity of cis-platinum. Clin. Pharmacol. Ther. 27:557-562, 1980.
357. Shilsky, R. L.; and Anderson, T. Hypomagnesemia and renal magnesium wasting in patients receiving cisplatin. Ann. Intern. Med. 90:929-931, 1979.
358. Guarino, A. M.; Miller, D. S.; Arnolds, S. T.; Pritchard, J. B.; Davis, R. D.; Urbanek, M. A.; Miller, T. J.; Litterst, C. L. Platinate toxicity: Past, present, and prospects. Cancer Treat. Rep. 63:1475-1483, 1979.
359. Litterst, C. L. Alteration in toxicity of cis-platinum. Toxicol. Appl. Pharmacol. 61: 99-108, 1981.
360. Vaziri, N. D.; Ness, R. L.; Fairshter, R. D.; Smith, W. R.; and Rosen, S. M. Nephrotoxicity of paraquat in man. Arch. Intern. Med. 139:172-174, 1979.
361. Spencer, A. G.; and Franglen, G. T. Gross amino-aciduria following a Lysol burn. Lancet 1:190-192, 1952.
362. Moss, A. H.; Gabow, P. A.; Kaehny, W. D.; Goodman, S. I.; Haut, L. L.; and Haussler, M. R. Fanconi's syndrome and distal renal tubular acidosis after glue sniffing. Ann. Intern. Med. 92:69-70, 1980.
363. Streicher, H. Z.; Gabow, P. A.; Moss, A. H.; Kono, D.; and Kaehny, W. D. Syndromes of toluene sniffing in adults. Ann. Intern. Med. 94:758-762, 1981.
364. Taher, S. M.; Anderson, R. J.; McCartney, R.; Popovtzer, M. M.; and Schrier, R. W. Renal tubular acidosis associated with toluene "sniffing." N. Engl. J. Med. 290:765-768, 1974.
365. Kroeger, R. M.; Moore, R. J.; Lehman, T. H.; Giesy, J. D.; and Skeeters, C. E. Recurrent urinary calculi associated with toluene sniffing. J. Urol. 123:89-91, 1980.
366. Hall, P. W.; Piscator, M.; Vasiljevic, M.; and Popovic, N. Renal function studies in individuals with the tubular proteinuria of endemic Balkan nephropathy. Q. J. Med. 41:385-393, 1972.
367. Radonic, M. Beta$_2$-microglobulin in Balkan endemic nephropathy. Pathol. Biol. 26: 317-320, 1978.
368. Riley, A. L.; Ryan, L. M.; and Roth, D. A. Renal proximal tubular dysfunction and paroxysmal nocturnal hemoglobinuria. Am. J. Med. 62:125-129, 1977.
369. Stark, H.; and Geiger, R. Renal tubular dysfunction following vascular accidents of the kidneys in the newborn period. J. Pediatr. 83:933-940, 1973.
370. Chisolm, J. J.; and Harrison, H. E. Aminoaciduria in vitamin D deficiency states in premature infants and older infants with rickets. J. Pediatr. 60:206-219, 1962.
371. Winberg, J.; and Bergstrom, T. Renal acidification defect in infants with mild deficiency rickets. Acta Paediatr. Scand. 54:139-148, 1965.
372. Guignard, J. P.; and Torrado, A. Proximal renal tubular acidosis in vitamin D deficiency rickets. Acta Paediatr. Scand. 62:543-546, 1973.
373. Teotio, M.; Teotia, S. P. S.; Sharma, N. L.; Singh, R.; Singh, R. K.; and Teotia, N. P. S. Renal acidification defect in vitamin-D deficiency rickets. Indian J. Med. Res. 62: 204-210, 1974.
374. Muldowney, F. P.; Freaney, R.; and McGeeney, D. Renal tubular acidosis and aminoaciduria in osteomalacia of dietary or intestinal origin. Q. J. Med. 37:517-539, 1968.
375. Chesney, R. W.; and Harrison, H. E. Fanconi syndrome following bowel surgery and hepatitis reversed by 25-hydroxycholecalciferol. J. Pediatr. 86:857-861, 1975.
376. Huguenin, M.; Schacht, R.; and David, R. Infantile rickets with severe proximal renal tubular acidosis, responsive to vitamin D. Arch. Dis. Child. 49:955-959, 1974.
377. Arnaud, C.; Maijer, R.; Reade, T.; Scriver, C. R.; and Whelan, D. T. Vitamin D dependency: An inherited postnatal syndrome with secondary hyperparathyroidism. Pediatrics 46:871-880, 1970.

378. Brooks, M. H.; Bell, N. H.; Love, L.; Stern, P. H.; Orfei, E.; Queener, S. F.; Hamstra, A. J.; and DeLuca, H. F. Vitamin-D-dependent rickets type II. N. Engl. J. Med. 298: 996-999, 1978.
379. Sockalosky, J. J.; Ulstrom, R. A.; DeLuca, H. F.; and Brown, D. M. Vitamin-D-resistant rickets: End-organ unresponsiveness to 1,25 $(OH)_2D_3$. J. Pediatr. 96:701-703, 1980.
380. Beer, S.; Tieder, M.; Kohelet, D.; Liberman, O. A.; Vure, E.; Bar-Joseph, G.; Gabizon, D.; Borochowitz, Z. U.; Varon, M.; and Modai, D. Vitamin D resistant rickets with alopecia: A form of end organ resistance to 1,25 dihydroxy vitamin D. Clin. Endocrinol. 14:395-402, 1981.
381. Phillips, M. E. Aminoaciduria—Its relationship to vitamin D and parathyroid hormone. CRC Crit. Rev.-Clin. Lab. Sci. 12:215-239, 1980.
382. Rampini, S.; Fanconi, A.; Illig, R.; and Prader, A. Effect of hydrochlorothiazide on proximal renal tubular acidosis in a patient with idiopathic "deToni-Debre-Fanconi syndrome." Helv. Paediatr. Acta 23:13-21, 1968.
383. Callis, L.; Castello, F.; Fortuny, G.; Vallo, A.; and Ballabriga, A. Effect of hydrochlorothiazide on rickets and on renal tubular acidosis in two patients with cystinosis. Helv. Paediatr. Acta 25:602-619, 1970.
384. Donckerwolcke, R. A.; Van Stekelenburg, G. J.; and Tiddens, H. A. Therapy of bicarbonate-losing renal tubular acidosis. Arch. Dis. Child. 45:774-779, 1970.
385. Van Biervliet, J. P. G. M.; Donckerwolcke, R. A. M. G.; Van Stekelenburg, G. J.; and Wadman, S. K. Sodium chloride restriction and extracellular fluid volume contraction in hyperphosphaturic vitamin D resistant rickets in the Lowe syndrome. Helv. Paediatr. Acta 30:365-375, 1975.
386. Arant, B. S.; Greifer, I.; Edelmann, C. M.; and Spitzer, A. Effect of chronic salt and water loading on the tubular defects of a child with Fanconi syndrome (cystinosis). Pediatrics 58:370-377, 1976.
387. Sebastian, A.; McSherry, E.; and Morris, R. C. Renal potassium wasting in renal tubular acidosis (RTA). J. Clin. Invest. 50:667-678, 1971.
388. Giebisch, G.; and Stanton, B. Potassium transport in the nephron. Ann. Rev. Physiol. 41:241-56, 1979.
389. Bovee, K. C.; Joyce, T.; Reynolds, R.; and Segal, S. The Fanconi syndrome in Basenji dogs: A new model for renal transport defects. Science 201:1129-1131, 1978.
390. Gray, R. W.; Omdahl, J. L.; Ghazarian, J. G.; and DeLuca, H. F. 25-Hydroxycholecalciferol-1-hydroxylase. Subcellular location and properties. J. Biol. Chem. 247: 7528-7532, 1972.
391. Brunette, M. G.; Chan, M.; Ferriere, C.; and Roberts, K. D. Site of 1,25 $(OH)_2$ vitamin D_3 synthesis in the kidney. Nature 276:287-289, 1978.
392. Akiba, T.; Endou, H.; Koseki, C.; and Sakai, F. Localization of 25-hydroxyvitamin D_3-1-alpha-hydroxylase activity in the mammalian kidney. Biochem. Biophys. Res. Commun. 94:313-318, 1980.
393. Kawashima, H.; Torikai, S.; and Kurokawa, K. Localization of 25-hydroxyvitamin D_3-1-alpha-hydroxylase and 24-hydroxylase along the rat nephron. Proc. Natl. Acad. Sci. U.S.A. 78:1199-1203, 1981.
394. Brewer, E. D.; Tsai, H. C.; Szeto, K. S.; and Morris, R. C. Maleic acid-induced impaired conversion of $25(OH)D_3$ to $1,25(OH)_2D_3$: Implications for Fanconi's syndrome. Kidney Int. 12:244-252, 1977.
395. Anderson, C.; and Danylchuk, K. D. Plasma levels of immunoreactive parathyroid hormone in dogs chronically exposed to low levels of cadmium chloride. J. Environ. Pathol. Toxicol. 2:1151-1159, 1979.
396. Feldman, S. L.; and Cousins, R. J. Influence of cadmium on the metabolism of 25-hydroxycholecalciferol in chicks. Nutr. Rep. Int. 8:251-260, 1973.

397. Gertner, J. M.; Brenton, D. P.; Dent, C. E.; Domenech, M. Treatment of the rickets of cystinosis with 1-alpha-hydroxycholecalciferol. Calif. Tissue Res. 521:63-67, 1977.
398. Etches, P.; Pickering, D.; and Smith, R. Cystinotic rickets treated with vitamin D metabolites. Arch. Dis. Child. 52:661-664, 1977.
399. Kitagawa, T.; Akatsuka, A.; Owada, M.; and Mano, T. Biologic and therapeutic effects of 1-alpha-hydroxycholecalciferol in different types of Fanconi syndrome. Contrib. Nephrol. 22:107-119, 1980.
400. Chesney, R. W.; Rosen, J. F.; Hamstra, A. J.; and DeLuca, H. F. Serum 1,25-dihydroxyvitamin D levels in normal children and in vitamin D disorders. Am. J. Dis. Child. 134:135-139, 1980.
401. Kruse, K.; and Bartels, H. Hypercalciuria in idiopathic Fanconi syndrome. Eur. J. Pediatr. 131:247-254, 1979.
402. Chesney, R. W.; Kaplan, B. S.; Phelps, M.; and DeLuca, H. F. Renal tubular acidosis does not alter circulating values of calcitriol. J. Pediatr. 104:51-55, 1984.
403. Gray, R. W.; Wilz, D. R.; Caldas, A. E.; and Lemann, J. The importance of phosphate in regulating plasma 1,25-$(OH)_2$-vitamin D levels in humans: Studies in healthy subjects, in calcium-stone formers and in patients with primary hyperparathyroidism. J. Clin. Endocrinol. Metab. 45:299-306, 1977.
404. Hughes, M. R.; Brumbaugh, P. F.; Haussler, M. R.; Wergedahl, J. E.; and Baylink, D. J. Regulation of serum 1-alpha, 25-dihydroxyvitamin D_3 by calcium and phosphate in the rat. Science 190:578-580, 1975.
405. Rader, J. I.; Baylink, D. J.; Hughes, M. R.; Safilian, E. F.; and Haussler, M. R. Calcium and phosphorus deficiency in rats: Effects on PTH and 1,25-dihydroxyvitamin D_3. Am. J. Physiol. 236:E118-E122, 1979.
406. Chesney, R. W.; Zimmerman, J.; Hamstra, A.; DeLuca, H. F.; and Mazess, R. B. Vitamin D metabolite concentrations in vitamin D deficiency. Am. J. Dis. Child. 135: 1025-1028, 1981.
407. Steendijk, R. The effect of a continuous intravenous infusion of inorganic phosphate on the rachitic lesions in cystinosis. Arch. Dis. Child. 36:321-324, 1961.
408. Salassa, R. M.; Power, M. H.; Ulrich, J. A.; and Hayles, A. B. Observations on the metabolic effects of vitamin D in Fanconi's syndrome. Proc. Mayo. Clin. 29:214-224, 1954.
409. Stanbury, S. W.; and Lumb, G. A. Metabolic studies of renal osteodystrophy. I. Calcium, phosphorus and nitrogen metabolism in rickets, osteomalacia and hyperparathyroidism complicating chronic uremia and in the osteomalacia of the adult Fanconi syndrome. Medicine 41:1-31, 1962.
410. Wasnich, R. D.; Benfante, R. J.; Yano, K.; Heilbrun, L.; and Vogel, J. M. Thiazide effect on the mineral content of bone. N. Engl. J. Med. 309:344-347, 1983.
411. Lemann, J.; Litzow, J. R.; and Lennon, E. J. The effects of chronic acid loads in normal man: Further evidence for participation of bone mineral in the defense against chronic acidosis. J. Clin. Invest. 45:1608-1614, 1966.
412. Cunningham, J.; Fraher, L. J.; Clemens, T. L.; Revell, P. A.; and Papapoulos, S. E. Chronic acidosis with metabolic bone disease. Effect of alkali on bone morphology and vitamin D metabolism. Am. J. Med. 73:199-204, 1982.
413. Kraut, J. A.; Gordon, E. M.; Ranson, J. C.; Horst, R.; Slatopolsky, E.; Coburn, J. W.; and Kurokawa, K. Effect of chronic metabolic acidosis on vitamin D metabolism in humans. Kidney Int. 24:644-648, 1983.
414. Lee, S. W.; Russell, J.; and Avioli, L. V. 25-Hydroxycholecalciferol to 1,25-dihydroxycholecalciferol: Conversion impaired by systemic metabolic acidosis. Science 195: 994-996, 1977.

415. Reddy, G. S.; Jones, G.; Kooh, S. W.; and Fraser, D. Inhibition of 25-hydroxyvitamin D_3-1-hydroxylase by chronic metabolic acidosis. Am. J. Physiol. 243:E265-E271, 1982.
416. Brenner, R. J.; Spring, D. B.; Sebastian, A.; McSherry, E. M.; Genant, H. K.; Palubinskas, A. J.; and Morris, R. C. Incidence of radiographically evident bone disease, nephrocalcinosis, and nephrolithiasis in various types of renal tubular acidosis. N. Engl. J. Med. 307:217-221, 1982.
417. Richards, P.; Chamberlain, M. T.; and Wrong, O. M. Treatment of osteomalacia of renal tubular acidosis by sodium bicarbonate alone. Lancet 2:994-997, 1972.
418. Holick, M. F.; Tavela, T. E.; Holick, S. A.; Schnoes, H. K.; DeLuca, H. F.; and Gallagher, B. M. Synthesis of 1-alpha-hydroxy[6-^{3}H] vitamin D_3 and its metabolism to 1-alpha,25-dihydroxy[6-^{3}H] vitamin D_3 in the rat. J. Biol. Chem. 251:1020-1024, 1976.
419. Brickman, A. S.; Coburn, J. W.; Friedman, G. R.; Okamura, W. H.; Massry, S. G.; and Norman, A. W. Comparison of effects of 1-alpha-hydroxyvitamin D_3 and 1,25-dihydroxy-vitamin D_3 in man. J. Clin. Invest. 57:1540-1547, 1976.
420. Harrison, H. E.; and Harrison, H. C. Dihydrotachysterol: A calcium active steroid not dependent upon kidney metabolism. J. Clin. Invest. 51:1919-1922, 1972.

15

Pathogenesis of the Fanconi Syndrome

HARVEY C. GONICK
Cedars-Sinai Medical Center and University of California at Los Angeles School of Medicine, Los Angeles, California

HERBERT J. KRAMER
University of Bonn, Bonn, Federal Republic of Germany

The preceding chapter has emphasized the generalized nature of the renal tubular transport dysfunction in the human Fanconi syndrome and has described the several clinical settings in which Fanconi syndrome is observed. However, clinical studies in humans do not permit elucidation of the underlying biochemical pathogenetic mechanisms. For this reason, various experimental animal models have been developed. In the discussion that follows, we shall describe first the experimental models and then, based on experimental observations in each of these models, develop a hypothesis to account for the fundamental pathophysiological defect in Fanconi syndrome.

I. EXPERIMENTAL MODELS

A. Maleic Acid Model

Physiological Observations

The maleic acid model of Fanconi syndrome was the first to be recognized and the most extensively used to explore the physiological, morphological, and biochemical correlates. In 1950, Berliner and colleagues (1) initially observed that when maleic acid was given intravenously to acidotic dogs the animals developed an alkaline urine, together with a diuresis of sodium, phosphate, glucose, and potassium, and a decreased Tm_{PAH}. Most subsequent studies have been performed in rats. Harrison and Harrison (2) found that the intraperitoneal injection of maleic acid neutralized with NaOH (maleate) into young rats fed a low-phosphate, high-calcium "rachitogenic diet" produced phosphaturia, glucosuria, and aminoaciduria, but decreased excretion of calcium and citrate. Individual amino acids identified by paper chromatography included leucine, iso-leucine, valine, methionine, histidine, alanine, and glutamic acid, indicating that the aminoaciduria was of a generalized nature. When maleate was injected on a daily basis, resistance to its effect developed rapidly with a decrease in phosphaturia and aminoaciduria observed by the third day; this maleate effect could be reelicited 5-7 days after cessation of injections.

Other investigators noted that the acute renal tubular effect of maleate was dose dependent. Harrison and Harrison (2) had employed a relatively low dose of 0.9 mmol maleate/kg body weight. Worthen (3) injected 3, 6, or 9 mmol maleate/kg intraperitoneally into adult male rats. The time of onset and the severity of tubular dysfunction roughly paralleled the amount of maleate given. The urinary abnormalities (glucosuria, aminoaciduria, proteinuria, polyuria, and increased urine pH) developed within 1 hr at the highest dose and within 2 hr at the lowest dose. Conversely, normal renal function returned within 24 hr in animals given the lowest dose, but it persisted up to 72 hr in animals given the largest dose. Schärer et al. (4) injected maleic acid subcutaneously into male rats at doses of 0.4, 0.9, 1.7, and 3.4 mmol/kg body weight and found a dose-related effect on urine volume but not on aminoaciduria. Only the rats given a dose of 3.4 mmol/kg showed consistent generalized aminoaciduria. Kramer and Gonick (5,6) injected adult female rats intraperitoneally with maleate at a low dose (1.5 mmol/kg) and a high dose (9 mmol/kg) and found dose-related changes in urine volume and sodium and calcium excretion. Both groups of animals demonstrated increases in urine volume, pH, glucosuria, and proteinuria within 15 min after injection (Fig. 1). The animals injected with 1.5 mmol/kg showed maximum alterations in renal function at 90 min and normal excretion patterns were observed after 8 hr; those injected with 9 mmol/kg showed maximal alterations sustained over a period of more than 2 hr, with abnormalities persisting well beyond 8 hr. Glomerular filtration rate remained normal at the low dose but was reduced to 30% of normal at the high dose, even when volume losses were replaced with saline. Animals given 1.5 mmol/kg maleate showed increased clearances of sodium, calcium, potassium, and phosphate, but magnesium clearance and urate clearance were unaltered.

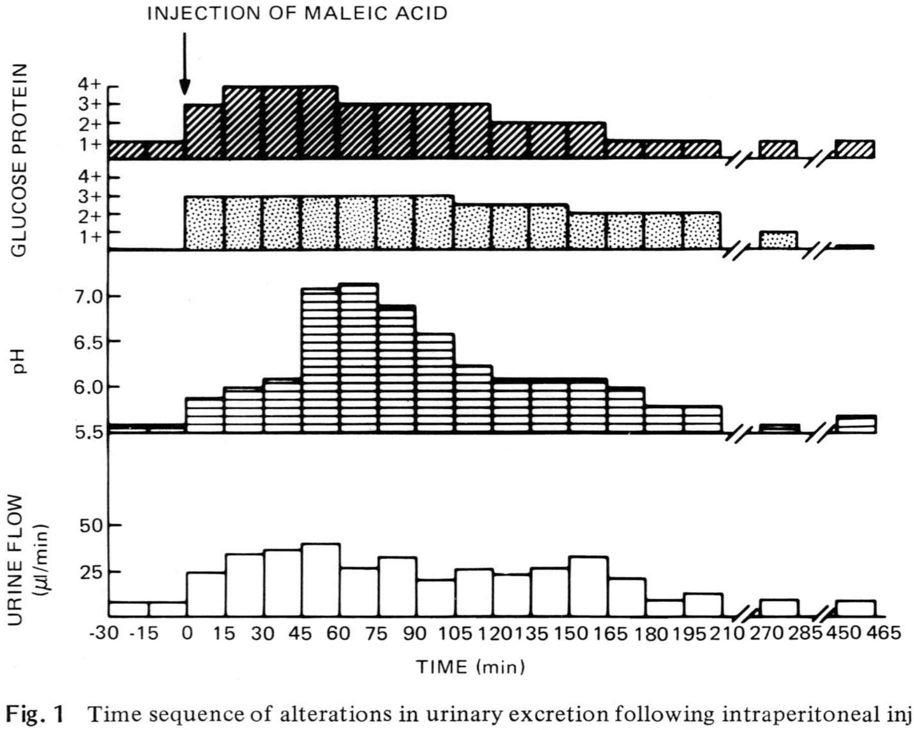

Fig. 1 Time sequence of alterations in urinary excretion following intraperitoneal injection of 1.5 mmoles of maleic acid per kg body weight. (From Ref. 6.)

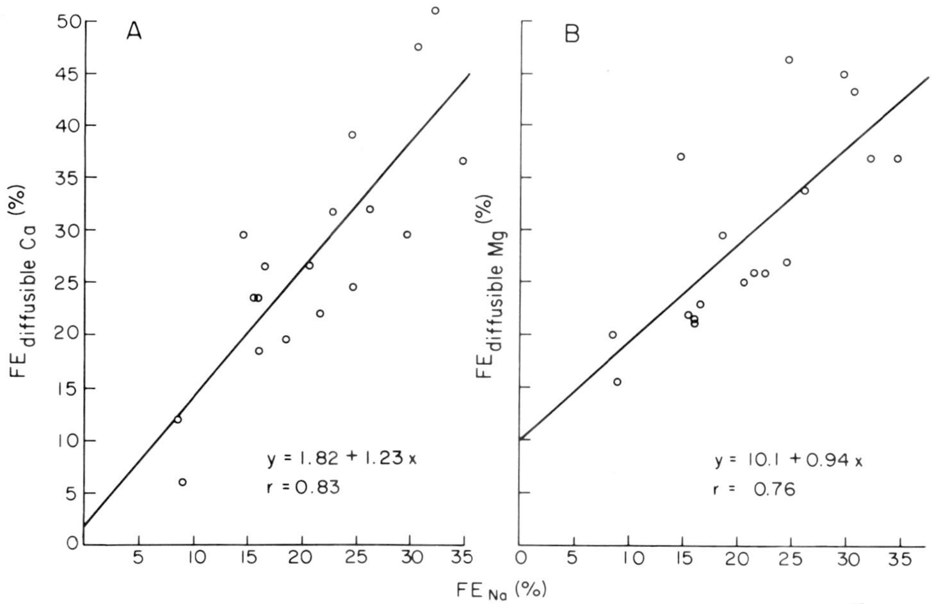

Fig. 2 Relationship between fractional excretion of calcium ($FE_{diffusible\ Ca}$) and fractional excretion of sodium (FE_{Na}) (A) and between fractional excretion of magnesium ($FE_{diffusible\ Mg}$) and FE_{Na} (B) in parathyroidectomized rats injected with 9.0 mmoles maleic acid per kg body weight. (From Ref. 6.)

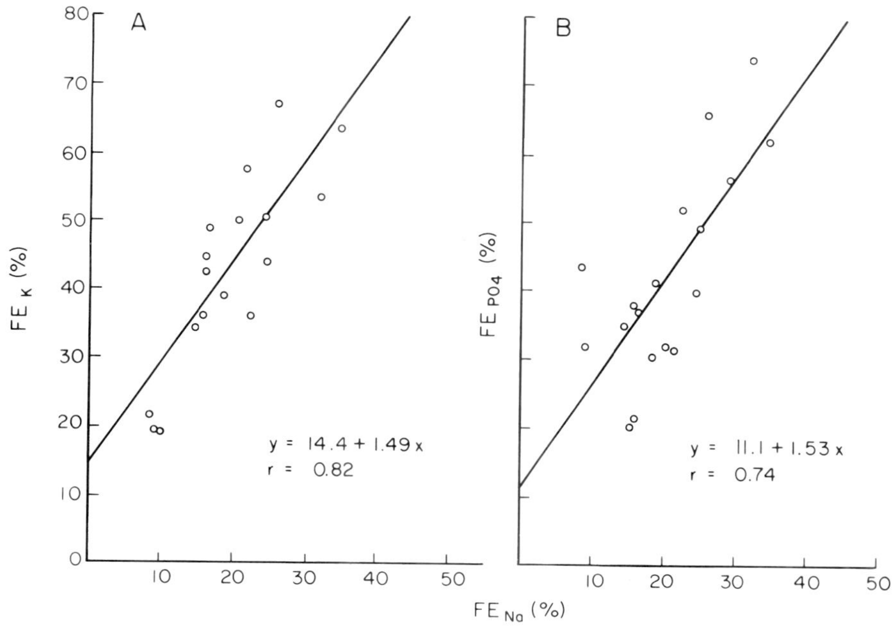

Fig. 3 Relationship between fractional excretion of potassium (FE_K) and fractional excretion of sodium (FE_{Na}) (A) and between fractional excretion of phosphate (FE_{PO_4}) and FE_{Na} (B) in parathyroidectomized rats injected with 9.0 mmoles maleic acid per kg body weight. (From Ref. 6.)

Animals given 9 mmol/kg maleate and volume-repleted with saline and parathyroidectomized to prevent parathyroid-mediated changes in phosphate handling showed increased clearances of sodium, calcium, potassium, phosphate, and magnesium, but not of urate. In this latter group of animals a significant correlation could be demonstrated between the fractional excretion of sodium and the fractional excretion of calcium, magnesium, potassium, phosphate, and urate (Figs. 2 and 3). As the slopes of the regression lines relating fractional excretion of sodium to the fractional excretion of calcium, magnesium, and urate were close to unity, these results were interpreted as demonstrating that maleic acid affected a common reabsorptive pathway for these ions. The slopes of the regression lines relating fractional excretion of sodium to the fractional excretion of potassium and phosphate were significantly greater than unity, implying, in the case of potassium, that the maleate-induced increase in

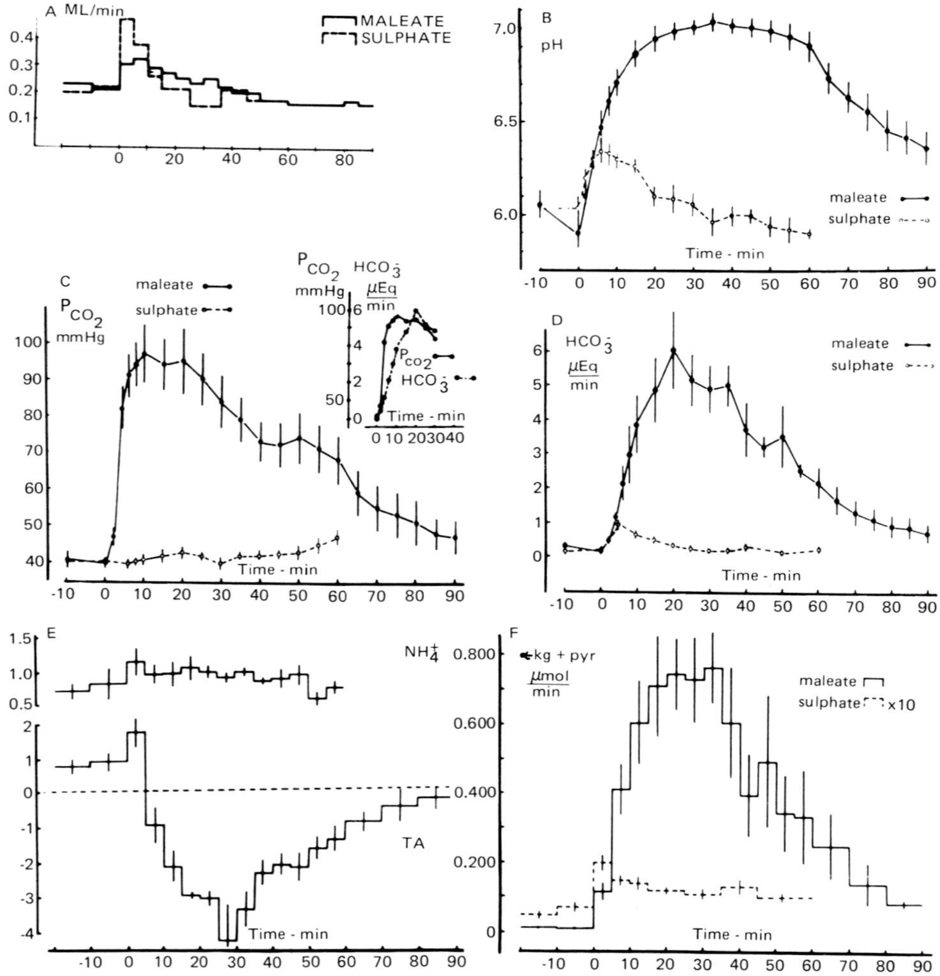

Fig. 4 Effects of maleate on urine flow (A), urine pH (B), urine PCO_2 (C), urine HCO_3^- excretion (D), titratable acid and NH_4^+ excretion in µmoles/min (E), and urine α-ketoacids excretion (F). In control experiments an equimolar dose of sodium sulfate was injected instead of maleate. (From Ref. 8.)

potassium excretion was due to enhanced distal tubular potassium secretion following increased distal delivery of sodium and impermeant anions. Such anions would include bicarbonate, α-ketoacids, citrate, and maleate, all of which have been shown to increase in the urine after maleate administration (7).

Gmaj et al. (7-10) have explored the effects of maleate on renal acidification mechanisms. These authors have emphasized that at low dosage (0.9 mmol/kg body weight) the most prominent effects of maleate in the rat are bicarbonate diuresis, ketoaciduria, and phosphaturia; glucosuria is mild and aminoaciduria is absent. In addition to the bicarbonaturia, rats given this dose of maleate also show a prompt increase in urine pH and PCO_2, but no change in ammonium excretion, and a decrease in titratable acid excretion (Fig. 4). The decrease in titratable acid excretion was less than would be predicted from the simultaneous increase in bicarbonate excretion as the buffering capacity was increased by the presence of maleate (pK 6.5) in the urine. Several observations suggested that the bicarbonaturia was due to a selective impairment of bicarbonate reabsorption by the proximal tubule, independent of any effect on the carbonic anhydrase system. First, carbonic anhydrase activity in erythrocyte-free kidney homogenates was unaffected in vitro by concentrations of maleate ranging from 5×10^{-4} mmol/liter to 5×10^{-2} mmol/liter. Secondly, the effects in vivo of maleate (2.5 mmol/kg) and acetazolamide (50 mg/kg) on bicarbonate reabsorption were additive, maleate inhibiting fractional bicarbonate reabsorption 25%, acetazolamide by 30%, and maleate plus acetazolamide by 54-72%. Both acetazolamide and maleate plus acetazolamide increased urine PCO_2 to approximately the same values. The high urinary PCO_2 was inferred to reflect increased secretion of H^+ by a functionally intact distal nephron, stimulated, like the increased secretion of K^+, by enhanced distal delivery of sodium and impermeant anions.

Similar findings were reported in the dog by Gougoux et al. (11), who also noted marked increases in sodium, potassium, and phosphate excretion without change in chloride excretion following maleate injection. Gmaj et al. (9) compared in the rat the effects of maleate with those of another metabolic inhibitor, arsenite, while Gougoux et al. (11) compared in the dog the effects of maleate or maleate plus acetazolamide with yet another metabolic inhibitor, malonate. Neither arsenite nor malonate affected bicarbonate reabsorption, although the arsenite had significant effects on sodium and chloride reabsorption. Thus, both authors argue that the effect of maleate on bicarbonate reabsorption cannot be ascribed simply to Krebs cycle inhibition or to an effect on the sodium-stimulated ATP-Na-K-ATPase transport system (see below), but rather to some alternative effect, e.g., inhibition of mitochondrial proton transport (10), altered permeability to anionic bicarbonate at the luminal membrane (backflux), or impaired anionic bicarbonate reabsorption (11). Al-Bander et al. (12) also examined the bicarbonaturic effect of maleate in dogs, employing fractional free water clearance (C_{H_2O}/GFR), fractional delivery of total solute (V/GFR), and fractional delivery of potentially reabsorbable solute ($[C_{Cl}+C_{H_2O}]$/GFR) to examine other aspects of tubular function. The maleate-induced increase in fractional excretion of bicarbonate was accompanied by increases in each of these parameters (Fig. 5). The effect was attenuated by acidosis and enhanced by increasing the plasma bicarbonate concentration. Although the absolute excretion of chloride decreased, the observed increase in C_{H_2O}/GFR was interpreted as indicating that maleate caused a decrease in proximal tubular reabsorption of sodium and chloride, as well as bicarbonate, with enhanced chloride reabsorption in the postproximal nephron. These observations could be considered to be compatible with the hypothesis that the bicarbonaturia, like other aspects of maleate-induced alterations in proximal tubular function, is secondary to an effect on sodium-linked tubular transport. However, conflicting results were reported by Brewer et al. (13), who combined clearance and micropuncture

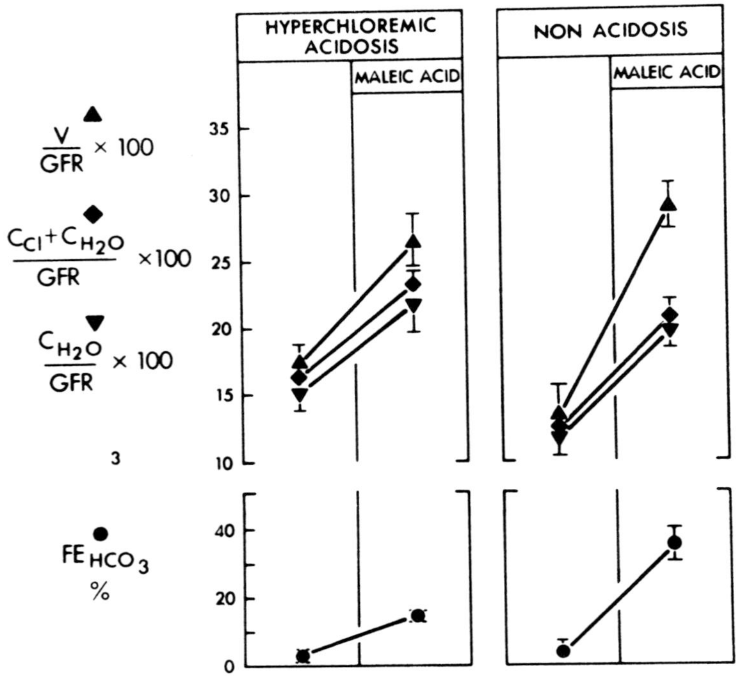

Fig. 5 Effect of administration of maleic acid on V/GFR, C_{H_2O}/GFR, (C_{Cl} + C_{H_2O})/GFR, and FE_{HCO_3} in 4 dogs undergoing water diuresis at normal plasma HCO_3^- concentration (right panel) and during hyperchloremic metabolic acidosis (left panel). In both sets of studies the same dose of maleic acid (0.4 mmoles/kg) was administered. (From Ref. 12.)

studies in rats to demonstrate that bicarbonate, but not chloride, reabsorption was decreased by maleate in the proximal tubule and fractional free water clearance was *decreased* rather than increased, implying that maleate affected reabsorption by the distal nephron as well as the proximal nephron.

Maleate has been shown to increase not only the clearances of electrolytes, glucose, and amino acids, but also of certain larger molecular weight substances. Asatoor et al. (14) demonstrated enhanced clearance of peptides as well as free amino acids in rats after the subcutaneous injection of 3.5 mmol maleate per kg body weight. The response was quantitatively different, however. Whereas total amino acid output increased 8 1/2 to 10 times control values, peptide excretion increased to only 1 1/3 to 1 9/10 times control values. Fujita and Itakura (15) reported that excretion of lysozyme, a low-molecular-weight protein, was increased following the intravenous injection in rats of 2 or 8 mmol/kg maleate and that fractional reabsorption of lysozyme was significantly correlated with fractional reabsorption of sodium, the slope of the regression line approximating unity. Christensen and Maunsbach (16) further explored the mechanism of maleate-induced lysozymuria by ultrastructural analyses. The digestion of reabsorbed lysozyme was reduced in renal cortical slices from maleate-treated rats as compared to normals and autoradiography revealed that the transport of lysozyme from endocytic vacuoles to lysosomes in proximal tubule cells was partially inhibited (Figs. 6a,b). Endocytic vacuoles rapidly accumulated in the apical cytoplasm, but apical tubules disappeared, indicating an altered recycling of membrane. The authors (16) concluded that maleate caused low-molecular-weight proteinuria via decreased tubular reabsorption accompanied by decreased transport of protein from endocytic vacuoles to lysosomes and subsequent low tubular protein catabolism.

Brewer et al. (17) have examined vitamin D metabolism in vitamin D-deficient rats and chicks injected with maleic acid. Conversion of radiolabeled 25(OH)D_3 to 1,25$(OH)_2$$D_3$ was impaired in the vitamin D-deficient rats as evidenced by a markedly reduced recovery of 1,25$(OH)_2$$D_3$ in kidney, small intestinal mucosa, and blood in maleate-treated rats as compared to controls. Similar findings were noted in the chicks. In addition, kidney homogenates and isolated renal tubules from vitamin D-deficient chicks showed diminished activity of 25-hydroxyvitamin D_3-1-hydroxylase after maleic acid was administered in vivo or added in vitro to the incubation medium. As this enzyme is restricted in location to the inner membrane of mitochondria of the proximal tubule (18), the impaired conversion of 25-(OH)D_3 may represent yet another example of an adverse effect of maleate on proximal tubular mitochondrial metabolism.

Popovtzer et al. (19) examined the effect of parathyroid hormone, calcitonin, dibutyryl cyclic AMP, and 25(OH)D_3 on the phosphaturia found in parathryoidectomized rats with maleate-induced Fanconi syndrome. Neither parathyroid hormone nor calcitonin affected the urinary excretion of cyclic AMP or phosphorus in these animals, and dibutyryl cyclic AMP failed to affect the phosphaturia. However, administration of 25(OH)D_3 to the maleate-treated rats significantly reduced the fractional excretion of phosphorus from 0.39 ± 0.03 to 0.23 ± 0.02, an action similar to the reported ability of vitamin D or its metabolites to decrease urinary losses of phosphorus in some patients with Fanconi syndrome (20-22). The authors postulate that the inhibition of accumulation of calcium in mitochondria of renal tubular cells in maleate-treated rats noted by previous investigators (10) may be reversed by vitamin D, leading to increased mitochondrial uptake of cytosolic calcium and phosphorus, thus reducing phosphaturia.

It has been suggested by some authors (23,24) that the intestine as well as the renal proximal tubule may show transport defects in some forms of Fanconi syndrome. Wapnir et al. (25) examined the possibility that intestinal transport of electrolytes, glucose, and amino acids and Na-K-ATPase activity in intestinal mucosa might be affected by maleate. Adult male rats were injected intraperitoneally with either 1.5 or 9.0 mmol maleate/kg body weight and jejunal transport was studied 30 min later, when glycosuria and proteinuria were evident. Intestinal sodium absorption and mucosal Na-K-ATPase activity were markedly impaired by maleate, but there was no dose-related effect on transport despite a greater inhibition of Na-K-ATPase activity at the 9.0 mmol/kg dose. Potassium secretion was also lower in the maleate-treated animals than in the controls, but intestinal transport of glucose and amino acids were unaffected.

Morphological Observations

Worthen (3) utilized light microscopy, phase microscopy, and electron microscopy to explore the tubular alterations in maleic acid-treated rats. In rats given 3, 6, or 9 mmol maleic acid/kg, the lesions were confined to the proximal tubule but the extent of abnormal changes was dose related. Distal tubules appeared normal. By light microscopy, the most significant changes in the proximal tubule were dilation and increased granularity. Phase and electron microscopy revealed coarsening of the brush border, with thickening and shortening of the microvilli and a loss of the delicate tubular structure. There was marked vacuolation of the area under the brush border and increased density of the basilar zone, with blurring of cytoplasmic details. The mitochondria appeared structurally normal but were crowded together,

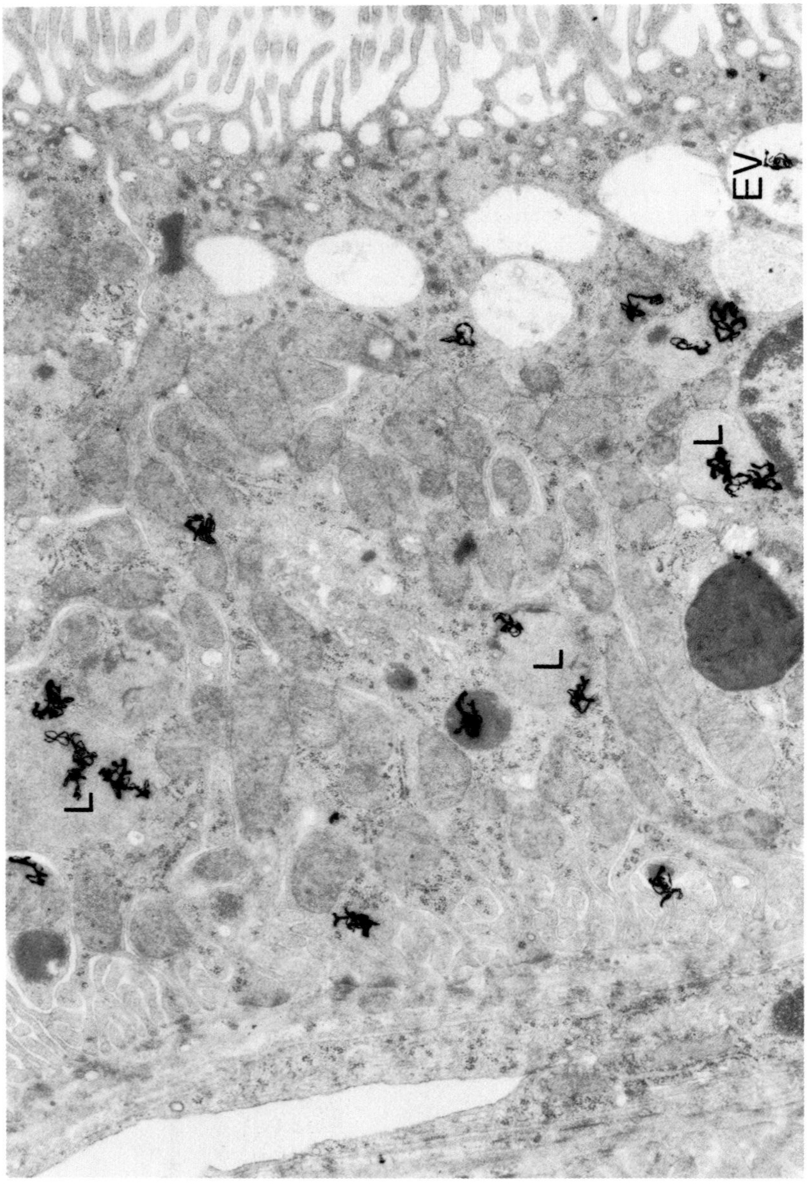

Fig. 6a Electron microscope autoradiograph of proximal tubule cells from a rat fixed by vascular perfusion 60 min after I.V. injection of labeled lysozyme. Five minutes before the injection of protein, the rat was injected with 0.9% sodium chloride (control). Most autoradiographic granules are located over lysosomes (L). A single granule can be seen over an endocytic vacuole (EV). (X 13,000.)

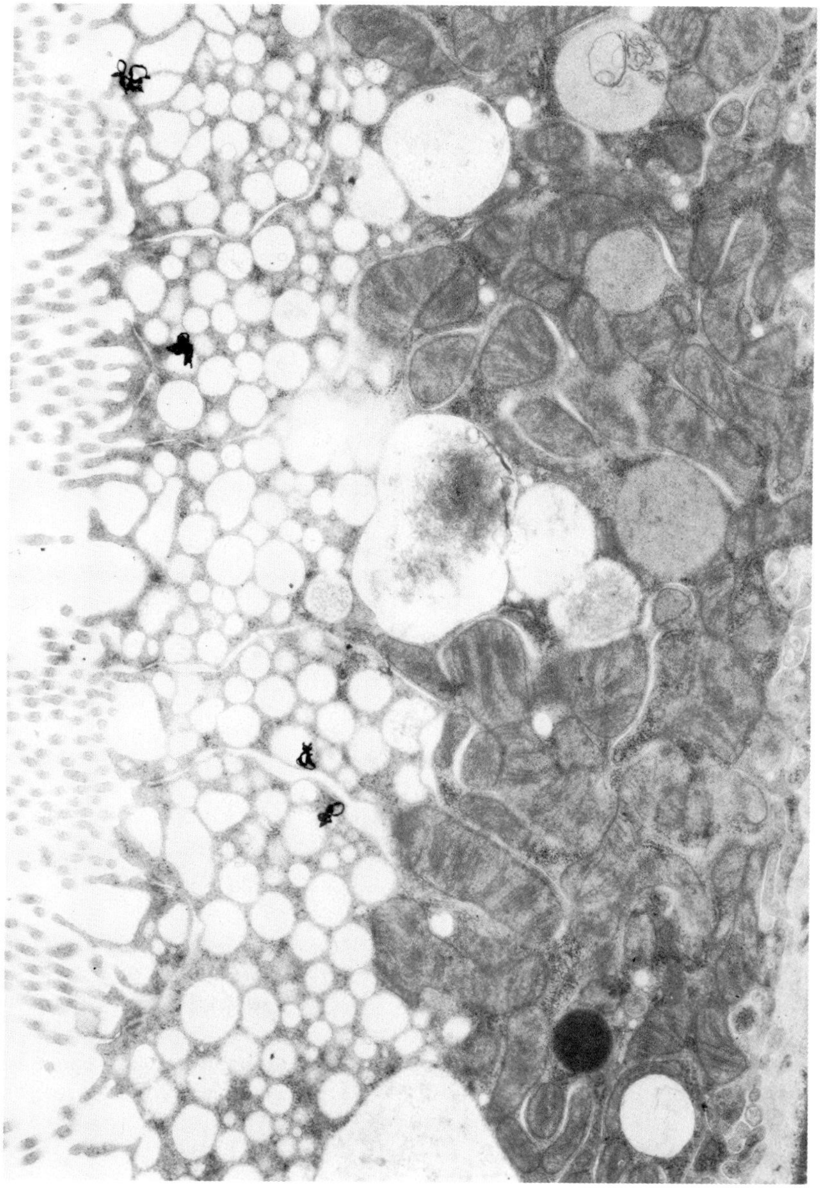

Fig. 6b Electron microscope autoradiograph of proximal tubule cells from a rat prepared as in Fig. 6a, but injected with sodium maleate, 3.5 mmol/kg body weight, instead of sodium chloride. All grains are located over endocytic vacuoles. (X 13,000.) (From Ref. 16.)

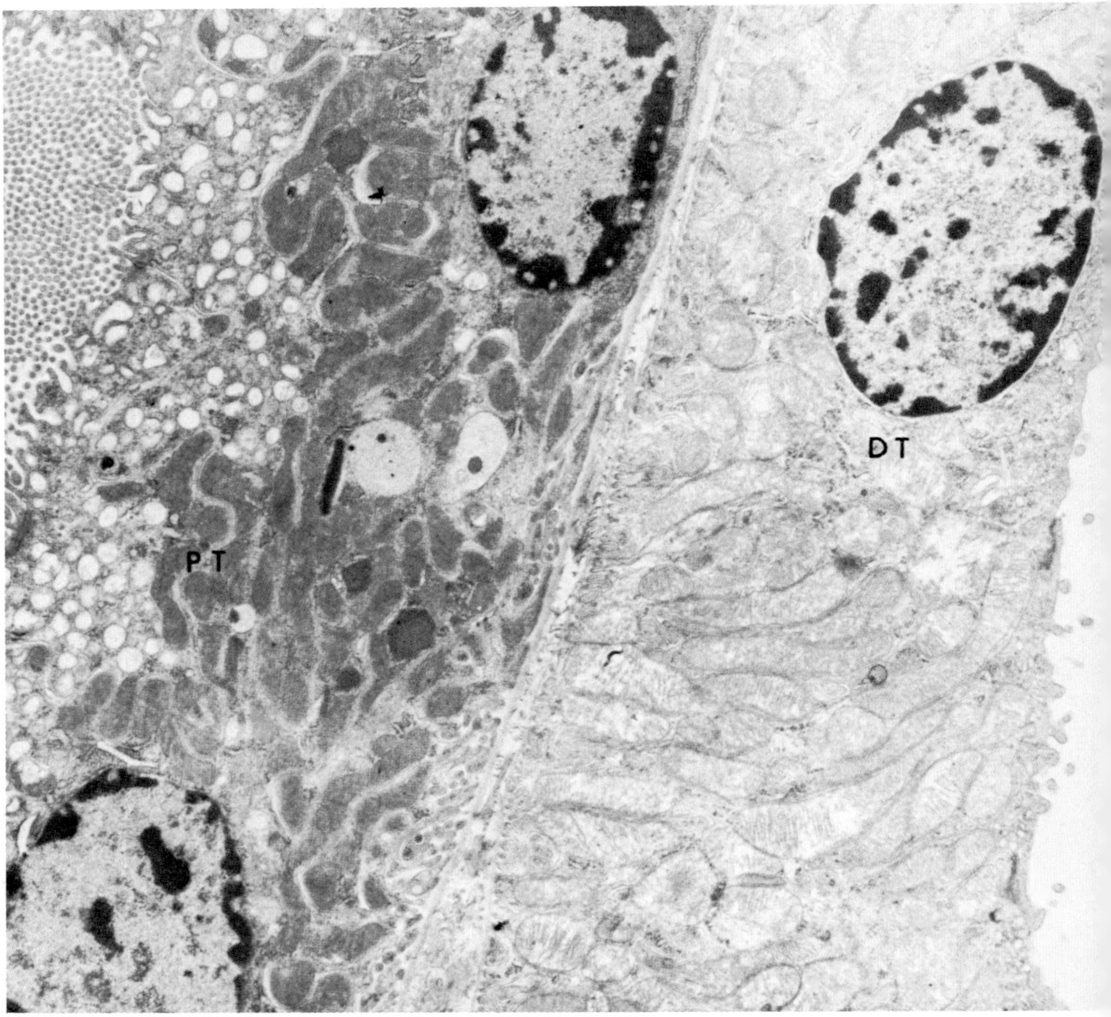

Fig. 7 Electron micrograph showing distal convoluted tubule (DT) and proximal convoluted tubule (PT) in rat receiving an injection of 9.0 mmol maleate/kg body weight. Distal cell cytoplasm is within normal limits and mitochondria show the normal degree of density of matrix and slight disruption of cristae. Proximal tubules show markedly increased mitochondrial density and granularity and increase of apical vacuolar and vesicular activity. Several dense microbodies are also recognized within the proximal tubule cell. The density of ribosomal bodies is apparent between the basal infolding which extends far into the cytoplasm. (From Ref. 28.)

and the basilar membranous infoldings were seen to be thickened and distorted by localized accumulations of fluid. Worthen interpreted these findings as suggestive for accumulation of reabsorbed material within the cell because of an inability of the cell to transport the substance through the cell and into the peritubular capillary. This interpretation was offered since similar findings had previously been noted in rats loaded with solutes such as glucose, sucrose, mannitol, and dextran, which entered the cell at a rate which exceeded the exit rate.

Subsequent authors have, in the main, verified Worthen's (3) findings. Schärer et al. (4) noted that rats treated with a very low dose of maleic acid (0.4 mmol/kg) showed no morphological alterations by light or electron microscopy in the proximal tubule, although aminoaciduria was present. Rats treated with 0.9, 1.7, or 3.4 mmol/kg showed proximal tubule alterations resembling those described by Worthen (3), except that mitochondrial changes were seen in rats given the two highest doses of maleic acid. The mitochondria were more globular than normal, the cristae were marginated and did not cross the mitochondria, and the matrices were rarefied. No lesions were noted in the glomeruli or the structure of the tubular basement membrane. In the rats treated with 3.4 mmol/kg of maleic acid, severe cellular damage of the distal tubule was noted, consisting of clumping of nuclear chromatin, blebbing of the apical portion of the cell, and swelling of the endoplasmic reticulum. Bergeron and Laporte (26) also noted a major modification of the relationship between mitochondria and the network of perimitochondrial membranes of *both* proximal and distal tubules within 24 hr after injection of maleate. These observations served as one of the cornerstones of the Bergeron hypothesis of altered membrane permeability as a cause of the transport defects in experimental Fanconi syndrome (27) (see below). In contrast, neither Rosen et al. (28) nor Verani et al. (29), were able to demonstrate abnormalities in distal tubular ultrastructure in rats treated with high doses of maleate (9 mmol/kg and 3.4 mmol/kg, respectively). An electron micrograph contrasting the appearance of the proximal tubule and adjacent distal tubule in a rat treated with 9 mmol/kg maleic acid is illustrated in Fig. 7, from Rosen et al. (28). A more detailed presentation of the proximal tubular changes noted by electron microscopy in kidneys of rats treated with an intermediate dose of maleic acid (1.7 mmol/kg) is shown in Figs. 8a and 8b, from Verani et al. (29).

Verani et al. (29) performed a systematic examination by light, transmission electron, and scanning electron microscopy to ascertain the site of morphological injury within the kidney after maleic acid administration. Evidence of injury was observed only in cells of the late pars convoluta and the pars recta in the medullary rays of the cortex and in the outer stripe of the medulla. The loops of Henle and distal convoluted tubules were normal except for the presence of granular and hyaline casts in the lumens. Collecting ducts in the outer medulla showed an increased number of dark cells per total cell population, which were thought to represent an adaptive response to the functional abnormalities of maleic acid-induced Fanconi syndrome, in particular to the osmotic diureses and/or hypokalemia, rather than to a cell injury phenomenon.

Biochemical Observations

Maleic acid is not found naturally in mammalian tissues, but it is a cis isomer of a known metabolite, fumaric acid. The first proton is dissociated readily from maleic acid (pKa_1 1.57), the second with difficulty (pKa_2 6.20). At pH 7.4, the major form of the molecule would be the dianion, with 2% as the monoanion, H-maleate, and a negligible amount as undissociated acid (30). Maleate can be metabolized by the mammalian kidney to CO_2 via

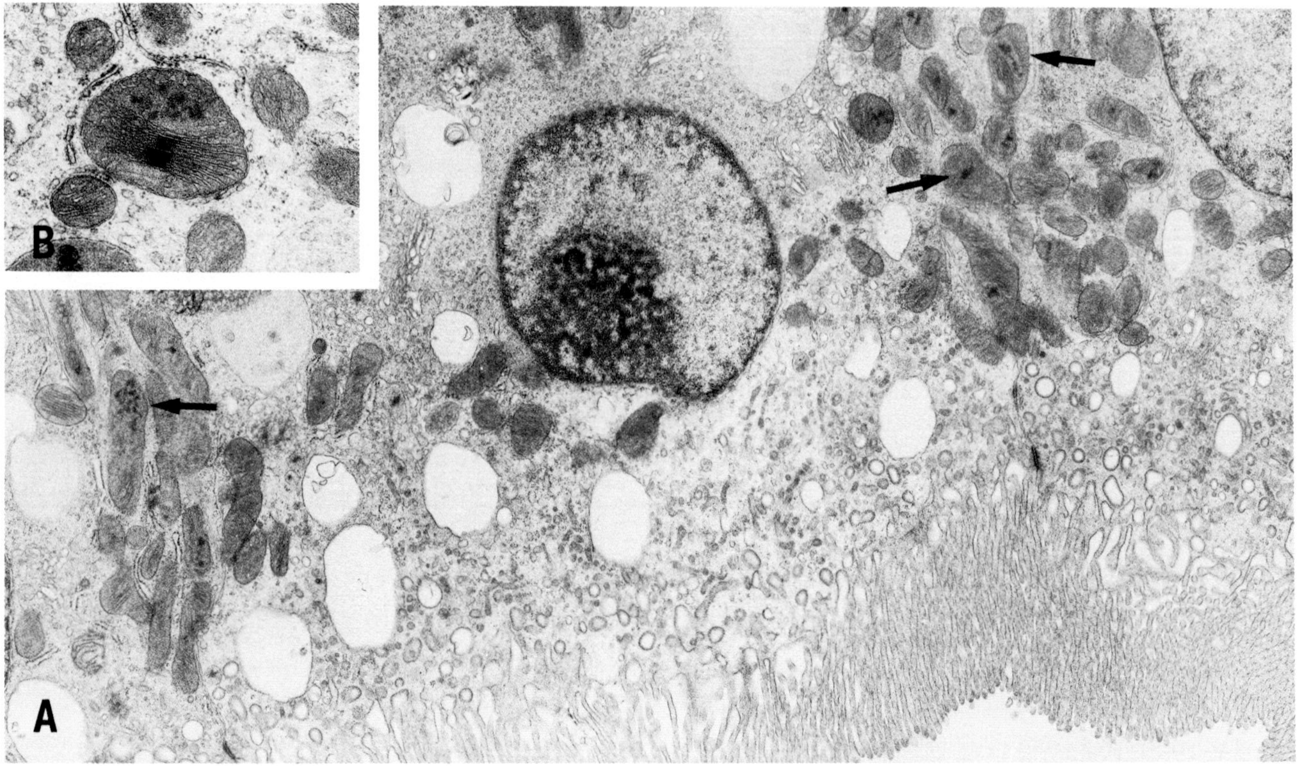

Fig. 8 Illustrations are taken from a rat kidney fixed at 24 hr after administration of maleic acid, 1.7 mmol/kg. (A) Electron micrograph of a proximal tubule that appeared normal by light microscopy. Microvilli and plasma membranes appear normal. Mitochondria contain numerous irregular densities (arrows) not seen in mitochondria of control animals. Dark and light lysosomes and lipid vacuoles are more numerous than in controls. Nucleolus is quite prominent in the nucleus of one cell. (X 18,000.) (B) High magnification view of mitochondria in one of the cells of the same tubule as shown in Fig. 8A. Cristal membranes are condensed, and irregular electron-dense material has accumulated within the mitochondrial matrix. (X 57,000.) (From Ref. 29.)

a malate hydratase-catalyzed conversion to D-malate, which then enters the citric acid cycle to form oxaloacetate (31,32); injected maleate also appears in urine as a poorly reabsorbable anion (7,8,30). Maleate readily reacts with thiols and chelates cations more strongly than fumarate. The selective toxicity of maleate toward renal tissue is partially related to the unique renal avidity for this compound, shared only, to a lesser extent, by the liver. When maleate was labeled with ^{14}C and a dose of 0.9 mmol/kg injected into rats, the biological half-life was found to be 23 min (30). During the first 60 min only the kidney had a tissue/plasma radioactivity ratio which exceeded unity and the concentration of radioactivity in the mitochondrial fraction of the kidney was about five times that of the supernatant from which the mitochondria were obtained.

Most of the information concerning the biochemical effects of maleate has emanated from a series of studies by Angielski, Rogulski, and their colleagues. Rogulski initially demonstrated a significant diminution in the content of both protein and nonprotein SH groups in kidney, but not liver, of maleate-treated rats (33). A decrease in nonprotein SH groups was observed in cytoplasmic, nuclear, and mitochondrial subcellular fractions of kidney, while a decrease in protein SH groups was observed only in the nuclear and mitochondrial fractions. In vitro, maleic acid bound nearly 90% of SH groups of cysteine during a 60-min incubation, but only 20% of SH groups of glutathione; the addition of kidney homogenate increased the efficiency of maleic acid binding to SH groups of glutathione to 70% (34). Maleate at concentrations below 1 mmol inhibited oxidation of α-ketoacids in isolated mitochondria of rat kidneys, but a 10 times higher concentration of maleate was required to inhibit citrate, malate, and pyruvate oxidation; succinate oxidation was not affected. These effects were not observed in liver mitochondria (35). In vivo, a dose of maleate exceeding 2.2 mmol/kg body weight was necessary to produce the tubular abnormalities and to affect ketoglutarate oxidation in kidney homogenates. No effect on ketoglutarate oxidation was seen at a dose of 1.7 mmol/kg, whereas 75% inhibition of ketoglutarate oxidation was observed when a dose of 2.6 mmol/kg was employed (36).

Although the mechanism of action of maleate appeared to be linked to its effect on oxidative decarboxylation of ketoglutarate, maleate had no direct effect on activity of purified ketoglutarate dehydrogenase (35,37), did not affect NADH oxidation by submitochondrial preparations, and, in mitochondrial preparations, did not affect the reduction of cytochrome *c* by NADH except in the presence of ketoglutarate (30). These observations suggested that maleate action does not concern the dehydrogenation of ketoglutarate or further steps of electron transfer, but may affect the direct metabolite of the carbon chain of ketoglutarate, succinyl-CoA, or the mitochondrial transport system. Studies by Pacanis et al. (38) demonstrated that maleate inhibited substrate-level phosphorylation linked to anaerobic dismutation of ketoglutarate in mitochondria, that phosphate and magnesium diminished this effect, and also that acetoacetate, malonate, and succinate, the substrates of CoA-transferase, relieved the inhibition of ketoglutarate metabolism by maleate in both respiring mitochondria and in an "anaerobic" system containing antimycin and rotenone. These results were considered to be consistent with the hypothesis that maleate-induced inhibition of ketoglutarate was linked to substrate-level phosphorylation and that the maleate action concerned succinyl-CoA synthetase or other reactions in which succinyl-CoA was involved. It was postulated that maleate could be an acceptor of CoA, forming maleyl-CoA as a trapping system, thus removing free CoA from the metabolic pool (Fig. 9). Direct measurements of total CoA content in kidney tissue of maleate-treated rats and in normal kidney mitochondria incubated in the presence of ketoglutarate and maleate revealed a highly significant decrease in total CoA, acid-soluble CoA, and CoA-SH. Acetoacetate not only abolished the inhibitory effect of maleate on oxidation of ketoglutarate but also prevented the decrease of CoA con-

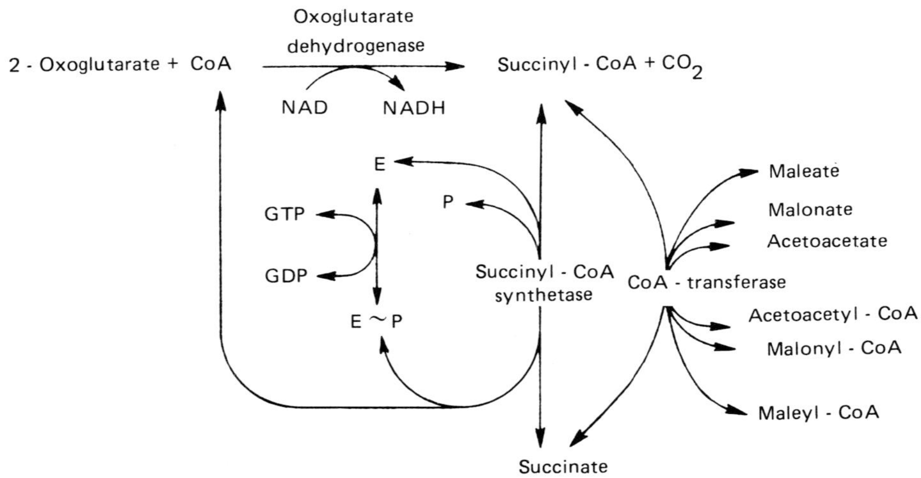

Fig. 9 The suggested mechanism of maleate action on 2-oxoglutarate metabolism. (From Ref. 38.)

tent (39). Succinyl-CoA formation from ketoglutarate in kidney mitochondria under conditions of anaerobic dismutation was found to be significantly diminished by maleate (39). Schärer et al. (4) were also able to demonstrate a 50% reduction of acetyl-CoA in the kidney of maleate-intoxicated rats. Thus, it appears that the major substrates for ATP synthesis via the Krebs cycle are diminished by maleate.

Changes in adenylate nucleotides in renal cortex produced by maleate administration (0.9 mmol/kg given intravenously) were measured directly by Angielski et al. (40). In confirmation of results reported earlier by Kramer and Gonick (5) and Schärer et al. (4), there was a significant (40%) reduction in cortical ATP, which appeared as early as 15 min after maleate injection and persisted throughout 60 min of observation. Levels of ADP and AMP increased, whereas inorganic phosphate was unchanged. In kidney cortex slices, maleate has been shown to stimulate glycolysis, resulting in increased conversion of glucose to lactate, but to inhibit gluconeogenesis, particularly from pyruvate (41). The sensitivity of pyruvate-related gluconeogenesis may be explained by the decrease in acetyl-CoA, which is required for activation of pyruvate carboxylase. Although these results in general might be interpreted to imply that the generation of ATP from succinyl-CoA could be the critical biochemical step affected by maleate, it was subsequently observed in rats given acetoacetate concomitantly with maleate that renal tubular dysfunction was aborted, but the reduction in kidney cortex ATP levels was unaffected (42), implying that maleyl-CoA per se may affect tubular function by an as yet undetermined mechanism (for further discussion, see Sects. II.A. and II.B.).

B. Cadmium Model

As reviewed in Ch. 14, nephrotoxicity due to cadmium exposure in the setting of industrial exposure or environmental pollution may result in renal tubular dysfunction consistent with the Fanconi syndrome. Clinical features requiring explanation via experimental models include: (1) the long lag period between initial exposure and the development of signs of renal disease; (2) the origin of the low-molecular-weight proteinuria (e.g., β_2-microglobulinuria), which is the first indicator of renal tubular damage after cadmium exposure; (3) the genesis of the bone disease which is a prominent feature of the full-blown cadmium pollution-related itai itai byo, or "ouch-ouch" disease.

Observations in the Kidney

The majority of the early studies on cadmium nephrotoxicity in animals focused on morphological alterations. Thus, Friberg examined the effects of prolonged exposure of rabbits to cadmium dust or to cadmium injections (43), and found that a chronic renal lesion was produced. Later, Bonnell et al. (44) carried out a similar series of experiments in rats given repeated intraperitoneal injections of cadmium for periods up to 12 months and found tubular atrophy and interstitial fibrosis to be the most prominent renal lesions. These lesions first appeared at 4 months and progressed with continuing cadmium dosing. The severity of the lesions was maximum at 5 and 6 months, irrespective of whether cadmium dosing was continued. In a parallel fashion, the cadmium concentration in the kidneys increased linearly for the first 3-4 months, after which a plateau was reached. Axelsson et al. (45) performed similar studies in rabbits, finding that mild alterations in proximal tubular epthelial cells occurred after 3-4 months of subcutaneous cadmium injections, progressing to more profound tubular changes after 6-7 months. There was evidence for regeneration of tubular epithelium in rabbits examined 7 months after cessation of cadmium injections although the extent of metal deposition, evaluated histochemically, remained constant. Metal deposits in this study and others, in which radioactive cadmium was employed (46), were located chiefly in the proximal tubules. Stowe et al. (47) demonstrated that long-term administration of cadmium in drinking water also produced interstitial renal cortical fibrosis in rabbits. In these studies, and in others (48), the toxic content of cadmium in renal cortex was found to range from 170 to 400 μg/g wet weight ($\sim$ 100 times normal). Of interest in both the experimental animal models and in human autopsy studies (48,49) is the observation that a concentration of cadmium in kidney cortex of about 200 μg/g wet weight appears to be a "saturation" level, which must be reached before morphological or physiological alterations occur, but which does not increase further despite continued exposure.

In the majority of experimental studies, glomeruli showed either slight or no apparent alterations and the collecting tubules were not detectably affected (43-45,47,49). Light microscopic changes were limited to alterations in the proximal tubules and interstitial fibrosis. Ultrastructural changes were confined to the cells of the proximal tubule (50,51). The size and number of lysosomes were increased. Mitochondria became oval or rounded, and increased in volume. Cristae were vesicular, shortened, and marginal. Other changes included an increase in microbodies, focal proliferation of smooth endoplasmic reticulum, appearance of intranuclear inclusions, and extensive loss of basal plasma membrane infoldings.

An experimental model of the Fanconi syndrome has been produced by repetitive injections of cadmium chloride at a dose of 0.6 mg/kg body weight in adult female rats (51). Glucosuria and aminoaciduria appeared abruptly after 3 weeks of injections (average total dose of cadmium 2.25 mg) and disappeared gradually over a 4-5-day period after discontinuation of injections (Fig. 10). At the height of glucosuria, the complete expression of the Fanconi syndrome was elicited, i.e., diuresis, glucosuria, aminoaciduria, proteinuria, and increased clearances of sodium, potassium, calcium, magnesium, phosphate, and urate (Table 1). Excretion of β_2-microglobulin also increased abruptly at this time (52). At the peak of the Fanconi syndrome, renal cortical ATP levels were decreased by 38% and cortex homogenate Na-K-ATPase activity was decreased by 60% (Fig. 11). Ultrastructural changes at this stage

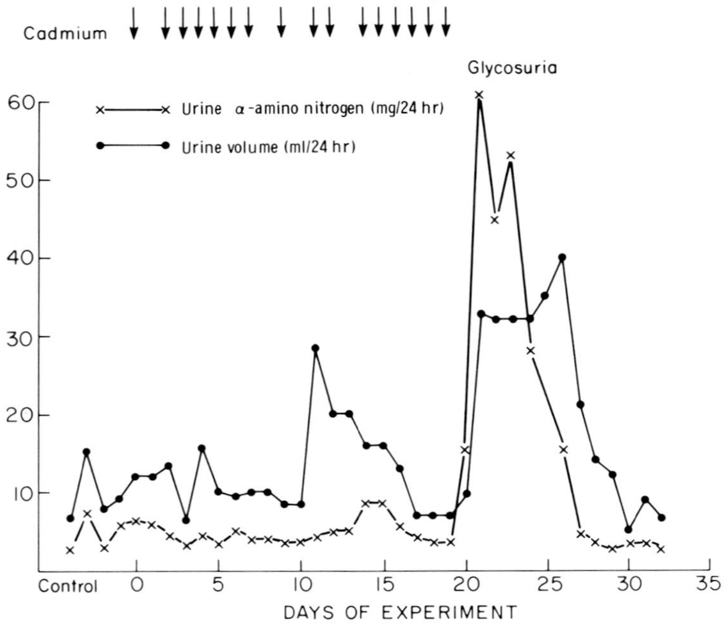

Fig. 10 Development of polyuria, aminoaciduria, and glycosuria in a representative animal after repetitive intraperitoneal injections of cadmium, 0.6 mg/kg body weight. Tubular dysfunction receded within 1 week of cessation of cadmium injections. (From Ref. 51.)

Table 1 Comparison of Renal Function in Control and Experimental Group II Animals (Mean ± SEM)

	Control group (n = 11)	Experimental group II (n = 7)
Urine volume, ml/day	12.3 ± 1.7	50.6 ± 7.6[b]
Urine glucose, mg/day	3.0 ± 0.6	143 ± 56[a]
Urine protein, mg/day	52 ± 10	143 ± 33[a]
Urine α-amino N, mg/day	3.7 ± 0.6	20.1 ± 3.4[b]
Na clearance, μl/min/100 g	4.2 ± 0.4	14.4 ± 1.5[b]
Fractional excretion, %	0.33 ± 0.04	4.4 ± 1.2[b]
K clearance, μl/min per 100 g	79.1 ± 9.5	139 ± 15.6[b]
Fractional excretion, %	6.1 ± 0.8	41.3 ± 11.7[b]
Ca clearance, μl/min per 100 g	9.3 ± 1.2	24.6 ± 4.2[b]
Fractional excretion, %	0.72 ± 0.10	7.7 ± 2.5[a]
P clearance, μl/min per 100 g	77.2 ± 14.6	95.3 ± 7.3
Fractional excretion, %	5.9 ± 1.1	27.7 ± 8.4[a]
Mg clearance, μl/min per 100 g	41.4 ± 3.7	63.1 ± 5.5[b]
Fractional excretion, %	3.3 ± 0.3	16.9 ± 4.0[b]
Urate clearance		
μl/min per 100 g	23.3 ± 3.9	19.5 ± 5.6
Fractional excretion, %	1.8 ± 0.3	5.3 ± 1.8

Comparison between control and experimental group: [a] $p < 0.05$.
[b] $p < 0.01$.
Source: Ref. 51.

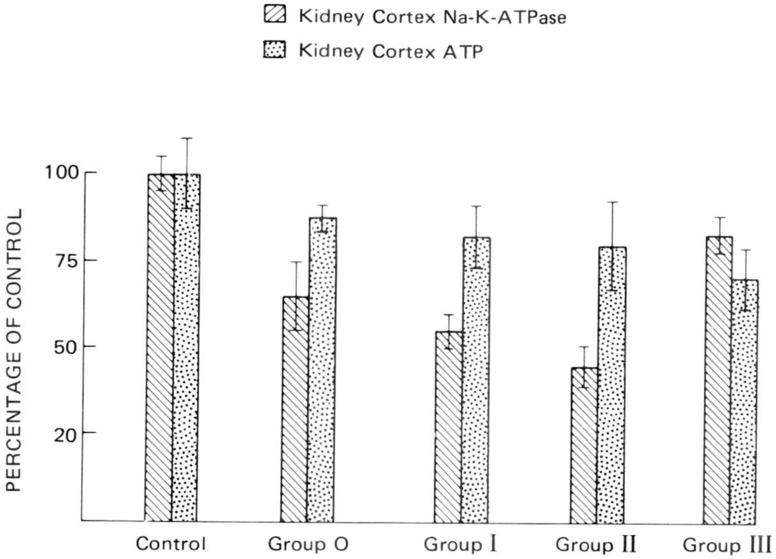

Fig. 11 Kidney cortex Na-K-ATPase activity and ATP concentration in control and experimental cadmium-treated animals. Group O = pre-Fanconi, average total dose of cadmium, 2.03 mg; group I = first day of tubular dysfunction consistent with Fanconi syndrome, average total dose of cadmium, 2.25 mg; group II = second day of Fanconi syndrome, no further cadmium injections; group III = third day of Fanconi syndrome, no further cadmium injections. Values are mean ± SEM. (Data from Ref. 51.)

paralleled the biochemical findings in that the mitochondria were dramatically altered in size and shape and there was extensive loss of the basal plasma membrane infoldings in Fanconi animals as contrasted to normal controls and to animals sacrificed just prior to onset of glucosuria ("pre-Fanconi") (Figs. 12a, b). Cadmium concentration in renal cortex increased 80-fold from control levels (to ~ 200 μg/g wet weight) in pre-Fanconi animals and remained at the same level in the Fanconi animals and in animals recovering from the Fanconi syndrome. This concentration of cadmium, which calculates as 3×10^{-3} mmol/liter if all of the metal is considered to be present in the ionized form, is 100-fold more than is necessary to inhibit Na-K-ATPase by 60%. These observations suggested that the majority of cadmium was present in a bound form, compartmentalized in a manner which prohibited enzyme inhibition.

Since the earliest work of Kägi and Vallee (53) it has been appreciated that cadmium exposure induces the formation of a low-molecular-weight metalloprotein, named metallothionein because of its high sulfhydryl content (principally as cysteine) and metal content (principally cadmium and zinc). Cadmium-metallothionein is initially synthesized within the liver, then transported to the kidney where it is completely filtered then reabsorbed in the proximal tubule by a saturatable mechanism (54). The kidney is much more susceptible to acute injury from cadmium given in conjunction with metallothionein (55) or cysteine (56) than from cadmium given in its inorganic form. Intravenously injected cadmium-thionein is rapidly taken up by the kidney and then the protein is degraded with liberation of the metal. The liberated cadmium is then incorporated into nascent chains of thionein within the kidney (57). There is some evidence that kidney metallothionein may differ slightly in composition

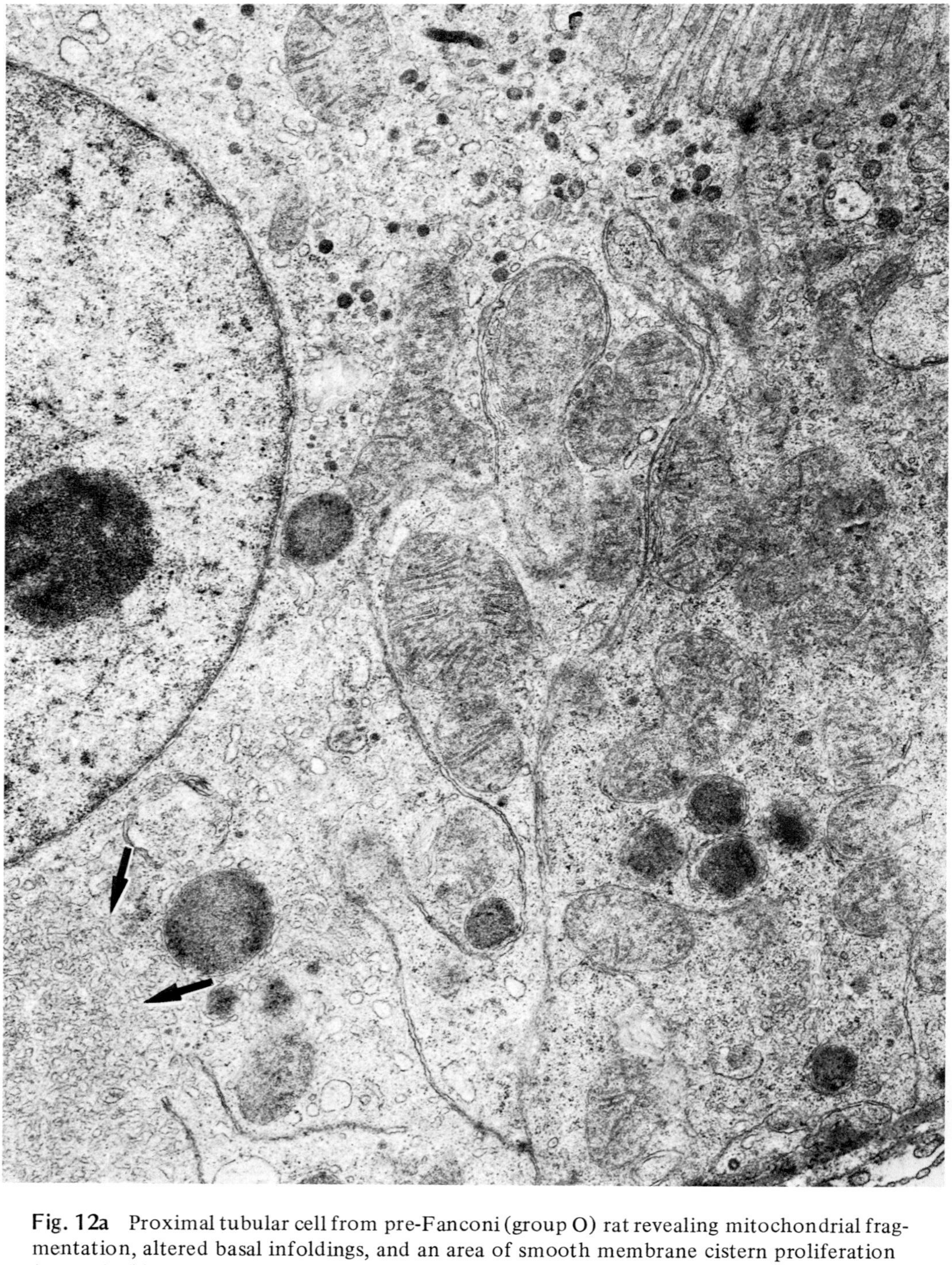

Fig. 12a Proximal tubular cell from pre-Fanconi (group O) rat revealing mitochondrial fragmentation, altered basal infoldings, and an area of smooth membrane cistern proliferation (arrows). (X 10,000.)

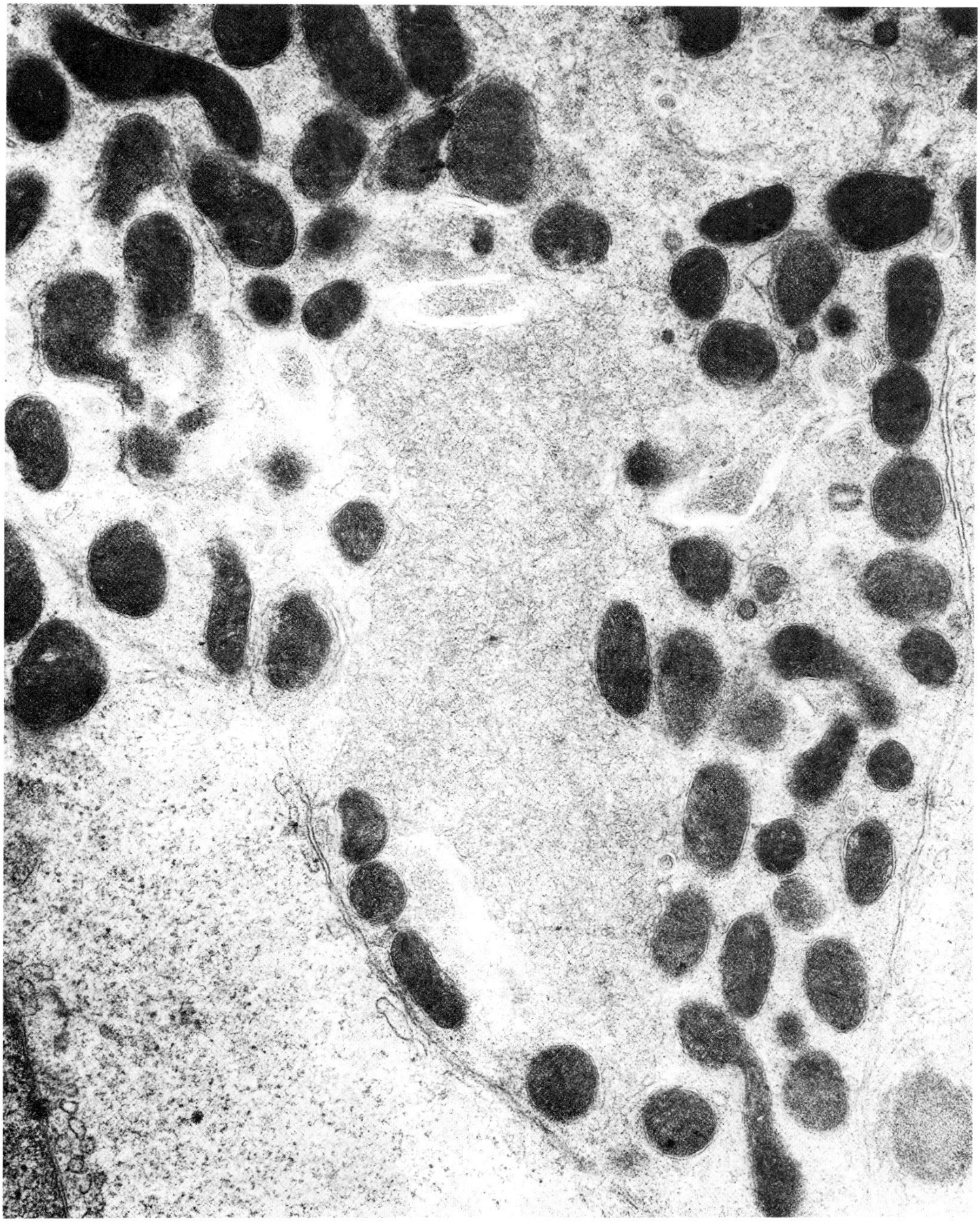

Fig. 12b Proximal tubular cell of rat sacrificed at height of Fanconi syndrome (Fanconi group II) showing massive smooth membrane proliferations and marked mitochondrial density, pleomorphism, and effacement of cristae pattern. (X 8,500.) (From Ref. 51.)

from liver metallothionein. The liver protein consists of two isometallothioneins, containing cadmium and zinc, while the kidney protein includes, in addition, a third isomer, which contains copper (58).

It would therefore appear likely that both the delayed onset of renal tubular dysfunction after initial exposure to cadmium and the saturation level of cadmium in renal cortex are related in some way to the interaction between cadmium and its binding protein, metallothionein. To explore the possibility that protein-binding of cadmium within the renal cortex conditioned the distribution of free cadmium within the mitochondrial and microsomal subcellular fractions, and thus inhibition of cadmium-sensitive enzymes within these cellular compartments, further studies incorporating radioactive $^{109}CdCl_2$ were done on the experimental rat model (59). The radioactive cadmium was injected into each animal just prior to sacrifice.

Blood, urine, and samples of liver, kidney cortex, and kidney medulla were removed for analysis of total cadmium content and the percent of radioactive cadmium present in each of the subcellular fractions of kidney cortex. As metallothionein is found in the soluble cytoplasmic fraction, high- and low-molecular-weight protein fractions were also separated from this fraction in liver and kidney cortex by Sephadex (dextran) G-75 column chromatography. The low-molecular-weight fraction was subsequently identified as metallothionein by further purification through Sephadex (dextran) G-50 chromatography and acrylamide gel electrophoresis. The purified protein had essentially the same amino acid composition and cadmium content as the metallothionein described by Winge and Rajagopalan (60). Of interest was the observation that serum cadmium increased slightly in both pre-Fanconi and Fanconi animals, but urinary cadmium was increased only in Fanconi animals, when α-amino nitrogen and β_2-microglobulin excretion also increased (Table 2), implying that the appearance of cadmiumuria in these experimental animals reflects renal tubular dysfunction rather than either increased filtered load or total body burden.

Analysis of liver and kidney cadmium content revealed that liver cadmium decreased significantly, while kidney cortex and kidney medulla cadmium increased significantly in the Fanconi as compared to pre-Fanconi animals (Fig. 13). When the subcellular distribution of cadmium isotope in kidney cortex was examined, the largest amount (91.7%) was found in the soluble cytoplasm fraction in control animals, with a very small percent remaining in nuclear, mitochondrial, and microsomal fractions. In the pre-Fanconi and Fanconi animals there was a progressive reduction in the cadmium present in the soluble cytoplasm fraction and a concomitant increase in the other subcellular fractions, particularly the microsomal fraction (Fig. 14). Sephadex (dextran) gel chromatography of the soluble cytoplasm fraction from liver and kidney cortex revealed that most of the cadmium isotope segregated with a low-molecular-weight protein, presumptively metallothionein, in the pre-Fanconi animals, whereas a greater proportion of the isotope was found with high-molecular-weight proteins in the Fanconi animals (Fig. 15). The results of this second study were in accord with the hypothesis that the Fanconi syndrome resulted after the cadmium-binding capacity of kidney cortex metallothionein was saturated, with the excess metal free to "spill over" from the soluble cytoplasm fraction to other subcellular fractions.

To further verify this hypothesis, rats were studied before, during, and after recovery from cadmium-induced Fanconi syndrome. The animals were sacrificed after 3, 6, 9, 14 (pre Fanconi), and 15 (Fanconi) injections of cadmium. In addition, a post-Fanconi group was sacrificed 7 days after resolution of tubular dysfunction. Cadmium content and Na-K-ATPase activity were measured both in kidney homogenates and microsomal fractions in each group. The relationship between microsomal cadmium and Na-K-ATPase activity determined in vivo in control, pre-Fanconi, Fanconi, and post-Fanconi animals (Fig. 16) was

Table 2 Comparison of Urine Volume, Cadmium, α-Amino Nitrogen, and $\beta 2$-Microglobulin Excretion in Control and Experimental Animals

	Urine volume ml/24 hr	Cadmium µg/24 hr	α-Amino nitrogen mg/24 hr	$\beta 2$-Microglobulin	
				µg/ml	µg/24 hr
Control	7.8 ± 0.6	0.30 ± 0.04	1.10 ± 0.17	0.22 ± 0.02	1.7 ± 0.2
Pre-Fanconi	13.9 ± 1.8^{a}	$0.31 \pm 1.06^{b,c}$	1.14 ± 0.13	0.40 ± 0.05^{a}	5.4 ± 0.7^{b}
Fanconi	$22.9 \pm 0.8^{b,c}$	$3.36 \pm 0.15^{b,c}$	$2.63 \pm 0.27^{a,c}$	$1.96 \pm 0.11^{b,c}$	$44.7 \pm 1.1^{b,c}$

[a]Comparison between control and experimental group $p < 0.01$
[b]Comparison between control and experimental group $p < 0.001$
[c]Comparison between pre-Fanconi and Fanconi group $p < 0.001$
Values are mean ± SEM n = 6 in all groups
Source: Ref. 52.

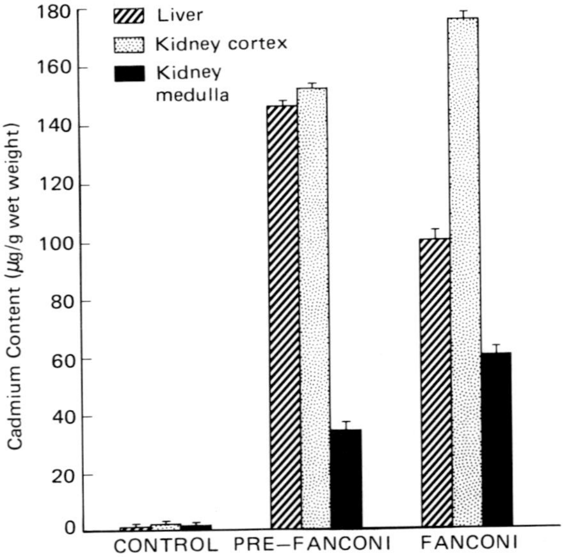

Fig. 13 Cadmium content of liver, kidney cortex, and kidney medulla of control and two experimental groups, pre-Fanconi sacrificed 2 days prior to development of glycosuria, and Fanconi, sacrificed at peak of renal tubular dysfunction. Values are mean ± SEM. n = 6 in each group. (From Ref. 52.)

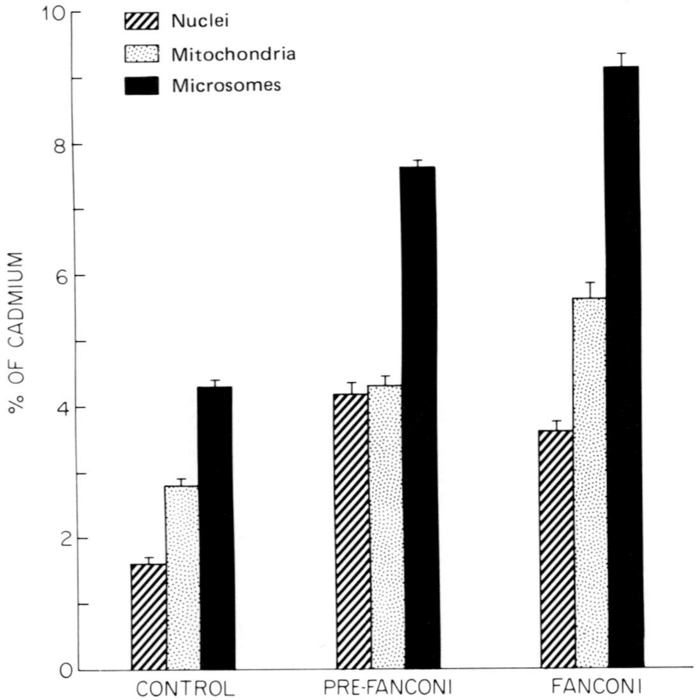

Fig. 14 Percentage distribution of radioactive cadmium in subcellular fractions in kidney cortex of control and experimental Fanconi animals. The soluble cytoplasm fraction, which contains the majority of the radioactive cadmium, is not displayed in order to magnify the changes in the remaining subcellular fractions. Values are mean ± SEM. n = 5 in each group. (From Ref. 52.)

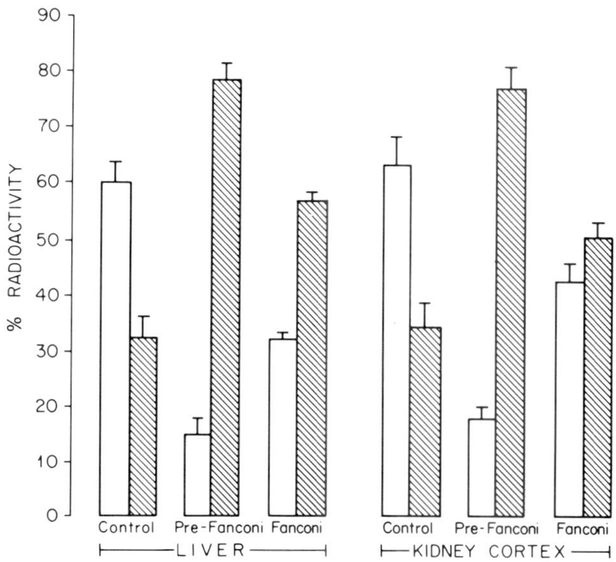

Fig. 15 Distribution of radioactive cadmium in high-molecular-weight (□) and low-molecular-weight (▧) proteins in the soluble cytoplasm of liver and kidney cortex of control and experimental Fanconi animals. Values are mean ± SEM. (From Ref. 59.)

compared with the in vitro titration curve of cadmium inhibition of microsomal Na-K-ATPase (Fig. 17). Only the Fanconi animals revealed a significant decrease in microsomal Na-K-ATPase activity. The 45% inhibition of microsomal Na-K-ATPase found in vivo, when cadmium concentration in this fraction was 4.9 μmol/mg protein, was precisely that predicted from the in vitro titration curve.

Metallothionein was measured in liver and kidney cortex homogenates in each group of animals by tracing metallothionein with radioactive mercury as described by Zelazowski et al. (61). Metallothionein concentration increased gradually from control values of 0.02 mg/g wet weight to a maximum of 2.90 mg/g wet weight in Fanconi animals, with relatively little further change in the post-Fanconi animals. The binding capacity for ^{109}Cd of purified metallothionein from kidney cortex in each group of animals was assessed by Scatchard plot analysis. The number of binding sites and dissociation constants were determined for both metallothionein and metal-free thionein. These measurements were essentially unchanged in animals sacrificed at 3, 6, 9, and 14 days and in Fanconi animals. The number of binding sites in thionein was approximately 7 g atoms/mol and in metallothionein was about 0.6 g atom/mol. The dissociation constant for thionein was 9×10^{-3} mol/liter and for metallothionein was 4×10^{-4} mol/liter. The cadmium and zinc content and the cadmium/zinc ratio were also determined in purified metallothionein from liver and kidney homogenates of pre-Fanconi and Fanconi animals. The results are displayed in Table 3. The most striking finding was a marked increase in the cadmium/zinc ratio in kidney metallo-

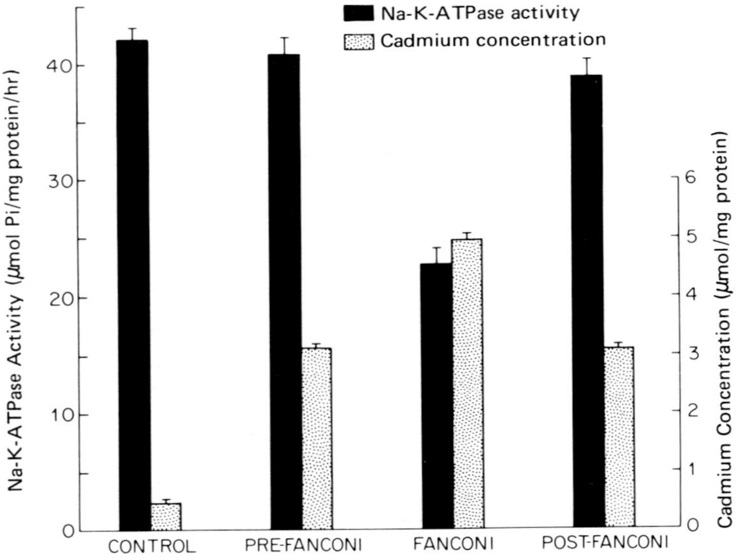

Fig. 16 Kidney microsomal Na-K-ATPase activity and cadmium concentration at various stages in the development of cadmium-induced Fanconi syndrome. Pre-Fanconi = 2 days prior to development of glycosuria. Fanconi = peak of renal tubular dysfunction. Post-Fanconi = 7 days after peak of renal tubular dysfunction. (From Ref. 52.)

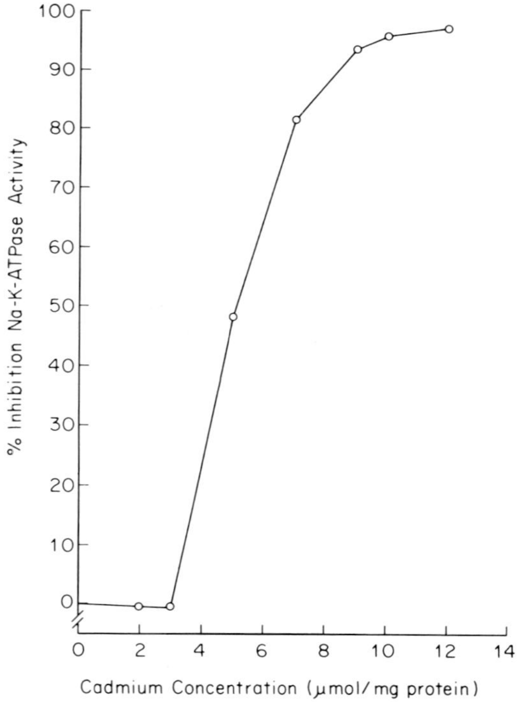

Fig. 17 Percent inhibition of kidney microsomal Na-K-ATPase activity by various concentrations of cadmium ion in the final incubate, calculated as μmol/cadmium per mg of protein in the microsomal fraction. Note that 45% inhibition of enzyme activity is achieved at a cadmium concentration of approximately 5 μmol/mg protein. (From Ref. 52.)

Table 3 Cadmium and Zinc Analysis in Purified Metallothionein (g atoms/mol)

	Liver			Kidney		
	Cadmium	Zinc	Cd/Zn Ratio	Cadmium	Zinc	Cd/Zn Ratio
Pre-Fanconi	4.91	1.88	2.6	4.65	1.55	3.0
Fanconi	6.27	0.51	12.0	6.07	0.12	50.0

Source: Ref. 52.

thionein from Fanconi animals (50 in Fanconi animals vs. 3 in pre-Fanconi). Thus, the previously observed saturation level of cadmium in kidney cortex and the long delay after exposure before development of Fanconi syndrome may be ascribed both to a limit in the kidney's capability of synthesizing metallothionein and the displacement by cadmium of zinc from common binding sites on the protein. The excess cadmium presented to the kidney spills over from the saturated protein-binding sites in the soluble cytoplasm to microsomal and mitochondrial fractions, where cadmium-sensitive enzyme systems are located. As will be discussed in a subsequent section, these findings support the concept that inhibition of the ATP-Na-K-ATPase transport system forms the metabolic basis for the inhibition of active transport in the proximal tubule in both experimental and human forms of the Fanconi syndrome.

Observations in Other Epithelial Tissues

Hillyard et al. (62,63) have utilized Ussing chambers to examine the effects of cadmium on short circuit current across various frog epithelial tissues. In frog skin, cadmium ion added to the outside Ringer's solution (apical surface) increased both potential difference and short circuit current. These effects were additive to the stimulation produced by vasopressin and by removal of calcium. There was no effect on short circuit current when cadmium ion was added to the inside Ringer's solution bathing the basal-lateral surface. This result was somewhat unexpected, since cadmium ion might be anticipated to inhibit Na-K-ATPase on the basal-lateral side of the cell, and in this manner to inhibit active transport and short circuit current. One possible explanation for this negative finding was that cadmium might be trapped in the dermal layers of the frog skin and therefore prevented from reaching the active transport sites in the epithelial cells. Another possibility was that there might be a barrier to the permeation of cadmium ion into or across the membranes of some epithelial cells and that this barrier could be overcome by supplying a carrier substance such as metallothionein or cysteine. Thus, the effects on short circuit current produced by cadmium ion alone, or cadmium in conjunction with an equimolar amount of cysteine, were studied in the isolated frog skin, isolated frog skin epithelium, large intestine, and urinary bladder. Cadmium ion alone inhibited short circuit current when added to the basal-lateral surface of frog urinary bladder and large intestine, but not frog skin or isolated frog skin epithelium. When cadmium and cysteine together were added to the apical surface of the frog skin, *inhibition* rather than stimulation of short circuit current was noted (Fig. 18). Cysteine was also found to affect the amount of cadmium (measured by cadmium isotope) remaining within the skin after the washout procedure. The results suggest that, as in the mammalian kidney, cadmium requires a carrier in order to effectively permeate frog skin, and thus to influence active transport by inhibiting the enzymatic mechanism for active transport. The urinary bladder and large intestine do not appear to require a carrier for cadmium permeation.

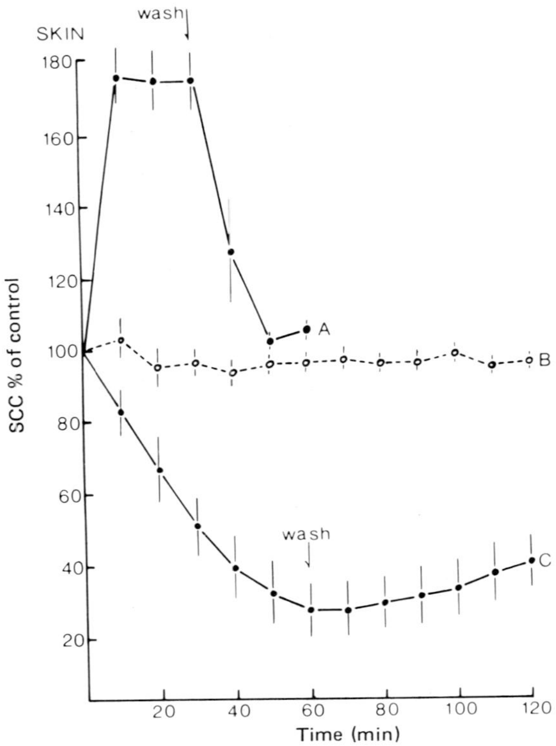

Fig. 18 Inhibition of SCC by equimolar (10^{-3} mol/liter) Cd^{2+} and cysteine added to the apical Ringer's solution (C) compared with the stimulation produced by 10^{-3} mol/liter Cd^{2+} alone (A). Cysteine alone (B) had no effect on SCC (n = 5). (From Ref. 63.)

Several studies have also addressed the effect of cadmium on calcium absorption by the small intestine. Hamilton and Smith (64) employed in vitro studies of calcium flux in sections of normal rat duodenum to evaluate the effect of preincubation with cadmium and found inhibition of the second phase, time-dependent uptake of calcium (which is influenced by vitamin D status and dietary levels of calcium) but no inhibition of initial rapid uptake of calcium. Sugawara (65) demonstrated that rats fed a diet containing 100 ppm of cadmium for 33 days showed diminished intestinal calcium absorption, as judged by blood levels of ^{45}Ca 1 hr after oral administration. Contrary results were reported by Yuhas et al (66), who failed to demonstrate an effect of 100 ppm cadmium given in drinking water for 13 weeks on in situ intestinal calcium absorption in rats. Chertak et al. (67), on the other hand, reported unequivocal effects of both acute and chronic cadmium exposure on calcium absorption by everted duodenal gut sacs from rats. An enteropathic lesion, structurally similar to that seen in human malabsorption syndromes, was described by Richardson and Spivey Fox (68) in the proximal small intestine of Japanese quail fed cadmium from hatching to 4 weeks of age. Valberg et al. (69) found that isolated loops of mouse small intestine perfused for 1 hr with either 100 μmol/liter $CdCl_2$ or cadmium-thionein showed a much more severe alteration in the absorptive cells when the cadmium-thionein solution was used.

The bone lesion of itai itai byo disease, reportedly osteomalacic, could in theory result from: (1) long-standing phosphate depletion secondary to the renal phosphaturic abnormality; (2) an effect of cadmium on vitamin D metabolism; (3) a direct effect of cadmium on intestinal absorption of calcium and/or phosphorus; or (4) a direct effect on bone metabolism. Attempts to explore the pathogenesis of the bone lesion in experimental animals have been hampered by difficulties in reproducing the osteomalacia. Although negative calcium balance has resulted from chronic feeding of cadmium to calcium-deprived rats (70) and the bones show decreased mineral ash and calcium content (70-74), the bone lesions, both radiologically and histologically, in general have been more compatible with osteoporosis than osteomalacia (71,73-75), although some authors have reported widened osteoid seams (72). The latter lesion was seen in calcium-deficient rats fed low levels of cadmium over a long period of time. Anderson and Danylchuk (76-78) studied the effects of chronic low-level cadmium intoxication on the Haversian remodeling system in skeletally mature littermate beagle dogs. When cadmium was administered at a dose of 25 ppm for 6 months, rib mid-shaft biopsies disclosed a significant decrease in activation frequency, radial closure rates, number of osteoid seams, and bone formation rates in the cadmium-treated animals. As plasma levels of immunoreactive parathyroid hormone and of 1,25-dihydroxycholecalciferol levels did not vary, the toxic effects of cadmium were thought to be exerted directly on bone. However, Feldman and Cousins (79) reported that in vitamin D-deficient chicks cadmium interfered with kidney mitochondrial production of 1,25-dihydroxycholecalciferol both in vitro and in vivo. Our laboratory (24) has shown that rats fed with 40 ppm cadmium in drinking water for 9 months after recovery from cadmium injection-induced Fanconi syndrome no longer have evidence of renal tubular dysfunction, but they show a mild osteoporotic lesion in ribs and decreased transport of calcium and phosphorus in duodenal and jejunal everted gut sacs. Calcium ATPase activity was reduced in duodenal homogenates and in bone metaphyses. Intestinal Na-K-ATPase activity, on the other hand, was unaffected by the prolonged cadmium exposure. Thus, the bone disease could be dissociated from renal tubular dysfunction, but it may have resulted from direct effects of cadmium on both intestinal and bone enzyme activity, affecting transport of calcium and phosphorus. The direct relevance of the bone disease found in experimental animals to human itai itai byo disease, however, remains obscure, as the advanced itai itai byo bone disease is found only in multiparous-aged women, suggesting that some feature of pregnancy is a necessary predisposing factor which has not yet been adequately addressed in the experimental model.

C. Degraded Tetracycline Model

A reversible Fanconi syndrome caused by outdated tetracycline was first reported in 1963 by Frimpter et al. (80), Ehrlich and Stein (81), Gross (82), and Rosenthal (83). The degradation product thought to be responsible for the tubular dysfunction was anhydro-4-epitetracycline, formed from the parent compound under the influence of heat, moisture, and low pH. This substance was subsequently employed to produce experimental Fanconi syndrome in rats and dogs (84-86). In the first study, Benitz and Diermeier (84) administered each of four test substances to rats by gavage as a single 1000 mg/kg dose. The substances included tetracycline, 4-epitetracycline, anhydrotetracycline, and anhydro-4-epitetracycline. Within the first 24-78 hr after dosing, only the animals receiving anhydro-4-epitetracycline consistently showed renal functional and morphological changes. The functional abnormalities included an increase in urinary glutamic-oxalacetic transaminase activity, proteinuria, glucosuria, and cellular debris in the urinary sediment. Morphological changes (light microscopy) consisted of renal edema and various degrees of cortical tubular necrosis. One dog given anhydro-4-epitetracycline in a dose of 10 mg/kg on the first day and 20 mg/kg on the second day became moribund and was found at autopsy to show severe cortical tubular necrosis. Other dogs given either tetracycline or anhydrotetracycline in the same dosage remained healthy.

Lowe et al. (85) administered anhydro-4-epitetracycline intravenously to rats in doses ranging from 1 to 12 mg/100 g body weight. The threshold dose was found to be 3 mg/100 g body weight. In rats receiving this dose or higher, glucosuria developed at 16 hr after injection and persisted for 5-6 days. Transient hemoglobinuria was also noted. Necrosis of proximal convoluted tubules became evident at 24 hr, the degree of necrosis being roughly proportional to the amount of drug administered. Regeneration of the necrotic tubules began at 2 days and was complete by 6 days. Loops of Henle, distal convoluted tubules, and collecting tubular cells remained normal throughout.

Lindquist and Fellers (86) explored the possibility that anhydro-4-epitetracycline produced the Fanconi syndrome by inhibiting oxidative energy metabolism, basing their postulate on earlier observations that tetracycline selectively accumulates in mitochondria of living renal cells (87) and may interfere with oxidative phosphorylation (88). They gave degraded tetracycline (containing anhydrotetracycline and anhydro-4-epitetracycline) intraperitoneally to rats in a dose of 2.5 mg/100 g body weight every 12 hr for up to 14 days. Animals injected with pure tetracycline served as controls. Rats given degraded tetracycline developed azotemia and increased clearances of α-amino nitrogen, phosphate, and glucose; changes were maximal at 7 days and returned toward normal by 14 days. At 7 days, severe alterations in proximal tubular morphology were also demonstrated in the rats treated with degraded tetracycline. Many tubules were dilated, lined by flattened basophilic epithelial cells which contained few stainable mitochondria and lacked brush borders. Mitochondrial changes, i.e., transformation of rod-shaped forms into short, swollen forms, occurred as early as 3 days, when tubules were normal in appearance. Oxidative enzyme activities were studied by histochemical techniques, using tetranitroblue tetrazolium as an electron receptor and indicator of enzyme activity. Activities of all the oxidative enzymes studied, including members of Embden-Meyerhof glycolysis, Krebs citric acid cycle, hexose monophosphate shunt, and β-oxidation of fatty acids, were moderately decreased within the first 24 hr with maximal changes seen at 7 days; enzyme activities returned toward normal by 14 days. As with the morphological alterations, the decrease in enzyme activity was confined to the convoluted and straight portions of the proximal convoluted tubules. In vitro studies confirmed that degraded tetracycline was a more potent inhibitor of mitochondrial respiration than pure tetracycline in whole kidney homogenates.

D. Spontaneous Fanconi Syndrome in Dogs

A spontaneous Fanconi syndrome, manifested by glycosuria, polyuria, electrolyte disturbances, and generalized debilitation was first reported in the basenji breed of dogs by Easley and Breitschwerdt (89); later Bovee et al. described abnormal reabsorption of several solutes in dogs of the basenji breed as well as in a Norwegian elkhound and a Shetland sheepdog (90-92). Renal clearance studies revealed reduced tubular reabsorption of glucose, phosphate, sodium, potassium, and uric acid. Excessive quantities of sugars, amino acids, and organic acids were also subsequently described in the urines of affected dogs. The renal clearance of bicarbonate was reduced in some dogs and was normal in others. Five of 10 dogs initially studied died within 90 days of diagnosis from acute renal failure, associated with profound dehydration, acidosis, and papillary necrosis. The other dogs remained stable for 18 months without treatment. Kidney tissue from autopsy or biopsy was examined in nine dogs. Histological results were very variable, ranging from normal findings to severe tubulointerstitial disease with tubular dilation, interstitial fibrosis and inflammation, and

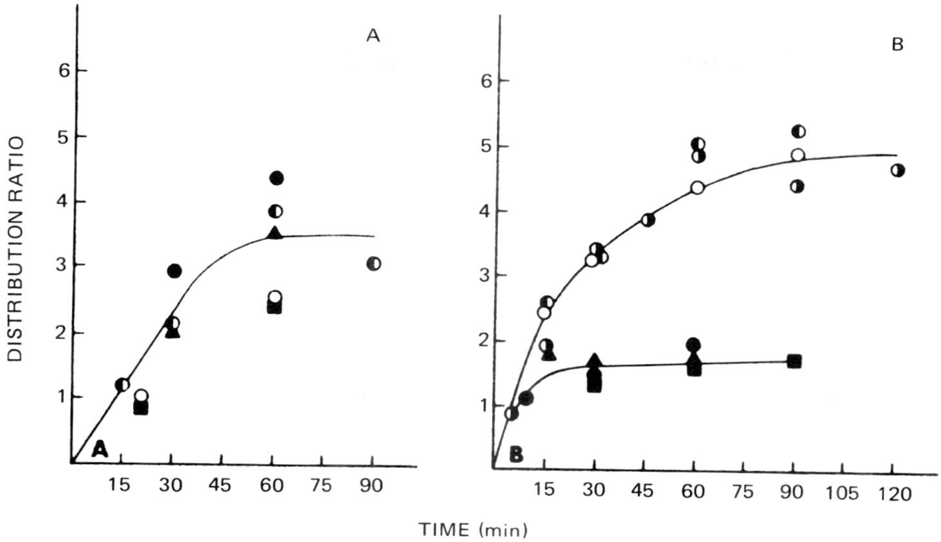

Fig. 19 The time course of accumulation of 0.065 mmol/liter α-aminoisobutyric acid (A) or 2.065 mmol/liter α-methyl-D-glucoside (B) by canine renal cortical slices. The slices were incubated in Krebs-Ringer bicarbonate at 37°C for the times indicated. Each point is the mean of at least triplicate determinations. ●, Basenji; ■, Elkhound; ▲, Shetland sheepdog; ○, ◐, ●, control normals. (From Ref. 90.)

glomerulosclerosis. Electron microscopy revealed no ultrastructural abnormalities in renal tubular cells other than enlargement and elongation of nuclei in basenji dogs. A heavy metal causation was ruled out by normal spectographic analyses of liver and kidney tissues from three of the dogs who died and by negative calcium ethylenediaminetetraacetic acid (EDTA) lead mobilization tests in four of the more stable dogs.

Transport studies were performed in renal cortical kidney slices from tissue removed at biopsy from Fanconi animals. As compared to normal controls, these slices showed reduced uptake of α-methyl-D-glucoside, a nonmetabolized sugar, and reduced uptake of the amino acids lysine and glycine, but not of aminoisobutyric acid (90,92) (Fig. 19). The slow initial uptake of α-methyl-D-glucoside in the tissue slices from Fanconi dogs was interpreted as indicating that the defect resides in the influx of sugar into the renal tubular cells.

II. THE BASIC PATHOPHYSIOLOGICAL DEFECT IN THE FANCONI SYNDROME

A. Alterations in the ATP-Na-K-ATPase Transport System

The compelling evidence for the primacy of the ATP-Na-K-ATPase transport system in providing the energy for the active transport of sodium in the kidney, and, in particular, the proximal tubule of the kidney, has been presented in detail in the first three chapters of this text. Some of the data will be reviewed briefly in order to set the stage for a discussion of the possibility that inhibition of this transport system is the predominant mechanism responsible for producing generalized inhibition of proximal tubular transport, i.e., the Fanconi syndrome.

In the intact isolated perfused rat kidney, addition of sufficient ouabain to completely inhibit kidney Na-K-ATPase reduces the reabsorption of filtered sodium by 50% whereas further addition of the metabolic inhibitors cyanide and iodoacetic acid blocks the remaining reabsorption of sodium (93). It has been calculated for the whole kidney that 40-50% of sodium transport is ouabain sensitive, i.e., Na-K-ATPase dependent, 20% is inhibitable by acetazolamide, i.e., bicarbonate driven, while less than 10% is mediated by an ATPase which is sodium- but not potassium-stimulated, and inhibited by ethacrynic acid rather than ouabain (94,95).

In the proximal tubule, one-third of sodium transport is Na-K-ATPase dependent, one-third is bicarbonate dependent, and one-third depends on passive physicochemical forces (95-98). The *exit* of sodium across the basal-lateral membrane occurs against an electrochemical potential difference, i.e., requiring energy, and is mediated predominantly by the Na-K-ATPase system (97,99,100). Despite the observation that Na-K-ATPase activity is lower in the proximal tubule than in other areas of the nephron (101), the specific activity of the enzyme per millimeter of transporting epithelium has been found to be more than sufficent to account for the active component of sodium reabsorption. Indeed, the relatively low level of Na-K-ATPase activity in the proximal tubule may account for its susceptibility to inhibition by various transport inhibitors.

The hydrolysis of adenosine triphosphate (ATP) constitutes that part of the coupling mechanisim which links the ion transfer by the transport ATPase to the metabolic rate in epithelia (102). Thus, Na-K-ATPase activity can be equated to the product of enzyme concentration, i.e., the number of functional enzyme sites, and the rate of ATP hydrolysis (103). The activity of this enzyme transport system can be modified not only by availability of substrate ATP but also by the quantity of activators or inhibitors present within the cell. Magnesium, for example, is a necessary and specific cofactor for the enzyme (104). In the proximal tubule, metabolic energy is derived almost exclusively from ATP produced by oxidative metabolism in the mitochondria via the citric acid cycle (105). In contrast to the renal medulla, where anaerobic metabolism predominates (103,106), the contribution of glycolysis to the basal metabolic rate is negligible (107,108). The substrates considered most important in the generation of ATP for active transport are glucose and lactate, while free fatty acid oxidation may provide further energy for synthetic processes within the epithelial cells of the proximal tubule (109).

As reviewed in the first three chapters, there is considerable in vitro and in vivo evidence indicating that the proximal tubular transport of several inorganic and organic solutes is linked to the active transport of sodium. Sodium "cotransport" systems for glucose, amino acids, and phosphate, and a sodium "countertransport" system for hydrogen ion have been described in isolated luminal membranes, while a sodium countertransport system for calcium has been found in isolated basal-lateral membranes (97). Micropuncture studies have revealed that inhibition of Na-K-ATPase activity by ouabain reduces not only the proximal tubular transport of sodium, but also the transport of aminoacids, glucose, phosphate, and calcium (110). In vivo, a link has also been noted between reduced renal tubular reabsorption of sodium and reduced reabsorption of calcium (111), magnesium (111), bicarbonate (112), and phosphate (113), following extracellular volume expansion, a maneuver which alters proximal tubular reabsorption both by changes in physical driving forces and by elaboration of natriuretic hormone, shown recently to be an inhibitor of renal Na-K-ATPase (114).

With these observations as a background, one might expect a reduction in the proximal tubular reabsorption of sodium as well as the reabsorption of those solutes normally linked to the transport of sodium under one or more of the following circumstances: (1) a change in the metabolic processes necessary to generate sufficient ATP to provide energy for active transport; (2) a change in electrochemical potential difference for sodium across the luminal cell border by reduction in the pumping activity at the exit site (i.e., Na-K-ATPase), by an alteration in permeability of the cell membrane, or both; (3) changes in the transport processes or coupled transport processes for the individual solutes. Based on these considerations, we should like to propose a model (Fig. 20) which advances the hypothesis that inhibition of the ATP-Na-K-ATPase transport system in the proximal tubule of the kidney is responsible for production of the Fanconi syndrome (115). This hypothesis requires that the various metabolic and transport inhibitors reported to be associated with either hereditary or acquired Fanconi syndrome result in a rate-limiting diminution in ATP synthesis, in Na-K-ATPase activity, or both. The discussion which follows will consider the experimental and clinical evidence supporting the concept that depletion of critical cofactors or an excessive accumulation of certain toxic inhibitors leads to the development of the Fanconi syndrome by reducing the activity of the ATP-Na-K-ATPase transport system below a threshold level.

Magnesium Depletion

Magnesium deficiency in man is known to affect renal function by increasing potassium clearance (116). In the rat, azotemia, proteinuria, aminoaciduria, and increased phosphate clearance have also been observed (117-120). Magnesium is an essential cofactor for many enzymes, including Na-K-ATPase. This enzyme requires the presence of magnesium for the formation of a Mg-ATP complex as the enzyme's substrate (104). Severe magnesium depletion or displacement of magnesium from the Mg-ATP complex, e.g., by calcium or heavy metals (Fig. 1), may therefore contribute to the development of a Fanconilike syndrome in some patients (23-115).

Hypercalcemia

Hypercalcemia in man is generally associated with increased urine flow and sodium excretion (121,122). This may be due to inhibition of Na-K-ATPase enzyme activity in the proximal tubule, the thick ascending limb of Henle's loop, the distal convolution, and the collecting

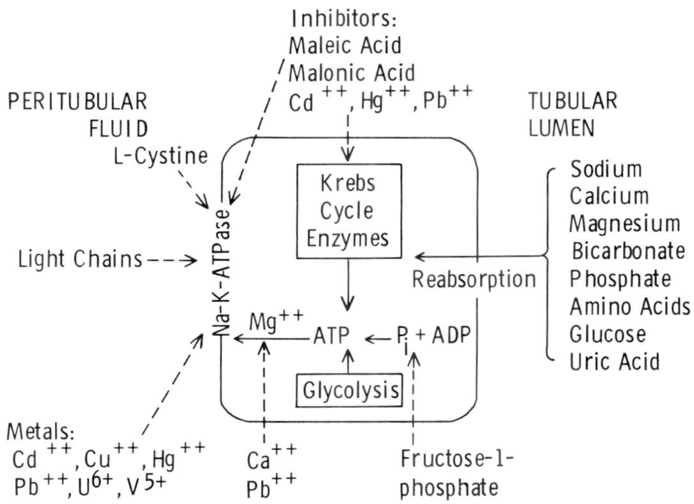

Fig. 20 Schema for the pathogenesis of Fanconi syndrome. *Dashed arrows* represent speculated site of action of transport or metabolic inhibitors. (From Ref. 115.)

duct. In some instances, the diuresis is sufficiently severe to cause extracellular fluid volume (ECFV) contraction with increased proximal tubular bicarbonate reabsorption. In contrast, high serum calcium concentrations in the presence of parathyroid hormone (PTH) and non-contracted ECFV may cause decreased proximal bicarbonate absorption (123). Sodium, calcium, and magnesium reabsorption in the proximal tubule as well may be decreased (124-126). In addition, hypercalcemia suppresses free water formation in the thick ascending limb by inhibiting NaCl reabsorption and also suppresses water reabsorption in the collecting duct, resulting in polyuria resistant to vasopressin (127).

Fresh kidney tissue contains about 1-3 mmol calcium per kg. In intact cells, however, a much lower cytoplasmic calcium concentration is maintained by the mitochondrial calcium pump. Therefore, under normal circumstances, calcium in the cell is mainly bound to mitochondria and to the nucleus, and the magnesium concentration is normally three to five times higher than that of calcium (104). Induction of hypercalcemia, however, leads to an increased content of calcium in kidney tissue, where it predominantly accumulates in the medulla. Increased cytoplasmic calcium inhibits phosphofructokinase and pyruvate kinase and may also inhibit Na-K-ATPase by the formation of a Ca-ATP complex. This Ca-ATP complex then competes with Mg-ATP as false substrate for the transport enzyme (104). Epstein and Whittam (104) have shown that a calcium concentration corresponding to 10% of that of magnesium inhibits Na-K-ATPase by 32% and Wheeler and Whittam (128) showed that a calcium concentration equal to 5% of the Mg-ATP concentration causes a 22% inhibition of this enzyme. Our own in vitro results show that 50% inhibition of renal Na-K-ATPase is achieved at a calcium concentration of 7×10^{-4} mol/liter (Table 4).

Phosphate Depletion

Clinical manifestations of phosphate depletion include renal tubular acidosis resulting from decreased bicarbonate reabsorption, hypercalciuria, hypermagnesiuria, and reduced glucose reabsorption (129). All these features may be an expression of proximal tubular dysfunction. In that part of the nephron in which transport essentially depends on energy derived from oxidative phosphorylation, inorganic phosphate is of crucial importance, since it may regulate the rate of mitochondrial respiration via its contribution to the phosphorylation potential ATP-ADP-P_i (130).

Table 4 Effects of Divalent Cations and of Uranium on Na-K-ATPase Activity in Homogenates of Rat Renal Cortex

Metal Salt	I_{50} (mol/liter)
$BaCl_2$	1×10^{-3}
$CaCl_2$	7×10^{-4}
$CdCl_2$	1×10^{-4}
$CuCL_2$	3×10^{-4}
$HgCl_2$	3×10^{-6}
$MnCl_2$	8×10^{-4}
$PbCl_2$	7×10^{-5}
$UO_2(C_2H_3O_2)_2$	2×10^{-4}
$ZnCl_2$	5×10^{-4}

Source: Kramer, H. J.; Gonick, H. C.; and Lu, E. (unpublished observations).

In experimental phosphate depletion no direct correlation between plasma P_i, tissue P_i, and ATP can be observed, since only prolonged severe phosphate depletion causes a fall in kidney ATP content. This may be due to the fact that a large portion of P_i can be stored in mitochondria. Also the continuing tubular reabsorption of P_i may help to prevent loss of P_i from cellular stores (131,132). In microperfusion studies, Brazy et al. (130) were able to demonstrate defective proximal tubular function and metabolism during removal of P_i from the tubular fluid, but not from the bath. Intracellular P_i is not only important for oxidative phosphorylation but also for glycolysis; P_i is a substrate for glyceraldehyde-3-phosphate dehydrogenase and for phosphofructokinase. Therefore, measures which enhance the incorporation of P_i into glycolytic substrates may rapidly impair function of the proximal tubule by deviating P_i from oxidative phosphorylation, whereas measures which decrease incorporation of P_i into glycolytic substrates allow more of the existing stores of P_i to be utilized in oxidative phosphorylation (130).

The defective fluid reabsorption and decreased oxygen consumption which follows the removal of P_i from the luminal fluid of isolated perfused proximal rabbit kidney tubules was not observed when glucose entry into the cell was simultaneously inhibited by phlorizin or by substituting the nonmetabolizable sugar α-methyl-D-glucopyranoside for glucose, or by inhibition of glycolysis with 2-deoxyglucose. Thus, glucose metabolism may interfere with the availability of intracellular P_i and, therefore, worsen the proximal tubular transport defect resulting from phosphate depletion (130). Similarly, an immediate fall in the intracellular concentration of P_i and of ATP occurs when kidney cells are exposed to fructose, which also may deviate P_i from oxidative phosphorylation to the glycolytic pathway (133) (see section Hereditary Fructose Intolerance below and Fig. 20).

Parathyroid Hormone

Secondary hyperparathyroidism due to malabsorption of vitamin D in an adult patient with cystic fibrosis was reported to be associated with a generalized Fanconi-type proximal tubular dysfunction (134). This included proximal renal tubular acidosis, aminoaciduria, and phosphaturia, while glycosuria was absent. Similar abnormalities, including glycosuria, were described in patients with osteomalacia of dietary or intestinal origin (20,135,136) and in patients with parathyroid adenomas (137). As PTH exerts a marked effect on proximal reabsorption of phosphate and reduces net volume reabsorption which also causes decreased sodium and chloride reabsorption, this tubular dysfunction may be due to the excessive secretion of PTH under such circumstances. The resulting phosphate depletion (see previous section) in these patients may, in addition, contribute to the defect by decreasing cellular generation of ATP and thereby worsening the tubular dysfunction. The observed defects in tubular function were corrected after treatment of these patients with vitamin D.

Heavy Metals

Cadmium

As discussed earlier, cadmium has been incriminated as a cause of Fanconi syndrome in humans, resulting from both occupational and environmental exposure (138-140). The evidence that protracted administration of cadmium can produce a reversible tubulointerstitial disease with generalized proximal tubular dysfunction has also been cited earlier. In rats given repetitive intraperitoneal injections of $CdCl_2$, renal cortical ATP levels were reduced by 38% and cortex homogenate Na-K-ATPase activity by 60% at the height of the Fanconi syndrome (51). The most convincing evidence that cadmium inhibition of Na-K-ATPase activity was intimately linked to the development of tubular dysfunction was the demonstration that renal microsomal Na-K-ATPase activity was reduced significantly (by 45%)

only in animals sacrificed at the height of the Fanconi syndrome and not in animals sacrificed either just prior to development of the Fanconi syndrome or shortly after recovery (see Fig. 16). Furthermore, the microsomal cadmium concentration found in the Fanconi animals (4.9 μmol/mg protein) was exactly the amount predicted by in vitro titration of renal microsomal Na-K-ATPase to result in this degree of inhibition of enzyme activity, whereas lower cadmium concentrations found in the microsomal fractions from pre-Fanconi and post-Fanconi animals (3 μmol/mg protein) did not inhibit Na-K-ATPase *in vitro* (115, 141) (see Fig. 17). The relative specificity of the inhibition of Na-K-ATPase by cadmium in this experimental model is suggested by the observation that in the animals with Fanconi syndrome there were no significant changes in activities of Mg-ATPase, of acid phosphatase, or of β-glucuronidase in renal cortex or medulla (51).

In vitro studies of renal Na-K-ATPase derived from dog kidney revealed that half-maximal inhibition (I_{50}) of Na-K-ATPase in microsomal fractions from outer and inner cortex and of outer medulla was achieved at $CdCl_2$ concentrations between 2.1 and 3.2×10^{-4} mol/liter (142). This inhibition was not affected by changing sodium or potassium concentrations in the incubate but was prevented by the addition of EDTA, a metal-chelating agent. Mg-ATPase from dog and human kidney was approximately 10 times less sensitive to $CdCl_2$ inhibition than was Na-K-ATPase. In whole kidney homogenates or microsomal fractions from guinea pig similar concentration of $CdCl_2$ were necessary for 50% inhibition of Na-K-ATPase. Enzyme derived from cat kidney showed less sensitivity to inhibition by cadmium, whereas renal Na-K-ATPase from rat, rabbit, mouse, and sheep was more sensitive, I_{50} occurring between 1.0 and 1.6×10^{-4} mol/liter (142) (Table 4). The cadmium I_{50} for human kidney microsomal Na-K-ATPase has been found to be 1.4×10^{-4} mol/liter (143). Tissue homogenates apparently do not contain substances which protect the enzyme from inhibition (143).

Na-K-ATPase activity and cellular metabolism are affected in tissues other than the kidney. In vitro studies of alveolar macrophage membrane ATPase showed 20.4% inhibition of Na-K-ATPase and 11.0% inhibition of Mg-ATPase by cadmium at a concentration of 5×10^{-4} mol/liter (144). Cadmium at a concentration of 5×10^{-5} mol/liter completely inhibited mitochondrial respiration and a concentration of 5×10^{-3} mol/liter almost completely inhibited cellular O_2 uptake in alveolar macrophages (144). A similar uncoupling effect of cadmium was reported for liver mitochondria, to which the metal is strongly bound in vitro. When cadmium was fed to rats for 60 days liver mitochondrial succinic oxidase activity and the P/O ratio were significantly reduced; however, with continued cadmium feeding for 335 days, these values normalized. Cadmium was also found to affect the Embden-Meyerhof pathway in rat liver (145).

Cadmium thus appears to affect transepithelial sodium transport by inhibiting Na-K-ATPase and by suppressing cellular metabolism, resulting in decreased availability of substrate ATP (Fig. 20).

Lead

In contrast to adults, in whom exposure to lead causes renal failure without typical proximal dysfunction (146), lead poisoning in young children has been reported to result in proteinuria, glycosuria, and aminoaciduria (147). To mimic this tubular transport defect in an experimental model, rats were fed a diet containing 1% lead as lead acetate. Toxic renal changes were found to be confined to the proximal tubule. In the subcellular fractions, the major portion of lead was found in the supernatant fraction, less in microsomes, and the smallest amount in mitochondria and nuclei (148). Only small amounts of lead are bound to metallothionein and this binding protein does not seem to play a major role in the detoxification process for lead (149). On the other hand, lead feeding results in the appearance of intranuclear inclusion bodies in the proximal tubule of the kidney. These inclusion bodies have been shown to consist of lead bound to a protein with a molecular weight of 27,000 daltons, serving to detoxify part of the administered lead as a nondiffusible nontoxic lead-protein complex (150). Other major histological changes in kidney tubules from lead-intoxicated rats include swelling of the mitochondria, which also show marginated cristae and a reduction in the granularity of the matrix (151).

In rats and guinea pigs fed a diet containing 0.1% lead acetate for up to 6 months kidney homogenates showed unaltered activities of succinate and lactate dehydrogenase and of cytochrome oxidase, but a significant reduction in malate and glutamate dehydrogenases (152). Glucose-6-phosphate dehydrogenase activity, in contrast, was significantly increased by chronic lead administration (153). Mitochondria of renal cortex from lead-treated rats showed a lower ADP/O ratio related to glucose oxidation in the kidney. There was a decreased rate of mitochondrial O_2 consumption and of ADP-stimulated respiration. This partial uncoupling of oxidative phosphorylation in mitochondria was reversible by EDTA (154).

Lead has a high affinity for sulfhydryl groups and, therefore, is likely to also affect the Na-K-ATPase enzyme. In vitro, lead has been shown to be an inhibitor of Na-K-ATPase of human erythrocyte membranes (155). Incubation for 40 min with 2.5×10^{-5} mol/liter $PbCl_2$ results in 100% inhibition of the enzyme. In microsomal fractions and tissue homogenates from human kidney 50% inhibition of Na-K-ATPase was achieved at a lead concentration of 6 to 8×10^{-5} mol/liter, and there was no evidence that tissue homogenates contain a protective protein against this inhibition (143). Mg-ATPase was 100-fold more resistant to inhibition by lead. The inhibition by lead is reversible and is reduced when the concentrations of sodium or ATP are increased, while an increase in Mg enhances the enzyme inhibition by lead. Thus, lead interacts with Na-K-ATPase at both the sodium-sensitive and the phosphate sites and, in addition, lead may chelate ATP to form a lead-ATP complex displacing Mg-ATP as substrate (143) (Fig. 20). As mentioned above, this chelation is reversible by increasing the concentration of ATP in the incubate. Similar, but less striking, results were found in studies of alveolar macrophage membrane, in which Na-K-ATPase was inhibited by 28% in the presence of 5×10^{-4} mol/liter lead, while Mg-ATPase was inhibited by 6.5% (144).

Our own studies of tissue homogenates of rat renal cortex revealed a 50% inhibition of Na-K-ATPase activity at a $PbCl_2$ concentration of 7×10^{-5} mol/liter (Table 4), which is similar to that described for human kidney Na-K-ATPase (143).

Thus, based on these metabolic and enzymatic effects of lead, it appears reasonable to speculate that the tubular transport defect observed in chronic lead poisoning, as in chronic cadmium poisoning, may be related to disturbances in the ATP-Na-K-ATPase transport system.

Copper

A tubular syndrome similar to the Fanconi syndrome has been reported in copper miners as well as in patients with Wilson's disease, a hereditary disorder in which copper accumulates in multiple organs, including the kidney (156).

When radiolabeled copper acetate is injected in rats it accumulates within a few hours in the liver, intestine, and kidney. Comparing the copper deposition in the brain, liver, and kidney, the latter organ contains the highest amount of this metal (157). Even more profound accumulation of copper was found in the kidney when the metal was fed together with glutathione. This accumulation was prevented by the administration of penicillamine.

In patients with Wilson's disease, copper accumulation is associated with marked fat deposition in the proximal convoluted tubule where also hydropic changes were noted; similar findings have not been seen in distal tubules (158). Kidneys of rats treated with copper acetate reveal lamellar structures of lipoid in lysosomes in the proximal tubular cells where, in addition, a loss of cristae and vacuolization of mitochondria occur (158). Zinc protects the experimental animal against copper intoxication by a mechanism which has not yet been delineated, but which might involve the induction of a copper-binding protein.

There are at present very little data on the effects of copper on metabolism or on Na-K-ATPase activity of the kidney. However, studies of the effects of copper on brain metabolism and ATPase activity have been performed both in vivo and in vitro. Thus, in vitro studies have shown that slices of cerebral tissue from guinea pig or pigeon do not show changes in respiration when copper concentration ranges from 0.12 to 3×10^{-4} mol/liter, but there is a significant decrease in tissue ATP concentration (from 1.80 to 1.11 μmol/g wet weight) at a copper concentration of 3×10^{-4} mol/liter (159). Similarly, it was demonstrated that while copper at a concentration of 0.2×10^{-3} mol/liter completely inhibited O_2 uptake and mitochondrial oxidation of pyruvate in crude brain homogenates and isolated brain mitochondria of the pigeon, it did not affect mitochondrial respiration in more intact tissue preparations, such as brain slices (160). This suggests the presence of other proteins in the intact tissue which protect mitochondria from the toxic effect of copper.

Since copper accumulates to a significantly greater amount in the ATPase-rich microsomal fraction than in mitochondria of the brain, it has been suggested that copper toxicity is related to its toxic effect on membrane ATPase rather than on mitochondrial respiration (161). Thus, copper was found to reversibly interact with chick brain Na-K-ATPase, which is inhibited by 50% in the presence of less than 1.4×10^{-6} mol/liter copper. At concentrations higher than 6×10^{-6} mol/liter copper induced an irreversible inhibition of the enzyme. Mg-ATPase is much less sensitive to this divalent cation; beef brain Mg-ATPase was inactivated only in the presence of 10^{-3} mol/liter copper (162). The Na-K-ATPase enzyme system appears to be partially protected by high ATP concentrations in the incubation medium. Inhibition of the enzyme was in addition completely reversed by the addition of L-phenylalanine, L-histidine, d-penicillamine, and L-cysteine. A noncompetitive inhibition by copper was observed with respect to ATP and potassium, but a competitive inhibition occurred with respect to sodium ions (163).

In vitro, both Na-K-ATPase and Mg-ATPase in microsomal fractions of brain tissue from guinea pig and pigeons were significantly inhibited by copper. In the guinea pig, 3×10^{-4} mol/liter copper inhibited Na-K-ATPase by 71% in tissue homogenates and by 65% in microsomal fractions (161). Others have found that microsomal ATPase from pigeon brain normally contains little Na-K-ATPase activity; maximum total ATPase inhibition (by 25%) occurred at a copper concentration of 4×10^{-5} mol/liter and no further inhibitory effect was observed by the addition of ouabain (159). The rat brain microsomal ATPase, in contrast, is more sensitive to ouabain and to copper than the pigeon brain and is inhibited by 41% at a copper concentration of 2×10^{-5} mol/liter and by 50% at a concentration of 10^{-5} mol/liter. This inhibition can be completely prevented by histidine-HC1 at a pH of 7.2 (164). Mg-ATPase appears to be little affected by copper at this concentration, although conflicting results have been reported (161,164). Mg-ATPase in erythrocyte ghosts was found to be activated by copper, while Na-K-ATPase was inhibited by 50% in the presence of 10^{-4} mol/liter copper (164). Copper was also reported to inhibit Na-K-ATPase of alveolar macrophages in vitro by 36.4% and Mg-ATPase by 30.3% at a concentration of 5×10^{-4} mol/liter (144). Rat kidney homogenate Na-K-ATPase was inhibited in vitro at 30%

at a copper concentration of 10^{-4} mol/liter; Mg-ATPase was inhibited by 18% at this copper concentration (165). Our own studies of rat renal cortex homogenate revealed a 50% inhibition of Na-K-ATPase at a copper concentration of 3×10^{-4} mol/liter (Table 4).

In summary, the effects of copper on tissue metabolism and enzyme activity suggest that the toxic action of copper on membrane ion transport is more likely related to its direct inhibition of the Na-K-ATPase enzyme than to a depletion in its cellular energy source, i.e., the availability of ATP (Fig. 20).

Mercury

Chronic intoxication with mercury has been reported to cause proximal tubular transport abnormalities. Mercury accumulates in the kidney, primarily in the renal cortex. The intracellular binding of mercury appears to depend on the type of mercury salt. Thus, mercuric chloride ($HgCl_2$) is predominantly (166), and mercuric acetate and phenylmercuric acetate (167) are, to a large degree, bound to metallothionein within the soluble fraction in the cytosol of the kidney. In contrast, methyl mercury, with its high lipid solubility, has only a very low affinity for metallothionein (168). Early after its administration methoxyethyl mercury acetate binds to a high-molecular-weight protein and less to metallothionein and a low-molecular-weight protein, respectively. However, with time the relative amount of mercury in the metallothionein fraction increases, thus permitting storage in a nontoxic form. Metallotheionein, however, has a limited binding capacity for mercury (169). Kidneys of animals fed this mercury compound are enlarged and the cortex shows grayish striation. Histological examination reveals tubular atrophy, degenerative changes, and dilatation of tubules with cortical interstitial cell infiltration and fibrosis (170).

Mercuric chloride has been found to be a potent inhibitor of Na-K-ATPase in microsomal fractions from the human kidney (the I_{50} ranges from 1 to 6×10^{-6} mol/liter). Tissue homogenates apparently contain protective substances which reduce the inhibitory action of $HgCl_2$. Since increasing sodium concentrations also reduces the enzyme inhibition by $HgCl_2$, it appears that mercury competes with sodium for the same enzyme site (143). Other effects of mercury compounds, e.g., of methyl mercury, include inhibition of the synthesis of macromolecules such as DNA, RNA, and protein within the kidney (171). They also have acute effects on glycolytic intermediates in the brain (172), cause a reduction of NADPH-specific glutathione reductase (173), and increase acid phosphatase activity (174).

The lethal effects of $HgCl_2$ in rats can be prevented by prior administration of spironolactone, which causes increased fecal and biliary excretion of mercury as well as enhanced transfer of mercury from plasma to the gut lumen (175,176). Spironolactone appears to have a general protective action against renal damage in this animal. Selenite as well has been shown to offer protection against chronic mercury toxicity in rats.

Mercury thus appears to affect transmembrane ion transport by a direct inhibition of the Na-K-ATPase transport enzyme as well as by disturbing cellular energy metabolism (Fig. 20).

Uranium

In experimental uranium intoxication the main site of injury is the proximal tubule, where swelling and necrosis of the epithelium occur (177,178). Minor degenerative changes such as vacuolization also appear. The terminal portion of the proximal tubule, particularly the pars recta, reveals necrosis and loss of nuclei. Less severe morphological changes are found in the distal nephron, with early regeneration of necrotic changes in this area. Variable interstitial inflammation occurs (179).

In vitro studies of the effects of this metal on ATPase have been performed with uranyl nitrate ($UO_2{}^{2+}$ or U^{6+}). Total ATPase and Na-K-ATPase in microsomal fractions from the dog kidney cortex and outer medulla as well as from brain and heart were similarly affected by uranium (I_{50} = 4 to 5 × 10^{-5} mol/liter), while the enzyme from the liver was less sensitive (I_{50} = 8 × 10^{-5} mol/liter). Tissue homogenates of kidney cortex and medulla required twice as much uranium for half-maximal inhibition of Na-K-ATPase as the microsomal fraction (I_{50} = 8 to 9 × 10^{-5} mol/liter), suggesting the presence of protective substances in the homogenate. The sensitivity of Mg-ATPase in microsomal fractions or tissue homogenates from kidney cortex was comparable to that observed for total ATPase or Na-K-ATPase (180).

Total ATPase of the whole kidney microsomal fraction from the rat revealed sensitivity to uranium which was similar to the dog (I_{50} = 7 × 10^{-5} mol/liter), while that from hamster, rabbit, and cat and from man was less sensitive (I_{50} = 1 × 10^{-4} mol/liter). Na-K-ATPase in homogenates of human kidney was even more resistant to this toxic substance (I_{50} = 2 × 10^{-4} mol/liter) (180). Mg-ATPase from human kidney microsomal fraction and tissue homegenate was 5.0 and 2.5 times less sensitive than was total ATPase or Na-K-ATPase, respectively. Changes in potassium concentration of the medium did not affect the enzyme inhibition by uranyl nitrate, which therefore appears to inhibit the enzyme at its sodium-sensitive site (180). Our own data revealed that the I_{50} for Na-K-ATPase in rat kidney cortex homogenate was 2 × 10^{-4} mol/liter (Table 4). No data are available concerning the effect of uranium on cellular metabolism.

Other Metals

Vanadium. Vanadium is found as vanadate in several organs, including the kidney, where it accumulates in the cortex and the proximal tubules at high concentrations sufficient to affect the Na-K-ATPase enzyme system (181). This metal was, therefore, suggested to act as a possible natural modulator of the renal regulation of the extracellular fluid volume. When administered parenterally to experimental animals vanadium increases urine flow and water excretion, induces a marked phosphaturia, depresses maximal glucose and bicarbonate absorption, and affects both free water absorption and free water clearance. Potassium excretion, however, remains unaltered. Vanadate therefore appears to act at both proximal and distal tubular sites (182). Vanadate has been shown to inhibit various ATPases including Na-K-ATPase (183), Ca-ATPase (184), HCO_3-ATPase (185), and a proton-ATPase (186). It also inhibits other enzymes such as adenylate kinase and phosphofructokinase, while stimulating adenylcyclase. However, phosphaturia resulting from I.V. administration of vanadate in the acutely thyroparathyroidectomized rat was not accompanied by increased renal cAMP excretion (182).

The inhibition of Na-K-ATPase by vanadate was first observed in vitro by Charney et al. (183), who recognized vanadate as an impurity of commercially available ATP, which resulted in decreased activity of the enzyme prepared from various tissues such as red cells and kidney tissue (187). In contrast to ouabain, which binds to the pump from the outside of the cell membrane, vanadate reversibly binds to the pump from the inside of the cell at the sodium-sensitive enzyme site. In addition, however, this metal may also facilitate the binding of ouabain to the pump (188). Vanadate is a 10-fold more potent inhibitor of renal Na-K-ATPase than is ouabain. Jorgensen found that 50% inhibition of the enzyme activity is achieved by approximately 5 × 10^{-7} mol/liter vanadate, and for comparison, by 5 × 10^{-6} mol/liter ouabain and by approximately 10^{-3} mol/liter ethacrynic acid, respectively (189). Mg-ATPase was found to be 1000-10,000 times more resistant to vanadate than was Na-K-ATPase (190).

Reducing agents such as ascorbic acid and citric acid decrease the inhibitory activity of the metal on Na-K-ATPase. Similarly, the in vivo regulation of Na-K-ATPase by vanadate may be influenced by glutathione, which might be anticipated to reduce vanadate to vanadyl, a compound having only a fraction of the inhibitory potency of vanadate. Intracellular ATP may also protect the enzyme, either by binding vanadate or by competing with vanadate for a mutual receptor of the Na-K-ATPase enzyme (190).

Platinum. Cisplatin (*cis*-diamminedichloroplatinum), a potent cytotoxic agent, may induce tubular defects, resulting in proteinuria, mild renal failure, and renal magnesium wasting (191). After intraperitoneal administration to experimental animals cisplatin is found in highest concentration in the corticomedullary region of the kidney. It binds to the cytosol fraction, nuclei, mitochondria, plasma membranes, and microsomes. Treatment of mice and rats with this agent results in dilatation mainly of proximal convoluted tubules. Early changes consist of cytoplasmic and mitochondrial vacuolization and loss of brush-border epithelium. In rats the acute administration of cisplatin induces focal necrosis in the proximal and distal tubules. Chronic treatment in addition causes tubular dilatation due to atrophic epithelium, interstitial edema, and lymphocytic infiltration, which later results in irreversible interstitial fibrosis and thickening of basement membrane accompanied by hyalinization of glomeruli (192).

No data on metabolic changes within the kidney are available at present, though the renal lesions closely resemble those of heavy metal intoxication. Platinum may interact with SH-groups of protein (enzymes) and has been shown to inhibit ATPases and other enzymes in vivo and in vitro (193). For human kidney renal microsomal ATPases (Na-K-ATPase, Mg-ATPase, and Ca-ATPase), I_{50} values for cisplatin were found to range from 6 to 8×10^{-4} mol/liter (194).

Chromium. Acute renal failure from heavy chromium exposure has been reported repeatedly, but tubular dysfunction, primarily tubular proteinuria and enzymuria, has been described in workers chronically exposed to chromium (195). Repeated intraperitoneal administration of potassium dichromate to rats experimentally induces a proximal tubular defect with proteinuria and glycosuria (196,197). Histologically the pathological changes in the kidney are confined to the proximal tubule, where vascular changes and lysosomes with phagocytosed material are found in the cytoplasm. The mitochondria are distorted and also show vacuolization. Microvilli and the basilar infoldings of the proximal convoluted tubule (which contain the Na-K-ATPase) are markedly changed or absent (198). These fine structural changes of the proximal tubule, without alterations in the brush border, suggest a defect at the basolateral membrane of the tubular epithelium as the site of the tubular transport defect induced by the administration of potassium dichromate. Unfortunately no in vitro or in vivo data are at present available regarding the effects of chromium on the ATP-Na-K-ATPase enzyme systen.

Gold. Gold administered for treatment of rheumatic disease is deposited within the kidney where it may affect kidney function either by immunologically mediated glomerular lesions or by toxic effects on tubular epithelium (199). This metal, like cadmium, stimulates the synthesis of a metallothioneinlike protein in the kidney, which thereby may protect the organ from cellular damage unless chronic exposure leads to excessive accumulation of gold. Gold administered to animals was found in the cytoplasm of renal cortical cells where it accumulates in lysosomes to form so-called aurosomes (200). Since gold has a high affinity for SH-groups, it seems likely that this metal would also inhibit the Na-K-ATPase enzyme. In vitro, kidney ATPase is very sensitive to gold. Total microsomal ATPase from dog kidney reveals an I_{50} ranging from 2×10^{-7} mol/liter to 1×10^{-6} mol/liter for the trivalent chlorauric acid ($HAuCl_4$), while tissue homogenates of whole kidney show an I_{50} ranging from 2×10^{-6} mol/liter to 2×10^{-5} mol/liter, of medulla at 2×10^{-5} mol/liter, and of cortex at 6×10^{-5} mol/liter. Human whole kidney homogenates are somewhat more sensitive and reveal an I_{50} at 6×10^{-6} mol/liter.

Monovalent gold (Au^+) (for example, administered as gold sodium thiomalate) is two to three times more potent as an inhibitor of Na-K-ATPase than is trivalent gold. The inhibitory effects of gold cannot be modified by changing the concentrations of sodium, potassium, magnesium, or ATP in the incubation medium (201).

Zinc. After injection of radiolabeled zinc chloride into rats, two-thirds of the zinc is found in the soluble cytoplasm of the kidney. Most of this is bound to proteins of higher molecular weight than that which binds cadmium, although part of the zinc administered is initially bound to metallothionein in the cytoplasm. This binding is less firm than that of cadmium and there may be an intracellular competition for binding sites among zinc, cadmium, and mercury. One-third of the zinc chloride in the kidney is found in other organelles, i.e., a small portion in nuclei, followed by mitochondria, and the remainder in the microsomes (202).

In vitro we have found that zinc chloride inhibits 50% of Na-K-ATPase derived from tissue homogenates of rat kidney cortex at a concentration of 5×10^{-4} mol/liter, which is in agreement with previous observations on the inhibition of Na-K-ATPase derived from alveolar macrophage membranes (144). Zinc has also been shown to block ADP stimulation of mitochondrial respiration, an effect which is reversible in the presence of EDTA (203).

As a means of comparing the relative toxicity of various divalent cations and also of uranium (U^{6+}) on renal Na-K-ATPase, we have previously studied the effects of the metal on the enzyme in tissue homogenates from rat renal cortex. The following metals are listed according to their relative ability to inhibit Na-K-ATPase in vitro: Hg > Pb > Cd > U > Cu > Zn > Ca > Mn > Ba. The approximate concentrations which induced 50% enzyme inhibition (I_{50}) are summarized in Table 4.

Hereditary Disorders

Various inherited metabolic diseases may be associated with the appearance of the renal Fanconi syndrome. These include galactosemia, hereditary fructose intolerance, and tyrosinemia. In all of these, the accumulation of toxic carbohydrate metabolites appears to be responsible for the tubular transport defect. The accumulation of L-cystine within the renal tubule is responsible for the transport defect in cystinosis, the hereditary disorder most commonly associated with Fanconi syndrome.

Galactosemia

Disturbances in galactose metabolism may result in the development of a Fanconi-like renal syndrome. The primary defect in galactosemia is a deficiency in galactose-1-phosphate uridyltranferase, which results in the accumulation of galactose-1-phosphate as a toxic metabolic intermediate (204). The sequence of toxic events or the direct target organelles within the cell are unknown.

Hereditary Fructose Intolerance

In hereditary fructose intolerance, the lack of aldolase B isoenzyme causes the accumulation of fructose-1-phosphate in the renal cortex, where this enzyme is of crucial importance. Fructose-1-phosphate is derived from D-fructose via the enzyme fructokinase. Its high rate of synthesis without further metabolism leads to rapid intracellular depletion of inorganic phosphate, accompanied by a decrease in extracellular phosphate concentration. Extra- and intracellular depletion of inorganic phosphate results in a decrease in the rate of ATP synthesis within the tubular cell. Phosphate depletion has been shown to significantly depress renal gluconeogenesis in isolated renal cortical tubules (i.e., glucose production from *a*-

ketoglutarate, malate, and pyruvate) by 50-65%, and to result in a decrease in ATP concentration from 18 to 1.6 μmol/g wet weight in kidney tissue (131,132). Fructose loading in the rat has been demonstrated to reduce renal cortical ATP content by 50% (from 2.46 to 1.26 μmol/g wet weight) when administered in amounts of 40 mmol/kg body weight, result- in a tissue concentration of fructose-1-phosphate of 6.5 μmol/g wet weight. Tissue concentration of AMP remained unaltered, while ADP concentration increased. However, in this animal model no functional defect mimicking the Fanconi syndrome was induced. The metabolic disturbances could be ameliorated by administration of inorganic phosphate and of adenine, respectively (133).

In patients with hereditary fructose intolerance, decreased intracellular ATP appears to become critical only in the presence of PTH , which by stimulating adenylate cyclase activity to form cAMP from ATP causes a further and functionally relevant depletion of cellular ATP concentration (205). This in turn suppresses the rate of oxidative phosphorylation in the mitochondria of proximal tubular cells. It is unknown whether the Na-K-ATPase enzyme system is affected in this disease.

Tyrosinemia

In type 1 tyrosinemia accumulation of tyrosine, *p*-hydroxy-phenyl-pyruvic acid, fructose, and fructose-1-phosphate occurs. Tubular transport defects may therefore be caused by mechanisms similar to those proposed in hereditary fructose intolerance. Alternatively, the accumulation of maleylacetoacetate (see also the section on maleic acid-induced Fanconi syndrome below), an intermediary of tyrosine metabolism, was proposed to be toxic (206).

Cystinosis

The infantile and adolescent forms of inherited cystinosis (Lignac-Fanconi syndrome), a rare autosomal recessive disorder, are often associated with the congenital renal Fanconi syndrome (207,208). Intracellular cystine is elevated, especially in the atrophic proximal tubules of the kidney, in which it is found as hexagonal cystine crystals (209). L-Cystine mainly accumulates in lysosomes. The exact pathophysiological biochemical events leading to the generalized proximal tubular defect, however, are as yet unknown. Since this renal lesion apparently cannot be induced experimentally simply by administration of L-cystine in excessive amounts into animals, no studies of the effects of L-cystine on cellular metabolism in vivo or in vitro nor of its effects on Na-K-ATPase in vivo are available. In vitro, however, we have previously shown that L-cystine inhibits Na-K-ATPase of tissue homogenates of rat renal cortex in a dose-dependent manner, with a maximum inhibition of 40% reached at concentrations between 10^{-6} and 10^{-5} mol/liter (5). We also observed an 89% inhibition of frog skin Na-K-ATPase after 1 hr of incubation with 10^{-3} mol/liter of L-cystine, which inhibited short-circuit current of the isolated frog skin by 39% and 47% at concentrations of 10^{-4} mol/liter and 10^{-3} mol/liter, respectively, when added to the outside bathing Ringer solution (210).

Multiple Myloma

It is well known that patients with multiple myeloma and light chain proteinuria are highly susceptible to progressive renal failure, but they may also demonstrate the features of renal Fanconi syndrome (211). In the reported cases the increased light chain exretion is almost invariably restricted to κ-chains, while λ-chain excretion is ordinarily normal or only slightly increased (212). Patients with renal tubular disease of other etiologies, in contrast, show a moderate increase in the excretion of both classes of light chains. Light chain proteins, which are nephrotoxic and accumulate in the proximal tubular epithelium as crystalline cytoplasmic inclusion bodies (23,213), have been shown in vitro experiments to inhibit *p*-aminohippurate (PAH) uptake by rabbit renal cortex slices (214).

To further explore this transport defect, plasma membranes from rat renal cortical tubules were incubated with κ-light chain from two patients with multiple myeloma. Light chain at concentrations of 10^{-4} and 10^{-5} mol/liter inhibited Na-K-ATPase by 100% and by 35%, respectively, but had no effect on Mg-ATPase (215). The authors mention that they observed comparable in vitro effects with the λ-light chain protein purified from the urine of a third patient. This finding contrasts with the above cited clinical observations, but it suggests that the physicochemical state of κ-chains may be more conducive toward reaching the site of Na-K-ATPase in the proximal tubule in vivo. In isolated cortical tubules light chain stimulated the maximum rate of glucose synthesis from lactate by 36% and increased ATP concentration by 27% (215). Analogous metabolic effects were obtained with ouabain at a concentration of 10^{-4} mol/liter, suggesting that light chain acted predominantly as an inhibitor of Na-K-ATPase, diminishing the rate of hydrolysis of substrate ATP. Since purified light chain did not affect sodium reabsorption by the isolated perfused rat kidney (216), it was suggested that its toxic effects may become manifest only after prolonged exposure.

Malonate

After administration of malonate to experimental animals, highest concentrations are found in the kidneys. Renal damage, however, occurs only from exceptionally high doses of malonate. Malonate causes a loss of cellular potassium with an equivalent rise in intracellular sodium. The effects of malonate on kidney function include reversible inhibition of active cellular uptake of PAH, which may be related to inhibition of renal succinate dehydrogenase and Krebs cycle function. Malonate was also reported to cause a diuresis and to depress the Tm for phosphate, but to affect the Tm of glucose only to a minor degree. Other studies showed that administration of malonate to water-loaded rats resulted in a systemic acidosis accompanied by an increased urinary excretion of sodium, potassium, phosphate, and titratable acid as well as a reduction in ammonia excretion (217). These features may point to a proximal tubular transport defect. It has been suggested that malonate acts by depressing aerobic metablism in general rather than to act on specific enzymes such as succinate dehydrogenase. This interference with the operation of the Krebs cycle would be anticipated to reduce the rate of ATP formation and, therefore, the availability of substrate for the Na-K-ATPase transport system.

Maleic Acid

The injection of maleic acid into dogs and rats is known to produce a generalized defect of renal tubular transport similar to the congenital or acquired renal Fanconi syndrome (1,2, 3,6,36) (see Sect. I.A.).

As reviewed earlier, a number of biochemical studies have been performed on this experimental model in an attempt to account for the pathogenesis of the renal tubular dysfunction. Angielski and Rogulski (36) found that maleate selectively accumulated within the kidney, particularly the renal cortex. The principal action appeared to be an inhibitory effect on renal mitochondrial Krebs cycle enzymes, limiting oxidative phosphorylation and, thus, presumably ATP synthesis (36). Rogulski (33) had initially postulated that maleate inhibits SH-enzymes in general. Subsequent studies have indicated that inhibition of SH-enzymes by maleate is selective, rather than generalized, as malate dehyrogenase and succinate dehydrogenase, both typical mitochrondrial SH-enzymes, are not inhibited, or only poorly inhibited, by maleate (5,217). The two groups of enzymes most strongly inhibited by maleate are transaminases and α-ketoacid oxidase (36,218,219).

Kidney homogenates from rats treated with maleic acid revealed a marked inhibition of the oxidation of ketogutarate, citrate, pyruvate, glutamate, and malate, in decreasing order, while the isolated mitochrondria revealed inhitibition of oxidation of α-ketoacids at maleate concentrations below 1 mmol/liter (36). Maleate inhibited phosphorylation with all substrates of tricarboxylic acid cycle tested except succinate (30). Inhibition of phosphorylation was always more pronounced than inhibition of oxygen uptake. It was proposed based on these studies of substrate phosphorylation that maleate interfered with succinyl-CoA metabolism (30,37). In presumed confirmation, measurements of CoA in kidney mitochrondria showed a 70% decrease in the presence of ketoglutarate and maleate. However, direct addition of CoA to disrupted mitochrondria failed to remove the inhibitory effect of maleate on ketoglutarate oxidation (30).

Szczepanska and Angielski (42) observed that infusion of acetoacetate into rats subsequently treated with maleate ameliorated the tubular dysfunction. They postulated that in animals treated with maleic acid, CoA is transferred by the enzyme, succinyl-CoA-transferase, from succinyl-CoA to maleic acid to form maleyl-CoA according to the reaction:

Succinyl-CoA + maleate > maleyl-CoA + succinate

The activated double bond of the maleyl moiety could then react with free SH-groups of CoA-SH, glutathione, and proteins to form respective addition products (220). Verification of this effect of maleate came from subsequent observations by Pacanis et al. (39) of a maleate-induced decrease in total CoA content of rat kidney mitochrondria both in vitro and in vivo. Acetoacetate (which is a physiological substrate for succinyl-CoA transferase, and can compete with maleate to prevent formation of maleyl-CoA), when added to mitochondria before maleate abolished its inhibitory effect on oxidation of 2-oxoglutarate, and prevented the decrease of CoA content. In the study by Szczepanska and Angielski (42), measurements of renal cortical ATP in vivo revealed that the 44% reduction in ATP content caused by maleic acid injection was unaltered by the simultaneous administration of acetoacetate. The authors of this report interpret their findings to indicate that either the decreased ATP level is not the cause of the decrease of tubular solute transport or that the measured total ATP content is not representative of the real level of ATP at the site of the cell where transport takes place. In favor of the likelihood that ATP content or the phosphorylation potential, ATP-ADP-P_i, may be a limiting factor in the tubular dysfunction caused by maleate are recent observations that phosphate loading attenuates maleic acid-induced bicarbonaturia in the dog (221).

In our own studies of the maleic acid model in rats, we have demonstrated parallel dose-dependent changes in renal tubular function, renal morphology, ATP content, and Na-K-ATPase activity (5). The functional and morphological changes have been described earlier. ATP concentrations in renal cortex 1 hr after the administration of 1.5 and 9.0 mmol maleate/kg body weight were reduced from 1.19 to 0.82 and 0.15 μmol/g wet weight, respectively, i.e., by 31 and 87% (5) (Fig. 21). Similarly, Schärer et al. (4) observed a decrease in rat renal cortical ATP content from 0.122 to 0.080 μmol/mg DNA, i.e., by 34%, following administration of 3.4 mmol of maleic acid/kg body weight.

In our experimental animals, renal cortical Na-K-ATPase activity was inhibited by 33 and 41%, respectively, after injection of 1.5 and 9.0 mmol maleic acid/kg body weight (Fig. 22). These findings were confirmed by Fujita and Itakura (15), who showed that injection of 2 mmol and 8 mmol maleic acid/kg body weight inhibited Na-K-ATPase of light microsomes from rat renal cortical tissue by 25 and 43%, respectively. In vitro, we have shown that maleic acid inhibits renal cortical Na-K-ATPase in a dose-dependent manner, when the compound is preincubated for 1 hr with rat renal cortex homogenized in sucrose-Tris-HCl buffer (5). At a maleic acid concentration of 10^{-3} mol/liter, the enzyme was inhibited by 64%. Frog skin Na-K-ATPase, exposed to maleic acid at this same concentration, is inhibited by 94% (210).

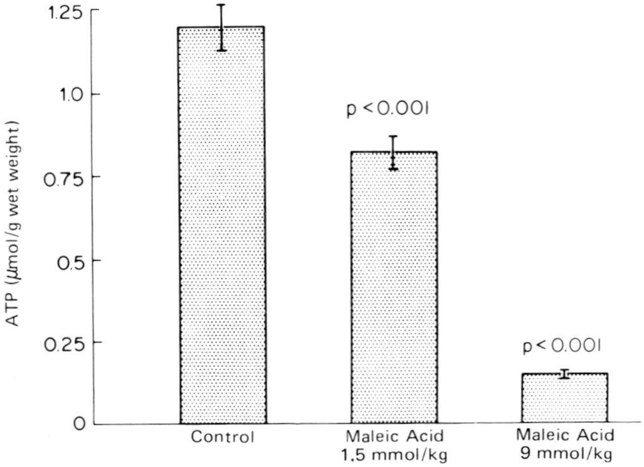

Fig. 21 ATP concentrations in renal cortical tissue after injection of maleic acid (1.5 or 9.0 mmol/kg body weight). Values are mean ± SEM. (From Ref. 5.)

Short circuit current, a measure of active transport in frog skin, is also inhibited by maleic acid in a reversible, dose-dependent manner, when this compound is added to the inside surface of the skin (site of the sodium pump) (210). Maleic acid at a concentration of 10^{-3} mmol/liter induced a 55% inhibition of short circuit current when added to the Ringer's solution bathing the inside surface of the skin. When the same concentration was added to the Ringer's solution bathing the outside (epithelial) surface of the skin, however, a slight *increase* in short circuit current of 18.4% was noted. These findings are compatible with maleic acid acting primarily as an inhibitor of active transport via inhibition of Na-K-ATPase, but also having a minor effect to increase epithelial cell permeability.

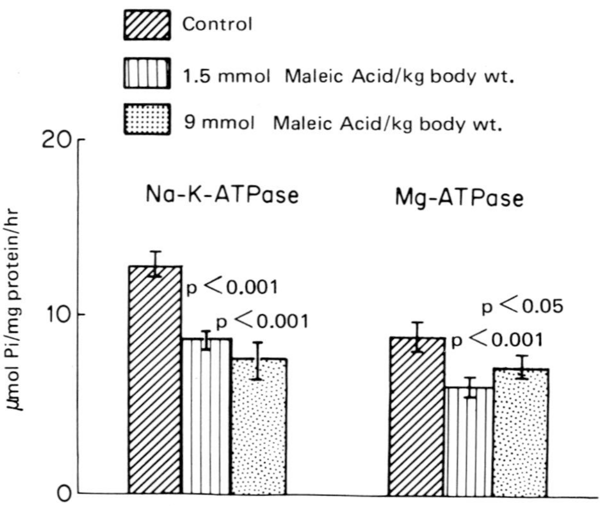

Fig. 22 Activity of Na-K-ATPase and Mg-ATPase in homogenates of renal cortex after injection of maleic acid (1.5 or 9.0 mmol/kg body weight). Values are mean ± SEM. (From Ref. 5.)

Quantitative Considerations

As many of the conditions affecting proximal tubular function, reviewed above, are associated with both reduced ATP synthesis and Na-K-ATPase inhibition, it is difficult to define that degree of reduction of either component of the ATP-Na-K-ATPase transport system which would become rate limiting in active transport. Cardiac glycosides, on the other hand, affect only Na-K-ATPase activity, and therefore it is reasonable to assume that the degree of inhibition of Na-K-ATPase following administration of the glycoside which results in a reduction of fractional sodium absorption may constitute a "threshold" effect. Nechay et al. (222) have demonstrated that chronic digitalization of dogs, which results in a 26-33% reduction in kidney microsomal Na-K-ATPase activity, fails to alter sodium handling. However, when ouabain is infused directly into the renal artery, Na-K-ATPase inhibition of greater than 40% results in reduced sodium and chloride absorption and a decrease in concentration and diluting ability (223). Other studies in the literature appear to support the contention that at least 40% of Na-K-ATPase activity must be inhibited before sodium absorption in intact or isolated kidneys or sodium efflux in isolated kidney cells is affected (Table 5).

With regard to kidney ATP content, the "threshold" level appears to be a 30-40% reduction before alteration in tubular transport are seen. Thus, when ATP depletion is induced in rat kidney cortex slices, by anaerobiosis or by inhibitors of oxidative phosphorylation (amobarbital [Amytal], dinitrophenol, oligomycin, and maleic acid), a reduction in ATP content by more than 40% is associated with decreased accumulation of α-aminoisobutyric acid, a measure of the active transport of amino acids (230). Infusion of the metabolic inhibitors cyanide or oligomycin into the renal artery of intact kidneys results in a significant depression of sodium absorption when tissue ATP content is reduced by 24.9 or 32.2% (231) (Table 6). In isolated perfused rabbit proximal tubules, a close correlation has been demonstrated between oxygen consumption, cellular ATP content, mitochondrial NAD redox state,

Table 5 Changes in Kidney Na-K-ATPase and Sodium Absorption as Reported or Approximated from Data in the Literature

% Inhibition of Na-K-ATPase	% Decrease in Na Absorption	Reference
A. Inhibition of total kidney Na-K-ATPase and sodium absorption by ouabain administered into the renal artery		
23	0	224
<25	0	225
37	5	224
42 (cortex) 54 (medulla)	10	226
53	9	224
73	61	227
75	40	228
81 (cortex) 75 (medulla)	35	98
83	25	224
B. Inhibition of Na-K-ATPase and ^{22}Na efflux from kidney plasma membranes and renal epithelial cell cultures by antibody against Na-K-ATPase		
83	30[a]	229

[a]% change in Na efflux.

Table 6 Changes in Renal ATP and Sodium Absorption as Reported or Approximated from Data in the Literature

A. Relation between renal ATP and sodium absorption following administration of the metabolic inhibitor into the renal artery

% Decrease in tissue ATP content	% Decrease in Na absorption	Inhibitor	Reference
24.9	5.5	Cyanide	231
32.2	6.9	Oligomycin	231

B. Relation between changes in ATP content in cortical tubule suspensions and fluid absorption by isolated perfused proximal convoluted tubules

% Decrease in tissue ATP content	% Decrease in fluid absorption		
31.4	40	Rotenone 10^{-7} mol/liter	232
73.8	100	Rotenone 10^{-6} mol/liter	232
94.4	93	Antimycin A 10^{-6} mol/liter	232

and sodium transport in the presence of inhibitors of mitochondrial oxidative phosphorylation (232). In these studies at least a 30% decrease in ATP levels is required before there is a measurable suppression of overall active tubular transport (Table 6).

Although the absorption of glucose, phosphate, and amino acids by the proximal renal tubule depend, at least in part, upon some function of sodium transport (97,110,233), inhibition of sodium transport is not uniformly associated with parallel degrees of inhibition of transport of these other substances. When sodium transport in the isolated perfused rabbit proximal tubule is partially blocked by arsenate, an uncoupler of oxidative phosphorylation (234), or by substitution of choline for intraluminal sodium (235), there is a more profound effect on phosphate transport than on glucose transport. The authors of these reports speculate that a significant portion of glucose absorption may occur independent of sodium transport and that the entry step for glucose may depend more on the transmembrane electrical potential than on the chemical gradient for sodium (234). Such considerations may pertain to the variability in alterations in discrete tubular function observed in Fanconi syndrome of differing etiologies.

In the two experimental models of Fanconi syndrome described earlier (maleic acid and cadmium), the cortical ATP levels and Na-K-ATPase activities were reduced below the threshold levels and all measured tubular functions were impaired, i.e., there was glucosuria and aminoaciduria in association with increased fractional excretion of sodium, phosphate, urate, calcium, magnesium, and potassium, and a metabolic acidosis, presumed to be on the basis of reduced bicarbonate reabsorption. Furthermore, the degree of tubular dysfunction in the maleic acid model was dose related, correlating with the amount of depression of renal cortical ATP content and inhibition of Na-K-ATPase activity (particularly the former). The implication of such observations is that toxins which affect both components of the ATP-Na-K-ATPase transport system to a significant degree may be more likely to cause profound changes in tubular function than toxins which selectively inhibit either ATP generation or Na-K-ATPase activity.

In conclusion, the evidence presented here suggests that impairment of the ATP-Na-K-ATPase transport system, through diminution in the availability of metabolic energy, a decrease in the active transcellular movement of sodium via Na-K-ATPase, or both, is the predominant biochemical mechanism responsible for the pathogenesis of the Fanconi syndrome. An alternative explanation of cell leakage (passive backflux) with enhanced efflux from the tubular epithelial cell is considered next.

B. Alterations in Membrane Permeability

The principal focus in the preceding section of this chapter has been on the possibility that inhibition of the sodium pump at the basolateral membrane or exit site, as manifested by inhibition of the ATP-Na-K-ATPase transport system, might account entirely for the generalized inhibition of proximal tubular dysfunction that constitutes the Fanconi syndrome. Bergeron et al. (27,236,237) and others have advanced an alternative hypothesis, namely, that altered membrane permeability, both in the proximal and distal tubule, is an important contributory factor to the pathophysiology of Fanconi syndrome. In 1971, Bergeron and Vadeboncoeur demonstrated by microinjection of L-leucine-^{3}H and inulin-^{14}C both into the lumen and into the peritubular capillaries of proximal convoluted tubules of rat kidney that maleate administration did not result in impaired entry of amino acid into the tubular cell, but rather to enhanced transtubular flux of amino acid in the direction of the tubular lumen (236). As the intracellular amino acid pool was also found to be decreased (236), Bergeron interpreted these findings as compatible with increased amino acid efflux from the cell secondary to increased membrane permeability. In a later study, Bergeron et al. (27) extended these observations with studies of amino acid, glucose, and phosphate transport in maleate-treated rats. Their experimental model was studied at 2 hr after injection of 0.9 mmol/kg maleate (after glucosuria had appeared) by means of microinjections of labeled amino acids, 3-O-methyl-D-glucose, and phosphate into proximal convoluted tubules of the kidney, stop-flow diuresis, and microperfusion of single nephrons. Their data indicated that in the accessible proximal tubule net influx of amino acids (L-proline, L-OH-proline, and glycine) remained normal in the maleate-treated animals as did entry of amino acids, glucose, and phosphate from the luminal side of the proximal tubule cell. However, as implied by stop-flow experiments which showed precedence of excretion of amino acids or phosphate over inulin, and stop-flow microperfusion experiments, which demonstrated both precedence and greater excretion of amino acid or glucose over inulin in treated animals as compared to controls, there was enhanced antiluminal movement of amino acids, glucose, and phosphate in the proximal distal tubule. Bergeron (27) has interpreted these findings as indicating normal luminal movement of all three molecular species into the proximal tubule that predominates and corrects the antiluminal movement there. However, increased antiluminal movement toward the apical side of an adjacent distal tubule cannot be corrected. Once in the lumen of the distal nephron, the molecules would be eliminated directly into the urine because (in contrast to the proximal tubule) reabsorption of sugars and amino acids does not occur at this site and reabsorption of phosphate is minimal. This hypothesis is illustrated diagramatically in Fig. 23a and 23b. The altered permeability could be related to modification of energetic processes (238) or to diminution in cytoplasmic ATP, as in vitro studies with other metabolic inhibitors such as 2,4-dinitrophenol have indicated that efflux phenomena are energy linked (239). Bergeron et al. also suggested that maleic acid may act as a chelator of divalent cations, such as calcium and magnesium, which are important in maintaining membrane stability (237). Finally, Günther et al. (240) have proposed that a maleate-induced reduction in renal glutathione (36), which in its reduced form protects the free SH-groups of the cell and helps to keep the structures of membranes in their normal shape (241), could be responsible for altered membrane function.

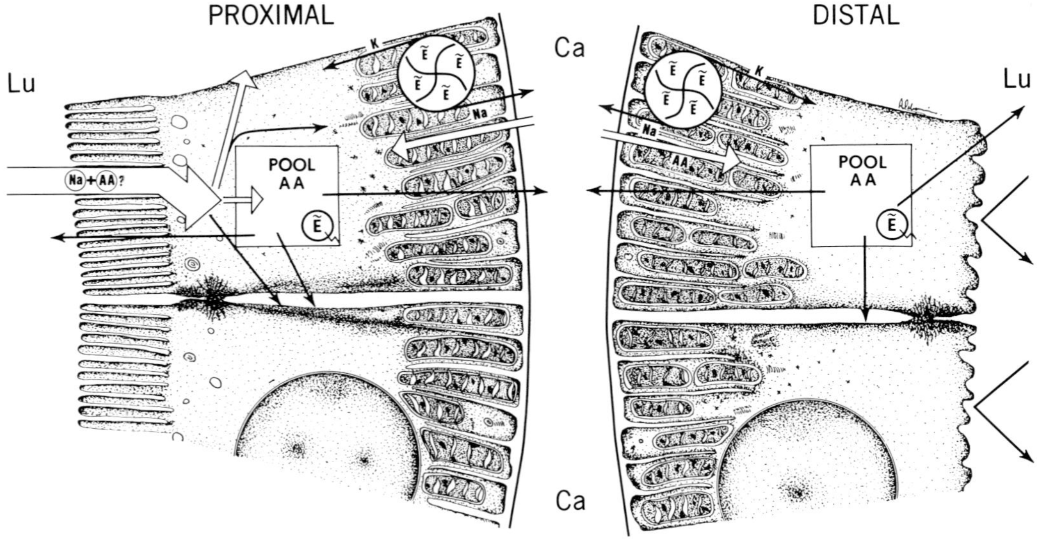

Fig. 23a A schematic representation of the movements of amino acids in the normal nephron. At the proximal tubule, amino acids gain access to the cell through the microvillosities of the apex or through the infoldings of the antiluminal membrane. Since there is an intracellular accumulation of amino acids against a concentration gradient, active transport has to be postulated. However, at the brush border, a carrier-mediated process might be facilitated by the sodium gradient as suggested by various authors. Efflux will take place at all membranes. At the distal tubule, similar amino acid movements (efflux and influx) are seen except that there is no entry of amino acids from the lumen. Lu, lumen; Ca, capillary, AA, amino acids; E, energy.

Apparent agreement with Bergeron's interpretations (27) came from subsequent micropuncture and microinjection studies by Maesaka and McCaffery (242) of rats treated with maleate (2.5 mmol/kg body weight). These authors demonstrated a segmental effect of maleate on tubular leakage of lissamine green from the late proximal tubule and of inulin from a site between the late proximal tubule and the superficial distal tubule. While single nephron GFR measured from the late accessible proximal tubule collections was unchanged from normal in the maleate-treated animals, whole kidney GFR was significantly reduced, presumably due to the more distal leakage of inulin. The net transport of sodium and phosphate by the late proximal tubule was also reduced. Although the authors (242) interpreted their data in favor of Bergeron's hypothesis that maleate alters solute transport by affecting membrane permeability, particularly in the distal nephron, without affecting active transport in the accessive proximal tubule, one criticism of this study is that all observations were made 20 hr after injection of maleate, when overt proximal tubular dysfunction has usually disappeared.

Günther et al. (240) also utilized micropuncture techniques to explore the Fanconi syndrome, but they focused their observations on rats studied 1-6 hr after injection of 1.7 mmol/kg body weight of maleic acid, when tubular dysfunction was still evident. As in the Maesaka and McCaffery studies (242), whole kidney GFR was markedly reduced, while single nephron GFR in intact nephrons was only slightly diminished; inulin leakage could not be demonstrated in these nephrons. Fractional excretion of amino acids (taurine, glycine,

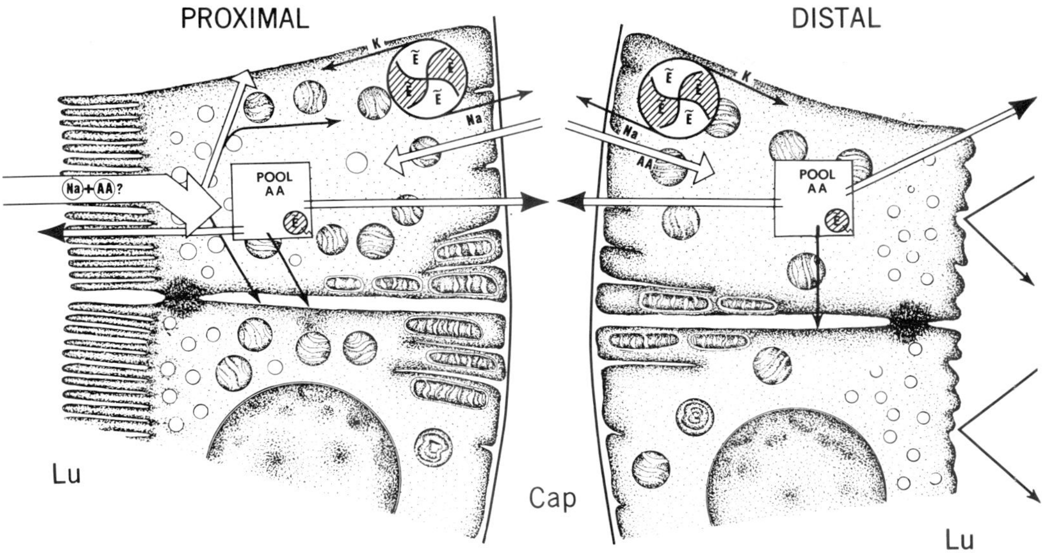

Fig. 23b In the maleic acid model, the cell structure is modified by intense vacuolization, globular and swollen mitochondria, and loss of the infoldings of the basal membrane. Intracellular accumulation of amino acid is decreased despite a rather normal entry at the luminal side. The efflux can be partially or totally corrected in the proximal nephron, since the reabsorption capacity of these cells is very high. At the distal sites, the efflux of molecules cannot be corrected, which will lead to their subsequent excretion. Abbreviations as in Fig. 23a. (From Ref. 27.)

alanine, and L-aspartate) was increased from 20-fold to 230-fold. The reabsorption of amino acids was found to be drastically reduced along the whole proximal tubule, caused by inhibition of the saturable reabsorption process rather than by enhanced back diffusion secondary to increased passive permeability. Micropuncture studies of rats by Brewer et al. (13), 2 hr after injection of 1.7 mmol/kg maleate, also demonstrated diminished reabsorption of sodium, phosphate, and bicarbonate in the late accessible proximal tubule. Bergeron's micropuncture data (27), showing normal reabsorption of solutes by the accessible proximal tubule are clearly different than the data of Günther et al. (240) and Brewer et al. (13). Furthermore, transport studied in the accessible portion of the proximal tubule (as performed by Bergeron [27]) may not be a valid assessment of function in those portions of the proximal tubule which are morphologically most abnormal in maleate-treated animals, namely the late pars convoluta and the pars recta (29). Indeed, the data of Günther et al. (240) revealed a significant reduction in net transport of amino acids between the late proximal tubule and early distal tubule, a segment that includes the late pars convoluta and pars recta. These authors (240) also demonstrated normal efflux of amino acids in the distal tubule. Thus, the evidence for enhanced distal tubular permeability as a primary cause of tubular dysfunction in the maleate-induced Fanconi syndrome must be regarded as questionable.

Studies of glucose transport in maleate-treated dogs at 30-60 min after injection by Wen (243) have shown that at "low dose" (0.15 mmol/kg), fractional transport of sodium, phosphate, and glucose is inhibited in the proximal tubule, while at "high dose" (0.30 mmol/kg) significant glycosuria, due to reduced net glucose reabsorption in the distal nephron, was also seen. These alterations in distal nephron transport could be compatible with either reduced active transport of glucose at this nephron site or to altered permeability with increased back flux. Silverman and Huang (244) also explored the mechanism of glycosuria in dogs given 2.2 mmol/kg of maleate 30 min prior to study. Selected reference indicators (metabolizable and nonmetabolizable sugars, phlorizin) were used to localize the dynamics between sugars and the "cytoplasmic" face of both brush-border and antiluminal membranes as well as the interactions of the exterior of these membrane surfaces. Maleic acid did not affect the interaction of glucose with the antiluminal membrane from the peritubular fluid surface and did not affect phlorizin binding (and thus, inferentially, glucose binding) at the urine (luminal) side of the brush-border. The glucosuria was found to be related to movement of cytoplasmic glucose back across the brush border into the urine, attributable either to partial inhibition of glucose movement from cytoplasm across the antiluminal membrane into blood or to movement of cytoplasmic glucose back across the luminal membrane into urine.

Several studies performed with kidney cortex slices, tubule fragments, and brush-border membrane vesicles have been cited as evidence for or against the membrane permeability hypothesis. To be compatible with this hypothesis, such studies should demonstrate that maleic acid should affect efflux of transported solutes rather than influx, or alternatively, should affect efflux preferentially over influx. Moreover, these studies should be performed with slices, tubule fragments, or membrane vesicles removed from maleate-treated animals with demonstrable renal tubular dysfunction rather than with normal tissue treated in vitro with maleate. In keeping with their earlier studies (see above), which have shown that it is the metabolite maleyl-CoA rather than maleate per se that affects the energetics of tubular transport, Hong Que and co-workers (245) showed that Na^+-dependent glucose and phenylalanine transport in brush-border membrane vesicles isolated from normal rat kidneys was not inhibited in vitro by 5 mmol/liter maleate added to the incubation medium. But when the membrane vesicles were isolated from kidney cortex slices which had been preincubated with maleate or from rats injected with 1.7 mmol/kg maleic acid, the Na^+-dependent transport of these solutes as well as Na^+ permeability were shown to be inhibited. In the slice experiments these effects were reversed by acetoacetate, indicating that the abnormalities were most likely produced by the metabolite maleyl-CoA. In contrast to these results, Silverman (246) was unable to demonstrate an effect of maleic acid on Na^+-dependent D-glucose uptake in brush-border membrane vesicles isolated from dogs pretreated with 2.2 mmol/kg maleic acid or in vesicles from normal dogs exposed in vitro to 9 mmol maleate. In two other animal models of the Fanconi syndrome, the syndrome occurring spontaneously in basenji dogs (92), and the Fanconi syndrome produced by anhydro-4-epi-tetracyline injection into rabbits (247), Na^+-dependent glucose uptake in brush-border basement membrane vesicles was impaired. In the latter model, paralleling the observations with maleate, incubation of brush-border membrane vesicles in vitro with the tetracycline metabolite failed to cause an alteration in glucose uptake.

Whether *the* basic pathophysiological defect in the Fanconi syndrome relates primarily to alterations in the ATP-Na-K-ATPase transport system, to alterations in membrane permeability, or to both, must remain a matter for fruitful debate and for further investigation. The weight of evidence at this juncture would appear to lean toward an interpretation that sodium-coupled transport at the brush-border of the proximal tubule is inhibited by intracytoplasmic accumulation of Na^+, secondary to impeded movement of Na^+ across the antiluminal membrane via the ATP-Na-K-ATPase transport system. Evidence for such an accumulation of intracellular Na^+ in the maleic acid model has been provided by Hong Que et al. (245). Enhanced permeability of the brush-border, perhaps also due to depleted cellular

ATP, may play an additional role in decreasing *net* transport of solutes across the proximal tubule.

Bergeron's permeability model serves a useful purpose in emphasizing the need to look at the distal nephron as an additional site of abnormal transport (27). Abnormalities of distal acidification and of concentrating ability have been described in the human Fanconi syndrome (23). An abnormality in concentrating ability has been described in the cadmium experimental model of the Fanconi syndrome (51) and in free water clearance in the maleic acid model (13), in the absence of ultrastructural changes in the distal nephron in either model. These latter observations in experimental animals, however, imply alterations in function of medullary, rather than cortical, distal nephron segments, where, according to the Bergeron hypothesis (27), permeability changes might be anticipated. Alternatively, a decrease in medullary Na-K-ATPase activity, as noted in the cadmium experimental model (51), would impair reabsorption of sodium chloride the thick ascending limb of Henle, and therefore could affect both concentrating and diluting ability.

Finally, it should be clearly stated that the maleic acid model of the Fanconi syndrome, although examined in the greatest detail, may be relatively unique. Conclusions based on studies of this model may not be entirely applicable to other forms of experimental or human Fanconi syndrome. One important distinction is that maleic acid acutely induces both renal tubular dysfunction and morphological alterations and these changes are reversible after withdrawal of the toxin. Other forms of the Fanconi syndrome, both genetic and acquired, are related to constant exposure to the offending toxin(s) and can lead to irreversible tubulointerstitial disease, progressing in some instances to end-stage renal failure. In either the human Fanconi syndrome, or the experimental counterparts, each identifiable toxin or metabolic aberration deserves independent investigation to ascertain the mechanism by which tubular function is disrupted.

REFERENCES

1. Berliner, R. W.; Kennedy, T. J.; and Hilton, J. G. Effect of maleic acid on renal function. Proc. Soc. Exp. Biol. Med. 75:791-794, 1950.
2. Harrison, H. E.; and Harrison, H. C. Experimental production of renal glycosuria, phosphaturia, and aminoaciduria by injection of maleic acid. Science 120:606-608, 1954.
3. Worthen, H. G. Renal toxicity of maleic acid in the rat. Enzymatic and morphologic observations. Lab. Invest. 13:791-801, 1963.
4. Schärer, K.; Yoshida, T.; Voyer, L.; Berlan, S.; Pietra, G.; and Metcoff, J. Impaired renal gluconeogenesis and energy metabolism in maleic acid-induced nephropathy in rats. Res. Exp. Med. 157:136-152, 1972.
5. Kramer, H. J.; and Gonick, H. C. Experimental Fanconi syndrome. I. Effect of maleic acid on renal cortical Na-K-ATPase activity and ATP levels. J. Lab. Clin. Med. 76:799-808, 1970.
6. Kramer, H. J.; and Gonick, H. C. Effect of maleic acid on sodium-linked tubular transport in experimental Fanconi syndrome. Nephron 10:306-319, 1973.
7. Gmaj, P.; Hoppe, A.; Angielski, S.; Rogulski, J.; and Metler, M. Effects of maleate on renal reabsorption of bicarbonate. In: Biochemical Aspects of Renal Function, edited by Angielski, S., and Dubach, U. C. Bern, Hans Huber, 1975, pp. 101-105.
8. Gmaj, P.; Hoppe, A.; Angielski, S.; and Rogulski, J. Acid-base behavior of the kidney in maleate-treated rats. Am. J. Physiol. 222:1182-1186, 1972.
9. Gmaj, P., Hoppe, A.; Angielski, S.; and Rogulski, J. Effects of maleate and arsenite on renal reabsorption of sodium and bicarbonate. Am. J. Physiol. 225:90-94, 1973.

10. Hoppe, A.; Gmaj, P.; Metler, M.; and Angielski, S. Additive inhibition of renal bicarbonate reabsorption by maleate plus acetazolamide. Am. J. Physiol. 231:1258-1262, 1976.
11. Gougoux, A.; Lemieux, G.; and Lavoie, N. Maleate-induced bicarbonaturia in the dog: A carbonic anhydrase-independent effect. Am. J. Physiol. 231:1010-1017, 1976.
12. Al-Bander, H. A.; Weiss, R. A.; Humphreys, M. H.; and Morris, R. C., Jr. Dysfunction of the proximal tubule underlies maleic acid-induced type II renal tubular acidosis. Am. J. Physiol. 243:F604-F611, 1982.
13. Brewer, E. D.; Senekjian, H. O.; Ince, A.; and Weinman, E. J. Maleic acid-induced reabsorptive dysfunction in the proximal and distal nephron. Am. J. Physiol. 245:F339-F344, 1983.
14. Asatoor, A. M.; Bending, M. R.; and Milne, M. D. Peptide excretion in experimental Fanconi syndrome in the rat. Clin. Sci. Molec. Med. 55:205-212, 1978.
15. Fujita, T.; and Itakura, M. Renal handling of lysozyme in experimental Fanconi syndrome. J. Lab. Clin. Med. 92:135-140, 1978.
16. Christensen, E. I.; and Maunsbach, A. B. Proteinuria induced by sodium maleate in rats: Effects on ultrastructure and protein handling in renal proximal tubule. Kidney Int. 17:771-787, 1980.
17. Brewer, E. D.; Tsai, H. C.; Szeto, K-S.; and Morris, R. C., Jr. Maleic acid-induced impaired conversion of 25 $(OH)D_3$ to $1,25(OH)_2D_3$: Implications for Fanconi's syndrome. Kidney Int. 12:244-252, 1977.
18. Akiba, T.; Endou, H.; Koseki, C.; and Sakai, F. Localization of 25-hydroxyvitamin D_3-1α-hydroxylase activity in the mammalian kidney. Biochem. Biophys. Res. Commun. 94:313-318, 1980.
19. Popovtzer, M. M.; Mehandru, S. K.; Saghafi, D.; and Blum, M. S. Antiphosphaturic action of 25(OH) vitamin D_3 in experimental Fanconi syndrome. Am. J. Physiol. 236: E90-E97, 1979.
20. Chesney, R. W.; and Harrison, H. E. Fanconi syndrome following bowel surgery and hepatitis reversed by 25-hydroxy-cholecalciferol. J. Pediatr. 86:857-861, 1975.
21. Milne, M. D.; Stanbury, S. W.; and Thomson, A. E. Observations on the Fanconi syndrome and renal hyperchloremic acidosis in the adult. Q. J. Med. 45:61-82, 1952.
22. Rodriguez-Soriano, J.; Houston, I. B.; Boichis, H.; and Edelman, C. M. Calcium and phosphorus metabolism in the Fanconi syndrome. J. Clin. Endocrinol. 28:1555-1563, 1968.
23. Lee, D. B. N.; Drinkard, J. P.; Rosen, V. J.; and Gonick, H. C. The adult Fanconi syndrome. Observations on etiology, morphology, renal function and mineral metabolism in three patients. Medicine 51:107-138, 1972.
24. Raghavan, S. R. V.; Walling, M.; Mills, B.; Mirra, J.; Hartenbower, D.; Coburn, J.; and Gonick, H. Dissociation of osteodystrophy from renal tubular dysfunction in cadmium-induced experimental Fanconi syndrome. Clin. Res. 25:139A, 1977.
25. Wapnir, R. A.; Exeni, R. A.; McVicar, M.; DeRosas, F. J.; and Lifshitz, F. Inhibition of sodium intestinal transport and mucosal (Na^+-K^+)-ATPase in experimental Fanconi syndrome. Proc. Soc. Exp. Biol. Med. 150:517-520, 1975.
26. Bergeron, M.; and Laporte, P. Effet membranaire du maleate au niveau du nephron proximal et distal. Rev. Can. Biol. 32:275-279, 1973.
27. Bergeron, M.; Dubord, L.; and Hausser, C. Membrane permeability as a cause of transport defects in experimental Fanconi syndrome. J. Clin. Invest. 57:1181-1189, 1976.
28. Rosen, V. J.; Kramer, H. J.; and Gonick, H. C. Experimental Fanconi syndrome. II. Effect of maleic acid on renal tubular ultrastructure. Lab. Invest. 28:446-455, 1973.
29. Verani, R. R.; Brewer, E. D.; Ince, A.; Gibson, J.; and Bulger, R. E. Proximal tubular necrosis associated with maleic acid administration to the rat. Lab. Invest. 46:79-88, 1982.
30. Angielski, S.; and Rogulski, J. Metabolic studies in experimental renal dysfunction resulting from maleate administration. In: Biochemical Aspects of Renal Function, edited by Angielski, S., and Dubach, U. C. Bern, Hans Huber, 1975, pp. 86-100.

31. Sachs, W. Evidence for the metabolism of maleic acid in dogs and human beings. Science 127:594, 1958.
32. Taggart, J. V.; Angielski, S.; and Morell, H. Complete oxidation of maleic acid via D(+)-malate in kidney. Biochim. Biophys. Acta 58:141-144, 1962.
33. Rogulski, J. The sulfhydryl groups of cellular fractions in the kidney of maleate-treated rats. Acta Biochim. Pol. 10:419-426, 1963.
34. Angielski, S.; and Rogulski, J. The influence of kidney homogenate upon the reaction between glutathione and maleic acid. Acta Biochim. Pol. 8:89-103, 1961.
35. Angielski, S. The effect and metabolism of maleic acid in the kidney. Acta Biol. Med. (Gdansk) 7:61-97, 1963.
36. Angielski, S.; and Rogulski, J. Effect of maleic acid on the kidney. I. Oxidation of Krebs cycle intermediates by various tissues of maleate-intoxicated rats. Acta Biochim. Pol. 9:357-365, 1962.
37. Rogulski, J.; Pacanis, A.; Adamowicz, W.; and Angielski, S. On the mechanism of maleate action on the rat kidney mitochondria. Effect on oxidative metabolism. Acta Biochim. Pol. 21:403-413, 1974.
38. Pacanis, A.; Rogulski, J.; Ledochowski, H.; and Angielski, S. On the mechanism of maleate action on rat kidney mitochondria. Effect on substrate-level phosphorylation. Acta Biochim. Pol. 22:1-10, 1975.
39. Pacanis, A.; Strzelecki, T.; and Rogulski, J. Effects of maleate on the content of CoA and its derivatives in rat kidney mitochondria. J. Biol. Chem. 256:13035-13038, 1981.
40. Angielski, S.; Pempkowiak, L.; Gmaj, P.; Hoppe, A.; and Nowicka, C. The effect of maleate and lithium on renal function and metabolism. In: Biochemical Aspects of Renal Function, edited by Angielski, S., and Dubach, U. C. Bern, Hans Huber, 1975, pp. 142-152.
41. Rogulski, J.; Pacanis, A.; Strzelecki, T.; Kaminska, E.; and Angielski, S. Effects of maleate on carbohydrate metabolism in rats. Am. J. Physiol. 230:1163-1167, 1976.
42. Szczepanska, M.; and Angielski, S. Prevention of maleate-induced tubular dysfunction by acetoacetate. Am. J. Physiol. 239:F50-F56, 1980.
43. Friberg, L. Health hazards in the manufacture of alkaline accumulators with special reference to chronic cadmium poisoning. Acta Med. Scand. 138(Suppl.):240, 1950.
44. Bonnell, J. A.; Ross, J. H.; and King, E. Renal lesions in experimental cadmium poisoning. Br. J. Industr. Med. 17:69-80, 1960.
45. Axelsson, B.; Dahlgren, S. E.; Piscator, M. Renal lesions in the rabbit after long-term exposure to cadmium. Arch. Environ. Health 17:24-28, 1968.
46. Berlin, M.; Hammarström, L.; and Maunsbach, A. Microautoradiographic localization of water-soluble cadmium in mouse kidney. Acta Radiol. 2:345-352, 1964.
47. Stowe, H. D.; Wilson, M.; and Goyer, R. A. Clinical and morphologic effects of oral cadmium toxicity in rabbits. Arch. Pathol. 94:389-405, 1972.
48. Roels, H.; Bernard, A.; Buchet, J. P.; Goret, A.; Lauwerys, R.; Chettle, D. R.; Harvey, T. C.; and Al-Haddad, I. Critical concentration of cadmium in renal cortex and urine. Lancet 1:221, 1979.
49. Friberg, L.; Piscator, M.; Nordberg, G. F.; and Kjellstrom, T. (Ed.) Cadmium in the Environment, 2nd ed., Cleveland, CRC Press, 1974.
50. Nishizumi, M. Electron microscopic study of cadmium nephrotoxicity in the rat. Arch. Environ. Health 24:215-225, 1972.
51. Gonick, H. C.; Indraprasit, S.; Rosen, V. J.; Neustein, H.; Van de Velde, R.; and Raghavan, S. R. V. Experimental Fanconi syndrome. III. Effect of cadmium on renal tubular function, the ATP-Na-K-ATPase transport system and and renal tubular ultrastructure. Miner. Electrolyte Metab. 3:21-35, 1980.
52. Gonick, H. C.; and Raghavan, S. R. V. Experimental cadmium-induced Fanconi syndrome. Proceedings of the IVth International Cadmium Conference, Munich, March 2-4, 1983, Cadmium Association, Cadmium Council, ILZRO, Inc.

53. Kägi, J. H. R.; and Vallee, B. L. Metallothionein: A cadmium and zinc-binding protein from equine renal cortex. J. Biol. Chem. 235:3460-3465, 1960.
54. Foulkes, E. C. Renal tubular transport of cadmium-metallothionein. Toxicol. Appl. Pharmacol. 45:505-512, 1978.
55. Nordberg, G. F.; Goyer, R. A.; and Nordberg, M. Comparative toxicity of cadmium-metallothionein and cadmium chloride on mouse kidney. Arch. Pathol. 99:1192-1197, 1975.
56. Gunn, S. A.; Gould, T. C.; and Anderson, W. A. D. Selectivity of organ response to cadmium injury and various protective measures. J. Pathol. Bacteriol. 96:89-96, 1968.
57. Cherian, M. G.; Goyer, R. A.; and Delaquerriere-Richardson, L. Cadmium-metallothionein-induced nephropathy. Toxicol. Appl. Pharmacol. 38:399-408, 1976.
58. Suzuki, K. T.; Motomura, T.; Tsuchiya, Y.; and Yamamura, M. Separation of metallothioneins in rat liver, kidney and spleen using SW and Sephadex columns. Analyt. Biochem. 107:75-85, 1980.
59. Raghavan, S. R. V.; and Gonick, H. C. Experimental Fanconi syndrome. IV. Effects of repetitive injections of cadmium on tissue distribution and protein-binding of cadmium. Miner. Electrolyte Metab. 3:36-43, 1980.
60. Winge, D. R.; and Rajagopalan, K. V. Purification and some properties of Cd-binding protein from rat liver. Arch. Biochem. Biophys. 153:755-762, 1972.
61. Zelazowski, A. J.; and Piotrowski, J. K. A modified procedure for determination of metallothionein-like proteins in animal tissues. Acta Biochem. Pol. 24:419-425, 1972.
62. Hillyard, S. D.; and Gonick, H. C. Effects of Cd^{++} on short-circuit current across epithelial membranes. I. Interactions with Ca^{++} and vasopressin on frog skin. J. Membr. Biol. 26:109-119, 1976.
63. Hillyard, S. D.; Sera, R.; and Gonick, H. C. Effects of Cd^{++} on short-circuit current across epithelial membranes. J. Membr. Biol. 46:283-294, 1979.
64. Hamilton, D. L.; and Smith, M. W. Inhibition of intestinal calcium uptake by cadmium and the effect of a low calcium diet on cadmium retention. Environ. Res. 15:175-184, 1978.
65. Sugawara, N. Inhibitory effect of cadmium on calcium absorption from the rat duodenum. Arch. Environ. Contam. Toxicol. 5:167-175, 1977.
66. Yuhas, E. M.; Miya, T. S.; and Schnell, R. C. Influence of cadmium on calcium absorption from the rat intestine. Toxicol. Appl. Pharmacol. 43:23-31, 1978.
67. Chertak, R. J.; Sasser, L. B.; Callaham, M. F.; and Jarboe, G. E. Influence of cadmium on the intestinal uptake and absorption of calcium in the rat. J. Nutr. 111:631-638, 1981.
68. Richardson, M. E.; and Spivey Fox, M. R. Dietary cadmium and enteropathy in the Japanese quail. Histochemical and ultrastructural studies. Lab. Invest. 31:722-731, 1974.
69. Valberg, L. S.; Haist, J.; Cherian, M. G.; Delaquerriere-Richardson, L.; and Goyer, R. A. Cadmium-induced enteropathy: comparative toxicity of cadmium chloride and cadmium-thionein. J. Toxicol. Environ. Health 2:963-975, 1977.
70. Kobayoshi, J. Effects of cadmium on calcium metabolism in rats. Trace Subst. Environ. Health 7:295-304, 1973.
71. Itokawa, Y.; Abe, T.; and Tanaka, S. Bone changes in experimental chronic cadmium poisoning. Arch. Environ. Health 26:241-244, 1973.
72. Itokawa, Y.; Abe, T.; Tabei, R.; and Tanaka, S. Renal and skeletal lesions in experimental cadmium poisoning. Histological and biochemical approaches. Arch. Environ. Health 28:149-154, 1974.
73. Itokawa, Y.; Nishino, K.; Takashima, M.; Nakata, T.; Kaito, H.; Okamoto, E.; Dayo, K.; and Kawamura, J. Renal and skeletal lesions in experimental cadmium poisoning in rats. Histology and renal function. Environ. Res. 15:206-217, 1978.

74. Nomiyama, K.; Nomiyama, H.; and Taguchi, T. No osteomalacia found in mice, rabbits and monkeys given cadmium for a prolonged period. In: Cadmium-Induced Osteopathy, edited by Shigematsu, I., and Nomiyama, K. Tokyo, Japan Public Health Association, 1980, pp. 51-53.
75. Furuta, H. Cadmium effects on bone and dental tissues of rats in acute and subacute poisoning. Experientia 34:1317-1318, 1978.
76. Anderson, C.; and Danylchuk, K. D. Effect of chronic low-level cadmium intoxication on the Haversian remodeling system in dogs. Calcif. Tissue Int. 27:121-126, 1979.
77. Anderson, C.; and Danylchuk, K. D. Effect of chronic low-level cadmium intoxication on the Haversian remodeling system in dogs: A reversible phenomenon. Calcif. Tissue Int. 27:121-126, 1979.
78. Anderson, C.; and Danylchuk, K. D. Plasma levels of immunoreactive parathyroid hormone in dogs chronically exposed to low levels of cadmium chloride. J. Environ. Pathol. Toxicol. 2:1151-1159, 1979.
79. Feldman, S. L.; and Cousins, R. J. Influence of cadmium on the metabolism of 25-hydroxycholecalciferol in chicks. Nutr. Rep. Int. 8:251-260, 1973.
80. Frimpter, G. W.; Timpanelli, A. E.; Eisemenger, W. J.; Stein, H. S.; and Ehrlich, L. I. Reversible "Fanconi syndrome" caused by degraded tetracycline. JAMA 184:125-127, 1963.
81. Ehrlich, L. I.; and Stein, H. S. Abnormal urinary findings following administration of Achromycin V. Pediatrics 31:339, 1963.
82. Gross, J. M. Fanconi syndrome (adult type) developing secondary to ingestion of outdated tetracycline. Ann. Intern. Med. 56:523-528, 1963.
83. Rosenthal, S. M. Abnormal urinary findings and Achromycin V. Pediatrics 31:697, 1963.
84. Benitz, K.-F.; and Diermeier, H. F. Renal toxicity of tetracycline degradation products. Proc. Soc. Exp. Biol. Med. 115:930-935, 1964.
85. Lowe, M. B.; Obst, D.; and Tap, E. Renal damage caused by anhydro-4-epi-tetracycline. Arch. Pathol. Lab. Med. 81:362-364, 1966.
86. Lindquist, R. R.; and Fellers, F. X. Degraded tetracycline nephropathy: Functional, morphologic, and histochemical observations. Lab. Invest. 15:864-876, 1966.
87. Du Buy, H. G.; and Showacre, J. L. Selective localization of tetracycline in mitochondria of living cells. Science 133:194-195, 1961.
88. Van Meter, J. C.; Spector, A.; Oleson, J. J.; and Williams, J. H. In vitro action of aureomycin on oxidative phosphorylation in animal tissues. Proc. Soc. Exp. Biol. Med. 81: 215-217, 1952.
89. Easley, J. R.; and Breitschwerdt, E. B. Glycosuria associated with renal tubular dysfunction in three basenji dogs. J. Am. Vet. Med. Assoc. 168:938-943, 1976.
90. Bovee, K. C.; Joyce, T.; Reynolds, R.; and Segal, S. Spontaneous Fanconi syndrome in the dog. Metabolism 27:45-52, 1978.
91. Bovee, K. C.; Joyce, T.; Blazer-Yost, B.; Goldschmidt, M. S.; and Segal, S. Characterization of renal defects in dogs with a syndrome similar to the Fanconi syndrome in man. J. Am. Vet. Med. Assoc. 174:1094-1099, 1979.
92. Bovee, K. C.; Anderson, T.; Brown, S.; Goldschmidt, M. H.; and Segal, S. Renal tubular defects of spontaneous Fanconi syndrome in dogs. In: Animal Models of Inherited Metabolic Diseases, edited by Desnick, R. C., and Patterson, D. F. New York, Liss, 1982, pp. 435-447.
93. Ross, B.; Leaf, A.; Silva, P.; and Epstein, F. H. Na-K-ATPase in sodium transport by the perfused rat kidney. Am. J. Physiol. 226:624-629, 1974.
94. Stoff, J. S.; and Epstein, F. H. Recent advances in renal tubular biochemistry. Physiol. Rev. 38:46-68, 1976.

95. Györy, A. Z.; Brendel, U.; and Kinne, R. Effect of cardiac glycosides and sodium ethacrynate on transepithelial sodium transport in *in vivo* micropuncture experiments and on isolated plasma membrane Na-K-ATPase in vitro of the rat. Pflugers Arch. 335:287-296, 1972.
96. Frömter, E.; Rumrich, G.; and Ullrich, K. J. Phenomenologic description of Na^+, Cl^-, and HCO^-_3 absorption from proximal tubules of the rat kidney. Pflugers Arch. 343: 189-220, 1973.
97. Kinne, R. Current concepts of renal proximal tubular function. Contr. Nephrol. 14: 14-24, 1978.
98. Toretti, J.; Hendler, E.; Weinstein, E.; Longnecker, R. E.; and Epstein, F. H. Functional significance of Na-K-ATPase in the kidney: Effects of ouabain inhibition. Am. J. Physiol. 222:1398-1405, 1972.
99. Heidrich, H.-G.; Kinne, R.; Kinne-Saffron, E.; and Hannig, K. The polarity of the proximal tubule cell in rat kidney: Different surface charges for the brush-border microvilli and plasma membranes from the basal infolding. J. Cell. Biol. 54:232-245, 1972.
100. Schmidt, U.; and Dubach, U. C. Na K stimulated adenosinetriphosphatase: Intracellular localisation within the proximal tubule of the rat nephron. Pflugers Arch. 330: 265-270, 1971.
101. Schmidt, U.; and Dubach, U. C. (eds.). Na-K-ATPase in the rat nephron related to sodium transport: Results with quantitative histochemistry. Part II. In: Recent Advances in Quantitative Histo- and Cytochemistry. Bern, Hans Huber, 1971, p. 320.
102. Mandel, L. J.; Lazaro, J.; and Balaban, R. S. Stoichiometry and coupling of active transport to oxidative metabolism in epithelial tissues. Am. J. Physiol. 240:F357-F371, 1981.
103. Kiil, F. Renal energy metabolism and regulation of sodium reabsorption. Kidney Int. 11:153-160, 1977.
104. Epstein, F. H.; and Whittam, R. The mode of inhibition by calcium of cell-membrane adenosine-triphosphatase activity. Biochem. J. 99:232-239, 1966.
105. Györy, A. Z.; Kinne, R.; and Moewes, B. Energy source for transepithelial sodium transport in rat renal proximal tubules. Pflugers Arch. 327:234-260, 1971.
106. Herms, W.; and Malvin, R. L. Effect of metabolic inhibitors on urine osmolality and electrolyte excretion. Am. J. Physiol. 204:1065-1070, 1963.
107. Lee, J. B.; Vance, V. K.; and Cahill, G. F. Metabolism of C^{14}-labelled substrates by rabbit cortex and medulla. Am. J. Physiol. 203:27 36, 1962.
108. Weinstein, S. W.; and Kloss, R. M. Micropuncture studies on energy metabolism and sodium transport in the mammalian nephron. Am. J. Physiol. 217:498-504, 1969.
109. Cohen, J. J. Metabolic support for renal sodium reabsorption. Med. Clin. North Am. 59:523-538, 1975.
110. Ullrich, K. J.; Capasso, G.; Rumrich, G.; Papavassiliou, F.; and Kloss, S. Coupling between proximal tubular transport processes. Studies with ouabain, SITS and HCO_3-free solutions. Pflugers Arch. 368:245-252, 1977.
111. Massry, S. G.; Coburn, J. W.; Chapman, L. W.; and Kleeman, C. R. The effect of NaCl infusion on urinary Ca^{++} and Mg^{++} during reduction in their filtered loads. Am. J. Physiol. 213:1218-1224, 1967.
112. Kurtzman, N. A. Regulation of renal bicarbonate reabsorption by extracellular volume. J. Clin. Invest. 49:586-594, 1970.
113. Massry, S. G.; Coburn, J. W.; and Kleeman, C. R. The influence of extracellular volume expansion on renal phosphate reabsorption in the dog. J. Clin. Invest. 48:1237-1245, 1969.
114. Hillyard, S. D.; Lu, E.; and Gonick, H. C. Further characterization of the natriuretic factor derived from kidney tissue of volume-expanded rats: Effects on short-circuit current and Na-K-ATPase activity. Circ. Res. 38:250-255, 1976.

115. Gonick, H. C. Pathophysiology of human proximal tubular transport defects. Klin. Wochenschr. 60:1201-1211, 1982.
116. Shils, M. E. Experimental human magnesium depletion. Medicine 48:61-85, 1969.
117. Greenberg, D. M.; Lucia, S. P.; and Tufts, E. V. The effect of magnesium deprivation on renal function. Am. J. Physiol. 121:424-430, 1938.
118. Ginn, H. E.; and Shanbour, L. L. Phosphaturia in magnesium-deficient rats. Am. J. Physiol. 212:1347-1350, 1967.
119. Mazzocco, V. E.; Lizarralde, G.; Flink, B.; and Jones, J. E. Generalized aminoaciduria in magnesium deficient rats. Proc. Soc. Exp. Biol. Med. 23:403-408, 1966.
120. Whang, R.; and Welt, L. G. Observations in experimental magnesium depletion. J. Clin. Invest. 42:305-313, 1963.
121. Benabe, J. E.; and Martinez-Maldonado, M. Hypercalcemic nephropathy. Arch. Intern. Med. 138:777-779, 1978.
122. Epstein, F. H. Calcium and the kidney. Am. J. Med. 45:700-714, 1968.
123. Crumb, C.; Martinez-Maldonado, M.; Eknoyan, G.; and Suki, W. N. Effects of volume expansion, purified parathyroid extract, and calcium on renal bicarbonate reabsorption in the dog. J. Clin. Invest. 54:1287-124, 1974.
124. DiBona, G. F. Effect of hypercalcemia on renal tubular sodium handling in the rat. Am. J. Physiol. 220:49-53, 1971.
125. Edwards, B. R.; Sutton, R. A. L.; and Kirks, J. H. Effect of calcium infusion on renal tubular reabsorption in the dog. Am. J. Physiol. 227:13-18, 1974.
126. Le Grimellec, F.; Roinel, N.; and Morel, F. Simultaneous Mg, Ca, P, Na, K, Na and Cl analysis in rat tubular fluid. III. During acute Ca plasma loading. Pflugers Arch. 346: 171-188, 1974.
127. Suki, W. N.; Eknoyan, G.; and Rector, F. C., Jr. The renal diluting and concentrating mechanism in hypercalcemia. Nephron 6:50-61, 1969.
128. Wheeler, K. P.; and Whittam, R. Structural and enzymic aspects of the hydrolysis of adenosine triphosphate by membranes of kidney cortex and erythrocytes. Biochem. J. 93:349-363, 1964.
129. Lee, D. B. N.; Brautbar, N.; and Kleeman, C. R. Disorders of phosphorus metabolism. In: Disorders of Mineral Metabolism, vol. 3, edited by Bronner, F., and Coburn, J. W. New York, Academic Press, 1981, pp. 83-421.
130. Brazy, P. C.; Gullans, S. R.; Mandel, L. J.; and Dennis, V. W. Metabolic requirement for inorganic phosphate by the rabbit proximal tubule. Evidence for a Crabtree effect. J. Clin. Invest. 70:53-62, 1982.
131. Kurokawa, K.; and Kreusser, W. J. Renal cell metabolism in phosphate depletion: Adenine nucleotide metabolism and gluconeogenesis. Curr. Probl. Nephrol. 8:337-342, 1977.
132. Kurokawa, K.; Dreusser, W. J.; and Massry, S. G. Phosphate depletion and adenine nucleotide metabolism in kidney and liver. Adv. Exp. Med. Biol. 103:217-338, 1978.
133. Morris, R. C.; Nigon, K.; and Reed, E. B. Evidence that the severity of depletion of inorganic phosphate determines the severity of the disturbance of adenine nucleotide metabolism in the liver and renal cortex of the fructose-loaded rat. J. Clin. Invest. 61: 209-220.
134. Scott, J.; Elias, E.; Moult, P. J. A.; Barnes, S.; and Wills, M. R. Rickets in adult cystic fibrosis with myopathy, pancreatic insufficiency and proximal renal tubular dysfunction. Am. J. Med. 63:488-492, 1977.
135. MacCuish, A. C.; Munro, J. F.; and Lamb, W. L. Reversible renal tubular defects in gluten enteropathy with osteomalacia. Br. Med. J. 2:343-344, 1970.
136. Muldowney, F. P.; Freaney, R.; and McGeeney, D. Renal tubular acidosis and aminoaciduria in osteomalacia of dietary or intestinal origin. Q. J. Med. 37:517-539, 1968.
137. Muldowney, F. P.; Carroll, D. V.; Donohoe, J. F.; and Freaney, R. Correction of renal bicarbonate wastage by parathyroidectomy. Q. J. Med. 40:487-498, 1971.

138. Adams, R. G.; Harrison, J. F.; and Scott, P. The development of cadmium-induced proteinuria, impaired renal function and osteomalacia in alkaline battery workers. Q. J. Med. 38:425-443, 1981.
139. Kazantzis, G.; Flynn, F. U.; Spowage, J. S.; and Trott, D. G. Renal tubular malfunction and pulmonary emphysema in cadmium pigment workers. Q. J. Med. 32:165-192, 1963.
140. Saito, H.; Shioji, R.; Hurukawa, Y.; Nagai, K.; Arikawa, T.; Saito, T.; Sasaki, Y.; Furuyma, T.; and Yoshinaga, K. Cadmium-induced proximal tubular dysfunction in a cadmium-polluted area. Contrib. Nephrol. 6:1-12, 1977.
141. Raghavan, S. R. V.; and Gonick, H. C. Cadmium (Cd)-induced Fanconi syndrome (FS): Parallel changes in Cd content and Na-K-ATPase activity of kidney microsomes. Abstract of the Proceedings of the VIIIth Annual Meeting of the American Society of Nephrology, 1975, p. 93.
142. Guarino, A. M.; Miller, D. S.; Arnold, S. T.; Pritchard, J. B.; Davis, R. D.; Urbanek, M. A.; Miller, T. J.; and Litterst, C. L. Platinate toxicity: Past, present, and prospects. Cancer Treat. Rep. 63:1475-1483, 1979.
143. Nechay, B. R.; and Saunders, J. P. Inhibitory characteristics of cadmium, lead, and mercury in human sodium and potassium dependent adenosine triphosphatase preparations. J. Environ. Pathol. Toxicol. 2:283-290, 1978.
144. Mustafa, M. G.; Cross, C. E.; Munn, R. J.; and Hardie, J. A. Effects of divalent metal ions on alveolar macrophage membrane adenosine triphosphatase activity. J. Lab. Clin. Med. 77:563-571, 1971.
145. Sporn, A.; Dinu, I.; and Stoenescu, L. Influence of cadmium administration on carbohydrate and cellular energetic metabolism in the rat liver. Rev. Roum. Biochim. 7:299-305, 1970.
146. Hong, C. D.; Hanenson, I. B.; Lerner, S.; Hammond, P. B.; Pesce, A. J.; and Pollak, V. E. Occupational exposure to lead: Effects on renal function. Kidney Int. 18:489-494, 1980.
147. Chisholm, J. J., Jr.; Harrison, H. C.; Eberlein, W. R.; and Harrison, H. E. Aminoaciduria, hypophosphatemia, and rickets in lead poisoning. A.M.A. Am. J. Dis. Child. 89:159-168, 1955.
148. Barltrop, D.; Barrett, A. J.; and Dingle, J. T. Subcellular distribution of lead in the rat. J. Lab. Clin. Med. 77:705-712, 1971.
149. Ulmer, D. D.; and Vallee, B. L. Effects of lead on biochemical systems. In: Trace Substances in Environmental Health, vol. II, edited by Hemphill, D. D. Columbia, Missouri, University Press, 1968, pp. 7-27.
150. Goyer, R. A.; May, P.; Cates, M. M.; and Krigman, M. R. Lead and protein content of isolated intranuclear inclusion bodies from kidneys of lead-poisoned rats. Lab. Invest. 22:245-251, 1970.
151. Goyer, R. A. The renal tubule in lead poisoning. I. Mitochondrial swelling and aminoaciduria. Lab. Invest. 19:71-77, 1968.
152. Secchi, G. C.; Alessio, L.; and Cirla, A. The effect of experimental lead poisoning on some enzymatic activities of the kidney. Clin. Chim. Acta 27:467-474, 1970.
153. Iannaccone, A.; Boscolo, P.; and Bombardieri, G. Comparative effects of experimental lead poisoning on enzymatic activities of kidney and liver in rat. Life Sci. 19:427-432, 1976.
154. Goyer, R. A.; Krall, A.; and Kimball, J. P. The renal tubule in lead poisoning. II. In vitro studies of mitochondrial structure and function. Lab. Invest. 19:78-83, 1968.
155. Gaspers, M. L.; and Siegel, G. J. Inhibition by lead of human erythrocyte ($Na^+ + K^+$)-adenosine triphosphatase associated with binding of ^{210}Pb to membrane fragments. Biochim. Biophys. Acta 600:27-35, 1980.
156. Reynolds, E. S.; Tannen, R. L.; and Tyler, R. The renal lesion in Wilson's disease. Am. J. Med. 40:518-527, 1966.

157. Owen, C. A.; and Hazelrig, J. B. Copper metabolism in the rat. Birth Defects Orig. Art. Series IV:1-7, 1968.
158. Yoshitoshi, Y.; Oda, T.; Yamane, Y.; Nagan, M.; Mori, K.; and Shikata, T. Renal lesions in Wilson's disease. Birth Defects Orig. Art. Series IV:104-108, 1968.
159. Epstein, P. S.; and McIlwain, H. Actions of cupric salts on isolated cerebral tissues. Proc. Roy. Soc. B. 166:295-302, 1966.
160. Peters, R.; and Walshe, J. M. Studies on the toxicity of copper. I. The toxic action of copper in vivo and in vitro. Proc. R. Soc. Lond. (Biol.) 166:173-284, 1966.
161. Peters, R.; Shorthouse, M.; and Walshe, J. M. Studies on the toxicity of copper. II. The behaviour of microsomal membrane ATPase of the pigeon's brain tissue to copper and some other metallic substances. Proc. R. Soc. Lond. (Biol.) 166:285-294, 1966.
162. Gibbs, R.; Roddy, P. M.; and Titus, E. Preparation, assay, and properties of an Na^+- and K^+-requiring adenosine triphosphatase from beef brain. J. Biol. Chem. 240:2181-2187, 1965.
163. Ting-Beall, H. P.; Clark, D. A.; Suelter, C. H.; and Wells, W. W. Studies on the interaction of chick brain microsomal (Na^+ K^+)-ATPase with copper. Biochim. Biophys. Acta 291:229-236, 1973.
164. Bowler, K.; and Duncan, C. J. The effect of copper on membrane enzymes. Biochim. Biophys. Acta 196:116-119, 1970.
165. Rifkin, R. J. *In vitro* inhibition of Na^+-K^+ and Mg^{2+} ATPases by mono, di- and trivalent cations. Proc. Soc. Exp. Biol. Med. 120:802-804, 1965.
166. Piotrowski, J. K.; Trojanowska, B.; Wisniewska-Knypl, J. M.; and Bolanowska, W. Mercury binding in the kidney and liver of rats repeatedly exposed to mercuric chloride. Induction of metallothionein by mercury and cadmium. Toxicol. Appl. Pharmacol. 27:11-19, 1974.
167. Ellis, R. W.; and Fang, S. C. The *in vivo* binding of mercury to soluble proteins of the rat kidney. Toxicol. Appl. Pharmacol. 20:14-21, 1971.
168. Chen, R. W.; Ganter, H. E.; and Hoekstra, W. G. Studies on the binding of methylmercury by thionein. Biochem. Biophys. Res. Commun. 51:383-390, 1973.
169. Helleberg, A.; and Gyrd-Hanen, N. Mercury binding in the kidney of rats exposed to methoxyethyl mercury. Acta Pharmacol. Toxicol. 38:384-288, 1976.
170. Gyrd-Hansen, N.; and Helleberg, A. Methoxyethyl mercury toxicity in pigs: Kidney function and mercury distribution. Acta Pharmacol. Toxicol. 38:229-240, 1976.
171. Brubaker, P. E.; Kein, R.; Herman, S. P.; Lucier, G. W.; Alexander, L. O.; and Long, M. D. DNA, RNA and protein synthesis in brain, liver and kidneys of asymptomatic methymercury-treated rats. Exp. Molec. Pathol. 18:263-280, 1973.
172. Paterson, R. A.; and Usher, D. R. The toxicity of methyl mercury on glycolytic intermediates and adenine nucleotides of rat brain. Life Sci. 10:121-128, 1971.
173. Pekkanen, T. J.; and Sandholm, M. Effect of experimental methyl mercury poisoning on activity of TPNH-specific glutathione reductase of rat brain and liver. Acta Vet. Scand. 13:14-19, 1972.
174. Taylor, N. S. Histochemical studies of nephrotoxicity with sublethal doses of mercury in rats. Am. J. Pathol. 46:1-21, 1965.
175. Haddow, J. E.; Fish, C. A.; Marshall, P. C.; and Lester, R. Biliary excretion of mercury enhanced by spironolactone. Gastroenterology 63:1053-1058, 1972.
176. Haddow, J. E.; and Marshall, P. Increased stool mercury excretion in the rat: The effect of spironolactone. Proc. Soc. Exp. Biol. Med. 140:707-709, 1972.
177. MacNider, W. B. A review of acute experimental nephritis. Physiol. Rev. 4:595-638, 1924.
178. Nomiyama, K.; and Foulkes, E. C. Some effects of uranyl acetate on proximal tubular functions in rabbit kidney. Toxicol. Appl. Pharmacol. 13:89-98, 1968.

179. Bowman, F. J.; and Foulkes, E. C. Effects of uranium on rabbit renal tubules. Toxicol. Appl. Pharmacol. 16:391-399, 1970.
180. Nechay, B. R.; Thompson, J. D.; and Saunders, J. P. Inhibition by uranyl nitrate of adenosine triphosphatases derived from animal and human tissues. Toxicol. Appl. Pharmacol. 53:410-419, 1980.
181. Balfour, W. E.; Grantham, J. J.; and Glynn, I. M. Vanadate-stimulated natriuresis in the rat. Nature (Lond) 275:768, 1978.
182. Westenfelder, C.; Hamburger, R. K.; and Garcia, M. E. Effect of vanadate on renal tubular function in rats. Am. J. Physiol. 240:F522-F529, 1981.
183. Charney, A. N.; Silva, P.; and Epstein, F. H. An *in vitro* inhibitor of Na-K-ATPase present in an adenosine triphosphate preparation. J. Appl. Physiol. 39:155-158, 1975.
184. O'Neal, S. G.; Rhoads, D. B.; and Racker, E. Vanadate inhibition of sarcoplasmic reticulum Ca^{2+}-ATPase and other ATPases. Biochem. Biophys. Res. Commun. 89:845-850, 1979.
185. Sabatini, S.; and Westenfelder, C. The effect of Na_3VO_4 on the anion-sensitive ATPase from renal cortex. Clin. Res. 28:460A, 1980.
186. Bowman, B. J.; and Slayman, C. W. The effects of vanadate on the plasma membrane ATPase of Neurospora crassa. J. Biol. Chem. 254:2928-2934, 1979.
187. Bond, G. H.; and Hudgins, P. M. Dog kidney (Na^+, K^+)-ATPase is more sensitive to inhibition by vanadate than human red cell (Na^+, K^+)-ATPase. Biochim. Biophys. Acta 646:479-482, 1981.
188. Hansen, O. Facilitation of ouabain binding to (Na^+ K^+) ATPase by vanadate at *in vivo* concentrations. Biochem. Biophys. Acta 568:265-269, 1979.
189. Jörgensen, P. L. Sodium and potassium ion pump in kidney tubules. Physiol. Rev. 60:864-917, 1980.
190. Nechay, B. R.; and Saunders, J. P. Inhibition by vanadium of sodium and potassium dependent adenosine triphosphatase derived from animal and human tissues. Environ. Pathol. Toxicol. 2:247-262, 1978.
191. Blachley, J. D.; and Hill, J. B. Renal and electrolyte disturbances associated with cisplatinum. Ann. Int. Med. 95:628-632, 1981.
192. Choie, D. D.; Longnecker, D. S.; and Del Campo, A. A. Acute and chronic cisplatin nephropathy in rats. Lab. Invest. 44:397-402, 1981.
193. Friedman, M. E.; and Melius, P. Interactions of cis- and trans-platinum (II) complexes with dehydrogenase enzymes in the presence of different mono- and polynucleotides: Evidence for a ternary complex. Bioinorganic Chem. 8:341-353, 1978.
194. Nechay, B. R. Personal communication.
195. Mutti, A.; Cavatorta, A.; Pedroni, C.; Borhi, A.; Giaroli, C.; and Franchini, I. The role of chromium accumulation in the relationship between airborne and urinary chromium in welders. Int. Arch. Occup. Environ. Health 43:123-133, 1979.
196. Biber, T. U. L.; Mylle, M.; Baines, A. D.; Gottschalk, C. W.; Oliver, J. R.; and MacDowell, M. C. A study of micropuncture and microdissection of acute renal damage in rats. Am. J. Med. 44:664-705, 1968.
197. Franchini, I.; Mutti, A.; Cavatorta, A.; Corradi, A.; Cosi, A.; Olivetti, G.; and Borghetti, A. Nephrotoxicity of chromium. Contr. Nephrol. 10:98-110, 1978.
198. Evan, A. P.; and Dail, W. G. The effects of sodium chromate on the proximal tubules of the rat kidney. Lab. Invest. 30:704-715, 1971.
199. Watanabe, I.; Whittier, F. C., Jr.; Moore, J.; and Cuppage, F. E. Gold nephropathy. Ultrastructural, fluorescence and microanalytic studies of two patients. Arch. Pathol. Lab. Med. 100:632-635, 1976.
200. Shaw, C. F.; Thompson, H. O.; Witkiewicz, P.; Satre, R. W.; and Siegesmund, K. Subcellular distribution of gold in rat renal cortex cells: Limitations of electron microscopy and subcellular fractionation techniques. Toxicol. App. Pharmacol. 61:349-357, 1981.

201. Nechay, B. R. Inhibition of adenosine triphosphatases by gold. Arthritis Rheum. 23: 464-470, 1980.
202. Shaikh, Z. A.; and Lucis, O. J. Cadmium and zinc binding in mammalian liver and kidneys. Arch. Environ. Health 24:419-425, 1972.
203. Brierley, G. P.; and Knight, V. A. Ion transport by heart mitochondria. X. The uptake and release of Zn^{++} and its relation to the energy-linked accumulation of magnesium. Biochemistry 6:3892-3901, 1967.
204. Beutler, E. Galactosemia. Am. J. Clin. Nutr. 21:923-925, 1968.
205. Morris, R. C. An experimental renal acidification defect in patients with fructose intolerance. I. Its resemblance to renal tubular acidosis. J. Clin. Invest. 47:1389-1398, 1968.
206. Lindblad, B.; Lindstedt, S.; and Steen, G. On the enzmatic defects in hereditary tyrosinemia. Proc. Natl. Acad. Sci. U.S.A. 74:4641-4645, 1977.
207. Beumer, H.; and Wepler, W. Uber die Cystinkrankheit der ersten Lebenszeit. Klin. Wochenschr. 16:8-10, 1937.
208. Schneider, J. A.; and Schulman, J. D. Cystinosis: A review. Metabolism 26:817-839, 1977.
209. Jackson, J. D.; Smith, F. G.; Litman, N. N.; Yuile, C. L.; and Latta, H. The Fanconi syndrome with cystinosis. Am. J. Med. 33:893-910, 1962.
210. Kramer, H. J.; and Burgard, U. G. Further studies on epithelial transport defect in experimental and human Fanconi syndrome. Effects of maleic acid and L-cystine on sodium transport and (Na^+ K^+)-ATPase of the isolated frog skin. Clin. Chim. Acta 55: 57-63, 1974.
211. Smithline, J.; Kassirer, J. P.; and Cohen, J. J. Light-chain nephropathy: Tubular dysfunction and light-chain proteinuria. N. Engl. J. Med. 294:71-74, 1976.
212. Maldonado, J. E.; Velosa, J. A.; Kyle, R. A.; Wagoner, R. D.; Holley, K. E.; and Salassa, R. M. Fanconi syndrome in adults. A manifestation of a latent form of myeloma. Am. J. Med. 58:354-364, 1975.
213. Costanza, D. J.; and Smoller, M. Multiple myeloma with Fanconi syndrome. Am. J. Med. 34:125-133, 1963.
214. Preuss, H. G.; Hammack, W. J.; and Murdaugh, H. V. The effect of Bence-Jones protein on the *in vitro* function of rabbit renal cortex. Nephron 5:210-216, 1967.
215. McGeoch, J.; Ledingham, J.; Smith, J. F.; and Ross, B. Inhibition of active-transport sodium-potassium-ATPase by myeloma protein. Lancet 2:17-18, 1978.
216. Falcone Smith, J. F.; Van Hegan, R. I.; Esnouf, M. P.; and Ross. B. D. Characteristics of renal handling of human immunoglobulin light chain by the perfused rat kidney. Clin. Sci. 57:113-120, 1979.
217. Webb, J. L. Enzyme and Metabolic Inhibitors, vol. II, New York, Academic Press, 1966, pp. 1-244.
218. Rogulski, J.; and Angielski, S. Effect of the maleic acid on the kidney. III. Succinate as hydrogen donor in the reductive amination in the rat kidney. Acta. Biochim. Pol. 10:125-132, 1963.
219. Rogulski, J.; and Angielski, S. Effect of maleic acid on the kidney. IV. Synthesis of amino acids in the kidney of maleate-treated rats. Acta Biochim. Pol. 10:133-139, 1963.
220. Pacanis, A.; and Rogulski, J. Studies on chemical and enzymatic synthesis of maleyl-CoA. J. Biol. Chem. 256:13030-13034, 1981.
221. Al-Bander, H.; Weiss, R. A.; Paulkert, T. T.; Morris, R. C.; and Humphreys, M. H. Phosphate loading attentuates the bicarbonaturia by maleic acid in the dog. Clin. Res. 29: 101A, 1981.
222. Nechay, B. R.; Jackson, R. E.; Ziegler, M. G.; Neldon, S. L.; and Thompson, J. D. Effects of chronic digitalization on cardiac and renal Na^+ and K^+-dependent adenosine triphosphatase activity and circulating catecholamines in the dog. Circ. Res. 49:655-660, 1981.

223. Nechay, B. R. Biochemical basis of diuretic action. J. Clin. Pharmacol. 17:626-641, 1977.
224. Nelson, J. A.; and Nechay, B. R. Effects of cardiac glycosides on renal adenosine triphosphatase activity and Na^+ reabsorption in dogs. J. Pharmacol. Exp. Ther. 175: 727-740, 1970.
225. Hook, J. B. A positive correlation between natriuresis and inhibition of renal Na-K-adenosine triphosphatase by ouabain. Proc. Soc. Exp. Biol. Med. 131:731-734, 1969.
226. Allen, J. C.; Martinez-Maldonado, M.; Ekonoyan, G.; Suki, N. N.; and Schwarts, A. Relation between digitalis binding *in vivo* and inhibition of sodium, potassium-adenosine triphosphatase in canine kidney. Biochem. Pharmacol. 20:73-80, 1971.
227. Segersted, D. M.; Lie, M.; and Kiil, F. Effect of ouabain on metabolic rate in renal cortex and medulla. Am. J. Physiol. 220:1488-1493, 1971.
228. Segersted, O. M.; Steen, P. A.; and Kiil, F. Energetics of tubular sodium reabsorption sensitive to ethacrynic acid and ouabain. Am. J. Physiol. 242:F254-F260, 1982.
229. Ebel, H.; Aulbert, E.; and Averdunk, R. Inhibition of renal (Na^+ K^+)-ATPase and cation transport by an antibody against NaI extracted kidney plasma membranes. Pflugers Arch. 370:269-276, 1977.
230. Rea, C.; and Segal, S. ATP content of rat kidney cortex slices: Relation to α-amino-isobutyric acid uptake. Kidney Int. 2:102-106, 1972.
231. Urbaitis, R. K.; and Kessler, R. H. Actions of inhibitor compounds on adenine nucleotides of renal cortex and sodium excretion. Am. J. Physiol. 220:1116-1123, 1971.
232. Fullans, S. R.; Brazy, P. C.; Soltoff, S. P.; Dennis, V. W.; and Mandel, L. J. Metabolic inhibitors: Effects on metabolism and transport in the proximal tubule. Am. J. Physiol. 243:F133-F140, 1982.
233. Ullrich, K. J.; Rumrich, G.; and Kloss, S. Transport of inorganic and organic substances in the renal proximal tubule. Klin. Wochenschr. 60:1165-1172, 1982.
234. Brazy, P. C.; Balaban, R. S.; Gullans, S. R.; Mandel, L. J.; and Dennis, V. W. Inhibition of renal metabolism. Relative effects of arsenate on sodium, phosphate, and glucose transport by the rabbit proximal tubule. J. Clin. Invest. 66:1211-1221, 1980.
235. Dennis, V. W.; and Brazy, P. C. Sodium, phosphate, glucose, bicarbonate and alanine interactions in the isolated proximal convoluted tubule of the rabbit kidney. J. Clin. Invest. 62:387-397, 1978.
236. Bergeron, M.; and Vadeboncoeur, M. Microinjections of L-leucine into tubules and peritubular capillaries of the rat. II. The maleic acid model. Nephron 8:367-374, 1971.
237. Bergeron, M.; Dubord, L.; Laporte, P.; Hausser, C.; and Alle-Ando, L. On the pathophysiology of Fanconi syndrome. In: Amino Acid Transport and Uric Acid Transport, edited by Silbernagel, S., Lang, F., and Greger, R. Stuttgart, Thieme, 1976, pp. 46-52.
238. Roth, K. S.; Hwang, S. M.; and Segal, S. Effect of maleic acid on the kinetics of α-methyl-D-glucoside uptake by isolated rat renal tubules. Biochim. Biophys. Acta 426:675-687, 1976.
239. Rosenberg, L. E.; Berman, M.; and Segal, S. Studies of the kinetics of amino acid transport, incorporation into protein and oxidation in kidney-cortex slices. Biochim. Biophys. Acta 71:664-675, 1963.
240. Gunther, R.; Silbernagl, S.; and Deetjen, P. Maleic acid induced aminoaciduria, studied by free flow micropuncture and continuous microperfusion. Pflügers Arch. 382: 109-114, 1979.
241. Flohe, L.; Gunzler, W. A.; and Ladenstein, R. Glutathione dependent enzymatic reactions. In: Glutathione: Metabolism and Function, edited by Arias, I. M., and Jacoby, W. B. New York, Raven, 1976, pp. 115-138.
242. Maesaka, J. E.; and McCaffery, M. Evidence for renal tubular leakage in maleic acid-induced Fanconi syndrome. Am. J. Physiol. 239:F507-F513, 1980.

243. Wen, S.-F. Micropuncture studies of glucose transport in the dog: Mechanism of renal glycosuria. Am. J. Physiol. 231:468-475, 1976.
244. Silverman, M.; and Huang, L. Mechanism of maleic acid-induced glucosuria in dog kidney. Am. J. Physiol. 231:1024-1032, 1976.
245. Hong Que, N. T.; Gmaj, P.; and Angielski, S. Uncoupling of Na^+-dependent solute transport in renal brush border membranes of maleate-treated rats. Acta Biochim. Pol. 29:275-287, 1982.
246. Silverman, M. The mechanism of maleic acid nephropathy: Investigations using brush border membrane vesicles. Membr. Biochem. 4:63-69, 1981.
247. Yanase, M.; Orita, Y.; Okada, N.; Nakanishi, T.; Horio, M.; Ando, A.; and Abe, H. Decreased Na^+-gradient-dependent D-glucose transport in brush-border membrane vesicles from rabbits with experimental Fanconi syndrome. Biochim. Biophys. Acta 733:95-101, 1983.

Index

A

B

C

G

H

I

O

P

R

S

T

U

V

W

Z